Gynecologic and Obstetric Pathology, Volume 1

Wenxin Zheng
Oluwole Fadare
Charles Matthew Quick
Danhua Shen
Donghui Guo
Editors

Gynecologic and Obstetric Pathology, Volume 1

Science Press
Beijing

Springer

Editors
Wenxin Zheng
Department of Pathology
Department of Obstetrics and Gynecology
University of Texas Southwestern Medical Center
Dallas, TX
USA

Charles Matthew Quick
Department of Pathology, College of Medicine
University of Arkansas for Medical Sciences
Little Rock, AR
USA

Donghui Guo
Department of Obstetrics and Gynecology
Tianjin Gynecologic and Obstetrics Central Hospital
Tianjin
China

Oluwole Fadare
Department of Pathology
University of California San Diego
San Diego, CA
USA

Danhua Shen
Department of Pathology
Peking University People's Hospital
Beijing
China

ISBN 978-981-13-3015-5 ISBN 978-981-13-3016-2 (eBook)
https://doi.org/10.1007/978-981-13-3016-2

This Springer imprint is published by the registered company Springer Nature Singapore Pte Ltd.
The registered company address is: 152 Beach Road, #21-01/04 Gateway East, Singapore 189721, Singapore

Foreword

The field of gynecologic and obstetric pathology is at a cross-roads. In the past decade we have begun to witness the departure of venerated contributors to this discipline and now we are being inundated with new information about pathogenesis that informs diagnostic expectations and patient outcome. The old model in which the next generation sits at the knee of the learned and patiently awaits their turn at the helm is rapidly fading. Succession is now not simply achieved by learning the old language but by speaking a new one.

The textbook *Gynecologic and Obstetrics Pathology*, edited by Drs. Zheng, Fadare, and Quick is emblematic of the sea change. We've all heard the joke about resorting to one's grandchild to solve a computer conundrum. How many of us turn to our younger colleagues to interpret emerging genomic information in the management of gynecologic cancer? An appreciation of such talent is crucial to our evolution as well as that of our discipline.

The senior editor in this project, Dr. Wenxin Zheng, has a long track record of innovation. With this has come a facility to recognize the most talented young clinician-investigators and to recruit them into this new textbook. Drs. Fadare and Quick as well as the younger chapter authors are well on their way, having already put us on notice that by their dedication, creativity and their role in discovery. Their input is what will keep this and subsequent editions at the forefront of pathology texts dedicated to women's health.

Energy and intellect drive discovery but experience is essential to provide a needed perspective when this information is transmitted to the practicing pathologist. The editors wisely balance the list of talented newcomers with recognized experts in the field. Together they provide the finer details of diagnosis and differential diagnosis while eliciting the nuances relevant to clinical management.

In the current world, where discoveries and their impact on practice can become global almost instantaneously, one does not need to travel far to realize that expertise in obstetric and gynecologic pathology is intercontinental. In recognizing this, Zheng et al. will also provide an edition written in Chinese, bringing this message to pathologists (and their patients) in countries where the language is read and spoken. To my knowledge, this book will be the first of its kind to accomplish this, creating a truly international presence that will place this first edition among the leading texts in the field. The editors and authors are to be commended for their contribution and I look forward to their success in opening a new chapter (and book!) in the history of the pathology of the female reproductive tract.

Christopher P. Crum
Division of Women's and Perinatal Pathology
Harvard Medical School, Brigham and Women's Hospital
Boston, MA, USA

Preface

Pathology of the female genital tract is complex, and encompasses a wide spectrum of neoplastic and non-neoplastic diseases of the gonads, reproductive ducts, secondary müllerian system, and external genitalia. Clinical practitioners in this discipline must therefore familiarize themselves with a broad spectrum of pathology, including skin-like diseases of the vulva, a myriad of peritoneal diseases, as well as conventional diseases of other female genital tract organs. This field progresses in a vibrant and dynamic academic environment in which diagnostic concepts continually evolve as our understanding of various disease processes improves over time. The contemporary gynecologic pathologist is in a unique position to recognize and define morphologic correlates to newly defined genomic profiles and individual gene mutations, assess whether they are likely to have diagnostic or prognostic significance for a given patient and/or her family, and broadly participate in the push towards increasingly personalized cancer care. These exciting trends notwithstanding, it remains true that definitive pathologic classification of gynecologic disease is still primarily based on the traditional pillars of surgical pathology, including gross pathology, morphologic assessment buttressed by immunophenotypic analysis where needed, and careful clinicopathologic correlation.

This book is envisioned as a "bridge" that acknowledges both of the aforementioned realities. It is designed to provide a broad coverage of diagnostic gynecologic and obstetric pathology, inclusive of both neoplastic and non-neoplastic diseases. The book is neither a dense and comprehensive treatise on every disease process nor is it a dry listing of relevant "facts" about each entity. Rather, it is best conceptualized as a large scale aggregation of the most up to date information in gynecologic pathology, all presented in a concise and narrative manner that is designed to be easily accessible to the general practitioner, specialist and student alike. An overt effort has been made to discuss each topic in a way that is maximally relevant to the diagnostic surgical pathologist, such that by reading any section should substantially increase the reader's confidence that the most germane clinicopathologic information on that entity has been reviewed before a diagnostic decision is made.

The material is organized into 36 chapters, representing the full spectrum of diagnostic gynecologic pathology. In addition to chapters on traditional topics in gynecologic pathology, there are individual chapters on site-specific carcinogenesis, gynecologic cytology, intraoperative consultation, endometriosis and development/maldevelopment of the female reproductive system, among others. Additionally, in a departure from most current texts, there are stand-alone chapters to provide intensive coverage of some traditionally under-covered topics, including melanocytic lesions of the female genital tract, non-neoplastic diseases of the endometrium, and vulvovaginal soft tissue lesions. Entities with a significant diagnostic component are presented, where feasible, divided into the following subsections: *Clinical features, Gross findings, Microscopic findings, Differential diagnosis, Biomarkers,* and *Genetic features.* As expected, not all entities or chapters lend themselves to this specific format, but most chapters are broadly structured based on these general themes. Microscopic findings are lavishly illustrated, and numerous tables help summarize pertinent points for easy reference. The overall objective of each chapter is to integrate traditional pathologic features, clinical features, where applicable, and current paradigms in disease classification into a format that can be readily applied in routine practice. These chapters are authored by over 50 physicians, most of whom are experienced subspecialty practitioners of clinical gynecologic pathology from around the world, and without whose expertise, dedication, and diligence this work would not have been possible. It is the sincere hope of the editors that all of those who are interested in gynecologic pathology—diagnostic pathologists, students, residents and investigators—will find this book tremendously useful.

The understanding of gynecologic disease involves pathologists and researchers from across oceans and all over the world, and to that end an exciting feature of this book is that it is written with a direct linkage to the second edition of the book "Gynecologic and Obstetric Pathology". The latter book is in Chinese, and is published by Science Press, Beijing, China. The current text is published in both English and Chinese, representing a collaborative effort by both publishers: Springer and Science Press. Although the titles and the number of chapters are identical in the two books, the authors of the chapters are different. Additionally, while the chapter outlines and some of the contents overlap, the two books do not represent a direct translation from one to the other. Rather, they are best considered complementary "sister" books. This results from Dr. Wenxin Zheng serving as the first editor-in-chief for both books. Considering this special and close relationship, the co-editors for the Chinese book, Drs. Danhua Shen and Donghui Guo, are listed as co-editors of the English version of this book, while Drs. Fadare and Quick are also listed as co-editors on the second edition of the Chinese book.

Dallas, TX — Wenxin Zheng
San Diego, CA — Oluwole Fadare
Little Rock, AR — Charles Matthew Quick

Acknowledgments

To my dear wife Wenda and my beloved family (Yuxin, Genfu, and Deshun) for their constant love and endless support! In memory of my parents Maoguan Zheng and Jinxian Wang as well as my ultimate mentor Dr. Stuart C. Lauchlan.

Wenxin Zheng

To my wife Abby for her love, encouragement, and inspiration, and to our beloved children Nathaniel, Darrell and Olivia for (mostly) putting up with the occasional absences that were required to do this.

Oluwole Fadare

To my everything, Shelly, and my wonderful children Dexter, Bernice, and Alice.

Charles Matthew Quick

To my beloved family members for their continuous support and care, and to all my colleagues who participated in editing this outstanding book. I am honored to be an editor for this prestigious book.

Danhua Shen

To my beloved family members for their constant support and care, and to Drs. Zhaoai Kong and Song Lin whose past instruction and training have been and continues to be invaluable.

Donghui Guo

The Editors would like to sincerely thank Dr. Christopher P. Crum, M.D. for serving as a senior consulting adviser for this book. Dr. Crum has made significant contributions to the field of gynecologic pathology and has trained innumerable residents and fellows, including many who have served as an author for this book. The quality of this work is in part attributable to his years of dedicated teaching and research in the field of gynecologic pathology.

Contents

About the Editors

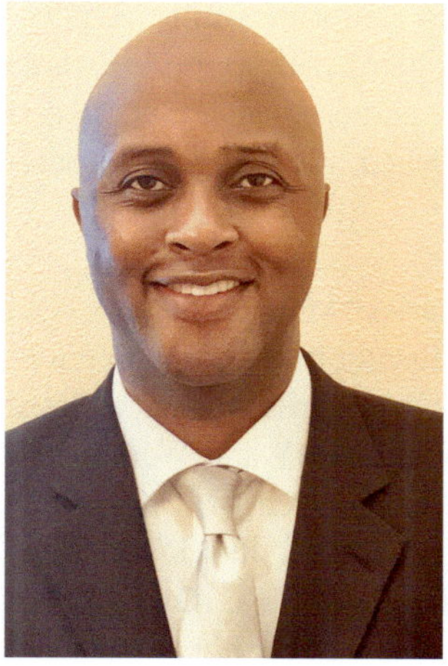

Oluwole Fadare Dr. Oluwole Fadare is a Professor of Pathology at the University of California San Diego School of Medicine (UCSD, San Diego, CA, USA), where he also serves as the Chief of Anatomic Pathology for the UCSD Health System and Director of the Gynecologic/Breast Pathology fellowship. Dr. Fadare completed a fellowship in breast and gynecologic pathology at the Yale University School of Medicine (New Haven, CT, USA) in 2005, and has spent his subsequent academic career focused on the pathologic aspects of women's health. Dr. Fadare has been the recipient of numerous prestigious awards, including most recently the 2018 Arthur Purdy Stout Prize from the Arthur Purdy Stout Society of Surgical Pathologists in recognition of "significant career achievements in Surgical Pathology by a Surgical Pathologist (less than 45 years old) whose publications have had a major impact on diagnostic pathology", a 2018 Stowell-Orbison Certificate of Merit from the United States and Canadian Academy of Pathologists (USCAP), and a 2017 Excellence in Mentoring Award from UCSD Health Sciences International "in recognition of a sustained commitment to helping create a cadre of global leaders in innovative academic medicine". Dr. Fadare has published more than 200 peer-reviewed articles in high impact scientific journals, predominantly centered on gynecologic pathology. Previous books edited or co-written include *Diagnosis of Neoplasia in Endometrial Biopsies: A Pattern-Based and Algorithmic Approach* (Cambridge University Press, 2014) and *Precancerous Lesions of the Gynecologic Tract: Diagnostic and Molecular Genetic Pathology* (Springer 2015). Dr. Fadare has served in various editorial capacities for over 80 journals, and is currently an editorial board member for the *International Journal of Gynecological Pathology, Human Pathology, Advances in Anatomic Pathology, Archives of Pathology and Laboratory Medicine, Archives of Medical Research*, and *Diagnostic Pathology*, among others. He is also active in various professional societies, and currently serves on the education committee for the International Society of Gynecologic Pathologists and on the membership committee for USCAP. Dr. Fadare's research has been clinical based, and has focused on integrating morphological, immunohistochemical and molecular aspects of gynecologic tract neoplasms to optimize diagnostic, prognostic and predictive patient care.

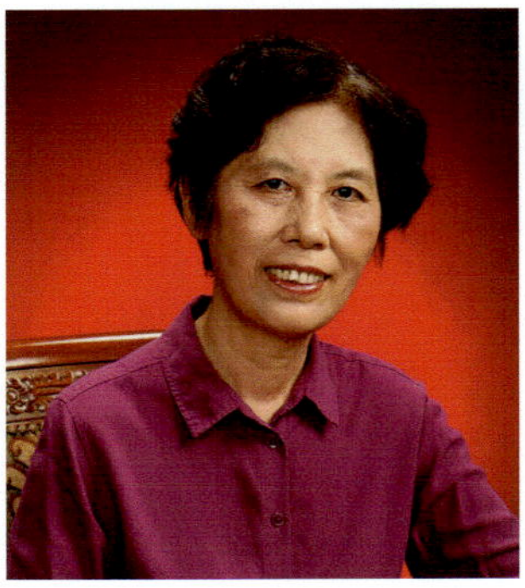

Donghui Guo Dr. Guo graduated from the Fourth Military Medical University of China in 1974, and is one of the top gynecologic pathologists in China. Mentored by Professor Song Lin in the early part of her career, Dr. Guo has practiced gynecologic pathology for more than 30 years. Dr. Guo served as Chairman in the Department of Pathology, Tianjin Central Hospital of Obstetrics and Gynecology for 10 years. She has mentored many graduate students, residents, and fellows with an interest in gynecologic pathology. Dr. Guo has served as a committee member as well as a well-recognized expert in gynecologic pathology for many professional societies in China. Dr. Guo has completed 4 major scientific achievements (please provide the details here) with multiple awards in Tianjin, China. Dr. Guo has authored and co-edited 5 pathology books and has published more than 30 peer-reviewed articles.

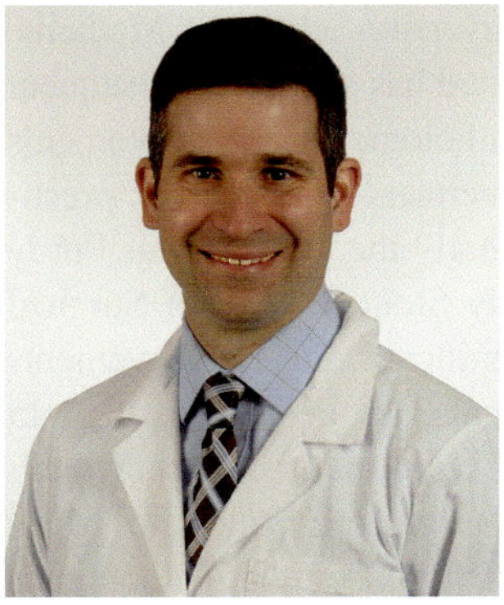

Charles Matthew Quick Dr. Charles "Matt"hew Quick is an associate professor and clinical educator in the Department of Pathology at UAMS in Little Rock, Arkansas. He completed fellowships in surgical pathology at UAMS and Women's & Perinatal pathology at Harvard Medical School, Brigham & Women's Hospital. Dr. Quick serves as the Director of Anatomic Pathology Sub-Specialty Practice, Gynecologic Pathology, and the Surgical Pathology Fellowship.

He has published numerous research publications and review articles, and has authored and co-edited multiple textbooks, including "High-Yield Pathology: Gynecologic and Obstetric Pathology." He loves all things teaching and gynecologic pathology related and has won numerous teaching awards for his medical student and resident education efforts, including UAMS's campus-wide "Chancellor's Award for Teaching Excellence." Dr. Quick is dedicated to expanding pathology education in medical school and has started numerous programs at UAMS to effect this change including the UAMS pathology interest group: SCOPE, a summer pathology preceptorship, and the integration of autopsy pathology into the first year gross anatomy course, earning him an Education Innovation award in 2015. His efforts have led to a dramatic increase in medical students choosing pathology as a career in the state of Arkansas.

Dr. Quick serves as an Ambassador for the United States and Canadian Academy of Pathology, and has taught numerous interactive microscopy courses for the USCAP at both annual meetings and the new teaching complex located in Palm Springs, California. He serves as the Gynecologic Pathology Course Director for the USCAP Interactive Microscopy Center. Dr. Quick's research interests include the study of endometrial precancers, vulvar squamous carcinogenesis and the impact of epithelial-mesenchymal transition on tumor behavior.

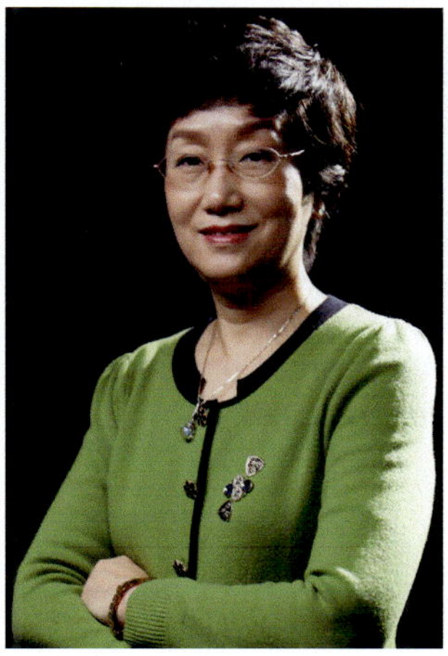

Danhua Shen Dr. Danhua Shen, Associate Professor of Pathology, is the Chairman of the Department of Pathology, People's Hospital of Peking University, China. Dr. Shen is one of the top gynecologic pathologists in China. In addition to her dedication to pathology diagnosis, Dr. Shen has participated in many research projects of *National Natural Science Foundation of China.* She is the head of the *Female Reproductive Diseases Group of the Pathology Branch of the Chinese Medical Association*, and serves as an executive committee member for many prestigious professional societies including the *Chinese Gynecologic Oncology Group, Chinese Society of Obstetrics and Gynecology*, and *Chinese Society of Colposcopy and Cervical Pathology*, etc. Dr. Shen is also an editorial board member for the *Journal of Chinese Pathology* and the *Chinese Journal of Obstetrics and Gynecology*, and the *Journal of Diagnostic Pathology*.

Dr. Shen has published more than 100 peer reviewed articles, and has been involved in seven clinical and pathological related monographs/books or book chapters either as an editor-in-chief or deputy editor-in-chief. Dr. Shen has also participated in many book translations in the field of Pathology and Obstetrics and Gynecology.

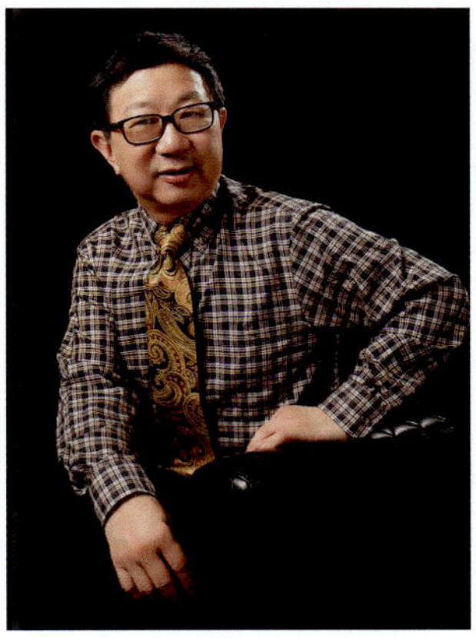

Wenxin Zheng Dr. Zheng is a tenured Professor in the Department of Pathology and the Department of Obstetrics and Gynecology at the University of Texas Southwestern Medical Center (UTSW). An internationally recognized gynecologic pathologist as well as active physician scientist, he specializes in all aspects of gynecologic pathology and holds the Mark and Jane Gibson Distinguished Professorship in Cancer Research. Dr. Zheng also serves as the Director of Gynecologic Pathology service and the Director of Gynecologic Pathology Fellowship at the UTSW Medical Center.

Dr. Zheng earned his medical degree at Shanghai Medical College Fudan University. He completed a residency in obstetrics and gynecology at the Hospital of Obstetrics and Gynecology in Shanghai and, later, a residency in anatomic and clinical pathology at New York Hospital-Cornell Medical Center. He received advanced training through a gynecologic pathology fellowship at Women & Infants Hospital of Rhode Island and a research fellowship in molecular reproductive medicine at Columbia University College of Physicians and Surgeons (New York).

Dr. Zheng runs an active consultation practice that receives material world wide. Dr. Zheng has published more than 180 peer-reviewed articles in high impact scientific journals, mostly in the field of gynecologic pathology. He has served in various editorial capacities for over 50 journals, and is currently an editorial board member for multiple journals in the biomedical sciences. His main research contributions include endometrial serous carcinogenesis and precancerous lesion endometrial glandular dysplasia, cell origin of low-grade ovarian serous carcinoma, molecular mechanism of progestin resistance in endometrial cancer and its precancers, hormonal etiology of ovarian epithelial cancers, and tubal contribution of ovarian endometriosis and its associated ovarian cancers. In addition, Dr. Zheng has created a novel approach called one-stop cervical care (OSCC) to diagnose and treat cervical pre-cancers. Dr. Zheng Loves teaching gynecologic pathology to residents and fellows and have taught numerous gynecologic pathology courses nationally and internationally.

Contributors

Isabel Alvarado-Cabrero Department of Pathology, Mexican Oncology Hospital, Mexico City, Mexico

Michaela Bártů First Faculty of Medicine, Institute of Pathology, Charles University and General University Hospital in Prague, Prague, Czech Republic

Diane Bruyere Laboratory of Experimental Pathology, GIGA-Cancer, University of Liege, Liege, Belgium

Katelynn Campbell University of Arkansas for Medical Sciences, Little Rock, AR, USA

M. Carolina Reyes Department of Pathology, Hospital of the University of Pennsylvania, Philadelphia, PA, USA

Diego H. Castrillon Department of Pathology, University of Texas Southwestern Medical Center, Dallas, TX, USA

Hao Chen Department of Pathology, University of Texas Southwestern Medical Center, Dallas, TX, USA

Kyle Devins Department of Pathology, Hospital of the University of Pennsylvania, Philadelphia, PA, USA

Michael DeWall Department of Pathology, University of Arkansas for Medical Sciences, Little Rock, AR, USA

Bojana Djordjevic Division of Anatomic Pathology, Sunnybrook Health Sciences Centre, Toronto, ON, Canada

Department of Laboratory Medicine and Pathobiology, University of Toronto, Toronto, ON, Canada

Pavel Dundr First Faculty of Medicine, Institute of Pathology, Charles University and General University Hospital in Prague, Prague, Czech Republic

Andrew Dunn Department of Pathology, University of Arkansas for Medical Sciences, Little Rock, AR, USA

Oluwole Fadare Department of Pathology, University of California San Diego, San Diego, CA, USA

Raji Ganesan Birmingham Women's Hospital, Birmingham, UK

Debra S. Heller Department of Pathology, Immunology and Laboratory Medicine, Rutgers New Jersey Medical School, Newark, NJ, USA

Michael Herfs Laboratory of Experimental Pathology, GIGA-Cancer, University of Liege, Liege, Belgium

Eric C. Huang Department of Pathology, University of Washington School of Medicine, Harborview Medical Center, Seattle, WA, USA

Susanne K. Jeffus Department of Pathology, University of Arkansas for Medical Sciences, Little Rock, AR, USA

Jennifer Kaley Department of Pathology, University of Arkansas for Medical Sciences, Little Rock, AR, USA

Dmitry V. Kazakov Medical Faculty in Pilsen, Sikl's Department of Pathology, Charles University in Prague, Pilsen, Czech Republic

Bioptical Laboratory, Pilsen, Czech Republic

Anastasia M. Konstantinova Department of Pathology, Clinical Research and Practical Center for Specialized Oncological Care, Saint-Petersburg, Russia

Medical Faculty, Department of Pathology, Saint-Petersburg State University, Saint-Petersburg, Russia

Department of Pathology, Saint-Petersburg Medico-Social Institute, Saint-Petersburg, Russia

Alizee Lebeau Laboratory of Experimental Pathology, GIGA-Cancer, University of Liege, Liege, Belgium

Mariah Zampieri Leivo Department of Pathology, University of California San Diego, San Diego, CA, USA

Anatomic Pathology Division, Department of Pathology, University of California San Diego Health, La Jolla, CA, USA

Michal Michal Medical Faculty in Pilsen, Sikl's Department of Pathology, Charles University in Prague, Pilsen, Czech Republic

Bioptical Laboratory, Pilsen, Czech Republic

Anne M. Mills Department of Pathology, University of Virginia, Charlottesville, VA, USA

Kristýna Němejcová First Faculty of Medicine, Institute of Pathology, Charles University and General University Hospital in Prague, Prague, Czech Republic

Carlos Parra-Herran Department of Laboratory Medicine and Pathobiology, University of Toronto, Toronto, ON, Canada

Sunnybrook Health Sciences Centre, Toronto, ON, Canada

Charles Matthew Quick Department of Pathology, University of Arkansas for Medical Sciences, Little Rock, AR, USA

Sara C. Shalin Department of Pathology, University of Arkansas for Medical Sciences, Little Rock, AR, USA

Department of Dermatology, University of Arkansas for Medical Sciences, Little Rock, AR, USA

Sharon J. Song Department of Pathology, Hospital of the University of Pennsylvania, Philadelphia, PA, USA

Simona Stolnicu Department of Pathology, University of Medicine and Pharmacy of Targu Mures, Targu Mures, Romania

Geok Chin Tan Universiti Kebangsaan Malaysia Hospital, Kuala Lumpur, Malaysia

Vighnesh Walavalkar Department of Pathology, UCSF School of Medicine, San Francisco, CA, USA

Anthony T. Williams Birmingham Women's Hospital, Birmingham, UK

Deyin Xing Department of Pathology, The Johns Hopkins University School of Medicine, Baltimore, MD, USA

T. Yee Khong SA Pathology, Women's and Children's Hospital, North Adelaide, Australia

University of Adelaide, Adelaide, Australia

Somaye Yeke Zare Department of Pathology, University of California San Diego, San Diego, CA, USA

Anatomic Pathology Division, Department of Pathology, University of California San Diego Health, La Jolla, CA, USA

Wenxin Zheng Department of Pathology, Obstetrics and Gynecology, University of Texas Southwestern Medical Center, Dallas, TX, USA

Development and Maldevelopment of the Female Reproductive System

1

Diego H. Castrillon

Abstract

The female reproductive tract has its embryological origins in the paired Müllerian ducts and their fusion to each other and the urogenital sinus. The Müllerian ducts give rise to the oviducts, uterus, and cervix, while the urogenital sinus forms the vagina and external genitalia. Primordial germ cells formed near the yolk sac migrate to colonize the gonadal ridge, where in females interactions between germ and somatic cells coalesce to create the functional ovarian units known as follicles.

A classical morphologic understanding of the embryology of these structures has served as the foundation for a general understanding of myriad conditions due to maldevelopment or malignant transformation. Increasingly, the molecular underpinnings of these complex underlying developmental transformations are being revealed, yielding deeper insights into the biological basis of female reproductive tract disease pathophysiology and also providing many useful markers, such as Sall4, Foxl2, Wt1, and Pax8, routinely used in clinical practice. In some cases, Müllerian maldevelopment syndromes such as Müllerian agenesis are now known to be caused by mutations in the genes encoding factors required for Müllerian duct development.

The once far-fetched idea that epithelial cells of the oviduct—not the ovary itself—are the origin of most "ovarian" carcinomas now has universal acceptance. Female reproductive tract malignancies of the cervix, uterus, and ovary recently believed to have disparate cellular/embryologic origins are now understood to have a shared origin in the epithelial lining of the Müllerian ducts. This insight rationalizes many prior observations, for example, that the diverse tumor histotypes common to the cervix, endometrium, or tubo-ovarian complex are encountered across each site. This chapter summarizes our understanding of female gonadal and reproductive tract development, with an emphasis on morphologic and molecular aspects that currently appear most relevant to disease pathophysiology.

Keywords

Primordial germ cells · Gonadal ridge · Sex determination · Müllerian duct · Maldevelopment · Female reproductive tract

1.1 Primordial Germ Cells: Formation and Migration

Four embryologically and anatomically distinct primordia form the female genital tract: (1) primordial germ cells, (2) the gonadal ridge, (3) the paired Müllerian ducts, and (4) the urogenital sinus. The initial formation of these primordia and subsequent developmental processes occur in coordinated steps throughout gestation (summarized in Table 1.1).

Germ cells, which ultimately give rise to gametes, are responsible for the transmission of genetic information and the propagation of species. Because of their relatively small numbers, their formation and preservation is of utmost biological importance. The initially formed germ cells are termed primordial germ cells (PGCs). In invertebrates such as the common fruit fly *Drosophila melanogaster*, PGCs are specified by cytoplasmic components known as the germplasm allocated to the posterior of the egg during oogenesis, and PGCs are the first cells formed in the embryo (preformation) [1]. In mice, humans, and other mammals, PGCs are formed much later in development by inductive processes requiring cell-cell interactions and external signals (epigenesis) [2]. Thus in mammals, the germ cell lineage (the "germline") is discontinuous.

D. H. Castrillon (✉)
Department of Pathology, University of Texas Southwestern Medical Center, Dallas, TX, USA
e-mail: Diego.Castrillon@UTSouthwestern.edu

W. Zheng et al. (eds.), *Gynecologic and Obstetric Pathology, Volume 1*, https://doi.org/10.1007/978-981-13-3016-2_1

Table 1.1 Development of the female reproductive tract

Weeks gestation (from ovulation)	Crown-rump length (mm)	Heel-toe length (mm)	Developmental event
3 weeks	2.5		Germline specification begins
4 weeks	3–5		Primordial germ cells are formed
5 weeks	7		Gonadal ridge formation
6 weeks	11		Müllerian ducts appear as funnel-shaped opening of coelomic epithelium (initiation phase)
7 weeks	18		Müllerian ducts migrate to about half distance to urogenital sinus
	23		Müllerian ducts extend caudally to near the urogenital sinus
8 weeks	30		Primordial germ cells colonize gonadal ridge
			Müllerian ducts begin midline fusion and make contact with urogenital sinus at the Müllerian tubercle
9 weeks	50		Müllerian ducts fuse (septum disappears); epithelium lining uterovaginal canal stratifies (1–2 cells layers thick)
10 weeks	60	2–5	Oogonia in leptotene prophase of meiosis I (initiation of meiosis in some oogonia continues to at least 16 weeks)
11 weeks	71	5–8	Bilateral sinovaginal bulbs (evagination of UGS) appear
	75		Vaginal plate first seen distinctly at 75 mm (complete at 140 mm; week 17)
14 weeks	110–140	15–17	Marked growth of caudal vagina
			Vaginal rudiment reaches level of vestibular glands; uterovaginal canal (15 mm total length) divisible into vagina (one-half), cervix (one-third), and corpus (one-sixth); boundaries ill-defined
			Endometrial and myometrial layers of uterus become apparent
			Solid epithelial precursors of anterior and posterior fornices appear
			Vagina shows epithelial squamous differentiation
15 weeks	130–140	18–21	Primordial follicle individualization begins and continues through first postnatal months
			Cervix about 5 mm long
			Fallopian tube begins active growth phase
			Vaginal plate extends to endocervical canal
16 weeks	142	21–24	Uterine/cervical glands begin as outpouchings of simple columnar epithelium
			Vaginal plate longest and begins to canalize
			Solid epithelial projections of anterior and posterior fornices demarcate cranial end of vagina
17 weeks	153–162	24–27	Palmate folds of cervix appear (forerunner adult cervix)
			Mucoid development of cervix begins. Estrogen-induced thickening of vaginal epithelium
19 weeks	177	31–33	Canalization of vaginal plate completed
			Uterine tube growth marked (~3 mm/week to week 34)
			Cervix about 10 mm long
22 weeks	208	40–43	Vagina completely formed
			Differentiation of uterine myometrium complete
24 weeks	215–295	47–49	Uterine fundus well defined, uterus assumes adult form, uterine body about 10 mm long
38 weeks	362		Birth
Postnatal			Meiosis and primordial follicle individualization continue and are completed within a few months to establish primordial follicle reserve

Landmarks in Müllerian tract adapted from Robboy SJ et al. 97:9 (2017) [80] with permission (Elsevier). Other landmarks from references as described in text

1.1.1 Germline Specification and Migration

Germline specification in humans begins at around the time of gastrulation, at the 3rd week of development, and PGCs are first observed during the 4th week of development in the extraembryonic yolk sac wall near the allantois (Fig. 1.1) [3]. PGCs are cytologically distinctive and significantly larger than the surrounding somatic cells, with a diameter of 25–30 μm. The initial complement of PGCs may be as few as 50–100 individual cells [3]. PGCs express alkaline phosphatase, which can be detected via a histochemical reaction [4]. They also express the cell surface receptor tyrosine kinase Kit (CD117) and other germ cell-specific markers [5]. Kit is required for PGC migration and survival [6]. PGCs can be identified in human embryos by immunostaining for Kit or the pan-germ cell marker Vasa (Fig. 1.2) [5]. Human PGCs also express pluripotency genes first turned on in embryonic stem cells, such as Oct4 [7] and Sall4 [8], which are sup-

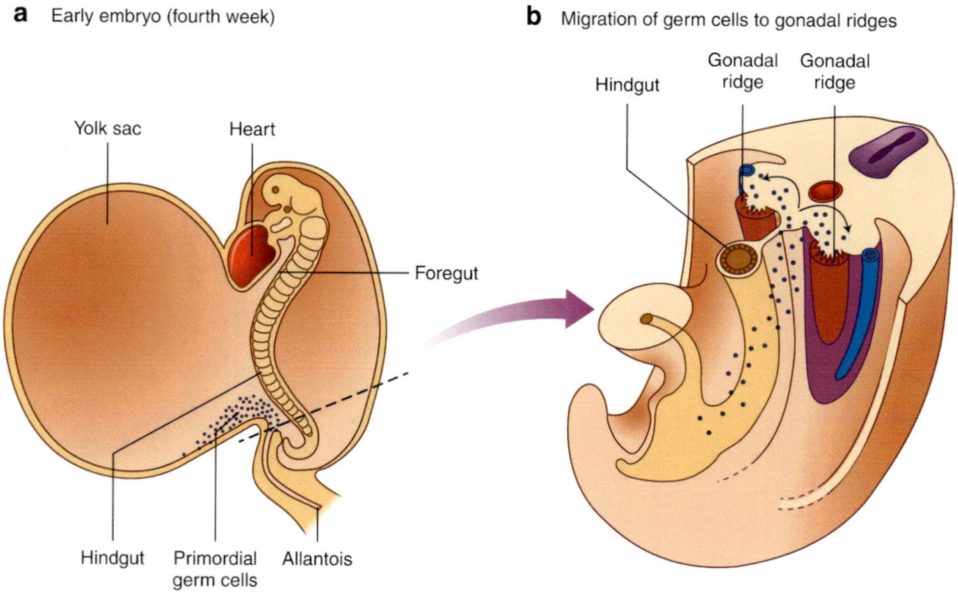

Fig. 1.1 Formation and migration of primordial germ cells (PGCs). (**a**) PGC formation in early embryo. (**b**) Migration through embryonic structures to eventual destination in bilateral gonadal ridges. Redrawn with permission from Mesiano S and Jones EE, Medical Physiology 3rd edition, Chapter 53 (2017) (Elsevier)

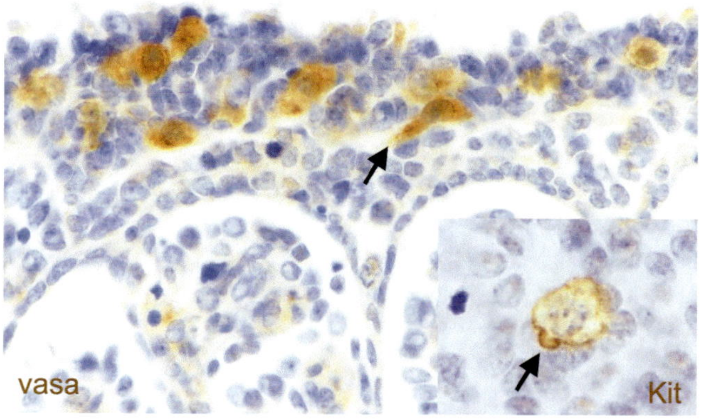

Fig. 1.2 Primordial germ cells migrating into gonadal ridge, human embryo at 8 weeks estimated gestational age. The top cell layers are part of the gonadal ridge; the subjacent tubules are part of the mesonephros (early excretory system that will degenerate). Inset: Kit immunostaining shows membrane localization in migratory PGC near gonadal ridge. Note pseudopodia (arrows)

pressed in somatic lineages. Therefore, Oct4 and Sall4 are useful as male and female germ cell markers throughout life, although they do exhibit some differences. In the neonatal ovary, Oct4 is expressed in oogonia but not in oocytes (i.e., in individualized primordial follicles, see discussion below), whereas Sall4 exhibits the opposite pattern (Fig. 1.3).

After their formation, PGCs begin a remarkable long-range migration from the yolk sac through various embryonic structures including the gut to eventually reach and colonize the gonadal primordium (the gonadal ridge) by 8 weeks gestational age (Fig. 1.1). During migration, PGC numbers expand mitotically, and the cells adopt an amoeboid shape with pseudopodia [3]. In females, PGCs that have colonized the gonadal ridge become round and are termed oogonia. The external signals and homing mechanisms guiding PGCs to the gonadal ridge are poorly understood but involve Kit ligand (aka stem cell factor) acting through the Kit cell surface receptor and cell adhesion molecules [9–11]. The existence of extragonadal germ cell tumors (i.e., sacrococcygeal or within the mediastinum or cranium) has been attributed to mismigration of PGCs during embryogenesis (see e.g., [12, 13]), but this intriguing notion remains unproven.

Due to the impracticability of studying early postimplantation human embryos, the molecular specification of PGCs has been most extensively explored in mice, although there has been an increasing focus on human studies. In mice, Bmp signals act through downstream Smad proteins to induce the expression of the transcriptional repressor Prdm1 in PGCs. Prdm1 robustly suppresses somatic gene expression (i.e., the expression of non-germline genes) and is critically required for mouse PGC development [14, 15]. Prdm1 is also induced in human PGCs and is required for their development. The secreted factor Wnt3 acting through the downstream transducer β-catenin is also involved in mouse and human PGC specification. However, while human and mouse PGC specification share many similarities, there are also salient molecular differences. For example, the lineage-specifying transcription factor Sox2 is required for PGC proliferation in mice, whereas human PGCs lack Sox2 but require Sox17 for their specification [16].

1.1.2 Epigenetic Reprogramming of the Germline

DNA methylation at cytosine residues in CpG dinucleotides (producing 5-methylcytosine or 5mC) is an important repressor of transcription in the genome. During mammalian development, epigenetic reprogramming occurs via global

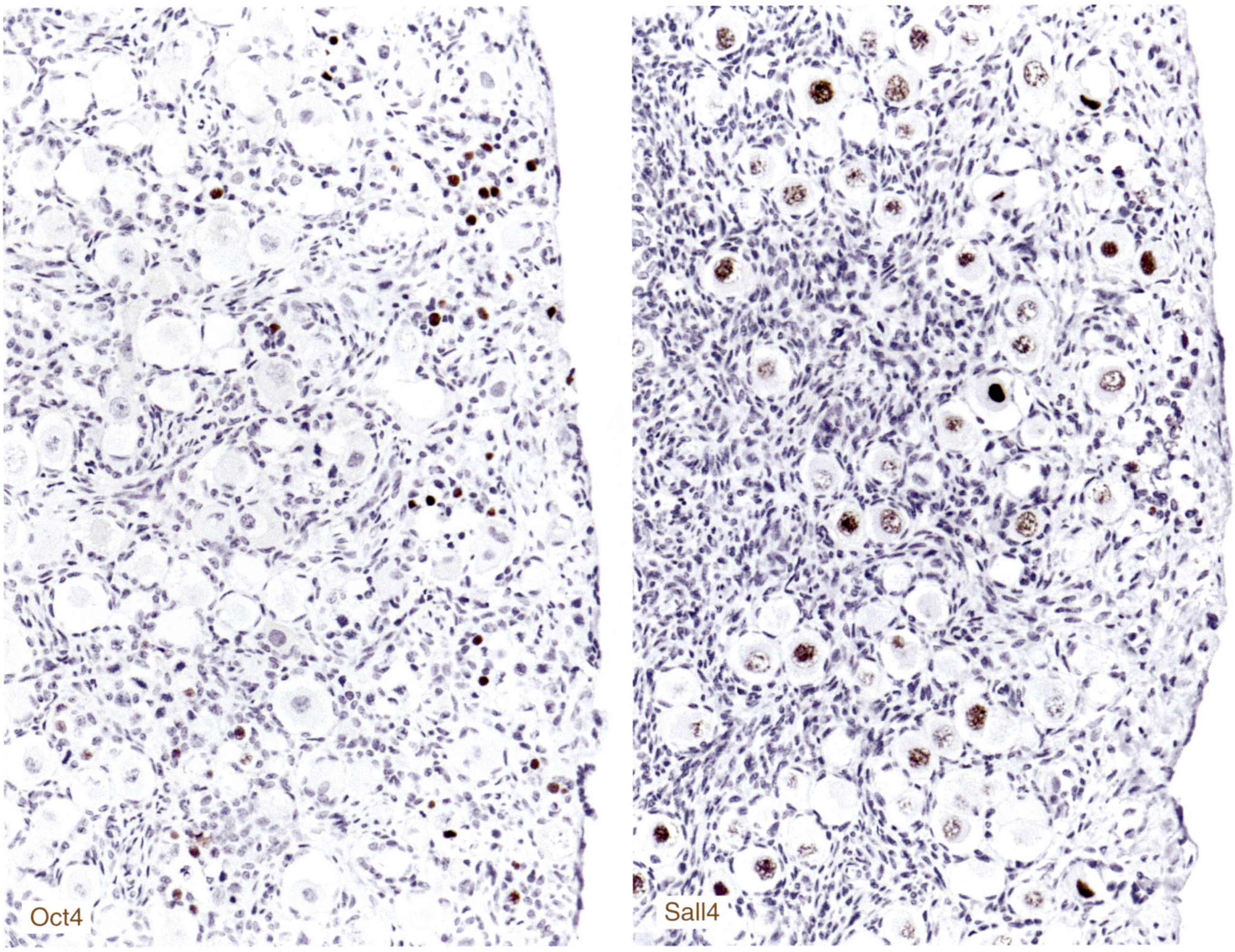

Fig. 1.3 Expression of Oct4 and Sall4 in the neonatal human ovary. Oct4 is highly expressed in oogonial clusters that have not yet individualized but not in individualized primordial oocytes, whereas Sall4 is expressed in the oocytes in fully individualized primordial follicles but not in the oogonia. Note nuclear localization for both markers

DNA demethylation, both (1) after fertilization in the zygote and (2) during early germline (i.e., PGC) development. DNA methylation, which is the basis of genomic imprinting (differential expression of alleles based on parent-of-origin), is generally stably inherited through cell divisions. Reprogramming in the zygote serves to erase epigenetic marks acquired from the gametes (except the marks on imprinted loci such as *CDKN1C*, which encodes p57KIP2) permitting the acquisition of totipotency. A key aspect of the developing germline is the resetting of the epigenome (i.e., genomic imprints) [17]. Such imprints are erased in PGCs of both sexes as they undergo genome-wide demethylation, X chromosome reactivation, and chromatin reorganization during migration and colonization of the gonadal ridge. This hypomethylation is believed to occur through a passive mechanism whereby Prdm1 and other factors repress the expression of the DNA methylases Dnmt3a and b. Consequently, both de novo and maintenance methylation is repressed, resulting in passive demethylation during DNA synthesis as PGCs proliferate. CpG methylation levels drop dramatically, and because of this hypomethylation, parental epigenetic memories are erased through secondary chromatin modifications including depletion of H3K9me2 repressive histone marks (Fig. 1.4). Other mechanisms also contribute to DNA demethylation in PGCs [16].

1.2 The Gonadal Ridges as the Origin of the Bipotential Gonads

The gonadal ridges (aka genital ridges) are the paired precursors (anlagen) of the gonads in both sexes. At around the 5th week of gestation, two small bulges form on the dorsal coelomic wall, lateral to the aorta and medial to the mesonephric duct (Fig. 1.1). The bulges consist of overlying coelomic epithelium (i.e., mesothelium) and the underlying mesenchyme

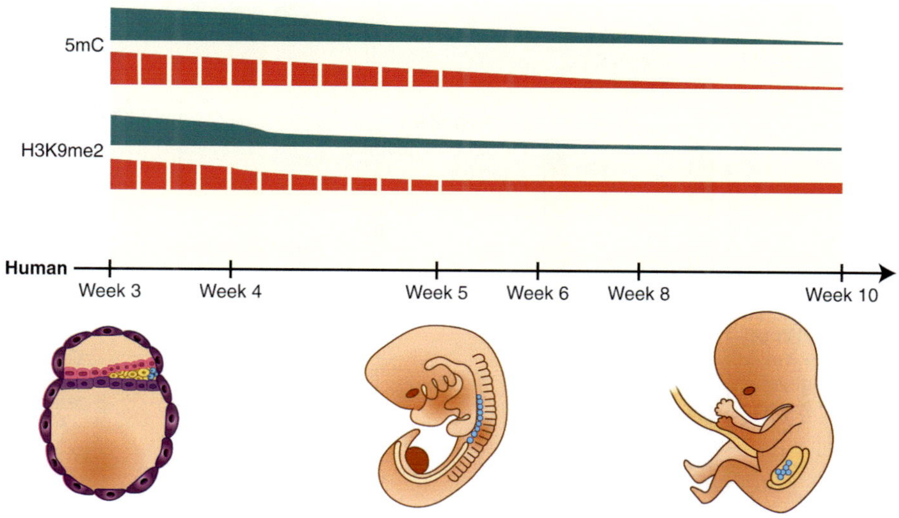

Fig. 1.4 PGCs are epigenetically programmed to reset genomic imprints during their development. Levels of DNA methylation (5-methylcytosine, 5mC) decrease due to a number of mechanisms. This alters various chromatin/histone marks such as H3K9me2 as well as others not shown. Redrawn with permission from Tang WW et al., Nature Review Genetics 17:585 (2016) [16] (Springer Nature)

[18]. The coelomic epithelium proliferates, and the basement membrane becomes fragmented, allowing the epithelial cells to migrate inward, an example of epithelial-mesenchymal transition (see section below on this subject). Prior to the arrival of PGCs, the gonad is histologically identical in both sexes (bipotential gonad), and the cells therein have the unique ability to differentiate into one of two functionally and morphologically distinct organs, an ovary or testis.

The embryologic cells of origin of the adult ovarian somatic cell types (granulosa and theca cells) remain the subject of some debate, and they may have more than one source [19, 20]. The signals that trigger and direct coelomic epithelium to proliferate and differentiate are unknown, but several transcription factors that are highly expressed in the bipotential gonad (Wt1, Sf1, Emx2, Lhx9, and Gata4) are required for formation of the gonadal ridge, among other embryological functions. Mice genetically engineered to be deficient for these factors fail to form gonadal ridges [21–24].

1.3 Sex Determination, Meiosis, and Early Gonadal Development

1.3.1 The Bipotential Gonads

Remarkably, the gonad is the only tissue in the mammalian body plan with two different potential developmental outcomes. In contrast, the development of other sexually dimorphic organs such as the male vs. female reproductive tract (discussed below) depends on the differentiation vs. regression of two entirely distinct precursor structures (the Müllerian vs. Wolffian ducts). Following the arrival of the PGCs, the bipotential gonad adopts two very different fates—testis or ovary—based on chromosomal sex (XX or XY). Subsequent sexual differentiation, including the acquisition of secondary sexual characteristics such as the development of external genitalia, is governed by what type of gonad develops in the embryo.

1.3.2 Sex Determination: Sry, Sox9, and the Male Pathway

The sex-determining region Y protein (encoded by the *Sry* gene on the Y chromosome) is a Sox (Sry-related HMG box) family transcription factor that is both necessary and sufficient to induce testis development [25]. The key and apparently only function of Sry is to induce expression of a second Sox family member gene, Sox9, which is autosomal (human chromosome 17). In XY gonads, Sox9 expression is increased, whereas the opposite occurs in XX gonads. The Sry-positive cells in XY gonads differentiate into Sertoli cells. It is currently thought that a precursor cell in the bipotential gonad differentiates into either Sertoli or granulosa cells dependent on the induction of Sox9 within these cells. Sox9 continues to be highly expressed in adult Sertoli cells and is a useful marker for Sertoli cells within the gonad. It is also believed that a second distinct type of precursor cell differentiates into either testicular Leydig or ovarian theca cells. The transcription factor Wt1, which also functions in MD development, promotes Sertoli cell differentiation and participates in the activation of Sry [26]. Once its expression is established, Sox9 initiates expression of downstream genes including anti-Müllerian hormone (AMH) (Fig. 1.5) [25]. Sox9 also antagonizes β-catenin, a key component of the ovary-determining pathway (see below) by transcriptional and other mechanisms [27, 28].

Deletion of Sox9 in the gonads of XY mice leads to the development of ovaries, and conversely, overexpression

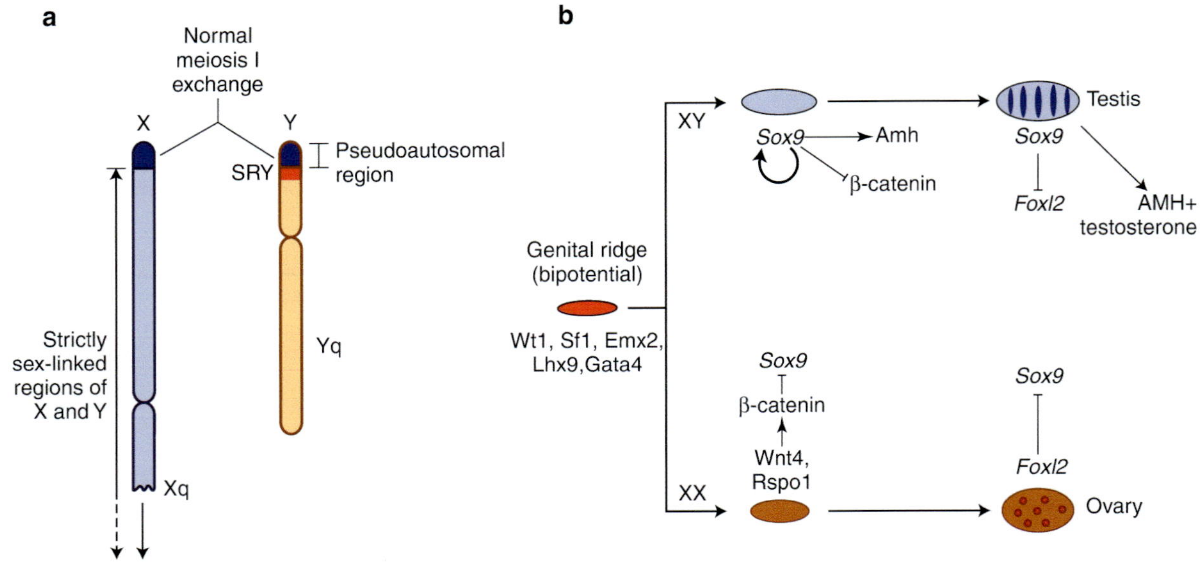

Fig. 1.5 The Y chromosome/SRY/Sox9 pathway of gonadal sex determination. (**a**) The Sry gene is Y-linked (exists only on Y chromosome) and resides on the p arm outside of the pseudoautosomal region. The pseudoautosomal regions are regions of homology on the X and Y chromosomes needed for pairing and crossing-over during meiosis. (**b**) Molecular pathway of gonadal sex determination. Factors required for genital (gonadal) ridge formation are on the left. Simplified male (XY) and female (XX) gonadal pathways are schematized. Redrawn with permission from Nussbaum Rl et al., Chapter 6, Genetics of Medicine, 8th edition (2016) (Elsevier); and Sekido R and Lovell-Badge R, Trends in Genetics, 25:19 (2009) [31] (Elsevier)

of Sox9 in the gonads of XX mice leads to the formation of testes. Thus, Sox9, like Sry, is both necessary and sufficient for testis differentiation. It is interesting to consider why Sox9 evolved as a necessary intermediate step versus a simpler mechanism requiring only Sry as the sole driver of sex determination. One attractive explanation is that Sox9 serves to amplify feeble signals from Sry. Due to the Y chromosome's lack of a homologous partner for crossing-over, the Y undergoes meiotic recombination with the X only in its small pseudoautosomal region, which is needed for X chromosome pairing during meiosis. This makes the Y vulnerable to accumulation of mutations at a much faster rate than the other chromosomes, leading to its biological and functional "enfeeblement" in the non-pseudoautosomal loci including the *Sry* locus over evolutionary timescales [29].

Once Sox9 expression is induced, Sox9 protein maintains its own expression in a robust feed-forward loop that no longer requires a sustained Sry signal. This secures an "all-or-none" binary decision for the appropriate gonadal cells to adopt a Sertoli vs. granulosa cell fate, thus ensuring either completely male or female sexual differentiation. The situation has been compared to "a short pulse from a relatively flimsy starter motor [Sry] which awakens a powerful engine that keeps itself running [Sox9]" [30]. Acquisition of secondary sex differentiation including the development of a male vs. female reproductive tract thus ultimately depends on the formation of Sertoli vs. granulosa cells. If Sertoli cells develop, they secrete factors that induce testicular differentiation, and the Sertoli cells together with Leydig cells produce factors that dictate all subsequent sex determination [31]. These factors are further discussed in the section below on Müllerian duct development.

As mentioned above, at around the time of PGC colonization of the gonadal ridge, the bipotential gonads begin to differentiate into testes in XY embryos and ovaries in XX embryos.

By mechanisms that are not well understood but that depend on a variety of cues including the vasculature, the Sertoli cells from discrete cords, or tubules that can easily be observed grossly by transillumination and are the precursors to the seminiferous tubules. The germ cells, now subjected to the sex-specific cues of their surroundings, adopt very different fates. The male germ cells become embedded within the tubules and enter a state of mitotic arrest; those that fail to become incorporated into the tubules are eliminated. In contrast, the ovaries remain relatively unstructured, containing interspersed somatic cells and oogonia [32].

1.3.3 Initiation of Meiosis in the Female Germline

While germ cells in the testis become mitotically arrested and do not initiate meiosis until puberty, the female germ cells initiate meiosis. In human oogonia, as in other mammals, the initiation of meiosis proceeds rather asynchronously; that is to say, meiosis is not triggered simultaneously

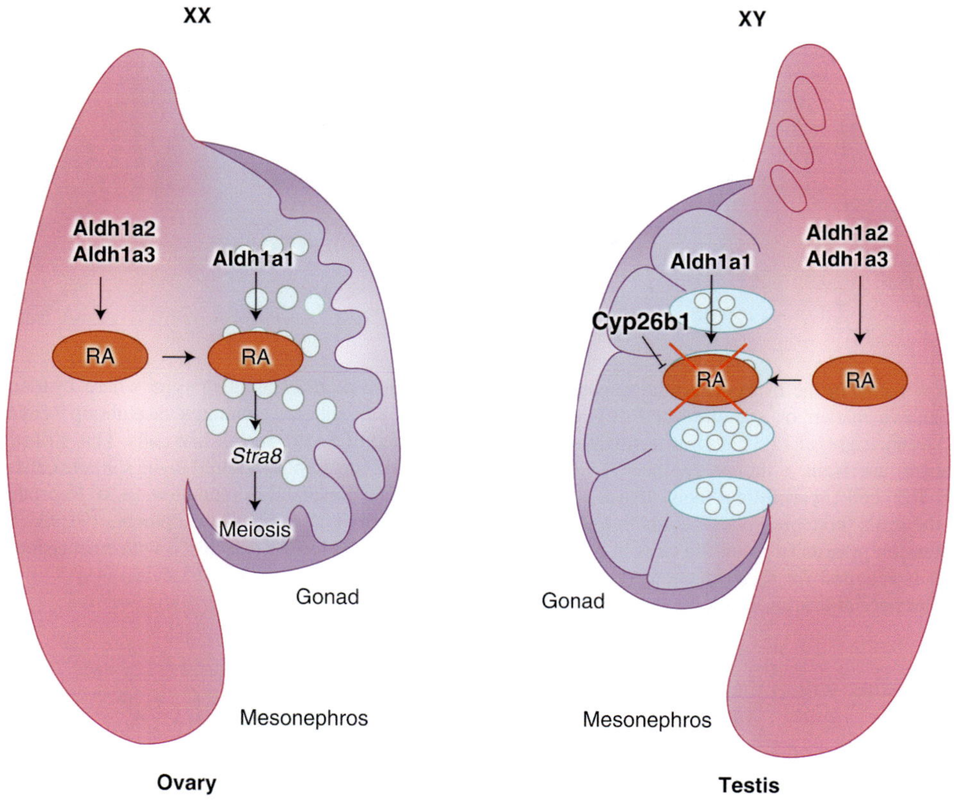

Fig. 1.6 Pathways of retinoic acid (RA) metabolism driving the initiation of meiosis in the XX (female) gonad. Expression of Cyp26b1 in the male gonad metabolizes RA, inhibiting the initiation of meiosis

in all oogonia. Oogonia in the initial leptotene prophase of meiosis I are first observed in embryos at 10–11 weeks gestation [33], but other oogonia continue proliferating and do not initiate meiosis until at least 16 weeks. Oogonia remain arrested in prophase I of meiosis for years or decades, until meiosis resumes following fertilization.

Entry into meiosis is the first outward sign that germ cells have initiated female development. This initiation of meiosis in females (and its absence in males) depends upon retinoic acid (RA) signaling. RA is a diffusible signal and the essential metabolite of vitamin A (retinol). RA acts through binding the retinoic acid receptor (RAR), leading to the control (repression or activation) of downstream genes whose regulatory control regions contain RAR binding sites [32]. Genes encoding the RA synthesis enzymes Aldh1a1, Aldh1a2, and Aldh1a3 are expressed in the gonad and developing mesonephros (part of the developing renal system) adjacent to the gonad, exposing the gonad to relatively high levels of RA. In the XX gonad, these high levels of RA induce the expression within germ cells of downstream RA target genes such as Stra8, leading to progression through meiosis. However, in the XY gonad, the expression within somatic cells of Cyp26b1, a RA-degrading enzyme of the P450 family, effectively degrades the RA signal, and meiosis is not initiated. Cyp26b1 is upregulated by Sox9, linking the sex determination pathway to the initiation of meiosis in germ cells (Fig. 1.6) [25, 32, 34].

1.3.4 Somatic Gonadal Differentiation: Foxl2, Granulosa Cells, and the Ovary-Determining Pathway

Another salient difference between the male and female germline is that while spermatogonia in early cords are individualized (i.e., physically separate from one another), the oogonial mitotic divisions preceding the initiation of meiosis occur with incomplete cytokinesis, leading to syncytial nests of female germ cells interconnected by intercellular bridges (ring canals). These oogonial nests, also known as cysts, are invested in somatic cells destined to become granulosa cells.

In humans, *Wnt4* and *Rspo1* loss-of-function mutations result in sex reversal in XX females, and both of these factors function by stabilizing β-catenin. Consistent with this idea, XY mice engineered to express a constitutively active form of β-catenin in the somatic cells of the gonad undergo ovarian development (sex reversal). This does not affect the initial upregulation of Sox9 in the gonad but interferes with maintenance of Sox9 expression. Thus, Wnt4, Rspo1, and

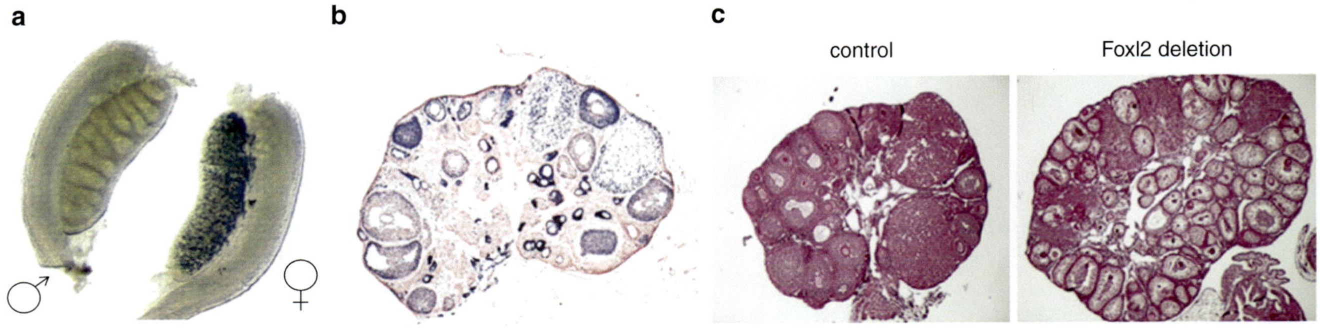

Fig. 1.7 Foxl2 is a key factor in the ovary-determining pathway. (**a**) Foxl2 is the earliest known marker of granulosa cell differentiation: mouse testis (left) and ovary (right) at 12.5 days postfertilization. These male and female gonads are from a mouse engineered to express β-galactosidase in Foxl2⁺ cells, permitting their visualization. No expression is seen in the testis (note presence of cords in testis but not ovary). (**b**) Foxl2 expression persists in granulosa cells in adult mouse ovary (blue stain) and is required for their function. (**c**) Deletion of Foxl2 in adult mice (after normal ovarian development has taken place) results in sex reversal phenotype where ovarian follicles are transformed into tubular structures resembling seminiferous tubules and comprised of Sox9⁺ Sertoli-like cells. This striking sex reversal shows that Foxl2 function is required in the somatic cells of the ovary to maintain female gonadal differentiation. (**a**, **b**) Reproduced with permission from Schmidt D et al., Development, 131:933 (2004) (Company of Biologists) [36]. (**c**) Reproduced with permission from Uhlenhaut NH et al., Cell 139:1130 (2009) (Elsevier) [41]

β-catenin function together within the gonad as "anti-testis" factors (Fig. 1.5) [25].

The forkhead transcription factor Foxl2 also serves an essential and evolutionarily conserved role in the establishment and continuation of ovarian fate [35]. Foxl2 is among the earliest genes induced in the developing ovary and is the earliest established marker of granulosa cell fate. In mouse XX gonads, Foxl2 is first expressed in the somatic cells surrounding germ cell nests of XX gonads at the time that cord-like structures are first formed in XY gonads (Fig. 1.7) [36]. The mechanisms underlying the induction of Foxl2 induction specifically within XX gonads and its lack thereof in XY gonads are not well understood. Later in development and in early postnatal mouse ovaries, Foxl2 expression occurs in both granulosa and interstitial cells, but decreases in the latter population with age (Fig. 1.7) [37]. This expression in both granulosa and interstitial ovarian cells also occurs in the human ovary (Fig. 1.8) and rationalizes the fact that Foxl2 is a sensitive and specific immunohistochemical marker of sex-cord stromal tumors in general, but is not specific for granulosa cell tumors [38].

Foxl2 is not required for the formation of the ovary in mice, as Foxl2-deficient mice develop ovaries. However, Foxl2-deficient female mice exhibit abnormal postnatal granulosa cell/follicular development, leading to defective follicles, massive follicular atresia, and premature ovarian failure and sterility [36, 39]. Interestingly, genes involved in the testis pathway are abnormally activated in Foxl2-deficient ovaries, indicating that Foxl2 represses the testicular gene expression program [40]. Foxl2 is also essential for the continued maintenance of granulosa cell fate in adult life. Bypassing this embryonic requirement for Foxl2 function in follicle formation through postnatal deletion of the *Foxl2* gene in adult mouse ovaries revealed a striking phenotype

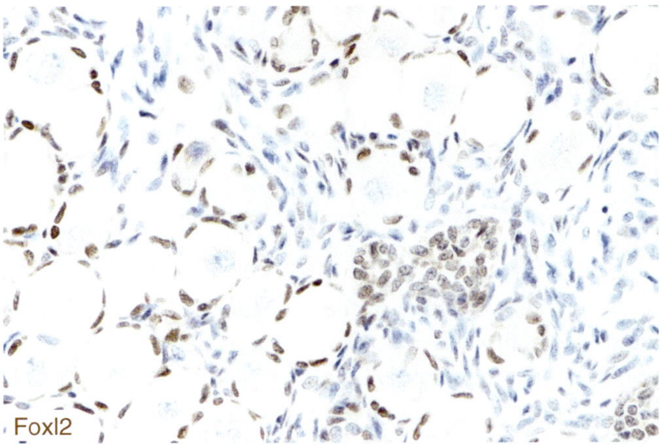

Fig. 1.8 Expression of Foxl2 in the human neonatal ovary. Expression is most prominent in the granulosa cells (at this stage almost all follicles are primordial and thus have a single layer of flattened granulosa cells) but there is also scattered expression in other ovarian mesenchymal cells

whereby all ovarian granulosa cells transdifferentiated into Sertoli-like cells (Fig. 1.7), with abnormal expression of Sox9 and AMH. This leads to conversion of the ovarian follicles into cord-like structures resembling testicular cords/seminiferous tubules, and testosterone levels similar to those of XY littermates. These results demonstrate that the ovarian vs. testicular somatic phenotype is actively maintained throughout female life by Foxl2 [41].

In humans, inherited loss-of-function mutations in the *Foxl2* gene do not lead to sex reversal, but rather to the autosomal dominant blepharophimosis-ptosis-epicanthus inversus syndrome (BPES), which is associated with eyelid malformations and premature ovarian failure (OMIM: 110100). In humans, as in mice, Foxl2 is expressed in the mesenchyme around the developing eyelid as well as granulosa cell precursors. The phenotype of Foxl2 mice, which also includes eyelid and craniofacial anomalies, thus closely matches that of the human syndrome, although in mice both alleles need to be inactivated for phenotypic expression, whereas BPES results from loss-of-function mutation of a single allele (haploinsufficiency) [35]. The heterozygous loss-of-function *FOXL2* mutations that lead to developmental defects in BPES thus contrast with the specific 402C→G (C134W) *FOXL2* gain-of-function mutation in ~90% of adult granulosa cell tumors [42, 43]. Despite its fundamental significance in ovarian development, studies to date have not systematically evaluated Foxl2 expression in the developing human ovary.

1.4 The Prenatal Ovary: Oocyte Death and Primordial Follicle Assembly and Dormancy

Following the establishment of testicular cords containing spermatogonia, the testis enters a state of relative dormancy. During late embryonic and postnatal development, as male germ cells remain in a state of quiescence, the general testicular anatomy is already established, and spermatogenesis is not initiated until puberty. In sharp contrast, late fetal and perinatal development is a particularly dynamic stage of ovarian differentiation characterized by striking cellular reorganizations that occur in conjunction with significant oocyte apoptosis, culminating in the formation of fully individualized and quiescent primordial follicles.

The primordial follicle is a minute, long-lived structure that remains quiescent until reawakening (a specific, gonadotropin-independent biological process described below). Primordial follicles are the reserve precursor pool for maturing follicles during reproductive life. Primordial follicles are produced only during embryogenesis in finite numbers, and hence their production and subsequent maintenance and preservation are of fundamental significance to female reproduction and fertility [44]. Thus, in this section, three intertwined subjects in ovarian development are discussed: oocyte apoptosis, primordial follicle formation/individualization, and primordial follicle reawakening.

1.4.1 Oogonial Nests and Their Breakdown

Following gonadal sex determination and establishment of ovarian fate, oogonia exist as syncytial nests (aka “cysts”) due to incomplete cytokinesis during the preceding oogonial mitotic divisions. The intercellular bridges also known as ring canals can be highlighted via immunolocalization of Tex14, a major protein component of the canals [45]. Ring canals mediate transport of organelles and other cytoplasmic factors among oogonia [46]. The oogonial chains linked by these intercellular bridges vary in size (i.e., number of physically linked oogonia) and exhibit diverse morphologies where each oogonium can be connected to one, two, or three other oogonia (Fig. 1.9).

The oogonial nests contain somatic cells that will become pregranulosa cells, a loose structural arrangement sometimes termed “ovigerous cords,” although these are not true cords as in the testis (Fig. 1.10) [47]. By a process that is not well understood, the somatic cells assist in the breakdown of the nests, and the oocytes become physically separated as the intercellular bridges are broken down, a process termed “cyst breakdown.” Apoptosis of individual oogonia (see below) may serve as another mechanism driving oogonial chain fragmentation. The oogonia, now oocytes, become enclosed in a thin squamoid layer of granulosa cell precursors termed pregranulosa cells (Fig. 1.10). Together, the primordial oocyte and its surrounding sheath of a single layer of flattened pregranulosa cells are termed the primordial follicle. This process of primordial follicle individualization begins at the 15th–16th week of gestation but occurs asynchronously and continues throughout fetal life and in the first postnatal months [48]. The primordial follicle thus individualized retains its shape and minute size until its reawakening. The signals that trigger individualization/cyst breakdown and control the timing of primordial follicle individualization remain enigmatic [49]. Although Kit is highly expressed in oogonia and primordial oocytes (Fig. 1.10) and is essential for primordial follicle reawakening (see below), primordial follicle individualization appears to be Kit-independent, as individualization occurs normally in mouse ovaries with Kit-deficient oogonia [50].

1.4.2 Oogonial Apoptosis

The number of germ cells in both ovaries reaches a peak of ~7,000,000 per ovary at around 5 months gestation. Thereafter, the number decreases to ~2,000,000 at birth (Fig. 1.11) [51]. Conventional apoptosis in situ assays such as TUNEL reveal an abundance of apoptotic oocytes during this period. Thus, after the initiation of meiosis and during the process of primordial follicle assembly, the majority of oogonia undergo programmed cell death (apoptosis). A number of hypotheses have been invoked to explain this massive apoptosis, such as culling of defective oocytes. For example, meiotic recombination involves the formation of numerous double-strand DNA breaks, a process that can lead to abnormal oocytes with meiotic pairing or recombination anomalies if some of the DNA breaks are not successfully repaired. In this scenario, apoptosis may eliminate defective oocytes to retain meiotically competent oocytes needed for later fertility [52]. Turner’s syndrome, due to deficiency of one X chromosome (XO), as well as chromosomal translocations involving the X or other chromosomes, may trigger oocyte loss and ovarian failure

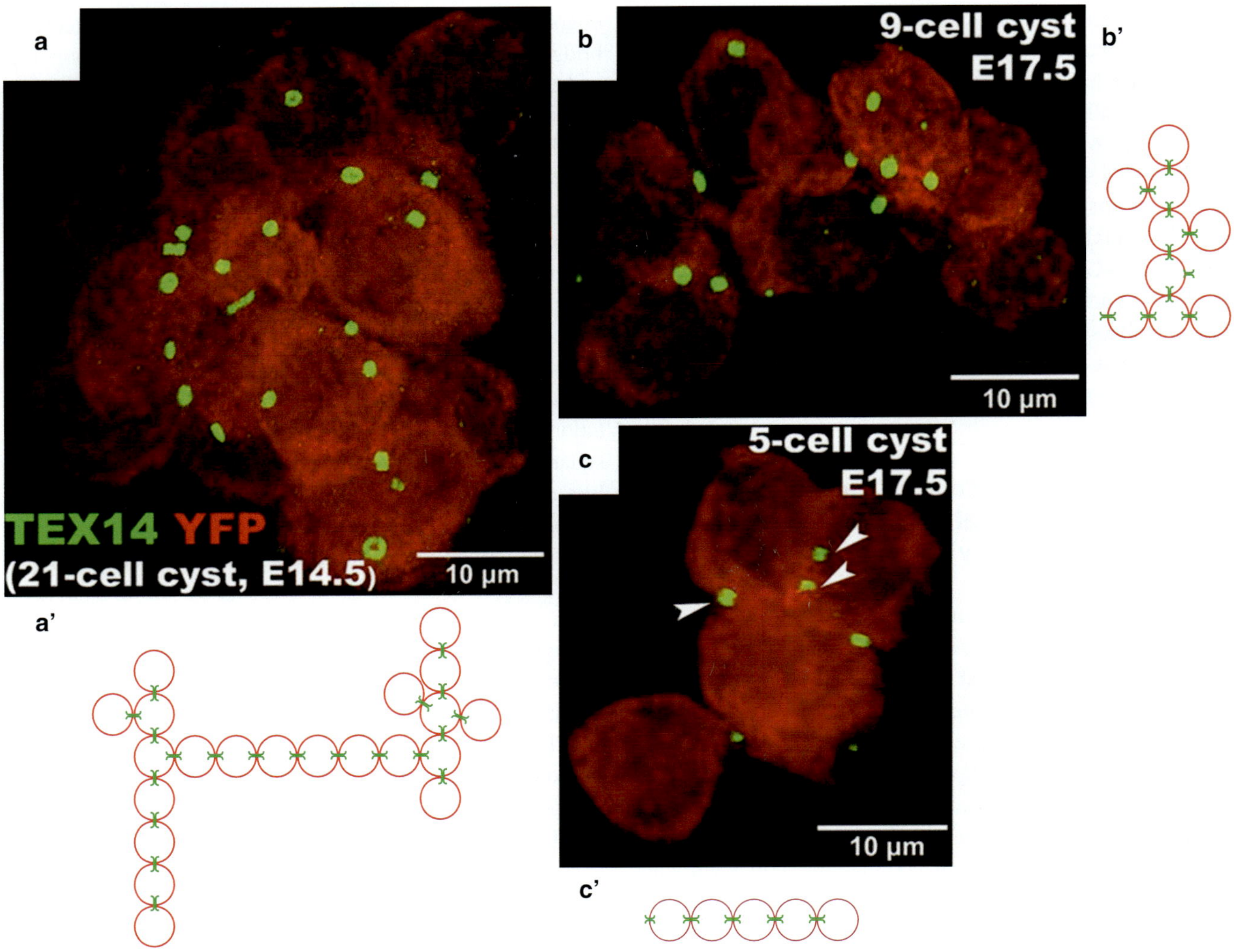

Fig. 1.9 Tex14, ring canals, and structure of oogonial cysts prior to their breakdown in mouse ovaries. Ring canals connecting oogonia are labeled by immunofluorescence of the ring canal component Tex14 (green). Examination of oogonial clusters at multiple planes of focus permits reconstructions of oogonial cyst structure. Cysts have complex patterns and are made of oogonia with one, two, or three bridges. Later, the bridges are broken down to give rise to fully individualized primordial follicles. (**a**) 21–cell oogonial cyst. (**b**) 9-cell cyst. (**c**) 5-cell oogonial cyst. Redrawn with permission from Lei L and Spradling AC, Science 352:2016 [46] (The American Association for the Advancement of Science). *E* embryonic day, *YFP* yellow fluorescent protein (expressed in oogonial cytoplasm)

(so-called gonadal dysgenesis) through such mechanisms [53]. Apoptosis could also serve to cull germ cells for reasons not directly related to meiosis. For example, in one mouse study, oogonia with the most cytoplasm/organelles selectively survived, while those that transferred their cytoplasmic contents into neighboring oogonia selectively underwent apoptosis [46]. If so, then some oogonia, in an act of self-sacrifice, "nurse" through their intercellular bridges other oogonia destined to survive. In any case, apoptosis appears to be one of the major mechanisms influencing the number of oocytes present at birth (the "endowment"). The number of primordial follicles (the "follicle reserve") is highest at birth but continues to fall throughout life until nearly depleted, signifying the menopause (Fig. 1.11) [54].

Molecular pathways that prevent or trigger apoptosis in female germ cells have been extensively investigated in mouse models. The Kit cell surface receptor and the PI3K/Akt pathway, which mediates PGC migration and survival, also has important roles in oocyte survival. Mice with mutations in PI3K pathway components (Akt1, Pdk1, and Kit) undergo increased oocyte apoptosis leading to gradual loss of all oocytes. This, together with the demonstration that PI3K/Akt pathway is the central pathway controlling reawakening (see next section), suggests that the PI3K/Akt pathway serves as a "rheostat" balancing and controlling both reawakening and apoptosis [44]. Other factors highly expressed in primordial oocytes, including p63, BCL2 (a member of the BH3 protein family of apoptosis regulators), and other BH3 proteins, also participate in oocyte apoptosis and play diverse roles in preventing vs. triggering apoptosis following exposure to chemotherapy, radiation, or environmental toxicants [55, 56]. Such mechanisms are likely

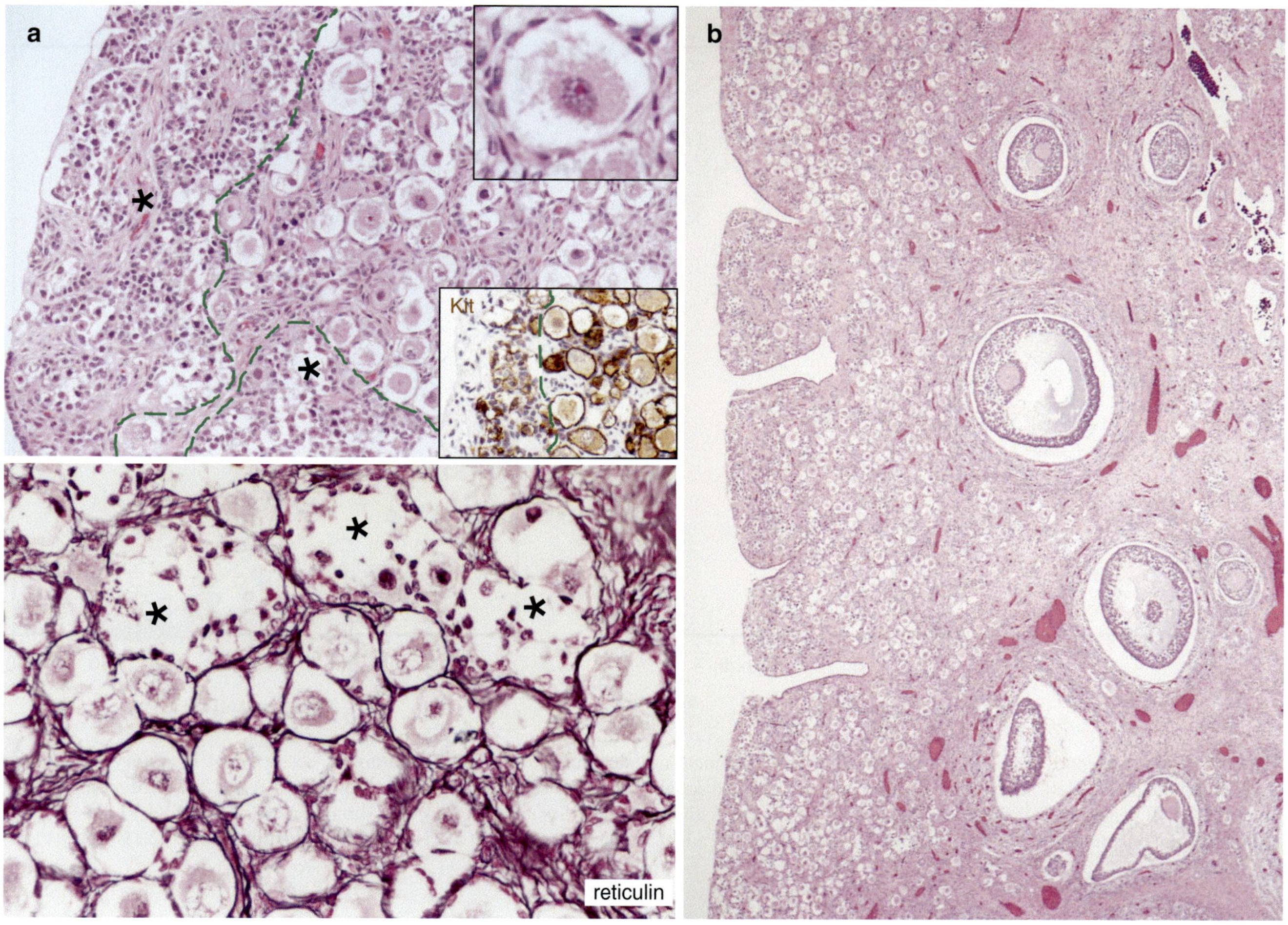

Fig. 1.10 Human neonatal ovary (term gestation). (**a**) Top panel, H&E showing admixture of oogonial cysts (also called ovigerous cords) made of oogonia and somatic cells (asterisks), and separate areas of fully individualized primordial follicles demarcated by green dashed line. Ring canals cannot be seen in H&E-stained sections. Top inset shows higher magnification of single primordial follicle with oocyte and surrounding layer of squamoid granulosa cells, also termed pregranulosa cells (oocytes exhibit retraction artifact following formalin fixation). Inset below is of Kit immunostain. Dashed line separates cysts (left) from primordial follicles (right); strong membrane-associated Kit is present in primordial follicles. Bottom panel, reticulin stain highlighting and surrounding oogonial cysts as well as individualized primordial follicles. (**b**) Lower magnification of same ovary shows many antral follicles, underscoring the striking asynchrony of ovarian follicle development at birth, and also that primordial follicle reawakening begins well before the onset of sexual maturity

important mediators of female reproductive function, because primordial oocyte apoptosis proceeds throughout life (albeit at a reduced rate), and this gradual loss culminates in the eventual depletion of primordial follicles and the menopause [44].

1.4.3 Defects in Primordial Follicle Formation and Relationship to Early Menopause Syndromes

Although idiopathic primary amenorrhea (PA) and idiopathic primary ovarian insufficiency (POI, also known as premature ovarian failure) are manifest later in life (at menarche or adulthood, respectively), these early menopause syndromes are briefly discussed here because reawakening occurs throughout reproductive life but begins during prenatal development. POI is defined as menopause prior to the age of 40 (average age at menopause is 51), and histologic studies have shown that the condition is due to depletion of primordial follicles. However, since histologic evaluation is not part of the clinical workup of PA or POI, these scenarios are rarely if ever encountered by surgical pathologists [44]. Also, PA and POI are disorders of primordial follicle formation or preservation with significant secondary aging disease phenotypes in adult women [57], but may have origins during prenatal development. While manifest at different ages (before or after puberty), the fundamental mechanism unifying PA and POI is accelerated primordial follicle depletion. Thus, PA (depletion of all pri-

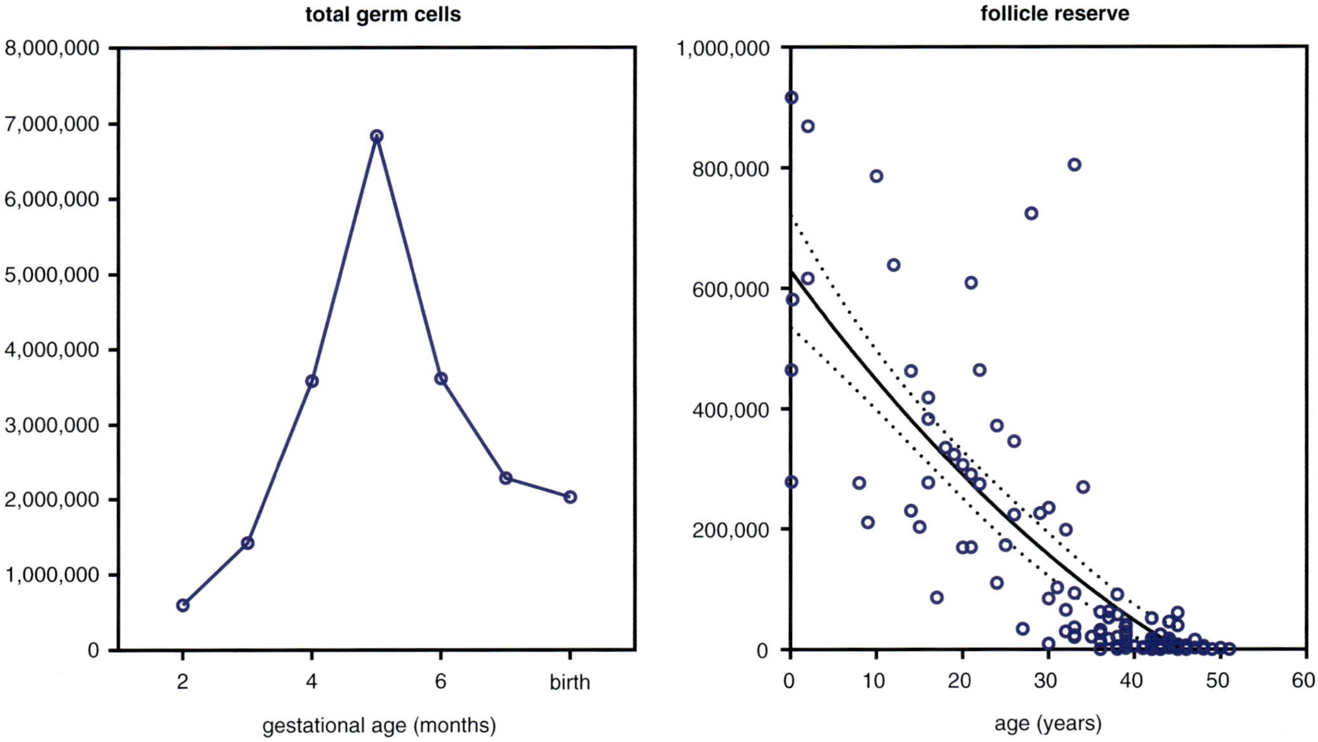

Fig. 1.11 Germ cell and follicle reserve counts in the ovary as function of developmental age. Left panel: total number of germ cells peaks at 5 months. Right panel: the follicle reserve (primordial follicles) is highest at birth, but oocyte apoptosis and reawakening contribute to gradual depletion, eventually resulting in cessation of ovulatory cycles (the menopause). Graphs drawn from data in Baker TG, Proceedings of the Royal Society of London B Biological Sciences 158:417 (1963) [51], and Hansen KR et al., Human Reproduction 23:699 (2008) [54]

mordial follicles prior to menarche) could be viewed as a more severe form of POI, but both conditions are likely to share common etiologies [44].

1.4.4 Reawakening of Primordial Follicles as the First Step of Ovarian Follicle Maturation

Primordial follicle reawakening, also termed follicle initiation or activation, is the metered process by which primordial follicles that would otherwise remain dormant for years or decades are selected from this long-lived reserve pool into the growing follicle pool (Fig. 1.12) [58]. Reawakening has been likened to grains of sand falling through an hourglass. At any instant (from birth to menopause), there is only a gradual trickle of primordial follicles undergoing reawakening. Reawakening is irreversible in that follicles that have initiated growth undergo atresia if not selected for subsequent stages of maturation [59]. The earliest morphologic hallmarks of reawakening are oocyte growth and transition of the flattened pregranulosa cells to a cuboidal shape, accompanied by brisk granulosa cell proliferation [59]. The age-dependent decrease of primordial follicle numbers is attributed to two distinct mechanisms: primordial oocyte apoptosis and reawakening, since each process effectively eliminates primordial follicles from the finite reserve pool. Thus, reawakening must be tightly controlled to ensure that some number of growing follicles are available during each estrus cycle but also forestall premature utilization and depletion of primordial follicles.

There is a frequent misconception that reawakening is triggered by pituitary gonadotropins, but this is clearly not the case (Fig. 1.12) [44]. Reawakening and early follicle maturation, unlike later stages of follicle maturation, are regulated within the ovary itself independent of pituitary gonadotropins, as evidenced by several observations: (1) reawakening occurs in only a small subset of primordial follicles in newborn mouse ovaries explanted and maintained in vitro (beyond the influence of pituitary gonadotropins) [60], (2) reawakening begins well before the onset of sexual maturity—indeed, as soon as some primordial follicles are formed (perinatally) in both mice and humans, and (3) the dynamics of reawakening are unaltered following hypophysectomy, treatment with exogenous gonadotropins, or in mice deficient for GnRH (gonadotropin-releasing hormone) [58, 61].

The entire process of follicle maturation from reawakening to ovulation can thus be divided into separate "stages," the first gonadotropin-independent and the second gonadotropin-dependent (Fig. 1.12). The final stages of

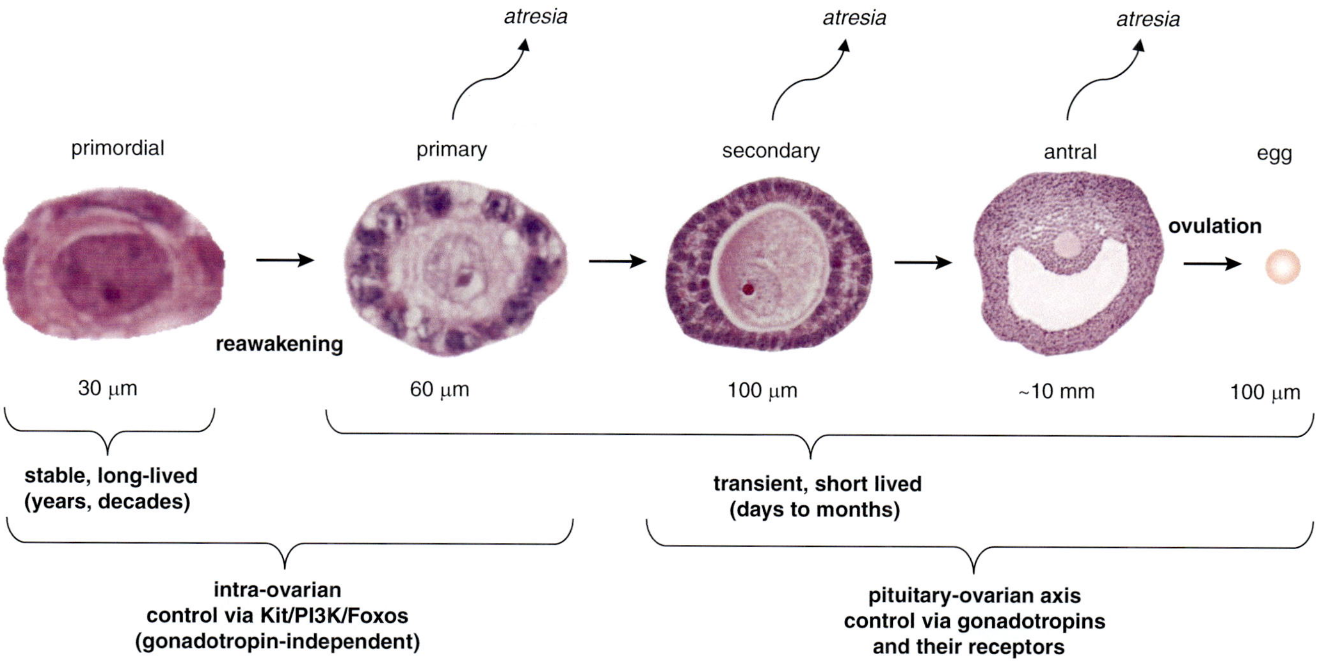

Fig. 1.12 Stages of follicular maturation with emphasis on differences between first step (reawakening) and subsequent maturation. Follicles are depicted (not to scale: approximate sizes shown below each follicle). Follicle growth is asynchronous, such that the adult ovary contains follicles at all stages. The vast majority of follicles are primordial, and only a very small percentage are growing at any instant. Reawakening is the regular, metered process by which individual primordial follicles are continually selected to begin maturation. It begins when the first primordial follicles become individualized (during fetal development). The earliest morphologic hallmarks of reawakening are oocyte growth, a change in granulosa cells from a flattened to a cuboidal shape, and granulosa cell proliferation. Whereas primordial follicles are long-lived, growing follicles are transient because those that do not progress undergo atresia. Primary follicles have initiated growth and undergone a transition from flattened to cuboidal granulosa cells but have only one layer of granulosa cells. Secondary follicles have two layers of granulosa cells, and antral follicles are large follicles with a chamber (antrum) in preparation for ovulation. From Saatcioglu HD et al., PLoS Genetics 12 (2016) (PLoS Open Access) [50]

maturation including ovulation that are gonadotropin-dependent proceed only after the establishment of the pituitary-ovarian axis at puberty. Whereas ovulation occurs every ~28 days in women, the entire process of follicle maturation (from reawakening to ovulation) takes at least 280 days, underscoring that reawakening and later stages of follicle maturation are uncoupled. Thus, the dominant follicle selected for ovulation is one that underwent reawakening many reproductive cycles earlier. For these reasons, growing follicles are readily identified in prepubertal human ovaries, even at birth (Fig. 1.10), but are destined to undergo atresia. Why nature employs such a seemingly wasteful process is a mystery, but is consistent with observed and significant decreases in primordial follicle numbers from birth to puberty (Fig. 1.11).

How reawakening is triggered in a single primordial follicle among many neighbors is unknown, but mouse studies have identified the transcription factor Foxo3 as the key switch controlling this process [62–64]. Foxo3 knockout mice undergo normal primordial follicle individualization, but then all of the primordial follicles undergo reawakening simultaneously, leading to ovarian hypertrophy (Fig. 1.13) [63, 64]. Thus, Foxo3 is a suppressor of reawakening. Initially, prior to follicle individualization, the Foxo3 protein is cytoplasmic, but becomes imported into the nucleus as individualization occurs. Foxo3 then remains in the nucleus, until reawakening occurs, when it shuttles back to the cytoplasm. This behavior is consistent with a switch mechanism where nuclear Foxo3 controls the primordial oocyte's quiescence.

Other studies have implicated Kit, which is highly expressed in primordial oocytes in mice and humans, as the upstream cell surface receptor controlling this process. Mice engineered to express a constitutively active form of Kit within oocytes also undergo global oocyte reawakening as soon as primordial follicle assembly is complete. Conversely, mice with oocyte-specific inactivation of Kit exhibit an opposite phenotype: complete failure of reawakening. In such mice, primordial follicles remain quiescent, leading to an unusual form of ovarian failure with abundant primordial follicles but no growing follicles. These reciprocal genetic experiments have proven that Kit is necessary and sufficient for reawakening (Fig. 1.13) [50]. Other genetic experiments in mice showed that Kit acts via the PI3K/Akt/Pten signaling pathway and that this pathway is the key mediator of pri-

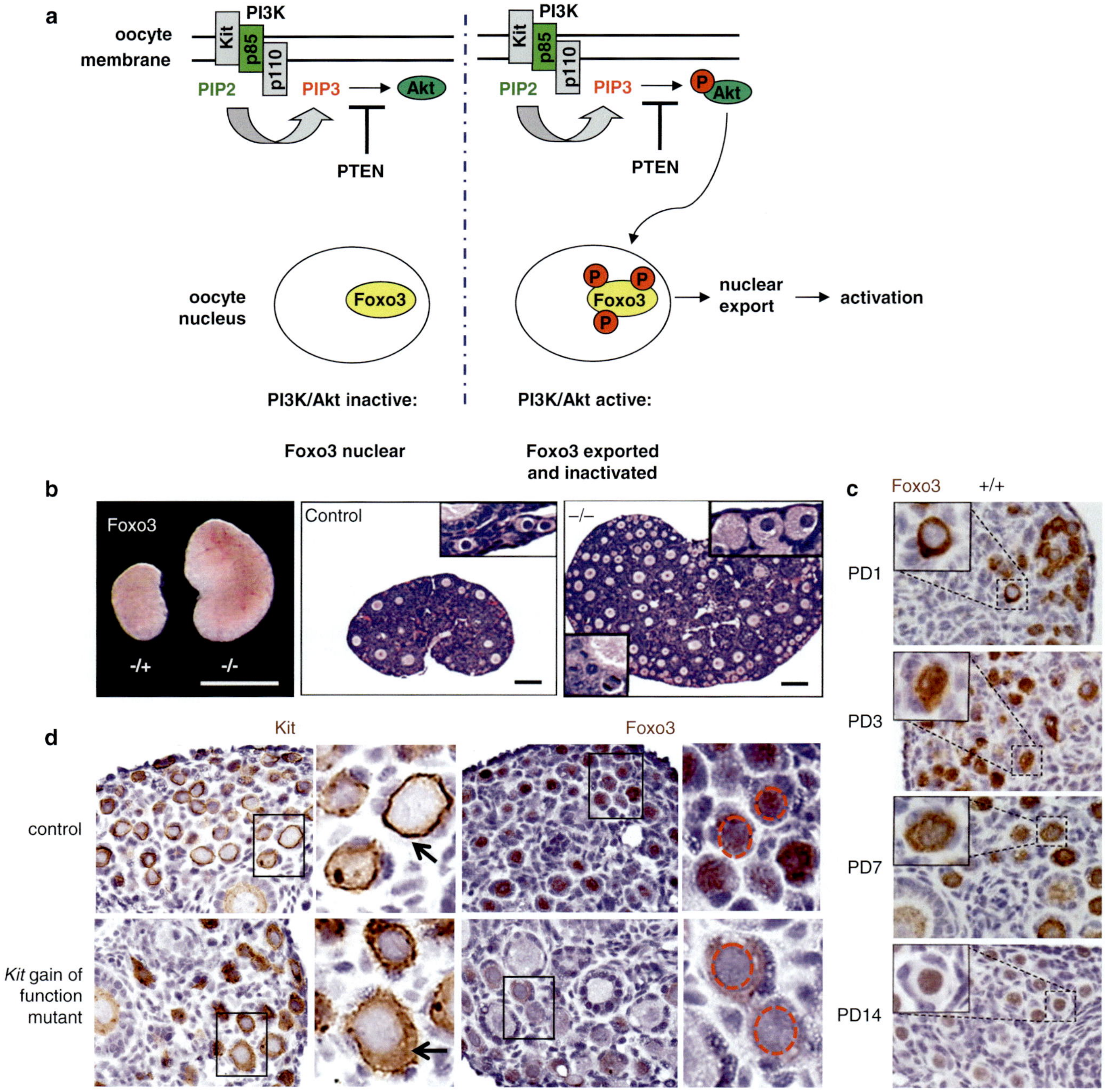

Fig. 1.13 Control of primordial follicle reawakening by Kit-Foxo3 axis. Panels are of ovaries from knockout or control mice. Antibodies are indicated in brown lettering. (**a**) Role of the receptor tyrosine kinase (RTK) Kit in regulating reawakening through PI3K/Akt pathway and ultimately Foxo3. It is notable that this pathway controls other aspects of female reproductive tract development and is the principal pathway mutated in endometrial cancer (e.g., Pten). (**b**) Foxo3 knockout results in global primordial follicle reawakening, resulting in ovarian hypertrophy. Such mice later undergo rapid depletion of their primordial follicle reserve, resulting in premature ovarian failure and small ovaries. (**c**) Foxo3 protein in normal mice is cytoplasmic in oogonial cysts but becomes nuclear after individualization; *PD* postnatal day. Foxo3 remains in primordial oocyte nucleus until reawakening, when it shuttles back to the cytoplasm (not shown). (**d**) Kit activating mutations also result in global reawakening phenotype. Kit expression is not affected by the mutation (arrows), but its activation results in increased PI3K/AKT signaling, Foxo3 nuclear export (red dashed circles), triggering primordial follicle reawakening. Images adapted with permission from Castrillon DH et al., Science 301:215 (2003) (The American Association for the Advancement of Science), John GB et al. 321:197 (2008) (Elsevier), and Saatcioglu HD et al. PLoS Genetics 12 (2016) (PLoS Open Access) [50, 62, 202]

mordial oocyte reawakening via Foxo3 [62–65]. Kit/PI3K/Akt signaling results in Akt-dependent Foxo3 phosphorylation and export from the nucleus into the cytoplasm, effectively turning Foxo3 off by preventing its control of transcription (Fig. 1.13) [64]. In humans, Foxo3 is not as highly expressed within oocytes, and the other Foxo factors Foxo1 and Foxo4 are believed to serve as a redundant network safeguarding reawakening [66]. It is notable that PI3K/Akt/Pten pathway serves multiple roles in MD and germ cell development and is the principal pathway mutated in endometrial carcinoma. Alterations in the genes encoding RTKs, PI3K subunits, AKT, PTEN, and the FOXOs represent the most frequent recurring mutations in endometrial cancer [67].

1.5 The Müllerian Ducts as Precursors of the Upper Female Reproductive Tract

1.5.1 Formation and Growth of the Müllerian Duct, and the Testicular Factors AMH and Testosterone in its Regression

The Müllerian (aka paramesonephric) ducts (MDs) are named after the German anatomist and embryologist Johannes Peter Müller. He was not the first to identify the MD as the embryologic precursor to the female reproductive tract, but Müller correctly emphasized its distinctiveness from the Wolffian duct (which gives rise to the male reproductive tract) and its tubal (i.e., luminal) nature [68, 69]. The morphologic steps of MD formation and development have been studied in human [70], diverse mammalian [71], and rodent species, with the mouse serving as the principal modern system for the identification and further investigation of the underlying molecular factors controlling these developmental processes [72]. The MDs give rise to the upper cervix, uterus, and oviducts, while the Wolffian (aka mesonephric) ducts (WDs) give rise to the male reproductive tract.

In male (XY) embryos, the Sox9-positive testicular Sertoli cells secrete anti-Müllerian hormone (AMH), a protein of the TGF-β family structurally related to inhibin and activin [73]. AMH acts in a paracrine manner to bind to Type I and II AMH receptors expressed in the MD mesenchyme to induce MD regression [74]. Another testicular hormone, testosterone (produced by Leydig cells), acts via androgen receptors expressed in the WD to inhibit WD regression. In female (XX) embryos, the absence of these testicular signals (AMH and testosterone) leads to the converse outcome: MD persistence and WD regression (Fig. 1.14). The transcription factor COUP-TFII functions within WD mesenchyme to actively eliminate the WD in females, but the nature of any crosstalk between COUP-TFII and the androgen receptor remains undefined [75]. Thus, the male and female reproductive tracts are derived from adjacent but distinct embryologic ducts (Müllerian vs. Wolffian) initially fully formed in both male and female embryos, but programmed to regress or persist in a mutually exclusive manner dependent upon chromosomal/gonadal sex (Fig. 1.14).

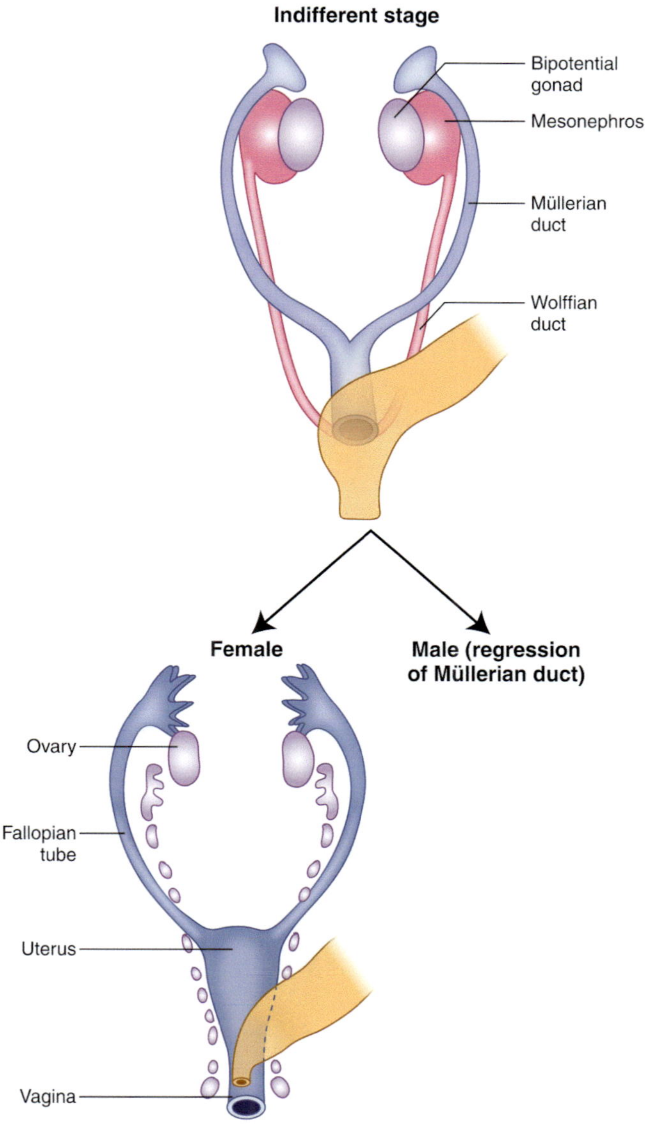

Fig. 1.14 Development of female reproductive tract from persistence of Müllerian duct and regression of Wolffian duct. Redrawn with permission from Bulun SE, Chapter 17, Williams Textbook of Endocrinology, 13th edition (2016) (Elsevier)

1.5.2 Dependence of Müllerian Duct Formation upon the Presence of Wolffian Duct

Although distinct structures, the MD and WD are developmentally interdependent [72, 76]. The WD forms first and then instructs multiple aspects of MD development. Ablation of the WD by diverse means (physical or genetic) results in secondary absence of the MD [77–79]. Three phases of MD formation have been described: initiation, invagination, and elongation (Fig. 1.15). Initiation begins at around week 6 of human development [80]. In the mouse, initiation is associated with expression of the homeobox transcription factor Lhx1 in a region of coelomic epithelium that will give rise to the MD. Lhx1 is also expressed in the WD epithelium and is required for initial development of the WD (Fig. 1.16). In Lhx1−deficient mouse embryos, a failure of WD formation leads secondarily to the cell non-autonomous loss of the MD. However, conditional Lhx1 inactivation specifically in MD epithelium leads to a block in MD duct elongation and uterine hypoplasia characterized by loss of the entire endometrium, demonstrating that Lhx1 also functions independently within the MD [81].

In the next phase of MD development, expression of the secreted protein Wnt4 from the Wolffian duct mesenchyme

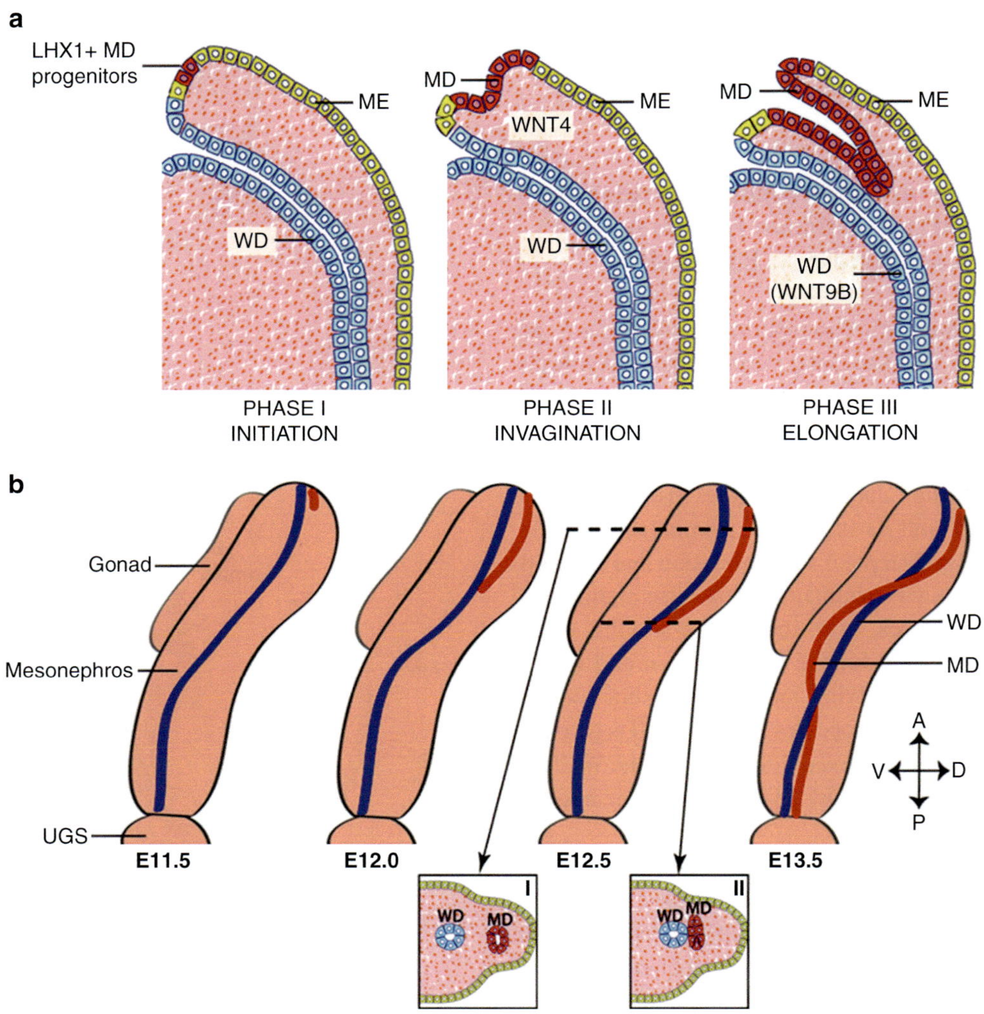

Fig. 1.15 Formation of the Müllerian duct (MD). (**a**) MD (red) formation occurs in three phases: initiation, invagination, and elongation. Initiation: MD progenitor cells in mesonephric epithelium (yellow) are specified and begin to express Lhx1. Invagination: In response to Wnt4 signaling from mesenchyme, Lhx1+ MD progenitor cells invaginate caudally into mesonephros towards the WD (blue). Elongation: The MD tip contacts the WD and elongates caudally in close proximity to the WD requiring Wnt9B signaling from the WD. (**b**) Beginning at embryo (E) day ~11.5 in mice, the MD invaginates and extends posteriorly guided by the WD. During elongation, mesenchymal cells separate the WD and MD anterior to the growing tip. However at the MD tip, the MD and WD are in contact. At ~E12.5, the MD crosses over the WD. Elongation is complete by ~E13.5 with the MDs reaching the UGS. *A* anterior (dorsal); *E* embryonic day in mouse, *D* dorsal, *ME* mesonephric epithelium, *MD* Müllerian duct, *P* posterior (caudal), *UGS* urogenital sinus, *V* ventral, *WD* Wolffian duct. Figure and text adapted with permission from Mullen RD and Behringer RR, Sexual Development, 8:281 (2014) (S. Karger AG, Basel)

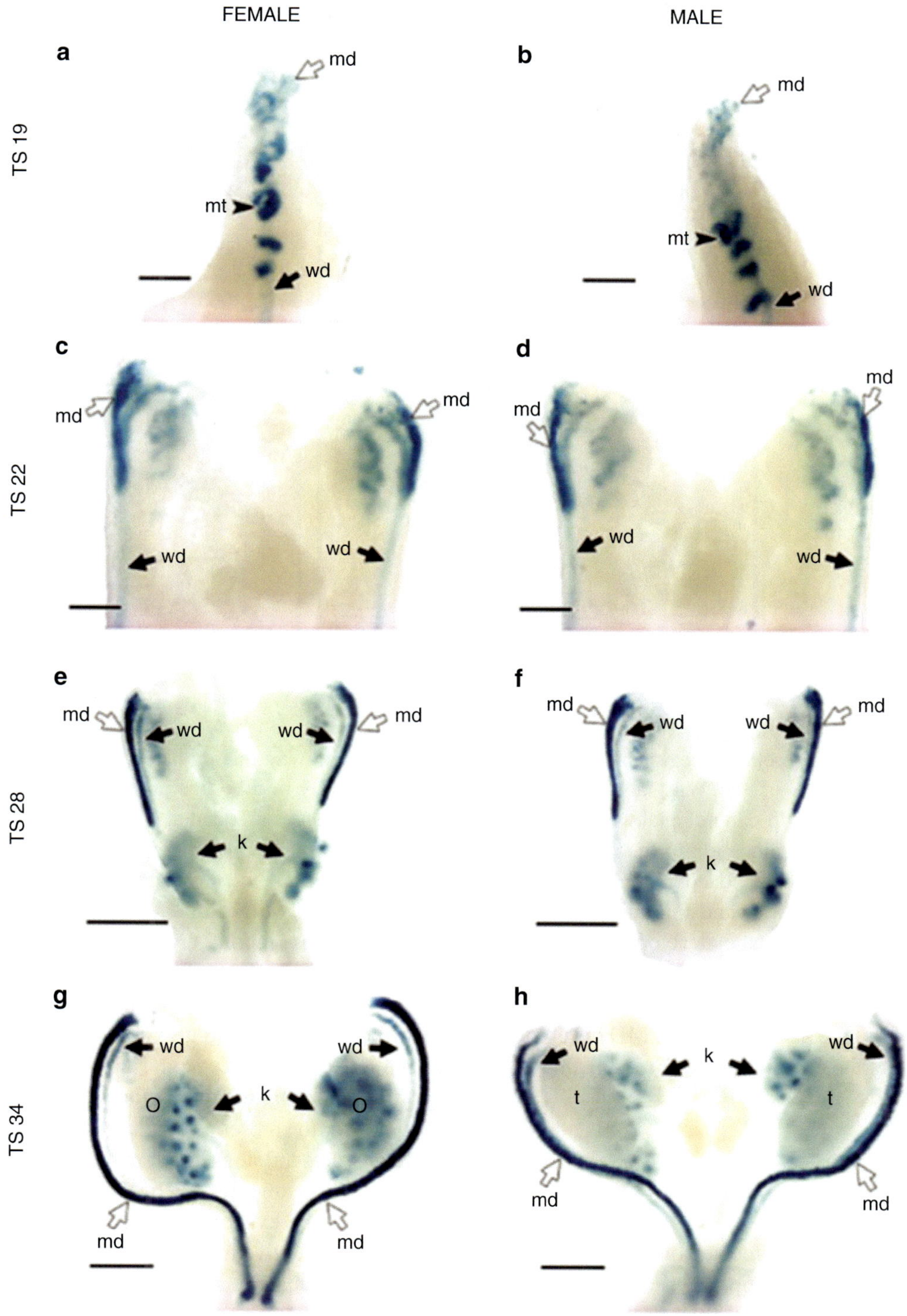

Fig. 1.16 Müllerian duct (MD) development. Images are from mice where a β-galactosidase gene was knocked into the Lhx1 gene. This permits visualization in whole mounts of cells expressing Lhx1 and therefore of Lhx1−expressing structures. The figure illustrates the utility of genetically engineered reporter mice to study MD development. Lhx1/β-galactosidase is strongly expressed in the MD and more weakly in the WD, permitting visualization of both the MD and WD. Lateral (**a**, **b**) and ventral (**c–h**) views are shown. *TS* tail somite (used for embryo staging). Müllerian duct precursor cells arise from the coelomic epithelium at TS19 in both females (**a**) and males (**b**). By TS22, both females (**c**) and males (**d**) have accomplished Müllerian duct invagination from the coelomic epithelium and contacted the Wolffian duct. The Müllerian duct has completed half of its elongation to the urogenital sinus at TS28 (**e**, **f**) and reached the urogenital sinus by TS34 (**g**, **h**). *k* kidney (metanephros), *md* Müllerian duct, *mt* mesonephric tubules, *o* ovary, *t* testis, *wd* Wolffian duct. Scale bar: 200 μM in **a–d**; 500 μM in **e–h**. Reproduced with permission from Orvis GD and Behringer RR, Developmental Biology 306:493 (2007) (Elsevier) [132]

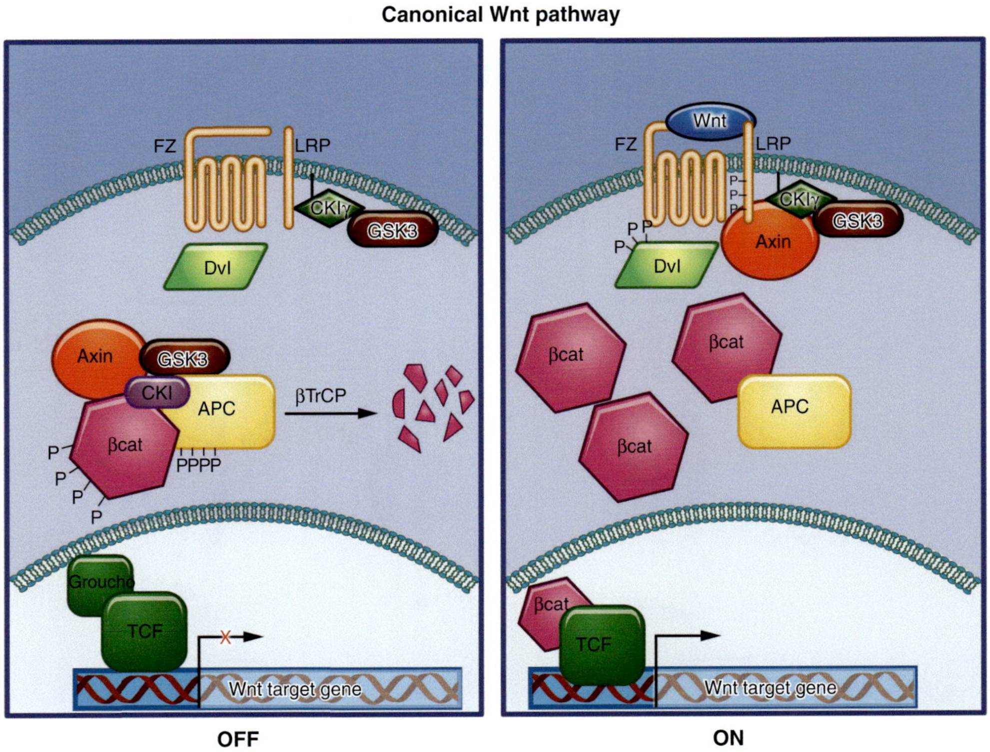

Fig. 1.17 The canonical Wnt/β-catenin signaling pathway controls many aspects of female reproductive tract development and malignant transformation. Wnts are secreted factors that act in a paracrine fashion and bind to Frizzled cell surface receptors. There are 19 human Wnt and 10 Frizzled genes, and their differential patterns of expression and combinatorial binding possibilities add significant complexity to studies of their interactions. Casein kinase I-γ (CKIγ), Dvl (Disheveled), and Groucho are additional components of this pathway. Redrawn with permission from Clevers H, Cell 127:469 (2006) [203]

signals the MD progenitor cells to begin invagination [78, 82]. Like all 19 members of the Wnt family, Wnt4 acts through the canonical Wnt/β-catenin pathway to stabilize β-catenin and permit its translocation to the nucleus, where β-catenin acts a transcriptional coactivator influencing cell fate specification, proliferation, and migration (Fig. 1.17). Wnt4 is highly expressed in the developing MD mesenchyme, and the MD fails to develop in both male and female Wnt4-deficient embryos [82, 83]. Other Wnt family members (Wnt5a, Wnt7a) are also essential in MD development, further highlighting the significance of Wnt signaling in MD development (discussed below).

1.5.3 Elongation of the Müllerian Duct

The final phase of MD development, elongation, commences when the invaginating MD tip physically contacts the WD. MD elongation proceeds adjacent to the WD caudally until the MD fuses with the urogenital sinus. During this process, the developing MD uses the WD as a "guide wire," and although the MD and WD epithelium come in direct contact without an intervening basement membrane, there is no mixing of MD and WD epithelial cells (Fig. 1.15) [84]. The WD is believed to guide elongation through secretion of Wnt9b from the WD [72]. MD elongation occurs as a result of proliferation of the MD epithelium. The PI3K/Akt pathway, the principal pathway misregulated in endometrial cancers and less frequently in tubo-ovarian cancers, influences the morphologic changes associated with MD elongation. PI3K/Akt pathway activation promotes cellular proliferation along the length of the MD, and facilitates breakdown of the basement membrane and extracellular matrix around the MD, which would otherwise inhibit migration [85].

In female embryos, after MD elongation is complete, the WD regresses due to the lack of AMH and testosterone, as described above. The regression is characterized by fragmentation of the WD, with subsequent loss of cells by apoptosis. Incomplete regression of the WD is common and accounts for the presence of minute mesonephric (Wolffian) remnants present along the female reproductive tract (cervix, broad ligament). Such Wolffian remnants in turn account for the existence of "mesonephric" tumors in the female reproductive tract (mesonephric hyperplasias/carcinomas and female adnexal tumors of Wolffian origin, aka FATWOs) [86]. The transcription factor Gata3 is selectively expressed in the developing Wolffian duct, where its expression is induced by Pax2/8. Gata3 expression is retained in Wolffian (mesonephric) rests but is more consistently retained in the lower versus the upper female reproductive tract (Fig. 1.18) likely accounting for observations that Gata3 is a reliable marker of lower (but not upper) female reproductive tract tumors with mesonephric differentiation [87–89].

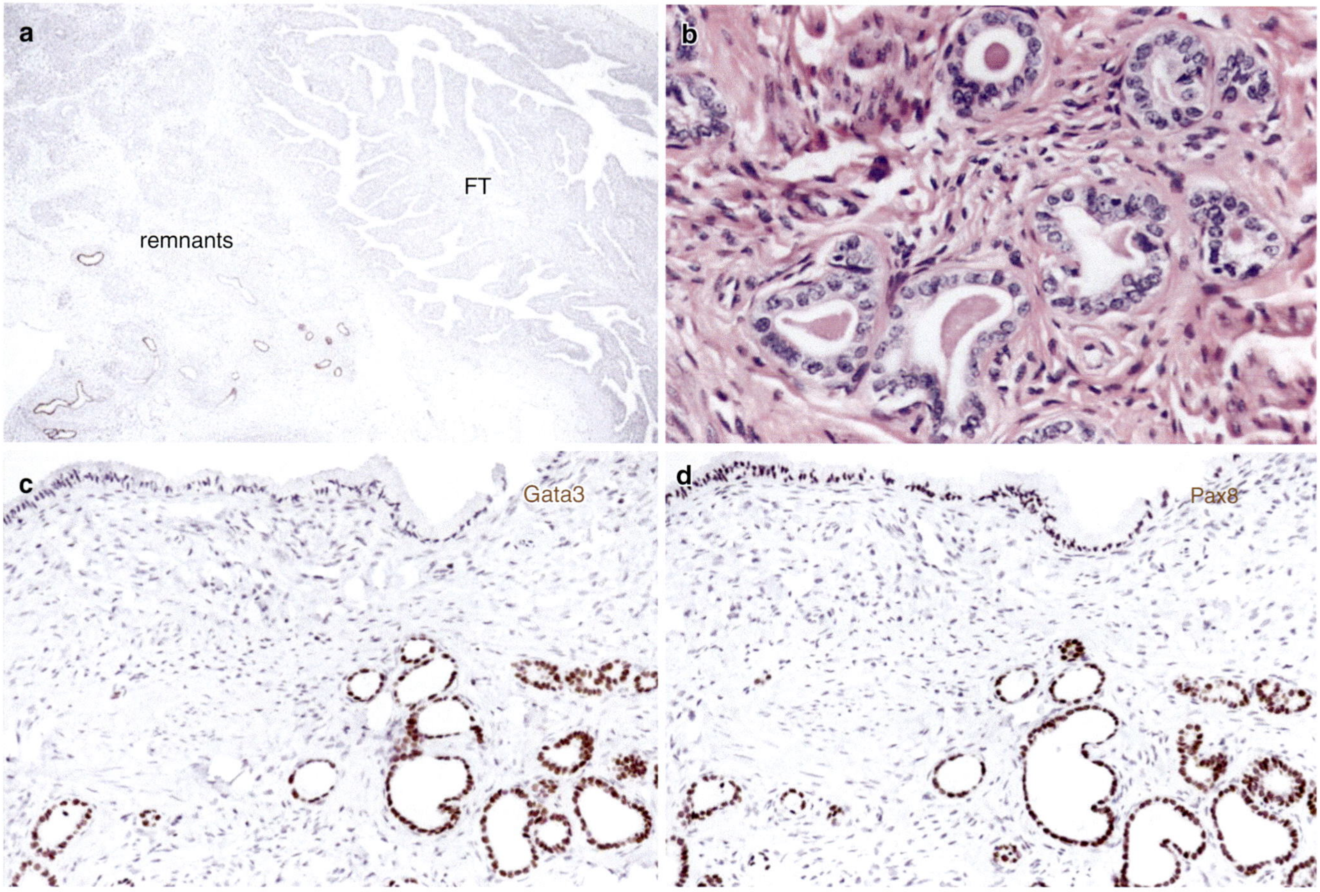

Fig. 1.18 Expression of Gata3 in human mesonephric remnants. (**a**) Fallopian tube (FT) and adjacent upper reproductive tract mesonephric remnants in neonate show only patchy expression of Gata3. (**b–d**) Mesonephric remnants in adult cervix (all panels from same individual). (**b**) Typical histologic appearance of cervical mesonephric remnants consisting of cuboidal non-ciliated epithelium with eosinophilic intraluminal secretions. (**c**) Mesonephric remnants but not adjacent endocervical epithelium are strongly Gata3 positive. (**d**) Mesonephric remnants are also strongly Pax8 positive consistent with essential roles of Pax8 in both Wolffian and Müllerian duct development as described in text

1.5.4 Pax2, Pax8, and Wt1 in Müllerian Duct Development

Other notable factors that serve as early MD lineage markers and play essential roles in MD development include the homeodomain transcriptional regulators Pax2 and Pax8. Pax2 is significantly expressed in both the WD and MD. The MD is lost secondarily in Pax2-deficient mice likely due an initial defect in WD elongation, but high Pax2 expression within the MD suggests that Pax2 also acts cell autonomously within the MD to promote MD formation and maintenance [79, 81, 90]. Pax8, like Pax2, is also highly expressed throughout the developing MD [82] (Fig. 1.19) and Pax8-deficient female mice are infertile with poorly developed MD remnants [91]. Pax2 and Pax8 are functionally redundant within the MD, with loss of one being partially compensated by the other, as is the case in other developmental processes in which these two factors cooperate [92, 93].

Wt1 (Wilms tumor suppressor gene 1) is a zinc finger transcription factor that regulates multiple aspects of urogenital development, in addition to being a canonical tumor suppressor gene. Inherited loss-of-function *Wt1* mutations result in genitourinary tract malformations such as WAGR syndrome (Wilms' tumor, aniridia, genitourinary anomalies, and retardation, OMIM: 612469) and a striking predisposition to Wilm's tumors following loss/mutation of the second allele (via the classic two-hit inactivation model for hereditary tumor suppressor gene mutations). Wt1 functions within the gonad and is required for gonad development where it participates in the activation of Sry in Sertoli cells [26]. In the MD, Wt1 serves an essential and specific function in MD regression by promoting the expression of Amhr2, the receptor for AMH [94]. Wt1 knockout mice have no kidneys, gonads, or adrenal glands, resulting in embryonic lethality. Embryological studies in mice have emphasized the expression and function of Wt1 in the relevant mesenchymal compartments in these tissues [26, 95]. The utility of Wt1 as an immunohistochemical

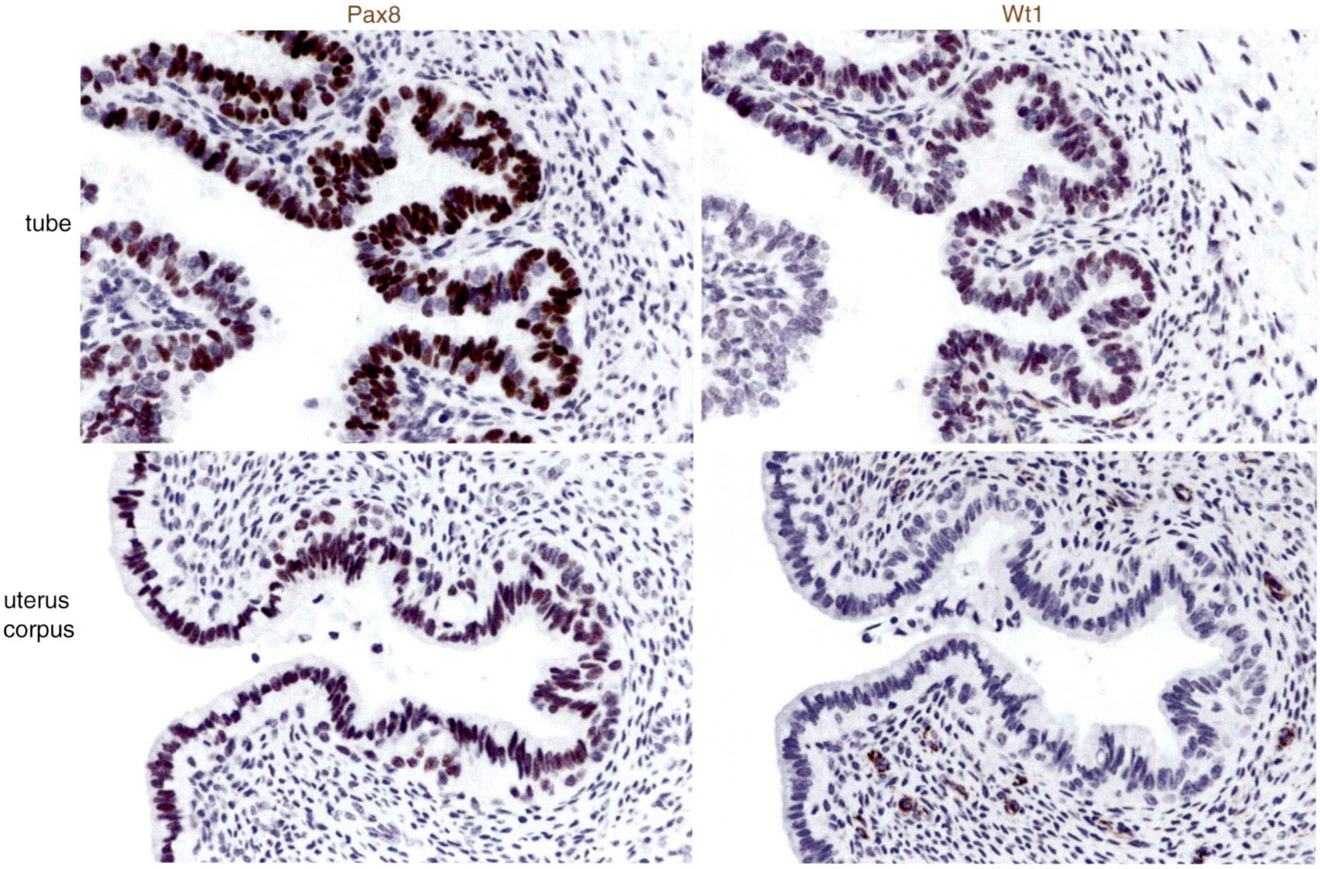

Fig. 1.19 Expression of Pax8 and Wt1 in the neonatal fallopian tube and uterine corpus. Whereas Pax8 is strongly expressed in both compartments, Wt1 is expressed in the tubal but not uterine epithelium

marker of Müllerian tubal epithelial differentiation in adult women is somewhat difficult to reconcile with mouse and human embryological data; e.g., Wt1 is reportedly not significantly expressed in developing mouse or human MD epithelium [95, 96]. Nonetheless, Wt1 is expressed in human adult tubal epithelium (Fig. 1.19) (but not in endometrium), rationalizing its value as a selective lineage marker for serous neoplasms of tubal (vs. uterine) origin [97–99].

1.5.5 Early Segmental Patterning of the Müllerian Ducts by the *Hoxa* Gene Cluster

The MD is initially structurally and histologically homogenous but becomes segmentally patterned into the upper vagina, cervix uteri, corpus uteri, and the fallopian tubes (FTs) in a process driven by a complex network of *HoxA* (homeobox transcriptional regulators) genes working in concert with *Wnt* genes. The 39 mouse/human *Hox* genes are organized into four clusters (*HoxA-D*) on different chromosomes, with each cluster composed of individual *Hox* genes in a contiguous array where *Hox* gene expression follows a sequential 3′–5′ order, with the 3′ genes being expressed earlier in development and more cephalad and the 5′ genes being expressed later in development and more caudal. In this manner, and through the transcriptional control of downstream targets, the *Hox* genes specify diverse aspects of embryonic segmental/axial patterning.

In the MD, four *HoxA* genes (*HoxA9, 10, 11, 13*) are transcribed in partially overlapping domains according to their 3′–5′ order. *HoxA9* is expressed in the more cephalad portions of the MD that will become the FT, *HoxA10* in a segment of the MD corresponding to the uterus, and *HoxA11* in a segment that will give rise to the uterus and cervix (Fig. 1.20). *HoxA13* is expressed in the ectocervix and upper vagina (there is no *HoxA12* gene in humans) [100]. These expression patterns of the four *HoxA* genes appear to be conserved in the mouse and human MD [101]. Knockout of the mouse *HoxA* genes results in corresponding regional defects in the female reproductive tract; e.g., *HoxA13*-null mice exhibit agenesis of the caudal portions of the MD [102], while *HoxA10* inactivation converts the cephalad portions of the uterus into an fallopian tube-like structure ("cephalization"), providing genetic demonstration that the spatial *HoxA* expression controls MD segmentation.

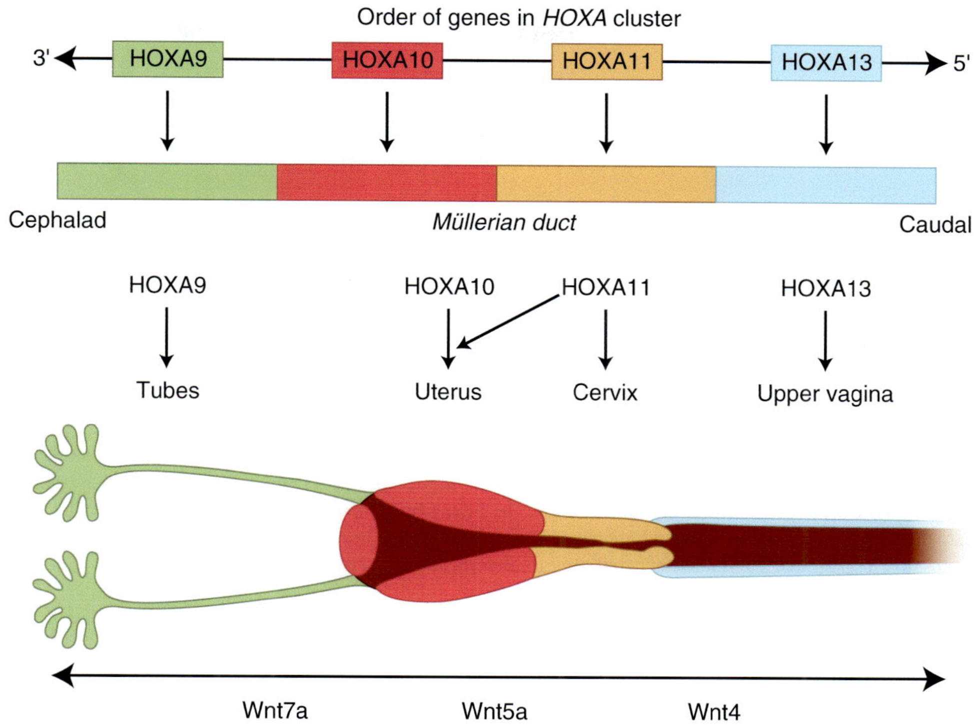

Fig. 1.20 Segmental specification of the Müllerian duct is dependent upon ordered spatial expression of the Hoxa gene cluster. Hoxa 13, Hoxa11, Hoxa10, and Hoxa9 are part of a gene cluster on chromosome 7. Their order on the chromosome corresponds to the spatial patterning of the MD in a caudal to cephalad direction. The Hoxa homeobox transcription factors work in concert with Wnt signaling in MD specification. Redrawn with permission from Du H and Taylor HS (2015) (Cold Spring Harbor Laboratory Press) [100]

1.5.6 p63 and Squamous Differentiation of the Müllerian Duct

The DNA-binding protein and transcriptional transactivator p63 (a homolog of the p53 tumor suppressor) is an early and ubiquitous marker of squamous differentiation in the embryo and is required for squamous differentiation in diverse anatomic sites. p63-deficient mice exhibit a striking absence of squamous epithelium in the vagina and cervix [103, 104]. p63 expression is retained in squamous epithelium throughout life and is a sensitive and useful marker of squamous differentiation [105]. The induction of p63 expression in vaginal and cervical epithelium depends upon the Bmp4-Smad activin A-Runx1 and Fgf7/10-Mapk pathways; when these pathways are genetically disrupted by conditional deletion of Smad4, Runx1, or Fgfr2, the epithelial cells of the vagina and cervix fail to express p63 and remain simple columnar [106–108].

1.5.7 Postnatal Development of the Müllerian Tract, Including Adenogenesis (Gland Formation)

The MDs are specified and then segmented in the embryo, but major maturational processes—most notably adenogenesis (the formation and development of glands from the original epithelial monolayer)—occur in the immediate postnatal period [109]. Adenogenesis also occurs in the endocervix, which in the adult contains a branching network of mucinous glands. Endocervical glands begin to form at 16 weeks gestation [80] and are well developed by the first year of life [110]. A comparable process of epithelial development and maturation (albeit one characterized by the formation of plicae instead of glands) also occurs in the fallopian tube [80]. However, adenogenesis has been most thoroughly investigated in the endometrium in animal models including rodents, sows, and ewes, with considerably less attention given to the process of glandular/plical maturation in the cervix and fallopian tube.

Mice and rats lack endometrial glands at birth, but epithelial invaginations or buds arise at regularly spaced intervals. The buds grow downward and branch, and the basic adult configuration of glands is established by postnatal day 15. Two noteworthy aspects of adenogenesis are that (1) it occurs in sexually immature animals well before puberty in the absence of steroid hormones and (2) the process of budding would appear to represent a form of controlled "invasion" with rapid growth and incursion of the MD epithelium into and throughout the underlying stroma. In sows and ewes, adenogenesis is also initiated at birth and largely completed within 2 months [109]. In humans, endometrial adenogenesis has been investigated histologically and begins at an earlier comparable developmental stage (prenatally, at 16 weeks gestation) [80]. Nonetheless, at birth human endometrial epithelium exhibits minimal complexity [111], with only superficial invaginations [110] demonstrating that adenogenesis also proceeds postnatally (Fig. 1.21), as in other mammals. The biomarkers and genes related to adenogenesis are described below.

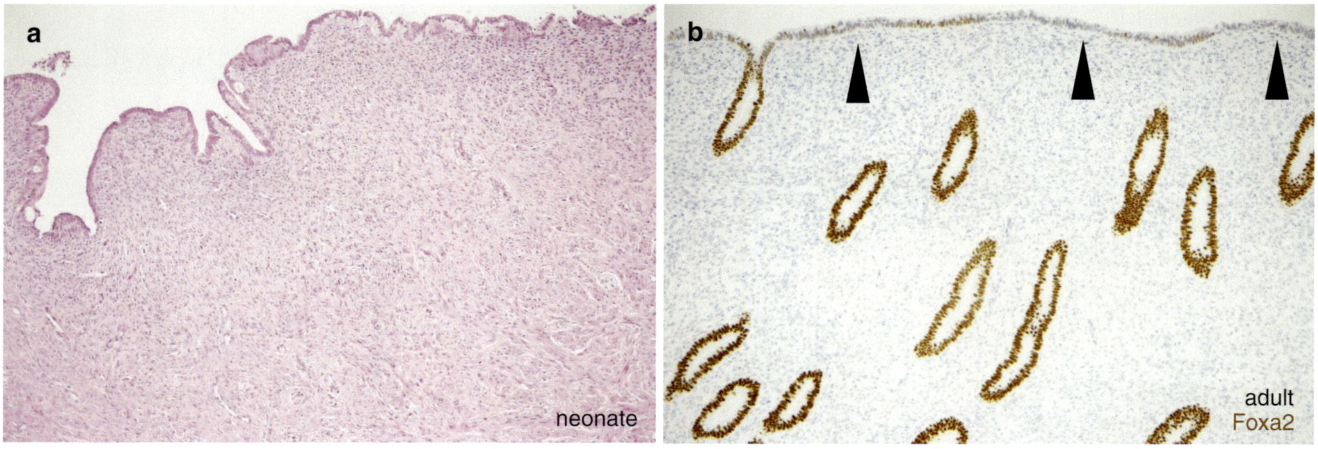

Fig. 1.21 Adenogenesis and Foxa2. (**a**) Neonatal human uterus shows slight invaginations but minimal gland formation. (**b**) Foxa2 immunohistochemistry of adult human endometrium shows strong nuclear expression in glandular but not surface epithelium (arrowheads), except in areas near the necks of glands. Mouse knockout studies have shown that this induction of Foxa2 expression is necessary for adenogenesis (gland formation); endometrial glands do not form in *Foxa2* knockout mice

1.5.8 The Ovarian Steroid Hormones Progesterone and Estrogen in Uterine Maturation

As presented in greater detail below, estrogen and progesterone govern essential uterine processes including cycling, menstruation, and pregnancy, but play more limited roles in early development. Estrogen is a potent mitogen in the adult endometrium (both stroma and epithelium), whereas progesterone potently counteracts the effects of estrogen by inhibiting proliferation and promoting differentiation. Within a few days of birth, rapid uterine epithelial proliferation is initiated, and this is intimately associated with epithelial budding and branching. The proliferation associated with adenogenesis (unlike that of cycling adult endometrium) is steroid hormone independent [112]; indeed, withdrawal from the high levels of progesterone to which the embryo is exposed during pregnancy appears to be the major cue instigating adenogenesis. Administration of a synthetic progesterone to neonatal ewes halts epithelial cell proliferation and permanently blocks adenogenesis, leading to the complete absence of endometrial glands in adult ewes and the inability to sustain a pregnancy [113]. Equivalent results have been obtained in mice [114, 115], arguing that (1) adenogenesis must occur during a limited (postnatal) developmental window, (2) progesterone withdrawal is the signal that triggers adenogenesis, and (3) endometrial glands serve essential functions in the establishment of pregnancy in diverse mammalian species.

1.5.9 Participation of Foxa2 in Uterine Adenogenesis

The forkhead transcription factor Foxa2 [116], which serves multiple roles in cell proliferation and development and is broadly expressed in epithelia in adults, has a central role in adenogenesis. In the adult uterus in diverse mammals including humans, Foxa2 is preferentially expressed in the uterine glandular vs. luminal epithelium, demonstrating that glandular and luminal epithelium are functionally and molecularly distinct (Fig. 1.21). Foxa2 expression in mouse endometrial epithelium is evident by postnatal day 6, when it begins marking the first invaginating buds and continues to be expressed in glands throughout life [117]. Uterine-specific ablation of Foxa2 in neonatal mice leads to the absence of uterine glands in adults with ensuing infertility, demonstrating that the induction of Foxa2 expression in the glandular epithelial cells is necessary for adenogenesis. Ablation of Foxa2 in adult mice (after adenogenesis is complete) leads to uteri with normal gland architecture but which cannot sustain pregnancy due to defective blastocyst implantation, showing that Foxa2 also continues to regulate uterine function and fertility in a cell-autonomous manner in concert with external (i.e., endocrine) control even after normal adenogenesis is complete [118]. It is also noteworthy that the *Foxa2* gene is a tumor suppressor in human endometrial cancer where loss-of-function mutations characterize >5% of cases [67].

1.5.10 Wnt and Hoxa Cooperation in MD Specification and Adenogenesis

Wnt and *HoxA* genes, which play important earlier roles in MD specification, also participate in postnatal maturation of the MD, including adenogenesis [72, 109]. Wnt7a is highly expressed throughout the developing MD epithelium but becomes restricted to the uterine and tubal epithelium postnatally, and Wnt7a-deficient female mice are infertile because of severe maldevelopment of the uterus and tubes [119, 120].

Wnt7a-deficient uteri are glandless, and the epithelium undergoes a conversion from columnar (endometrioid) to squamous (stratified) epithelium (i.e., resembling normal, more caudal, ectocervical/vaginal epithelium, or "caudalization"). This demonstrates that the Wnt/β-catenin pathway also contributes to the specification of the diverse epithelial cell types in different anatomical regions of the mature female reproductive tract. The oviducts in Wnt7a-deficient mice show defective coiling, but the epithelium does not undergo cell-type conversion [119, 120]. Wnt7a expression in MD epithelium is completely suppressed by progestin treatment, and Wnt7a is necessary for the maintenance of HoxA10 and HoxA11 expression in the MD [120], providing a link between progesterone and the Wnt/HoxA genes (Fig. 1.20). Other Wnts such as Wnt4 and Wnt5a are also expressed in the MD and contribute to MD development [72, 120]. Wnt4 is expressed in endometrial stroma [121], and postnatal Wnt4 ablation renders female mice infertile with reductions in uterine gland numbers and conversion of uterine endometrial epithelium to squamous epithelium [122], similar to the phenotype in *Wnt7a*-deficient uteri. One emergent theme is that the multiple factors needed early in MD development for specification are reutilized during adult physiologic control and function. Another is that the stroma provides essential inductive signals controlling both epithelial differentiation and function.

1.5.11 Wnt Action Through Frizzled Receptors and the Canonical β-Catenin Pathway

The multiplicity of *Wnt* genes expressed in the MD and later in the mature female reproductive tract, together with their diverse functional studies, highlights the considerable redundancies and partially overlapping functions among the Wnts. In the canonical Wnt pathway, secreted Wnts act in a paracrine fashion or across short distances through Frizzled transmembrane receptors. There are 10 mammalian *Frizzled* genes (*Frizzled1–10*), which, like the Wnts, are expressed in complex and partially overlapping domains. Wnt and Frizzled genes thus form a complex network of interactions. Determinants of Wnt-Frizzled specificity are poorly understood, and the large number of combinations of potential ligand/receptor interactions greatly complicates analyses of the specific roles of individual Wnts and Frizzled receptors [123]. Irrespective of such considerations, Wnt binding to Frizzled receptor acts in the canonical pathway to stabilize and activate β-catenin (Fig. 1.17). In the absence of bound Wnt, the Axin, Gsk3-β, and Apc (adenomatous polyposis coli) proteins, together known as the "destruction complex," degrades β-catenin via ubiquitination/proteasomal targeting. However, Wnt binding to Frizzled inactivates the complex, permitting β-catenin to accumulate and localize in the nucleus where it forms complexes with Tcf/Lef transcription factors to activate specific programs of gene expression and induce Wnt target gene expression [124]. Thus, β-catenin is the central effector and target of canonical Wnt signaling.

1.5.12 β-Catenin in Müllerian Duct Development

Concordantly, as an effector of Wnt4, 5a, 7a, and other Wnts expressed in either the MD epithelium or mesenchyme, β-catenin is critical for many aspects of MD development. Stabilization of β-catenin (constitutive activation) via genetic means (deletion of exon 3 containing the motifs required for β-catenin degradation) in the developing mouse MD mesenchyme resulted in infertility, absence of the fallopian tube, and a hypotrophic uterus with severe gland defects. Alterations within uterine epithelium include decreased proliferation and delayed uterine gland formation [125]. In contrast, postnatal ablation of β-catenin (i.e., functional inactivation) in both the epithelium and mesenchyme resulted in a dramatic conversion of the uterine endometrioid columnar epithelium to squamous epithelium, akin to the "caudal shift" observed in Wnt7a- and Wnt4-deficient uteri [126]. Thus, β-catenin signaling within the epithelium/stroma is essential for normal MD development and female reproductive tract function including the specification of epithelial cell fate. Once again, it is noteworthy that this pathway essential for MD development is also frequently misregulated in cancers of the MD later in life, particularly in endometrial cancers. For example, the *Ctnnb1* gene encoding β-catenin is mutated in 30% of endometrioid adenocarcinomas [67]. β-catenin misregulation including mutation likely underlies the common phenomenon of squamous differentiation (e.g., squamous morules) in endometrial cancers or precursor lesions [127].

1.5.13 Adenomyosis and Possible Basis in β-Catenin Abnormalities During Development

It is remarkable that during adenogenesis, the invasive growth of epithelium is programmed to halt at the endo-myometrial interface and not extend into the myometrium. The molecular basis of this restriction is unknown but must reflect "anti-invasion" signals in the myometrium, "pro-invasion" signals in the endometrial stroma, or both. Adenomyosis, an extremely common condition in adult women associated with pain, subfertility, and abnormal uterine bleeding, results from ectopic islands of endometrium (typically endometrial glands and endometrial-type stroma) within the myometrium. In some women, adenomyosis can be extensive and infiltrate throughout the uterus, leading to severe uterine hypertrophy and pain requiring hysterectomy for definitive treatment. The etiology and biological basis of adenomyosis remain unknown [128], but may result from abnormal adenogenesis. Adenomyosis has been observed in mice following constitutive genetic activation of β-catenin in the uterine mesenchymal compartment [129], pointing to abnormal Wnt/β-catenin signaling as one potential cause for this condition. While endometrial cancer can arise within adenomyosis, adenomyosis is not associated with a significantly increased risk of endometrial cancer [130, 131].

1.5.14 Epithelial-Mesenchymal and Mesenchymal-Epithelial Transitions in the Müllerian Duct

The initial step in MD formation, as introduced above, is the invagination of a few cells of coelomic epithelium to form first a bud, and then a distinct duct. The cells forming this duct are entirely epithelial in character morphologically, but express vimentin in addition to classical epithelial markers (cytokeratins) [132]. Vimentin is generally considered a mesenchymal marker but is not entirely specific as such since endometrial and tubal epithelia (unlike most epithelia) strongly express vimentin [133, 134]. Another interpretation is that these MD-derived epithelia, unlike most epithelia, retain some mesenchymal characteristics. Thus, vimentin expression in the developing MD could be viewed as evidence for a "mesoepithelial character" of the MD epithelium, but if so, then this is also true of the adult endometrial and tubal epithelium (vimentin is not expressed in cervical squamous or endocervical epithelium) [133]. The early steps of MD invagination thus appear to represent an epithelial-mesenchymal transition, since the coelomic epithelium does not express vimentin [132]. Interestingly, MD regression (which occurs in males only) may represent a continuation of this initial epithelial-mesenchymal transition. During MD regression, the basement membrane surrounding the MD epithelium is dissolved, and the epithelial cells adopt mesenchymal morphology and become incorporated into the surrounding mesenchyme [135]. In lineage tracing studies in mice, the endometrial epithelial and stromal compartments retain separate identities during normal cycling; surprisingly, after postpartum regeneration, a subset of endometrial stromal cells differentiate into endometrial epithelial cells that subsequently persist and are long-lived [136]. These results imply some degree of developmental plasticity and the potential for epithelium-mesenchymal and mesenchymal-epithelial transitions during MD development and subsequent physiologic functions.

As discussed earlier, the MD mesenchyme (i.e., stroma) is not a passive bystander in the process of MD specification and segmentation but rather specifies differentiation of the overlying epithelium. In classic experiments where mesenchymal and epithelial cells were isolated in pure form from the neonatal mouse vagina or uterus and subsequently mixed (homo- or heterotypically) and implanted into female hosts, epithelial differentiation (vaginal vs. uterine) of the resulting organoids depended upon the origin of the underlying mesenchyme. Such heterotopic induction and plasticity were observed only with neonatal mouse tissues; after 9 days of age, the epithelium became unresponsive to heterotypic induction, indicating that specification had already occurred [137]. These results demonstrated that the mesenchyme induces differentiation of the overlying epithelium. It is now known that these inductive properties depend upon the expression of Hox genes in the mesenchyme controlling in turn the secretion of specific Wnt proteins [72].

1.6 Müllerian Duct Fusion and Septal Regression

The uterus is formed by the fusion of lower segments of the bilateral MDs. This process begins at around the 8th week (when the MDs make contact with the urogenital sinus, see below) and is completed by the 9th week. The MDs are initially separated by intervening mesenchyme, which eventually disappears, leaving the basement membranes of the paired MDs in direct contact. The intervening basement membranes then disappear, the right and left Müllerian ducts come into direct contact, and the epithelia fuse in a caudal to cranial "zipping together" [80]. By this time, the septum has been resorbed and has disappeared, yielding a single uterine cavity (Fig. 1.22). The uterine muscular layer is formed by the 14th week; the endometrial and myometrial layers can be distinguished at this time. By the 22nd week, the differentiation of the myometrium is complete. The uterus has assumed its adult form with a well-defined fundus by the 24th week [80]. Uterine development at birth is thus anatomically complete, but the endometrial glands are immature (i.e., adenogenesis is not yet complete as discussed above), and the uterine body is still significantly smaller than the cervix. After the maturation of the uterus in puberty, the size ratio of the uterine body and cervix is reversed [80]. This relative growth and remodeling of the uterus as a consequence of ovarian steroid hormones results in ectropion or the migration of the cervical squamocolumnar junction from a more internal (and colposcopically unevaluable) location to a position beyond the cervical os. Exposure of the everted endocervical epithelium to the vaginal environment leads to p63-driven squamous metaplasia of the endocervical mucinous epithelium [138]. The endometrium of neonates can be influenced by maternal hormones and can exhibit proliferative or secretory changes.

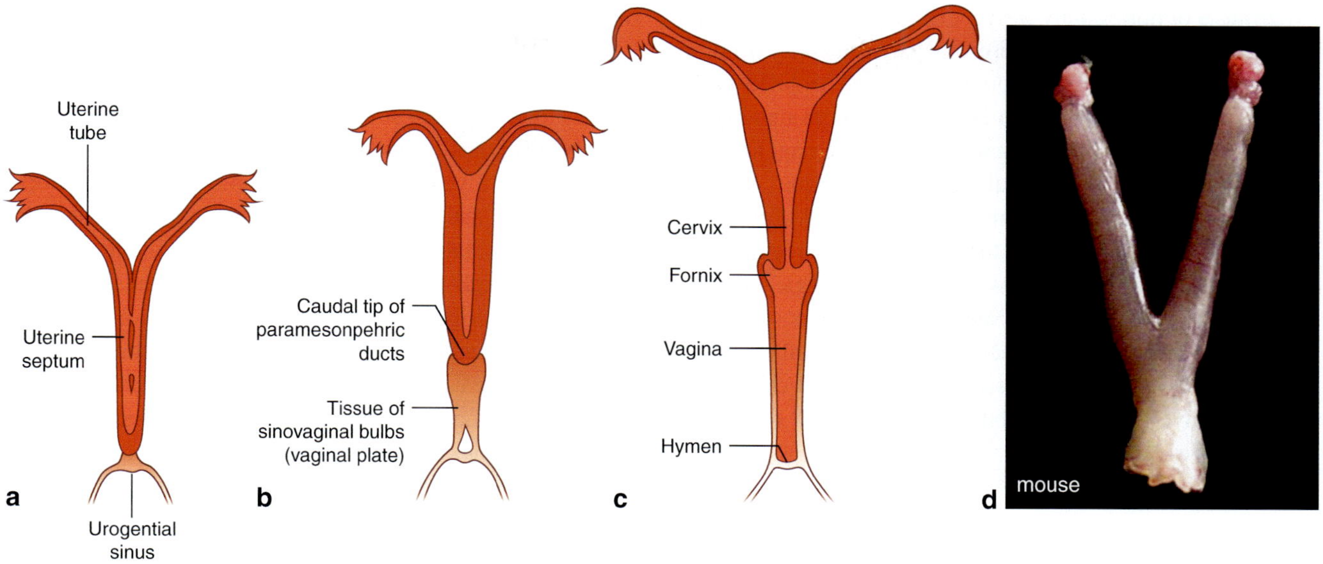

Fig. 1.22 Uterine fusion and septal regression. (**a**) 9 weeks. The uterine septum is regressing. (**b**) 3rd month. Note the vaginal plate is present as solid tube. (**c**) Neonate. Redrawn with permission from Sadler TW, Chapter 16, Langman's Medical Embryology, 12th edition (Wolters Kluwer). (**d**) Normal mouse uterus, where Müllerian duct fusion is minimal and limited to the caudal end, resulting in two uterine horns

Uterine anatomy varies in mammalian species because of vast differences in the extent of MD fusion. In rodents including mice, fusion of the MDs is minimal and occurs only in the caudal portion of the MDs, resulting in a duplex uterus consisting of two long uterine horns (Fig. 1.22). In humans and other primates, the fusion extends more rostrally, resulting in a simplex uterus with a single uterine cavity [139]. Perhaps because mice undergo minimal MD fusion and none at the level of the uterus, the molecular mechanisms underlying Müllerian duct fusion and septal regression are poorly understood. However, some insights have come from genetic and other observational studies of human Müllerian congenital anomalies (discussed below).

1.7 Urogenital Sinus as Precursor to External Genitalia, Fusion to the Müllerian Ducts, and Origin of Vaginal Epithelium

At week 8, around the time that the MDs make their midline fusion, the caudal ends of the MDs make contact with the urogenital sinus at the Müllerian tubercle (Fig. 1.22). The urogenital sinus provides the basis for the development of the urethra and external genitalia. Based on classic studies grounded on H&E stained sections, the vaginal epithelium has been proposed to be derived from both the Müllerian (upper vagina) and urogenital sinus epithelium (lower vagina). More recently, developmental studies of human embryos studied immunohistochemical expression of Pax2 and Foxa1, which are dichotomously expressed in Müllerian and urogenital sinus epithelium. Initially, the vaginal plate appears as a solid tube of squamous epithelium surrounded by mesenchyme. The vaginal plate begins to cavitate and canalize by the 16th week, and this process is completed by the 19th week. In studies of multiple human embryos from 12 to 21 weeks, epithelial Pax2 expression was present from the cervix to the uterus, with Foxa1 expression from the introitus to the fornices up to the cervix. These newer data support the proposal that the entire vaginal epithelium is derived from urogenital sinus epithelium and argue against a dual origin [80, 140]. However, the question is unresolved. On one hand, lineage tracing studies to definitively address this question are not feasible in humans, and on the other, lineage tracing studies from mammalian model systems may not be directly applicable to humans, since some significant molecular/morphological differences in sexual development have been noted across species. Thus, it may prove difficult to establish definitively the embryological origin (urogenital sinus vs. MD) of the upper vagina in humans.

1.8 Maldevelopment of the Vulva

1.8.1 Clitoromegaly

Clitoromegaly is the most common developmental abnormality of female external genitalia. It is usually a manifestation of virilization syndromes and disorders of sexual development, which can result from congenital adrenal hyperplasia or hormonally active virilizing tumors of ovarian or adrenal origin. However, clitoromegaly can rarely occur in isolation (unexplained clitoromegaly). Such isolated cases have multiple causes and can be due to benign underlying neoplasms (pseudoclitoromegaly) such as hemangioma or neurofibroma [141]. Clitoral hypertrophy can be the presenting sign of neurofibromatosis [142, 143]. Epidermal inclusion cysts (sometimes in the setting of ritual female circumcision [144]) are the most common etiologic basis of pseudoclitoromegaly [145]. Such cases can be surgically treated by partial clitoral resection or transclitoral resection of the underlying tumor. Persistent unexplained congenital clitoromegaly is also a rare but well-recognized feature in premature girls [146].

1.8.2 Labial Fusion

Labial fusion is an abnormality that occurs most commonly between the ages of 2 and 7 years and may be caused by inflammation and low prepubertal estrogen levels, but other factors may be involved. It is hypothesized that overactivation of macrophages and inflammation leads to fibrosis and deposition of collagen with scarring. Labial fusion can be asymptomatic or result in urinary incontinence, urinary tract infections, or vaginitis. Treatments include topical estrogens and surgery [147]. Labial fusion can also occur as a nondevelopmental disorder in adult females, for example, in association with lichen sclerosus [148].

1.8.3 Imperforate Hymen

Imperforate hymen is the most common congenital abnormality of the vagina, with an incidence of 1/2000. The internal genitalia are usually normal. This condition is commonly missed during the neonatal period and usually discovered at menarche (10–18 years of age) because of retained menstruation and abdominal pain that becomes unendurable after a few cycles. An abdominal mass can be palpated if the obstruction has been long-standing. The obstruction results in the accumulation of blood in the vaginal vault (hematocolpos) and the uterus (hematometra). The diagnosis is made by visual examination, which shows an imperforate hymen that is bulging or bluish, with confirmation by ultrasound evaluation. Delays in treatment can result in retrograde menstruation, endometriosis, pelvic adhesions, infections, bilateral hydronephrosis, and other conditions that could cause infertility or represent acute emergencies. Imperforate hymen sometimes presents in prepubertal girls or newborns with an accumulation of mucoid material (mucocolpos). The treatment is surgical (hymenotomy) [149–151].

1.8.4 Childhood Asymmetric Labia Major Enlargement

This distinctive lesion, sometimes termed prepubertal vulvar fibroma [152], has been described in prepubertal girls ranging from 3 to 13 years of age. The lesions are grossly poorly circumscribed with consistency similar to surrounding tissue, resulting in labia major enlargement and the impression of a mass, typically unilateral. Histologically, the lesions are poorly circumscribed and consist of normal vulvar soft tissue with predominance of a bland fibrous component. Limited follow-up is consistent with a benign condition; thus, surgical treatment is not necessary. In patients followed by observation, the lesions are noted to wax and wane in size. The etiology is unknown, but may reflect an asymmetric hormonal response by vulvar soft tissue, which expresses estrogen receptor [153].

1.8.5 Rare Conditions

Double vulva, consisting of complete or partial duplication of the vulva (sometimes with duplication of vagina, uterus, or bladder), has been reported as an extremely rare condition (less than 20 cases in the literature); the biological basis is unknown [154]. Congenital absence of the clitoris has also been described in isolated case reports [155].

1.9 Maldevelopment of the Vagina

As discussed above, the vagina has classically been considered to have a dual embryological origin with the upper third of Müllerian origin and the lower portion being of urogenital sinus (UGS) origin. Recent studies based on Pax2 and Foxa1 expression have suggested that the entire vagina is derived from the UGS [80, 140], but such expression patterns are insufficient to establish cell lineage relationships.

One proposed classification scheme for the complex vaginal malformations discussed below, based on anatomical and clinical criteria, is summarized in Table 1.2 [156].

1.9.1 Vaginal Agenesis, Atresia, and Transverse/Longitudinal Septum

Vaginal malformations are complex and can occur in isolation or in association with a highly variable spectrum of abnormalities in Müllerian and/or genitourinary development. Vaginal agenesis refers to the complete lack of a vagina, whereas vaginal atresia refers to the absence of a segment of vagina. Most cases of vaginal agenesis occur in association with the Mayer-Rokitansky-Kuster-Hauser (MRKH)

Table 1.2 Classification scheme for vaginal malformations

Type	Malformation	Subtype	Characteristics	
I	Agenesis Complete lack of vagina	IA	Associated with uterine agenesis (MRKH)	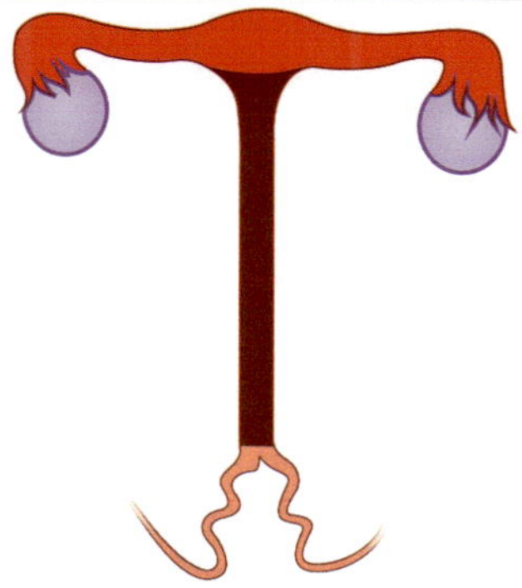
		IB	Isolated	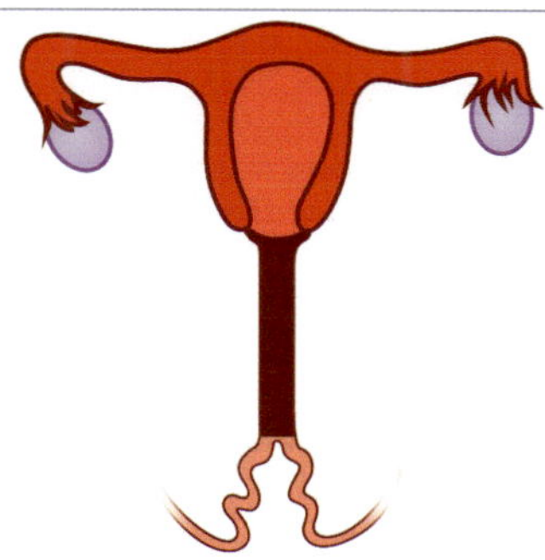
II	Atresia Absence of a tract of vagina	IIA	Proximal	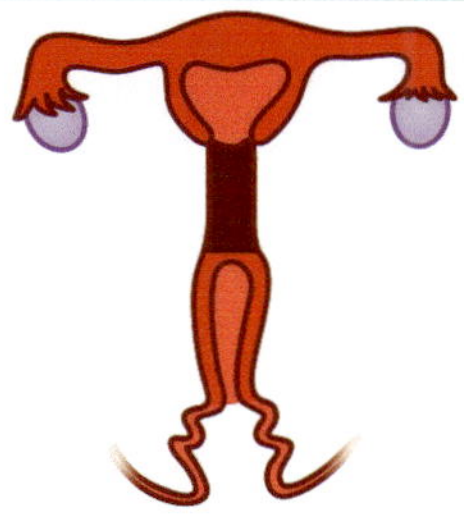
		IIB	Distal	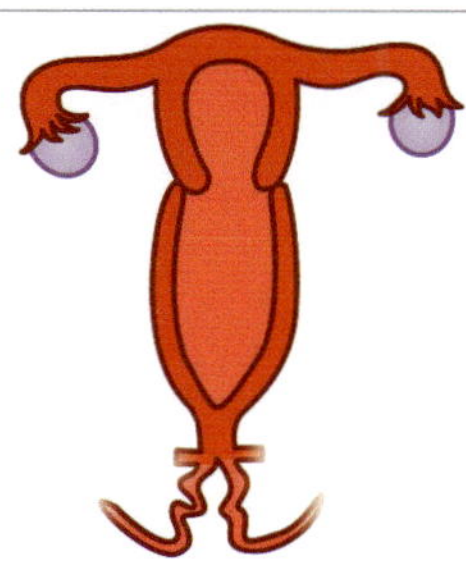

(continued)

Table 1.2 (continued)

Type	Malformation	Subtype	Characteristics	
III	Atresia with fistula, persistent UGS Persistent UGS with atresia of distal third of vagina	IIIA	Proximal fistula (above the urethral sphincter) high UGS	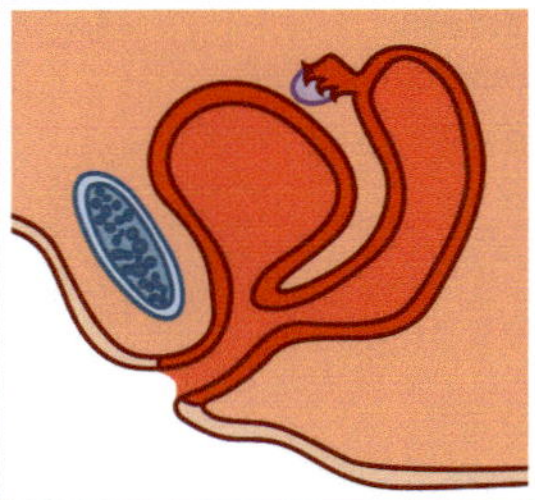
		IIIB	Distal fistula (under the urethral sphincter) low UGS	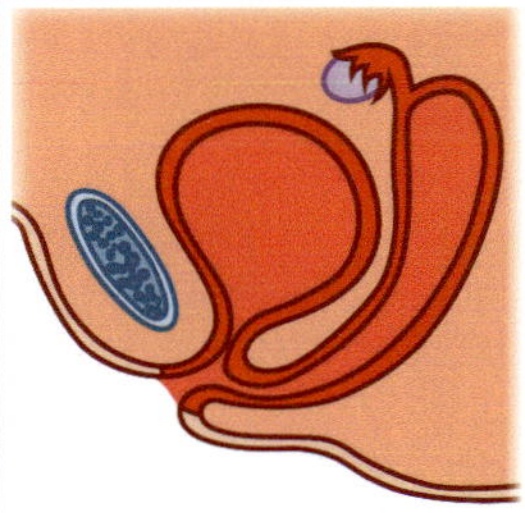
IV	Atresia as diaphragm Small transverse atresic tract of vagina as a diaphragm, that can be located along all the length of vagina, mostly proximal	IVA	Transverse septum • Complete • Incomplete	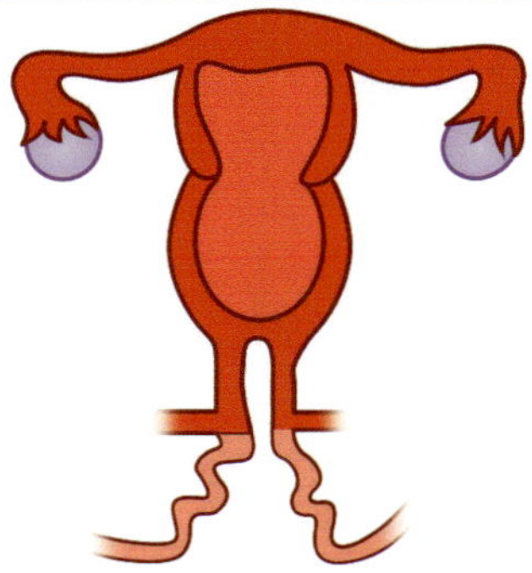
		IVB	Imperforate hymen	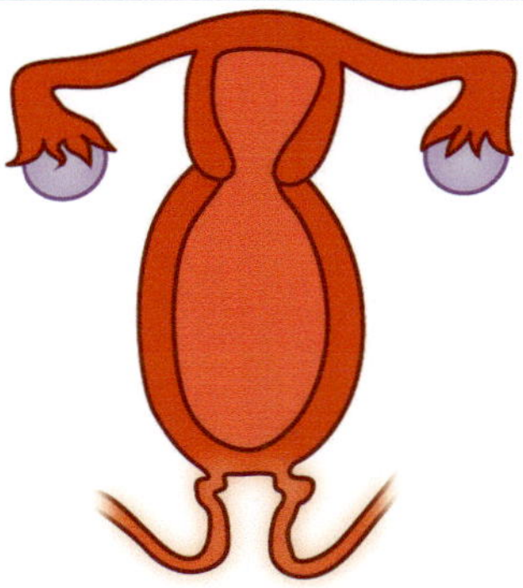

Table 1.2 (continued)

Type	Malformation	Subtype	Characteristics	
V	Duplication	VA	Complete duplication (development of two vaginas, in absence of intestinal anomalies)	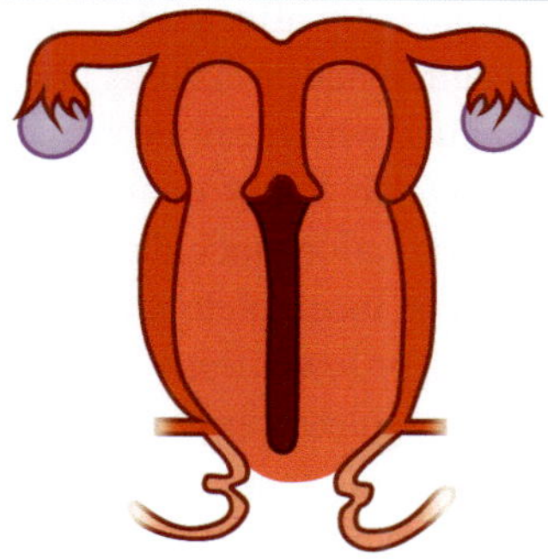
		VB	Longitudinal septum (divides vagina into two hemivaginas; one of them can be atresic in its distal tract)	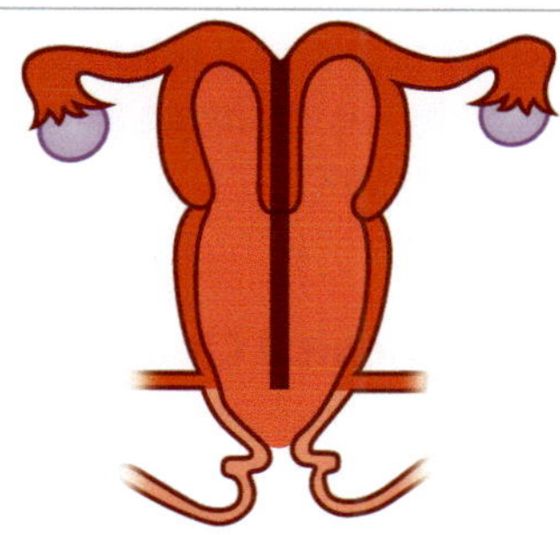
VI	Cloaca Communication of urinary tract, internal genitalia, and rectum into the urethra	VI		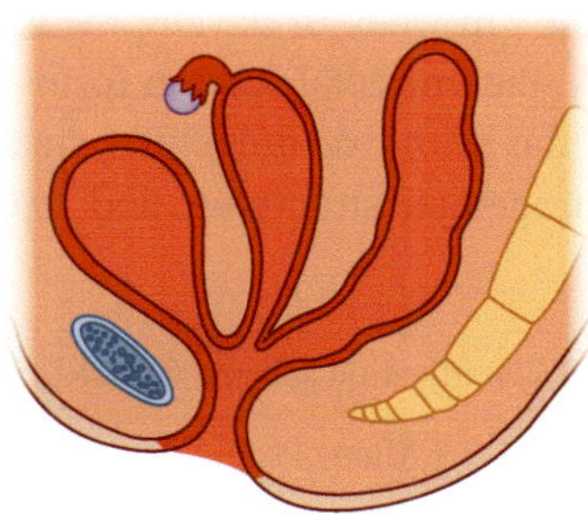

From Ruggeri G et al., Pediatric Surgery International 28:797 (2012) [156], reproduced with permission (Elsevier) syndrome. MRKH is discussed in the section below on maldevelopment of the uterus, since the uterus is the Müllerian structure principally affected in MRKH.

Some vaginal malformations are associated with urethrovaginal fistulas, which can occur either below or above the urethral sphincter. Other common types of developmental vaginal malformations include transverse septum, which can be complete or incomplete and may lie at the level of the upper, middle, or lower third of the vagina. The clinical presentation of complete transverse septum can resemble that of imperforate hymen, including hematocolpos [157] or mucocolpos [158]. Longitudinal septum can manifest as the development of two vaginas (duplication) and is frequently diagnosed at puberty for hematocolpos [156]. Vaginal septum is ostensibly due to abnormal canalization of the vaginal plate, which begins as a solid tube of squamous epithelium surrounded by mesenchyme and canalizes in the 16th–19th week of development.

1.9.2 Congenital Cloaca

Congenital cloaca (aka persistent cloaca) refers to a rare anomaly (1 in 20,000 live births) where a female infant is born with a single orifice in the perineum, which communicates with the urethra, vagina, and rectum. In human embryology, the cloaca is an expansion of the hindgut formed around the 5th week of development. Normally, in the 5th–6th week, the urorectal septum forms and partitions the cloaca into the primitive urogenital sinus (UGS), which gives rise to urogenital structures, and the rectum. The surgical repair of these severe defects with the goal of restoring bowel, urinary, and sexual function is a significant challenge [159, 160].

1.10 Maldevelopment of the Uterus

Developmental abnormalities of the proximal Müllerian structures are frequent in the general population. The prevalence is estimated at 5%, but this includes a high prevalence of arcuate-shaped uterus, which can be considered a normal anatomic variant [161]. Most cases are sporadic, but familial recurrences occur. There is evidence of genetic causality for mutations in a small number of loci including *HOXA13*, *WNT9B*, and *HNF1B*. Nonetheless, only a small percentage of cases (<10%) can be attributed to hereditary factors [162] and a much lower percentage to specific genetic mutations. The modest <5% risk in first-degree relatives [162] and reports of discordant phenotypes in monozygotic twins [76, 163] support the notion that epigenetic or environmental factors underlie most of these congenital malformations.

Uterine malformations include a broad spectrum of anomalies. Classification systems group these complex malformations according to the anatomical components and defects in formation or fusion of the Müllerian ducts or septal absorption. The ESHRE/ESGE classification system, proposed by the European Society of Human Reproduction and Embryology (ESHRE) and the European Society for Gynaecological Endoscopy (ESGE), was recently developed in an effort to simplify and minimize subjectivity (Table 1.3, Fig. 1.23) [164]. Cervical and vaginal malformations are classified inde-

Table 1.3 Classification scheme (ESHRE/ESGE) for congenital anomalies of the female reproductive tract

	Main class	Main subclass	Coexistent subclass
	Uterine anomaly		Cervical/vaginal anomaly
Class 0	Normal uterus		*Cervix*
			C0 normal
Class I	Dysmorphic uterus	(a) T-shaped	*C1 septate*
		(b) Infantilis	*C2 double "normal"*
Class II	Septate uterus	(a) Partial	*C3 unilateral aplasia/dysplasia*
		(b) Complete	*C4 aplasia/dysplasia*
Class III	Dysfused uterus (including dysfused "septate")	(a) Partial	
		(b) Complete	*Vagina*
Class IV	Unilaterally formed uterus	(a) Rudimentary horn with cavity (communicating or not)	*V0 normal vagina*
			V1 longitudinal non-obstructing vaginal septum
		(b) Rudimentary horn without cavity/aplasia (no horn)	*V2 longitudinal obstructing vaginal septum*
Class V	Aplastic/dysplastic	(a) Rudimentary horn with cavity (bi- or unilateral)	*V3 transverse vaginal septum/imperforate hymen*
		(b) Rudimentary horn without cavity (bi- or unilateral)/aplasia	*V4 vaginal aplasia*
Class VI	Unclassified malformations		

Reproduced from Grimbizis GF et al., Gynecologic Surgery 10:800 (2013) [164] (Springer Nature Open Access)

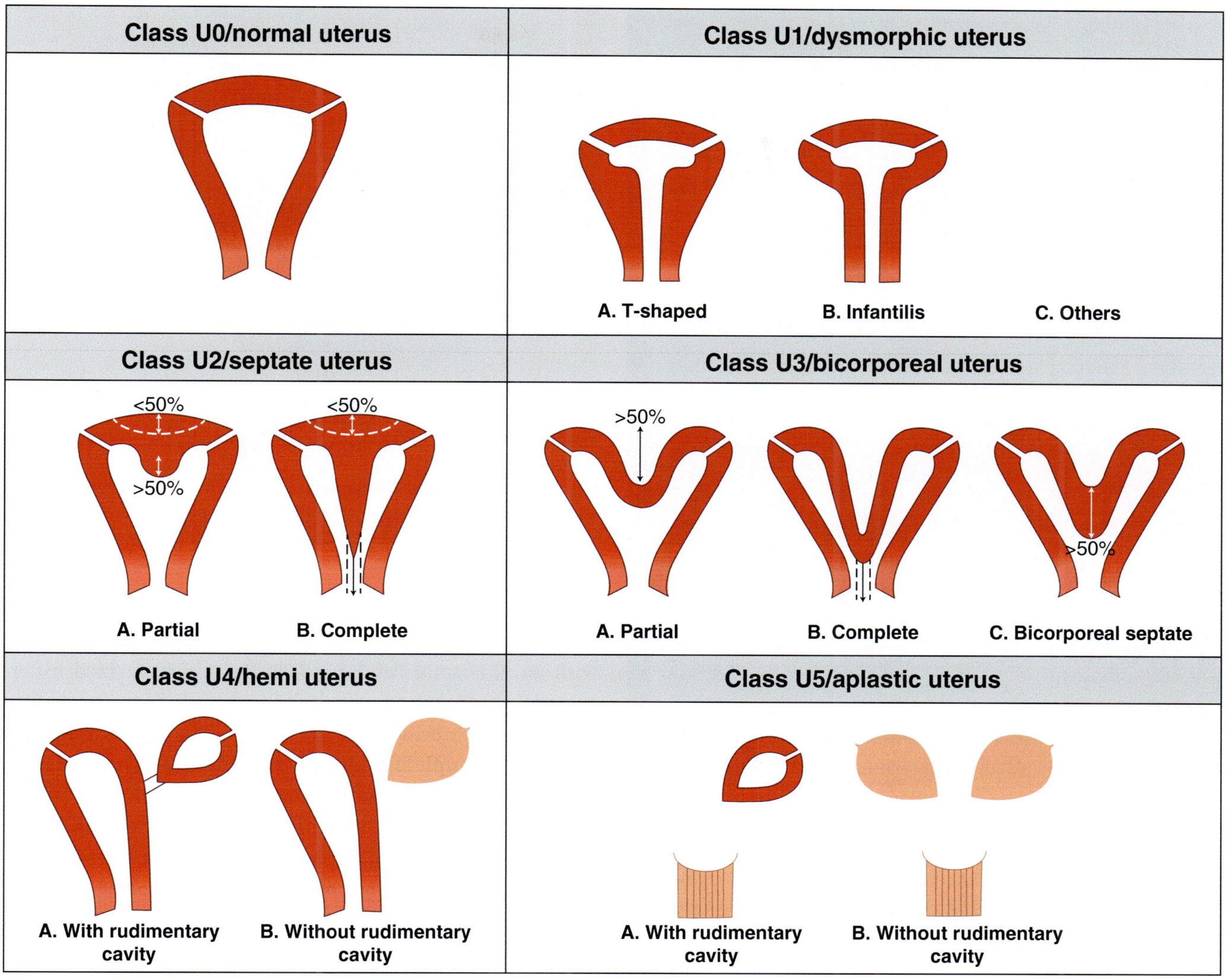

Fig. 1.23 Classification scheme (ESHRE/ESGE) for congenital anomalies of the female reproductive tract. Reproduced from Grimbizis GF et al., Gynecologic Surgery 10:800 (2013) (Springer Nature Open Access) [164]

pendently because cervicovaginal anomalies can occur independently or in combination with uterine/tubal anomalies [164]. Alternative schemes include the American Society for Reproductive Medicine (ASRM) classification; the relative merits of these systems have been debated [165–167].

1.10.1 Aplastic Uterus: Mayer-Rokitansky-Kuster-Hauser Syndrome (MRKH)

At the most severe end of the spectrum is congenital absence of the uterus, known as aplastic uterus (Class U5). This condition is typically diagnosed during late adolescence, often coming to clinical attention because of primary amenorrhea. Mayer-Rokitansky-Kuster-Hauser syndrome (MRKH, OMIM: 277000), sometimes shortened to MRK or MR syndrome, is defined as congenital absence of the uterus and cervix, with a shortened, blind-ending vagina. In some cases, there are uterine or tubal remnants with or without a rudimentary cavity (Fig. 1.24) [164]. Height and secondary female sexual characteristics including external genitalia are normal. Cases are further categorized as Type 1 (no other significant congenital malformations) or Type 2 (significant congenital abnormalities that can include genitourinary or musculoskeletal abnormalities, as well as hearing loss and cardiac complications) [168]. MRKH is also referred to in the literature as Müllerian agenesis, Müllerian aplasia, uterine agenesis, or congenital absence of the uterus [76].

1.10.2 Less Severe Variants: Dysmorphic, Septate, Bicorporeal, and Hemi-Uterus

Dysmorphic uterus (Class U1) incorporates cases with a normal uterine silhouette but with an abnormal shape of the uterine cavity (excluding septa). Class U1a refers to a

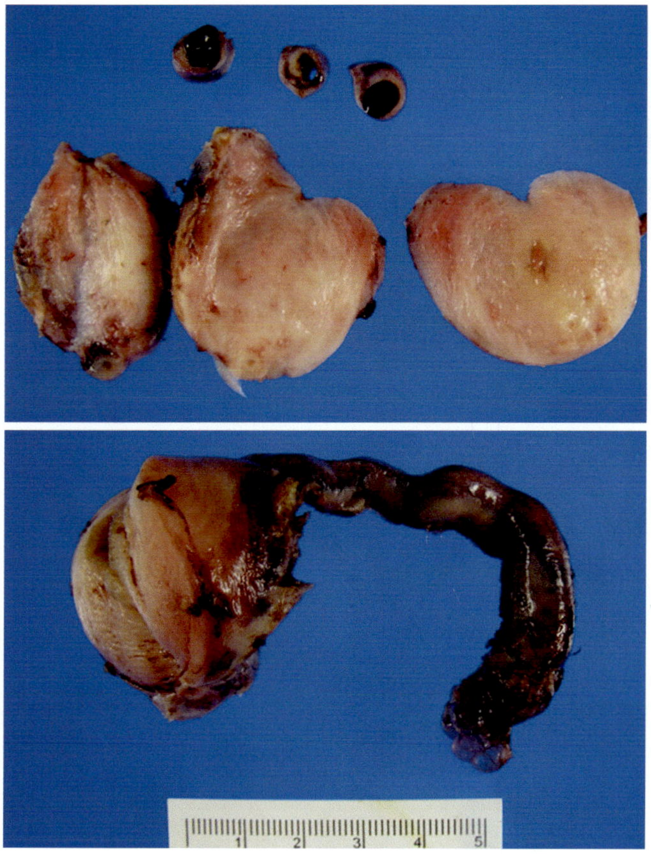

Fig. 1.24 Left fallopian tube and uterine horn remnant in 14 y/o girl with Müllerian agenesis (Mayer-Rokitansky-Kuster-Hauser syndrome/ MRKH) . Only a very rudimentary cavity is present in the uterine horn remnant (top panel, right). Images courtesy of Drs. Amanda Strickland and Dinesh Rakheja (UT Southwestern)

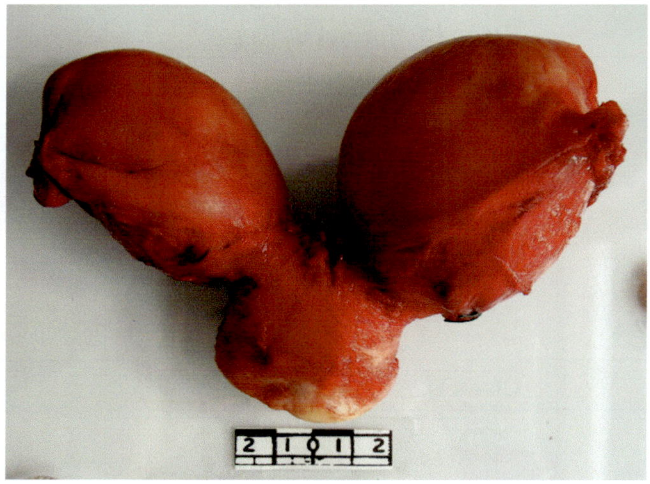

Fig. 1.25 Bicorporeal uterus (Class U3) with double cervix and two well-defined uterine horns. Reproduced with permission from Zheng W, Chapter 1, Obstetric and Gynecologic Pathology, 1st edition (2013) (Science Press)

T-shaped uterus with a narrow uterine cavity due to thickened lateral walls. Class U1b, or uterus infantilis, is characterized by a narrow uterine cavity without lateral wall thickening. Class U1c includes all other minor deformities of the uterine cavity including those with an inner indentation at the fundal midline level of <50% of the uterine wall (i.e., myometrial) thickness. Dysmorphic uteri are usually small in size [164] and are associated with a lower incidence of clinical pregnancy and live births [169]. Of note, arcuate uterus, a mildly variant shape of the uterus characterized by mild thickening (<50%) of the uterine wall, is not included in the ESHRE/ESGE classification system. Arcuate uterus is considered a normal variant, and the clinical value of the distinction is questionable: reproductive outcomes appear normal [164, 169].

Septate uterus (Class U2) includes only patients with a normal uterine silhouette and abnormal regression of the midline septum, leading to an internal indentation (septum) >50% of the uterine thickness. The septum can partially (U2a) or completely (U2b) divide the uterine cavity. In some cases the septum can extend to the cervix and/or vagina [164].

Bicorporeal uterus (Class U3) is defined as a uterus with an abnormal fundal silhouette, characterized by an external indentation at the fundal midline involving >50% of the uterine wall thickness. This indentation can partly or completely divide the uterus. A completely bicorporeal uterus can be associated with a double cervix (previously known as uterine didelphys) or a single cervix (previously known as bicornuate uterus); see Fig. 1.25 for example of Class U3 bicorporeal uterus. Vaginal septal defects can also occur, more commonly when a double cervix is present. In the ESHRE/ESGE classification, bicorporeal uteri with single or double cervix are classified together as Class U3b (bicorporeal uterus, complete) in an attempt to create a more functional and accurate definition category, whereas in previous classification schema (ASRM), bicornuate and didelphys uteri were classified separately [76].

Hemi-uterus (Class U4) describes a uterus with a rudimentary endometrial cavity due to unilateral uterine/ Müllerian development (i.e., unilateral Müllerian agenesis). The contralateral part is either incompletely formed or absent altogether. In Class U4a, there is a rudimentary cavity on the defective side that may or may not communicate with the contralateral horn; in class U4b, there is no rudimentary cavity [164].

1.10.3 Uterus-Like Mass

Uterus-like mass is a rare phenomenon (about 30 cases reported) whereby an extrauterine mass comprised of smooth muscle surrounding a central endometrial-lined cavity is identified, typically within the pelvis [170, 171]. These masses resemble uterine "organoids." Anatomic locations are varied and include the broad ligament, adnexa, and liver, and can occur in XY males, resulting in a wide range of clinical presentations [172, 173]. Cases are frequently associated with endometriosis and, more rarely, with developmental anomalies such as neural tube defects [174]. In sporadic cases, uterus-like mass has been associated with endometrioid or clear cell adenocarcinoma [175, 176]. Uterus-like mass has been termed endomyometrosis in some reports [173], and the etiology is uncertain [177].

1.10.4 Genetic Basis of Uterine Developmental Anomalies

Numerous genes have been identified as potential candidates; however, in many cases pathogenicity is not well established. Furthermore, although they provide intriguing links between human and mouse development, all of the variants described below are rare and account for only a small percentage of uterine anomalies. As described earlier, differential spatial expression of the *HoxA* gene cluster (*HoxA9*, *10*, *11*, and *13*) during embryogenesis segments the MD into the cervix, uterus, and fallopian tubes, and segmentation defects have been documented in mouse mutants. In humans, *HoxA13* loss-of-function mutations have been identified as the cause of hand-foot-genital syndrome (OMIM: 140000). This hereditary condition is autosomal dominant and is associated with small feet, abnormal thumbs, genitourinary abnormalities, and uterine anomalies due to various defects of Müllerian duct fusion or septal regression. The mutation is inherited in an autosomal dominant fashion because of haploinsufficiency; i.e., the syndrome results from the inactivation of a single allele [178, 179]. *HoxA10* and *HoxA11* mutations have also been reported in women with uterine anomalies [76, 180, 181].

Wnt7A homozygous mutations result in a range of limb malformations and abnormal genitourinary/Müllerian development including uterine/vaginal agenesis (OMIM: 276820) [76, 182]. *Wnt4* and *Wnt9B* have been analyzed in series of patients with MRKH syndrome and other Müllerian anomalies. Several heterozygous missense variants were identified, implicating the mutations as pathogenic, but additional data is needed to establish the pathogenicity of these rare variants. [76].

Mutations in *Hnf1β* (hepatocyte nuclear factor-1β, also known as *Tcf2*) result in renal cysts and diabetes syndrome (RCAD, OMIM: 137920), an autosomal dominant syndrome characterized by abnormal renal development, diabetes, and abnormal Müllerian development including vaginal aplasia and aplastic uterus (MRKH). The condition results from mutation of a single allele; i.e., the autosomal dominant pattern of inheritance is due to haploinsufficiency. The Hnf1β protein is a POU domain transcription factor strongly expressed in the developing Wolffian and Müllerian ducts [183] and is required for normal expression of Wnt9b and Pax8 [184]. *Hnf1β* mutations occur in women with uterine plus renal malformations, but appear rare or absent in women with isolated uterine anomalies [76]. Interestingly, Hnf1β protein is overexpressed in most clear cell adenocarcinomas of the ovary and uterus, making it a useful immunohistochemical marker to distinguish clear cell adenocarcinoma from its histologic mimics. The biological basis of such overexpression in clear cell adenocarcinomas and the significance of this phenomenon vis-à-vis the role of Hnf1β in MD development are unclear [185].

1.11 Maldevelopment of the Fallopian Tube and Ovary

Unilateral absence of the fallopian tube is rare and can be associated with infertility; usually the ipsilateral ovary is also absent [186–189]. Also rare but well documented is the presence of an accessory fallopian tube with fimbria [190], which can sometimes undergo torsion [191]. In one patient, three tubes were present on the right side; the main tube was normal in size and anatomy, whereas the other two accessory tubes were thin but with fimbriated ends [192]. Accessory fallopian tube can be associated with infertility [193]. It has been suggested that "congenital" absence of the tube and ovary might be due to ovarian torsion and subsequent infarction and thus might not represent a congenital abnormality [194]. Undescended ovary (ovarian maldescent) has also been described as an unusual cause of infertility and occurs when the upper pole of the ovary is above the pelvic brim; it is associated with a small infundibulopelvic ligament, an elongated utero-ovarian ligament, and an elongated fallopian tube. Ovarian maldescent does not preclude fertility [195].

1.12 Diethylstilbestrol and Female Reproductive Tract Anomalies

Diethylstilbestrol (DES) was an orally active estrogen prescribed in pregnancy to prevent miscarriages. It was used beginning in the 1940s, and in 1947 the U.S. Food and Drug Administration approved the use of DES to prevent miscarriage. Tragically, the drug was prescribed without strong evidence of clinical benefit, and in 1953, a large blinded control study found DES to be ineffective in the prevention of premature births. Despite this and subsequent studies that also failed to show clinical benefit, DES continued to be prescribed in the United States until 1971 and in European countries until the late 1970s [196]. In 1971, exposure to DES during fetal development was shown to be strongly associated with vaginal clear cell adenocarcinoma, an otherwise rare malignancy [197], and prescription of the drug was discontinued.

DES is a synthetic estrogen five times more potent than estradiol. It is believed to have diverse effects on gene expression, but its mode of action as a teratogen remains poorly understood. Among other effects, exposure of the developing female reproductive tract to DES represses expression of HoxA10 [198].

The incidence of clear cell adenocarcinoma was only 0.1% in women exposed to DES in utero (DES daughters)—but other teratogenic effects were much more common. DES daughters have a high incidence (40%) of vaginal adenosis—the abnormal presence of glandular epithelium in the vagina. DES also resulted in a high incidence of Müllerian duct abnormalities including vaginal septae, and dysmorphic or septate uterus [199]. Women exposed to DES had a relative risk of 1.3 of never becoming pregnant [200]. Due to the cessation of the drug in 1971, the diagnosis of new DES-associated malignancies or structural defects in DES daughters in current clinical practice is now unlikely. However, the long-term effects are unknown and may include an increased incidence of breast cancer [201].

References

1. Dansereau DA, Lasko P. The development of germline stem cells in Drosophila. Methods Mol Biol. 2008;450:3–26. https://doi.org/10.1007/978-1-60327-214-8_1.
2. Kumar DL, DeFalco T. Of mice and men: in vivo and in vitro studies of primordial germ cell specification. Semin Reprod Med. 2017;35(2):139–46. https://doi.org/10.1055/s-0037-1599085.
3. De Felici M. Origin, migration, and proliferation of human primordial germ cells. In: Coticchio G, Albertini DF, De Santis L, editors. Oogenesis. London: Springer; 2013. p. 19–38. https://doi.org/10.1007/978-0-85729-826-3.
4. McKay DG, Hertig AT, Adams EC, Danziger S. Histochemical observations on the germ cells of human embryos. Anat Rec. 1953;117(2):201–19.
5. Castrillon DH, Quade BJ, Wang TY, Quigley C, Crum CP. The human VASA gene is specifically expressed in the germ cell lineage. Proc Natl Acad Sci U S A. 2000;97(17):9585–90. https://doi.org/10.1073/pnas.160274797.
6. De Felici M. Regulation of primordial germ cell development in the mouse. Int J Dev Biol. 2000;44(6):575–80.
7. Mollgard K, Jespersen A, Lutterodt MC, Yding Andersen C, Hoyer PE, Byskov AG. Human primordial germ cells migrate along nerve fibers and Schwann cells from the dorsal hind gut mesentery to the gonadal ridge. Mol Hum Reprod. 2010;16(9):621–31. https://doi.org/10.1093/molehr/gaq052.
8. Eildermann K, Aeckerle N, Debowski K, Godmann M, Christiansen H, Heistermann M, Schweyer S, Bergmann M, Kliesch S, Gromoll J, Ehmcke J, Schlatt S, Behr R. Developmental expression of the pluripotency factor sal-like protein 4 in the monkey, human and mouse testis: restriction to premeiotic germ cells. Cells Tissues Organs. 2012;196(3):206–20. https://doi.org/10.1159/000335031.
9. Mamsen LS, Brochner CB, Byskov AG, Mollgard K. The migration and loss of human primordial germ stem cells from the hind gut epithelium towards the gonadal ridge. Int J Dev Biol. 2012;56(10–12):771–8. https://doi.org/10.1387/ijdb.120202lm.
10. Hoyer PE, Byskov AG, Mollgard K. Stem cell factor and c-Kit in human primordial germ cells and fetal ovaries. Mol Cell Endocrinol. 2005;234(1–2):1–10. https://doi.org/10.1016/j.mce.2004.09.012.
11. Tanaka SS, Yamaguchi YL, Tsoi B, Lickert H, Tam PP. IFITM/Mil/fragilis family proteins IFITM1 and IFITM3 play distinct roles in mouse primordial germ cell homing and repulsion. Dev Cell. 2005;9(6):745–56. https://doi.org/10.1016/j.devcel.2005.10.010.
12. Chaganti RS, Rodriguez E, Mathew S. Origin of adult male mediastinal germ-cell tumours. Lancet. 1994;343(8906):1130–2.
13. Sanchez A, Amatruda JF. Zebrafish germ cell Tumors. Adv Exp Med Biol. 2016;916:479–94. https://doi.org/10.1007/978-3-319-30654-4_21.
14. Yamashiro C, Hirota T, Kurimoto K, Nakamura T, Yabuta Y, Nagaoka SI, Ohta H, Yamamoto T, Saitou M. Persistent requirement and alteration of the key targets of PRDM1 during primordial germ cell development in mice. Biol Reprod. 2016;94(1):7. https://doi.org/10.1095/biolreprod.115.133256.
15. Ohinata Y, Payer B, O'Carroll D, Ancelin K, Ono Y, Sano M, Barton SC, Obukhanych T, Nussenzweig M, Tarakhovsky A, Saitou M, Surani MA. Blimp1 is a critical determinant of the germ cell lineage in mice. Nature. 2005;436(7048):207–13. https://doi.org/10.1038/nature03813.
16. Tang WW, Kobayashi T, Irie N, Dietmann S, Surani MA. Specification and epigenetic programming of the human germ line. Nat Rev Genet. 2016;17(10):585–600. https://doi.org/10.1038/nrg.2016.88.
17. Clark AT. DNA methylation remodeling in vitro and in vivo. Curr Opin Genet Dev. 2015;34:82–7. https://doi.org/10.1016/j.gde.2015.09.002.
18. Satoh M. Histogenesis and organogenesis of the gonad in human embryos. J Anat. 1991;177:85–107.
19. Liu C, Peng J, Matzuk MM, Yao HH. Lineage specification of ovarian theca cells requires multicellular interactions via oocyte and granulosa cells. Nat Commun. 2015;6:6934. https://doi.org/10.1038/ncomms7934.
20. Karl J, Capel B. Sertoli cells of the mouse testis originate from the coelomic epithelium. Dev Biol. 1998;203(2):323–33. https://doi.org/10.1006/dbio.1998.9068.
21. Hu YC, Okumura LM, Page DC. Gata4 is required for formation of the genital ridge in mice. PLoS Genet. 2013;9(7):e1003629. https://doi.org/10.1371/journal.pgen.1003629.
22. Miyamoto N, Yoshida M, Kuratani S, Matsuo I, Aizawa S. Defects of urogenital development in mice lacking Emx2. Development. 1997;124(9):1653–64.
23. Birk OS, Casiano DE, Wassif CA, Cogliati T, Zhao L, Zhao Y, Grinberg A, Huang S, Kreidberg JA, Parker KL, Porter FD, Westphal H. The LIM homeobox gene Lhx9 is essential for mouse gonad formation. Nature. 2000;403(6772):909–13. https://doi.org/10.1038/35002622.
24. Kreidberg JA, Sariola H, Loring JM, Maeda M, Pelletier J, Housman D, Jaenisch R. WT-1 is required for early kidney development. Cell. 1993;74(4):679–91.
25. Eggers S, Ohnesorg T, Sinclair A. Genetic regulation of mammalian gonad development. Nat Rev Endocrinol. 2014;10(11):673–83. https://doi.org/10.1038/nrendo.2014.163.
26. Hastie ND. Wilms' tumour 1 (WT1) in development, homeostasis and disease. Development. 2017;144(16):2862–72. https://doi.org/10.1242/dev.153163.
27. Topol L, Chen W, Song H, Day TF, Yang Y. Sox9 inhibits Wnt signaling by promoting beta-catenin phosphorylation in the nucleus. J Biol Chem. 2009;284(5):3323–33. https://doi.org/10.1074/jbc.M808048200.

28. Lin YT, Capel B. Cell fate commitment during mammalian sex determination. Curr Opin Genet Dev. 2015;32:144–52. https://doi.org/10.1016/j.gde.2015.03.003.
29. Hughes JF, Page DC. The biology and evolution of mammalian Y chromosomes. Annu Rev Genet. 2015;49:507–27. https://doi.org/10.1146/annurev-genet-112414-055311.
30. Koopman P. The curious world of gonadal development in mammals. Curr Top Dev Biol. 2016;116:537–45. https://doi.org/10.1016/bs.ctdb.2015.12.009.
31. Sekido R, Lovell-Badge R. Sex determination and SRY: down to a wink and a nudge? Trends Genet. 2009;25(1):19–29. https://doi.org/10.1016/j.tig.2008.10.008.
32. Spiller C, Koopman P, Bowles J. Sex determination in the mammalian germline. Annu Rev Genet. 2017;51:265–85. https://doi.org/10.1146/annurev-genet-120215-035449.
33. Kurilo LF. Oogenesis in antenatal development in man. Hum Genet. 1981;57(1):86–92.
34. Kashimada K, Svingen T, Feng CW, Pelosi E, Bagheri-Fam S, Harley VR, Schlessinger D, Bowles J, Koopman P. Antagonistic regulation of Cyp26b1 by transcription factors SOX9/SF1 and FOXL2 during gonadal development in mice. FASEB J. 2011;25(10):3561–9. https://doi.org/10.1096/fj.11-184333.
35. Crisponi L, Deiana M, Loi A, Chiappe F, Uda M, Amati P, Bisceglia L, Zelante L, Nagaraja R, Porcu S, Ristaldi MS, Marzella R, Rocchi M, Nicolino M, Lienhardt-Roussie A, Nivelon A, Verloes A, Schlessinger D, Gasparini P, Bonneau D, Cao A, Pilia G. The putative forkhead transcription factor FOXL2 is mutated in blepharophimosis/ptosis/epicanthus inversus syndrome. Nat Genet. 2001;27(2):159–66. https://doi.org/10.1038/84781.
36. Schmidt D, Ovitt CE, Anlag K, Fehsenfeld S, Gredsted L, Treier AC, Treier M. The murine winged-helix transcription factor Foxl2 is required for granulosa cell differentiation and ovary maintenance. Development. 2004;131(4):933–42. https://doi.org/10.1242/dev.00969.
37. Mork L, Maatouk DM, McMahon JA, Guo JJ, Zhang P, McMahon AP, Capel B. Temporal differences in granulosa cell specification in the ovary reflect distinct follicle fates in mice. Biol Reprod. 2012;86(2):37. https://doi.org/10.1095/biolreprod.111.095208.
38. Al-Agha OM, Huwait HF, Chow C, Yang W, Senz J, Kalloger SE, Huntsman DG, Young RH, Gilks CB. FOXL2 is a sensitive and specific marker for sex cord-stromal tumors of the ovary. Am J Surg Pathol. 2011;35(4):484–94. https://doi.org/10.1097/PAS.0b013e31820a406c.
39. Uda M, Ottolenghi C, Crisponi L, Garcia JE, Deiana M, Kimber W, Forabosco A, Cao A, Schlessinger D, Pilia G. Foxl2 disruption causes mouse ovarian failure by pervasive blockage of follicle development. Hum Mol Genet. 2004;13(11):1171–81. https://doi.org/10.1093/hmg/ddh124.
40. Ottolenghi C, Omari S, Garcia-Ortiz JE, Uda M, Crisponi L, Forabosco A, Pilia G, Schlessinger D. Foxl2 is required for commitment to ovary differentiation. Hum Mol Genet. 2005;14(14):2053–62. https://doi.org/10.1093/hmg/ddi210.
41. Uhlenhaut NH, Jakob S, Anlag K, Eisenberger T, Sekido R, Kress J, Treier AC, Klugmann C, Klasen C, Holter NI, Riethmacher D, Schutz G, Cooney AJ, Lovell-Badge R, Treier M. Somatic sex reprogramming of adult ovaries to testes by FOXL2 ablation. Cell. 2009;139(6):1130–42. https://doi.org/10.1016/j.cell.2009.11.021.
42. Shah SP, Kobel M, Senz J, Morin RD, Clarke BA, Wiegand KC, Leung G, Zayed A, Mehl E, Kalloger SE, Sun M, Giuliany R, Yorida E, Jones S, Varhol R, Swenerton KD, Miller D, Clement PB, Crane C, Madore J, Provencher D, Leung P, DeFazio A, Khattra J, Turashvili G, Zhao Y, Zeng T, Glover JN, Vanderhyden B, Zhao C, Parkinson CA, Jimenez-Linan M, Bowtell DD, Mes-Masson AM, Brenton JD, Aparicio SA, Boyd N, Hirst M, Gilks CB, Marra M, Huntsman DG. Mutation of FOXL2 in granulosa-cell tumors of the ovary. N Engl J Med. 2009;360(26):2719–29. https://doi.org/10.1056/NEJMoa0902542.
43. Buza N, Wong S, Hui P. FOXL2 mutation analysis of ovarian sex cord-stromal tumors: genotype-phenotype correlation with diagnostic considerations. Int J Gynecol Pathol. 2018;37(4):305–15. https://doi.org/10.1097/PGP.0000000000000426.
44. Sullivan SD, Castrillon DH. Insights into primary ovarian insufficiency through genetically engineered mouse models. Semin Reprod Med. 2011;29(4):283–98. https://doi.org/10.1055/s-0031-1280914.
45. Greenbaum MP, Yan W, Wu MH, Lin YN, Agno JE, Sharma M, Braun RE, Rajkovic A, Matzuk MM. TEX14 is essential for intercellular bridges and fertility in male mice. Proc Natl Acad Sci U S A. 2006;103(13):4982–7. https://doi.org/10.1073/pnas.0505123103.
46. Lei L, Spradling AC. Mouse oocytes differentiate through organelle enrichment from sister cyst germ cells. Science. 2016;352(6281):95–9. https://doi.org/10.1126/science.aad2156.
47. Konishi I, Fujii S, Okamura H, Parmley T, Mori T. Development of interstitial cells and ovigerous cords in the human fetal ovary: an ultrastructural study. J Anat. 1986;148:121–35.
48. Sforza C, Vizzotto L, Ferrario VF, Forabosco A. Position of follicles in normal human ovary during definitive histogenesis. Early Hum Dev. 2003;74(1):27–35.
49. Pepling ME. Follicular assembly: mechanisms of action. Reproduction. 2012;143(2):139–49. https://doi.org/10.1530/REP-11-0299.
50. Saatcioglu HD, Cuevas I, Castrillon DH. Control of oocyte reawakening by Kit. PLoS Genet. 2016;12(8):e1006215. https://doi.org/10.1371/journal.pgen.1006215.
51. Baker TG. A quantitative and cytological study of germ cells in human ovaries. Proc R Soc Lond B Biol Sci. 1963;158:417–33.
52. Tilly JL. Commuting the death sentence: how oocytes strive to survive. Nat Rev Mol Cell Biol. 2001;2(11):838–48. https://doi.org/10.1038/35099086.
53. Qin Y, Jiao X, Simpson JL, Chen ZJ. Genetics of primary ovarian insufficiency: new developments and opportunities. Hum Reprod Update. 2015;21(6):787–808. https://doi.org/10.1093/humupd/dmv036.
54. Hansen KR, Knowlton NS, Thyer AC, Charleston JS, Soules MR, Klein NA. A new model of reproductive aging: the decline in ovarian non-growing follicle number from birth to menopause. Hum Reprod. 2008;23(3):699–708. https://doi.org/10.1093/humrep/dem408.
55. Livera G, Petre-Lazar B, Guerquin MJ, Trautmann E, Coffigny H, Habert R. p63 null mutation protects mouse oocytes from radio-induced apoptosis. Reproduction. 2008;135(1):3–12. https://doi.org/10.1530/REP-07-0054.
56. Hutt KJ. The role of BH3-only proteins in apoptosis within the ovary. Reproduction. 2015;149(2):R81–9. https://doi.org/10.1530/REP-14-0422.
57. Rafique S, Sterling EW, Nelson LM. A new approach to primary ovarian insufficiency. Obstet Gynecol Clin North Am. 2012;39(4):567–86. https://doi.org/10.1016/j.ogc.2012.09.007.
58. McGee EA, Hsueh AJ. Initial and cyclic recruitment of ovarian follicles. Endocr Rev. 2000;21(2):200–14. https://doi.org/10.1210/edrv.21.2.0394.
59. Peters H, Byskov AG, Himelstein-Braw R, Faber M. Follicular growth: the basic event in the mouse and human ovary. J Reprod Fertil. 1975;45(3):559–66.
60. Eppig JJ, O'Brien M, Wigglesworth K. Mammalian oocyte growth and development in vitro. Mol Reprod Dev. 1996;44(2):260–73. https://doi.org/10.1002/(SICI)1098-2795(199606)44:2<260::AID-MRD17>3.0.CO;2-6.

61. Peters H, Byskov AG, Lintern-Moore S, Faber M, Andersen M. The effect of gonadotrophin on follicle growth initiation in the neonatal mouse ovary. J Reprod Fertil. 1973;35(1):139–41.
62. Castrillon DH, Miao L, Kollipara R, Horner JW, DePinho RA. Suppression of ovarian follicle activation in mice by the transcription factor Foxo3a. Science. 2003;301(5630):215–8. https://doi.org/10.1126/science.1086336.
63. John GB, Shirley LJ, Gallardo TD, Castrillon DH. Specificity of the requirement for Foxo3 in primordial follicle activation. Reproduction. 2007;133(5):855–63. https://doi.org/10.1530/REP-06-0051.
64. John GB, Gallardo TD, Shirley LJ, Castrillon DH. Foxo3 is a PI3K-dependent molecular switch controlling the initiation of oocyte growth. Dev Biol. 2008;321(1):197–204. https://doi.org/10.1016/j.ydbio.2008.06.017.
65. Reddy P, Liu L, Adhikari D, Jagarlamudi K, Rajareddy S, Shen Y, Du C, Tang W, Hamalainen T, Peng SL, Lan ZJ, Cooney AJ, Huhtaniemi I, Liu K. Oocyte-specific deletion of Pten causes premature activation of the primordial follicle pool. Science. 2008;319(5863):611–3. https://doi.org/10.1126/science.1152257.
66. Tarnawa ED, Baker MD, Aloisio GM, Carr BR, Castrillon DH. Gonadal expression of Foxo1, but not Foxo3, is conserved in diverse Mammalian species. Biol Reprod. 2013;88(4):103. https://doi.org/10.1095/biolreprod.112.105791.
67. Cancer Genome Atlas Research N, Kandoth C, Schultz N, Cherniack AD, Akbani R, Liu Y, Shen H, Robertson AG, Pashtan I, Shen R, Benz CC, Yau C, Laird PW, Ding L, Zhang W, Mills GB, Kucherlapati R, Mardis ER, Levine DA. Integrated genomic characterization of endometrial carcinoma. Nature. 2013;497(7447):67–73. https://doi.org/10.1038/nature12113.
68. Müller JP. Bildungsgeschichte der Genitalien, vol. xviii, 152 p. Düsseldorf: Arnz; 1830.
69. Adelmann HB, editor. Marcello Malpighi and the evolution of embryology, Cornell publications in the history of science, vol. 4. Ithaca: Cornell University Press; 1966. p. 1851–901
70. Hashimoto R. Development of the human Mullerian duct in the sexually undifferentiated stage. Anat Rec A Discov Mol Cell Evol Biol. 2003;272(2):514–9. https://doi.org/10.1002/ar.a.10061.
71. Vigier B, Picard JY, Bezard J, Josso N. Anti-Mullerian hormone: a local or long-distance morphogenetic factor? Hum Genet. 1981;58(1):85–90.
72. Mullen RD, Behringer RR. Molecular genetics of Mullerian duct formation, regression and differentiation. Sex Dev. 2014;8(5):281–96. https://doi.org/10.1159/000364935.
73. Josso N, di Clemente N, Gouedard L. Anti-Mullerian hormone and its receptors. Mol Cell Endocrinol. 2001;179(1–2):25–32.
74. Klattig J, Englert C. The Mullerian duct: recent insights into its development and regression. Sex Dev. 2007;1(5):271–8. https://doi.org/10.1159/000108929.
75. Zhao F, Franco HL, Rodriguez KF, Brown PR, Tsai MJ, Tsai SY, Yao HH. Elimination of the male reproductive tract in the female embryo is promoted by COUP-TFII in mice. Science. 2017;357(6352):717–20. https://doi.org/10.1126/science.aai9136.
76. Jacquinet A, Millar D, Lehman A. Etiologies of uterine malformations. Am J Med Genet A. 2016;170(8):2141–72. https://doi.org/10.1002/ajmg.a.37775.
77. Gruenwald P. The relation of the growing müllerian duct to the wolffian duct and its importance for the genesis of malformations. Anat Rec. 1941;81:1–19.
78. Kobayashi A, Shawlot W, Kania A, Behringer RR. Requirement of Lim1 for female reproductive tract development. Development. 2004;131(3):539–49. https://doi.org/10.1242/dev.00951.
79. Torres M, Gomez-Pardo E, Dressler GR, Gruss P. Pax-2 controls multiple steps of urogenital development. Development. 1995;121(12):4057–65.
80. Robboy SJ, Kurita T, Baskin L, Cunha GR. New insights into human female reproductive tract development. Differentiation. 2017;97:9–22. https://doi.org/10.1016/j.diff.2017.08.002.
81. Huang CC, Orvis GD, Kwan KM, Behringer RR. Lhx1 is required in Mullerian duct epithelium for uterine development. Dev Biol. 2014;389(2):124–36. https://doi.org/10.1016/j.ydbio.2014.01.025.
82. Vainio S, Heikkila M, Kispert A, Chin N, McMahon AP. Female development in mammals is regulated by Wnt-4 signalling. Nature. 1999;397(6718):405–9. https://doi.org/10.1038/17068.
83. Prunskaite-Hyyrylainen R, Skovorodkin I, Xu Q, Miinalainen I, Shan J, Vainio SJ. Wnt4 coordinates directional cell migration and extension of the Mullerian duct essential for ontogenesis of the female reproductive tract. Hum Mol Genet. 2016;25(6):1059–73. https://doi.org/10.1093/hmg/ddv621.
84. Kurita T. Developmental origin of vaginal epithelium. Differentiation. 2010;80(2–3):99–105. https://doi.org/10.1016/j.diff.2010.06.007.
85. Fujino A, Arango NA, Zhan Y, Manganaro TF, Li X, MacLaughlin DT, Donahoe PK. Cell migration and activated PI3K/AKT-directed elongation in the developing rat Mullerian duct. Dev Biol. 2009;325(2):351–62. https://doi.org/10.1016/j.ydbio.2008.10.027.
86. Devouassoux-Shisheboran M, Silver SA, Tavassoli FA. Wolffian adnexal tumor, so-called female adnexal tumor of probable Wolffian origin (FATWO): immunohistochemical evidence in support of a Wolffian origin. Hum Pathol. 1999;30(7):856–63.
87. Labastie MC, Catala M, Gregoire JM, Peault B. The GATA-3 gene is expressed during human kidney embryogenesis. Kidney Int. 1995;47(6):1597–603.
88. Grote D, Souabni A, Busslinger M, Bouchard M. Pax 2/8-regulated Gata 3 expression is necessary for morphogenesis and guidance of the nephric duct in the developing kidney. Development. 2006;133(1):53–61. https://doi.org/10.1242/dev.02184.
89. Howitt BE, Emori MM, Drapkin R, Gaspar C, Barletta JA, Nucci MR, McCluggage WG, Oliva E, Hirsch MS. GATA3 is a sensitive and specific marker of benign and malignant Mesonephric lesions in the lower female genital tract. Am J Surg Pathol. 2015;39(10):1411–9. https://doi.org/10.1097/PAS.0000000000000471.
90. Atsuta Y, Takahashi Y. Early formation of the Mullerian duct is regulated by sequential actions of BMP/Pax2 and FGF/Lim1 signaling. Development. 2016;143(19):3549–59. https://doi.org/10.1242/dev.137067.
91. Mittag J, Winterhager E, Bauer K, Grummer R. Congenital hypothyroid female pax8-deficient mice are infertile despite thyroid hormone replacement therapy. Endocrinology. 2007;148(2):719–25. https://doi.org/10.1210/en.2006-1054.
92. Batista MF, Lewis KE. Pax2/8 act redundantly to specify glycinergic and GABAergic fates of multiple spinal interneurons. Dev Biol. 2008;323(1):88–97. https://doi.org/10.1016/j.ydbio.2008.08.009.
93. Bouchard M, de Caprona D, Busslinger M, Xu P, Fritzsch B. Pax2 and Pax8 cooperate in mouse inner ear morphogenesis and innervation. BMC Dev Biol. 2010;10:89. https://doi.org/10.1186/1471-213X-10-89.
94. Klattig J, Sierig R, Kruspe D, Besenbeck B, Englert C. Wilms' tumor protein Wt1 is an activator of the anti-Mullerian hormone receptor gene Amhr2. Mol Cell Biol. 2007;27(12):4355–64. https://doi.org/10.1128/MCB.01780-06.
95. Armstrong JF, Pritchard-Jones K, Bickmore WA, Hastie ND, Bard JB. The expression of the Wilms' tumour gene, WT1, in the developing mammalian embryo. Mech Dev. 1993;40(1–2):85–97.
96. Parenti R, Perris R, Vecchio GM, Salvatorelli L, Torrisi A, Gravina L, Magro G. Immunohistochemical expression of Wilms' tumor protein (WT1) in developing human epithelial and mesen-

chymal tissues. Acta Histochem. 2013;115(1):70–5. https://doi.org/10.1016/j.acthis.2012.04.006.
97. Shimizu M, Toki T, Takagi Y, Konishi I, Fujii S. Immunohistochemical detection of the Wilms' tumor gene (WT1) in epithelial ovarian tumors. Int J Gynecol Pathol. 2000;19(2):158–63.
98. Kommoss F, Faruqi A, Gilks CB, Lamshang Leen S, Singh N, Wilkinson N, McCluggage WG. Uterine serous carcinomas frequently metastasize to the fallopian tube and can mimic serous tubal intraepithelial carcinoma. Am J Surg Pathol. 2017;41(2):161–70. https://doi.org/10.1097/PAS.0000000000000757.
99. Nafisi H, Ghorab Z, Ismill N, Dube V, Plotkin A, Han G, Cesari M, Lu FI, Saad R, Khalifa M, Nofech-Mozes S. Immunophenotypic analysis in early Mullerian serous carcinogenesis. Int J Gynecol Pathol. 2015;34(5):424–36. https://doi.org/10.1097/PGP.0000000000000179.
100. Du H, Taylor HS. The role of Hox genes in female reproductive tract development, adult function, and fertility. Cold Spring Harb Perspect Med. 2015;6(1):a023002. https://doi.org/10.1101/cshperspect.a023002.
101. Taylor HS, Vanden Heuvel GB, Igarashi P. A conserved Hox axis in the mouse and human female reproductive system: late establishment and persistent adult expression of the Hoxa cluster genes. Biol Reprod. 1997;57(6):1338–45.
102. Warot X, Fromental-Ramain C, Fraulob V, Chambon P, Dolle P. Gene dosage-dependent effects of the Hoxa-13 and Hoxd-13 mutations on morphogenesis of the terminal parts of the digestive and urogenital tracts. Development. 1997;124(23):4781–91.
103. Yang A, Schweitzer R, Sun D, Kaghad M, Walker N, Bronson RT, Tabin C, Sharpe A, Caput D, Crum C, McKeon F. p63 is essential for regenerative proliferation in limb, craniofacial and epithelial development. Nature. 1999;398(6729):714–8. https://doi.org/10.1038/19539.
104. Ince TA, Cviko AP, Quade BJ, Yang A, McKeon FD, Mutter GL, Crum CP. p63 Coordinates anogenital modeling and epithelial cell differentiation in the developing female urogenital tract. Am J Pathol. 2002;161(4):1111–7. https://doi.org/10.1016/S0002-9440(10)64387-8.
105. Crum CP, McKeon FD. p63 in epithelial survival, germ cell surveillance, and neoplasia. Annu Rev Pathol. 2010;5:349–71. https://doi.org/10.1146/annurev-pathol-121808-102117.
106. Kurita T, Mills AA, Cunha GR. Roles of p63 in the diethylstilbestrol-induced cervicovaginal adenosis. Development. 2004;131(7):1639–49. https://doi.org/10.1242/dev.01038.
107. Laronda MM, Unno K, Ishi K, Serna VA, Butler LM, Mills AA, Orvis GD, Behringer RR, Deng C, Sinha S, Kurita T. Diethylstilbestrol induces vaginal adenosis by disrupting SMAD/RUNX1-mediated cell fate decision in the Mullerian duct epithelium. Dev Biol. 2013;381(1):5–16. https://doi.org/10.1016/j.ydbio.2013.06.024.
108. Terakawa J, Rocchi A, Serna VA, Bottinger EP, Graff JM, Kurita T. FGFR2IIIb-MAPK activity is required for epithelial cell fate decision in the lower Mullerian duct. Mol Endocrinol. 2016;30(7):783–95. https://doi.org/10.1210/me.2016-1027.
109. Cooke PS, Spencer TE, Bartol FF, Hayashi K. Uterine glands: development, function and experimental model systems. Mol Hum Reprod. 2013;19(9):547–58. https://doi.org/10.1093/molehr/gat031.
110. Valdes-Dapena MA. Uterine development in late Fetal life, infancy, and childhood. In: Norris HJ, Hertig AT, Abell MR, editors. The uterus. Monographs in pathology. Baltimore: Williams & Wilkins; 1973. p. 40–67.
111. Fluhmann CF. The developmental anatomy of the cervix uteri. Obstet Gynecol. 1960;15:62–9.
112. Ogasawara Y, Okamoto S, Kitamura Y, Matsumoto K. Proliferative pattern of uterine cells from birth to adulthood in intact, neonatally castrated, and/or adrenalectomized mice, assayed by incorporation of [125I]iododeoxyuridine. Endocrinology. 1983;113(2):582–7. https://doi.org/10.1210/endo-113-2-582.
113. Gray CA, Taylor KM, Ramsey WS, Hill JR, Bazer FW, Bartol FF, Spencer TE. Endometrial glands are required for preimplantation conceptus elongation and survival. Biol Reprod. 2001;64(6):1608–13.
114. Filant J, Spencer TE. Endometrial glands are essential for blastocyst implantation and decidualization in the mouse uterus. Biol Reprod. 2013;88(4):93. https://doi.org/10.1095/biolreprod.113.107631.
115. Cooke PS, Ekman GC, Kaur J, Davila J, Bagchi IC, Clark SG, Dziuk PJ, Hayashi K, Bartol FF. Brief exposure to progesterone during a critical neonatal window prevents uterine gland formation in mice. Biol Reprod. 2012;86(3):63. https://doi.org/10.1095/biolreprod.111.097188.
116. Friedman JR, Kaestner KH. The Foxa family of transcription factors in development and metabolism. Cell Mol Life Sci. 2006;63(19–20):2317–28. https://doi.org/10.1007/s00018-006-6095-6.
117. Dunlap KA, Filant J, Hayashi K, Rucker EB 3rd, Song G, Deng JM, Behringer RR, DeMayo FJ, Lydon J, Jeong JW, Spencer TE. Postnatal deletion of Wnt7a inhibits uterine gland morphogenesis and compromises adult fertility in mice. Biol Reprod. 2011;85(2):386–96. https://doi.org/10.1095/biolreprod.111.091769.
118. Kelleher AM, Peng W, Pru JK, Pru CA, DeMayo FJ, Spencer TE. Forkhead box a2 (FOXA2) is essential for uterine function and fertility. Proc Natl Acad Sci U S A. 2017;114(6):E1018–26. https://doi.org/10.1073/pnas.1618433114.
119. Parr BA, McMahon AP. Sexually dimorphic development of the mammalian reproductive tract requires Wnt-7a. Nature. 1998;395(6703):707–10. https://doi.org/10.1038/27221.
120. Miller C, Sassoon DA. Wnt-7a maintains appropriate uterine patterning during the development of the mouse female reproductive tract. Development. 1998;125(16):3201–11.
121. Hayashi K, Yoshioka S, Reardon SN, Rucker EB 3rd, Spencer TE, DeMayo FJ, Lydon JP, MacLean JA 2nd. WNTs in the neonatal mouse uterus: potential regulation of endometrial gland development. Biol Reprod. 2011;84(2):308–19. https://doi.org/10.1095/biolreprod.110.088161.
122. Franco HL, Dai D, Lee KY, Rubel CA, Roop D, Boerboom D, Jeong JW, Lydon JP, Bagchi IC, Bagchi MK, DeMayo FJ. WNT4 is a key regulator of normal postnatal uterine development and progesterone signaling during embryo implantation and decidualization in the mouse. FASEB J. 2011;25(4):1176–87. https://doi.org/10.1096/fj.10-175349.
123. Wang Y, Chang H, Rattner A, Nathans J. Frizzled receptors in development and disease. Curr Top Dev Biol. 2016;117:113–39. https://doi.org/10.1016/bs.ctdb.2015.11.028.
124. MacDonald BT, Tamai K, He X. Wnt/beta-catenin signaling: components, mechanisms, and diseases. Dev Cell. 2009;17(1):9–26. https://doi.org/10.1016/j.devcel.2009.06.016.
125. Stewart CA, Wang Y, Bonilla-Claudio M, Martin JF, Gonzalez G, Taketo MM, Behringer RR. CTNNB1 in mesenchyme regulates epithelial cell differentiation during Mullerian duct and postnatal uterine development. Mol Endocrinol. 2013;27(9):1442–54. https://doi.org/10.1210/me.2012-1126.
126. Jeong JW, Lee HS, Franco HL, Broaddus RR, Taketo MM, Tsai SY, Lydon JP, DeMayo FJ. beta-catenin mediates glandular formation and dysregulation of beta-catenin induces hyperplasia formation in the murine uterus. Oncogene. 2009;28(1):31–40. https://doi.org/10.1038/onc.2008.363.
127. Saegusa M, Okayasu I. Frequent nuclear beta-catenin accumulation and associated mutations in endometrioid-type endometrial and ovarian carcinomas with squamous differentiation. J Pathol. 2001;194(1):59–67. https://doi.org/10.1002/path.856.

128. Abbott JA. Adenomyosis and abnormal uterine bleeding (AUB-A)-pathogenesis, diagnosis, and management. Best Pract Res Clin Obstet Gynaecol. 2017;40:68–81. https://doi.org/10.1016/j.bpobgyn.2016.09.006.
129. Oh SJ, Shin JH, Kim TH, Lee HS, Yoo JY, Ahn JY, Broaddus RR, Taketo MM, Lydon JP, Leach RE, Lessey BA, Fazleabas AT, Lim JM, Jeong JW. beta-Catenin activation contributes to the pathogenesis of adenomyosis through epithelial-mesenchymal transition. J Pathol. 2013;231(2):210–22. https://doi.org/10.1002/path.4224.
130. Gun I, Oner O, Bodur S, Ozdamar O, Atay V. Is adenomyosis associated with the risk of endometrial cancer? Med Glas (Zenica). 2012;9(2):268–72.
131. Vercellini P, Parazzini F, Oldani S, Panazza S, Bramante T, Crosignani PG. Adenomyosis at hysterectomy: a study on frequency distribution and patient characteristics. Hum Reprod. 1995;10(5):1160–2.
132. Orvis GD, Behringer RR. Cellular mechanisms of Mullerian duct formation in the mouse. Dev Biol. 2007;306(2):493–504. https://doi.org/10.1016/j.ydbio.2007.03.027.
133. Castrillon DH, Lee KR, Nucci MR. Distinction between endometrial and endocervical adenocarcinoma: an immunohistochemical study. Int J Gynecol Pathol. 2002;21(1):4–10.
134. Nucci MR, Castrillon DH, Bai H, Quade BJ, Ince TA, Genest DR, Lee KR, Mutter GL, Crum CP. Biomarkers in diagnostic obstetric and gynecologic pathology: a review. Adv Anat Pathol. 2003;10(2):55–68.
135. Allard S, Adin P, Gouedard L, di Clemente N, Josso N, Orgebin-Crist MC, Picard JY, Xavier F. Molecular mechanisms of hormone-mediated Mullerian duct regression: involvement of beta-catenin. Development. 2000;127(15):3349–60.
136. Huang CC, Orvis GD, Wang Y, Behringer RR. Stromal-to-epithelial transition during postpartum endometrial regeneration. PLoS One. 2012;7(8):e44285. https://doi.org/10.1371/journal.pone.0044285.
137. Cunha GR. Stromal induction and specification of morphogenesis and cytodifferentiation of the epithelia of the Mullerian ducts and urogenital sinus during development of the uterus and vagina in mice. J Exp Zool. 1976;196(3):361–70. https://doi.org/10.1002/jez.1401960310.
138. Chang AR. 'Erosion' of the uterine cervix; an anachronism. Aust N Z J Obstet Gynaecol. 1991;31(4):358–62.
139. Kobayashi A, Behringer RR. Developmental genetics of the female reproductive tract in mammals. Nat Rev Genet. 2003;4(12):969–80. https://doi.org/10.1038/nrg1225.
140. Cunha GR, Kurita T, Cao M, Shen J, Robboy S, Baskin L. Molecular mechanisms of development of the human fetal female reproductive tract. Differentiation. 2017;97:54–72. https://doi.org/10.1016/j.diff.2017.07.003.
141. Jesus LE, Camelier P, Bastos J, Tome AS, Dekermacher S. Clitoral abnormalities in the absence of virilization: etiology and treatment strategies. Urology. 2016;88:170–2. https://doi.org/10.1016/j.urology.2015.10.020.
142. Griebel ML, Redman JF, Kemp SF, Elders MJ. Hypertrophy of clitoral hood: presenting sign of neurofibromatosis in female child. Urology. 1991;37(4):337–9.
143. Sutphen R, Galan-Gomez E, Kousseff BG. Clitoromegaly in neurofibromatosis. Am J Med Genet. 1995;55(3):325–30. https://doi.org/10.1002/ajmg.1320550316.
144. Rouzi AA, Sindi O, Radhan B, Ba'aqeel H. Epidermal clitoral inclusion cyst after type I female genital mutilation. Am J Obstet Gynecol. 2001;185(3):569–71. https://doi.org/10.1067/mob.2001.117660.
145. Hughes JW, Guess MK, Hittelman A, Yip S, Astle J, Pal L, Inzucchi SE, Dulay AT. Clitoral epidermoid cyst presenting as pseudoclitoromegaly of pregnancy. AJP Rep. 2013;3(1):57–62. https://doi.org/10.1055/s-0033-1334461.
146. Williams CE, Nakhal RS, Achermann JC, Creighton SM. Persistent unexplained congenital clitoromegaly in females born extremely prematurely. J Pediatr Urol. 2013;9(6 Pt A):962–5. https://doi.org/10.1016/j.jpurol.2013.03.001.
147. Mayoglou L, Dulabon L, Martin-Alguacil N, Pfaff D, Schober J. Success of treatment modalities for labial fusion: a retrospective evaluation of topical and surgical treatments. J Pediatr Adolesc Gynecol. 2009;22(4):247–50. https://doi.org/10.1016/j.jpag.2008.09.003.
148. Ziglioli F, Fornia S, Ciuffireda M, Meli S, Dinale F, Simonazzi M, Cortellini P. Lichen sclerosus: a review of literature and a case of an atypic surgical treatment. Acta Biomed. 2011;82(1):51–7.
149. Dietrich JE, Millar DM, Quint EH. Obstructive reproductive tract anomalies. J Pediatr Adolesc Gynecol. 2014;27(6):396–402. https://doi.org/10.1016/j.jpag.2014.09.001.
150. Olive DL, Henderson DY. Endometriosis and mullerian anomalies. Obstet Gynecol. 1987;69(3 Pt 1):412–5.
151. Loscalzo IL, Catapano M, Loscalzo J, Sama A. Imperforate hymen with bilateral hydronephrosis: an unusual emergency department diagnosis. J Emerg Med. 1995;13(3):337–9.
152. Iwasa Y, Fletcher CD. Distinctive prepubertal vulval fibroma: a hitherto unrecognized mesenchymal tumor of prepubertal girls: analysis of 11 cases. Am J Surg Pathol. 2004;28(12):1601–8.
153. Vargas SO, Kozakewich HP, Boyd TK, Ecklund K, Fishman SJ, Laufer MR, Perez-Atayde AR. Childhood asymmetric labium majus enlargement: mimicking a neoplasm. Am J Surg Pathol. 2005;29(8):1007–16.
154. Khunda S, Nakash A. Double vulva. J Obstet Gynaecol. 1999;19(1):94–5. https://doi.org/10.1080/01443619966155.
155. Bellemare S, Dibden L. Absence of the clitoris in a 13-year-old adolescent: medical implications for child and adolescent health. J Pediatr Adolesc Gynecol. 2005;18(6):415–8. https://doi.org/10.1016/j.jpag.2005.09.011.
156. Ruggeri G, Gargano T, Antonellini C, Carlini V, Randi B, Destro F, Lima M. Vaginal malformations: a proposed classification based on embryological, anatomical and clinical criteria and their surgical management (an analysis of 167 cases). Pediatr Surg Int. 2012;28(8):797–803. https://doi.org/10.1007/s00383-012-3121-7.
157. Wang J, Ezzat W, Davidson M. Transverse vaginal septum. A case report. J Reprod Med. 1995;40(2):163–6.
158. Rana A, Manandhar B, Amatya A, Baral J, Gurung G, Giri A, Giri K. Mucocolpos due to complete transverse septum in middle third of vagina in a 17-year-old girl. J Obstet Gynaecol Res. 2002;28(2):86–8.
159. Pena A. Cloaca—historical aspects and terminology. Semin Pediatr Surg. 2016;25(2):62–5. https://doi.org/10.1053/j.sempedsurg.2015.11.002.
160. Gupta A, Bischoff A, Pena A, Runck LA, Guasch G. The great divide: septation and malformation of the cloaca, and its implications for surgeons. Pediatr Surg Int. 2014;30(11):1089–95. https://doi.org/10.1007/s00383-014-3593-8.
161. Chan YY, Jayaprakasan K, Zamora J, Thornton JG, Raine-Fenning N, Coomarasamy A. The prevalence of congenital uterine anomalies in unselected and high-risk populations: a systematic review. Hum Reprod Update. 2011;17(6):761–71. https://doi.org/10.1093/humupd/dmr028.
162. Hammoud AO, Gibson M, Peterson CM, Kerber RA, Mineau GP, Hatasaka H. Quantification of the familial contribution to mullerian anomalies. Obstet Gynecol. 2008;111(2 Pt 1):378–84. https://doi.org/10.1097/01.AOG.0000267219.10869.9f.
163. Duru UA, Laufer MR. Discordance in Mayer-von Rokitansky-Kuster-Hauser syndrome noted in monozygotic twins. J Pediatr Adolesc Gynecol. 2009;22(4):e73–5. https://doi.org/10.1016/j.jpag.2008.07.012.

164. Grimbizis GF, Gordts S, Di Spiezio Sardo A, Brucker S, De Angelis C, Gergolet M, Li TC, Tanos V, Brolmann H, Gianaroli L, Campo R. The ESHRE-ESGE consensus on the classification of female genital tract congenital anomalies. Gynecol Surg. 2013;10(3):199–212. https://doi.org/10.1007/s10397-013-0800-x.
165. Ludwin A, Martins WP, Nastri CO, Ludwin I, Coelho Neto MA, Leitao VM, Acien M, Alcazar JL, Benacerraf B, Condous G, De Wilde RL, Emanuel MH, Gibbons W, Guerriero S, Hurd WW, Levine D, Lindheim S, Pellicer A, Petraglia F, Saridogan E. Congenital Uterine Malformation by Experts (CUME): better criteria for distinguishing between normal/arcuate and septate uterus? Ultrasound Obstet Gynecol. 2018;51(1):101–9. https://doi.org/10.1002/uog.18923.
166. Ludwin A, Ludwin I, Kudla M, Kottner J. Reliability of the European Society of Human Reproduction and Embryology/European Society for Gynaecological Endoscopy and American Society for Reproductive Medicine classification systems for congenital uterine anomalies detected using three-dimensional ultrasonography. Fertil Steril. 2015;104(3):688–97 e688. https://doi.org/10.1016/j.fertnstert.2015.06.019.
167. Kives S. Müllerian anomaly classification systems. In: Pfeifer SM, editor. Congenital Müllerian anomalies: diagnosis and management. Cham: Springer International Publishing; 2016. p. 3–12. https://doi.org/10.1007/978-3-319-27231-3_1.
168. Bombard DS 2nd, Mousa SA. Mayer-Rokitansky-Kuster-Hauser syndrome: complications, diagnosis and possible treatment options: a review. Gynecol Endocrinol. 2014;30(9):618–23. https://doi.org/10.3109/09513590.2014.927855.
169. Prior M, Richardson A, Asif S, Polanski L, Parris-Larkin M, Chandler J, Fogg L, Jassal P, Thornton JG, Raine-Fenning NJ. Outcome of assisted reproduction in women with congenital uterine anomalies: a prospective observational study. Ultrasound Obstet Gynecol. 2018;51(1):110–7. https://doi.org/10.1002/uog.18935.
170. Kaufman Y, Lam A. The pelvic uterus-like mass--a primary or secondary Mullerian system anomaly? J Minim Invasive Gynecol. 2008;15(4):494–7. https://doi.org/10.1016/j.jmig.2008.03.002.
171. Cozzutto C. Uterus-like mass replacing ovary: report of a new entity. Arch Pathol Lab Med. 1981;105(10):508–11.
172. Sopha SC, Rosado FG, Smith JJ, Merchant NB, Shi C. Hepatic uterus-like mass misdiagnosed as hepatic abscess. Int J Surg Pathol. 2015;23(2):134–9. https://doi.org/10.1177/1066896914534465.
173. Gonzalez RS, Vnencak-Jones CL, Shi C, Fadare O. Endomyometriosis ("uterus-like mass") in an XY male: case report with molecular confirmation and literature review. Int J Surg Pathol. 2014;22(5):421–6. https://doi.org/10.1177/1066896913501385.
174. Kakkar A, Sharma MC, Garg A, Goyal N, Suri V, Sarkar C, Mahapatra AK. Uterus-like mass in association with neural tube defect: a case report and review of the literature. Pediatr Neurosurg. 2012;48(4):240–4. https://doi.org/10.1159/000348811.
175. Rahilly MA, al-Nafussi A. Uterus-like mass of the ovary associated with endometrioid carcinoma. Histopathology. 1991;18(6):549–51.
176. Nakakita B, Abiko K, Mikami Y, Kido A, Baba T, Yoshioka Y, Yamaguchi K, Matsumura N, Konishi I. Clear cell carcinoma arising from a uterus-like mass. Pathol Int. 2014;64(11):576–80. https://doi.org/10.1111/pin.12218.
177. Seki A, Maeshima A, Nakagawa H, Shiraishi J, Murata Y, Arai H, Kubochi K, Kuramochi S. A subserosal uterus-like mass presenting after a sliding hernia of the ovary and endometriosis: a rare entity with a discussion of the histogenesis. Fertil Steril. 2011;95(5):1788 e1715–89. https://doi.org/10.1016/j.fertnstert.2010.11.051.
178. Mortlock DP, Innis JW. Mutation of HOXA13 in hand-foot-genital syndrome. Nat Genet. 1997;15(2):179–80. https://doi.org/10.1038/ng0297-179.
179. Jorgensen EM, Ruman JI, Doherty L, Taylor HS. A novel mutation of HOXA13 in a family with hand-foot-genital syndrome and the role of polyalanine expansions in the spectrum of Mullerian fusion anomalies. Fertil Steril. 2010;94(4):1235–8. https://doi.org/10.1016/j.fertnstert.2009.05.057.
180. Cheng Z, Zhu Y, Su D, Wang J, Cheng L, Chen B, Wei Z, Zhou P, Wang B, Ma X, Cao Y. A novel mutation of HOXA10 in a Chinese woman with a Mullerian duct anomaly. Hum Reprod. 2011;26(11):3197–201. https://doi.org/10.1093/humrep/der290.
181. Liatsikos SA, Grimbizis GF, Georgiou I, Papadopoulos N, Lazaros L, Bontis JN, Tarlatzis BC. HOX A10 and HOX A11 mutation scan in congenital malformations of the female genital tract. Reprod Biomed Online. 2010;21(1):126–32. https://doi.org/10.1016/j.rbmo.2010.03.015.
182. Schinzel A. Phocomelia and additional anomalies in two sisters. Hum Genet. 1990;84(6):539–41.
183. Coffinier C, Barra J, Babinet C, Yaniv M. Expression of the vHNF1/HNF1beta homeoprotein gene during mouse organogenesis. Mech Dev. 1999;89(1–2):211–3.
184. Lokmane L, Heliot C, Garcia-Villalba P, Fabre M, Cereghini S. vHNF1 functions in distinct regulatory circuits to control ureteric bud branching and early nephrogenesis. Development. 2010;137(2):347–57. https://doi.org/10.1242/dev.042226.
185. Lim D, Ip PP, Cheung AN, Kiyokawa T, Oliva E. Immunohistochemical comparison of ovarian and uterine endometrioid carcinoma, endometrioid carcinoma with clear cell change, and clear cell carcinoma. Am J Surg Pathol. 2015;39(8):1061–9. https://doi.org/10.1097/PAS.0000000000000436.
186. Pabuccu E, Kahraman K, Taskin S, Atabekoglu C. Unilateral absence of fallopian tube and ovary in an infertile patient. Fertil Steril. 2011;96(1):e55–7. https://doi.org/10.1016/j.fertnstert.2011.04.027.
187. Rapisarda G, Pappalardo EM, Arancio A, La Greca M. Unilateral ovarian and fallopian tube agenesis. Arch Gynecol Obstet. 2009;280(5):849–50. https://doi.org/10.1007/s00404-009-1018-z.
188. Tanaka Y, Koyama S, Kobayashi M, Kubota S, Nakamura R, Isobe M, Shiki Y. Complex Mullerian malformation without any present classification: unilateral ovarian and tubal absence with an arcuate uterus. Asian J Endosc Surg. 2013;6(1):55–7. https://doi.org/10.1111/j.1758-5910.2012.00159.x.
189. Mylonas I, Hansch S, Markmann S, Bolz M, Friese K. Unilateral ovarian agenesis: report of three cases and review of the literature. Arch Gynecol Obstet. 2003;268(1):57–60. https://doi.org/10.1007/s00404-002-0451-z.
190. Gandhi KR, Siddiqui AU, Wabale RN, Daimi SR. The accessory fallopian tube: a rare anomaly. J Hum Reprod Sci. 2012;5(3):293–4. https://doi.org/10.4103/0974-1208.106344.
191. Rottenstreich M, Smorgick N, Pansky M, Vaknin Z. Isolated torsion of accessory fallopian tube in a young adolescent. J Pediatr Adolesc Gynecol. 2016;29(4):e57–8. https://doi.org/10.1016/j.jpag.2016.03.003.
192. Ucar MG, Ilhan TT, Gul A, Korkutan C, Celik C. Patient with three fallopian tubes at right adnexa. J Clin Diagn Res. 2017;11(2):QJ03–4. https://doi.org/10.7860/JCDR/2017/22713.9263.
193. Narayanan R, Rajeev MA. Duplication of the fallopian tube. J Hum Reprod Sci. 2008;1(1):35–6.
194. Liu Q, Liu HQ, Jiang YY, Sun XB. Is unilateral uterine adnexa absence a congenital developmental abnormality or posteriority? Summary of 39 cases and literature review. Arch Gynecol Obstet. 2013;288(3):555–61. https://doi.org/10.1007/s00404-013-2891-z.
195. Verkauf BS, Bernhisel MA. Ovarian maldescent. Fertil Steril. 1996;65(1):189–92.
196. Veurink M, Koster M, LT B. The history of DES, lessons to be learned. Pharm World Sci. 2005;27(3):139–43. https://doi.org/10.1007/s11096-005-3663-z.

197. Herbst AL, Ulfelder H, Poskanzer DC. Adenocarcinoma of the vagina. Association of maternal stilbestrol therapy with tumor appearance in young women. N Engl J Med. 1971;284(15):878–81. https://doi.org/10.1056/NEJM197104222841604.
198. Ma L, Benson GV, Lim H, Dey SK, Maas RL. Abdominal B (AbdB) Hoxa genes: regulation in adult uterus by estrogen and progesterone and repression in mullerian duct by the synthetic estrogen diethylstilbestrol (DES). Dev Biol. 1998;197(2):141–54. https://doi.org/10.1006/dbio.1998.8907.
199. Kaufman RH, Adam E, Binder GL, Gerthoffer E. Upper genital tract changes and pregnancy outcome in offspring exposed in utero to diethylstilbestrol. Am J Obstet Gynecol. 1980;137(3):299–308.
200. Goldberg JM, Falcone T. Effect of diethylstilbestrol on reproductive function. Fertil Steril. 1999;72(1):1–7.
201. Swan SH. Intrauterine exposure to diethylstilbestrol: long-term effects in humans. APMIS. 2000;108(12):793–804.
202. John GB, Shidler MJ, Besmer P, Castrillon DH. Kit signaling via PI3K promotes ovarian follicle maturation but is dispensable for primordial follicle activation. Dev Biol. 2009;331(2):292–9. https://doi.org/10.1016/j.ydbio.2009.05.546.
203. Clevers H. Wnt/beta-catenin signaling in development and disease. Cell. 2006;127(3):469–80. https://doi.org/10.1016/j.cell.2006.10.018.

Noninfectious Inflammatory Disorders of the Vulva

2

Sara C. Shalin

Abstract

A myriad of diseases that affect the skin can involve the perigenital regions, including the vulvar skin and mucosa. Some of these processes may mimic neoplastic lesions, while others may increase the risk of developing neoplasia or may indicate a risk for subsequent disease/malignancy. Many processes carry substantial morbidity and will affect the patient's quality of life. Familiarity with the histologic spectrum of inflammatory processes involving the vulva will allow for appropriate treatment and further triage/screening of patients. This chapter provides a framework by which to recognize many of these inflammatory dermatoses, discusses the clinical presentations, associated conditions, histopathologic findings and differential diagnoses, and suggests practical ways in which to handle biopsies provided with minimal clinical information.

Keywords

Inflammatory · Contact dermatitis · Lichen simplex chronicus · Psoriasis · Lichen planus · Lichen sclerosus · Plasma cell vulvitis · Pemphigus · Pemphigoid · Hidradenitis · Pyoderma

2.1 Introduction

Many of the same diseases that affect skin can also involve vulvar skin and mucosa. Some of these processes may mimic neoplastic lesions, while others may increase the risk of developing neoplasia or may indicate a risk for subsequent disease/malignancy. Many processes carry substantial morbidity and will affect the patient's quality of life. Familiarity with the histologic spectrum of inflammatory processes involving the vulva will allow for appropriate treatment and further triage/screening of patients.

Dermatopathologists generally search for inflammatory reaction patterns to help classify cutaneous rashes (Table 2.1). The same inflammatory reaction patterns will be seen in the vulvar region, with some occasional but important differences. This chapter provides a framework by which to recognize many (although not all!) of the inflammatory dermatoses which may affect vulvar skin and mucosa.

Inflammatory reaction patterns encompass entities which affect predominantly the epidermis (spongiotic and psoriasiform patterns and some blistering diseases), the junction of the epidermis and dermis (lichenoid and interface dermatoses as well as some blistering diseases), or the dermis (granulomatous, vasculopathic, and perivascular). A number of diseases may manifest in the vulnerable vulvar region clinically as ulceration (Tables 2.2 and 2.3); such entities are given consideration in the ensuing chapter so that specific diagnoses may be suggested to the treating clinician rather than the nonspecific diagnosis of ulcer. Still other dermatologic conditions affecting the vulva may be due to inflammation of the hair follicle or sweat gland apparatus. Recognition of the inflammatory reaction pattern is generally the first clue to establishing a diagnosis. This chapter will give the reader the tools to recognize the reaction patterns in vulvar biopsies, discover salient histologic features of particular disease entities, and practical advice for the handling of both straightforward and complex vulvar biopsies of inflammatory disease.

S. C. Shalin (✉)
Department of Pathology, University of Arkansas for Medical Sciences, Little Rock, AR, USA

Department of Dermatology, University of Arkansas for Medical Sciences, Little Rock, AR, USA
e-mail: SCShalin@uams.edu

W. Zheng et al. (eds.), *Gynecologic and Obstetric Pathology, Volume 1*, https://doi.org/10.1007/978-981-13-3016-2_2

Table 2.1 Inflammatory reaction patterns and disease examples that may involve the vulva

Spongiotic	Psoriasiform (acanthotic)	Lichenoid and interface	Blistering and acantholytic	Granulomatous	Vasculopathic	Folliculocentric/ follicular occlusion
Allergic contact dermatitis	Psoriasis	Lichen planus	Pemphigus vulgaris	Crohn disease	Behcet disease	Hidradenitis suppurativa
Irritant contact dermatitis	Lichen simplex chronicus	Lichen sclerosus (et atrophicus)	Pemphigus vegetans	Sarcoidosis	Zoon vulvitis	Fox–Fordyce disease
Atopic dermatitis	Reiter syndrome	Fixed drug eruption	Linear IgA bullous dermatosis		Pyoderma gangrenosum	
Tinea (see chapter on infectious diseases)		Erythema multiforme/ Stevens Johnson syndrome/toxic epidermal necrolysis	Cicatricial pemphigoid			
Candida (see chapter on infectious diseases)		Graft-versus-host disease	Papular acantholysis of the vulvocrural folds			
Amicrobial pustulosis of the folds		Lupus erythematosus	Hailey–Hailey disease			
Inverse psoriasis		Plasma cell (Zoon) vulvitis	Darier disease			
			Herpes simplex virus infection (see chapter on infectious diseases)			
			Acute spongiotic dermatitis			
			Bullous fixed drug eruption			
			Stevens Johnson Syndrome/ Toxic Epidermal Necrolysis			

Entities in red font are diseases that are typically classified with a different reaction pattern but based on location or acuity may present with a less classic reaction pattern. See text for full details

Table 2.2 Diseases to consider that present with vulvar ulceration

Common disease involving vulva, ulceration is common presentation	Common disease involving vulva, ulceration is a rare presentation	Rare disease involving vulva, ulceration is a common presentation	Rare disease involving vulva, ulceration is a rare presentation
Lichen planus	Allergic or irritant contact dermatitis	Crohn disease	Reiter syndrome
	Lichen sclerosus	Behcet disease	Graft-versus-host disease
	Psoriasis	Pyoderma gangrenosum	
		Pemphigus vulgaris	
		Plasma cell (Zoon) vulvitis	
		Fixed drug eruption	

Table 2.3 Seeing past vulvar ulceration: clues to a more precise diagnosis

Disease presenting with ulceration	Clues to diagnosis (not always present)
Lichen planus (erosive variant)	Most commonly involves inner aspects of labia minora Presence of lichenoid band of inflammation in adjacent intact epithelium Oral and cutaneous involvement
Lichen sclerosus	Eosinophilic homogenization of collagen in areas without ulcer Focal basal vacuolar change Lymphocyte predominant infiltrate, infiltrating between thickened collagen bundles
Allergic or irritant contact dermatitis	Clinical history of contact with offending agent
Pemphigus vulgaris	Suprabasilar acantholysis in areas of intact epithelium Often oral and possibly cutaneous involvement Positive direct and/or indirect immunofluorescence studies

(continued)

Table 2.3 (continued)

Disease presenting with ulceration	Clues to diagnosis (not always present)
Crohn disease	Presence of gastrointestinal disease Dermal granulomas Eosinophils may favor Crohn disease over sarcoidosis
Behcet disease	Oral ulcers present Evidence of vasculitis (predominantly lymphocytic) Absence of lichenoid inflammation in adjacent intact epithelium
Pyoderma Gangrenosum	Neutrophilic dermatosis Negative special stains for organisms Pathergy present Healing with cribriform scarring Association with rheumatologic disease, inflammatory bowel disease, or lymphoproliferative disease
Psoriasis	Ulcerations and fissures limited to skin folds Presence of more conventional and classic psoriatic plaques on other body surfaces Typically bilateral and symmetric
Plasma cell (Zoon) vulvitis	Involves mucosa (labia minora, introitus) Plasma-cell-rich infiltrate Diamond-shaped keratinocytes in attenuated epithelium
Graft-versus-host disease	Involves mucosa May mimic lichen sclerosus or lichen planus History of transplant

2.2 Spongiotic Reaction Pattern

2.2.1 Eczematous Dermatitis: Contact (Allergic and Irritant) and Atopic Dermatitis

The term "eczematous dermatitis" encompasses a spectrum of inflammatory diseases linked by a spongiotic reaction pattern. Eczematous dermatitis can include irritant contact dermatitis (ICD), allergic contact dermatitis (ACD), and atopic dermatitis (AD), among others. Eczematous dermatitis is not unique to the vulva as it commonly affects cutaneous skin, but it represents some of the most commonly encountered vulvar dermatoses. The exact prevalence is unknown, with some sources citing 15–30% of women being affected [1]. However, as these conditions may be established relatively confidently through clinical history and physical exam, biopsies of these entities may be less common than other vulvar dermatoses such as lichen sclerosus, lichen simplex chronicus, and lichen planus [2–4].

Allergic contact dermatitis (ACD) is a type IV hypersensitivity reaction. As such, it requires sensitization to an allergen through penetration of the stratum corneum. The sensitizing agent, generally a low molecular weight, lipid-soluble molecule, interacts with endogenous proteins to release a cascade of cytokines and chemokines that activate dendritic cells which drain to regional lymph nodes to stimulate and expand T cell populations [5, 6]. Reexposure to the allergen elicits the cutaneous reaction clinicians appreciate as an allergic contact dermatitis. The delay between exposure and presentation (often at least several days) may preclude the determination of the precise allergen. ACD generally occurs in predisposed individuals, which means that reactions to various substances may be idiosyncratic and unpredictable between women. This is in contrast to irritant contact dermatitis, in which an irritant generally produces the same reaction in women with sufficient exposure. ACD may be particularly common in the vulva due to constant moisture and friction at these sites. Estrogen deficiency may further disrupt the epidermal barrier and allow for easier penetration of allergens into the skin [7].

Irritant contact dermatitis (ICD) is an immediate reaction to an irritating agent and does not require prior sensitization. ICD can be directly cytotoxic to keratinocytes or can disrupt the normal lipid barrier of the skin [6]. Given the moist environment of the vulva, vulvar skin and mucosa is particularly susceptible to ICD.

Atopic dermatitis (AD) of the vulva is seen in genetically predisposed individuals with a history of atopic dermatitis on other body sites. The presence of this chronic inflammatory skin condition should not exclude a practitioner from considering a superimposed ACD or ICD, as these can exist together.

Careful history and physical exam is often sufficient to suggest the diagnosis. Common irritants include body fluids (urine, feces, semen, and some vaginal discharges), soaps and detergents, sanitary pads, feminine hygiene products, and topical medications. Vigorous scrubbing of the vulvar skin can also damage the epithelial barrier and be an irritant in itself. Common allergens implicated in ACD include topical antibiotics (neomycin), topical anesthetics (benzocaine), fragrance, and nickel [6]. In one study of vulvar ACD specifically, 39% of women with vulvar pruritus symptoms had a relevant positive patch test, with fragrances, topical medications, and preservatives representing the most frequently encountered allergens [8]; another similar study most frequently implicated topical pharmaceutical agents as relevant allergens [9].

2.2.1.1 Clinical Features

Eczematous dermatoses present clinically in a similar manner, although presentation will depend on the degree and duration of exposure to the irritant or allergen. Irritant der-

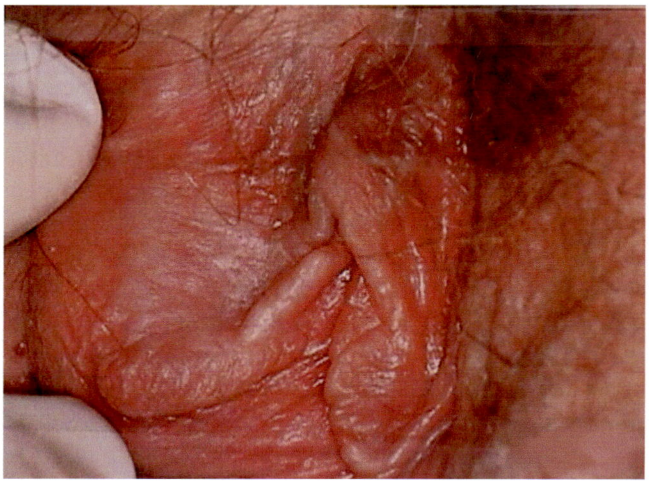

Fig. 2.1 Chronic spongiotic dermatitis. The vulvar skin shows thickened plaques and erythema. Photo provided courtesy of previous edition in Chinese (Science Press, Beijing, China)

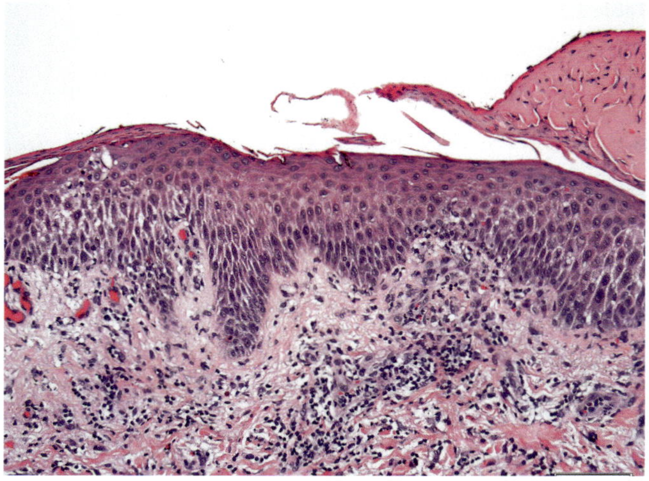

Fig. 2.2 Spongiotic dermatitis. There is increased intraepidermal edema, parakeratosis, and serum crust. There is exocytosis of a few lymphocytes into the epidermis, and a dermal infiltrate consisting of lymphocytes and eosinophils

matitis more commonly elicits complaints of burning, stinging, and pain, whereas patients with allergic contact and atopic dermatitis more often complain of pruritus [10]; however, there may be considerable overlap. Patients with seborrheic dermatitis and atopic dermatitis typically have skin lesions not limited to the vulvar area.

Allergic or irritant dermatitis will present as erythematous to edematous patches and plaques with maceration, erosion, and vesiculation in severe and/or acute cases. Contact dermatitis may be suspected by sparing of the skin folds, which may be protected from exposure to the allergen or irritant. Generally, early lesions are well demarcated, while subacute and chronic contact dermatitis becomes more poorly demarcated and scaly. With increasing chronicity, the skin becomes lichenified, with thickened, edematous plaques that display increased skin markings (Fig. 2.1). Hyperpigmentation is not infrequent, particularly in skin of color, and excoriations may attest to the clinical complaints of itching [6].

Identification of the offending contact allergens is paramount, as treatment relies on removal of the irritant or allergen. In general, recommendations begin with gentle vulvar hygiene, cessation of all fragrance-containing products, and cessation of all topical anesthetics and antibiotics. Bland petroleum jelly as a topical emollient is frequently recommended [6].

2.2.1.2 Histopathologic Features

Similar to the clinical presentation of eczematous dermatoses, the microscopic features are similar regardless of the precise etiology but depend greatly on the duration and severity of the symptoms. In general, distinction between ICD, ACD, AD, and other entities with the spongiotic reaction pattern is not possible on histologic grounds alone. All eczematous dermatoses are manifest by spongiotic dermatitis. The term "spongiosis" refers to the presence of epidermal edema, leading to increased apparent space between adjacent keratinocytes (Fig. 2.2).

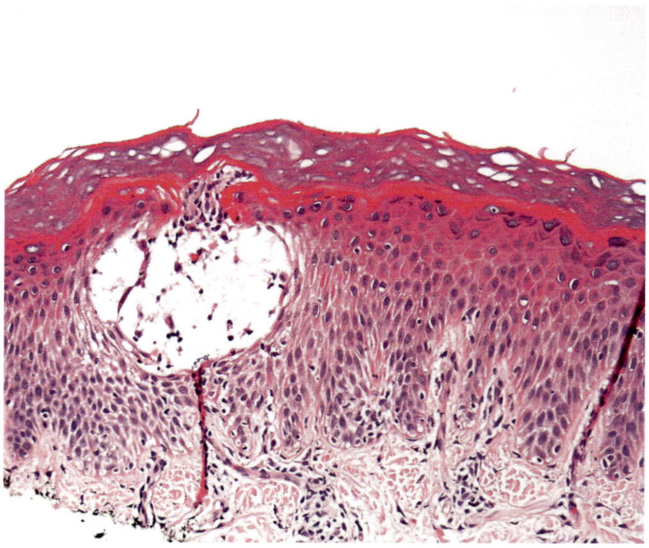

Fig. 2.3 Spongiotic dermatitis. A Langerhans cell microabscess in the epidermis is characteristic, with surrounding epidermal edema. Langerhans cell microabscesses are associated with, but not entirely specific for, allergic contact dermatitis

Early or acute eczematous dermatitis shows abundant intracellular edema; in some instances, this marked spongiosis can lead to mechanical failure of keratinocyte adhesion complexes (desmosomes) and the appearance of an intraepidermal vesicle or blister. Exocytosis, or the movement of lymphocytes into the epidermis, frequently accompanies spongiosis. Similarly, the presence of clusters of intraepidermal Langerhans cells (normal residents of the epidermis in single numbers) is a frequent finding and reflects the antigen processing inherent in these conditions. Langerhans cell microabscesses have been described as a common feature (Fig. 2.3) with a positive predictive value of 78% for ACD in one study

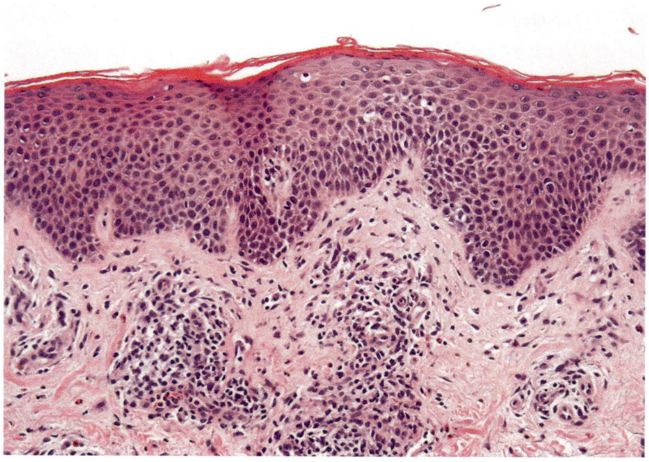

Fig. 2.4 Mild spongiotic dermatitis. There is slight acanthosis, mild epidermal edema, and parakeratosis. The dermal infiltrate shows a mix of lymphocytes and eosinophils

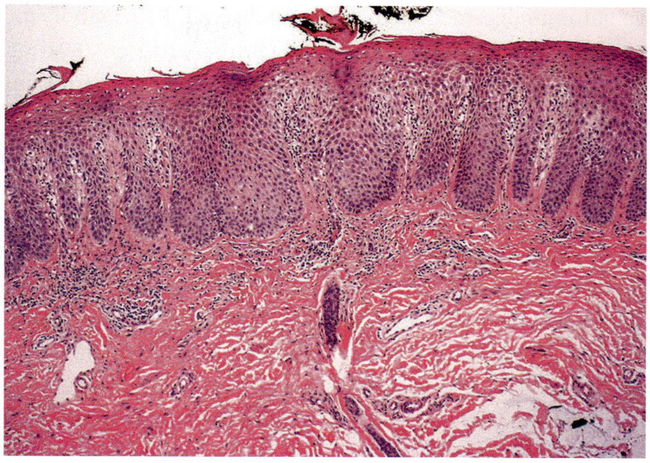

Fig. 2.5 Chronic spongiotic dermatitis. With time and continued stimulation, spongiotic dermatitis becomes chronic, characterized by more acanthosis and less spongiosis. Parakeratosis is still often seen. Photo provided courtesy of previous edition in Chinese (Science Press, Beijing, China)

[11], but they are not unique to ACD and may be seen in other spongiotic dermatoses, albeit somewhat less commonly [12]. Some authors suggest that the presence of keratinocyte necrosis may suggest specifically an irritant contact dermatitis [6, 13], while other studies have not found this to be a specific differentiating feature [11, 12]. In addition to marked spongiosis, early and acute eczematous processes will show minimal acanthosis and focal parakeratosis (Fig. 2.4). Parakeratosis, or the retention of keratinocyte nuclei beyond the granular layer, reflects an impaired keratinocyte maturation sequence and is seen in a wide variety of inflammatory, premalignant, and malignant processes. In early or acute spongiotic dermatitis, parakeratosis may be accompanied by a serum-rich and neutrophilic crust on the epithelial surface. Within the dermis, there is generally edema and a perivascular inflammatory infiltrate comprised of lymphocytes, histiocytes, and a variable number of eosinophils. While eosinophils have traditionally been associated with allergic contact dermatitis, their presence was not more common in patients with a positive patch test compared to those with a negative patch test [11]. The presence of eosinophils, while not particularly useful in differentiating between causes of spongiotic dermatitis, may be useful in excluding other inflammatory dermatoses as they are notably absent to very rare in entities such as psoriasis, lichen planus, and connective tissue disease [14, 15]. Neutrophils may be seen, particularly if there is epidermal erosion or ulceration nearby. Plasma cells are not typically part of the inflammatory infiltrate in spongiotic dermatitis. However, it should be remembered that plasma cells are a normal component of perigenital sites and therefore a few plasma cells within the infiltrate may be permissible on vulvar skin and mucosa [1]. The presence of spongiosis centered on the hair follicle with parakeratosis specifically concentrated on the lip of the follicle (so-called "shoulder parakeratosis") can suggest the possibility of seborrheic dermatitis.

With time and continued exposure to the inciting agent, the histopathologic features of spongiotic dermatitis change. In response to continued stimulus, the skin attempts to strengthen its barrier function by thickening. Acanthosis and parakeratosis become prominent, and spongiosis becomes less prominent (Fig. 2.5). Frequently there may be superimposed changes of lichenification (lichen simplex chronicus) due to rubbing and scratching by the patient in response to pruritus. Lichenification may be recognized by an increased granular layer (or formation of a thin granular layer on what should be normal mucosal epithelium), dermal or subepithelial fibrosis, and pigment (melanin) drop out into the superficial dermis.

In summary, spongiotic dermatitis represents a commonly encountered inflammatory reaction pattern. The exact etiology may not be determined on histology alone and always require correlation with the clinical presentation. It is this author's practice to sign out reports as "Spongiotic Dermatitis" with a comment that the features would be compatible with allergic or irritant contact dermatitis, atopic dermatitis, or other spongiotic processes.

2.2.1.3 Immunohistochemical Features

Immunohistochemical stains are not required to diagnose the spongiotic reaction pattern. As a superficial fungal infection (both dermatophyte and *Candida* sp.) may elicit a spongiotic reaction pattern, periodic acid-Schiff (PAS) or Grocott's methenamine silver (GMS) special stain is recommended as an ancillary test in the diagnosis of a spongiotic dermatitis.

2.2.1.4 Differential Diagnosis

The histologic differential diagnosis of spongiotic dermatitis can include blistering disorders, infection, and a drug eruption.

Spongiosis should be distinguished from acantholysis (see subsequent section on pemphigus) which may indicate an autoimmune-mediated blistering disease. In acantholysis, the desmosome complex failure is a primary process, leading to intraepidermal blistering, and the keratinocyte cytoplasm often retracts or collapses around the nucleus resulting in a rounded cell appearance. In contrast, vesiculation due to spongiosis results from keratinocytes being stretched to their limits until the edema overwhelms the desmosome complex. As a result, spongiosis can be suspected by angulated cytoplasmic fragments and a stellate, rather than rounded, cell shape. However, in cases in which a primary blistering disease is a consideration and definitive distinction between spongiosis and acantholysis is not possible, direct immunofluorescence studies will be necessary to exclude or confirm the possibility. Hailey–Hailey disease, an inherited genodermatosis characterized by defective desmosomal complexes resulting in extensive acantholysis of the epidermis, may be suspected when extensive acantholysis is seen in the absence of serum crusting, spongiosis, or significant dermal inflammation.

Infections may also mimic ACD, ICD, AD, and other spongiotic processes. Dermatophyte and Candida infections should be excluded through the use of GMS and/or PAS special stains. Herpetic infections may elicit a robust intraepidermal vesiculation and thereby mimic an acute spongiotic process; identification of the characteristic viral cytopathic effect will confirm this diagnosis.

Drug eruptions may sometimes result in identical histopathologic features as eczematous dermatoses. Careful correlation with clinical medication history is required.

Lastly, eczematous dermatitis may sometimes mimic other inflammatory dermatoses, namely early lichen sclerosus, a fixed drug eruption, or psoriasis. Moreover, superimposed ACD or ICD on one of these other inflammatory processes is always a possibility, particularly as patients try topical medications or home remedies either as directed by their physician or as an attempt to self-treat their skin disease. The most accurate diagnosis is made through a careful consideration of both clinical and histopathologic features.

2.3 Psoriasiform (Acanthotic) Reaction Pattern

2.3.1 Lichen Simplex Chronicus

Lichen simplex chronicus (LSC) is a histologic manifestation of excessive rubbing and scratching and is not a diagnosis in and of itself. LSC may be the end result of any inflammatory process that causes pruritus but it may also result from primary scratching without an identifiable underlying inflammatory process (i.e., idiopathic and/or neurodermatitis). LSC is a relatively frequent diagnosis in vulvar biopsies in general [3, 4], and was the most common diagnosis (26% of cases) in patients biopsied due to vulvar itching [16]. Pruritus is therefore the most common clinical symptom reported by patients with LSC. LSC indicates the presence of an itch-scratch cycle, in which itching precipitates scratching, and the scratching precipitates epidermal disruption that releases mediators that induce additional itching. The scratching and rubbing may be done consciously, unconsciously, or subconsciously, and will frequently occur during sleep [1, 17]. Histologic features of LSC may therefore be seen in isolation (for idiopathic or primary processes) or superimposed on other reaction patterns. In one study of vulvar biopsies, slightly more than 10% of vulvar biopsies showed two or more diagnosable processes; LSC was the second diagnosis in nearly all of these cases [3].

2.3.1.1 Clinical Features

LSC on the vulva may be recognized by thickened, erythematous plaques and papules, often with surface scaling. Lichenification refers to the presence of increased skin markings on the skin surface. Pigmentary changes (hyper- or hypopigmentation) are not infrequent. LSC most typically affects the vulvar regions surfaced by keratinizing squamous epithelium (as opposed to mucosal surfaces), namely the labia majora, peri-anal areas, and mons pubis [1]. Excoriations adjacent to the areas of lichenification will often be present.

The clinical differential diagnosis of LSC includes other inflammatory, infectious, and neoplastic vulvar skin conditions, and therefore skin biopsy is a common technique to establish the diagnosis and rule out other, more serious underlying conditions.

Treatment of LSC involves addressing any underlying inflammatory process, but ultimately requires breaking of the itch-scratch cycle. Topical steroids or steroid sparing agents may be helpful [18], but recurrences are not uncommon.

2.3.1.2 Histopathologic Features

LSC is classified by the International Society for the Study of Vulvovaginal Diseases (ISSVD) as having an "acanthotic" pattern [19]; dermatopathologists also often refer to this pattern as "psoriasiform." As may be inferred by this classification, LSC is characterized by thickening of the entire epidermis (acanthosis), generally in an irregular way. Irregular acanthosis means that the normal rete ridge pattern is expanded, but not in a uniform fashion (in contrast to psoriasis, which tends to demonstrate regular epidermal hyperplasia). Hyperkeratosis and hypergranulosis are seen at the surface, with parakeratosis a more variable finding (Fig. 2.6). Zones of pale keratinocytes have been reported in about three-quarters of vulvar LSC biopsies and were noted to be statistically more common in LSC than in other vulvar dermatoses examined [3]. Within the dermis, LSC generally shows papillary dermal fibrosis, with collagen fibers often

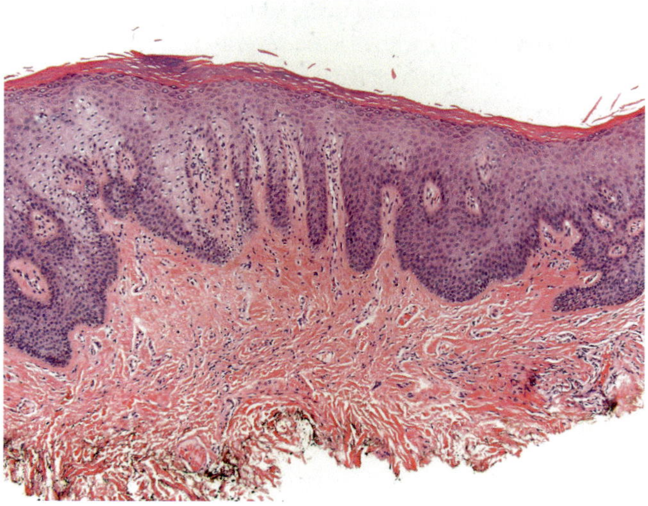

Fig. 2.6 Lichen simplex chronicus. The biopsy shows irregular acanthosis, hypergranulosis, and hyperkeratosis. There is minimal inflammation in the dermis

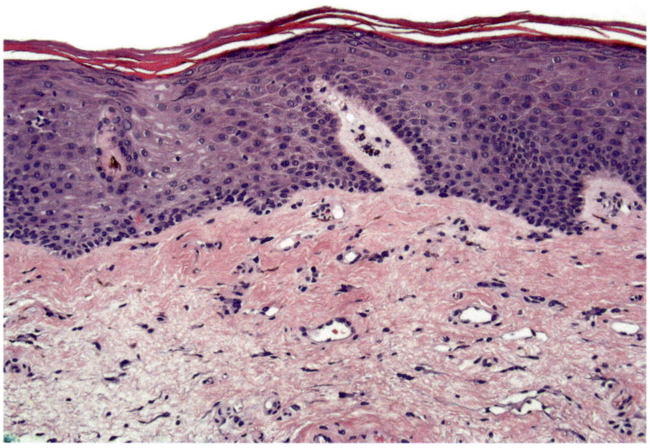

Fig. 2.7 Lichen simplex chronicus. On vulvar skin and mucosa in particular, the findings of lichen simplex chronicus may be subtle. Here there is slight acanthosis and a hint of an increased granular layer. There is slight melanin drop out in the subepithelium and a few multinucleate stromal cells

arranged in a characteristic vertical orientation in between dermal papillae; however, this feature has been suggested as less reproducible in biopsies from the vulvar region [3]. Instead of vertically oriented fibrosis, prominent stromal fibroblasts, including multinucleate forms (Fig. 2.7), have been suggested as a helpful clue to the diagnosis and were seen in more than half of biopsies in one histopathologic study of vulvar LSC [3]. There may be scant perivascular lymphocytes and a prominent vascularity in the superficial dermis. Of note, just because the name says "lichen" does not imply the necessity of a lichenoid pattern of inflammation. In fact, LSC as a primary process generally lacks a robust inflammatory infiltrate and the inflammation is not usually "band-like" in the superficial dermis. Melanin dropout (pigment incontinence) may also be seen as a result of chronic rubbing.

2.3.1.3 Immunohistochemical Features

As with eczematous dermatoses, immunohistochemical stains are generally not required in the diagnosis of LSC. Similar to eczematous dermatoses, performance of PAS or GMS special stains to exclude a fungal infection is recommended routinely. If pale intraepidermal keratinocytes are prominent, the pathologist may toy with the possibility of extramammary Paget disease. This diagnosis can be excluded with a small panel of immunohistochemical stains: generally Paget disease is cytokeratin 7, CAM 5.2, and mucicarmine positive, while LSC should be negative for these markers.

2.3.1.4 Differential Diagnosis

As previously mentioned, LSC may be an end result or a superimposed pattern on many inflammatory or preneoplastic conditions. Detection of even slight amounts of spongiosis, parakeratosis, or dermal eosinophils may suggest the possibility of a spongiotic dermatitis as the underlying process, and a diagnosis of "spongiotic dermatitis with secondary changes of lichenification" may be a more helpful diagnosis to treating clinicians than simply "lichen simplex chronicus." Detection of prominent dyskeratosis may suggest one of the diagnoses with a lichenoid pattern of inflammation. If the epidermal hyperplasia appears more regular in nature, with areas of granular layer loss and intraepidermal neutrophils, then psoriasis should be a preferred consideration. The presence of keratinocyte atypia is unusual in LSC. The presence of keratinocyte atypia should warrant careful examination to exclude a subtle high grade squamous intraepithelial neoplasia (VIN usual type) or differentiated vulvar intraepithelial neoplasia (d-VIN) with superimposed LSC. Overall, in the author's experience, the diagnosis of LSC is reserved for biopsies in which histologic features are limited to acanthosis, hyperkeratosis, hypergranulosis, papillary dermal fibrosis, and nonspecific chronic inflammation. The presence of any other histologic feature generally prompts a comment about the likelihood of secondary changes of lichen simplex chronicus complicating the diagnosis of another primary process.

2.3.2 Psoriasis

Psoriasis is a common skin condition which relatively uncommonly affects the vulvar skin and mucosa. The prevalence of psoriasis differs among demographic groups (being more common in adults than in children) and among geographic regions (being more common in countries more distant from the equator) [20]. Estimations of the prevalence range from approximately 0.5 to 8%, depending on the population sampled [20–22]. Most patients present in early adulthood, and women may present at a slightly earlier age than men [22]. Genital involvement is estimated to occur in about 30–40% of patients with psoriasis [23], and 2–5% of patients with psoriasis are estimated to have exclusive involvement of the genital skin [24]. Vulvar psoriasis seems to present in a similar age group of patients [21]. Children may also present with psoriasis and are more likely than adults to report a family history of the disease [21]. Classic psoriasis presents with a symmetric eruption of dry scaly plaques on the extensor surfaces. Inverse psoriasis refers to a distribution of lesions that affects the body folds (axillae, groin, umbilicus, inframammary creases, and antecubital and popliteal fossae). Inverse psoriasis does not always (but may) indicate the presence of genital psoriasis [25].

The pathogenesis of psoriasis is complex and multifactorial, and thorough discussion is beyond the scope of this chapter. Genetic and epigenetic events result in an autoinflammatory disorder skewed toward the Th-1 and Th-17 immune responses. The resultant altered immunity results in a hyperproliferative state of the epidermis, corresponding with the histologic elements of acanthosis and parakeratosis, and the clinical perception of scaly plaques.

Genetic susceptibility definitely plays a role in development of psoriasis. About 30% of patients with the disease have an affected first-degree relative [22]. Several genetic loci linked to familial cases of psoriasis have been documented, the most strongly linked being PSORS1, located on chromosome 6p. The various psoriasis susceptibility loci that have been found in genetic linkage studies encompass genes important for Th1 cell differentiation, Th17 cell differentiation, interferon signaling, keratinocyte growth, and antigen presentation [26]. Expression of the major histocompatibility complex (MHC) class I allele HLA-Cw6 is strongly linked to psoriasis and is encoded near the PSORS1 locus [22, 26]. Epigenetic alterations also seem to play a role in development of psoriasis, with research focusing on the role of posttranslational histone modifications, DNA methylation, and microRNAs [26].

Regardless of genetic influences, patients with psoriasis demonstrate altered immune responses. Induction of a Th-17 immune response is mediated by interleukin (IL)-23 and TNF-α release. IL-23 release stimulates differentiation of naïve T-cells to Th-17 type helper T-cells [27]. Th-17 cells then elicit a cascade of cytokines (notably including IL-17) that act on keratinocytes of the epidermis to become hyperproliferative [26] as well as feeding back to reactivate and amplify the cytokine cascade. IL-17 is also important in the recruitment of neutrophils and the upregulation of antimicrobial peptides that play a role in pathogenesis [27]. Psoriasis also shows features of a Th-1 immune response, with interferon-γ, IL-2, and IL-12 notably increased in the serum of patients with psoriasis and correlating with disease severity [22, 26].

Patients with psoriasis have a higher incidence of Crohn disease, type 2 diabetes and the metabolic syndrome, and depression [22, 25]. Patients also have a slightly increased risk of developing lymphoproliferative diseases (which may in part be related to risks imparted by systemic treatment for the disease) [25, 28].

Treatment of psoriasis depends on disease severity. Gentle skin care regimens are advised, and skin lesions may be treated with topical corticosteroids and steroid sparing agents such as calcineurin inhibitors or topical vitamin D analogues. Skin atrophy and fragility due to prolonged corticosteroid use is a particular problem in the treatment of genital skin [24], and many of the topical preparations used elsewhere on the body may be irritating to vulvar skin [21]. Systemic therapies are utilized for psoriasis refractory to topical treatments or when there is considerable body surface involvement. Systemic therapies target the cytokines known to be elevated in patients with psoriasis and broadly include TNF-α inhibitors, IL-12 and IL-23 inhibitors, and IL-17 inhibitors [26].

2.3.2.1 Clinical Features

The clinical appearance of lesions of genital psoriasis depends on the precise anatomic area involved, corresponding with the transition in this region from stratified squamous to mucosal type epithelium. Familiarity with the variation in presentation can aid diagnosis (Fig. 2.8). One study noted that of a cohort

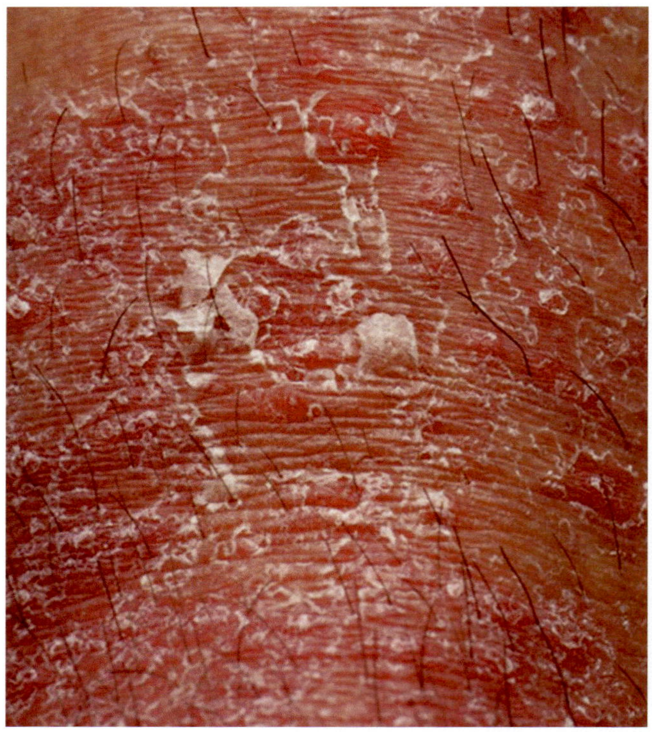

Fig. 2.8 Psoriasis. The lesion shows salmon colored, erythema, thin plaques and multiple scaly lesions in the vulvar region (Courtesy of Dr. Kenneth Hatch, University of Arizona)

of patients ultimately diagnosed with vulvar psoriasis at a vulvar specialty clinic, only 12% of the patients had been referred with a provisional diagnosis of psoriasis [21]. The mons pubis will show lesions resembling classic psoriasis vulgaris, with scaly salmon-colored, raised plaques that typically lack ulceration [21]. Involvement of the labia majora shows a more variable presence of scale, increased erythema, and occasionally erosions and ulceration [1, 21]. Vulvar regions of the inner labia majora, labia minora, and clitoris will lack scale and typically consist of well-demarcated erythematous to shiny plaques [21–23]. The inguinal folds often show symmetric, bright erythema without any scaling and a higher propensity for erosive and ulcerative lesions [1]. The vagina is generally not involved by psoriasis, so vaginal lesions should prompt consideration of other inflammatory disorders [21–23]. Of note, vulvar discomfort, including burning sensation and pruritus, is common in patients with psoriasis, even if there are no discernable skin/mucosal lesions [29]. In one study specifically of vulvar psoriasis, nearly 95% of women reported itching as a significant symptom [21].

Psoriasis is generally diagnosed on clinical exam. Examination of other body sites may reveal the classic silvery, dry scaly plaques distributed symmetrically on the extensor surfaces (knees, elbows, scalp). Examination of the gluteal cleft may reveal well-demarcated erythema. Nail involvement is a frequent finding in psoriasis, characterized by oil spots, pitting, and distal onycholysis (lifting of the nail plate from the nail bed) [22, 24]. Pustular lesions may be seen, particularly on the palms and soles, but pustules in the vulvar regions are distinctly uncommon [22]. Vulvar psoriasis is rarely unilateral in distribution [21].

The clinical differential diagnosis includes infectious etiologies (superficial fungal infections to include *Candida* sp., and dermatophyte/tinea), chronic spongiotic dermatoses (irritant and allergic contact dermatitis), lichen simplex chronicus, fixed drug eruptions, and even malignancies such as extramammary Paget disease [21]. Nonresponsiveness to antifungals and negative cultures can help exclude infectious etiologies. Biopsy is strongly recommended for patients who are not responsive to usual treatments to exclude extramammary Paget disease. Distinguishing psoriasis from irritant or allergic contact dermatitis may best be accomplished through clinical exam and history.

2.3.2.2 Histopathologic Features

The histologic features of vulvar psoriasis vary depending on the precise anatomic site involved and biopsied. The classically described histopathologic features of psoriasis as seen on other cutaneous sites may be seen on the hair-bearing sites of the mons pubis and labia majora; however, the features may be less specific and more variable on mucosal sites and the intertriginous folds of the female genitalia. One study suggested that biopsy should be performed predominantly to rule out other pathologies such as Paget disease and lichen sclerosus rather than as a means to confirm the diagnosis, noting that none of the five biopsies from patients with clinically diagnosed psoriasis demonstrated the "typical" features associated with the disease [21].

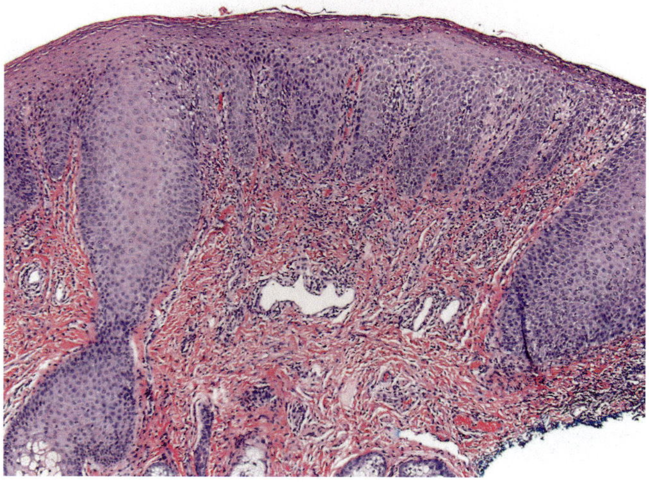

Fig. 2.9 Psoriasis. Low-power magnification shows regular epidermal hyperplasia with parakeratosis and intraepidermal neutrophils. Spongiosis is not prominent

Classic psoriasis, and thus its histologic appearance in biopsies of the external vulva and mons pubis, is characterized by regular epidermal hyperplasia, loss of the granular layer, and confluent parakeratosis (Fig. 2.9). Regular epidermal hyperplasia (or acanthosis) means that all rete ridges are elongated to a similar degree (as opposed to the irregular acanthosis that typifies lichen simplex chronicus). Neutrophils migrate into the epidermis, forming small aggregates known as spongiform pustules in the stratum spinosum and stratum corneum. Blood vessels in the superficial dermis are dilated and prominent within the dermal papillae. There is typically a scant perivascular lymphocytic infiltrate in the dermis. Eosinophils are typically absent, although they may be more common in biopsies from children [1] and a recent study suggests they may be more common in inverse psoriasis specifically [30]. Biopsies from mucosal sites or the intertriginous folds are more likely to show spongiosis, generally have less pronounced acanthosis, and the acanthosis may more often be irregular rather than regular [30]. Spongiosis may also be more prominent in early lesions of psoriasis (Fig. 2.10). In the author's experience, biopsies from the vulvar region are often not specific for psoriasis, but the possibility may be included in the differential diagnosis of a vulvar biopsy with slight acanthosis, spongiosis, and parakeratosis. In the absence of detailed clinical information and images, these biopsies are often reported as "Psoriasiform and spongiotic dermatitis," with a differential diagnosis including chronic spongiotic processes and psoriasis.

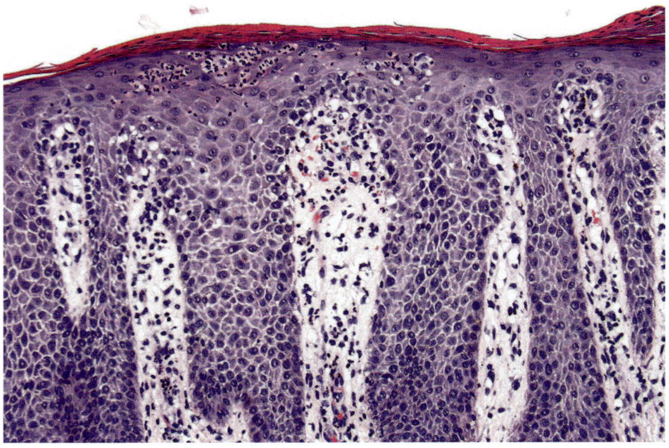

Fig. 2.10 Psoriasis. High-power magnification shows spongiform pustules, confluent parakeratosis, and suprapapillary thinning. This biopsy also shows a degree of spongiosis, which is more commonly seen in vulvar biopsies of psoriasis

The epidermis in psoriasis is hyperproliferative, and the normal sequence of keratinocyte maturation is sped up in psoriasis. Both cell cycle time and time for keratinocytes to transit from the basal layer to the top of the spinous layer is markedly accelerated [27]. As such, the presence of basilar mitotic figures (and occasionally suprabasally) is not an uncommon feature in psoriasis. The presence of basal mitoses should not be mistaken as a marker of a premalignancy/vulvar intraepithelial neoplasia.

2.3.2.3 Immunohistochemical Features

Particularly when the features of psoriasis are not classic, special stains to exclude a superficial fungal infection are recommended. These special stains would be reasonable even in the setting of otherwise classic psoriasis to exclude a secondary superimposed infection. Other ancillary testing is typically not indicated. Immunohistochemical evaluation of the proteins expressed in psoriatic plaques [31] or in the immune infiltrate [32] of psoriasis biopsies has indicated some differences compared to normal or other inflammatory skin diseases; however, to the author's knowledge, no assay is universally useful or routinely used in clinical practice to differentiate psoriasis from other cutaneous inflammatory conditions.

2.3.2.4 Differential Diagnosis

The histologic differential diagnosis includes fungal infection, chronic spongiotic dermatoses, lichen simplex chronicus, and Reiter syndrome. Fungal infection is easily excluded through the use of special stains PAS and/or GMS. Chronic spongiotic dermatoses (including atopic dermatitis, allergic or irritant contact dermatitis) may have considerable histologic overlap with psoriasis. The presence of abundant dermal eosinophils may somewhat favor contact or other spongiotic dermatitis, as large numbers of eosinophils are not typically induced in the Th1 and Th17 immune response that typifies psoriasis. Seborrheic dermatitis can involve the vulva and has considerable histologic overlap with psoriasis, but spongiosis preferentially involving hair follicle epithelium and parakeratosis adjacent to the follicle openings have been suggested as differentiating clues in seborrheic dermatitis. Lichen simplex chronicus classically shows irregular rather than regular epidermal hyperplasia. Reiter syndrome is rare but may be histologically identical to psoriasis and requires specific knowledge of the clinical presentation.

2.3.3 Reiter Syndrome

Another consideration when encountering a psoriasiform reaction pattern would be Reiter syndrome (reactive arthritis). This rare syndrome is characterized by the classic triad of urethritis, conjunctivitis, and arthritis. Pustular psoriasis-like lesions are also a commonly reported sign, historically referred to as keratoderma blennorrhagica. The syndrome is uncommon in females, and the presence of all of the classic signs is not required for diagnosis, thus leading to an atypical presentation. This atypical presentation may be more common in female patients [33], and vulvar involvement is exceptionally reported.

Reiter syndrome has been linked to genetic predisposition in patients possessing the antigen HLA B27 as well as infectious etiologies. The incidence of detection of the HLA B27 antigen is reported in as high as 90% of cases of Reiter syndrome, although the antigen may be less commonly detected in female patients [33]. This genetic disposition, when coupled with a urogenital or enteric infection, is thought to result in disease manifestation, with development of cross-reacting immune complexes [1]. Infections caused by *Chlamydia*, *Neisseria*, *Ureaplasma*, *Yersinia*, *Campylobacter*, *Shigella*, and *Salmonella* sp. have all been implicated as preceding infections in Reiter syndrome.

2.3.3.1 Clinical Features

The classic description of Reiter syndrome is the triad of urethritis, conjunctivitis, and arthritis, arising in young adult male patients. Females are less commonly affected but may have cervicitis. Arthritis typically involves the heels, knees, and back joints [34]. This differs from the arthritis associated with psoriasis, which more commonly involves the small joints of the hands. Mucocutaneous ulcerations may be present, and may precede the development of the other salient features of the disease.

Cutaneous lesions present as psoriatic, hyperkeratotic plaques in a similar distribution as psoriasis. Perigenital lesions and mucosal lesions are often ulcerative with exudative surface. Vulvar ulcerations have been described as shallow, sometimes rimmed by small papules arranged in a circular (annular) configuration [34]. Linear, rather than annular, ulcerations have also been described [33]. Verrucous lesions and pustules have also been described [1].

The clinical differential diagnosis of the mucocutaneous lesions typically includes pustular psoriasis or sexually transmitted diseases presenting with genital ulceration. Psoriasis typically does not involve the cervix, so cervical involvement would support Reiter syndrome over psoriasis, as would the previously mentioned distribution of joints affected by arthritic symptoms [34]. Sexually transmitted diseases such as lymphogranuloma venereum could be considered in the setting of vulvar ulceration and recent genital infection; this entity typically presents with lymphadenitis and the absence of extragenital manifestations, which is uncommon in Reiter syndrome [33].

Treatment regimens vary, and topical steroids, methotrexate, and retinoids all have been reported as being therapeutic.

2.3.3.2 Histopathologic Features

Biopsies from vulvar lesions show features similar to psoriasis. Epidermal acanthosis, hypogranulosis with diffuse parakeratosis, suprapapillary thinning, and intraepidermal neutrophilic microabscesses are typically seen. Pustules may be present. One author noted pseudoepitheliomatous hyperplasia with deep dermal pustules/microabscesses [33].

2.3.3.3 Immunohistochemical Features

Ancillary tests suggested in the workup of possible Reiter syndrome include a PAS stain to exclude a superficial fungal infection. Urethral or genital cultures or polymerase chain reaction may detect the presence of an infectious disease, which may be supportive of the disease as well [33].

2.3.3.4 Differential Diagnosis

The histopathologic differential diagnosis with the classically described features would include psoriasis, and distinction of the two entities may be impossible on histologic grounds alone. The presence of pseudoepitheliomatous hyperplasia in one reported case led to consideration of pemphigus vegetans; direct immunofluorescence studies were negative to help exclude this possibility [33].

There are no histopathologic features that are pathognomonic or specific for Reiter syndrome. Pathology reports should emphasize that the features may be supportive of the diagnosis assuming the clinical impression supports the diagnosis of Reiter syndrome. Ultimately, however, the diagnosis is a clinical one, although it may be suggested by the astute pathologist if he/she is provided with sufficient clinical information.

2.4 Lichenoid and Interface Reaction Pattern

2.4.1 Lichen Planus

Lichen planus (LP) is a relatively common condition that may affect both skin and mucosa of adults. It is estimated to be the cause of approximately 1% of dermatology visits. A subset of patients with LP will have mucosal disease, with oral cavity (tongue, buccal mucosa, gingiva) being the most commonly affected mucosal site, and mucosal LP may exist in the absence of cutaneous LP. At least half and up to three-quarters of patients with oral LP will also have genital disease [23, 35], and patients with vulvar LP are more likely to have oral involvement than cutaneous involvement [36]. The true incidence of vulvar involvement by LP is unknown; this is due to delays in diagnosis, occasional absence of symptomatology, and nonspecific clinical and histologic presentations. LP may present on the vulva in one of three forms: classic, hypertrophic, and erosive. Classic LP is similar to cutaneous disease and is generally more straightforward to diagnose. Hypertrophic LP is unusual but documented on vulvar skin [37]. Erosive LP is unique to mucosal sites (including vulva and vagina) and carries particular morbidity, including impairment in sexual relations, dyspareunia, scarring with stenosis, and a small but real increased risk of developing cancer.

LP affects perimenopausal or postmenopausal adults, generally presenting in the fifth or sixth decade of life. In one large series, the mean age of presentation of vulvar LP was 57 years (range 23–87) [36] and 55 years (range 12–87) in another [38]. Presentation during childhood is rare. LP is generally believed to be an autoimmune chronic disease mediated by cytotoxic T lymphocytes to a yet undiscovered antigen [35, 39]. Cytotoxic damage to keratinocytes is the basis of the histologic features seen in LP. The cytokine profile in LP is generally a Th-1 phenotype [40].

Patients with cutaneous LP have an increased incidence of hepatitis types B and C; this association has not been detected in patients with vulvar LP, at least in a few European-based studies [36, 41]. In contrast, patients with vulvar (specifically erosive) LP have been shown to have a higher incidence of associated autoimmune disorders than in a control population. In a large case-controlled series, nearly one-third of patients with erosive LP (29%) had at least one autoimmune-associated disease, including thyroid disease, vitiligo, alopecia areata, celiac disease, and rheumatoid arthritis [42].

Patients with LP are at an increased risk to develop squamous cell carcinoma (SCC) at some sites of involvement, particularly of the lip, tongue, oral cavity, esophagus, larynx, and vulva, but notably not in cutaneous skin [43]. Cancer risk in the vulva is generally an increased likelihood of developing SCC, which is unrelated to human papillomavirus infection [44, 45]. Although overall a rare phenomenon, vulvar SCC arises in older women, on mucosal (non-hair-bearing) surfaces of the vulva, and may be solitary or multifocal. In the largest series of vulvar SCC arising in LP (38 patients), SCC arose in the setting of erosive LP in one-third of patients and nonerosive LP in the remaining two-thirds of patients. Differentiated vulvar intraepithelial neoplasia (d-VIN) was present in the excision specimen in 22 of 38 patients, likely representing a precursor lesion [45]. SCC arising in the setting of vulvar LP is aggressive, with a large subset of patients demonstrating lymph node metastasis at presentation, high rates of recurrence, and 30% disease-related mortality [45].

Treatment of LP involving the vulva includes strategies designed to decrease symptoms and prevent scarring sequelae. Full resolution of lesions is difficult, and the disease generally runs a chronic course. Management generally involves high potency topical steroids and topical steroid-sparing agents such as tacrolimus, with progression to systemic immunosuppressive agents for refractory disease. Surgical management may be required if adhesions, stenosis, or significant scarring develop. Regular interval follow-up visits are important for surveillance given the increased risk of SCC, and biopsy is recommended for any nonhealing vulvar lesions [35, 36, 38, 46, 47].

2.4.1.1 Clinical Features

The majority of patients with vulvar LP present with complaints of soreness, burning, and pain; about half of patients may also report pruritus [47]. The symptoms reported may reflect the types of lesions the patients have, as classic LP lesions may be asymptomatic or pruritic, hypertrophic lesions tend to be itchy, and erosive lesions are painful [35]. Physical examination should not be limited to the genital skin; patients with LP usually have oral disease and may have cutaneous lesions. Hair involvement (scarring alopecia as lichen planopilaris or frontal fibrosing alopecia) and nail involvement may also be seen.

Classic LP presents as a papulosquamous disorder. Lesions consist of flat topped erythematous to violaceous papules and plaques surfaced by fine white lines called "Wickham's striae." Cutaneous lesions of LP usually involve the flexor surfaces of the extremities. When the vulva is involved, the labia majora and the interlabial sulci may show papules of LP, whereas the labia minora and clitoral hood will show flatter lesions with a white reticular network on the surface [35] (Fig. 2.11). Classic LP may clinically mimic lichen simplex chronicus, lichen sclerosus, and allergic or irritant contact dermatoses.

Erosive LP occurs on the mucosal aspect of the vulva and is usually painful. Erosive LP presents as glazed/shiny erythema that easily bleeds with any kind of manipulation. This erythema may be surrounded by a lace-like, white reticular and slightly hyperkeratotic border. Identification of this characteristic border is helpful in clinically suspecting the diagnosis, although it is not always present. Erosions are generally well demarcated and involve the inner aspect of the labia minora, the introitus, and vestibule [23, 36, 47, 48]. Over time, scarring can lead to obliteration of normal vulvar and vaginal architecture; the clitoral hood and labia may appear resorbed, there may be fusion of labia, and there may be stenosis of the vaginal opening [47]. Vaginal involvement is common in patients with erosive vulvar LP [49]. Patients with vaginal LP may present with a desquamative inflammatory vaginitis, complaining of symptoms such as irritation, painful sexual intercourse, and pain with increased vaginal secretions [50]. Nine diagnostic criteria for vulvar erosive LP have been proposed by a series of experts and include clinical signs, symptomatology, and histologic features (Table 2.4); fulfillment of three criteria is required for diagnosis [51].

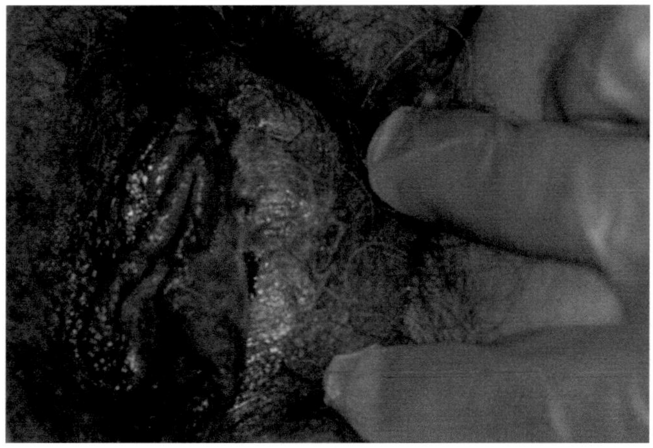

Fig. 2.11 Lichen planus. The labia are surfaced by a flat-topped lavender to white plaque with a white reticular network on the surface. Photo provided courtesy of previous edition in Chinese (Science Press, Beijing, China)

Hypertrophic LP rarely presents in the vulva, but when seen, lesions will be verrucous and hyperkeratotic. Clinically, hypertrophic LP lesions will mimic condyloma or other squamous intraepithelial neoplasia, so biopsy is warranted to confirm the diagnosis.

The clinical differential of LP, particularly the erosive variant, includes lichen sclerosus (LS), graft-versus-host disease, immunobullous diseases (mucous membrane pemphigoid or pemphigus vulgaris), acute irritant or allergic contact dermatitis, infections (particularly candidiasis or herpes virus), and vulvar intraepithelial neoplasia [35, 36]. LS has significant clinical and histologic overlap, and some important distinguishing features are included in Table 2.5. Clinically, mucosal LP is more likely to involve the inner aspect of the labia and patients often have nongenital involvement (most often oral erosions and ulcerations) than LS. It should be noted that LP and LS can coexist [52].

Table 2.4 Diagnostic criteria in the diagnosis of vulvar erosive lichen planus

1. Clinical signs: Well-demarcated erosions or glazed erythema present at vaginal introitus
2. Clinical signs: Hyperkeratotic white border around erythematous areas/erosions ± identifiable Wickham's striae on skin
3. Symptoms: Pain or burning
4. Clinical signs: Scarring and/or loss of normal vulvar architecture
5. Clinical signs: Vaginal inflammation
6. Clinical signs: Involvement of other mucosal sites
7. Histologic features: Well-defined inflammatory band involving the dermal–epidermal junction
8. Histologic features: Inflammatory band predominantly composed of lymphocytes
9. Histologic features: Basal layer degeneration (Civatte bodies, basal layer keratinocyte death, abnormal keratinization)

Adapted from *Simpson RC, Thomas KS, Leighton P, and Murphy R. Diagnostic criteria for erosive lichen planus affecting the vulva: an international electronic-Delphi consensus exercise. Br J Dermatol. 2013 Aug;169(2):337–43*

Table 2.5 Clinical and histologic features to distinguish lichen planus from early lichen sclerosus

	Lichen planus	Lichen sclerosus
Age at presentation	Adults (peri- and postmenopausal)	Children and adults
Site of vulvar involvement	Inner aspects of labia minora Can involve vagina (erosive variant)	Outer aspects of labia minora, perianal skin Does not involve vagina
Associated symptoms	Burning, ulcerations, and pain > pruritus	Pruritus
Helpful clinical clues	White, reticular border around erosions Sometimes hyperkeratotic	Atrophic or hyperkeratotic, figure of eight/hourglass appearance, purpuric
Associated disease	Oral or cutaneous LP, autoimmune disease	Autoimmune disease Extragenital involvement unusual
Epidermal changes	Squamatization of basal epithelium Angulated, "saw-tooth" rete ridge pattern Hypergranulosis (wedge shaped) Less common exocytosis	No squamatization of basal epithelium Attenuated rete ridge pattern ± hypergranulosis Exocytosis of lymphocytes
Basement membrane zone changes	Obscuring inflammation No basement membrane thickening	± obscuring inflammation Thickened basement membrane
Superficial dermal changes	No homogenization of dermal collagen Preservation of elastic fibers (usually) Cytoid bodies and melanophages	Homogenization of dermal collagen (papillary dermal tips) Loss of elastic fibers Subepithelial edema Hemorrhage and hemosiderin occasionally

Graft-versus-host disease may be clinically indistinguishable from LP, but will arise in the unique setting of prior hematopoietic stem cell transplantation. Immunobullous diseases, infection, and neoplastic processes can be readily distinguished from LP through biopsy.

Given the importance (for management and prognosis) in distinguishing between LP and LS, and given the clinical overlap of LP with preneoplastic and neoplastic entities, biopsies are frequently useful and necessary in the workup of a patient with presumed vulvar LP. Ideally, the biopsy should encompass non-eroded/ulcerated skin to decrease the chances of detecting nonspecific features of inflamed ulceration [50]. The best location to take a biopsy to confirm the diagnosis is the lacy border showing Wickham striae; however, this border may not be clinically evident [36]. If autoimmune blistering diseases are being considered in the clinical differential diagnosis, additional samples for direct immunofluorescence (submitted in Michel's or Zeus medium) should be included.

2.4.1.2 Histologic Features

LP is the prototypic example of a lichenoid inflammatory reaction pattern. The histologic features of cutaneous LP are reproducible and recognizable. Erosive LP may have less specific histologic features, particularly when the epidermis is ulcerated. Familiarity with the spectrum of patterns seen may increase the diagnostic yield. In one study of 38 women with clinically confirmed vulvar LP and biopsies available, biopsy results were supportive of the diagnosis in 25 (biopsies were classified as "diagnostic" in 18 and "consistent with" in 7). The remainder of patients had nonspecific features on biopsy [36]. This further underscores this difficulty in correctly diagnosing mucosal LP.

The classic histologic features of LP include wedge-shaped hypergranulosis, angulated or serrated rete ridges (often referred to as "saw-tooth"), and a lichenoid band of inflammation in the superficial dermis which obscures the normal dermal–epidermal interface (Fig. 2.12a, b). Lymphocytes may be seen moving into the epidermis (exocytosis), and cytotoxicity to keratinocytes is evidenced by apoptotic, brightly eosinophilic keratinocytes (Civatte bodies) interspersed within the epidermis, but favoring the basal epithelial layer. Cytoid bodies are clumps of brightly eosinophilic material (degenerated keratin fragments from dying keratinocytes) that deposit in the superficial dermis. The dermal infiltrate is composed predominantly of lymphocytes, although a minor plasma cell cohort is permissible. On mucosal sites, the abovementioned features may be subtle or absent. Mucosa normally lacks a granular layer, so presence of a slight acquired granular layer on mucosa may be a histologic clue to the diagnosis. Epithelium may be attenuated and parakeratosis alternating with slight hyperkeratosis may be seen [39] (Fig. 2.13). The presence of eroa

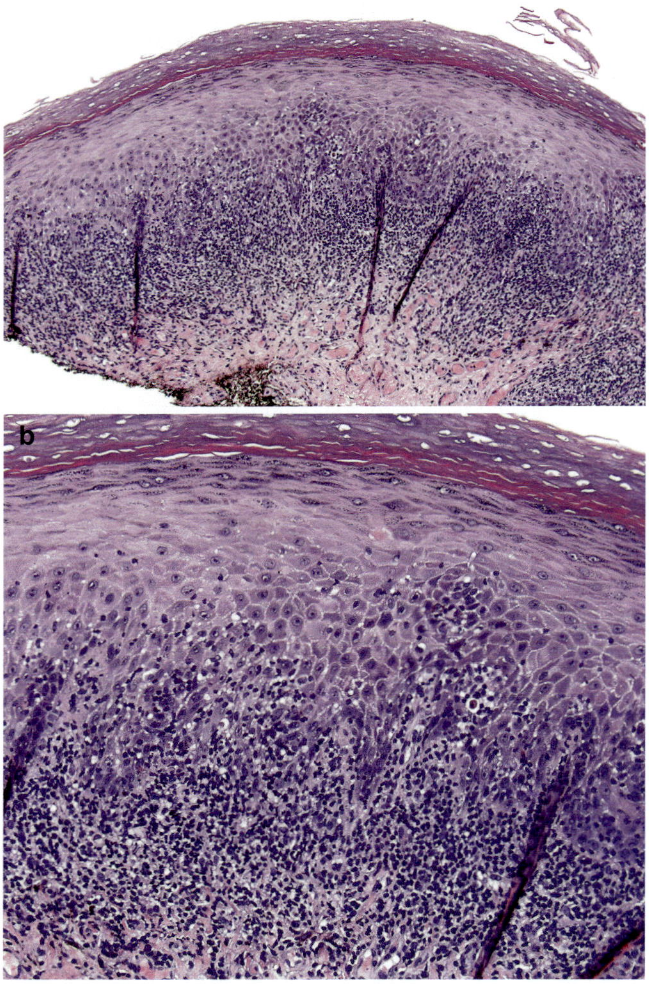

Fig. 2.12 Lichen planus. (**a**) Low-power magnification shows hyperkeratosis, hypergranulosis, and a band of inflammation that obscures the dermal–epidermal junction. (**b**) Higher power magnification demonstrates the saw tooth like rete ridge pattern, scattered dying keratinocytes approximated along the basal epidermis, and a vague "wedge-shape" can be appreciated in the hypergranulosis

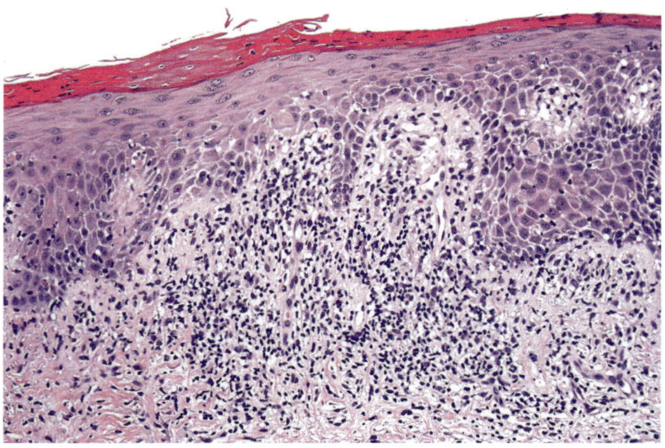

Fig. 2.13 Lichenoid dermatitis suggestive of lichen planus. There is parakeratosis with a hint of a granular layer. There is slight angulation of rete ridges with dying keratinocytes along the basilar epithelium

sion or ulceration with reepithelialization may result in reactive epithelial atypia, evidenced by nuclear enlargement, pleomorphism, and hyperchromasia. Basilar mitotic figures should not be increased and should not be atypical (if noted) [53].

2.4.1.3 Immunohistochemical Features

Ancillary testing is generally not required in the workup of LP. Direct immunofluorescence studies will be negative for any basement membrane zone or intercellular staining with immunoglobulin. However, fibrin may be apparent along the dermal–epidermal junction, and cytoid bodies may react with IgM and be visualized as small immunoreactive clumps in the superficial dermis. Ancillary stains may be useful to exclude infectious etiologies. Immunophenotyping of the inflammatory infiltrate within LP and LS has not shown any significant and distinguishing features and is therefore not useful in differentiating these two entities [54].

2.4.1.4 Differential Diagnosis

Histologic distinction between LP and early LS is known to be difficult (Table 2.5). Basal keratinocyte squamatization, hypergranulosis, pointed (rather than effaced) rete ridges, and cytoid bodies are all seen much more frequently in LP than in early LS [54]. Another study examining histologic features specifically of vulvar LP noted the relative rarity of these features [2]. One study has also suggested that wiry fibrosis and eosinophils within the infiltrate may favor LS over LP [3], and another study noted that the presence of basement membrane thickening, ectatic superficial dermal blood vessels, and early subtle sclerosis were helpful in discriminating between LS (where the features were seen) and LP (where the features were absent) [2]. Elastic fiber loss in the subepithelial space has been suggested as a helpful and differentiating feature in the diagnosis of LS [54], but other authors have reported similar elastic fiber loss in LP as well [2]. Ultimately, if a confident diagnosis cannot be made, the diagnosis of "lichenoid mucositis" may be made, with a comment detailing that the differential diagnosis includes both LP and the inflammatory phase of early LS (see further discussion in section and images below). It should be noted that LP and LS can coexist [52].

Besides LS, other histologic considerations within the differential diagnosis of LP include infection, other ulcerative diseases such as Behcet or Crohn disease, plasma cell (Zoon) vulvitis, and differentiated vulvar intraepithelial neoplasia (d-VIN). Infections (most commonly Candidiasis, herpes virus, and syphilis) may be excluded through the use of ancillary special or immunohistochemical stains. Other ulcerative conditions may show nonspecific ulceration or epithelial erosion, and both Behcet and Crohn disease may have oral involvement as well. Presence of a portion of intact epidermis to evaluate for the characteristic lichenoid infiltrate or vacuolar changes and cytotoxic damage to the epithelium that would characterize erosive LP is the most helpful way to differentiate these disorders. While LP and plasma cell vulvitis share a dense band-like infiltrate, LP generally shows a lymphocyte predominant infiltrate, and the presence of Civatte bodies in LP will be a distinguishing feature not seen in plasma cell vulvitis [55]. In one series comparing the two entities, the presence of Civatte bodies, lymphocyte predominance, and an accentuation of the granular layer were all noted in LP but lacking in plasma cell vulvitis [55]. D-VIN is a precursor of vulvar squamous cell carcinoma. D-VIN is unrelated to human papilloma virus infection and is thought to arise through a p53-dependent pathway. D-VIN is recognized by elongated, sometimes anastomosing rete ridges, with keratinocyte atypia (atypical mitotic figures, dyskeratosis, nuclear enlargement, and prominent nucleoli) restricted to the basal layer. Although parakeratosis is present, the squamous epithelium appears overall mature and may be confused with reactive epithelial atypia on low-power evaluation. By immunohistochemistry, d-VIN often shows diffuse confluent staining for p53 (basal and suprabasilar layer only) but rarely exhibits a null pattern of reactivity (no p53 staining) compared to weak patchy (wild type) staining of non-lesional epithelium. However, inflammation and stress can prolong the half-life of the p53 protein and result in a positive staining pattern. Therefore, a positive p53 stain should be interpreted in the proper clinical and histomorphologic context. Not surprisingly, studies are mixed with regard to the utility of p53 staining as an adjunct in distinguishing reactive atypia in erosive LP from d-VIN, with some studies indicating negative patterns of staining [54], while others have reported confluent p53 positivity in a subset of biopsies of erosive LP [53].

2.4.2 Lichen Sclerosus

Lichen sclerosus (LS) is a relatively common disorder that most commonly involves genital skin, including vulvar skin and mucosa. Women are affected much more commonly than men. Estimated to represent less than 1% of patients referred to a dermatologist [56] but at least one-third of cases seen at a vulvar specialty clinic [57], LS commonly presents as genital pruritus, discomfort, and dyspareunia. The disease is chronically progressive, and, if untreated over time, LS leads to significant alteration and scarring of the genital architecture.

In contrast to LP, LS demonstrates a broad age range of presentation. Although overall rarely diagnosed in children, LS represents approximately one-fifth of the vulvar complaints in prepubertal girls [58], and childhood LS is estimated to represent between 9% and 15% of all LS cases [59, 60]. Postmenopausal women make up the second, bimodal peak in incidence of LS, but occurrence during reproductive years may also be seen.

The exact mechanism for the development of LS is not known, although an autoimmune mechanism directed against antigens in the lower epidermis has been proposed [56, 61, 62]. Chronic irritation from exposure to urine has been suggested as a contributing factor [56]. Infectious triggers have been investigated, and *Borrelia burgdorferi* has been isolated from a substantial subset of LS biopsies in Europe but not in the United States [56].

Patients with LS have been shown to have a higher incidence of associated autoimmune disorders than in control populations [56, 60]. In a large case-controlled series, nearly one-third of patients with LS (28%) had at least one autoimmune-associated disease, including thyroid disease, vitiligo, alopecia areata, celiac disease, and rheumatoid arthritis [42].

The diagnosis of LS carries with it an associated risk of developing squamous cell carcinoma. The risk of developing carcinoma is estimated at 2–5%, with differentiated vulvar intraepithelial neoplasia (d-VIN) thought to represent an important precursor lesion (see differential diagnosis section below). The average time between diagnosis of LS and diagnosis of squamous cell carcinoma is 18 years [56]. Importantly, LS and the associated risks of dysplasia and carcinoma are unrelated to infection with human papillomavirus [63].

Management of patients diagnosed with LS is multifactorial. Vulvar self-examination and routine gynecologic examination is important. Management consists of avoidance of irritants, topical emollients, and ultrapotent topical corticosteroids. Steroid-resistant LS has been managed with calcineurin inhibitors, topical retinoids, and photodynamic therapy [56]. Early diagnosis, early treatment, and treatment compliance have all been associated with improved symptomatology, decreased scarring, and prevention of disease progression [56]. Given the risk of progression to squamous cell carcinoma, routine examination and low threshold for biopsy is mandatory.

2.4.2.1 Clinical Features

Characterized clinically by white, parchment paper-like atrophy and obliteration of normal vulvar landmarks (Fig. 2.14), LS imparts considerable morbidity to patients. LS has a fairly classic clinical appearance when well established in the course of the disease; early manifestations may be more difficult to discern as there may be overlap with other entities. LS occurs most commonly on the labia majora and labia minora but also frequently involves the clitoris and perineum. In contrast to lichen planus, the vagina and cervix are not involved by LS. Classic descriptors of the appearance of well-established LS include "figure of eight," which refers to the combined involvement of the labia minora and majora, clitoris and clitoral hood, perineum, and perianal areas [56]. Lesions initially appear as ivory to white (or porcelain), flat-topped lichenoid papules. Lesions may be single and small or can involve the entire vulva and extend to involve the perineal area and inner thighs [60]. With time, the cutaneous appearance becomes more atrophic, hypopigmented, and sclerotic. Secondary fissuring, erosions, ulcerations, and lichenifica-

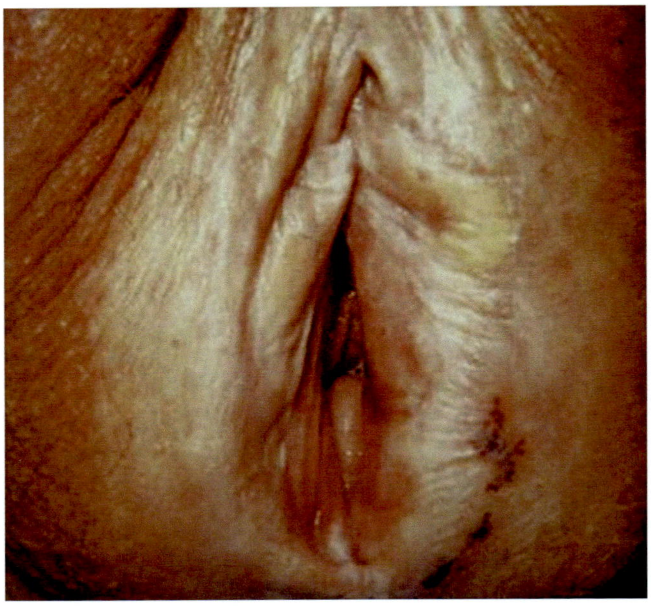

Fig. 2.14 Lichen sclerosus (well developed). White atrophic plaques encircling the vulva and obliterating normal vulvar architecture is present. There is hemorrhage into the plaques (bottom right)

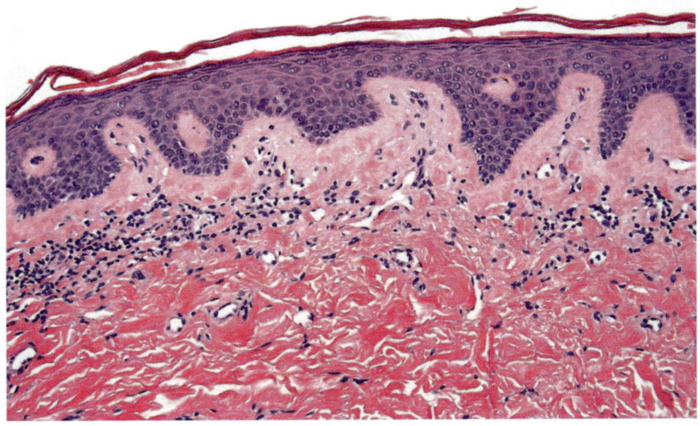

Fig. 2.15 Lichen sclerosus. The epidermal architecture is relatively preserved but there is papillary dermal homogenization with a slight band of lymphocytes in the dermis

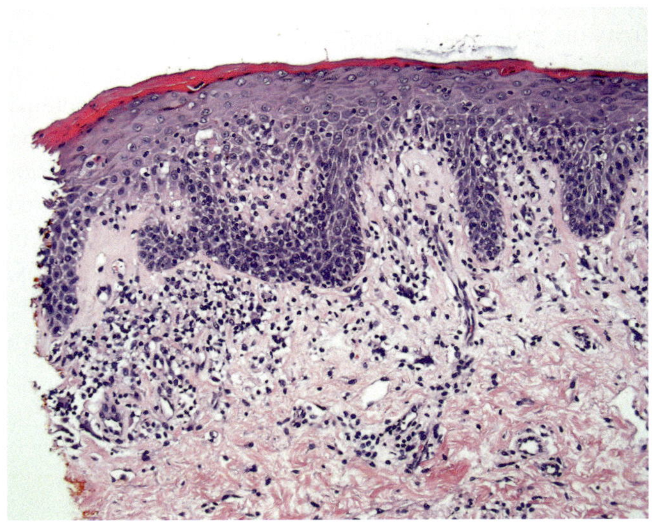

Fig. 2.16 Inflammatory phase of lichen sclerosus. There is vacuolar interface change with occasional dyskeratosis in the epidermis. There is very focal homogenized collagen in the papillary dermal tips (upper right), which suggests early lichen sclerosus

tion are not uncommon. Vascular fragility may give rise to purpura and ecchymoses. Fissures and ulcerations may occur in the interlabial sulci or in the perineum [56]. Pigmentary alterations are not uncommon, and hyperpigmentation from vulvar hypermelanosis may be mistaken for a melanocytic neoplasm [61]. Over time, there may be distortion of regional anatomy, with resorption and fusion of the labia minora, stenosis of the vaginal introitus, and entrapment of the clitoris [56].

Although LS may occur at extragenital sites, extragenital manifestations are not common, and disease is often restricted to the vulva. Examination of nongenital skin may therefore be unrevealing. Oral disease or nail abnormalities are not typically seen, in contrast to lichen planus.

The appearance of thick and irregular white plaques or new ulcers and erosions in a patient with LS may herald the presence of an associated squamous cell carcinoma and should prompt biopsy [60], although the hypertrophic variant of LS may also have this clinical appearance [62].

2.4.2.2 Histologic Features

LS has a range of histologic features depending on the time course in which it is biopsied. Early in the disease, there is a lichenoid band of inflammation aligning along the dermal–epidermal junction. As the disease becomes more established, this band of inflammation is pushed down into the deep papillary/superficial reticular dermis and replaced by increasing amounts of the diagnostic hyalinized eosinophilic collagen. The spectrum of changes that may be encountered in LS is detailed below.

Early LS

Biopsies of early LS show a blend of a lichenoid and vaguely psoriasiform inflammatory reaction pattern. The lichenoid infiltrate is composed predominantly of lymphocytes and may be mild (limited to perivascular inflammation and lymphocyte scatter between collagen bundles) to band-like. There may be vacuolar interface alteration involving basilar keratinocytes, and occasional dyskeratosis may be noted. The epidermis in LS may be atrophic, and there is often overlying hyperkeratosis. Requisite for the diagnosis of LS is the deposition of homogenized eosinophilic papillary dermal collagen (Fig. 2.15). This material may be only very focal (or not at all visible) in very early cases of LS

(Fig. 2.16), and thus diagnosis at this early stage may be difficult. When sclerosis is not prominent or even absent (estimated in one study to occur in about 40% of biopsies of LS), the most helpful clues to arriving at the correct diagnosis include minute foci of homogenized tissue in dermal papillae, marked thickening of individual papillary dermal collagen fibers, and thickening of the papillary dermis as a whole, with lymphocytes aligned linearly between wiry collagen fibers [3, 64]. Basement membrane zone thickening has been suggested as a clue helpful to differentiate LS (present) from LP (absent) [54]. Of note, some authors have suggested that even lesions of long clinical standing may demonstrate this psoriasiform and lichenoid pattern, and thus designation of "early" LS may be misleading [62, 64]. Biopsies demonstrating the features described above may have significant histologic overlap with other entities. It may therefore be necessary (and in the patient's best interest [2]) to avoid assigning a definitive diagnosis if there are insufficient features for an unequivocal diagnosis. Reports may be signed out as "Lichenoid dermatitis," with a comment indicating that the differential includes the early inflammatory phase of LS, as well as other entities such as lichen planus, fixed drug eruption, or even spongiotic dermatitis.

Late LS

Biopsies of established LS have relatively classic and distinctive features. The epidermis may be atrophic or acanthotic, and there may be subtle basal vacuolar change along the dermal–epidermal junction. There is often compact hyperkeratosis and follicular hyperkeratosis. The rete ridges of the epidermis often become effaced, which ultimately can result in detachment of the epidermis from the dermis. In one large series evaluating LS, approximately 60% of cases were found to have the characteristic broad papillary dermal homogenization [64]. This altered dermal collagen lacks cellularity and appears amorphous. Blood vessels may become fixed within the sclerosis, resulting in fragility and easy disruption with subsequent hemorrhage (Fig. 2.17). Evidence of remote hemorrhage may be seen in scattered hemosiderin laden macrophages in the dermis.

Pushed down below the sclerotic papillary dermal collagen is generally a lymphocyte-rich infiltrate. Sparse perivascular and interstitial lymphocytes or a dense band of lymphocytes may be seen. Eosinophils are never a large component of the infiltrate, but may be seen, possibly indicating an associated hypersensitivity component [3]. Together, all of these features impart a zonal appearance to the biopsy that has been termed the red, white, and blue sign (Fig. 2.18): epidermis (pink or red), band of sclerosis (white), and band of inflammation (blue).

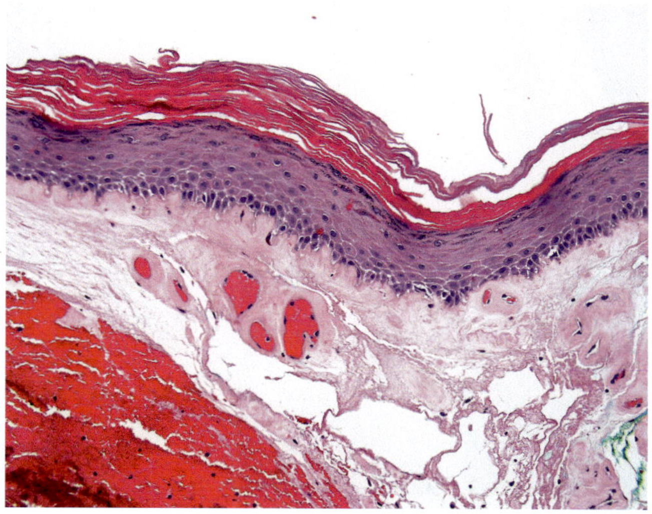

Fig. 2.17 Long-standing lichen sclerosus. There is attenuation of the epidermal rete ridge pattern, hyperkeratosis, and a broad band of homogenized dermal collagen with entrapped dilated vessels. Inflammation is minimal

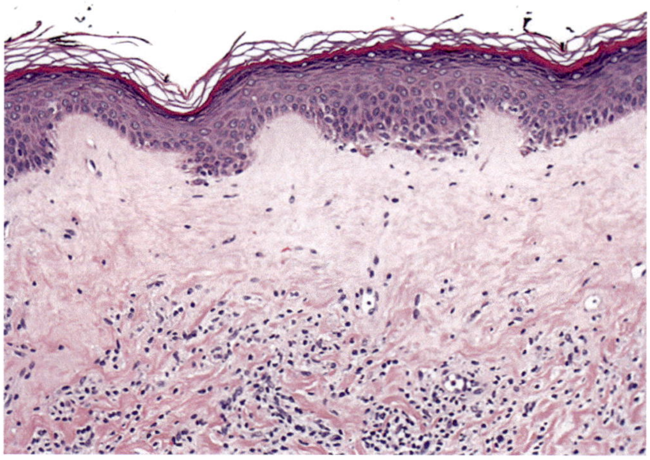

Fig. 2.18 Lichen sclerosus: the red, white, and blue sign. The zonal appearance in classic lichen sclerosus shows epidermis (pink or red) on top of a band of sclerosis (white) with underlying band of inflammation (blue). Photo provided courtesy of previous edition in Chinese (Science Press, Beijing, China)

Hypertropic LS

The hypertrophic variant of LS may have epidermal thickening (acanthosis), hypergranulosis, and orthokeratosis rather than the more usual epidermal atrophy (Fig. 2.19). This may in part arise due to repetitive rubbing and scratching of lesions of LS. While dyskeratosis and parakeratosis in such specimens are permissible and do not seem to pose an increased risk of progression to SCC, hypertrophic LS should not show nuclear atypia, basal cell crowding and disarray, or increased mitotic activity [62]. Parakeratosis, when seen, is often present in vertical columns. Hypertrophic LS is less likely to have obvious, well-defined dermal sclerosis and may appear more fibrotic.

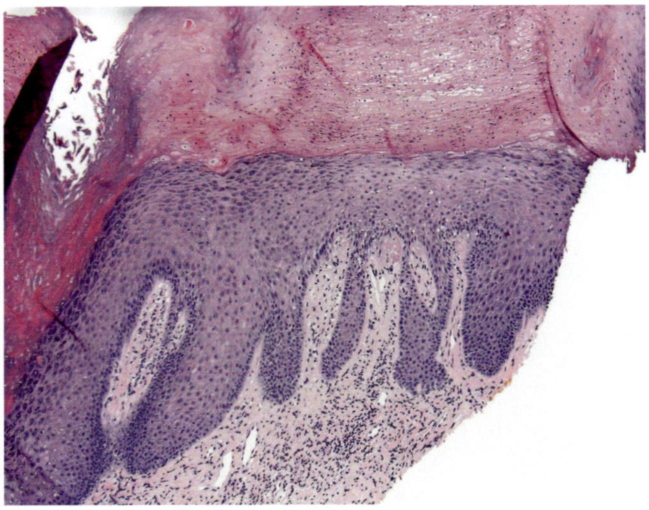

Fig. 2.19 Hypertrophic lichen sclerosus. Marked epithelial hyperplasia, columns of parakeratosis, and focal homogenization of collagen in papillary dermal tips

2.4.2.3 Immunohistochemical Features

Immunohistochemical staining is not required for the diagnosis of LS. Special stains may be utilized if there are features that suggest the possibility of coexistent infection. The use of elastic tissue stains may be helpful to establish loss of papillary dermal elastic fibers. In the author's experience, and as might be expected, the most robust loss of elastic fibers is seen in established lesions, where the diagnosis is less often in question. Immunohistochemical studies have identified a Th1 cytokine profile in the inflammatory milieu of LS (increased staining for IFN-γ, TNF-α, IL-1, CD25, IL-11a), but these stains are not routinely used in establishing the diagnosis and patterns are shared with other inflammatory disorders [65]. Tissue matrix metalloproteinases (MMP) and their inhibitors have been investigated as important to the collagen remodeling and sclerosis that occurs in LS, and MMP 2 and 9 have been shown to be increased by immunohistochemistry in biopsies of LS [66].

2.4.2.4 Differential Diagnosis

The differential diagnosis of LS varies depending on whether one is considering an early or established lesion. Early LS and lichen planus (LP) have considerable overlap both histologically and clinically and comprise one of the most important differentials. Histologic distinction between early LS and LP is known to be difficult (Table 2.5). Basal keratinocyte squamatization, hypergranulosis, pointed (rather than effaced) rete ridges, and cytoid bodies are all seen much more frequently in LP than in early LS [54]. However, another study examining histologic features specifically of vulvar LP noted the relative rarity of these features [2]. It has been suggested that wiry fibrosis and eosinophils within the infiltrate may favor LS over LP [3], and the presence of basement membrane thickening, ectatic superficial dermal blood vessels, and early subtle sclerosis have been described as helpful in discriminating between LS (where the features were seen) and LP (where the features were absent) [2]. Elastic fiber loss in the subepithelial space has been suggested as a helpful and differentiating feature in the diagnosis of LS [54], but other authors have reported similar elastic fiber loss in LP as well [2, 64]. Melanophages may be more common in LP than in LS [64]. Ultimately, if a confident diagnosis cannot be made, the diagnosis of "lichenoid dermatitis/mucositis" may be made, with a comment detailing that the differential diagnosis includes both LP and the inflammatory phase of early LS.

Other entities within the differential diagnosis of early LS include psoriasis, lichen simplex chronicus (LSC), irritant or allergic contact dermatitis, candidiasis, and mycosis fungoides (cutaneous T-cell lymphoma). Psoriasis and LSC in particular have considerable overlap with the hypertrophic variant of LS. Careful examination for the subtle, early papillary dermal homogenization will secure the appropriate diagnosis of LS. LSC generally lacks a lichenoid infiltrate in the dermis and the columns of vertical parakeratosis that can be seen in hypertrophic LS [62]. Psoriasis demonstrates suprapapillary thinning, hypogranulosis, and intraepidermal neutrophils. Irritant or allergic contact dermatitis shows less pronounced and less regular epidermal hyperplasia, more spongiosis and a polymorphous infiltrate in the dermis. Mycosis fungoides generally lacks dyskeratosis within the epidermis and in the best case scenario will show lymphocyte atypia.

The histologic differential diagnosis of established LS includes other sclerosing disorders of the skin, namely morphea, radiation dermatitis, and sclerodermoid graft-versus-host disease. Morphea is a sclerosing disorder of the reticular dermis and subcutis, in contrast to the sclerosis of the papillary dermis that typifies LS. In morphea, swollen collagen bundles replace adnexal structures and infiltrate into the subcutis, without an increase in the number of fibroblasts. Chronic radiation dermatitis has considerable overlap with LS but in general tends to have less inflammation, prominent dilated vessels, and stellate hyperchromatic fibroblasts. Radiation dermatitis can also extend more deeply into the reticular dermis than LS. Sclerodermoid graft-versus-host disease may be virtually indistinguishable although may extend more deeply into the reticular dermis and arises in the specific clinical setting of a prior hematopoietic stem cell transplant.

When evaluating a biopsy for LS, care should be taken to evaluate for the possibility of coexistent or background differentiated vulvar neoplasia (d-VIN). d-VIN is a precursor of vulvar squamous cell carcinoma (SCC). d-VIN is unrelated to human papilloma virus infection and is thought to arise through a p53-dependent pathway. d-VIN is recognized by elongated, sometimes anastomosing rete ridges, with keratinocyte atypia (atypical mitotic figures, dyskeratosis, nuclear enlargement, and prominent nucleoli) restricted to the basal layer. Although parakeratosis is present, the squamous epithelium appears overall mature and may be confused with reactive epithelial atypia on low-power evaluation. Retrospective review of a cohort of biopsies from patients with LS who ultimately progressed to SCC led to revised diagnoses of d-VIN in 42%, leading authors to speculate that d-VIN is underdiagnosed in biopsies of LS [67]. The authors also noted that in biopsies from patients whose biopsies showed LS without meeting criteria for d-VIN but who ultimately progressed to squamous cell carcinoma, parakeratosis, dyskeratosis, hyperplasia, and basal cell atypia were more often noted [67], although this conclusion has been called into question by another study [62]. Of note, by immunohistochemistry, d-VIN often shows diffuse confluent staining for p53 (basal and suprabasilar layer only) but rarely exhibits a null pattern of reactivity (no p53 staining) compared to weak patchy (wild type) staining of non-lesional epithelium. However, inflammation and stress can prolong the half-life of the p53 protein and result in a positive staining pattern [68]. Therefore, a positive p53 stain should be interpreted in the proper clinical and histomorphologic context.

2.4.3 Plasma Cell (Zoon) Vulvitis

Plasma cell vulvitis (PCV) has also been named Zoon vulvitis or vulvitis plasmacellularis. First described as a disorder affecting mucosal surfaces of the uncircumcised penis (Zoon balanitis), subsequent reports documented similar presentations and corresponding histologic features at other mucosal sites, including the vulva. The term "idiopathic lymphoplasmacellular mucositis-dermatitis" has been proposed as a unifying terminology for similar conditions now reported on virtually all mucosal sites [55]. PCV has been suggested to represent a mucosal reaction pattern to chronic irritation, moisture, and friction [69]. Poor hygiene and perspiration have also been proposed as predisposing factors and at least one author has postulated an autoimmune reaction to a yet unidentified mucosal antigen [70].

The disorder most often presents in middle age females but wide ranges of age presentation have been reported [69, 71]. There is frequently a significant (several year) delay in diagnosis, speculated to be due to a combination of patient factors and unfamiliarity of physicians with the condition [71].

PCV is thought to be idiopathic and patients generally lack associated diseases or syndromes, although rarely PCV has been reported in the setting of autoimmune polyglandular endocrine failure [70], hypothyroidism [72], and lichen sclerosus [73]. PCV does not seem to indicate a risk of transformation to or subsequent development of squamous cell carcinoma.

Treatment of PCV is often difficult. Topical steroids have been suggested as beneficial [72, 74], as has imiquimod [73]. In some patients, lesions persist over years but slow resolution without treatment is possible [1].

2.4.3.1 Clinical Features

Patients present most often complaining of pruritus, burning, and dyspareunia; however, a minority of patients may be asymptomatic [69, 71]. Patient-reported symptoms are frequently severe and may affect quality of life [71].

Clinically, lesions may present singly or as multiple bright red, red-orange to red-brown, well-circumscribed glistening or shiny erythematous macules or patches [69, 71] (Fig. 2.20). Erosions, epithelial friability, and the presence of pinpoint "cayenne pepper" petechial spots may sometimes be seen and are supportive of the diagnosis. Only mucosal-lined vulvar surfaces are involved, with one series reporting sites of common involvement to include (in order of decreasing frequency) the introitus, inner face of the labia minora, the periurethral area, vulvar vestibule, and clitoris [71]. Multifocal involvement of the vulva does not necessarily correlate with increasing severity of symptoms.

The clinical differential diagnosis may include squamous intraepithelial neoplasia, squamous cell carcinoma, extramammary Paget disease, blistering disorders, infectious etiologies, erosive lichen planus, and fixed drug eruption. Given this differential diagnosis, clinicians should have a low

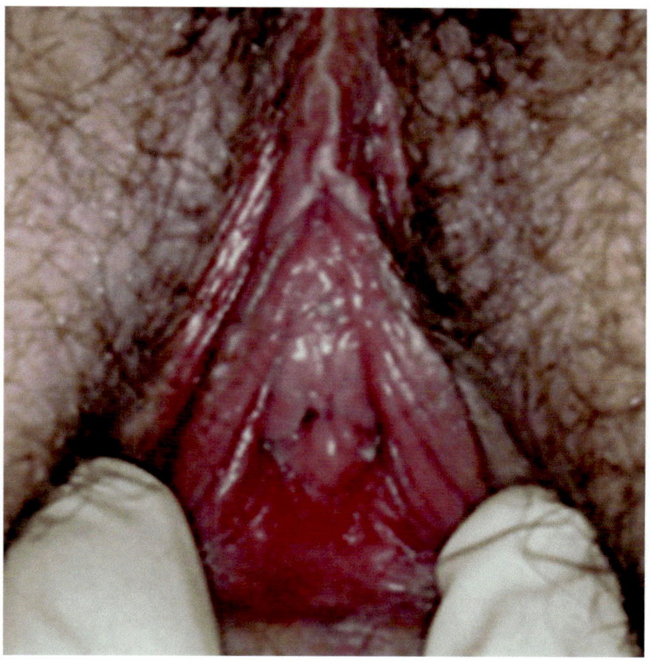

Fig. 2.20 Plasma cell vulvitis. A glistening red patch on vulvar mucosa. Photo provided courtesy of previous edition in Chinese (Science Press, Beijing, China)

threshold for biopsy, which will readily be able to ascertain the presence or absence of cancer. Distinction between other entities which have some histologic overlap are discussed further in the section below.

2.4.3.2 Histopathologic Features

Low-power histopathologic examination reveals an attenuated mucosal epithelium with a dense band of inflammation obscuring the mucosal/submucosal junction. Epithelial atrophy is seen commonly (in approximately two-thirds of cases), but occasionally acanthosis can be present [55] (Fig. 2.21). Erosion of the epithelium is more often visualized than frank ulceration (Fig. 2.22). Higher power examination may show focal vacuolar change at the mucosal-submucosal junction, exocytosis of neutrophils into the epithelium, and diamond- or "lozenge"-shaped keratinocytes in the suprabasal layer (Fig. 2.23). The lozenge-shaped keratinocyte was defined as a diamond-shaped suprabasilar keratinocyte that is wider than it is tall [55]. The frequency of identifying these distinctive keratinocytes in PCV ranges from rare to approximately 50% [55, 75]. Within the dermis/submucosa of PCV, there is consistently a dense band-like infiltrate rich in plasma cells. Admixed neutrophils, eosinophils, lymphocytes, and mast cells may be present, but the majority of the cells (greater than or equal to 50%) should be plasma cells. Intermediate numbers of plasma cells (25–50%) with additional supportive histologic features and a congruent clinical impression are permissible, but fewer than 25% plasma cells has generally been found to be nonspecific and site related and thus should draw into question the diagnosis of PCV [75]. Erythrocyte extravasation and hemosiderin deposition is a frequently identified feature, leading some authors to postulate a relationship to pigmented purpura and lichen aureus in particular [69]. Vasculature may be prominent with dilated vessels, and fibrosis may be appreciated [55, 74]. Occasionally, mucinous metaplasia has been reported in the epithelium, which can lead to erroneous diagnosis of extramammary Paget disease if the pathologist is unaware of this phenomenon in PCV [76]. Mucinous metaplasia, when present in PCV, shows a uniform replacement of the normal epithelium, no cytologic atypia, and no pagetoid spread of mucin-containing cells, thus helping to differentiate it from Paget disease [76].

In reality, all of the above-described features may not be identified. The most consistently present features of PCV

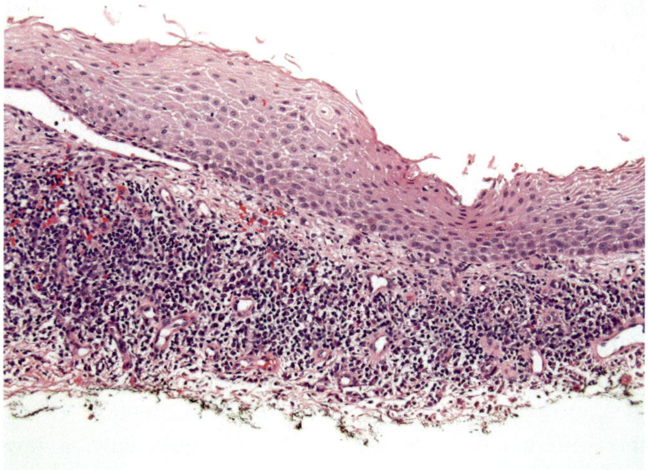

Fig. 2.21 Plasma cell vulvitis. Mucosal epithelium with an underlying band of inflammation rich in plasma cells is present. Dermal hemorrhage can also be appreciated

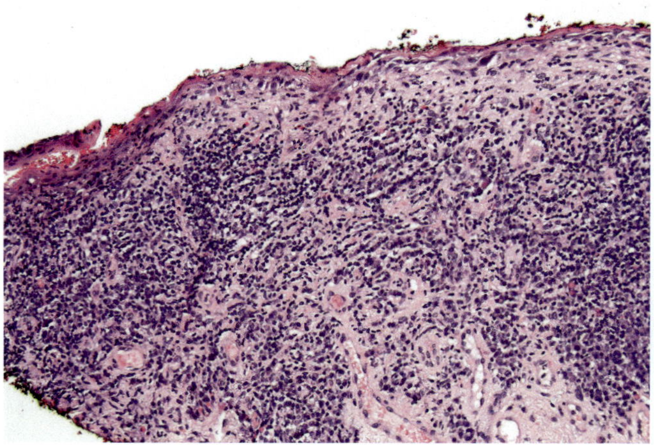

Fig. 2.22 Plasma cell vulvitis. Mucosal erosion or ulceration is commonly present in plasma cell vulvitis. The inflammatory infiltrate in the dermis is almost exclusively plasma cells

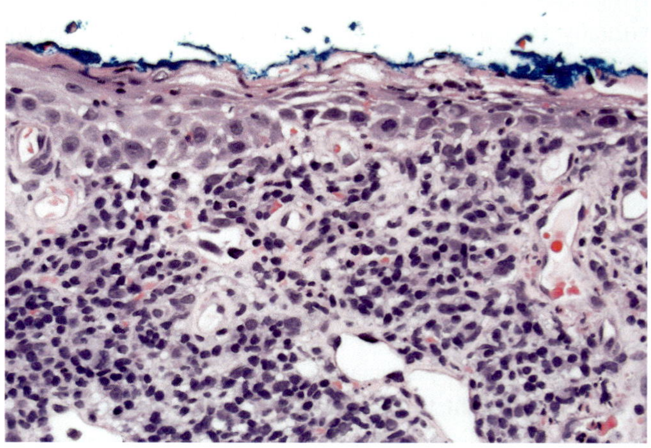

Fig. 2.23 Plasma cell vulvitis. High-power magnification reveals occasional "lozenge-shaped" keratinocytes, suprabasilar keratinocytes wider than they are tall

include the dense band of polyclonal plasma cells admixed with other inflammatory cell types and erythrocyte extravasation with hemosiderin deposition. More variable in their presence, but helpful features when present, include the distinctive lozenge-shaped keratinocytes and epithelial erosion or ulcer [55, 75].

2.4.3.3 Immunohistochemical Features

Ancillary testing in the evaluation of PCV involves exclusion of infectious etiologies. This may be accomplished by immunohistochemical staining for herpes virus and treponemal organisms, and PAS or GMS stains to exclude a fungal infection. An iron stain (Prussian blue or Perl's) may be useful to confirm the impression of hemosiderin deposition but is not requisite. If there is histologic concern for a plasma cell neoplasm, immunohistochemical stains or in situ hybridization should reveal a polytypic mix of kappa- and lambda-expressing light chains.

2.4.3.4 Differential Diagnosis

The histologic differential diagnosis includes lichen planus, other lichenoid dermatoses, infections (syphilis, Lyme, and herpes, among others), and contact dermatitis.

While lichen planus and PCV share a dense band-like infiltrate, lichen planus generally shows a lymphocyte predominant infiltrate, and the presence of Civatte bodies in lichen planus will be a distinguishing feature not seen in PCV [55]. In one series comparing the two entities, the presence of Civatte bodies, lymphocyte predominance, and an accentuation of the granular layer were all noted in lichen planus but lacking in PCV [55].

Syphilis typically demonstrates a plasma-cell-rich infiltrate. This possibility can and should be excluded with immunohistochemistry for *Treponema pallidum* and recommendations to the clinician to correlate with serological and laboratory data.

In cases with intermediate numbers of plasma cells (20–50%) and the absence of readily identifiable hemosiderin deposition, it may be more prudent to offer a descriptive diagnosis of lichenoid mucositis with a differential diagnosis to include PCV, lichen planus, fixed drug eruption, or a lichenoid contact reaction.

2.4.4 Other Diseases with a Lichenoid and Interface Pattern

Other diseases may demonstrate a lichenoid or interface inflammatory reaction pattern. They are mentioned here briefly for completeness. Histologically they may demonstrate identical features ranging from focal interface alteration and rare dyskeratosis to full thickness epidermal necrosis with a variable dermal infiltrate.

2.4.4.1 Erythema Multiforme, Stevens Johnson Syndrome, and Toxic Epidermal Necrolysis

Entities such as erythema multiforme (EM), Stevens Johnson syndrome (SJS), and toxic epidermal necrolysis (TEN) exist on a clinical spectrum defined by the clinical appearance, the involvement of mucosal surfaces, and the percent of body area affected by blistering or desquamation. EM is a rash with targetoid to blistering appearing clinical lesions and may be precipitated by infection (herpes virus or *Mycoplasma* infections are classic offenders) or by exposure to a drug. SJS and TEN are life-threatening blistering disorders often due to an adverse drug effect, presenting clinically with widespread erythema progressing to desquamation of the skin and mucosa. About 75% of patients with TEN will have genital lesions, with the vulva involved more often than the vagina [77]. Significant loss of full thickness epidermis puts affected patients at risk for water loss, temperature instability, and infection, which comprises the major causes of morbidity and mortality. The vulva may be involved in EM, SJS, or TEN, but as there is usually other skin and mucosal involvement, it would be an unusual choice to biopsy the vulva to establish the diagnosis [23]. EM is generally self-limited, and SJS/TEN are treated supportively after removal of any identifiable inciting drug. Long-term scarring sequelae may result from severe SJS and TEN, but fortunately is seen in only a minority of patients [77]. Adenosis (the presence of glandular epithelium in the surface epithelium) has been reported following SJS and TEN [78, 79].

2.4.4.2 Graft-Versus-Host Disease

Graft-versus-host disease (GVHD) arises in the setting of post hematopoietic stem cell transplant and may be acute (fewer than 100 days after transplant) or chronic (greater than 100 days after transplant). It results when donor lymphocytes recognize the host tissue as foreign and generally affects the skin, gastrointestinal tract, liver, and lung. Genital involvement is estimated to occur in approximately one-quarter to one-half of patients with GVHD [80, 81], although the disease is often under-recognized despite its considerable impact on patients' quality of life [82]. Most gynecologic complications arise between 7 months to 1 year after transplant, presenting with symptoms that include vulvar dryness, irritation and pain, and dyspareunia [1, 80]. Clinically, genital involvement by GVHD presents on a spectrum with erythema in mild cases and labial fusion, scarring and vaginal stenosis in severe cases. The vulva is usually affected before the vagina. Individual lesions can mimic both lichen sclerosus and lichen planus clinically, as pale, hypopigmented atrophic plaques or white reticulated patches, respectively [82]. Ulcerations, fissuring, and erosive plaques are signs of greater severity. While vulvar GVHD usually arises in concert with extragenital manifestations, rarely genital GVHD may occur in isolation [82].

Early detection and treatment with topical immunosuppressants and estrogens decrease the long-term severe sequelae [83]. Routine gynecological exams are of importance as posttransplant patients are at increased risk of human papilloma virus and subsequent cervical cancer. Use of immunosuppressive therapy also predisposes patients to other genital infections, such as herpes virus and *Candida* [82].

2.4.4.3 Fixed Drug Eruption

Fixed drug eruption (FDE) is a peculiar specific drug reaction whereby systemic ingestion of a drug leads to a reproducible mucocutaneous reaction. Clinically, one or several well-demarcated annular plaques appear after ingestion of a triggering drug, most often anti-inflammatory drugs (nonsteroidal anti-inflammatory drugs), antibiotics, and sedatives [23]. Any mucosal or cutaneous site may be involved, with women having a high incidence of FDE on distal extremities, while men have a high rate of FDE on genital skin and mucosa [84]. Genital sites are thought to comprise about 20% of FDEs [23]. Vulvar involvement is not uncommon, with both vulvar keratinized skin and mucosa being affected by FDE. In one series of vulvar FDE, women ranged in age from 15 to 84 at presentation [85]. Classically, FDE presents as round erythematous lesions, but on the vulva lesions may be bilaterally symmetric, erosive and non-pigmenting making it more difficult to recognize [1, 85]. FDE is usually locally symptomatic, with patients complaining of intense itching, stinging, or burning at the site of inflammation [23].

FDE is a Type IV hypersensitivity reaction, so the first presentation of FDE may be several weeks after exposure to an offending drug, but subsequent drug exposures shorten the latency to lesion development. In one study, lesions appeared on average 2 days after exposure to the drug [84]. With removal of the drug, the inflammation dissipates but classically leaves residual hyperpigmentation; however, post-inflammatory hyperpigmentation is less common in the vulva [85]. Reexposure to the drug results in inflammation in the same anatomic location as previously. Overall, a high index of suspicion is required to diagnose FDE as the clinical signs and histology may be relatively nonspecific, post-inflammatory pigmentation may not be present in the vulva, and a link to the offending medication may not be recognized. Once identified as a FDE, treatment involves removal of the triggering drug.

2.4.4.4 Histologic Features

The histopathologic features for EM, SJS, TEN, GVHD, and FDE are remarkably similar and thus considered together. They also show histologic overlap with previously discussed entities such as early lichen sclerosus, lichen planus, and plasma cell vulvitis. There is vacuolar interface dermatitis with orthokeratosis (parakeratosis is generally absent). Dying keratinocytes are peppered throughout the epidermis. The degree of dyskeratosis may range from focal and only apparent upon careful, high power evaluation (as in low-grade, acute GVHD) to moderate (as in classic examples of EM and FDE) (Fig. 2.24) to extensive (as in classic SJS/TEN). In low-grade acute GVHD, dyskeratosis may be very focal; more severe clinical examples are associated with more extensive cytotoxicity to keratinocytes. Satellite cell necrosis (the presence of lymphocytes surrounding a dying keratinocyte in the epidermis) is a buzzword for GVHD, but the finding is not specific nor always identified. With sufficient damage to keratinocytes, there may be formation of a subepidermal blister and full thickness necrosis of the epidermis (Fig. 2.25). Complete loss of the epidermis may lead to an appearance of nonspecific ulceration with or without

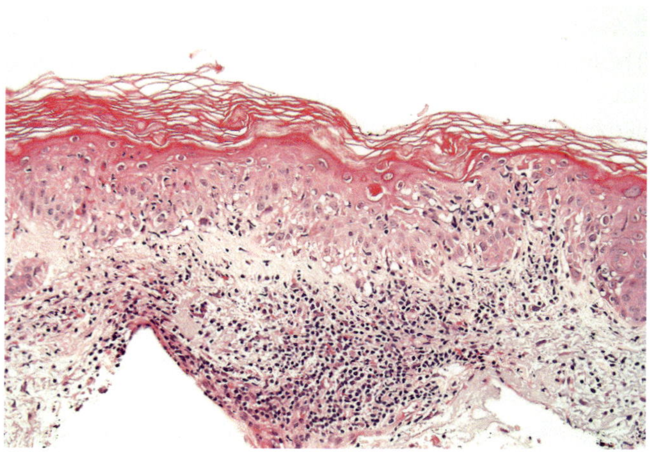

Fig. 2.24 Interface dermatitis. This is an example of erythema multiforme, showing dyskeratosis at all levels of the epidermis, orthokeratosis, and a moderate dermal inflammatory infiltrate

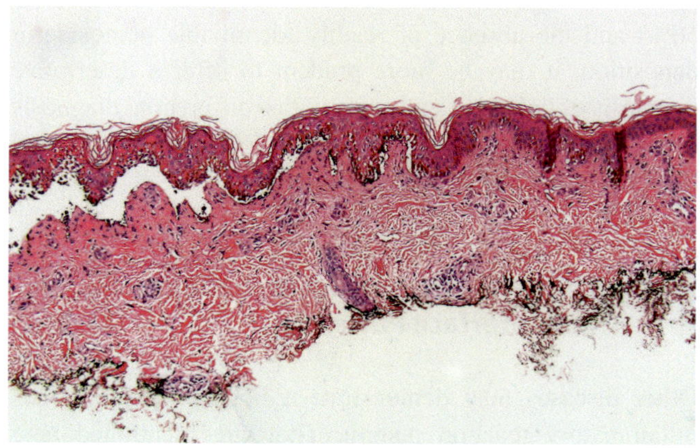

Fig. 2.25 Interface dermatitis. Cytotoxic damage to the epidermis has resulted in a subepidermal blister in this case of Stevens Johnson syndrome/toxic epidermal necrolysis. The dermis is almost devoid of inflammation

dermal inflammation. Nonspecific and nondiagnostic biopsies are common in vulvar FDE [85].

Within the dermis of these entities there may be sparse to robust inflammatory infiltrate. SJS/TEN and GVHD tend to have a sparse inflammatory dermal infiltrate. EM generally has more inflammation and FDE, particularly if active, has a more florid mixed inflammatory infiltrate comprised of lymphocytes, histiocytes, eosinophils, and neutrophils. The infiltrate in FDE can extend more deeply than EM and other lichenoid/interface dermatoses. The paradoxical presence of orthokeratosis (signifying acute onset) at the same time melanophages are prominent in the dermis (suggesting chronicity) is sometimes a clue to FDE, although in the vulva these changes may not be present as post-inflammatory pigmentation is usually minimal or absent at this site (Fig. 2.26).

Of note, in EM/SJS/TEN, the degree of epidermal damage and inflammation does not always correlate with the clinical severity of disease; this author has seen full thickness epidermal necrosis in EM and only moderate dyskeratosis in biopsies clinically compatible with TEN. In the author's opinion, the best way to handle such biopsies is to report "Interface dermatitis, compatible with the clinical spectrum of EM/SJS/TEN." Similarly, a biopsy of GVHD can support the diagnosis but is rarely in and of itself fully diagnostic. Acute GVHD and adverse drug reactions have both clinical and histologic overlap and no histologic features have been determined to definitively distinguish between the two. The diagnosis of FDE can be made fairly confidently if there is a clinical impression of a fixed plaque that becomes inflamed with ingestion of an offending agent coupled with the above-described histology, but as mentioned above, this scenario may be uncommon at genital sites.

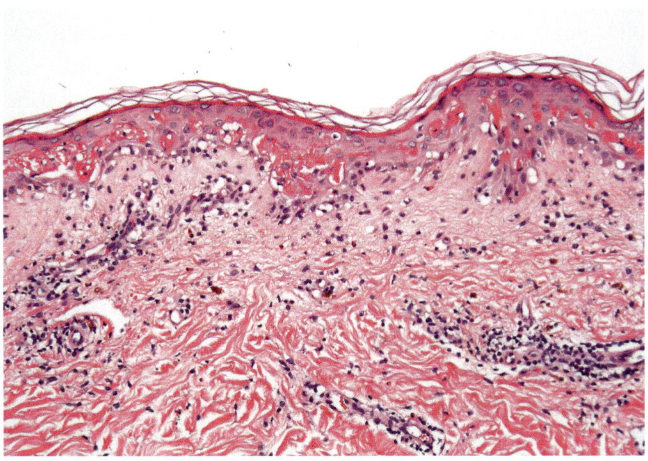

Fig. 2.26 Interface dermatitis. In this example of a fixed drug reaction, you can appreciate numerous dying keratinocytes in the epidermis. There is a sparse dermal infiltrate including neutrophils and eosinophils, and you can also appreciate some sparse melanin pigment in the dermis. Often fixed drug eruptions are more inflammatory than this case

2.4.4.5 Differential Diagnosis

The differential diagnoses for these entities include lichen planus, the inflammatory phase of lichen sclerosus, plasma cell vulvitis, and autoimmune-mediated blistering disorders. In lichen planus, dying keratinocytes are generally confined to the lower levels of the epidermis, and the infiltrate is brisk, with saw-tooth rete ridges and overlying hypergranulosis. The inflammatory phase of lichen sclerosus may have considerable overlap, but if homogenization of dermal collagen can be identified, even focally, the diagnosis can be favored. Lichen sclerosus also less likely presents as erosive or blistering plaques, so clinical impression may be useful if available in parsing out the differential. Plasma cell vulvitis will have a plasma-cell-rich infiltrate without epidermal necrosis or dyskeratosis. Autoimmune blistering diseases will show blister formation (intra- or subepidermal) without interface dermatitis or dyskeratosis. Positive direct immunofluorescence studies are useful to confirm the diagnosis (see Sect. 2.5).

2.5 Blistering Diseases and Acantholytic Disorders Affecting the Vulva

Blistering diseases and acantholytic processes generally result from a defect in normal adhesion between keratinocytes. The adhesion between keratinocytes and the dermis may also be abnormal and result in a blistering process. Most acquired blistering diseases affecting the vulva are in the pemphigus family of diseases (including pemphigus vulgaris and pemphigus vegetans, both discussed more in depth below) and are autoimmune-mediated with targets against cell–cell adhesion molecules. Blistering diseases can also result in subepithelial blisters, as in mucous membrane (cicatricial) pemphigoid or linear IgA bullous dermatosis. Acantholytic disorders are generally inherited due to a genetic defect in similar proteins involved in cellular adhesion. Pertinent details distinguishing diseases with a blistering reaction pattern are detailed in Table 2.6.

2.5.1 Intraepidermal Blistering Diseases: Pemphigus Vulgaris, Pemphigus Foliaceous, and Pemphigus Vegetans

Pemphigus vulgaris (PV) and its related variants pemphigus foliaceous (PF) and pemphigus vegetans (PVeg) are diseases with considerable morbidity which greatly affect patient's quality of life. Vulvar involvement, including the vulvar skin and mucosa, is relatively common in patients with PV and PVeg, whereas PF only rarely involves genital mucosa. The genital tract is thought to be the second most affected site (after oral mucosa) in PV, found in approximately one-third

Table 2.6 Blistering disorders affecting the vulva

Disorder	Clinical presentation	Autoimmune mediated?	Histologic features	Direct immunofluorescence results
Pemphigus Vulgaris	Flaccid blisters and erosions Mucous membrane involvement common	Yes	Suprabasilar acantholysis (intraepidermal blister)	Intercellular staining of keratinocytes by IgG and C3
Pemphigus Foliaceous	Superficial erosions of cutaneous skin; mucous membrane involvement unusual	Yes	Acantholysis in the corneal or granular layer	Intercellular staining of keratinocytes by IgG and C3
Pemphigus Vegetans	Verrucous plaques with maceration in intertriginous areas	Yes	Intraepidermal blister with acanthosis and eosinophilic microabscesses; acantholysis may be only focal	Intercellular staining of keratinocytes by IgG and C3
Mucous Membrane Pemphigoid	Tense blisters on an erythematous base Healing with scarring Vulvar involvement common, along with oral and conjunctiva	Yes	Subepidermal blister with eosinophils Subepithelial scarring possible	Linear IgG and C3 deposited along basement membrane zone
Bullous pemphigoid	Tense blisters on an erythematous base Vulvar involvement unusual	Yes	Subepidermal blister with eosinophils	Linear IgG and C3 deposited along basement membrane zone
Linear IgA bullous dermatosis	Annular lesions clustered with rimming by blisters or crusting	Yes	Subepidermal blister with neutrophils	Linear IgA (±C3) deposited along basement membrane zone
Hailey–Hailey disease	Intertriginous papules and plaques with maceration and erosion	No	Full thickness epidermal acantholysis; dyskeratosis unusual	Negative
Darier disease	Hyperkeratotic papules on face, chest, neck, back, ears, and groin	No	Acantholysis and dyskeratosis; corps ronds and grains; involvement of follicles	Negative
Papular Acantholytic Dykeratosis	Keratotic lesions limited to vulvar folds and upper thighs	No	Can look like Hailey Hailey disease or Darier disease	Negative

to one-half of patients with the disease [86–88]. Rarely, vulvar involvement by PV may be the sole manifestation of the disease [89]. Patients present in adulthood, with mean age of presentation generally in the early 40s to early 50s [86, 88, 90]. In some studies, women are slightly more commonly affected [90], while other studies note similar incidences in men and women [88].

Desmosomes are a multi-protein complex located on cell surface membranes designed to ensure that keratinocytes stay connected to their neighbors. Pemphigus is an acquired, autoimmune-mediated blistering disease due to autoantibodies targeting the desmoglein proteins of the desmosome. Desmoglein 3 is the main target in PV and PVeg, while desmoglein 1 is the main target in PF. IgG autoantibodies against this/these protein(s) are generated, leading to an incompetent connection to adjacent keratinocytes and altered subsequent downstream signaling [91]. This altered downstream signaling may involve further destruction of the desmosomal protein complex [91]. The resultant loss of cell–cell adhesion results in acantholysis and an intraepidermal blister that is visualized histologically. Desmoglein 3 in particular is highly expressed in mucosal epithelium, which is why patients with PV almost always have mucosal involvement. Desmoglein 1 has lower expression in mucosal epithelium, resulting in less frequent mucosal involvement in PF.

Patients with PV (and to a much lesser degree PF) may be susceptible to infection and subsequent mortality given the loss of their protective epidermal layer. Management is complex and usually requires long-term corticosteroid treatment. As chronic steroid use is limited by a high-risk profile and side effects, additional adjuvant therapeutics may also be employed with some degree of benefit. These medications include azathioprine and cyclophosphamide (which have a steroid sparing effect), intravenous immunoglobulin (which helps with rapid, early control of disease), and mycophenolate mofetil (which seems to lengthen the time to disease relapse) [92]. Topical epidermal growth factor has been shown to help with healing of mucosal erosions [92]. Other topical treatments include soaking baths with antiseptic additives and topical corticosteroids [88].

2.5.1.1 Clinical Features

The most commonly affected gynecologic sites in pemphigus are the labia minora, labia majora, the vagina, and less commonly the cervix or clitoris [86, 87]. Lesions present as relatively superficial but painful erosions distributed on the vulvar

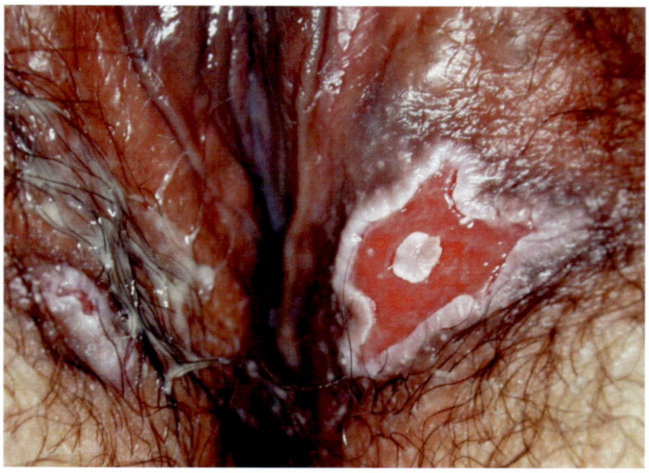

Fig. 2.27 Pemphigus vulgaris. Superficial erosions on the vulvar skin and mucosa. Photo provided courtesy of previous edition in Chinese (Science Press, Beijing, China)

skin and mucosa (Fig. 2.27). The presence of flaccid blisters may be a clue to the diagnosis but may be difficult to detect as they are generally easily ruptured leading to the more commonly visualized erosions. If there is vaginal involvement, the patient may present with a desquamative inflammatory vaginitis, complaining of symptoms such as irritation, painful sexual intercourse, and pain with increased vaginal secretions [50].

Lesions of PVeg have a verrucous or vegetative appearance. They are usually multiple in number, and clear evidence of a blister may be lacking. Lesions may appear macerated and become superinfected [89, 93].

Clinical exam should focus on evaluation of other mucosal sites for erosions and blisters. The oral cavity is almost always involved in PV, and about half of patients will have involvement of nasal mucosa. The sites of frequent cutaneous involvement include the face, scalp, and trunk [90]. Patients with PF have superficial erosions of the cutaneous skin and are less likely to involve genital mucosa. Patients with PVeg may have involvement of other intertriginous sites such as the inframammary folds or the axilla, as well as the mucosal involvement as seen in PV [94].

The clinical differential diagnosis of PV includes erosive lichen planus, Behcet disease, infections, and mucous membrane pemphigoid. The clinical differential diagnosis for PVeg includes infectious entities, including sexually transmitted diseases, some of the inherited acantholytic disorders (namely Hailey–Hailey disease and acantholytic dermatosis of the genital-crural region), noncontiguous/"metastatic" Crohn disease, and pyodermatitis vegetans. Clinical history and physical exam will help discern all of the body sites affected by disease and any associated symptoms and signs. Tissue cultures are helpful when the differential diagnosis includes infection. Biopsy is generally helpful in confirming the diagnosis of an autoimmune blistering disorder, particularly if a second sample is submitted in Michel's solution (not formalin!) for direct immunofluorescence studies.

2.5.1.2 Histologic Features

Biopsy should try to encompass non-eroded/ulcerated skin to decrease the chances of detecting nonspecific features of inflamed ulceration [50]. Whenever a blistering disease is suspected, it is recommended that a second biopsy of non-affected or perilesional skin be taken for direct immunofluorescence studies. This second biopsy should be submitted in an isotonic transport media that will stabilize proteins for immunofluorescence, such as Michel's solution or Zeus media. If such a media is not available, the biopsy can be submitted in saline but processing will need to occur within 2 days to prevent false negative results. Processing of specimens submitted in Michel's solution for direct immunofluorescence is generally recommended to occur within 5 days of biopsy, but studies have shown long-term (6 months) preservation of reproducible results [95].

Microscopically, PV demonstrates acantholysis of keratinocytes, resulting in an intraepidermal blister. Acantholysis can be recognized by the rounded borders of the keratinocytes. When the desmosomal protein complex fails, the cytoplasm tends to contract into the cell, resulting in a rounded epithelial cell with eosinophilic cytoplasm but preserved and intact nucleus. In contrast, a dyskeratotic keratinocyte may have pink and rounded cytoplasm but generally shows brighter dense pink cytoplasm and a pyknotic nucleus. Moreover, a blister resulting from spongiosis (edema) rather than acantholysis tends to show stellate looking (rather than uniformly rounded) keratinocytes as the desmosome proteins are still functional in spongiotic disorders and serve as the glue keeping keratinocytes adherent to one another. PV classically shows acantholysis that is most prominent in the spinous layers just above the basal layer, resulting in the so-called "suprabasilar" pattern of acantholysis (Fig. 2.28). This is due to the fact that desmoglein 3 is expressed in a gradient, with highest concentration in the suprabasilar keratinocytes. The autoantibodies generated in PV do the most damage to this area of the epithelium. In contrast, desmoglein 1 has higher expression in the superficial most layers of the epidermis, including the granular layer, and so the acantholysis that is observed in PF is typically in the superficial-most portions of the epidermis. Acantholysis in both variants may involve skin appendages, and acantholysis detected along the hair follicle epithelium may be a good clue to the diagnosis [96]. The preservation of intact basal keratinocytes with rounded cell borders in PV can lead to a pattern reminiscent of a row of tombstones [1]. Within the dermis, there is typically a moderately brisk inflammatory infiltrate comprised of lymphocytes, eosinophils, and neutrophils. Acantholytic cells may be detected on Pap smears and are recognized by their

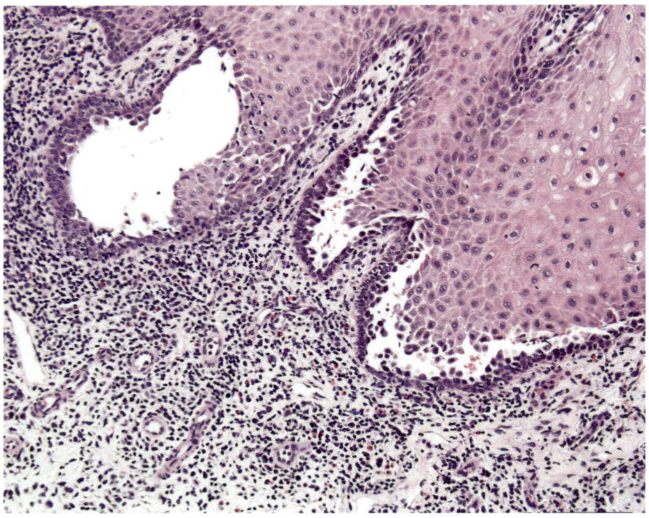

Fig. 2.28 Pemphigus vulgaris. Mucosal epithelium demonstrating suprabasilar acantholysis. The dermis shows a mixed infiltrate including eosinophils

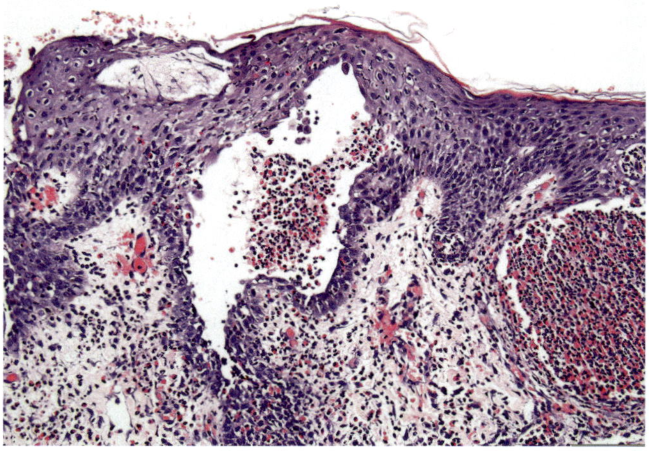

Fig. 2.29 Pemphigus vegetans. Acanthotic epidermis with large, intraepidermal eosinophilic microabscesses. Acantholysis can be appreciated at the edges of the microabscess

high nuclear-to-cytoplasm ratio but uniform, hypochromatic nucleus with small nucleoli [86, 87]. It is important to know the patient's disease to prevent misinterpretation of these findings as dysplasia [87].

PVeg has additional and often quite striking histologic features. Epidermal hyperplasia, which can be so exuberant as to be classified as pseudoepitheliomatous, correlates with the vegetative and verrucous appearance of clinical lesions. Eosinophilic microabscesses within the epidermis are also seen (Fig. 2.29). The acantholytic cells that identify the disease as pemphigus are often located within and therefore obscured by these intraepidermal eosinophilic microabscesses. Pathologists should be familiar with the expected histologic findings of PVeg so that this constellation of features prompts careful evaluation for acantholysis.

2.5.1.3 Immunohistochemical Features

While the histologic features of pemphigus are generally fairly diagnostic on routine examination, direct immunofluorescence studies provide an important adjunct test to definitively confirm the diagnosis. Application of fluorescent-conjugated antibodies to immunoglobulins will result in a characteristic pattern of staining matching the normal expression pattern of the target antigen, namely desmoglein 3 in PV. IgG and C3 decorate the cell membrane of keratinocytes (Fig. 2.30), with most prominent staining in the lower levels of the epithelium in PV. IgA is less commonly deposited [96, 97]. This intercellular pattern of staining has been described as "lace-like" or "fishnet-like." Usually the deposition is linear, as if a fine-tip marker is outlining each keratinocyte; however, a subset of patients will show a granular deposition pattern [97]. If a biopsy is encountered that does not show epidermis, a search for any hair follicles within the biopsy may provide the needed information, as follicular epithelium will show the same intercellular pattern of staining.

Other ancillary tests are not required for the diagnosis of PV. However, indirect immunofluorescence studies may provide information regarding disease activity. Indirect immunofluorescence is performed by incubating patient serum (containing the circulating autoantibodies) on a "normal" skin substrate (typically monkey esophagus is the preferred substrate). Serial dilutions of the serum can provide an estimated autoantibody titer, and high titers tend to correlate with severe disease [1, 86].

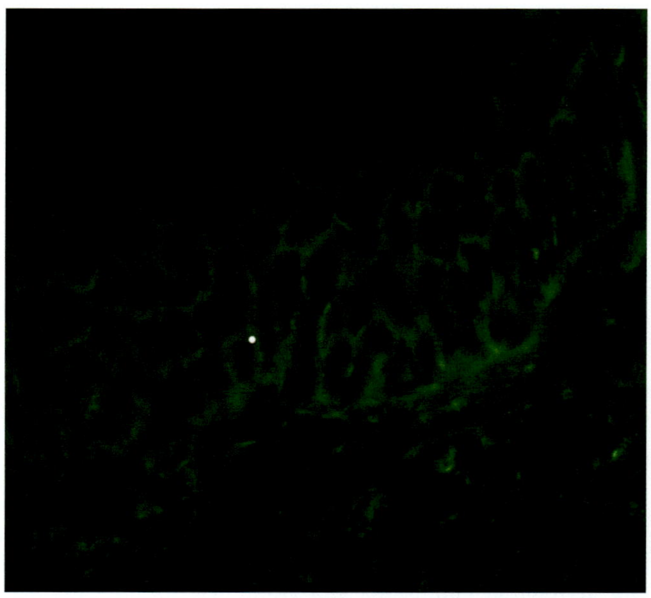

Fig. 2.30 Pemphigus. Intercellular deposition of IgG and C3 are seen in the pemphigus family of diseases

2.5.1.4 Differential Diagnosis

The histologic differential diagnosis of PV includes Hailey–Hailey disease, Darier disease, herpetic infection, and papular acantholytic dyskeratosis. Hailey–Hailey disease, Darier disease, and papular acantholytic dyskeratosis will also show variable degrees of acantholysis without (Hailey–Hailey) or with (Darier) dyskeratosis. Importantly, direct immunofluorescence studies will be negative in these inherited acantholytic disorders. Herpes virus infection usually shows the characteristic viral cytopathic effect of cellular molding, chromatin margination, and multinucleation and can be detected by immunohistochemical staining. Importantly, the topical anesthetic EMLA has been reported to cause intraepidermal acantholysis and can thus mimic pemphigus as well [98].

The histologic differential diagnosis of PF would include other diseases with more superficial blisters, including impetigo, staph-scalded skin, and tinea. Infectious stains coupled with cultures, negative immunofluorescence, and clinical history should help resolve this differential.

The histologic differential diagnosis of PVeg often includes infectious entities. Special stains for organisms and cultures are essential to detect the etiologic organisms. PVeg shares virtually identical histologic features with pyodermatits vegetans, a disease with strong association to inflammatory bowel disease. Microscopically, pyodermatitis vegetans shows the same pseudoepitheliomatous hyperplasia with eosinophilic microabscesses, but will have a negative direct immunofluorescence study [99, 100].

Subepidermal blistering diseases such as mucous membrane pemphigoid and bullous pemphigoid may enter the differential diagnosis, either clinically or histologically. These disorders, which occasionally involve the vulva, are characterized by tense (rather than flaccid) blisters on an erythematous base and are due to autoantibodies generated against proteins in the hemidesmosome complex that links basal keratinocytes to the dermis. Microscopically, the blister split occurs at the junction of the epidermis/epithelium and dermis/subepithelium, rather than the intraepidermal blister that occurs in the pemphigus family of diseases. Mucous membrane pemphigoid and bullous pemphigoid have positive direct immunofluorescence findings as well, but immunoreactants (usually IgG and C3) are localized to the basement membrane zone in a linear distribution rather than the intercellular pattern seen in pemphigus.

2.5.2 Subepithelial Blistering Disease: Mucous Membrane Pemphigoid, Bullous Pemphigoid, and Linear IgA Bullous Dermatosis

Subepidermal/subepithelial blistering diseases, similar to the pemphigus family, are generally autoimmune mediated. The pemphigoid family of diseases, including mucous membrane pemphigoid (MMP) and bullous pemphigoid (BP), may occasionally involve the vulva, and are characterized by tense (rather than flaccid) blisters on an erythematous base. These diseases are due to autoantibodies (predominantly of the IgG subtype) generated against proteins in the hemidesmosome complex that links basal keratinocytes to the dermis. Linear IgA bullous dermatosis (LIGABD) and chronic bullous disease of childhood (CBDC) are likely the same disease presenting along a spectrum, with the age of presentation being the biggest difference between these two entities. Both LIGABD and CBDC arise from autoantibodies generated to similar antigens as in BP and MMP, but the antibodies are of the IgA subtype.

BP is one of the more common autoimmune-mediated blistering diseases and most often arises in older adults. BP uncommonly involves mucosal or genital surfaces, estimated around 10% of patients with the disease. A subset of BP arises in childhood however, and these children may have exclusively vulvar involvement [1, 101]. MMP affects preferentially mucosal sites such as conjunctiva, and oral and genital mucosa. MMP is also termed "cicatricial pemphigoid" due to the propensity for scarring sequelae of the disease. Older females are most commonly affected, with the vulva being a frequent site of involvement (in contrast to BP) [89]. The criteria for diagnosis of MMP include blisters on mucous membranes and positive direct immunofluorescence studies as described below [102]. LIGABD (or CBDC when occurring in children) is a relatively unusual blistering disease. When occurring in adults, middle age to older adults are affected and there is a slight predilection for the disease to occur in women [1]. LIGABD is often related to recent antibiotic usage (particularly vancomycin) [96]. CBDC typically presents in prepubertal children (with average age in the range of 4–6 years old) as blistering genital lesions that evolve to more widespread cutaneous involvement. Resolution is generally self-limited over a few months or years and is generally resolved by onset of puberty [1, 103]. CBDC occurs with equal frequency in children of both sexes and all races and is the most common acquired autoimmune blistering disease in childhood [104].

In all of these entities, autoimmunity against proteins making up the hemidesmosome—the protein complex that links the basal keratinocyte to the collagen framework of the superficial dermis—characterizes the disease. BP is characterized by autoantibodies generated to the BP230 (BPAg1, a plakin) or BP180 (BPAg2, also known as collagen XVII) protein antigens of the hemidesmosome [96, 105]. The autoantibodies in MMP are generated to a variety of hemodesmosomal proteins, including BP230, BP180, as well as laminin332, and $\alpha 6\beta 4$ integrin [105]. LIGABD and CBDC generate an IgA autoantibody to fragments of the BP180 protein (collagen XVII), most commonly to the 97 and 120 kD fragments [104].

Similar to the pemphigus family of disease, these subepidermal blistering diseases are managed with aggressive immunosuppression, using corticosteroids and steroid sparing agents. Prednisone, cyclophosphamide, azathioprine, and mycophenolate mofetil have all been shown to have utility in the treatment of BP and MMP [102]. Rarely, mild or localized disease may be successfully managed with topical treatment alone [106]. LIGABD and CBDC may be managed with dapsone. MMP in particular, requires coordinated management with ophthalmologists and gastroenterologists or otolaryngologists due to the propensity for ocular, laryngeal, and esophageal involvement and the risk of scarring sequelae.

2.5.2.1 Clinical Features

BP rarely involves the vulva, although rare reports document convincing cases of exclusively vulvar involvement [101, 107]. BP presents as tense blisters on an erythematous base, most often involving the trunk and flexural sites. Blisters may be preceded by a nonspecific urticarial phase, in which clinical lesions are eczematous or urticarial-appearing. The mucosa is rarely involved. Blisters resolve without scarring. Patients often complain of pruritus.

MMP not uncommonly involves vulvar skin and mucosa, with the labia majora and minora both affected. Clinically, lesions resemble those seen in BP, with tense blisters arising on an erythematous base. However, in contrast to BP, scarring is a common sequelae as blisters resolve. Conjunctival and oral mucosal involvement is commonly also present upon examination.

LIGABD and CBDC have similar clinical appearances. Lesions are often annular or targetoid, with small clusters of blisters aligned along the perimeter. This has been often referred to as "clusters of jewels" or "string of pearls" sign [104]. The blisters, which are tense as in BP and MMP, may have serous or hemorrhagic fluid in them. The genital region is often involved (particularly in children), but the extremities, face (peri-oral), and rarely mucosa may also be involved by lesions. Complete skin examination and further workup is paramount, particularly as CBDC involving the vulva may be initially mistaken for childhood sexual abuse [106]. Healing of blisters often leaves pigmentary alteration but no scarring [104]. Clinical symptoms may include burning or itching, or they may be absent.

2.5.2.2 Histologic Features

Microscopically, the blister split for these diseases occurs at the junction of the epidermis/epithelium and dermis/subepithelium, rather than the intraepidermal blister that occurs in the pemphigus family of diseases. This subepidermal/subepithelial blister lacks epidermal necrosis and/or dyskeratosis. In BP, the blister cavity classically demonstrates an eosinophil-rich infiltrate. This eosinophil-rich infiltrate is also present in the dermis. BP should not show scarring in the dermis. In MMP, the blister cavity generally shows fewer inflammatory cells than in BP (Fig. 2.31). Neutrophils predominate in early blisters, with eosinophils and lymphocytes recruited in older blisters [106]. In some biopsies, scarring or dermal fibrosis may be evidence of a previous blistering episode. LIGABD and CBDC show identical histology, characterized by a subepidermal blister with a neutrophil-rich infiltrate in the blister cavity and superficial dermis. Neutrophils will often be aligned along the dermal–epidermal junction, often contiguously, but sometimes in a discontinuous pattern which will histologically mimic dermatitis herpetiformis.

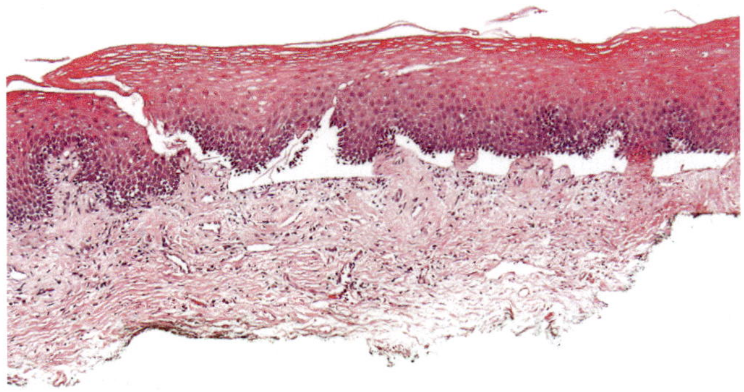

Fig. 2.31 Mucous membrane (cicatricial) pemphigoid. The mucosa demonstrates a subepithelial blister with minimal inflammation in the blister cavity or submucosa

2.5.2.3 Immunohistochemical Features

Direct immunofluorescence studies are imperative to confirm the diagnoses of MMP, BP, and LIGABD. In contrast to the intercellular pattern seen in pemphigus, these diseases have linear deposition of immunoreactants along the dermal–epidermal junction: in MMP and BP these immunoreactants are usually IgG and C3, and in LIGABD/CBDC the main immunoreactant is IgA (with C3 deposition also seen as a secondary immunoreactant) [96]. Direct immunofluorescence studies have been shown to have both a high sensitivity (nearly 91%) and a high specificity (98%) in the diagnosis of BP [108]; as such, most cases of suspected BP are captured through histology and direct immunofluorescence.

However, indirect immunofluorescence studies may also be of value in the diagnosis of subepidermal blistering diseases. The salt-split skin method involves inducing a subepidermal blister in normal skin substrate and incubating with patient serum. In the salt split skin test, autoantibodies will bind to either the epidermal side (the "roof") or the dermal side (the "floor") of the blister. This pattern provides information regarding the exact location of the split within the hemidesmosomal complex and shows high specificity (although relatively low sensitivity) in the diagnosis of BP [108]. In BP, the antigens targeted are relatively superficial in the lamina lucida of the basement membrane zone, and therefore autoantibodies localize to the roof/epidermal side of the blister. This is in contrast to similar diseases such as epidermolysis bullosa acquisita (see differential diagnosis below), where the autoantibody is generated to an antigen in the superficial dermis, so the immunoreactants in the salt split skin test localize to the floor/dermal side of the blister.

The salt split skin concept can be exploited by immunohistochemical staining for collagen type IV (basement membrane collagen) in formalin-fixed patient biopsies. As the blister in BP generally occurs at a relatively superficial location in the hemidesmosome, collagen IV will stain the floor/dermal side of the blister. In epidermolysis bullosa acquisita, the blister roof/epidermal side will be stained by collagen IV [96].

Due to the varied nature of the autoantibody targets in MMP and their different location within the hemidesmosome complex, the abovementioned indirect studies and collagen IV staining may not be as helpful in confirming the diagnosis.

The indirect immunofluorescence studies using monkey esophagus as a substrate has historically been less useful in the diagnosis and management of the pemphigoid family than in the pemphigus family of disease. False negative results are frequently reported in BP and sensitivities are relatively low [108]. However, some authors suggest that testing for subclasses of IgG (rather that IgG as a whole) can improve the detection capabilities [109].

Immunoblotting of patient serum may also rarely be used in the diagnostic workup. Target antigens, which define the disease, are identified by molecular weight, and thus the exact target antigen (ex BP180 or BP230) can be identified. Immunoblotting has largely given way to less technically demanding techniques such as ELISA (enzyme-linked immunosorbent assay) designed to detect specific, commonly targeted antigens. ELISA assays show overall moderate sensitivity but high specificity in the diagnosis of BP [108].

2.5.2.4 Differential Diagnosis

The pemphigus family of diseases can be distinguished from the pemphigoid family of diseases by the presence of an intraepidermal, rather than a subepidermal, blister. The location of the blister formation and the distribution of immunoreactivity with direct immunofluorescence is distinctive.

Subepidermal or subepithelial blisters may also result from cytotoxic damage to the epidermis, as seen in robust examples of interface dermatitis. As such, bullous examples of lichen planus, fixed drug eruption, and Stevens Johnson syndrome/toxic epidermal necrolysis may sometimes mimic the pemphigoid diseases. Any of these interface dermatoses should show individual necrotic keratinocytes and vacuolar changes at the dermal–epidermal junction. The edge of a blister is the best place to appreciate these changes.

Well-established, advanced lichen sclerosus may sometimes induce an artifactual subepidermal blister due to marked dermal sclerosis. This should not be interpreted as a superimposed, secondary autoimmune blistering disease. Negative direct immunofluorescence studies coupled with a homogenized papillary dermal collagen framework and attenuated rete ridge pattern would support a diagnosis of lichen sclerosus over a true blistering disease.

Additional subepidermal blistering diseases that have histologic overlap with both BP and MMP include epidermolysis bullosa acquisita (EBA) and pemphigoid gestationis. EBA occurs in a similar demographic of patients (older to elderly adults) as BP and is often more refractory to treatment. Autoantibodies are generated against collagen VII, which is present as an anchoring fibril in the superficial dermis. Disruption at this site will frequently result in scarring as blisters resolve. This propensity for scarring is similar to MMP. Classically, the blisters in EBA are pauci-inflammatory, but inflammatory cells (eosinophils or neutrophils) may be present in a subset of cases. Although direct immunofluorescence studies show linear IgG and C3 along the basement membrane zone (identical to BP and MMP), the target of the autoantibodies is to a more deeply located antigen (collagen VII). As a result, indirect salt-split skin will show deposition of immunoreactivity along the dermal side (the floor) of the blister, which is in contrast to the pattern of epidermal deposition in most cases of BP. Pemphigoid gestationis is essentially the development of BP during pregnancy (most often the second or third trimester) [96]. Histologic features and direct immunofluorescence studies are identical to BP, and thus accurate diagnosis relies on knowledge of the patient's pregnancy status.

The primary histologic differential diagnosis of LIGABD and CBDC is dermatitis herpetiformis. Also characterized by a subepidermal blister, neutrophils aligned along the dermal–epidermal junction, and deposition of IgA along the basement membrane zone, dermatitis herpetiformis shares many histologic features of LIGABD and CBDC. However, the dermal neutrophils in dermatitis herpetiformis tend to cluster in the papillary dermal tips, whereas in LIGABD and CBDC, the neutrophils are generally dispersed continuously along the dermal–epidermal junction. The IgA deposition seen on direct immunofluorescence in dermatitis herpetiformis is more granular and patchy than the linear deposition seen in LIGABD and CBDC. However, clinical presentation is also helpful in the distinction: dermatitis herpetiformis essentially never involves the vulvar skin (preferring instead extensor surfaces) and has a strong association with celiac disease.

2.5.3 Hailey–Hailey Disease, Darier Disease, and Papular Acantholytic Dyskeratosis

Hailey–Hailey Disease (HHD), Darier Disease (DD), and Papular Acantholytic Dyskeratosis (PAD) are all united by the common presence of the histologic feature of acantholysis. As previously mentioned, acantholysis is the dissociation of keratinocytes due to insufficient cell–cell adhesion. These genodermatoses are distinguished clinically by their distribution of lesions and presence/absence of a family history of similar rashes. Although HHD and DD are inherited diseases, presentation may not occur until early adulthood.

HHD, also known as benign familial pemphigus, is an inherited genodermatosis transmitted in an autosomal dominant manner. The genetic defect is a mutation in *ATP2C1*, which encodes a calcium pump involved in maintaining normal cell–cell adhesion [96]. As there is incomplete penetrance, not all patients will report a family history. Patients with HHD generally present in the second to fourth decade of life with pruritic intertriginous papules and plaques. Erosion and maceration is common, leaving patients susceptible to secondary bacterial, fungal, or viral (particularly herpetic) infection. A case report exists regarding the development of squamous cell carcinoma in a patient with HHD without other predisposing or contributable factors [110]; this occurrence seems the exception and not the rule. The clinical manifestations may have a waxing and waning course, with exacerbations from hot weather and increased friction and ultimate improvement with age [1, 96].

DD, also known a keratosis follicularis, is another inherited genodermatosis. This disease, also inherited in an autosomal dominant fashion with incomplete penetrance, is due to a mutation in *ATP2A2*, which—similar to HHD—encodes a calcium pump integral to desmosome integrity. Patients generally present in mid to late childhood (often around puberty) with hyperkeratotic papules distributed on the face, chest, neck, back, ears, and groin. Similar to HHD, these lesions are prone to secondary infection.

PAD, which has been variably termed papular acantholytic dermatosis of the genital-crural (or vulvar-crural) folds or papular genitocrural acantholysis, is a third example of an acantholytic dermatosis affecting vulvar skin. These lesions have clinical and histologic overlap with both HHD and DD, but lesions are generally limited to the genital folds and may extend to the upper thighs. Family history is uncommonly reported. Some studies have shown genetic similarity to HHD or DD [111, 112], lending support to the idea that PAD may be a localized variant or mosaic expression of HHD or DD.

Management for all of these acantholytic processes is similar, with ablative therapies (cryosurgery, laser, excision, or electrocautery) being common. Topical steroids, topical antibiotics to minimize infectious complications, and retinoids have also been utilized as therapies [113].

2.5.3.1 Clinical Features

Patients with HHD present with eroded or macerated plaques in the axillae, inguinal folds, vulva, perineum, neck, and inframammary folds. True blisters are generally not visible, but skin is typically erythematous, eroded, and crusted. Verrucous papules are another reported clinical presentation; this presentation may mimic condylomas [114]. An accompanying foul odor may point to secondary infection of lesions [1]. Evidence of associated lichenification attests to the pruritic nature of lesions [115].

Patients with DD demonstrate skin lesions in a seborrheic distribution (face, neck, ears, chest, back, and groin). Skin lesions are verrucous and keratotic papules that have a rough appearance and feel and often coalesce into papillomatous plaques [116]. The color of lesions ranges from flesh colored to yellow to red to brown. In addition to skin lesions, nail dystrophy is frequent. Similar to HHD, lesions may be foul smelling due to secondary infection.

The lesions in patients with PAD are localized to the perigenital region. Lesions are described as distinct white to flesh colored papules most often occurring on the labia majora [117]. Most often lesions are asymptomatic, but may occasionally cause itching or burning.

Clinical distinction between these three disorders may be difficult. The distribution of lesions and a positive family history are some of the most helpful distinguishing features. In the absence of family history, distinction may be more difficult. Clinically, in theory, PAD is more likely than HHD to present as asymptomatic distinct papules, whereas HHD is generally pruritic and painful with more vesiculation [113]. Other entities within the clinical differential (particularly with the isolated lesions seen in PAD) include fungal and viral infections [115] and genital warts [114].

2.5.3.2 Histologic Features

Microscopic evaluation of HHD reveals an acanthotic epidermis with acantholysis likened to a "dilapidated brick wall." The entire span of the epidermis may show breakdown between keratinocytes, in contrast to the suprabasilar accentuation of acantholysis in pemphigus vulgaris (Fig. 2.32). Adnexal structures (hair follicles) generally do not show acantholysis, and classically there is minimal dyskeratosis, with corps ronds and grains usually absent. There may be slight to moderate inflammation in the dermis (particularly when secondarily infected), as well as surface erosion or ulceration with serum crusting.

Biopsies from DD show a combination of both acantholysis and dyskeratosis. There is often a thick layer or column of parakeratosis overlying the lesions (Fig. 2.33). Dyskeratosis is manifest by corps ronds (rounded acantholytic cells with a round nucleus surrounded by a pale halo) and grains (basophilic cells with hyperchromatic, elongated/flattened nuclei, usually in the granular layer). Acantholysis is most promi-

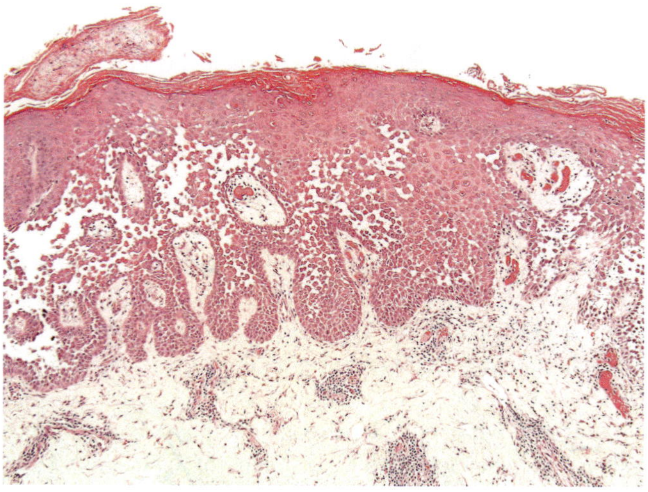

Fig. 2.32 Hailey–Hailey disease. The epidermis is acanthotic with prominent acantholysis but minimal dyskeratosis, recapitulating a "dilapidated brick wall"

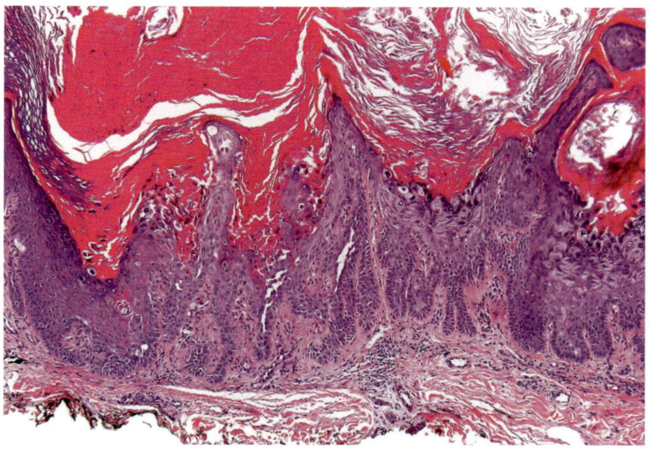

Fig. 2.33 Darier disease. Acantholysis and dyskeratosis is prominent within a papillomatous and acanthotic epidermis

nent in the suprabasilar layer, and all of the diagnostic features may be seen involving hair follicles. Typically there is scant dermal inflammation, unless there is secondary infection.

The histologic features of PAD may resemble either HHD or DD, and sometimes there may be features of both diseases in one biopsy specimen [113, 115, 118, 119]. The acantholysis in PAD may be more focal than in HHD [1].

Importantly, all three of these disorders should have negative direct immunofluorescence studies. Ancillary studies that may be performed in addition to direct immunofluorescence include stains for infectious organisms, should there be a histologic concern for secondary infection by bacterial, fungal, or viral (particularly herpetic) organisms.

The entities discussed above need to be differentiated from one another, and this is best accomplished through clinical–pathologic correlation. Predominant acantholysis without dyskeratosis and the correct distribution of lesions and/or family history favors HHD. Prominent dyskeratosis with corps ronds and grains and the correct distribution of lesions and/or family history favors DD. The other major histologic differential is pemphigus. Lesions of pemphigus are generally acquired and often (but not always!) present in an older cohort. Histologically, pemphigus generally shows suprabasilar acantholysis without significant dyskeratosis and will have positive direct immunofluorescence studies. If clinical history is not available, if there is histologic overlap with the different disorders discussed herein, and/or if direct immunofluorescence was not submitted, it may be prudent to sign out reports as "Acantholytic dermatosis (with or without dyskeratosis)" and give a differential that may variably include HHD, DD, PAD, or pemphigus. If pemphigus is within the differential diagnosis, direct immunofluorescence studies would be recommended as a follow-up test.

2.6 Granulomatous Reaction Pattern

2.6.1 Crohn Disease of the Vulva

Crohn disease (CD) involving the vulvar skin and mucosa is rare, but it is likely under-recognized and underreported. CD is a granulomatous process that affects the gastrointestinal (GI) tract, but may affect skin outside of the GI tract. CD may directly extend from the GI tract to the skin, presenting most often as fistulous tracts, or may present as discrete skin lesions. Referred to by some as "metastatic" lesions, this cutaneous involvement is perhaps more accurately referred to as noncontiguous involvement by CD [120].

Approximately one-third of patients with GI CD disease will have extracutaneous manifestations, including joint (arthritis), oral (aphthous ulcers), ocular (uveitis), and cutaneous lesions [120]. Cutaneous manifestations of CD include pyoderma gangrenosum, erythema nodosum, and noncontiguous cutaneous CD. Crohn disease in the vulva may precede the diagnosis of GI Crohn disease up to 50% of the time, depending on the study cited [120–122], and it may be possible to have CD limited to the vulva. In a single institution study of vulvar CD, the average age of presentation was 28 [120], while comprehensive literature reviews of CD of the vulva cite median presentation around age 34 [121, 123].

The precise pathogenesis of cutaneous CD remains unclear. Type IV hypersensitivity reactions, immune complex deposition, cross-reactivity between skin and gastrointestinal antigens, and genetic predispositions have all been proposed as possible mechanisms [124]. Cell-mediated immunity is thought to play a role as well in the development of granulomas specifically.

Depending on the presentation, clinical workup may require imaging to assess for enterocutaneous fistula formation. Therapeutic options include topical steroids, antibiotics, and TNF-α inhibitors, with surgical treatments reserved for refractory cases [120–123].

2.6.1.1 Clinical Features

Vulvar CD may present in several different and distinct manners. Although typically asymptomatic, patients may complain of pain/discomfort and less commonly pruritus. Labial edema is the most commonly observed manifestation, seen in approximately two-thirds of patients. This swelling is often asymmetrical and erythematous and may be the only physical finding. Ulcerations, often described as "knife-like" [121, 125] and of variable depth and distribution are also frequently encountered. Mass-forming lesions and abscesses are yet other presentations that may be encountered [1, 120]. Bulbous lesions clinically concerning for condylomata have also been detailed in the literature [121, 126] (Fig. 2.34).

The clinical differential diagnosis for vulvar CD includes infectious processes (namely a variety of sexually transmitted infections), hidradenitis suppurativa, pyoderma gangrenosum, and neoplastic entities. As such, a biopsy may be taken to help clarify the diagnosis.

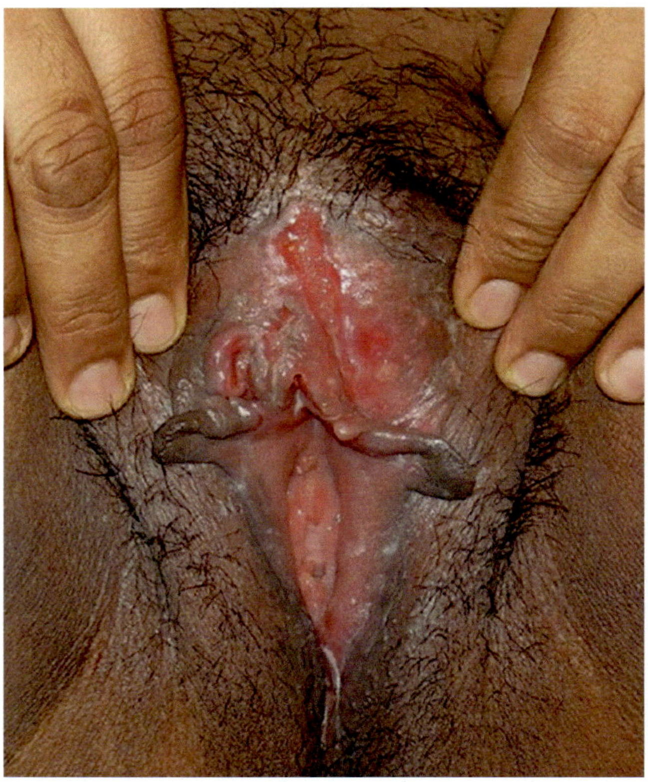

Fig. 2.34 Crohn disease involving the vulva. Edema and asymmetric ulcerations are present. Photo provided courtesy of previous edition in Chinese (Science Press, Beijing, China)

2.6.1.2 Histologic Features

The classically described histologic pattern of cutaneous CD is a noncaseating granulomatous dermatitis (Fig. 2.35). The granulomas are epithelioid, variably loose to tight, without central necrosis or suppuration, and multinucleated giant cells and a rim of associated lymphocytes may be present. Granulomas may be closely aligned to the dermal–epidermal junction, but may be located deep in the subcutis as well [124]. The presence of eosinophils was seen in two-thirds of cases (Fig. 2.36), and seems to be a distinguishing feature from sarcoidosis, which typically lacks eosinophils [124]. Granulomatous vasculitis and granulomatous lymphangitis have also been described [127].

However, while granulomatous inflammation is a distinctive and recognizable histologic feature of cutaneous CD, at

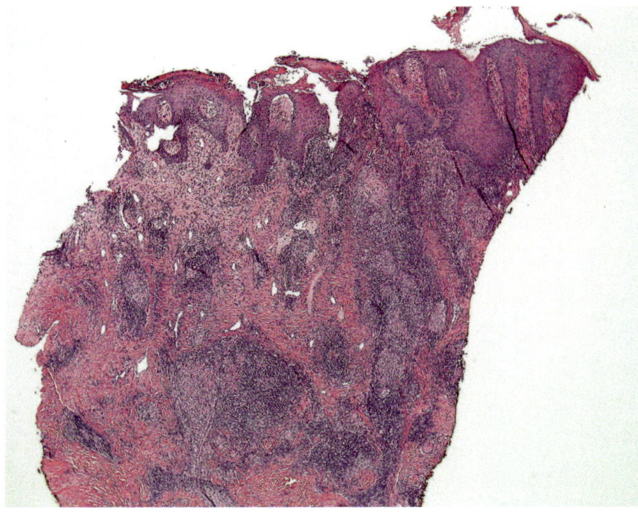

Fig. 2.35 Crohn disease. The epidermis is thickened and the dermis shows a noncaseating granulomatous dermatitis

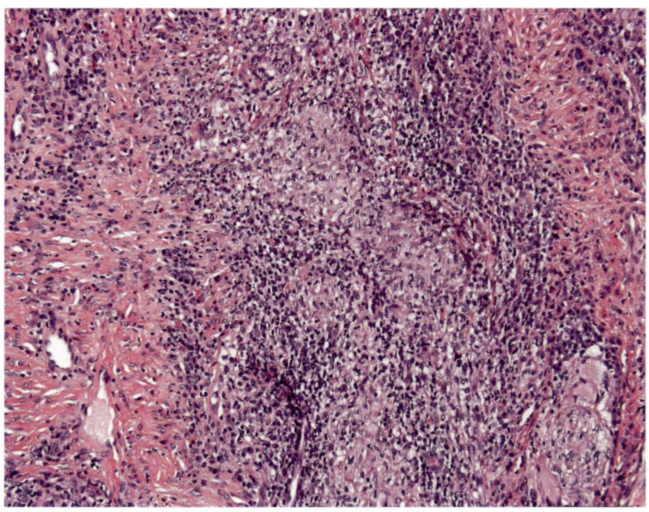

Fig. 2.36 Crohn's disease. Higher magnification shows noncaseating granulomas in the dermis with surrounding admixed eosinophils

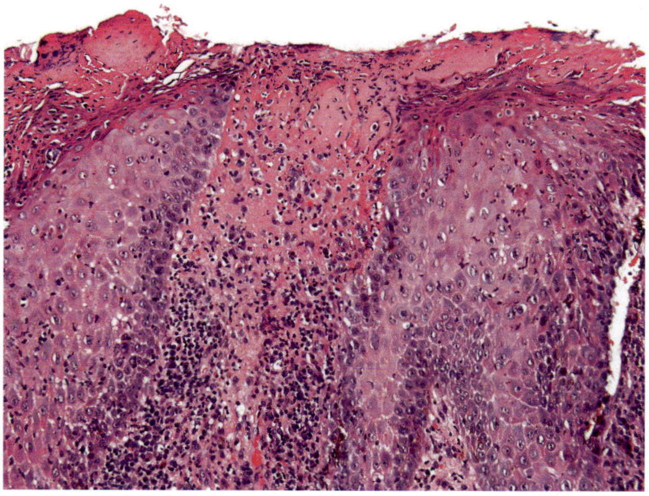

Fig. 2.37 Crohn disease. There is often surface ulceration or erosion, even in the absence of dermal granulomas

least one study suggested that granulomas are not requisite to make a diagnosis of noncontiguous/metastatic CD. In a single institutional study of clinically confirmed vulvar CD, only 38% of patient biopsies showed granulomatous inflammation, suggesting that requiring granulomas for a diagnosis of vulvar CD may be overly restrictive and thereby miss the diagnosis in a large subset of cases [126]. Another case series noted that two-thirds to three-quarters of patients with vulvar CD had biopsies which confirmed the diagnosis by documentation of granulomatous inflammation [120], suggesting the absence of such inflammation in the remaining patient biopsies.

Additional features seen in cutaneous CD include ulceration, lichenoid inflammation, and lymphatic dilatation. Ulceration of the epidermis is often appreciated in biopsies of cutaneous CD, corresponding to the frequently observed clinical ulceration, and may be present alone or with other inflammatory features (Fig. 2.37). Lichenoid inflammation may be seen with or without a granulomatous infiltrate [124, 126]. Dilated lymphatic spaces, thought to be a result of fibrosis from GI surgeries or from persistent chronic inflammation, have been documented and may prove to be an important clue to the diagnosis as it is less commonly described in entities that may be within the histologic differential diagnosis [126, 127]. Notably, a subset of patients demonstrated vulvar dysplasia or carcinoma on biopsy (particularly seen in the bulbous and exophytic lesions), further supporting the need for biopsy in these cases [126].

2.6.1.3 Immunohistochemical Features

Ancillary testing in cutaneous CD plays a minimal role. There are no diagnostic immunohistochemical stains. Special stains to include deep fungal and mycobacterial infections are generally performed as part of the workup, as with most granulomatous infiltrates confronting a pathologist.

2.6.1.4 Differential Diagnosis

Cutaneous CD may have histologic overlap with other ulcerating diseases such as hidradenitis suppurativa and pyoderma gangrenosum as well as infectious entities and granulomatous processes such as sarcoidosis. Hidradenitis, discussed below, presents with a rich, neutrophil-predominant inflammatory infiltrate centered around disrupted hair follicles and sweat glands. Pyoderma gangrenosum, as will be discussed later in this chapter, may be associated with inflammatory bowel disease, but involvement of the vulva is unusual. Infectious etiologies should be excluded with use of relevant special stains for organisms. Particularly as granulomatous diseases may herald a mycobacterial or deep fungal infection, acid fast and PAS or GMS stains are requisite to include infectious etiologies. Cultures and molecular techniques, coupled with a high index of suspicion, may be necessary to exclude some infections, particularly entities such as lymphogranuloma venererum, which may have nonspecific histologic features (coupled with characteristic lymphadenopathy) and negative special stains for organisms. Vulvar sarcoidosis may have considerable histologic overlap with CD and would be in the histologic differential diagnosis, particularly when granulomas are present and if the patient is presenting with vulvar disease alone in the absence of GI symptoms. Eosinophil-rich infiltrates are said to favor CD over sarcoidosis, and ulceration is common in CD but unusual in sarcoidosis [1, 124].

2.7 Vasculopathic Reaction Pattern

2.7.1 Behcet Disease

Behcet disease (BD) is a systemic disease that affects multiple organs and elicits considerable morbidity for patients. Considered by many to be an autoinflammatory disease requiring a genetic predisposition coupled with some exogenous triggering event, BD was initially characterized by the triad of oral, genital, and ocular lesions [128]. BD is now known to involve other organ systems, resulting in articular, neurologic, gastrointestinal, and cardiovascular signs and symptoms [128, 129]. Pulmonary artery aneurysm is a source of considerable morbidity and mortality. Involvement of the central nervous system and the ocular system generally predicts prognosis [128]. Expansion of spectrum of disease has led some authors to prefer that it be referred to as Behcet syndrome, as the constellation of features affecting different subgroups of patients may vary considerably [130].

BD is relatively rare in the United States and Western European countries. It has a higher prevalence in the Mediterranean, Central Asia, and the Far East, with Turkey having the highest incidence of affected patients, averaging approximately 400 per 100,000 in a few studies [129, 130].

BD affects men and women at similar frequencies, with an age of onset ranging from the mid-20s to mid-30s. Multiple studies have documented a more severe disease course in men, with higher rates of visceral involvement, morbidity, and mortality [128, 129, 131]. Women more often demonstrate genital ulcers and erythema nodosum and overall have been shown to have a better prognosis than their male counterparts [128]. Disease severity also seems to vary by geography, with milder disease reported in non-endemic regions such as the United States [130].

Proposed diagnostic criteria by an international Behcet disease study group include recurrent (>3 episodes per year) oral ulcers and two of the following minor criteria: recurrent genital ulceration, uveitis, cutaneous lesions, and/or a positive pathergy test [132]. Pathergy refers to the development of a hypersensitive clinical response to relatively minor trauma; typically, a papule or pustule develops in response to a minor skin irritation. The pathergy test used in the diagnosis of BD involves skin puncture with a sterile needle and evaluation for formation of an erythematous papule or pustule after 24–48 h and has a specificity of 87% and sensitivity of 60% for BD [1, 129]. One study found a positive test in nearly 60% of patients [131].

The pathogenesis of BD is complex and still under investigation. Currently, most experts believe BD results from a complex interplay between genetic predisposition, the activated immune system, and the possible contribution of infectious triggers. The presence of HLA-B51 allele of the major histocompatibility complex (MHC) class I has been strongly linked to BD in multiple studies [129, 130, 133] and has been estimated to account for about 20% of the genetic susceptibility to BD [129]. HLA-B51 genotype was noted to confer an increased risk of venous thrombosis [133]. Other MHC class I variants have also been investigated with regard to their relationship to various disease manifestations in BD [129, 133], as well as other genes encoding cytokines or regulators of cytokines [129]. Epigenetic events, particularly methylation (resulting in transcriptional silencing) of genes that affect T-helper cell function, have been proposed to play a role in BD [130]. Activation of Th-1 and Th-17 immune responses are thought to mediate much of the organ damage in BD, with cytokines related to these types of responses (IL-2, IFNγ, IL-6, IL-23, and others) being elevated in patients with BD [129, 130]. Hyper-activation of these immune responses may result from cross-reactivity with an infectious antigen, and innumerable viruses, bacteria, and mycobacteria have been proposed as inciting infectious agents in BD [129].

Treatment of BD requires a multidisciplinary approach, particularly when there is widespread organ involvement. Treatment is generally individualized and based on the severity of symptoms and organs involved [130]. Genital ulcerations in particular are generally treated with topical corticosteroid or steroid-sparing agents, systemic immunosuppressants such as corticosteroids, azathioprine, and cyclosporine, thalidomide, and colchicine [129, 130]. Anti-TNF-α therapies are commonly employed for visceral organ involvement [129].

2.7.1.1 Clinical Features

Ulcerations (both genital and oral) are generally some of the first manifestations of the disease and may be the only manifestations in up to one-half of patients [131] (Fig. 2.38a, b). Genital ulcers are typically large and deep, involve the labia majora, and heal over the course of several weeks with scarring. Lesions are generally large (often exceeding 1 cm in size), "punched out" appearing, and have a sharp border [129]. Ulcers may worsen in pregnancy [129]. Involvement of the cervix and vagina should prompt consideration of other ulcerative conditions as ulcerations at these sites are unusual in BD [130].

Diagnosis of BD remains predominantly a clinical one, and diagnostic laboratory tests are lacking. Biopsy may be supportive but is rarely specific. Additional skin examination should reveal the presence (or at least a history) of multiple, recurrent, painful mouth ulcers; the absence of mouth ulcerations strongly argues against a diagnosis of BD as this is a major criteria for diagnosis of the syndrome [130]. Erythema nodosum (painful subcutaneous nodules, frequently on the lower legs) may be seen in a subset of patients. Folliculitis or acneiform-like lesions are also relatively common cutaneous findings [129], and may be related to the pathergy that frequently is documented in BD [134].

The clinical differential diagnosis of genital ulcers in BD include infectious diseases (including herpes simplex virus, syphilis, chancroid, and lymphogranuloma venereum), ulcerative lichenoid processes such as fixed drug eruption, erosive lichen planus, or erythema multiforme, malignancy, and many of the other diseases discussed in this chapter than can present with genital ulceration [129].

2.7.1.2 Histopathologic Features

Biopsies of the ulcers in BD are relatively nonspecific. Ulcer with fibrin deposition along the dermal–epidermal junction is characteristic, with underlying mixed inflammation (Fig. 2.39). Neutrophils may predominate in early lesions, with transition to more lymphocytes, histiocytes, and plasma cells over time [1]. Vascular damage is a frequently documented event and fibrin rimming vascular walls may be seen (Fig. 2.40). Lymphocytic vasculitis (Fig. 2.41) has been suggested as being more common than a leukocytoclastic vasculitis [1]; however, distinction between a primary leukocytoclastic vasculitis and secondary neutrophilic inflammation of vessels in an ulcer bed can be difficult if not impossible.

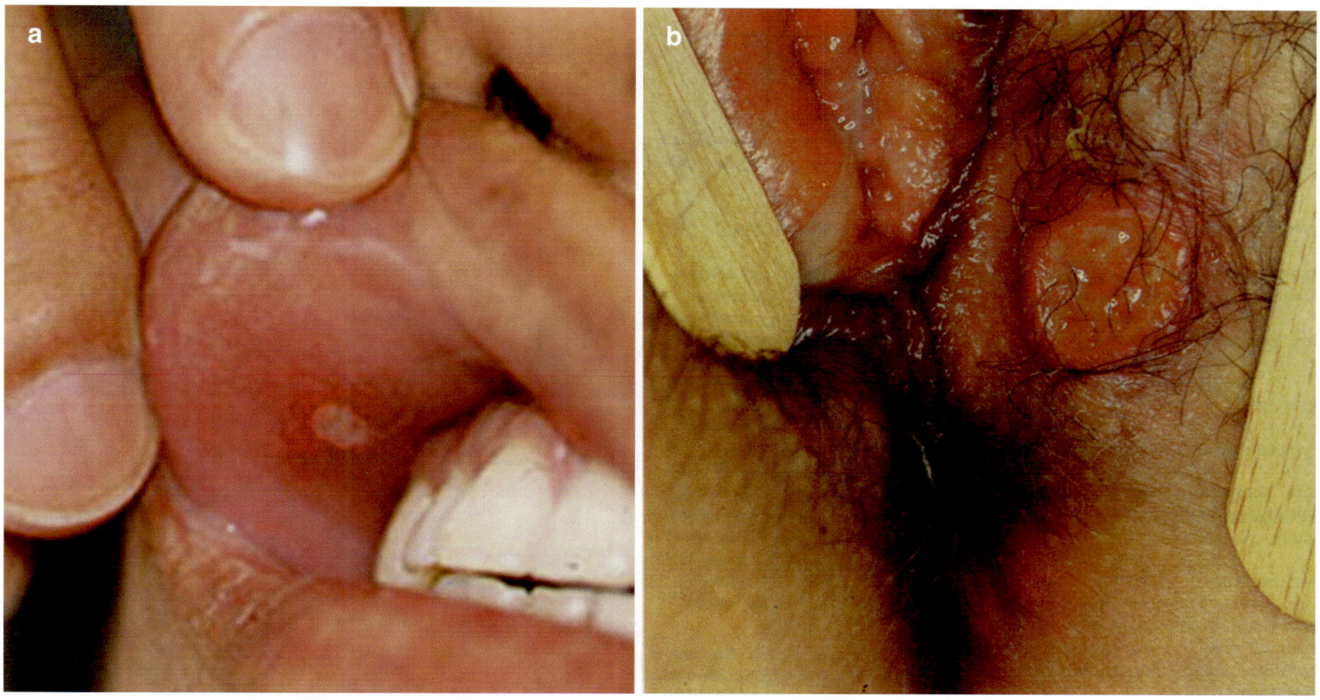

Fig. 2.38 Behcet's disease. (**a**) Oral ulcers are invariably part of the disease manifestations. (**b**) Ulceration of the labia majora is large and deep. Photo provided courtesy of previous edition in Chinese (Science Press, Beijing, China)

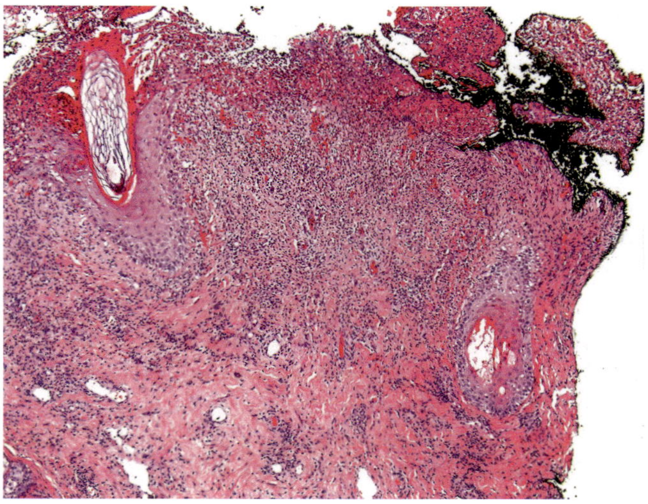

Fig. 2.39 Behcet disease. Surface ulceration with dermal inflammation is nonspecific but commonly seen in BD

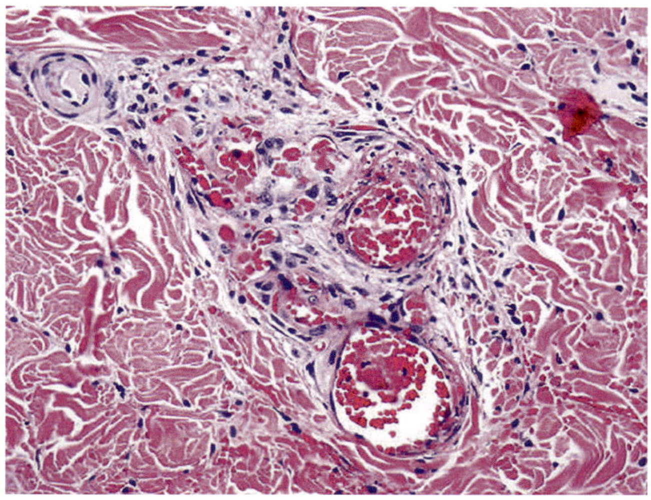

Fig. 2.40 Behcet disease. Vascular damage may be seen, with fibrin rimming vascular walls. Photo provided courtesy of previous edition in Chinese (Science Press, Beijing, China)

2.7.1.3 Immunohistochemical Features

Ancillary testing performs a limited role in the workup of possible BD. Stains to exclude identifiable infectious etiologies are recommended.

2.7.1.4 Differential Diagnosis

The histologic differential diagnosis includes ulcers from other localized and systemic diseases. It is important for biopsy specimens to include some portion of intact epidermis to evaluate for the characteristic lichenoid infiltrate or vacuolar changes and cytotoxic damage to the epithelium that would characterize erosive lichen planus, fixed drug eruption, or erythema multiforme. Herpetic ulcers may be differentiated from those occurring in BD by recognition of nuclear molding, chromatin margination, and multinucleation in the adjacent epidermal keratinocytes; immunohistochemical stains for the viral antigens may be useful if viral cytopathic effect is not readily identified. Pyoderma gangrenosum may show ulcer with underlying zonal inflammation. Crohn disease can present with ulcerations and may

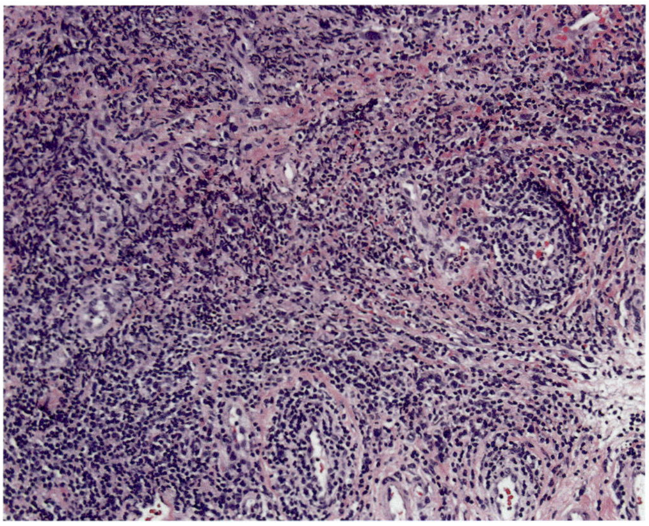

Fig. 2.41 Behcet disease. A lymphocytic vasculitis may be more common than a neutrophilic (leukocytoclastic) vasculitis. Note the layers of lymphocytes concentrically surrounding the vessels in this image

lack the characteristic and historically disease-defining granulomas, thus closely mimicking BD; the similarities between Crohn and Behcet disease in terms of clinical and histologic presentation and organ involvement have led to speculation about disease overlap [135].

Although the histopathologic features in BD are nonspecific, biopsies may be particularly useful to exclude other entities within the clinical differential. Autoimmune-mediated blistering disorders are often histologically distinct (and will show positive direct immunofluorescence studies), and malignancies can generally be detected with adequate sampling.

2.7.2 Pyoderma Gangrenosum

Pyoderma gangrenosum (PG) is a neutrophilic dermatosis that presents as nonhealing, sterile ulcerations. Ulcerations expand outward, are nonresponsive to antibiotics, and typically worsen rather than improve with surgical intervention due to pathergy. The vulva is rarely involved by PG; however, familiarity with the entity is important for clinicians and pathologists to prevent misdiagnosis and mistreatment. It can be misdiagnosed as infection (including necrotizing fasciitis), leading to inappropriate surgical intervention and subsequent long-term scarring sequelae [136, 137].

PG may present within any age group; vulvar involvement by PG is limited to case reports, with patients presenting anywhere from the late teens to late 70s [138–141]. PG has important associations with a variety of other diseases, and it is estimated that systemic disease association is present in approximately half of cases of PG [138]. The most common associations include rheumatologic disease, inflammatory bowel disease, or lymphoproliferative disorders.

PG is a diagnosis of exclusion and ruling out other causes of ulceration through careful history and physical exam, tissue cultures, and laboratory studies is imperative.

Treatment usually requires initiation of high dose topical and/or systemic corticosteroids or other immunosuppressive medications, although some lesions may be refractory to treatment. Debridement or surgical management should be avoided as it generally worsens the condition.

2.7.2.1 Clinical Features

Vulvar involvement by PG presents as large, painful ulcers, classically with a violaceous to gun-metal gray raised edge or rolled border [138, 141]. Ulcers often have jagged, irregular borders and may be surfaced by a purulent exudate and frank necrosis. Ulcers may also be multifocal and are often described as being "punched out" [138].

Patients may report that the lesion began as a small erythematous pustule or nodule which then ulcerated and expanded over time. Minimal trauma may further worsen the ulcer or precipitate new ones, a phenomenon known as pathergy. Lesions are generally exquisitely tender, with patients often reporting pain that seems out of proportion to exam findings [142]. With treatment and time, the ulcers flatten and heal leaving atrophic scars that have been described as cribriform.

The ulcerative variant of PG is most common; however, vegetative, bullous, and pustular variants are also reported [142].

The clinical differential diagnosis of PG is infection, other noninfectious ulcerating diseases such as Behcet syndrome, and less commonly malignancy [141]. For vulvar lesions, infections from numerous organisms may be considered. For the diagnosis of PG, a full infectious workup should be negative. Biopsy can support the diagnosis of PG, but the histologic features are not specific for the diagnosis. Biopsy will also help to rule out specific infectious etiologies or malignancy. The optimal biopsy technique to evaluate a patient with possible PG is via an incisional biopsy that encompasses the inflamed, rolled edge of the ulcer [142].

2.7.2.2 Histopathologic Features

Microscopically, biopsies of PG demonstrate an ulcer with underlying dense dermal inflammation (Fig. 2.42). As PG is a neutrophilic dermatosis, the dermis is filled predominantly with neutrophils, and vasculitis should be absent. There may be necrosis of the dermal collagen and leukocytoclasis (fragmented neutrophil debris). This histologic appearance will mimic an infectious abscess. There are no diagnostic features to confirm PG. However, if the rolled border of the ulcer has been appropriately sampled, the pathologist will be able to visualize "undermining" of the ulcer, that is, extension of the neutrophilic infiltrate under the edges of the ulcer bed and extending radially away from the ulcer. There have been some papers which suggest that very early lesions of PG may have a lymphocyte—rather than neutrophil—predominant inflammatory infiltrate [143].

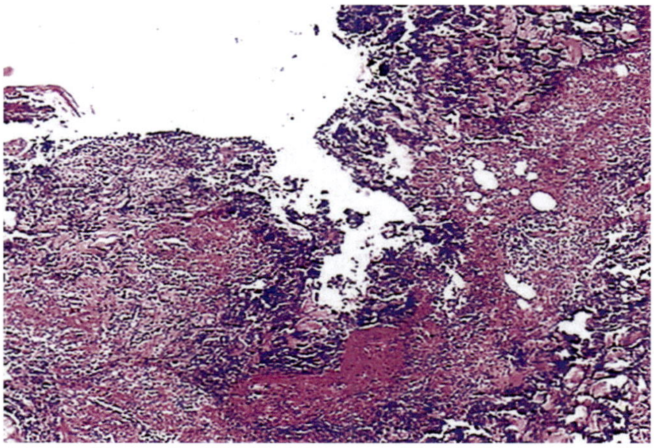

Fig. 2.42 Pyoderma gangrenosum. Histologic features are relatively nonspecific, showing ulceration with undermined borders and dermal neutrophils. Photo provided courtesy of previous edition in Chinese (Science Press, Beijing, China)

2.7.2.3 Immunohistochemical Features and Differential Diagnosis

Ancillary testing is necessary to exclude infectious etiologies, which comprises the major histologic differential diagnosis. Special stains (Gram, PAS, GMS, and Fite or Ziehl-Neelsen) should be negative for bacterial, fungal, and mycobacterial organisms, respectively. If the above histologic features are present and stains for infectious organisms are negative, it is the author's habit to make a diagnosis of "Neutrophilic dermatosis," with a comment suggesting that if infectious etiologies have been excluded clinically and through microbial culture methods, then the features would be compatible with a clinical diagnosis of PG.

2.8 Folliculocentric/Follicular Occlusion Reaction Pattern

2.8.1 Fox–Fordyce Disease

Fox–Fordyce Disease (FFD) is a follicular-based dermatosis thought to be due to obstruction of the apocrine sweat duct, which empties directly into the hair follicle (as opposed to eccrine sweat ducts which empty directly onto the skin surface). FFD is also commonly referred to as "apocrine miliaria." As might be expected based on the presumed pathogenesis, this disease manifests in skin regions containing apocrine sweat glands, namely the genital skin, axillae, and areola. Exacerbation of disease occurs with activities that induce sweating including exercise, warm weather, sexual activity, and other physical or emotional stressors [144, 145]. The disease was first described in 1902 by Drs. Fox and Fordyce. A strong role for a hormonal influence can be argued, as this dermatosis occurs predominantly in women of reproductive age (up to 90% of cases are thought to arise in this population [145]). Fluctuations with menstruation and improvement during pregnancy, with oral contraceptive use, and after menopause also lend credence to the role of hormones in the pathophysiology of the disease [144].

The pathogenesis, as alluded to above, is thought to be initiated by plugging of the hair follicles. This plugging (correlating histologically with follicular hyperkeratosis) allows for accumulation of the mucin and lipid-rich apocrine sweat secretions which are then eliminated through the follicular epithelium and may incite an inflammatory response. Histiocytes phagocytose the material, imparting a foamy appearance that correlates with the xanthomatous infiltrate frequently seen in biopsies [146, 147].

2.8.1.1 Clinical Features

The hallmark presentation of FFD is relapsing and recurring pruritus of skin regions characterized by the presence of apocrine glands. While the axilla is most commonly involved, vulvar involvement alone has also been described [148]. Patients generally present with a history of itching in the axilla and perigenital regions. The clinical history will often reveal exacerbations during summer months, perimenstrually, and/or after exercise. Examination reveals small (1–3 mm), smooth, uniform, and equidistant follicular-based papules in the axillae and on the groin and areola (Fig. 2.43).

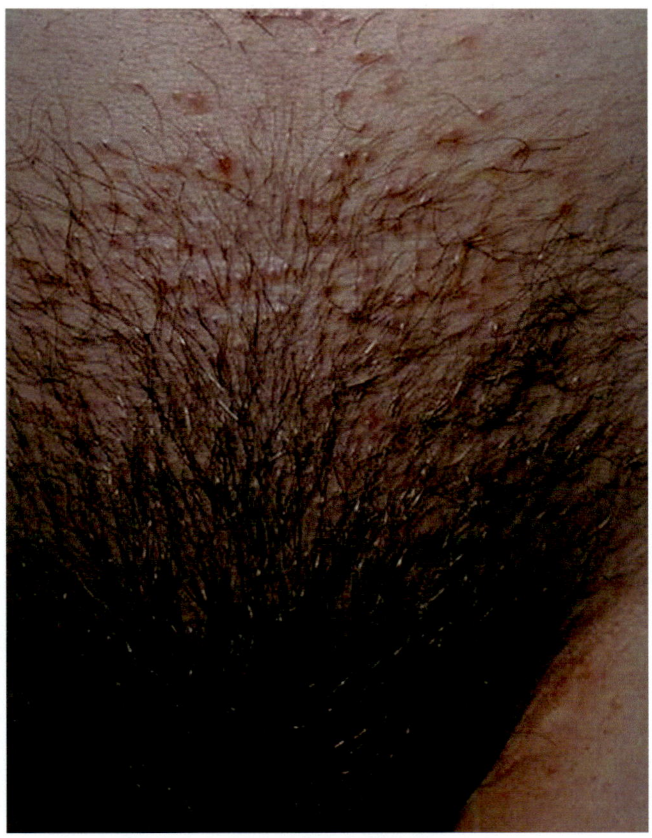

Fig. 2.43 Fox–Fordyce disease. Physical examination reveals follicular-based, uniform flesh-colored papules on mons pubis and external vulva. Photo provided courtesy of previous edition in Chinese (Science Press, Beijing, China)

The color of the lesions range from flesh colored to slightly erythematous to faintly yellow [146], and most papules lack an associated hair shaft [144].

Notably, although a hormonal influence is presumed based on the demographic patterns of affected patients, laboratory studies have not documented any consistent abnormalities in patients with FFD [144], and therefore are not indicated in the workup of this entity. The diagnosis is typically made clinically, although occasionally biopsy may be necessary to support the diagnosis and exclude other similarly appearing entities such as folliculitis (including acneiform eruptions and hidradenitis), lichen amyloidosis, lichen nitidus, and eruptive syringomas [145, 148].

Treatment of FFD is notoriously difficult. Avoidance of sweating may minimize exacerbations. Topical therapies including corticosteroids, retinoids, benzoyl peroxide, calcineurin inhibitors, and antibiotics are all mainstays of treatment. Systemic therapies include retinoids and oral contraceptive pills. Surgical excision or electrocautery have been reported in treatment-refractory cases [144, 145, 148].

2.8.1.2 Histopathologic Features

Early reports of the histology of FFD focused on the presence of a "retention vesicle" in the hair follicle in the region where the apocrine duct exits into the hair follicle (Fig. 2.44). Subsequent studies have expanded the features associated with the disease [146] and have abolished the requirement of a retention vesicle to be diagnostic. Some series have not convincingly identified retention vesicles in any cases [147]. As such, histopathologic examination of clinically presumed FFD may show a variety of features, many of which may be subtle. A nonspecific but nonetheless helpful clue will be the low-power observation of dilated apocrine glands [149]; however, this observation requires a punch biopsy as apocrine glands generally are not sampled in shave biopsies (Fig. 2.45). Most commonly observed and more specific features include spongiosis (edema) of the follicular infundibulum, follicular hyperkeratosis (follicular plugging by keratin), and dilation of the follicular infundibulum [146, 147, 150, 151] (Fig. 2.46). More contemporary series in the literature have focused on the presence of perifollicular foamy histiocytes, which in some cases may be subtle [145], and in other cases may be robust enough to form a frankly xanthomatous appearing zone [147, 151]. This perifollicular histiocytic infiltrate may also include lymphocytes and mast cells [147]. A less commonly observed feature is dyskeratosis within the follicular epithelium [146], which was seen in approximately one-quarter of cases in one study [147]. Cornoid lamellation (a narrow, vertical column of parakeratosis) and vacuolar changes in the epidermis have also been described occasionally [146] but were not seen in any of the seven cases examined of the largest series to date [147]. As the features may be subtle, serial sections may be necessary to find the described features that support the diagnosis;

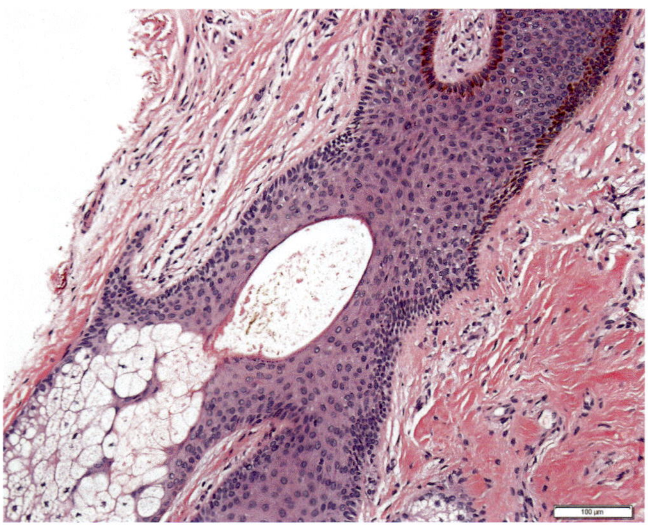

Fig. 2.44 Fox–Fordyce disease. A "retention vesicle" is seen in the follicle in the region where the apocrine duct enters the hair follicle

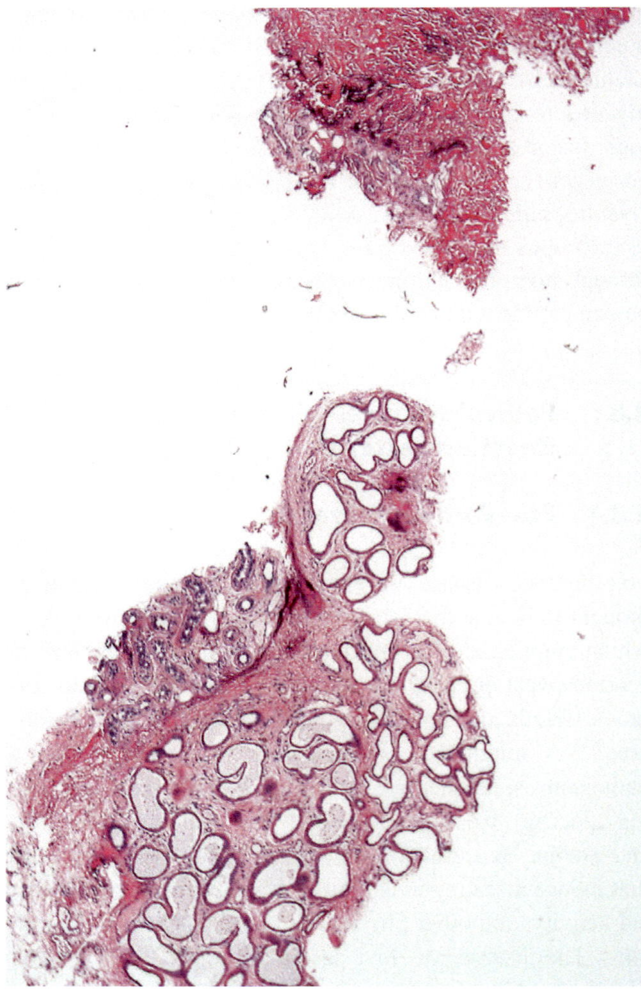

Fig. 2.45 Fox–Fordyce disease. Apocrine glands are often dilated, but not always sampled

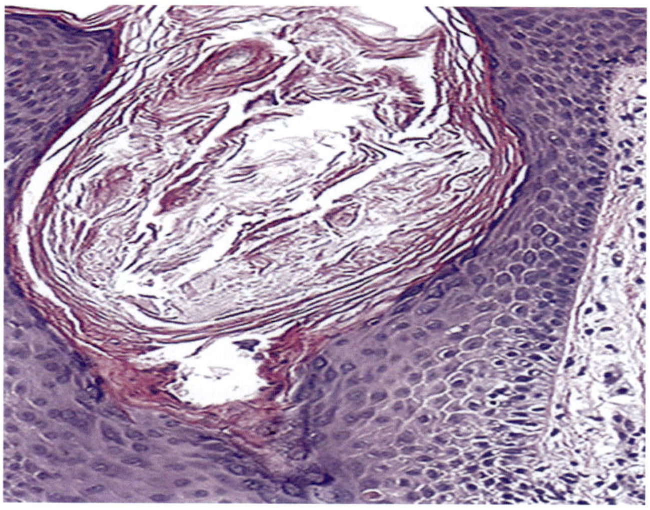

Fig. 2.46 Fox–Fordyce disease. The hair follicle is expanded and plugged by keratin (follicular hyperkeratosis). Photo provided courtesy of previous edition in Chinese (Science Press, Beijing, China)

alternatively, transverse sectioning (rather than the classical vertical sectioning of punch biopsies) can allow for evaluation of all hair follicles in the biopsy at once and has been advocated as the optimal method for diagnosis of FFD [150].

2.8.1.3 Immunohistochemical Features

Ancillary studies are not required to make the diagnosis. CD68 immunostaining will amplify subtle perifollicular histiocytes [145, 147]. The presence of PAS-positive, diastase-resistant material in the perifollicular zones has been used to support the notion that the perifollicular xanthomatous cells contain apocrine sweat secretions [151], but this finding has not been duplicated in other studies or cases [147, 149].

2.8.1.4 Differential Diagnosis

The histologic differential diagnosis includes xanthoma variants, granulomatous rosacea, and granulomatous perifolliculitis [147]. Xanthomas, which may occasionally involve similar sites as FFD, classically do not show preferential perifollicular location but are more interstitial. Serum lipid testing would reveal abnormalities in the case of xanthoma but would be expected to be normal in FFD. Granulomatous rosacea and granulomatous perifolliculitis would be unusual in the sites affected by FFD and are also typified by a granulomatous appearance that is less xanthomatous and may include multinucleated giant cells.

2.8.2 Hidradenitis Suppurativa

Hidradenitis suppurativa (HS) is a complex disease causing considerable morbidity for patients due to disabling pain and scarring. It is a chronic disease with episodic flaring. Patients are typically misdiagnosed in early stages of the disease, experience frequent delays in diagnosis, and often are inadequately managed by physicians unfamiliar with treating HS. The disease presents more commonly in females than in males (ratio 3:1) as painful inflammatory nodules in the intertriginous skin folds. Between 1 and 4% of the population may be affected by HS [125, 152]. The disease usually presents after puberty and often remits after menopause, which supports assertions of a hormonal role in the disease.

The pathogenesis of HS is related primarily to hair follicle abnormalities; however, factors such as the immune system, hormonal effects, diet and obesity, and external factors such as smoking all have been found to play a role in the development of the disease. The term "hidradenitis" is somewhat misleading as the sweat glands are not the source of the disease. In fact, HS is considered to be one of four diseases within the "follicular occlusion tetrad"—the others being acne conglobata, pilonidal cysts, and dissecting cellulitis [153]. All of these entities are linked by a similar pathogenic mechanism, namely, the obstruction of hair follicles, leading to occlusion, rupture, and recruitment of inflammatory cells. One of the first histologic changes in HS is hyperplasia and hyperkeratosis of the follicle in the region of the infundibulum (near the opening to the surface) [154]. As the follicles become hyperproliferative, sebum production may be increased [125] and occlusion of the follicle opening may occur. Ultimately, the expanded follicles rupture, spilling sebum, hair shafts, and any resident bacteria into the dermis and eliciting a robust inflammatory reaction. Defective immune responses to common skin flora may heighten the inflammatory response and prevent resolution of inflammation [153]. Over time, deep-seated ruptured follicles can form epithelial sinuses which can coalesce to form draining sinus tracts and nodules that characterize the disease.

HS can be seen in association with inflammatory bowel disease (both Crohn disease and ulcerative colitis), spondyloarthropathies linked to HLA B27, and pyoderma gangrenosum [153]. The association of HS with the metabolic syndrome has been a source of recent research focus [152].

Treatment of HS involves multidisciplinary care. Supportive care, medical management, and surgical excisions may all play a role through the duration of this chronic disease [125]. Current efforts involve increasing awareness of the disease to allow for earlier diagnosis to prevent long-term scarring sequelae. Chronic lymphedema and development of squamous cell carcinoma due to persistent inflammation are rare complications [152].

2.8.2.1 Clinical Features

HS presents with inflammatory lesions in the axillary, inguinal, anogenital, and inframammary skin folds. Patients will report recurring, waxing, and waning skin infections involving these regions. Skin lesions are generally tender and painful, and may prompt presentation to emergency departments rather than a primary care or gynecologic care center [125] (Fig. 2.47).

Physical examination during an acute episode may reveal large erythematous papules and nodules with fluctuance or bogginess distributed in the intertriginous sites. Acne-like lesions and pustules may be readily evident, as may ulcers and erosions. So-called "tombstone comedones" are characteristic of the disease. Inflammatory nodules may drain purulent, seropurulent, malodorous, and/or bloody fluid. Evidence of chronicity of the disease will be atrophic or hypertrophic scars, strictures, and contractures in these same areas [125]. Vulvar edema may be present as a result of inflammation elsewhere in the perigenital region.

Full body examination to include other sites that HS typically involves is imperative. Lymphadenopathy may sometimes be present as a result of the marked inflammation.

The clinical differential diagnosis of vulvar inflammatory nodules will include infections (including bacterial, mycobacterial, deep fungal, chronic herpetic, and other sexually transmitted infections), noncontiguous Crohn disease, and carcinoma. Cultures for microbial organisms are important to exclude infectious etiologies (whether primary or secondary). A skin biopsy (see histologic features below) is not always required to diagnose HS, but will be essential to exclude other more nefarious diagnoses.

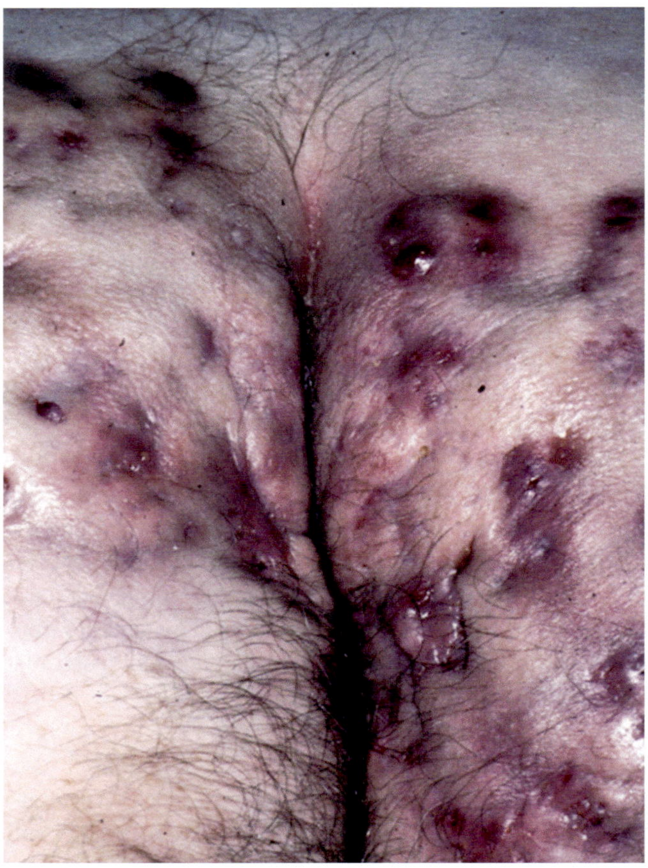

Fig. 2.47 Hidradenitis suppurativa. The vulva shows multiple erythematous and boggy lesions (Courtesy of Dr. Kenneth Hatch, University of Arizona)

2.8.2.2 Histopathologic Features

Skin biopsy is not requisite for a diagnosis of HS, and the features may differ depending on the stage and severity of the patient's disease.

Early lesions have been described as having both epidermal and follicular hyperplasia, perifolliculitis at the level of the infundibulum, and accumulation of keratin debris within the dilated follicle (follicular hyperkeratosis). These features were more common than actual follicular rupture or a neutrophilic-rich infiltrate, both of which were seen in only a quarter of early cases [155]. Follicular rupture and neutrophilic margination was postulated to be a later event in the sequence of lesional development (Figs. 2.48 and 2.49).

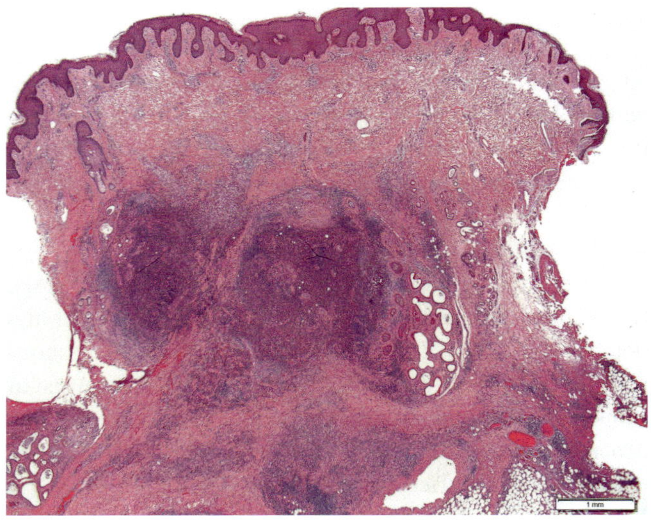

Fig. 2.48 Hidradenitis suppurativa. Scanning magnification shows a pan dermal infiltrate that destroys adnexal structures

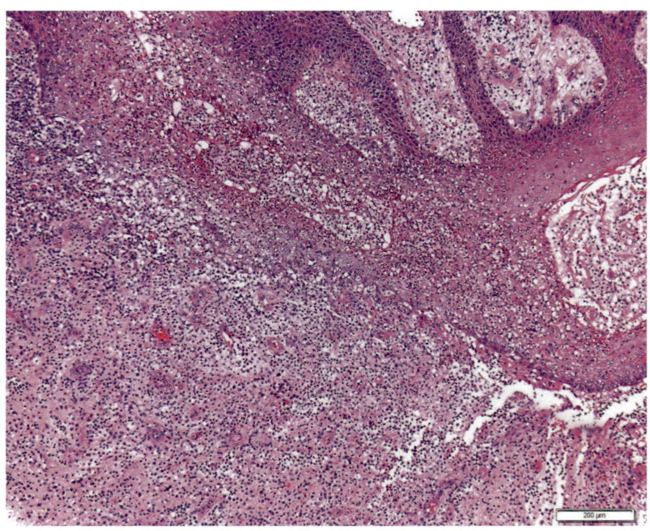

Fig. 2.49 Hidradenitis suppurativa. Follicular destruction and rupture mediated by neutrophils is commonly seen

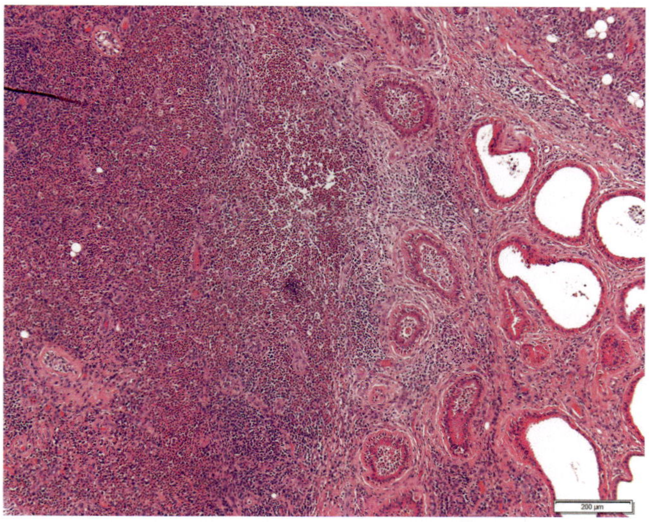

Fig. 2.50 Hidradenitis suppurativa. Less commonly, apocrine glands are invaded and destroyed by inflammation

Apocrine gland inflammation was seen in approximately half of cases [155] (Fig. 2.50), once again emphasizing that the term "hidradenitis" can be a misnomer.

The histologic features in well-established lesions (as may be seen in patients being surgically managed) are not particularly specific to the disease. However, the features seen are fairly characteristic and related to the pathogenesis. Dilated and ruptured hair follicles and follicular cysts are seen, with surrounding mixed inflammation and dermal fibrosis. Inflammation tends to be composed of neutrophils, lymphocytes, admixed polytypic plasma cells, histiocytes, and mast cells. Naked hair shafts surrounded by a granulomatous reaction and epithelial-lined sinus tracts are possible [156].

2.8.2.3 Immunohistochemical Features and Differential Diagnosis

The histologic differential diagnosis may include infection or nonspecific ruptured folliculitis. Special cytochemical or immunohistochemical stains to exclude infection may be useful, although microbial cultures will always provide a more sensitive mechanism to detect organisms. The presence of discrete, noncaseating granulomas may provide a clue to a diagnosis of metastatic/noncontiguous Crohn disease.

If tissue is provided without accompanying clinical information, it may be impossible to provide an outright diagnosis of HS. However, the astute pathologist, when confronted with a vulvar biopsy showing scarring, inflammation, and ruptured pilosebaceous units, may be able to suggest the possibility of HS.

Acknowledgements The author thanks Dr. Susi Jeffus for her generous editorial assistance during the preparation of this chapter.

References

1. Hoang MP, Selim MA. Vulvar pathology. 1st ed. New York: Springer; 2015.
2. Niamh L, Naveen S, Hazel B. Diagnosis of vulval inflammatory dermatoses: a pathological study with clinical correlation. Int J Gynecol Pathol. 2009;28:554–8.
3. Chan MP, Zimarowski MJ. Vulvar dermatoses: a histopathologic review and classification of 183 cases. J Cutan Pathol. 2015;42:510–8.
4. O'Keefe RJ, Scurry JP, Dennerstein G, et al. Audit of 114 non-neoplastic vulvar biopsies. Br J Obstet Gynaecol. 1995;102:780–6.
5. Koppes SA, Engebretsen KA, Agner T, et al. Current knowledge on biomarkers for contact sensitization and allergic contact dermatitis. Contact Dermatitis. 2017;77:1–16.
6. Schlosser BJ. Contact dermatitis of the vulva. Dermatol Clin. 2010;28:697–706.
7. Warner N, Salvaggio HL, Zaenglein AL. JAAD Grand Rounds quiz. An erosive vulvar rash. J Am Acad Dermatol. 2013;68:350–2.
8. O'Gorman SM, Torgerson RR. Allergic contact dermatitis of the vulva. Dermatitis. 2013;24:64–72.
9. Nardelli A, Degreef H, Goossens A. Contact allergic reactions of the vulva: a 14-year review. Dermatitis. 2004;15:131–6.
10. Pichardo-Geisinger R. Atopic and contact dermatitis of the vulva. Obstet Gynecol Clin N Am. 2017;44:371–8.
11. Rosa G, Fernandez AP, Vij A, et al. Langerhans cell collections, but not eosinophils, are clues to a diagnosis of allergic contact dermatitis in appropriate skin biopsies. J Cutan Pathol. 2016;43:498–504.
12. Willis CM, Young E, Brandon DR, et al. Immunopathological and ultrastructural findings in human allergic and irritant contact dermatitis. Br J Dermatol. 1986;115:305–16.
13. Taylor RM. Histopathology of contact dermatitis. Clin Dermatol. 1986;4:18–22.
14. Rosa G, Fernandez AP, Schneider S, et al. Eosinophils are rare in biopsy specimens of psoriasis vulgaris. J Cutan Pathol. 2017;44:1027–32.
15. Sharon VR, Konia TH, Barr KL, et al. Assessment of the 'no eosinophils' rule: are eosinophils truly absent in pityriasis lichenoides, connective tissue disease, and graft-vs.-host disease? J Cutan Pathol. 2012;39:413–8.
16. Ozalp SS, Telli E, Yalcin OT, et al. Vulval pruritus: the experience of gynaecologists revealed by biopsy. J Obstet Gynaecol. 2015;35:53–6.
17. Lynch PJ, Moyal-Barracco M, Scurry J, et al. 2011 ISSVD Terminology and classification of vulvar dermatological disorders: an approach to clinical diagnosis. J Low Genit Tract Dis. 2012;16:339–44.
18. Chibnall R. Vulvar pruritus and lichen simplex chronicus. Obstet Gynecol Clin N Am. 2017;44:379–88.
19. Lynch PJ. 2006 International Society for the Study of Vulvovaginal Disease classification of vulvar dermatoses: a synopsis. J Low Genit Tract Dis. 2007;11:1–2.
20. Parisi R, Symmons DP, Griffiths CE, et al. Global epidemiology of psoriasis: a systematic review of incidence and prevalence. J Invest Dermatol. 2013;133:377–85.
21. Kapila S, Bradford J, Fischer G. Vulvar psoriasis in adults and children: a clinical audit of 194 cases and review of the literature. J Low Genit Tract Dis. 2012;16:364–71.
22. Griffiths CE, Barker JN. Pathogenesis and clinical features of psoriasis. Lancet. 2007;370:263–71.
23. Andreassi L, Bilenchi R. Non-infectious inflammatory genital lesions. Clin Dermatol. 2014;32:307–14.
24. Guerrero A, Venkatesan A. Inflammatory vulvar dermatoses. Clin Obstet Gynecol. 2015;58:464–75.

25. Omland SH, Gniadecki R. Psoriasis inversa: a separate identity or a variant of psoriasis vulgaris? Clin Dermatol. 2015;33:456–61.
26. Woo YR, Cho DH, Park HJ. Molecular mechanisms and management of a cutaneous inflammatory disorder: psoriasis. Int J Mol Sci. 2017;18:2684.
27. Ogawa E, Sato Y, Minagawa A, et al. Pathogenesis of psoriasis and development of treatment. J Dermatol. 2018;45:264–72.
28. Geller S, Xu H, Lebwohl M, et al. Malignancy risk and recurrence with psoriasis and its treatments: a concise update. Am J Clin Dermatol. 2018;19:363–75.
29. Zamirska A, Reich A, Berny-Moreno J, et al. Vulvar pruritus and burning sensation in women with psoriasis. Acta Derm Venereol. 2008;88:132–5.
30. Chau T, Parsi KK, Ogawa T, et al. Psoriasis or not? Review of 51 clinically confirmed cases reveals an expanded histopathologic spectrum of psoriasis. J Cutan Pathol. 2017;44:1018–26.
31. Kocak M, Bozdogan O, Erkek E, et al. Examination of Bcl-2, Bcl-X and bax protein expression in psoriasis. Int J Dermatol. 2003;42:789–93.
32. Moy AP, Murali M, Kroshinsky D, et al. Immunologic overlap of helper T-cell subtypes 17 and 22 in erythrodermic psoriasis and atopic dermatitis. JAMA Dermatol. 2015;151:753–60.
33. Lotery HE, Galask RP, Stone MS, et al. Ulcerative vulvitis in atypical Reiter's syndrome. J Am Acad Dermatol. 2003;48:613–6.
34. Edwards L, Hansen RC. Reiter's syndrome of the vulva. The psoriasis spectrum. Arch Dermatol. 1992;128:811–4.
35. Lewis FM, Bogliatto F. Erosive vulval lichen planus—a diagnosis not to be missed: a clinical review. Eur J Obstet Gynecol Reprod Biol. 2013;171:214–9.
36. Kirtschig G, Wakelin SH, Wojnarowska F. Mucosal vulval lichen planus: outcome, clinical and laboratory features. J Eur Acad Dermatol Venereol. 2005;19:301–7.
37. Job AM, Kaimal S. Lichen planus hypertrophicus of the vulva—a rare entity. Int J STD AIDS. 2017;28:1048–50.
38. Cooper SM, Haefner HK, Abrahams-Gessel S, et al. Vulvovaginal lichen planus treatment: a survey of current practices. Arch Dermatol. 2008;144:1520–1.
39. Lewis FM. Vulval lichen planus. Br J Dermatol. 1998;138:569–75.
40. Terlou A, Santegoets LA, van der Meijden WI, et al. An autoimmune phenotype in vulvar lichen sclerosus and lichen planus: a Th1 response and high levels of microRNA-155. J Invest Dermatol. 2012;132:658–66.
41. Cooper SM, Kirtschig G, Jeffery KJ, et al. No association between hepatitis B or C viruses and vulval lichen planus in a UK population. BJOG. 2004;111:271–3.
42. Cooper SM, Ali I, Baldo M, et al. The association of lichen sclerosus and erosive lichen planus of the vulva with autoimmune disease: a case-control study. Arch Dermatol. 2008;144:1432–5.
43. Halonen P, Jakobsson M, Heikinheimo O, et al. Cancer risk of lichen planus: a cohort study of 13,100 women in Finland. Int J Cancer. 2018;142:18–22.
44. Ball R, Ball KM, Reutter J. Epithelial vulvar neoplasms and their changing classification. Semin Cutan Med Surg. 2015;34:199–205.
45. Regauer S, Reich O, Eberz B. Vulvar cancers in women with vulvar lichen planus: a clinicopathological study. J Am Acad Dermatol. 2014;71:698–707.
46. Cooper SM, Wojnarowska F. Influence of treatment of erosive lichen planus of the vulva on its prognosis. Arch Dermatol. 2006;142:289–94.
47. Mauskar M. Erosive Lichen Planus. Obstet Gynecol Clin N Am. 2017;44:407–20.
48. Fruchter R, Melnick L, Pomeranz MK. Lichenoid vulvar disease: a review. Int J Womens Dermatol. 2017;3:58–64.
49. Helgesen AL, Gjersvik P, Jebsen P, et al. Vaginal involvement in genital erosive lichen planus. Acta Obstet Gynecol Scand. 2010;89:966–70.
50. Murphy R. Desquamative inflammatory vaginitis. Dermatol Ther. 2004;17:47–9.
51. Simpson RC, Thomas KS, Leighton P, et al. Diagnostic criteria for erosive lichen planus affecting the vulva: an international electronic-Delphi consensus exercise. Br J Dermatol. 2013;169:337–43.
52. Day T, Moore S, Bohl TG, et al. Comorbid vulvar lichen planus and lichen sclerosus. J Low Genit Tract Dis. 2017;21:204–8.
53. Day T, Bowden N, Jaaback K, et al. Distinguishing erosive lichen planus from differentiated vulvar intraepithelial neoplasia. J Low Genit Tract Dis. 2016;20:174–9.
54. Fung MA, LeBoit PE. Light microscopic criteria for the diagnosis of early vulvar lichen sclerosus: a comparison with lichen planus. Am J Surg Pathol. 1998;22:473–8.
55. Brix WK, Nassau SR, Patterson JW, et al. Idiopathic lymphoplasmacellular mucositis-dermatitis. J Cutan Pathol. 2010; 37:426–31.
56. Fistarol SK, Itin PH. Diagnosis and treatment of lichen sclerosus: an update. Am J Clin Dermatol. 2013;14:27–47.
57. Ball SB, Wojnarowska F. Vulvar dermatoses: lichen sclerosus, lichen planus, and vulval dermatitis/lichen simplex chronicus. Semin Cutan Med Surg. 1998;17:182–8.
58. Fischer G, Rogers M. Vulvar disease in children: a clinical audit of 130 cases. Pediatr Dermatol. 2000;17:1–6.
59. Vilano SE, Robbins CL. Common prepubertal vulvar conditions. Curr Opin Obstet Gynecol. 2016;28:359–65.
60. Smith YR, Haefner HK. Vulvar lichen sclerosus: pathophysiology and treatment. Am J Clin Dermatol. 2004;5:105–25.
61. Murphy R. Lichen sclerosus. Dermatol Clin. 2010;28:707–15.
62. Weyers W. Hypertrophic lichen sclerosus with dyskeratosis and parakeratosis—a common presentation of vulvar lichen sclerosus not associated with a significant risk of malignancy. Am J Dermatopathol. 2013;35:713–21.
63. Aide S, Lattario FR, Almeida G, et al. Epstein-Barr virus and human papillomavirus infection in vulvar lichen sclerosus. J Low Genit Tract Dis. 2010;14:319–22.
64. Weyers W. Hypertrophic lichen sclerosus sine sclerosis: clues to histopathologic diagnosis when presenting as psoriasiform lichenoid dermatitis. J Cutan Pathol. 2015;42:118–29.
65. Farrell AM, Dean D, Millard PR, et al. Cytokine alterations in lichen sclerosus: an immunohistochemical study. Br J Dermatol. 2006;155:931–40.
66. de Oliveira GA, de Almeida MP, Soares FA, et al. Metalloproteinases 2 and 9 and their tissue inhibitors 1 and 2 are increased in vulvar lichen sclerosus. Eur J Obstet Gynecol Reprod Biol. 2012;161:96–101.
67. van de Nieuwenhof HP, Bulten J, Hollema H, et al. Differentiated vulvar intraepithelial neoplasia is often found in lesions, previously diagnosed as lichen sclerosus, which have progressed to vulvar squamous cell carcinoma. Mod Pathol. 2011;24: 297–305.
68. Liegl B, Regauer S. p53 immunostaining in lichen sclerosus is related to ischaemic stress and is not a marker of differentiated vulvar intraepithelial neoplasia (d-VIN). Histopathology. 2006;48:268–74.
69. Li Q, Leopold K, Carlson JA. Chronic vulvar purpura: persistent pigmented purpuric dermatitis (lichen aureus) of the vulva or plasma cell (Zoon's) vulvitis? J Cutan Pathol. 2003;30:572–6.
70. Salopek TG, Siminoski K. Vulvitis circumscripta plasmacellularis (Zoon's vulvitis) associated with autoimmune polyglandular endocrine failure. Br J Dermatol. 1996;135:991–4.
71. Virgili A, Corazza M, Minghetti S, et al. Symptoms in plasma cell vulvitis: first observational cohort study on type, frequency and severity. Dermatology. 2015;230:113–8.
72. Kavanagh GM, Burton PA, Kennedy CT. Vulvitis chronica plasmacellularis (Zoon's vulvitis). Br J Dermatol. 1993;129:92–3.

73. van Kessel MA, van Lingen RG, Bovenschen HJ. Vulvitis plasmacellularis circumscripta in pre-existing lichen sclerosus: treatment with imiquimod 5% cream. J Am Acad Dermatol. 2010;63:e11–3.
74. Bharatia PR, Pradhan AM, Zawar VP. Plasma cell vulvitis. Indian J Sex Transm Dis. 2015;36:185–7.
75. Virgili A, Levratti A, Marzola A, et al. Retrospective histopathologic reevaluation of 18 cases of plasma cell vulvitis. J Reprod Med. 2005;50:3–7.
76. Thomson MA, Carr RA, Ganesan R, et al. Extensive mucinous metaplasia of the vulva arising within Zoon's vulvitis. Br J Dermatol. 2007;156:750–2.
77. Meneux E, Paniel BJ, Pouget F, et al. Vulvovaginal sequelae in toxic epidermal necrolysis. J Reprod Med. 1997;42:153–6.
78. Noel JC, Buxant F, Fayt I, et al. Vulval adenosis associated with toxic epidermal necrolysis. Br J Dermatol. 2005;153:457–8.
79. Bonafe JL, Thibaut I, Hoff J. Introital adenosis associated with the Stevens-Johnson syndrome. Clin Exp Dermatol. 1990;15:356–7.
80. Ciavattini A, Clemente N. Female genital tract chronic graft-versus-host disease: review of the literature. Anticancer Res. 2015;35:13–7.
81. Smith Knutsson E, Bjork Y, Broman AK, et al. Genital chronic graft-versus-host disease in females: a cross-sectional study. Biol Blood Marrow Transplant. 2014;20:806–11.
82. Kornik RI, Rustagi AS. Vulvovaginal graft-versus-host disease. Obstet Gynecol Clin N Am. 2017;44:475–92.
83. Zantomio D, Grigg AP, MacGregor L, et al. Female genital tract graft-versus-host disease: incidence, risk factors and recommendations for management. Bone Marrow Transplant. 2006;38:567–72.
84. Brahimi N, Routier E, Raison-Peyron N, et al. A three-year-analysis of fixed drug eruptions in hospital settings in France. Eur J Dermatol. 2010;20:461–4.
85. Fischer G. Vulvar fixed drug eruption. A report of 13 cases. J Reprod Med. 2007;52:81–6.
86. Kavala M, Topaloglu Demir F, Zindanci I, et al. Genital involvement in pemphigus vulgaris (PV): correlation with clinical and cervicovaginal Pap smear findings. J Am Acad Dermatol. 2015;73:655–9.
87. Akhyani M, Chams-Davatchi C, Naraghi Z, et al. Cervicovaginal involvement in pemphigus vulgaris: a clinical study of 77 cases. Br J Dermatol. 2008;158:478–82.
88. Malik M, Ahmed AR. Involvement of the female genital tract in pemphigus vulgaris. Obstet Gynecol. 2005;106:1005–12.
89. Bohl TG. Vulvar ulcers and erosions—a dermatologist's viewpoint. Dermatol Ther. 2004;17:55–67.
90. Esmaili N, Chams-Davatchi C, Valikhani M, et al. Pemphigus vulgaris in Iran: a clinical study of 140 cases. Int J Dermatol. 2007;46:1166–70.
91. Spindler V, Eming R, Schmidt E, et al. Mechanisms causing loss of keratinocyte cohesion in pemphigus. J Invest Dermatol. 2018;138:32–7.
92. Atzmony L, Hodak E, Gdalevich M, et al. Treatment of pemphigus vulgaris and pemphigus foliaceus: a systematic review and meta-analysis. Am J Clin Dermatol. 2014;15:503–15.
93. Saldanha CS, Shenoy MM, Shanthala PR, et al. Multiple vegetating lesions over the genitalia. Diagnosis: pemphigus vegetans. Indian J Dermatol Venereol Leprol. 2015;81:325–6.
94. Jain V, Jindal N, Imchen S. Localized pemphigus vegetans without mucosal involvement. Indian J Dermatol. 2014;59:210.
95. Vaughan Jones SA, Salas J, McGrath JA, et al. A retrospective analysis of tissue-fixed immunoreactants from skin biopsies maintained in Michel's medium. Dermatology. 1994;189(Suppl 1):131–2.
96. Wick MR. Bullous, pseudobullous, & pustular dermatoses. Semin Diagn Pathol. 2017;34:250–60.
97. Diercks GF, Pas HH, Jonkman MF. Immunofluorescence of autoimmune bullous diseases. Surg Pathol Clin. 2017;10:505–12.
98. Lewis FM, Agarwal A, Neill SM, et al. The spectrum of histopathologic patterns secondary to the topical application of EMLA(R) on vulvar epithelium: clinicopathological correlation in three cases. J Cutan Pathol. 2013;40:708–13.
99. Nigen S, Poulin Y, Rochette L, et al. Pyodermatitis-pyostomatitis vegetans: two cases and a review of the literature. J Cutan Med Surg. 2003;7:250–5.
100. Carvalho S, Sanches M, Alves R, et al. Pyodermatitis vegetans of the vulva. Dermatol Online J. 2016;22(6).
101. Farrell AM, Kirtschig G, Dalziel KL, et al. Childhood vulval pemphigoid: a clinical and immunopathological study of five patients. Br J Dermatol. 1999;140:308–12.
102. Goldstein AT, Anhalt GJ, Klingman D, et al. Mucous membrane pemphigoid of the vulva. Obstet Gynecol. 2005;105:1188–90.
103. Hamann ID, NC H, Hunter JA. Chronic bullous dermatosis of childhood: relapse after puberty. J R Soc Med. 1995;88:296P–7P.
104. Mintz EM, Morel KD. Clinical features, diagnosis, and pathogenesis of chronic bullous disease of childhood. Dermatol Clin. 2011;29:459–62, ix.
105. Mihalyi L, Kiss M, Dobozy A, et al. Clinical relevance of autoantibodies in patients with autoimmune bullous dermatosis. Clin Dev Immunol. 2012;2012:369546.
106. Hoque SR, Patel M, Farrell AM. Childhood cicatricial pemphigoid confined to the vulva. Clin Exp Dermatol. 2006;31:63–4.
107. Urano S. Localized bullous pemphigoid of the vulva. J Dermatol. 1996;23:580–2.
108. Sardy M, Kostaki D, Varga R, et al. Comparative study of direct and indirect immunofluorescence and of bullous pemphigoid 180 and 230 enzyme-linked immunosorbent assays for diagnosis of bullous pemphigoid. J Am Acad Dermatol. 2013;69:748–53.
109. Jankaskova J, Horvath ON, Varga R, et al. Increased sensitivity and high specificity of indirect immunofluorescence in detecting IgG subclasses for diagnosis of bullous pemphigoid. Clin Exp Dermatol. 2018;43:248–53.
110. Holst VA, Fair KP, Wilson BB, et al. Squamous cell carcinoma arising in Hailey-Hailey disease. J Am Acad Dermatol. 2000;43:368–71.
111. Pernet C, Bessis D, Savignac M, et al. Genitoperineal papular acantholytic dyskeratosis is allelic to Hailey-Hailey disease. Br J Dermatol. 2012;167:210–2.
112. Knopp EA, Saraceni C, Moss J, et al. Somatic ATP2A2 mutation in a case of papular acantholytic dyskeratosis: mosaic Darier disease. J Cutan Pathol. 2015;42:853–7.
113. Hadjicharralambous E, Diamond S, Mehregan D. Papular acantholytic dyskeratosis of vulva in setting of Hailey-Hailey. Int J Dermatol. 2017;56:e126–8.
114. Langenberg A, Berger TG, Cardelli M, et al. Genital benign chronic pemphigus (Hailey-Hailey disease) presenting as condylomas. J Am Acad Dermatol. 1992;26:951–5.
115. Wieselthier JS, Pincus SH. Hailey-Hailey disease of the vulva. Arch Dermatol. 1993;129:1344–5.
116. Salopek TG, Krol A, Jimbow K. Case report of Darier disease localized to the vulva in a 5-year-old girl. Pediatr Dermatol. 1993;10:146–8.
117. Baliu-Pique C, Iranzo P. Papular acantholytic dyskeratosis of the vulva in a woman with benign familial pemphigus. Actas Dermosifiliogr. 2017;108:78–9.
118. Cooper PH. Acantholytic dermatosis localized to the vulvocrural area. J Cutan Pathol. 1989;16:81–4.
119. Wong TY, Mihm MC Jr. Acantholytic dermatosis localized to genitalia and crural areas of male patients: a report of three cases. J Cutan Pathol. 1994;21:27–32.
120. Laftah Z, Bailey C, Zaheri S, et al. Vulval Crohn's disease: a clinical study of 22 patients. J Crohns Colitis. 2015;9:318–25.
121. Barret M, de Parades V, Battistella M, et al. Crohn's disease of the vulva. J Crohns Colitis. 2014;8:563–70.

122. Boxhoorn L, Stoof TJ, de Meij T, et al. Clinical experience and diagnostic algorithm of vulval Crohn's disease. Eur J Gastroenterol Hepatol. 2017;29:838–43.
123. Andreani SM, Ratnasingham K, Dang HH, et al. Crohn's disease of the vulva. Int J Surg. 2010;8:2–5.
124. Emanuel PO, Phelps RG. Metastatic Crohn's disease: a histopathologic study of 12 cases. J Cutan Pathol. 2008;35:457–61.
125. Stewart KMA. Challenging ulcerative vulvar conditions: hidradenitis suppurativa, Crohn disease, and aphthous ulcers. Obstet Gynecol Clin North Am. 2017;44:453–73.
126. Foo WC, Papalas JA, Robboy SJ, et al. Vulvar manifestations of Crohn's disease. Am J Dermatopathol. 2011;33:588–93.
127. Ishida M, Iwai M, Yoshida K, et al. Metastatic Crohn's disease accompanying granulomatous vasculitis and lymphangitis in the vulva. Int J Clin Exp Pathol. 2013;6:2263–6.
128. Tursen U, Gurler A, Boyvat A. Evaluation of clinical findings according to sex in 2313 Turkish patients with Behcet's disease. Int J Dermatol. 2003;42:346–51.
129. Bulur I, Onder M. Behcet disease: new aspects. Clin Dermatol. 2017;35:421–34.
130. Yazici H, Seyahi E, Hatemi G, et al. Behcet syndrome: a contemporary view. Nat Rev Rheumatol. 2018;14:107–19.
131. Gurler A, Boyvat A, Tursen U. Clinical manifestations of Behcet's disease: an analysis of 2147 patients. Yonsei Med J. 1997;38:423–7.
132. International Study Group for Behcet's Disease. Criteria for diagnosis of Behcet's disease. Lancet. 1990;335:1078–80.
133. Kaya TI, Dur H, Tursen U, et al. Association of class I HLA antigens with the clinical manifestations of Turkish patients with Behcet's disease. Clin Exp Dermatol. 2002;27:498–501.
134. Maia S, Martins A, Santos C, et al. Genital ulcers: do not forget Behcet disease. BMJ Case Rep. 2012;2012.
135. Kim ES, Chung WC, Lee KM, et al. A case of intestinal Behcet's disease similar to Crohn's colitis. J Korean Med Sci. 2007;22:918–22.
136. Wong WW, Machado GR, Hill ME. Pyoderma gangrenosum: the great pretender and a challenging diagnosis. J Cutan Med Surg. 2011;15:322–8.
137. Slocum AMY. A surgeon's nightmare: pyoderma gangrenosum with pathergy effect mimicking necrotising fasciitis. BMJ Case Rep. 2017;2017.
138. Sau M, Hill NC. Pyoderma gangrenosum of the vulva. BJOG. 2001;108:1197–8.
139. Reed BG, Shippey S, Kremp A, et al. Vulvar pyoderma gangrenosum originating from a healed obstetric laceration. Obstet Gynecol. 2013;122:452–5.
140. Sripathi H, Rao R, Prabhu S, et al. Pyoderma gangrenosum affecting the vulva. Indian J Dermatol Venereol Leprol. 2008; 74:506–8.
141. Valmadre S, Gee A, Dalrymple C. Pyoderma gangrenosum of the vulva. Aust N Z J Obstet Gynaecol. 2002;42:548–9.
142. Dabade TS, Davis MD. Diagnosis and treatment of the neutrophilic dermatoses (pyoderma gangrenosum, Sweet's syndrome). Dermatol Ther. 2011;24:273–84.
143. Brooklyn T, Dunnill G, Probert C. Diagnosis and treatment of pyoderma gangrenosum. BMJ. 2006;333:181–4.
144. Yost J, Robinson M, Meehan SA. Fox-Fordyce disease. Dermatol Online J. 2012;18:28.
145. Kao PH, Hsu CK, Lee JY. Clinicopathological study of Fox-Fordyce disease. J Dermatol. 2009;36:485–90.
146. Boer A. Patterns histopathologic of Fox-Fordyce disease. Am J Dermatopathol. 2004;26:482–92.
147. Bormate AB Jr, Leboit PE, McCalmont TH. Perifollicular xanthomatosis as the hallmark of axillary Fox-Fordyce disease: an evaluation of histopathologic features of 7 cases. Arch Dermatol. 2008;144:1020–4.
148. Gurusamy L, Jegadeesan M, Jayakumar S. Fox-Fordyce disease of the vulva. Indian J Sex Transm Dis. 2016;37:65–7.
149. Macarenco RS, Garces SJ. Dilation of apocrine glands. A forgotten but helpful histopathological clue to the diagnosis of axillary Fox-Fordyce disease. Am J Dermatopathol. 2009;31: 393–7.
150. Stashower ME, SJ K, Turiansky GW. Fox-Fordyce disease: diagnosis with transverse histologic sections. J Am Acad Dermatol. 2000;42:89–91.
151. Brau Javier CN, Morales A, Sanchez JL. Histopathology attributes of Fox-Fordyce disease. Int J Dermatol. 2012;51:1313–8.
152. Ergun T. Hidradenitis suppurativa and the metabolic syndrome. Clin Dermatol. 2018;36:41–7.
153. Scheinfeld N. Diseases associated with hidranitis suppurativa: part 2 of a series on hidradenitis. Dermatol Online J. 2013;19: 18558.
154. Schneider MR, Paus R. Deciphering the functions of the hair follicle infundibulum in skin physiology and disease. Cell Tissue Res. 2014;358:697–704.
155. von Laffert M, Stadie V, Wohlrab J, et al. Hidradenitis suppurativa/acne inversa: bilocated epithelial hyperplasia with very different sequelae. Br J Dermatol. 2011;164:367–71.
156. Martorell A, Garcia-Martinez FJ, Jimenez-Gallo D, et al. An update on hidradenitis suppurativa (part I): epidemiology, clinical aspects, and definition of disease severity. Actas Dermosifiliogr. 2015;106:703–15.

3 Infectious Disorders of the Lower Genital Tract

Somaye Yeke Zare, Mariah Zampieri Leivo, Hao Chen, and Vighnesh Walavalkar

Abstract

Infectious diseases of the lower female genital tract include a variety of bacterial, viral, fungal, and parasitic infections that are commonly, but not exclusively, sexually transmitted. Sexually transmitted diseases (STDs) are a global public health issue and have serious impact on health care costs in the United States. The Centers for Disease Control and Prevention announced increasing numbers of reported STDs in recent years. Chlamydia, gonorrhea, and especially syphilis rates have increased dramatically over the past few years. Most infections of the lower female genital tract are diagnosed clinically, and tissue biopsies are rarely performed; however, it is important to be familiar with these entities and their histopathologic features to avoid misdiagnosis of these rather common infections. This chapter reviews clinical and pathologic presentations of common infections of the lower female genital tract, and incorporates the latest guidelines available for each entity. Human papillomavirus infection is briefly discussed under common sexually transmitted infections and generalized genital warts in patients with immunosuppression, and further reviewed in detail in other chapters. It also includes rare entities in the United States that should be considered in the differential diagnosis of patients with human immunodeficiency virus infection and vulvovaginal involvement by systemic infections in immunosuppressed individuals.

S. Y. Zare (✉) · M. Z. Leivo
Department of Pathology, University of California San Diego, San Diego, CA, USA
e-mail: syekezare@ucsd.edu

H. Chen
Department of Pathology, University of Texas Southwestern Medical Center, Dallas, TX, USA

V. Walavalkar
Department of Pathology, UCSF School of Medicine, San Francisco, CA, USA
e-mail: Vighnesh.Walavalkar@ucsf.edu

Keywords

Infectious diseases · Genital ulcers · Sexually transmitted disease · Discharge · Transmission

3.1 Common Sexually Transmitted Infections

3.1.1 *Trichomonas vaginalis*

Trichomoniasis is the most common nonviral sexually transmitted disease (STD), caused by a motile flagellate parasitic protozoan, *Trichomonas vaginalis* (*T. vaginalis*) [1]. The parasite is typically pyriform, although in vivo amoeboid forms are occasionally identified. It has four anterior flagella, plus one recurrent flagellum that forms the undulating membrane [2, 3]. *T. vaginalis* infection only occurs in humans, and is more common in women, with estimated prevalence of 3.1% among women of reproductive age in the United States [4]. Higher rates of *T. vaginalis* infections have been reported among women 40 years and older (>11%). The infection is more prevalent among women with other STDs and human immunodeficiency virus (HIV)-infected individuals [5, 6].

Trophozoites of *T. vaginalis* are transmitted through sexual intercourse and attach to the mucosal surfaces of the lower urogenital tract. The organisms colonize the mucosa and release proteinases resulting in desquamation of the vaginal and cervical epithelia [7]. Trichomoniasis is associated with adverse outcomes of pregnancy, such as preterm labor or delivery of a low-birth weight infant [1, 5]. In addition, *T. vaginalis* may increase women's risk of HIV acquisition and transmission [8].

Clinical features: The infection manifests with vulvovaginal pruritus and irritation, as well as frothy or yellow-green vaginal discharge. Cervical examination may reveal signs of cervicitis with punctate friability (strawberry cervix).

W. Zheng et al. (eds.), *Gynecologic and Obstetric Pathology, Volume 1*, https://doi.org/10.1007/978-981-13-3016-2_3

Multiple studies have indicated that nearly half of the infected women are asymptomatic [3, 5, 7].

Diagnostic methods: Diagnosis can be made through a variety of techniques such as wet mount microscopy, culture, rapid antigen tests, polymerase chain reaction, and nucleic acid amplification test [1, 3]. Pap smears are not considered appropriate diagnostic or screening tests for *T. vaginalis* because of their poor sensitivity; however, if the organism is identified on liquid-based cervical smears, the specificity is high [8, 9].

Microscopic findings: On histologic sections, the findings are nonspecific. The morphologic findings on cytology smears include identification of the pear-shaped organisms with eosinophilic cytoplasmic granules and eccentrically located vesicular nuclei (Fig. 3.1), clusters of neutrophils (polyballs), reactive nuclear changes with small perinuclear halos, and attachment of *T. vaginalis* to squamous cells [10, 11]. *Leptothrix* may be seen in association with *T. vaginalis* [11].

Management: Concurrent treatment of the patient and all sex partners is curative and reduces transmission. First-line therapy consists of a single dose of metronidazole or tinidazole, as recommended by the United States Centers for Disease Control and Prevention (CDC) [12].

3.1.2 Molluscum Contagiosum

Molluscum contagiosum is a viral infection caused by a double-stranded DNA virus of the Poxviridae family, *Molluscum contagiosum virus* (MCV). There are four known genotypes of MCV; type 1 is the most common form in healthy humans. The disease is more prevalent in children, transmitted by direct skin contact, and usually affects the exposed areas [13, 14]. In healthy young adults the disease is often transmitted sexually and lesions initially appear in genital area. However, the virus may be transmitted by casual contact or self-inoculation. Among HIV positive population, molluscum contagiosum is more common and can present as widespread lesions [13, 15].

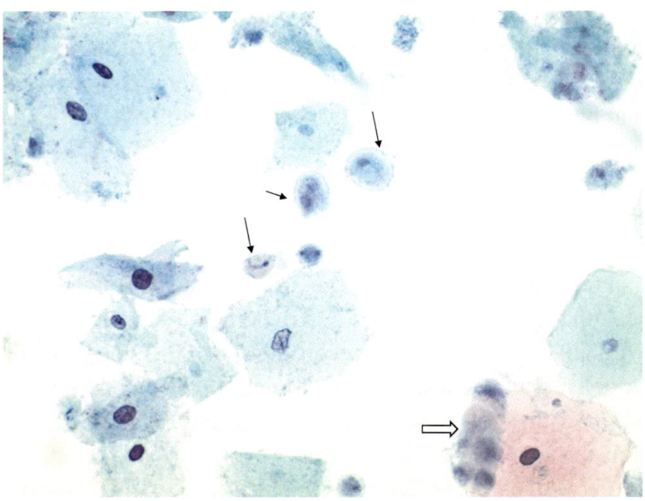

Fig. 3.1 Papanicolaou-stained liquid-based smear depicts *T. vaginalis*, pear-shaped organisms with eosinophilic cytoplasmic granules and eccentric nucleus (arrows) and attachment of the organisms to squamous cells (white arrow)

Clinical features: MCV primarily infects the skin and follicular epithelium, presenting with single or multiple lesions in the epidermis. The lesions manifest as flesh-colored, raised, umbilicated papules or nodules (Fig. 3.2). Diagnosis is usually made by identification of skin lesions. Immunocompromised patients may present with atypical features including giant lesions (>1 cm), verrucous papules, or clusters of hundreds of small lesions [15, 16].

Microscopic Findings: Histologically, the molluscum lesions are characterized by lobulated endophytic hyperplasia of the epithelium with acanthotic epidermis. Eosinophilic intracytoplasmic inclusions, known as molluscum bodies or Henderson-Patterson bodies, are result of virus replication within the cytoplasm. As the inclusions enlarge, they compress the nucleus of infected cells to the periphery and acquire a basophilic appearance (Fig. 3.2) [17]. The epidermis ruptures as a result of pressure due to underlying proliferation and produces the characteristic white-yellow core. The surrounding dermis is relatively unremarkable with little or no inflammatory reaction; rarely the lesion ruptures in dermis and triggers an inflammatory response.

3.1.3 Herpes Simplex Virus

Genital herpes is a widespread sexually transmitted disease. It is the most common cause of genital ulcers in the United States, and is caused by the human *herpes simplex virus* (HSV). HSV is a double-stranded DNA virus from ubiquitous Herpesviridae family, and has two distinct types based on different envelope protein and antigen properties. Both types can cause genital herpes, a lifetime incurable infection. HSV-2 is the major cause of genital herpes; however, increasing numbers of genital ulcerations that are caused by HSV-1 in developed countries have been reported [18, 19]. The virus is transmitted through direct mucocutaneous contact with herpetic lesions or exposure to mucosal secretions during periods of viral shedding. Transmission occurs not only when lesions are visible, but also when lesions are not clinically apparent [20]. Asymptomatic viral shedding in the absence of detectable lesions is responsible for up to 70% of all HSV-2 infections [21]. A considerable number of HSV-2 seropositive individuals do not have a history of symptomatic genital herpes. Transmission of HSV from mother to child during pregnancy is uncommon and usually occurs at the time of labor and delivery; however, new infections acquired late in pregnancy carry a high risk for transmission to neonate [22].

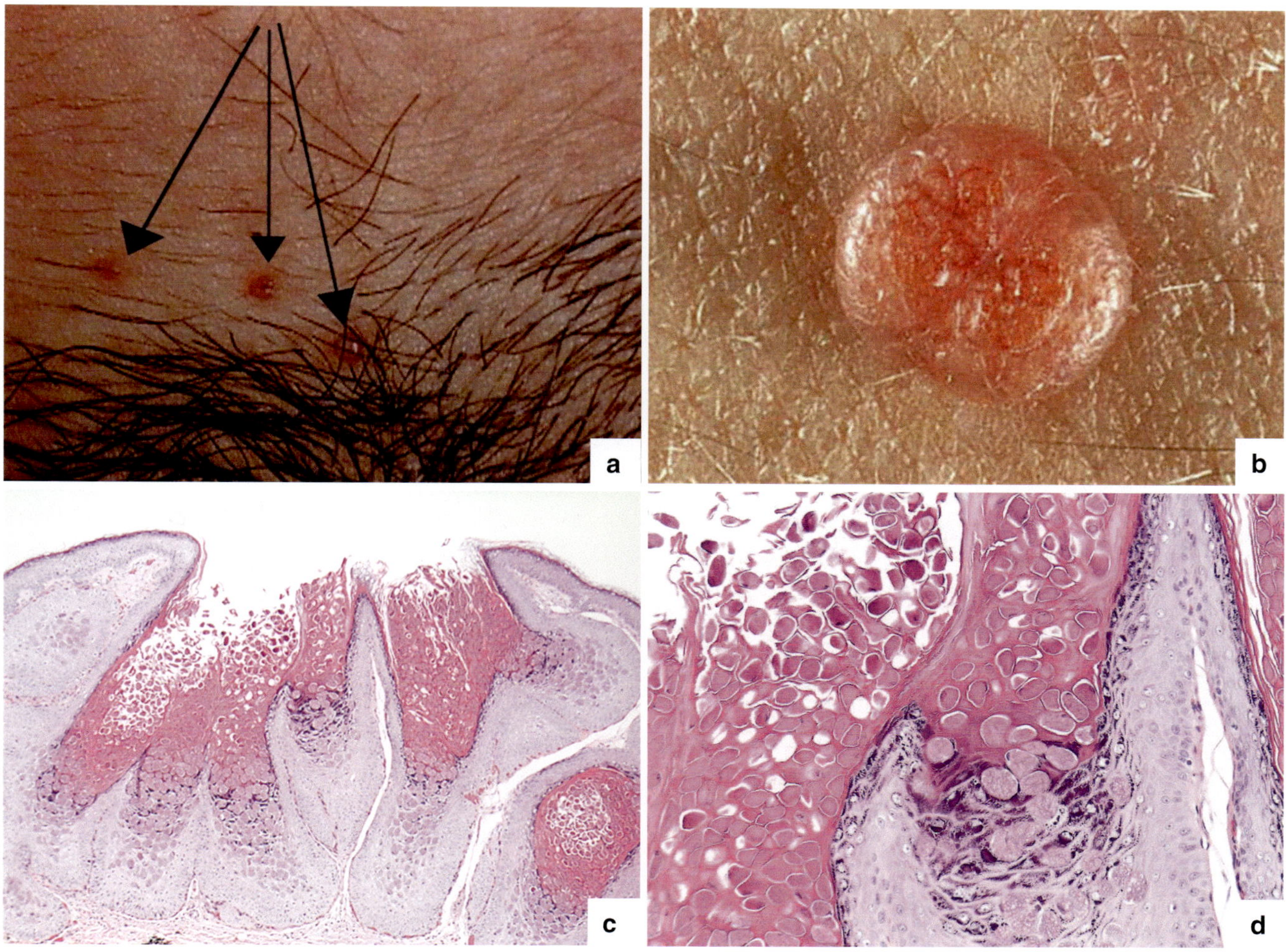

Fig. 3.2 Molluscum contagiosum: (**a**, **b**) Single or multiple flesh-colored, raised, umbilicated papules or nodules. Microscopic findings characterized by (**c**) lobulated crater-shaped hyperplasia of the epithelium and inclusions of *Molluscum contagiosum virus*. Infected cells reveal (**d**) eosinophilic intracytoplasmic inclusions (molluscum bodies or Henderson-Patterson bodies) that displace the nucleus to the periphery

Clinical features: Primary infections are usually asymptomatic and manifest with localized pain, tingling, or burning sensation at the site of exposure. Prodrome of systemic symptoms including headache, fever, malaise, dysuria, and lymphadenopathy is common. The virus damages the epithelium at the exposure site, causing eruption of vesicles within days. The vesicles rupture, resulting in erosion and ulceration, which heal without leaving scar. The virus travels by sensory nerve axons to the sacral ganglion and remains latent for the life of the host. Spontaneous or stress induced periodic reactivation of the virus manifests as mucocutaneous lesions [23]. HSV-1 induced infections are usually milder and recur 1–2 times a year, compared with HSV-2 infection causing 4–6 episodes of recurrence per year [19, 22]. Immunocompromised patients have an increased risk for extensive and recurrent HSV infection. Atypical presentations of genital herpes, including persistent ulcers and verrucous lesions, have been described in immunocompromised individuals [22, 24]. Another less common presentation of HSV in patients with immunodeficiency, known as "knife-cut sign," appears as linear ulcers and fissures in intertriginous areas, such as the inguinal region, vulva, and other areas with folds [25]. Genital herpes is a common infection among human immunodeficiency virus type 1 (HIV-1)-infected patients, ranging from 50% to 90% in different affected populations [24]. Individuals with HSV infection are more prone to acquisition of HIV infection. HSV-2 prevents an effective immune response at the site of entry; furthermore complex interactions between HSV and host can affect HIV-1 replication [26].

Microscopic findings: The histology of herpes infections is very distinctive. Acantholysis, spongiosis, and ballooning degeneration of keratinocytes form intraepidermal and subepidermal vesicles. The keratinocyte nuclei show ground-glass appearance of nucleus with peripheral condensation of chromatin. Multinucleated cells show "molding" nuclei. The

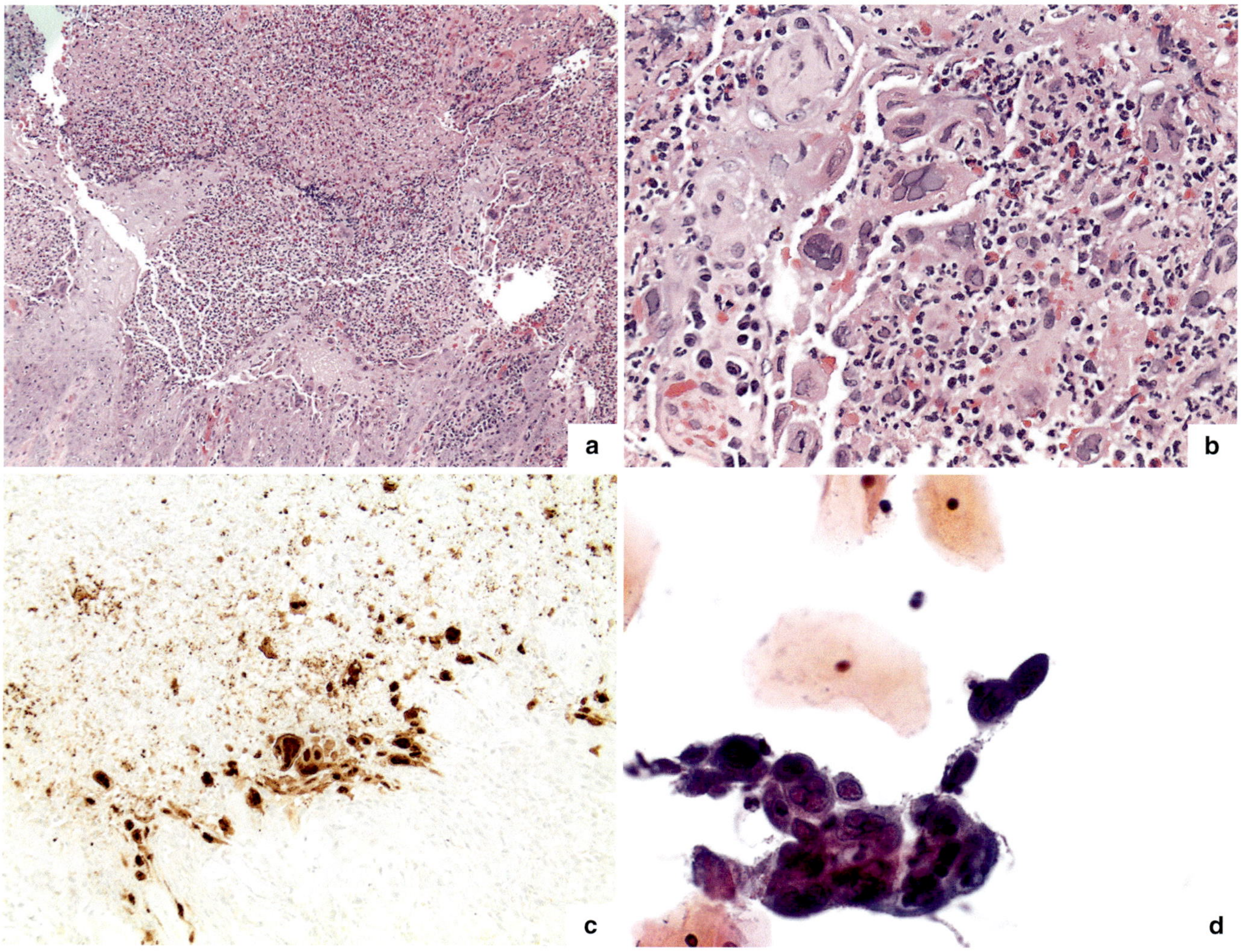

Fig. 3.3 *Herpes simplex virus* infection: (**a**) Low power view of a herpetic ulcer, epithelial ulceration with multinucleated keratinocytes. (**b**) Intranuclear inclusions show ground-glass appearance, margination of chromatin, multinucleation, and nuclear molding. (**c**) Immunohistochemical stain for HSV2 highlights virus-infected cells. (**d**) Papanicolaou-stained smear portrays the classic "3 Ms" herpes cytopathic effect

dermis shows polymorphous inflammation and leukocytoclastic vasculitis may be present. In late stages, vesicles rupture resulting in epithelial ulceration and crust [27]. Exophytic masses involving genital area associated with immunocompromised patients show pseudoepitheliomatous hyperplasia and can mimic cancer [28]. On cytology smears, herpes cytopathic effects present with the classic "3 Ms": multinucleation, molding, and margination of chromatin (Fig. 3.3). Nuclei have a ground glass appearance due to accumulation of viral particles and eosinophilic intranuclear (Cowdry A) inclusions surrounded with a clear halo are variably present [11].

Diagnostic methods: Diagnosis is made by nucleic acid amplification methods, including PCR assays or viral culture. Serologic tests that detect antibodies are available, but are not sensitive for differentiating acute and chronic infection. Direct immunofluorescence antigen staining is not recommended due to low sensitivity [23].

Differential diagnosis: Although HSV is the most common cause of genital ulcers in the United States, other ulcerative genital disease and the coexistence of other STDs must be considered. Other infectious etiologies such as chancroid and syphilis can be in differential diagnosis (Table 3.1). Noninfectious etiologies such as aphthous ulcers, Behçet syndrome, Stevens–Johnson syndrome, and Crohn's disease can cause vulvar ulcers. Clinical presentation, involvement of other sites, and clinical course of the lesions, as well as laboratory tests are helpful in differentiating herpes from these systemic diseases [27, 29].

Management: Antiviral treatment of HSV infection with nucleoside analogues does not cure the infection, but rather aims for reducing recurrence and the risk of transmission. Treatment of recurrent episodes decreases the length of outbreaks and the severity of symptoms [23]. Daily dose of valacyclovir results in significant reduction in recurrence and viral shedding [28].

Table 3.1 Ulcerative infections of the vulva

Disease	Etiology	Characteristics of the ulcers	Regional adenopathy	Histology of vulvar lesions	Diagnosis/ancillary methods	Treatment
Herpes Simplex Virus	HSV-1 and HSV-2	Painful multiple small vesicles that evolves into ulcers	Occasional tender adenopathy	Ballooning degeneration of keratinocytes and epidermal vesicles. "3 Ms": Multinucleation, molding, and margination of chromatin.	Detection of viral DNA by PCR or viral culture	Nucleoside analogues (e.g., acyclovir, valacyclovir)
Primary Syphilis/ Chancre	*Treponema pallidum*	Painless usually single non-purulent ulcer with well-defined elevated borders	Non-tender adenopathy	Endothelial swelling and proliferation with dense lymphoplasmocytic inflammation. Endarteritis obliterans may be present.	Dark field microscopy, serologic testing, PCR. Silver stain or immunohistochemistry of fixed tissue	Benzathine penicillin
Chancroid	*Haemophilus ducreyi*	Painful coalescent purulent ulcers with ragged poorly-defined borders	Tender, usually unilateral adenopathy, may suppurate	Ulcer with fibrinopurulent material, lymphoplasmocytic inflammation and granulation tissue. "School of fish" refers to the parallel chains of bacteria seen on cytology.	Culture of lesions. Giemsa or Gram stain detects the bacteria.	Azithromycin or ceftriaxone
Granuloma inguinale	*Klebsiella granulomatis*	Painless usually single hypervascular ulcer with elevated borders and a friable bleeding base	None. Pseudobuboes may be present	Pseudoepitheliomatous hyperplasia, granulation tissue with prominent vascularization and dense mixed inflammatory cell infiltrate	Warthin–Starry or Giemsa stains depict Donovan bodies	Doxycycline
Lymphogranuloma venereum	*Chlamydia trachomatis* (serotype L1–3)	Painless papule becoming an ulcer, that usually goes unnoticed	Tender usually bilateral adenopathy, may suppurate	Lymphoplasmocytic infiltrate, small foci of necrosis, and granulation tissue. Lymph nodes reveal stellate abscesses surrounded by epithelioid cells and histiocytes	Culture, direct immunofluorescence, or nucleic acid detection	Doxycycline

3.1.4 Gonorrhea

Clinical features: Gonorrhea is a common sexually transmitted infection caused by *Neisseria gonorrhea*, a gram-negative diplococcus. Gonorrhea is the second most commonly reported communicable disease [30]. Gonorrhea in women presents with urethritis, cervicitis, and vaginitis; however, a significant number of infected women are asymptomatic [30, 31]. The symptomatic patients present with pruritus, mucopurulant discharge, and urinary symptoms. Clinical exam may show friable cervix [31]. The infection can involve Bartholin's glands, resulting in abscess formation [32]. Co-infection with *Chlamydia* is common. It is important to screen the women at high risk for STDs for gonorrhea because asymptomatic infections are common. Untreated gonorrhea, including asymptomatic infections, can progress to pelvic inflammatory disease and complications such as infertility and ectopic pregnancy [33].

Diagnostic methods: Microscopic findings are nonspecific as gonorrhea is not associated with marked inflammation [34]. Diagnosis can be made through a variety of techniques; by identifying intracellular organisms in gram-stained cervical smears, culture, and detection of antigen or nucleic acid in the sample. Nucleic acid amplification test (NAAT) has the highest sensitivity for detecting *Neisseria gonorrhea* [30]. Patients are treated by simultaneous ceftriaxone and azithromycin administration according to the current CDC guidelines [30].

3.1.5 Syphilis

Syphilis is a worldwide chronic infectious disease caused by spirochete *Treponema pallidum.* The primary mode of transmission is by sexual contact followed by vertical transmission from infected mother to child [35, 36]. Repeated oscillation in incidence of syphilis in the United States has been observed since 1940s, when penicillin was used to treat syphilis [37]. The rate of infection varies by population subgroups and is more common among people with limited access to health care and individuals with high-risk sexual behavior [35].

Clinical features: Acquired syphilis is divided into four stages (primary, secondary, latent, and tertiary), each present with different clinical manifestations. Venereal syphilis is acquired by direct penetration of spirochetes to the mucosa or skin during sexual contact [38]. The primary stage presents with a single chancre at the site of inoculation after an incubation period ranging from 10 to 90 days (an average of 3 weeks after exposure). Some cases show multiple primary lesions. The chancre in women most often occurs on the vulva, perineum, cervix, or oral mucosa and may be accompanied by painless regional lymphadenopathy. The skin lesion typically becomes indurated and progresses to a painless and non-purulent ulcer with clean base which heals spontaneously within 4–6 weeks [39, 40].

If untreated, *T. pallidum* disseminates throughout the body by hematogenous spread during the primary stage. Manifestations of secondary syphilis usually occur within 6–8 weeks of resolution of primary lesions [41]. Secondary syphilis may involve any organ but most commonly presents with disseminated heterogeneous mucocutaneous rash. The classic presentation includes generalized macular and papulosquamous skin eruption accompanied with systemic symptoms and generalized lymphadenopathy. Genital lesions are more common in women and range from macules and ulcerations to fleshy verrucous papules known as condylomata lata [40]. A variety of uncommon presentations such as nodular lesions and malignant lues (ulceronodular lesions) have been described [42–44].

In untreated patients, the lesions resolve over several weeks and the infection enters an asymptomatic "latent" stage. A subset of patients with latent infection progress to tertiary syphilis which may present with cardiovascular syphilis, neurosyphilis, and involvement of the skin, bones, or viscera with gumma [45, 46]. Vertical transmission of *T. pallidum* from mother to fetus may occur during pregnancy at any stage of infection, resulting in stillbirth or congenital syphilis. Syphilis and HIV coinfection is common, and the two diseases affect each other in several ways [47]. Clinical course of syphilis can be accelerated by HIV and result in atypical presentations and syphilis infection increases the risk of HIV transmission by breaking skin and mucosal barrier and increasing viral shedding [48–50].

Microscopic findings: Most primary lesions exhibit prominent endothelial swelling and proliferation with perivascular lymphoplasmacytic inflammation. The endothelial hyperplasia can result in endarteritis obliterans and subsequent ulceration. Epidermal hyperplasia and acanthosis is common [40, 51]. Secondary syphilis can demonstrate with a variety of histologic findings. Most cases show endarteritis, endothelial swelling, and interstitial and perivascular infiltrate in the dermis composed of lymphocytes, plasma cells, macrophages, and some neutrophils (Fig. 3.4). The epidermis shows variety of changes such as parakeratosis, exocytosis, spongiosis, and most frequently acanthosis [51–53]. Secondary syphilis skin lesions can demonstrate prominent lichenoid or psoriasiform features [54]. Condylomata lata show pronounced epithelial hyperplasia, elongated rete ridges, neutrophil exocytosis, and perivascular lymphoplasmacytic inflammation [54, 55]. Follicular microabscesses and pustules characterized by folliculocentric neutrophilic inflammation as well as patchy alopecia can occur [27]. Tertiary syphilis lesions often demonstrate dense lymphocytic and plasma cell infiltration of the dermis, granulomatous inflammation, and endarteritis obliterans [46, 54]. Silver stain or immunohistochemistry can be used to confirm the presence of Treponema within and around dermis vessels and in dermal–epidermal junction in primary and secondary stage lesions, and less commonly tertiary lesions. Nontreponemal spirochetes can cause false positive results [56].

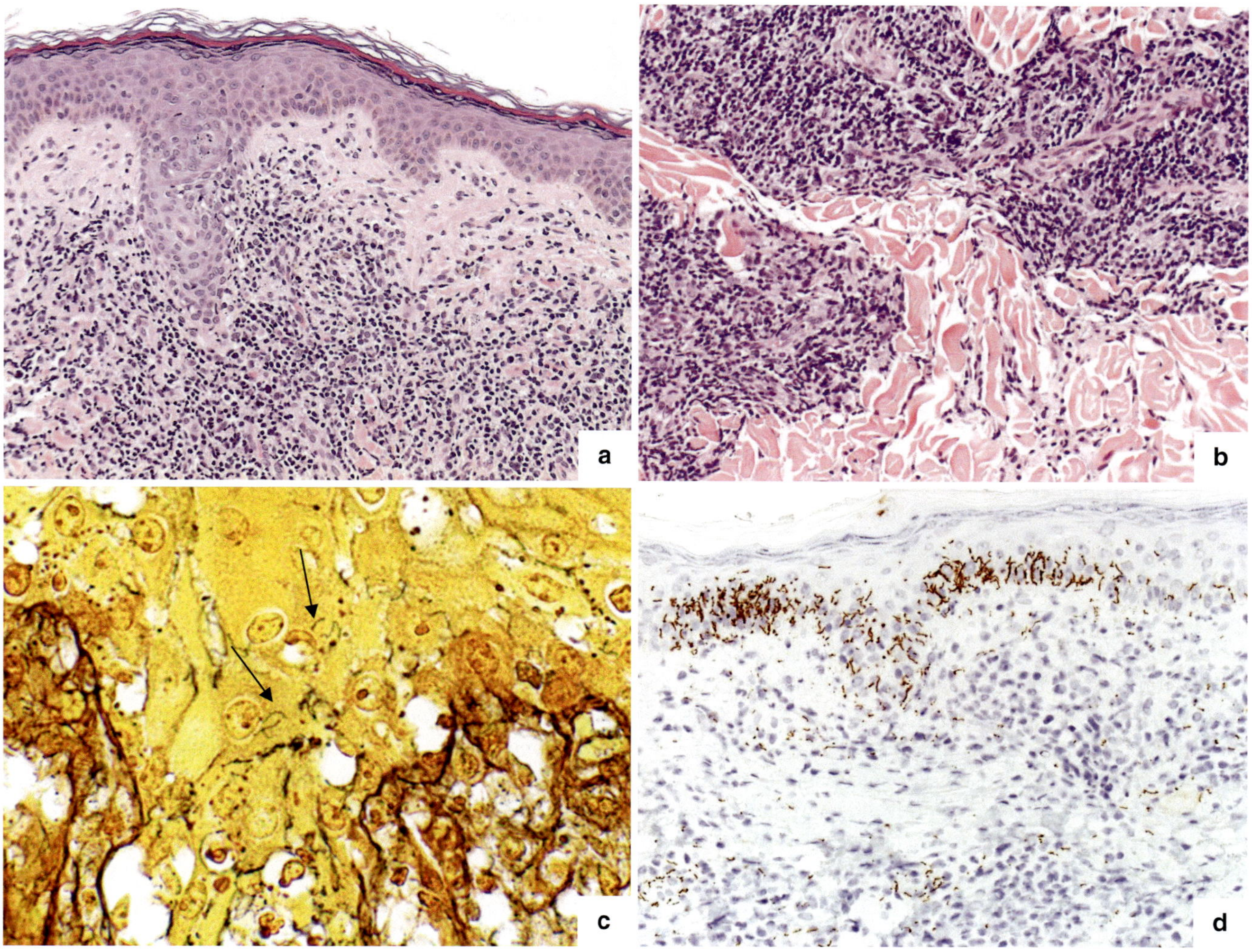

Fig. 3.4 Secondary syphilis: (**a**) Epidermal hyperplasia, acanthosis, and spongiosis with lymphoplasmacytic infiltrate in dermis. (**b**) Dermis demonstrates interstitial and perivascular lymphoplasmacytic infiltrate and vascular endothelial swelling and proliferation. (**c**) Warthin–Starry silver stain highlights spirochetes (arrows). (**d**) Immunohistochemical stain for *Treponema* highlights numerous spirochetes (Courtesy of Dr. Brian Hinds)

Diagnostic methods: Diagnosis can be made by detection of *T. pallidum* with dark field microscopy of primary or secondary lesions. Serologic testing is the main laboratory diagnostic method for secondary, latent, and tertiary syphilis; divided into non-treponemal and treponemal tests. Non-treponemal tests include the Venereal Disease Research Laboratory (VDRL) and the Rapid Plasma Reagin (RPR) which are useful for screening. Treponemal tests are used for confirming the infection and include the serum fluorescent treponemal antibody absorption test (FTA-ABS) and the microhemagglutination test for *T. pallidum* (MHA-TP) [39, 40]. Molecular detection of *T. pallidum* by PCR analysis have been developed and validated by some laboratories to detect the organism in serum, cerebrospinal fluid, amniotic fluid, lesion exudate, and fixed tissues [56, 57].

Differential diagnosis: Syphilis is called "great imitator" because it mimics the signs and symptoms of so many other diseases. Differential diagnoses of genital lesions in early syphilis include other infectious genital ulcer disease (chancroid, granuloma inguinale, lymphogranuloma venereum, and herpesvirus) Although, endothelial proliferation and perivascular lymphoplasmocytic inflammation are helpful hints to the diagnosis of syphilis. Secondary syphilis lesions can mimic inflammatory dermatoses such as lichen planus, eczema, psoriasis, and drug eruptions; however, involvement of deep dermis and predominance of plasma cells in the infiltrate is a clue for considering syphilis [41, 52]. In some cases dense inflammatory infiltrate may resemble lymphoma, but mixed population of inflammatory cells are in favor of a non-neoplastic process. Zoon's vulvitis (plasmacytosis mucosae), a chronic inflammatory disease of unknown origin, demonstrates a band-like, dense mucosal infiltration of plasma cells admixed with lymphocytes and dilated dermal vessels. The absence of pronounced superficial and deep perivascular inflammation and vascular endothelial proliferation is helpful in differentiating these entities [27]. Condylomata lata can mimic verruca vulgaris and other conditions with epidermal hyperplasia. Granulomatous inflammation in later stages may simulate granuloma annulare, or other granulomatous diseases such as leprosy, tuberculosis, or sarcoidosis [27].

Management: According to CDC guidelines, primary, secondary, or early latent syphilis is cured by single intramuscular injection of long-acting Benzathine penicillin G (2.4 million units). Three doses of long-acting Benzathine penicillin G, administered intramuscularly at weekly intervals, are recommended for treatment of late latent syphilis. Treatment will kill the syphilis bacterium and prevent further damage, but will not repair existing damages [58].

3.1.6 Chancroid

The prevalence of chancroid has declined in the United States, but still occurs in developing countries. It is caused by the fastidious gram-negative coccobacillus called *Haemophilus ducreyi* [59, 60]. The transmission occurs by sexual contact and the incubation period is approximately 10 days [61, 62].

Clinical features: Clinically, it presents as tender erythematous papule that progresses into pustular stage, and then rupture to form single or multiple small genital ulcers (measuring 1–2 mm in diameter) that are painful, soft with purulent exudate, and can form coalescent lesions with ragged borders. Association with tender, suppurative, usually unilateral, inguinal lymphadenopathy (buboes formation) reinforces the diagnosis. The genital ulcers seen in chancroid can increase the transmission and acquisition of HIV infection, like in infections by herpes and syphilis. Differential diagnosis includes syphilis and herpes simplex [60, 62, 63].

Diagnostic methods: The diagnosis of chancroid is challenging, and the definitive diagnosis is achieved by identification of *H. ducreyi* on culture, which is considered the "gold standard" method. Multiplex PCR is not FDA approved, but available and validated in clinical laboratories [63].

Microscopic findings: Histology of the ulcers exhibit three distinct zones, from surface to depth, as follows: exuberant necrosis intermixed with neutrophils, erythrocytes, and fibrin; granulation tissue associated with degeneration and thrombosis of vessels; and dense lymphoplasmacytic infiltrate in the deep dermis (Fig. 3.5). Giemsa or gram stains may identify the bacteria at the surface of the lesion. Cytologic features of the ulcer's exudate may show the bacteria in parallel chains ("school of fish") [61, 62].

Management: Patients are treated with antibiotics, and azithromycin and ceftriaxone regimen offers the advantage of single-dose therapy [60, 64].

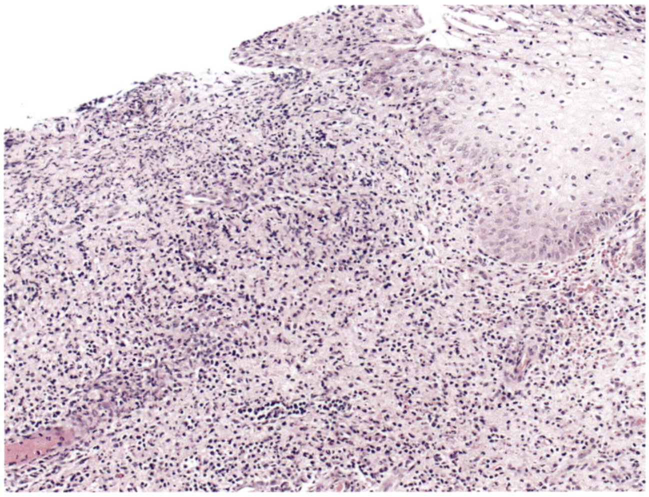

Fig. 3.5 Chancroid ulcer with superficial fibrinopurulent exudate and necrotic debris associated with acute and chronic inflammatory cell infiltrate in dermis

3.1.7 Granuloma Inguinale (Donovanosis)

Klebsiella granulomatis (known as *Calymmatobacterium granulomatis*) is an intracellular gram-negative bacillus causative agent of granuloma inguinale (also called donovanosis or granuloma venereum). It is endemic in some tropical and developing areas, and very rare in the United States [65].

Clinical features: The disease presents as genital ulcers on vulva, vagina, or cervix that are painless, highly vascular ("beefy red appearance") with rolled borders, and a friable bleeding base. Regional inguinal adenopathy is usually absent; however, subcutaneous granulomas (pseudobuboes) might occur. The incubation period is 1 week to 1 month after exposure. In addition to sexual contact, fecal contamination of the vulva or vagina has also been implicated. The ulcers can present in association with other sexually transmitted diseases or develop secondary superimposed bacterial infections. The lesions can spread and affect adjacent skin of perineum, thighs, and lower abdomen, and in severe cases may cause disfiguration of the genitals [59, 61, 62, 65].

Diagnostic methods: Smears of the lesion, stained by Wright or Giemsa, show mononuclear cells with numerous intracytoplasmic encapsulated ovoid bacteria (Donovan bodies). *K. granulomatis* is difficult to culture and the required specialized media is not available routinely. There are no FDA-cleared molecular tests for the detection of *K. granulomatis* DNA, but laboratories have developed and validated such tests. [63].

Microscopic findings: Histology of the lesion reveals an ulcer with central fibrinous exudate and necrosis, surround by pseudoepitheliomatous hyperplasia, underlay by granulation tissue with prominent vascularization and dense mixed inflammatory cell infiltrate (plasma cells and macrophages, predominantly). Histology sections stained with Warthin–Starry or Giemsa stains depict Donovan bodies found intracellularly (vacuoles of histiocytes) or extracellularly, which may appear as coccoid, coccobacillary, or bacillary organisms. The bipolar staining of the silver preparations confers the "safety pin" appearance of the bacteria. Electron microscopy may identify the organism within the phagosomes of macrophages [59, 62, 66].

Differential diagnosis includes nonhealing ulcers of squamous cell carcinoma, other STDs (chancroid, syphilis, and herpesvirus), infections caused by intracellular organism that affect histiocytes (leishmaniasis, histoplasmosis, and rhinoscleroma).

Management: The Centers for Disease Control and Prevention and the 2016 European guideline on donovanosis recommend treatment with azithromycin for at least 3 weeks and until all lesions have completely healed [59, 62, 65, 66].

3.1.8 Lymphogranuloma Venereum

Lymphogranuloma venereum (LGV) or lymphogranuloma inguinale is caused by the serotypes L1, L2, and L3 of *Chlamydia trachomatis*, an obligatory intracellular gram-negative bacterium [67]. The disease is more common in men, frequently found in tropical and subtropical areas of the world [68–70]. This sexual transmitted disease has a triphasic clinical presentation. The primary infection, after an incubation period of 3–30 days, presents with genital small painless papules, which become self-limiting ulcers, and frequently goes unnoticed. The secondary infection, after a few weeks, presents with regional lymphadenopathy and sometimes constitutional symptoms. The inguinal lymph nodes are more commonly involved in men, given the lymphatic drainage of the vagina and cervix is to the retroperitoneal rather than the inguinal lymph nodes. The "groove sign," thought to be pathognomonic for LGV, refers to the presence of adenopathy above and below the inguinal ligament, occurs in 10–20% of cases. The lymph nodes become enlarged, tender (buboes formation), and may develop draining sinuses. The third phase of the disease, more common in women, consists of chronic pelvic lymphangitis with fibrosis of the genital tract that can lead to lymphatic obstruction, causing elephantiasis of the genitalia, fistulas, and strictures of vagina and rectum [62, 67, 71].

Diagnostic methods: The diagnosis of LGV is difficult given lack of specific clinical presentation and standardized laboratory assays for this pathogen. The clinical suspicion, epidemiologic information, and exclusion of other entities can guide the diagnosis. Specimens from infected sites can be tested for *C. trachomatis* by culture, direct immunofluorescence, or nucleic acid detection. PCR-based genotyping can be used to differentiate LGV from non-LGV *C. trachomatis*, but it is time consuming and not widely available. Chlamydia serology may help reach the diagnosis, but lacks specificity [72].

Microscopic Findings: The ulcers are rarely biopsied, given the absence of clinical presentation. Histology demonstrates dense underlying lymphoplasmocytic infiltrate, small foci of necrosis, and granulation tissue. The involved lymph nodes develop stellate abscesses with coalescence of necrotic foci surrounded by poorly formed palisade of epithelioid cells and histiocytes. Sinus formation also occurs. In later lesions, there is variable fibrosis. *C. trachomatis* has been identified by numerous stains in inguinal lymphadenitis as intravacuolar organisms in macrophages (measuring 0.2–2.0 μm in diameter) [59, 71].

Different diagnosis includes other causes of inguinal adenopathy in association with genital ulcers (syphilis, HSV-2, and chancroid) or without ulcers (suppurative lymphadenitis caused by bacteria, cat-scratch disease, bubonic plague, tuberculous lymphadenitis, HIV infection, and lymphoma, among others) [59, 71].

Management: Medical therapy includes antibiotics (doxycycline is recommended), and aspiration of buboes to prevent the formation of sinus tract formation [67, 71].

3.1.9 Chlamydial Infection

Chlamydial infection is the most common sexually transmitted bacterial infection in the United States, caused by *Chlamydia trachomatis*, a gram-negative obligate intracellular pathogen [73]. *C. trachomatis* may involve lower urogenital tract (mainly endocervical mucosa), resulting in cervicitis, urethritis, and Bartholin's glands infection [74]. Symptomatic infections present with mucopurulent vaginal discharge and dysuria, although the infection is often asymptomatic. Untreated infection may result in pelvic inflammatory disease and its associated complications, including infertility and ectopic pregnancy, even when the infection is asymptomatic [75, 76].

The microscopic findings are nonspecific, showing chronic inflammation and reactive changes in epithelial cells. In some cases, lymphoid follicles with well-formed germinal centers are reported [34]. Immunoperoxidase staining for *C. trachomatis* can identify endocervical cells containing chlamydial bodies [77]. Diagnosis is made by isolation of *C. trachomatis* through culture or by detection of antigen or nucleic acid in first-catch urine or vaginal/cervical swab specimens. NAATs have the highest sensitivity, therefore are the recommended tests for detecting *C. trachomatis* infection. The current CDC guidelines recommend antibiotics treatment by a single dose azithromycin or 7 days of doxycycline [73].

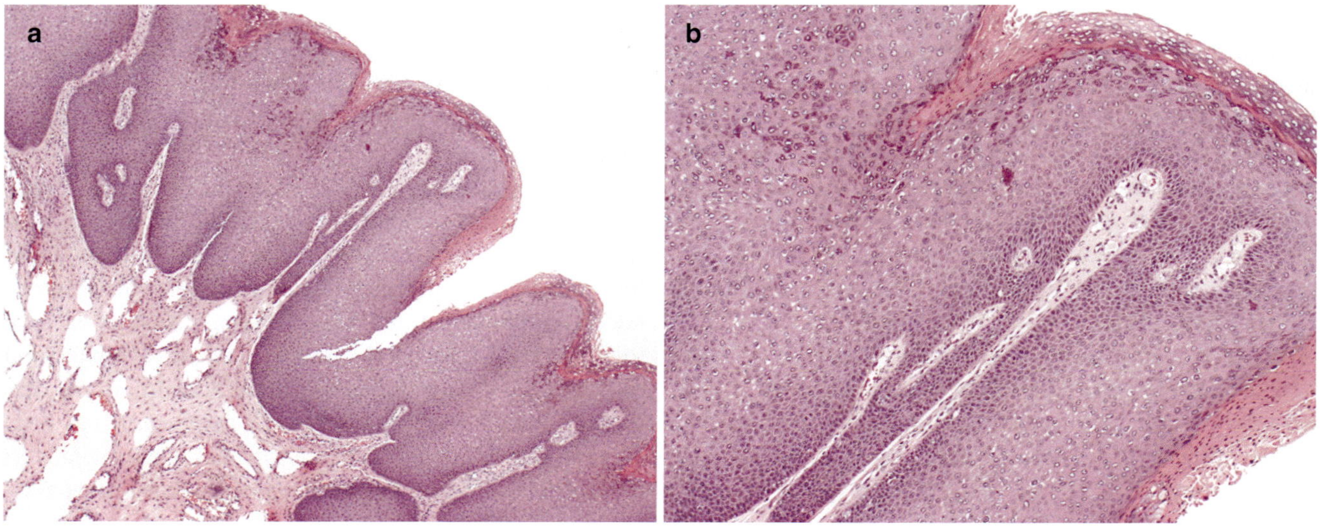

Fig. 3.6 Condylomata acuminatum: (**a**) Hyperplastic epidermis with acanthosis, parakeratosis, papillomatosis, prominent granular layer, and numerous koilocytes. (**b**) The koilocytes show irregular and wrinkled nuclei

3.1.10 Human Papillomavirus

Human Papillomavirus (HPV) infection is one of the most common sexually transmitted diseases and is responsible for a large number of anogenital cancers and warts in the United States [78]. Most sexually active individuals become infected with HPV and the course of the disease is usually asymptomatic and self-limited. Numerous subtypes of the virus have been identified which are further classified as oncogenic (e.g., high-risk, HPV types 16 and 18) and nononcogenic (e.g., low-risk, HPV types 6 and 11). Vulvar HPV-related lesions will be briefly discussed in this chapter, and other HPV-associated diseases will be further detailed in other chapters. Common manifestations of HPV infection in vulvar region include condyloma acuminatum (HPV types 6, 11), verruca vulgaris (HPV type 2), and giant condyloma (discussed under Sect. 3.5) [54, 59, 78].

3.1.10.1 Condyloma Acuminatum

Condyloma acuminata are common lesions of the vulva, vagina, and perianal region in adults, most commonly associated with HPV 6 or 11. Transmission is by skin-to-skin contact, including sexual intercourse or any other contact involving the genital area, even in the absence of visible warts [78].

Clinical features: Codyloma acuminatum presents as single or multiple lesions (filiform, plaque-like, or flat) that are flesh-colored or pigmented, and may extend to the perineum and perianal areas. Condyloma acuminatum are usually painless, unless involved by secondary infection [54, 59, 78].

Microscopic findings: Condyloma acuminatum shows papillomatous epidermal hyperplasia with hyperkeratosis, parakeratosis, accentuation of the granular layer, prominent fibrovascular cores, and basal cell hyperplasia. The surface of the lesion may display koilocytosis with squamous cells showing binucleation or multinucleation, perinuclear vacuolization and irregular nuclear contour. Chronic inflammatory infiltrate may be present. Peculiar histologic findings are seen in condylomata treated with resin of podophyllin. The squamous epithelium can show nuclear enlargement, increased number of mitosis, apoptotic keratinocytes, and pallor of superficial cells (Fig. 3.6) [54, 59, 79].

Diagnostic methods: Diagnosis is usually made by clinical inspection. Biopsy can confirm the diagnosis, and it is indicated in immunocompromised patients, lesions that worsen during therapy, and concerning atypical lesions that are pigmented, indurated, ulcerated, fixed to the underlying tissue, and easily bleed [78].

Differential diagnosis: includes vulvar intraepithelial neoplasia, which shows prominent nuclear atypia (including nuclear pleomorphism and hyperchromasia), increased number of mitotic figures throughout the epithelium, and minimal maturation. Verrucous carcinoma is another differential diagnosis and displays minimal cytologic atypia, no koilocytosis, abundant keratin between papillae, and broad-based rete ridges with pushing margins. Long-standing condylomata lesions may lack koilocytosis and can resemble seborrheic keratosis [54, 59, 62]. Papillary immature metaplasia (PIM) has been described in the squamous columnar junction of the anus and cervix, and is a type of exophytic low-grade squamous intraepithelial lesion. However, it distinguishes from condyloma acuminatum by the presence of immature squamous cells on the surface of the filiform papillary projections of the lesion. PIM can be easily misdiagnosed as high-grade squamous intraepithelial lesion

(HSIL) and awareness of this entity should be acknowledged. PIM lacks the nuclear atypia and conspicuous mitotic activity seen in HSIL. Immunostain for p16 is usually diffusely positive in HSIL, and negative in PIM [79–81].

Management: depends on the extent of the disease and identification of pathologic precancerous lesions. Certain antiviral therapy is not recommended, given that most lesions are self-limited. Excision, cryotherapy, and other types of ablation can be used. Lesions may also involute spontaneously within 1 year [78].

3.1.10.2 Verruca Vulgaris

Verruca vulgaris or common warts are usually seen in children and young adult and present as solitary, sometimes multiple, flesh-colored excrescences. They are usually asymptomatic, but can elicit pruritus, irritation, or bleeding. Microscopically, verruca vulgaris show a classic filiform surface architecture with parakeratosis, orthokeratosis, and hypergranulosis underlying a bland squamous epithelium with prominent papillary dermal vessels. The diagnosis is usually clinical. HPV genotyping can be used to differentiate verruca vulgaris from condyloma acuminatum in genital warts found in children, to assess for sexual abuse. The lesions can be excised or ablated (e.g., cryotherapy and electrocauterization) [54, 59].

3.1.11 Human Immunodeficiency Virus

The integrity of the vulvar and vaginal mucosal barrier is crucial in preventing pathogen invasion. The cellular immunity, microbiota, and mucus are some of the elements that maintain the intactness of tissue barrier. Mucosal inflammation increases the risk of HIV infection by elevating pro-inflammatory cytokines that disrupt the mucosa via neutrophil proteases activity, and increasing frequency of CD4+ T-cells, which are target cells of the virus. There is a high epidemiological association of STDs and HIV acquisition. Although the pathogenesis is unclear, HIV infection alters the integrity of the mucosal barrier and plays a role in acquisition of other STDs. Loss of Th17 cells is hypothesized to cause damage of the tight epithelial barrier allowing microbial translocation. In addition, HIV is capable of inducing inflammation by stimulating cells of the innate and adaptive immune system. Dysbiosis can also affect the immune cells in the mucosal surface and drive HIV infection. HIV-associated vulvar ulcers, without involvement of other pathogens are rare and few cases reported in literature describe the link between idiopathic vulvar ulcers and HIV infection that clinically present as multiple painful aphthous ulcers [59, 82–85].

3.2 Common Infections Not Typically Linked to Sexually Transmitted Diseases

3.2.1 Candida

Vulvovaginal Candidiasis (VVC) is a common infection of female genital tract. *Candida albicans*, an opportunistic yeast and a part of gastrointestinal tract flora, is responsible for 90% of VVCs [86]. Most of the remaining cases are caused by *C. glabrata* and *C. tropicalis* which are more resistant to treatment. Approximately 20–30% of asymptomatic women are carriers of candida in their lower genital tract. Epidemiologic data is limited due to the availability of over the counter treatment, yet it is estimated that up to 75% of women are affected at least once during their lives. Nearly 5–8% of women of reproductive age have recurrent vulvovaginal candidiasis [87].

VVC is not a sexually transmitted disease, but is more common in women who are sexually active. Risk factors for candida vulvovaginitis include pregnancy, diabetes mellitus, immunosuppression (e.g., HIV disease), and broad-spectrum antibiotic use [88, 89]. Menopausal women who receive exogenous estrogen replacement therapy are at higher risk of vulvovaginal candidiasis [90]. Studies have suggested that individuals with genetic factors such as nonsecretor phenotype of the ABO-Lewis blood group are at higher risk for recurrent VVCs [87, 91].

Clinical features: VC manifests by vulvar erythema, itching, irritation, and abnormal "cheese-like" or watery vaginal discharge. The infection can also result in candida intertrigo in inguinal region characterized by red lesions without central clearing and satellite rashes [91, 92].

Microscopic findings: On cytology smears, Candida organisms appear as eosinophilic yeast and pseudohyphae. Spearing of squamous cells, as if skewered by the pseudohyphae, is a frequent finding [11]. Histologic examination of vulva may show epidermal spongiosis, acanthosis, hyperkeratosis, and parakeratosis with subcorneal neutrophilic pustules (Fig. 3.7). Candida hyphae, pseudohyphae, and yeasts are highlighted by fungal stains (Grocott-Gomori methenamine silver stain or periodic acid–Schiff) in keratin layer [27].

Diagnostic methods: Diagnosis is based on identifying the organism by wet preparation, potassium hydroxide microscopy, culture, or molecular DNA detection of Candida [86, 88]. The patients are treated by short-course topical azole drugs [89].

3.2.2 Dermatophytosis

Tinea cruris (jock itch) is a superficial dermatophyte infection involving groin, inner thighs, perianal area, and rarely vulva. *Trichophyton rubrum* is the most common causative

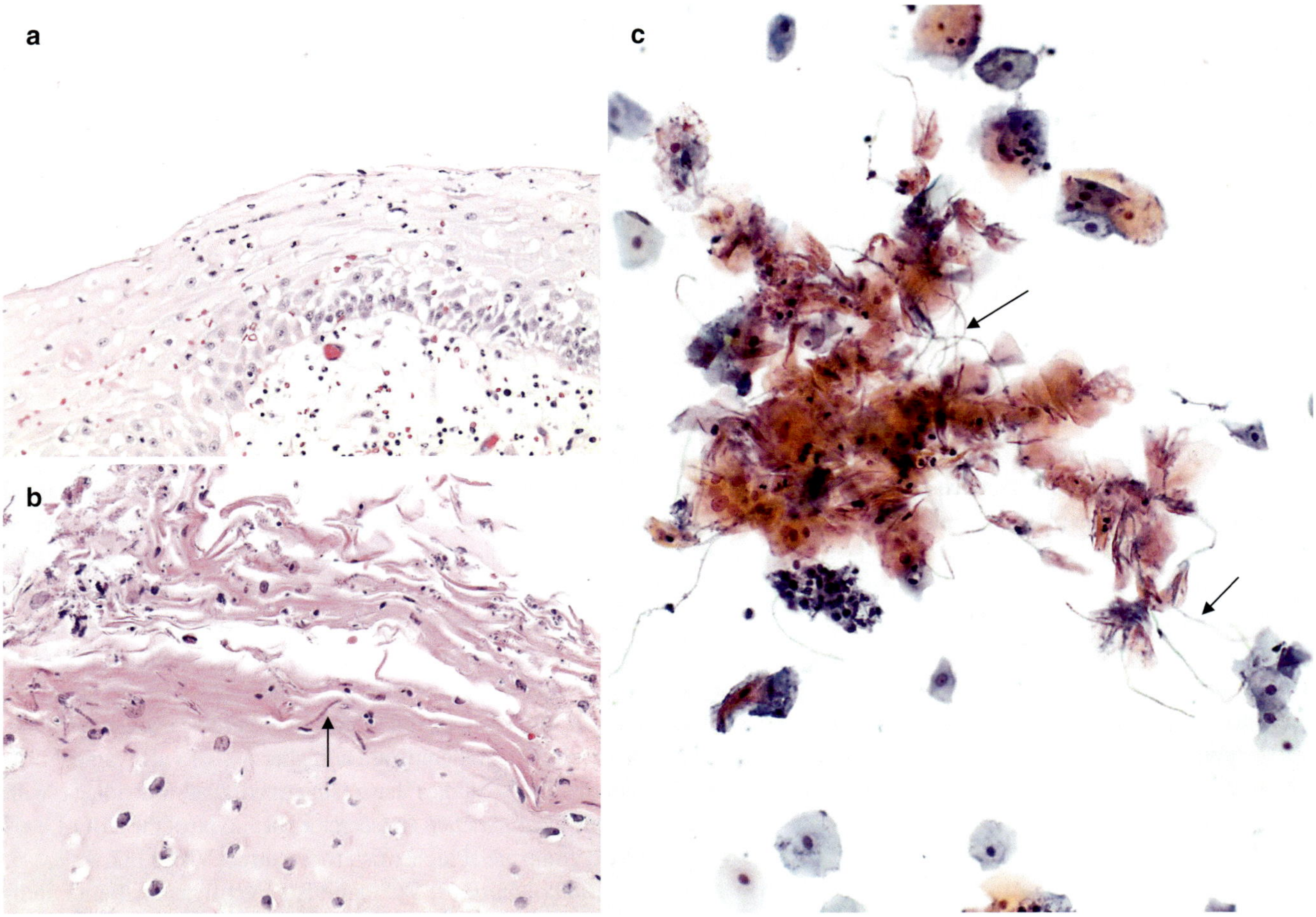

Fig. 3.7 Vulvovaginal candidiasis: (**a**) Vulvar epidermal spongiosis and associated dermal edema with *Candida* organisms and neutrophils in epidermis. (**b**) Epidermal parakeratosis with *Candida* pseudohyphae (arrow) and yeast in the thickened keratin layer. (**c**) Papanicolaou-stained cervical smear shows *Candida* pseudohyphae (arrow) and spearing of squamous cells

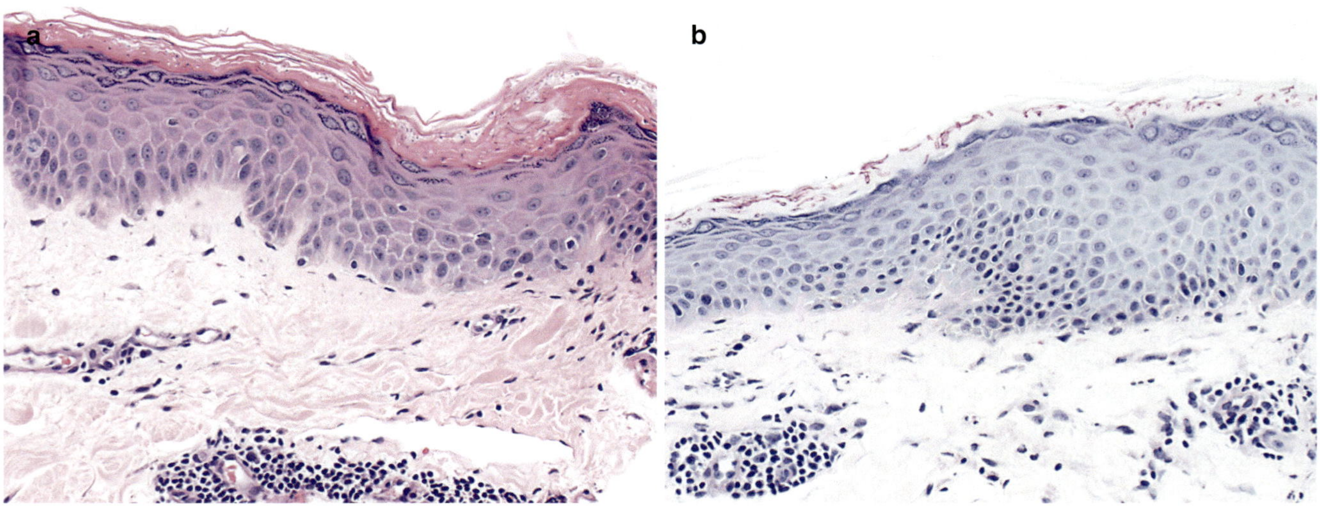

Fig. 3.8 Dermatophytosis: Epidermal hyperkeratosis and parakeratosis with fugal organisms in the thickened keratin layer on hematoxylin & eosin (**a**) and periodic acid–Schiff (**b**) stains

organism [93]. The patient presents with pruritic, sharply demarcated, discolored rashes with erythematous scaly borders, and sometimes with vesicles and pustules [94]. Biopsy findings are usually nonspecific, showing epidermal acanthosis, parakeratosis, spongiosis, and fungal yeast and hyphae (Fig. 3.8) [27]. Contact with contaminated fomites, tight clothing, and conditions such as excessive sweating and obesity that provide increased temperature and moisture in skin folds are predisposing factors [95]. Tinea cruris can often be diagnosed by a KOH preparation or culture. This infection usually responds to topical treatment, but oral antifungals may be indicated for extensive disease [93].

Deep dermatophytosis of the vulva is a rare infection mainly caused by *T. mentagrophytes* and *Microsporum canis*, most commonly affecting patients using topical steroids. Dermatophyte infection of the hair follicle and dermis evolves into scaly, erythematous plaques in vulva. The lesions may result in kerion formation or nodular granulomatous perifolliculitis, known as Majocchi's granuloma. Biopsy shows inflammation, granulomatous perifolliculitis, or cellulitis and abscess formation with or without fungal hyphae [96–98].

3.2.3 Bacterial Vaginosis

Bacterial vaginosis (BV) is the most common vaginal infection in women of reproductive age, affecting up to 29% of women in the United States. It is a polymicrobial syndrome caused by shift in vaginal microbial flora as a result of reduction in the normal Lactobacilli and overgrowth of anaerobic and facultative bacteria [99]. Molecular-based techniques have identified multiple bacterial vaginosis-associated agents including *Gardnerella* species, *Mobiluncus* species, *Atopobium* species, and *Mycoplasma hominis* [100]. Recent studies confirm the key role of *Gardnerella vaginalis* (GV) in pathogenesis of BV [101].

The exact etiology and epidemiology of BV is not clear and the role of sexual transmission is debated, although considerable evidence shows a significant association between BV and sexual activity with new and multiple partners [102]. Recent studies have emphasized on the sexual transmission of GV and suggest BV is started when GV adheres to host epithelium and creates a biofilm community in the vaginal environment [101]. BV is a risk factor for acquiring various sexually transmitted diseases and increases the risk of pelvic inflammatory disease, preterm labor, chorioamnionitis, and endometritis [99]. Importantly, BV has been associated with an increased risk of HIV acquisition and transmission. Studies have shown that interaction between epithelial cells and BV-associated species resulted in upregulation of cytokines and secretion of HIV-enhancing proteins that increases susceptibility to HIV infection [103, 104].

Clinical features: The infection presents with thin, malodorous vaginal discharge without typical signs of inflammation. Many affected women are completely asymptomatic [102].

Microscopic findings: On cytology smears (Fig. 3.9), BV present with squamous cells covered by small coccobacilli obscuring the cell edges, known as clue cells. Lactobacilli are usually absent and background is clean in liquid-based smear, given no to minimal inflammatory response [11].

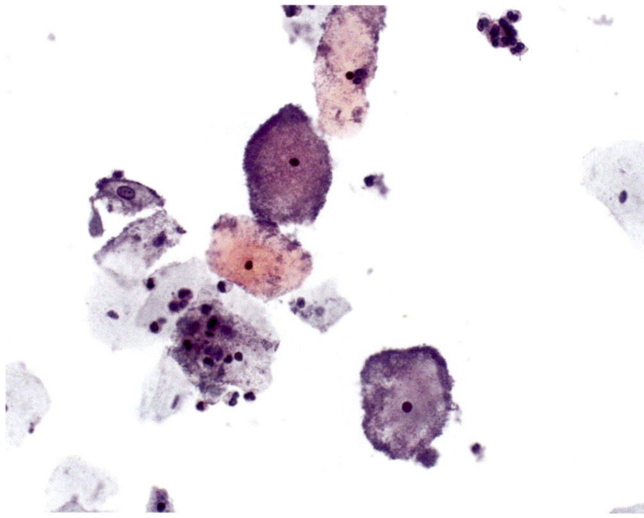

Fig. 3.9 Liquid-based preparation reveal squamous cells covered with coccobacilli ("clue cells") suggestive of bacterial vaginosis

Diagnostic methods: The diagnosis is usually made by applying clinical criteria, measuring vaginal fluid pH (>4.5), a positive whiff test (production of a fishy odor after adding 10% potassium hydroxide to vaginal fluid), gram stain (substitution of gram-positive rods and lactobacilli by gram-negative and gram-variable organisms), or molecular DNA detection [105].

3.2.4 Folliculitis and Other Bacterial Infections of Skin and Soft Tissue

Hair bearing skin of labia majora and pubic area can be involved by superficial and deep folliculitis secondary to bacterial infection of the hair follicles by *Staphylococcus aureus*. Trauma due to removing hair by shaving or waxing and wearing tight underwear are predisposing factors. The clinical and histologic appearance are similar to folliculitis from other body sites, presenting with papules, pustules, and granulomatous inflammation (Fig. 3.10) [98]. Other less common pathogens include *Pseudomonas aeruginosa* (hot tub folliculitis), *Malassezia*, and dermatophytes [106–108]. Exfoliative toxins of *S. aureus* can result in vesicles and blisters in genital area [98].

Vulvar cellulitis is bacterial infection of the dermis, usually caused by Streptococci group A and *S. aureus*, which affects the dermis in high-risk individuals including women with diabetes mellitus, obesity, pregnancy, and immunosuppression. This condition is often associated with fever, malaise chills, and nausea. Vulvar abscess formation often occurs due to progression of skin and hair follicle infections. These infections are often polymicrobial and Methicillin-resistant *Staphylococcus aureus* (MRSA) is the most common pathogen, isolated in 43–64% of cultures [32, 109–114]. Necrotizing fasciitis (or Fournier's gangrene) is a life-threatening progression of vulvar cellulitis that causes extensive necrosis of the

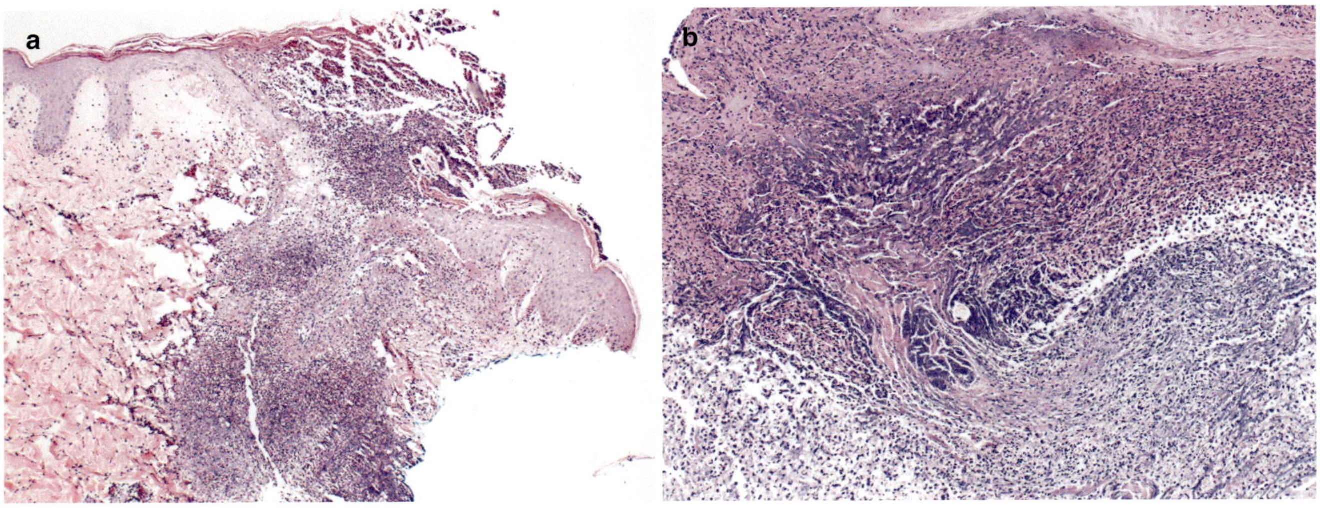

Fig. 3.10 (**a**, **b**) Folliculitis demonstrates mixed acute and chronic inflammation surrounding hair follicle with superficial ulcer

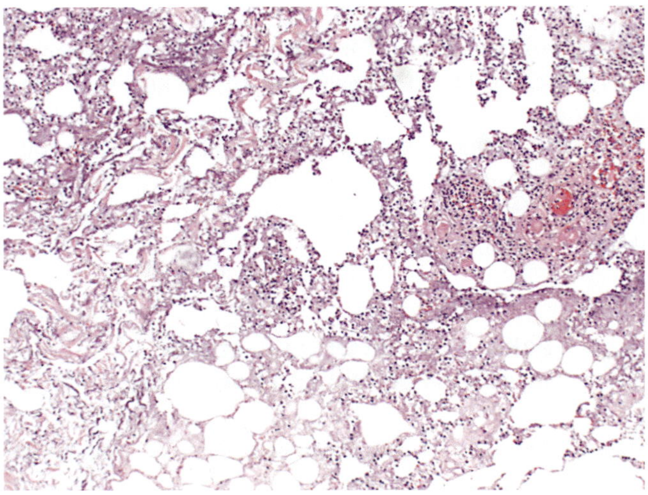

Fig. 3.11 Necrotizing fasciitis shows extensive necrosis with fascia involvement, abscess formation, vasculitis, and microvascular thrombosis

subcutaneous tissue. Tissue debridement and surgical reconstruction are the most important course of treatment. Histopathologic examination (Fig. 3.11) shows extensive necrosis with fascia involvement, abscess formation, vasculitis, and microvascular thrombosis [110, 114].

Bartholin gland obstruction and abscess formation affects approximately 2% of women. The infection is caused by mixed vaginal flora (*Bacteroides, Escherichia coli, S. aureus*) in nearly 80% of the cases; however, *Neisseria gonorrhoea* and rarely *Chlamydia* can cause this infection [32]. This condition presents with painful unilateral erythematous swelling in the vaginal introitus, and sometimes purulent discharge [32].

Periclitoral abscess is a rare condition with only few cases reported in literature. A significant number of these cases have occurred after local procedures, mostly after female circumcision [115–117]. In such cases, abscess formation is due to infected postsurgical inclusion cysts or less likely hematomas [116, 118]. Spontaneous periclitoral abscess formation without any previous surgery has been reported; however, due to rarity of this condition, association with specific causes and pathogens is unknown [116].

3.3 Infestations

3.3.1 Pediculosis Pubis

Pediculosis pubis (crab lice) is a highly contagious infestation caused by parasite *Phthirus pubis*. The disease is typically transmitted sexually; however, indirect infection through contact with infested objects is possible. Thirty percent of patients will have coexisting sexually transmitted disease. The crab louse is not a vector for systemic disease and commonly causes local symptoms by infesting pubic hair [119, 120].

Patients' main complaint is of itch in the pubic area. The affected skin can show red papules at the site of lice bites (Fig. 3.12). The host DNA can be extracted from lice [119]. Light blue-gray macules (maculae ceruleae) on the lower abdomen and thighs are characteristic findings of established infestation due to deep dermal hemosiderin deposition. Secondary superimposed infection may occur as a result of scratching. The diagnosis is made by spotting the lice and nits (eggs) attached to the genital area hair (Fig. 3.12) [119–122].

3.3.2 Scabies

Scabies is a contagious skin infestation caused by a human mite, *Sarcoptes scabiei* var. *hominis*. The mite burrows into

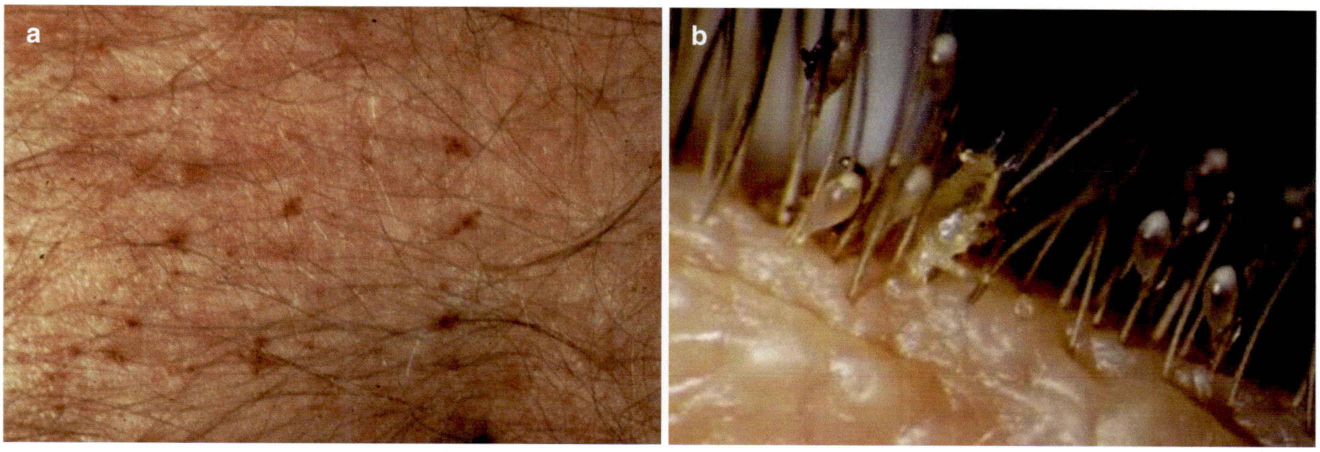

Fig. 3.12 Pediculosis pubis: (**a**) The affected skin shows red papules at the site of lice bites. (**b**) Lice and nits (eggs) attach to the genital area hair

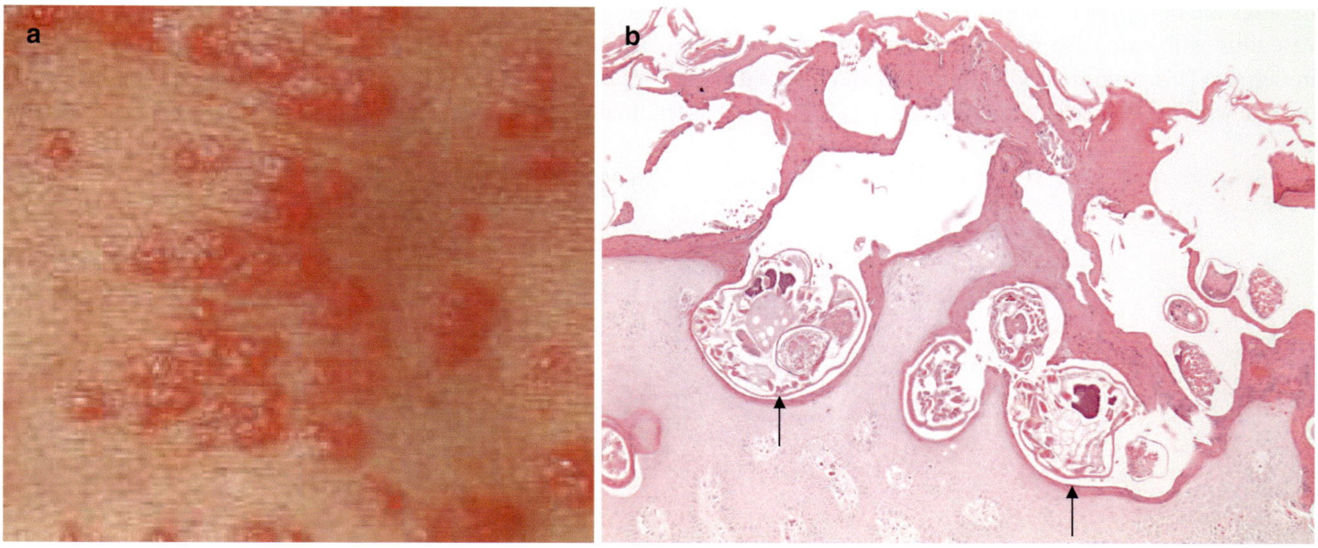

Fig. 3.13 Scabies: (**a**) The patient presents with pruritic papular rash or eczematous lesions. (**b**) Hyperparakeratotic, acanthotic epidermis with scabies mites (arrow)

and lives in the stratum corneum of the skin, commonly in finger webs and wrists. Involvement of genitalia usually presents with intensely pruritic papular rash or eczematous lesions. The parasite is usually transmitted by direct skin-to-skin contact, but infection by infested bedding or cloths is possible. The diagnosis of scabies can sometimes be confirmed microscopically by presence of mites, eggs, or fecal material in skin biopsy or scraping. Skin biopsy (Fig. 3.13) usually demonstrates features of hypersensitivity dermatitis with epidermal spongiosis and perivascular inflammation in dermis, composed of lymphocytes and eosinophils [122, 123]. Crusted scabies, formerly known as Norwegian scabies, is a severe form of infestation usually seen in immunocompromised patients and rarely involves vulvar region. Patients characteristically develop generalized thick, hyperkeratotic lesions simulating psoriasis, drug eruptions, and eczemas [124].

3.4 Other Rare Infections

3.4.1 Epstein-Barr Virus

Genital ulceration is rarely caused by primary *Epstein–Barr virus* (EBV) infection. This condition, known as Lipschütz's ulcer, is a non-sexually transmitted disease and primarily affects adolescent females (mean age of 14.5 years). Although several reports have outlined EBV shedding from genital tract secretions following acute systemic infection, genital ulceration caused by EBV are rarely described [125].

Patients typically present with one or multiple very painful ulcers, with purple-red irregular edges and clean or fibrinous base involving labia minora. Lymphadenopathy distant from the site of ulceration is common. Urinary symptoms such as dysuria and urine retention may be caused by the ulcers. Preceding prodromal systemic symptoms such as fatigue, headache, and low-grade fever are common and the majority of patients develop symptoms of mononucleosis [126]. The vulvar ulceration are more likely a manifestation of viremia and circulating infected B lymphocytes. The pathophysiology of ulceration is not clear; some believe a cytotoxic immune response to immune complex deposition triggers a type III hypersensitivity reaction, while others propose the ulcers are a manifestation of direct damage by EBV replication in the keratinocytes [125, 127]. Differential diagnoses include ulcerative STDs including HSV, chancroid, and syphilis.

Diagnosis is mainly clinical and based on excluding other causes of genital ulceration; confirmation can be made by detection of EBV-DNA by PCR examination of vulvar swabs or serologic evidence of acute EBV infection. The histologic findings are nonspecific, showing ulceration and underlying vasculitis with extensive mixed inflammatory cell infiltrate in dermis. This condition is self-limiting and ulcers usually resolve within 2–6 weeks without scarring [125].

3.4.2 Cytomegalovirus

Human *Cytomegalovirus* (CMV), a member of Herpesviridae family, is a ubiquitous virus that affects most of the world population. Immunocompetent hosts are generally asymptomatic or present with mononucleosis syndrome; however, it can cause life-threatening disease in immunocompromised patients. Like other members of Herpesviridae family, CMV establishes a lifelong latent infection of the host [128]. CMV can be identified in the cervix of up to 29% of women with normal cervical smears. The rate of CMV DNA detection in the cervical secretions has been as high as 66% in HIV-infected women [129, 130]. Symptomatic CMV infections of female genital tract are rare. Cases with anogenital ulcers and erosions have been reported in both healthy and immunocompromised patients [131, 132].

Histologically CMV is diagnosed by characteristic enlarged cells with large eosinophilic nuclear inclusions surrounded by a clear halo (owl's eye) and intracytoplasmic granulations (Fig. 3.14). CMV inclusions are mainly found in the endocervical glandular epithelial cells and also in

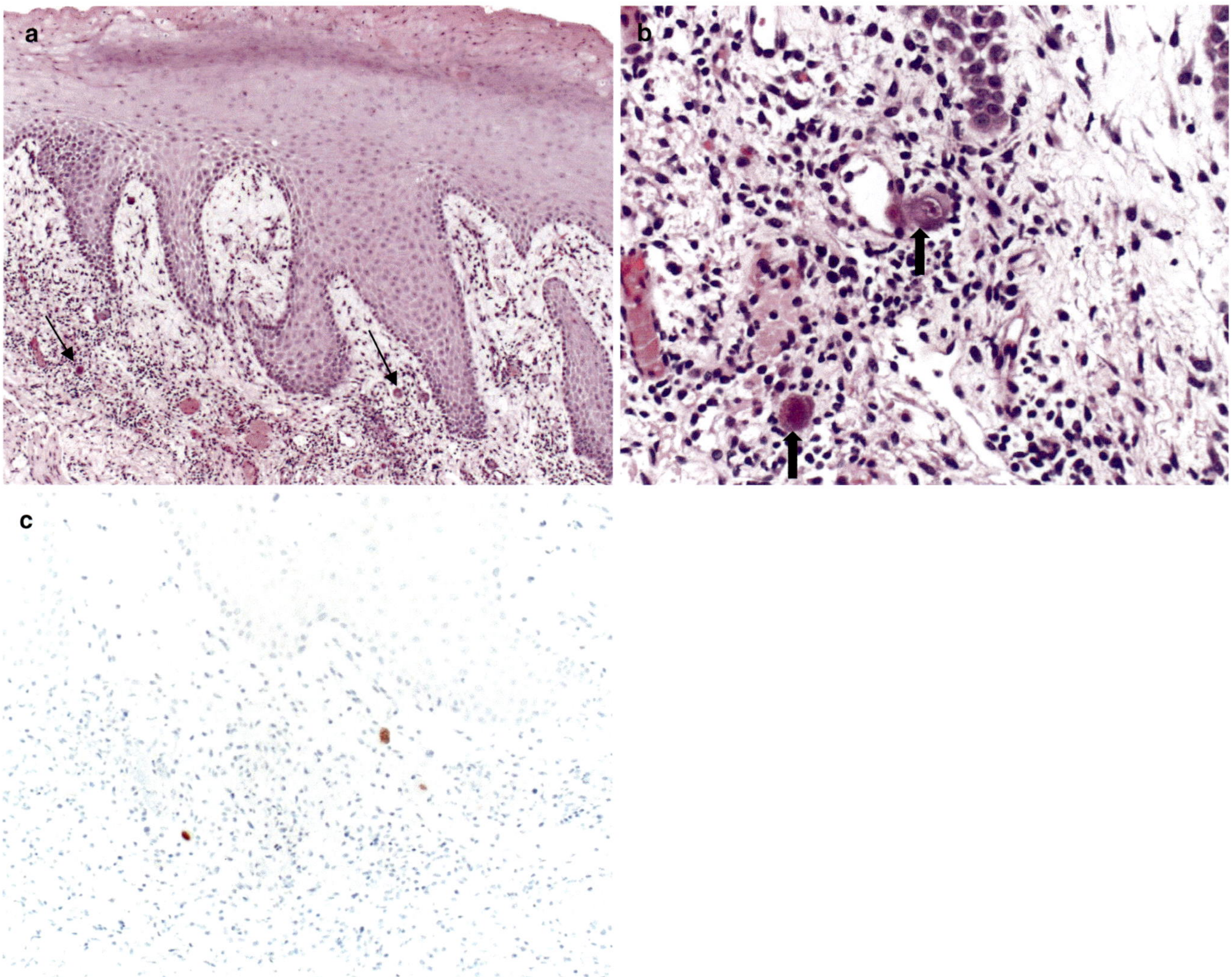

Fig. 3.14 *Cytomegalovirus*: (**a**) Epidermal hyperkeratosis and acanthosis with CMV inclusions in dermal vessels (arrows). (**b**) Characteristic "owl's eye" inclusions in infected endothelial cells (arrow). (**c**) Immunohistochemical stain for CMV highlights the infected cells

endothelial and mesenchymal cells [132]. In addition, CMV inclusions have rarely been detected in cervical smears [129]. When detected on cervical smears, CMV-infected cells are usually endocervical cells with characteristic large central eosinophilic inclusion with a prominent halo and small cytoplasmic basophilic inclusions [11].

3.4.3 Schistosomiasis

Schistosomiasis is an endemic parasitosis of countries in Africa, Middle East, South America, and Southeast Asia. *Schistosoma haematobium*, *S. japonicum*, and *S. mansoni* are the main species that infect humans, and are specific to certain geographic areas. The disease is acquired percutaneously by infection with cercariae found in contaminated freshwater of endemic areas. The inoculation of the cercariae can cause acute symptoms such as local dermatitis, and systemic prodromal symptoms, e.g., fever, headache, and cough. The adult schistosomes reside inside blood vessels of the human host's body, and are usually seen in the superior mesenteric veins, the venous plexus of bladder, and rectal venules. The worm is able to move to different venous sites, and produces numerous eggs that can surface through the lumen of the intestines or the bladder urothelium, and be expelled. The eggs can also travel to different sites of the body and cause serious pathologies [133, 134].

Infection of the lower female genital tract by schistosomiasis may present as dermatitis of the vulvar skin caused by inoculation of the cercariae, or by an inflammatory reaction around the trematode's eggs. Clinical presentation includes papules, plaques, ulcers, and/or extensive wart-like lesions that can be very similar to condyloma acuminata [59, 135, 136]. Schistosomiasis also affects the uterine cervix and causes rubbery papules, sandy patches, and neovascularization on the surface of the cervix. Histologically, the lesion encompasses mixed inflammatory cell infiltrate with neutrophils and eosinophils, worms or often calcified ova with adjacent granulomatous reaction, occasionally necrosis, and dense fibrosis (Fig. 3.15) [59]. In addition to biopsy of the lesions, the diagnosis can be made by detection of eggs in urine or feces, or serology testing. The later test has its limitations and cannot distinguish resolved versus active infection [133]. Female genital schistosomiasis has been proposed as a risk factor for HIV infection. However, no study was able to demonstrate a clear causality between the two entities, and confounding factors can also play a role in this association. Treatment of choice is the anti-helminthic praziquantel [133, 137–140].

3.4.4 Varicella Zoster

Varicella zoster virus (VZV) is a double-stranded DNA neurotropic human virus from Herpesviridae family. Primary

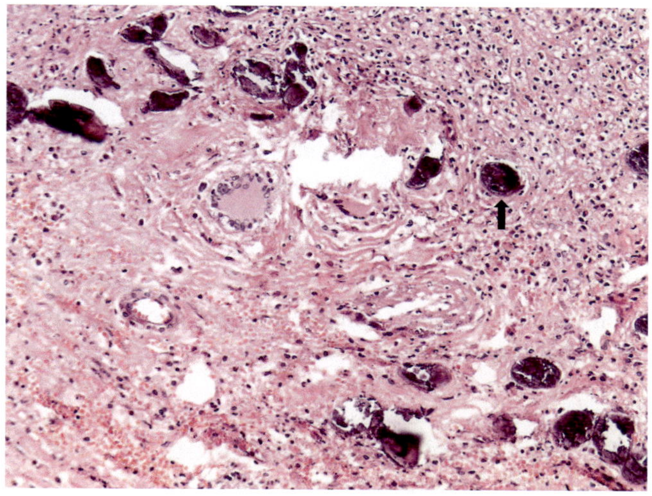

Fig. 3.15 Calcified *Schistosoma* ova (arrow) with adjacent mixed inflammatory cell infiltrate and multinucleated giant cells

infection with VZV causes chicken pox, a self-limited childhood disease presenting with disseminated vesicular rashes and fever. Shingles or herpes zoster is a result of reactivation of latent VZV, which establishes a dormant state in nerve ganglia after primary infection. Reactivation of VZV usually occurs in older adults and immunocompromised individuals, due to decreased immunity to the virus [141, 142].

Isolated herpes zoster of vulva is a rare cause of genital ulcers, triggered by reactivation of the VZV residing in sacral sensory ganglia [143, 144]. Lesions present with a prodrome of pain or burning sensation, followed by clusters of painful vesicles, pustules, and erosions in a dermatomal distribution. The lesions may be confused with herpes simplex; however, vulvar zoster is unlikely to recur in the same location or cross the midline. Post-herpetic neuralgia is a common complication and should be considered in vulvodynia patients [145]. Diagnosis can be made by detection of VZV from the lesions with culture, PCR, or direct Immunofluorescence assays (DFA). Biopsy samples are rarely taken which shows changes similar to HSV infection. Immunohistochemical staining can differentiate varicella zoster from herpes zoster.

3.4.5 Malakoplakia

Malakoplakia is an uncommon chronic inflammatory process, first described by Michaelis and Gutmann in 1902, which most commonly affects the urinary tract mucosa [146]. Female genital tract malakoplakia is rare and most reported cases describe vaginal involvement [146–148]. The pathogenesis of malakoplakia has not been fully elucidated, but several factors including microorganisms, abnormal immune response, and impaired macrophage function have been implicated [149]. *Escherichia coli* is found in majority of the cases; however, several organisms such as *Mycobacterium tuberculosis*, *Proteus*, and *Staphylococcus aureus* have been implicated [149].

Malakoplakia can present as mucosal plaques, nodules, and mass-like lesions which in some cases can mimic tumor [146, 148]. Microscopic examination shows sheets of large, granular histiocytes with eosinophilic to vacuolated cytoplasm containing granular basophilic periodic acid Schiff-positive, diastase-resistant inclusions and calcified Michaelis–Gutmann bodies. Michaelis–Gutmann bodies often exhibit a targetoid appearance and stain positively by Von Kossa (calcium) stain [149].

3.5 Vulvar Infections Associated with Immunosuppression

3.5.1 Generalized Genital Warts in Patients with Immunosuppression

Condylomata acuminata or anogenital warts are caused by HPV (90% is due to types 6 or 11) [78]. Patients with HIV infection or other causes of immunosuppression are prone to develop numerous and extensive lesions that are also more resistant to standard therapies [114, 150–152]. The reduction of CD8+ cytotoxic T-lymphocyte reactivity to HPV oncoproteins E6 and E7 (cell-mediated immunity) leads to inadequate elimination of the virus. Both transplant recipients and HIV-infected patients have been found to have a higher prevalence of high-risk HPV types. HIV patients have in particular HPV-16 type in their condylomata, which can be associated with foci of high-grade squamous intraepithelial lesions [59, 78, 114, 152].

Physical examination is sufficient for the diagnosis; however, biopsy of suspected wart can be used to confirm diagnosis and rule out malignancy. The histology of condilomata is the same as the lesions seen in immunocompetent individuals, and show acanthosis, dyskeratosis, parakeratosis, hyperkeratosis, papillomatosis, and a prominent granular layer. Koilocytosis is present in the superficial epithelial cells, and binucleated and multinucleated squamous cells are frequent findings (Fig. 3.6). Immunosuppressed patients are more likely to progress with dysplasia and invasive squamous cell carcinoma, regardless of the lesion's site (vulva, vagina, cervix, anus, or perineal skin). Other type of malignant transformation of HPV infection to be considered in immunosuppressed population, although very rare, is giant condyloma acuminatum or Buschke–Lowenstein tumor (BLT), which is a low-grade squamous cell carcinoma that manifest as a large exophytic mass that can form fistulas, abscesses, and local neoplastic invasion. Histologically, BLT is very similar to condylomata, but tends to infiltrate deeper tissue layers with pushing infiltrating pattern. Malignant transformation to invasive carcinoma is determined by the presence of numerous mitotic figures and frank invasion. The CDC supports course of treatment for all patient with HPV infection, irrespective of their immune status [59, 62, 78, 153].

3.5.2 Tuberculosis

Tuberculosis rarely involves the lower female genital tract. The disease may affect the vulva, vagina, and cervix directly by coitus of a partner with genitourinary tuberculosis, or indirectly by secondary spread of tuberculosis from other sites. The most common primary source of the infection is pulmonary tuberculosis. However, genital tuberculosis of different sites such as fallopian tube and endometrium can also disseminate to the lower genital tract. Genital tuberculosis should be considered in patients with immunosuppression and latent tuberculosis, as well as in patients with active disease. Special attention should be drawn to immunocompromised patients with HIV infection, diabetes mellitus, corticosteroid use, end-stage renal disease, and to the patients treated by tumor necrosis factor-alpha inhibitors [59, 154].

Given the indolent course of the disease, the mycobacterium can reside in the tissue for an extended period before leading to clinical manifestation. Diagnosis can be made histologically with classical presentation of caseating granulomas characterized by central caseous necrosis, epithelioid histiocytes, and giant cells (Fig. 3.16). Ziehl–Neelsen stain can demonstrate the acid-fast *Mycobacterium tuberculosis*. Unfixed specimen should be considered for microbiologic testing. According to the patient's immune response, caseous necrosis may be absent and the differential diagnosis includes foreign body giant cell granulomas (usually secondary to surgical procedures), lymphogranulomas venereum, schistosomiasis, sarcoidosis, granulomatous syphilis, and invasive cervical cancer. Diagnostic tests used for systemic tuberculosis, e.g., interferon-gamma assay, can also aid in the diagnosis of genital tuberculosis. Antituberculous therapy for genital disease follows the same guidelines used for pulmonary tuberculosis [154].

3.5.3 Bacillary Angiomatosis

Bacillary angiomatosis (BA) is caused by two closely related gram-negative coccobacilli, *Bartonella henselae* and *Bartonella quintana*, and occurs primarily in immunocompromised patients. We are aware of three cases of vulvar BA reported in the literature. Clinical presentation is similar to BA cutaneous lesions of other sites, and appear as red-purple nodules with vascular formation that easily bleed with trauma. Histologic examination reveals vascular proliferations that are lined by prominent epithelioid endothelial cells in a background of lymphocytes, histiocytes, and neutro-

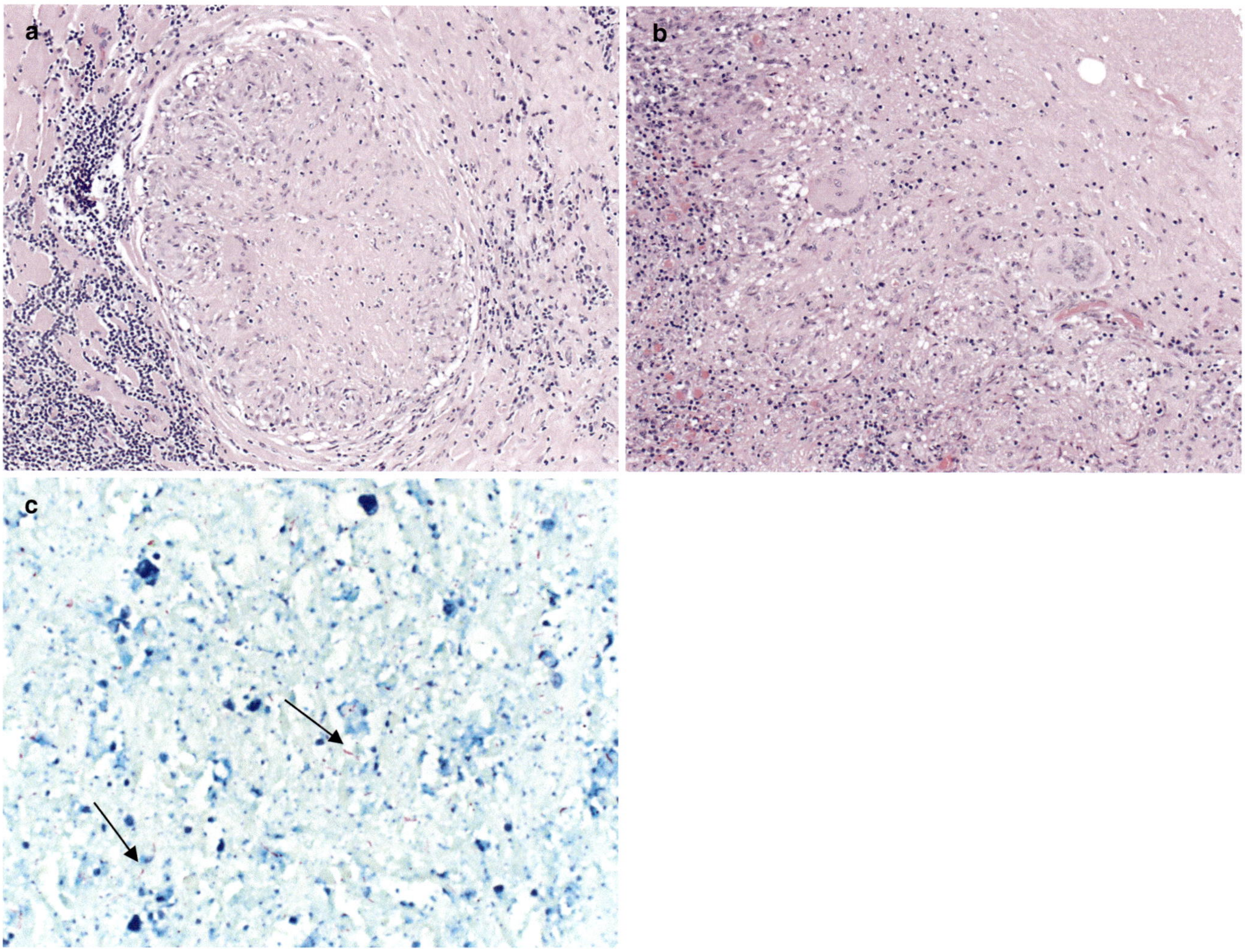

Fig. 3.16 Tuberculosis involving dermis. (**a**, **b**) Caseating granulomas reveal central caseous necrosis, epithelioid histiocytes, and multinucleated giant cells. (**c**) AFB stain highlights mycobacteria in the granuloma (arrows)

phils. Giemsa, Warthin–Starry, or Grocott-Gomori methenamine silver stain demonstrates hazy clumps of bacteria that characterize bacillary angiomatosis. Immunohistochemical techniques, culture, and polymerase chain reaction based methods have also been used to identify the organisms [62, 155–157]. Several antibiotics are effective against Bartonella infections, and macrolides are commonly used. Different diagnosis includes other vascular lesions such as pyogenic granuloma, Kaposi sarcoma, and cherry angioma, among others [62, 155].

References

1. Meites E. Trichomoniasis: the "neglected" sexually transmitted disease. Infect Dis Clin N Am. 2013;27(4):755–64.
2. Benchimol M. Trichomonads under microscopy. Microsc Microanal. 2004;10(5):528–50.
3. Schwebke JR, Burgess D. Trichomoniasis. Clin Microbiol Rev. 2004;17(4):794–803, table of contents.
4. Sutton M, Sternberg M, Koumans EH, McQuillan G, Berman S, Markowitz L. The prevalence of Trichomonas vaginalis infection among reproductive-age women in the United States, 2001–2004. Clin Infect Dis. 2007;45(10):1319–26.
5. Meites E, Gaydos CA, Hobbs MM, Kissinger P, Nyirjesy P, Schwebke JR, et al. A review of evidence-based care of symptomatic Trichomoniasis and asymptomatic Trichomonas vaginalis infections. Clin Infect Dis. 2015;61(Suppl 8):S837–48.
6. Van Der Pol B. Clinical and laboratory testing for Trichomonas vaginalis infection. J Clin Microbiol. 2016;54(1):7–12.
7. Harp DF, Chowdhury I. Trichomoniasis: evaluation to execution. Eur J Obstet Gynecol Reprod Biol. 2011;157(1):3–9.
8. Aslan DL, Gulbahce HE, Stelow EB, Setty S, Brown CA, McGlennen RC, et al. The diagnosis of Trichomonas vaginalis in liquid-based Pap tests: correlation with PCR. Diagn Cytopathol. 2005;32(6):341–4.
9. Lara-Torre E, Pinkerton JS. Accuracy of detection of Trichomonas vaginalis organisms on a liquid-based papanicolaou smear. Am J Obstet Gynecol. 2003;188(2):354–6.
10. Noel JC, Engohan-Aloghe C. Morphologic criteria associated with Trichomonas vaginalis in liquid-based cytology. Acta Cytol. 2010;54(4):582–6.
11. Nayar R, Wilbur DC. The Bethesda system for reporting cervical cytology: definitions, criteria, and explanatory notes. Cham:

Springer; 2015. Available from: SpringerLink. Restricted to UC campuses https://doi.org/10.1007/978-3-319-11074-5.
12. Centers for Disease Control and Prevention, National Center for HIV/AIDS, Viral Hepatitis, STD, and TB Prevention, Division of STD Prevention. Trichomoniasis.
13. Shisler JL. Immune evasion strategies of molluscum contagiosum virus. Adv Virus Res. 2015;92:201–52.
14. Smith KJ, Yeager J, Skelton H. Molluscum contagiosum: its clinical, histopathologic, and immunohistochemical spectrum. Int J Dermatol. 1999;38(9):664–72.
15. Tyring SK. Molluscum contagiosum: the importance of early diagnosis and treatment. Am J Obstet Gynecol. 2003;189(3 Suppl):S12–6.
16. Gur I. The epidemiology of Molluscum contagiosum in HIV-seropositive patients: a unique entity or insignificant finding? Int J STD AIDS. 2008;19(8):503–6.
17. Ishikawa MK, Arps DP, Chow C, Hocker TL, Fullen DR. Histopathological features of molluscum contagiosum other than molluscum bodies. Histopathology. 2015;67(6):836–42.
18. Chentoufi AA, Benmohamed L. Mucosal herpes immunity and immunopathology to ocular and genital herpes simplex virus infections. Clin Dev Immunol. 2012;2012:149135.
19. Fatahzadeh M, Schwartz RA. Human herpes simplex virus infections: epidemiology, pathogenesis, symptomatology, diagnosis, and management. J Am Acad Dermatol. 2007;57(5):737–63; quiz 64–6.
20. Stanberry L, Cunningham A, Mertz G, Mindel A, Peters B, Reitano M, et al. New developments in the epidemiology, natural history and management of genital herpes. Antivir Res. 1999;42(1):1–14.
21. Money D, Steben M. No. 207-Genital herpes: gynaecological aspects. J Obstet Gynaecol Can. 2017;39(7):e105–e11.
22. Johnston C, Corey L. Current concepts for genital herpes simplex virus infection: diagnostics and pathogenesis of genital tract shedding. Clin Microbiol Rev. 2016;29(1):149–61.
23. Beauman JG. Genital herpes: a review. Am Fam Physician. 2005;72(8):1527–34.
24. Strick LB, Wald A, Celum C. Management of herpes simplex virus type 2 infection in HIV type 1-infected persons. Clin Infect Dis. 2006;43(3):347–56.
25. Cohen PR. The "knife-cut sign" revisited: a distinctive presentation of linear erosive herpes simplex virus infection in immunocompromised patients. J Clin Aesthet Dermatol. 2015;8(10):38–42.
26. Desai DV, Kulkarni SS. Herpes simplex virus: the interplay between HSV, host, and HIV-1. Viral Immunol. 2015;28(10):546–55.
27. Robboy SJ. Robboy's pathology of the female reproductive tract. 2nd ed. Edinburgh: Churchill Livingstone/Elsevier; 2009. p. xxxviii, 1066 p.
28. Tangjitgamol S, Loharamtaweethong K, Thawaramara T, Chanpanitkitchot S. Vulvar pseudoepitheliomatous hyperplasia associated with herpes simplex virus type II mimicking cancer in an immunocompromised patient. J Obstet Gynaecol Res. 2014;40(1):255–8.
29. Groves MJ. Genital herpes: a review. Am Fam Physician. 2016;93(11):928–34.
30. Centers for Disease Control and Prevention, National Center for HIV/AIDS, Viral Hepatitis, STD, and TB Prevention, Division of STD Prevention. Gonorrhea. Available from: https://www.cdc.gov/std/tg2015/gonorrhea.htm.
31. Miller WC, Ford CA, Morris M, Handcock MS, Schmitz JL, Hobbs MM, et al. Prevalence of chlamydial and gonococcal infections among young adults in the United States. JAMA. 2004;291(18):2229–36.
32. Bora SA, Condous G. Bartholin's, vulval and perineal abscesses. Best Pract Res Clin Obstet Gynaecol. 2009;23(5):661–6.
33. LeFevre ML, US Preventive Services Task Force. Screening for chlamydia and gonorrhea: U.S. Preventive Services Task Force recommendation statement. Ann Intern Med. 2014;161(12):902–10.
34. Kiviat NB, Paavonen JA, Wolner-Hanssen P, Critchlow CW, Stamm WE, Douglas J, et al. Histopathology of endocervical infection caused by Chlamydia trachomatis, herpes simplex virus, Trichomonas vaginalis, and Neisseria gonorrhoeae. Hum Pathol. 1990;21(8):831–7.
35. Peeling RW, Hook EW 3rd. The pathogenesis of syphilis: the Great Mimicker, revisited. J Pathol. 2006;208(2):224–32.
36. Radolf JD, Deka RK, Anand A, Smajs D, Norgard MV, Yang XF. Treponema pallidum, the syphilis spirochete: making a living as a stealth pathogen. Nat Rev Microbiol. 2016;14(12):744–59.
37. Shockman S, Buescher LS, Stone SP. Syphilis in the United States. Clin Dermatol. 2014;32(2):213–8.
38. Lafond RE, Lukehart SA. Biological basis for syphilis. Clin Microbiol Rev. 2006;19(1):29–49.
39. Carlson JA, Dabiri G, Cribier B, Sell S. The immunopathobiology of syphilis: the manifestations and course of syphilis are determined by the level of delayed-type hypersensitivity. Am J Dermatopathol. 2011;33(5):433–60.
40. Singh AE, Romanowski B. Syphilis: review with emphasis on clinical, epidemiologic, and some biologic features. Clin Microbiol Rev. 1999;12(2):187–209.
41. Baughn RE, Musher DM. Secondary syphilitic lesions. Clin Microbiol Rev. 2005;18(1):205–16.
42. Balagula Y, Mattei PL, Wisco OJ, Erdag G, Chien AL. The great imitator revisited: the spectrum of atypical cutaneous manifestations of secondary syphilis. Int J Dermatol. 2014;53(12):1434–41.
43. Cid PM, Cudos ES, Zamora Vargas FX, Merino MJ, Pinto PH. Pathologically confirmed malignant syphilis using immunohistochemical staining: report of 3 cases and review of the literature. Sex Transm Dis. 2014;41(2):94–7.
44. Requena CB, Orasmo CR, Ocanha JP, Barraviera SR, Marques ME, Marques SA. Malignant syphilis in an immunocompetent female patient. An Bras Dermatol. 2014;89(6):970–2.
45. Bittencourt Mde J, Brito AC, Nascimento BA, Carvalho AH, Drago MG. Nodular tertiary syphilis in an immunocompetent patient. An Bras Dermatol. 2016;91(4):528–30.
46. Rocha N, Horta M, Sanches M, Lima O, Massa A. Syphilitic gumma—cutaneous tertiary syphilis. J Eur Acad Dermatol Venereol. 2004;18(4):517–8.
47. Karp G, Schlaeffer F, Jotkowitz A, Riesenberg K. Syphilis and HIV co-infection. Eur J Intern Med. 2009;20(1):9–13.
48. Stevenson J, Heath M. Syphilis and HIV infection: an update. Dermatol Clin. 2006;24(4):497–507, vi.
49. Tobian AA, Quinn TC. Herpes simplex virus type 2 and syphilis infections with HIV: an evolving synergy in transmission and prevention. Curr Opin HIV AIDS. 2009;4(4):294–9.
50. Zetola NM, Klausner JD. Syphilis and HIV infection: an update. Clin Infect Dis. 2007;44(9):1222–8.
51. Engelkens HJ, ten Kate FJ, Vuzevski VD, van der Sluis JJ, Stolz E. Primary and secondary syphilis: a histopathological study. Int J STD AIDS. 1991;2(4):280–4.
52. Abell E, Marks R, Jones EW. Secondary syphilis: a clinico-pathological review. Br J Dermatol. 1975;93(1):53–61.
53. Flamm A, Parikh K, Xie Q, Kwon EJ, Elston DM. Histologic features of secondary syphilis: a multicenter retrospective review. J Am Acad Dermatol. 2015;73(6):1025–30.
54. Brown L. Pathology of the vulva and vagina. London: Springer, 2013. Available from: SpringerLink. Restricted to UC campuses https://doi.org/10.1007/978-0-85729-757-0.
55. Pandhi RK, Singh N, Ramam M. Secondary syphilis: a clinicopathologic study. Int J Dermatol. 1995;34(4):240–3.
56. Buffet M, Grange PA, Gerhardt P, Carlotti A, Calvez V, Bianchi A, et al. Diagnosing Treponema pallidum in secondary syphilis by PCR and immunohistochemistry. J Invest Dermatol. 2007;127(10):2345–50.

57. Grange PA, Gressier L, Dion PL, Farhi D, Benhaddou N, Gerhardt P, et al. Evaluation of a PCR test for detection of treponema pallidum in swabs and blood. J Clin Microbiol. 2012;50(3):546–52.
58. Centers for Disease Control and Prevention, National Center for HIV/AIDS, Viral Hepatitis, STD, and TB Prevention, Division of STD Prevention. Syphilis. Available from: https://www.cdc.gov/std/syphilis/default.htm.
59. Blaustein A, Kurman RJ, Ronnett BM. Blaustein's pathology of the female genital tract. 6th ed. New York: Springer; 2011. 1246 p.
60. Centers for Disease Control and Prevention, National Center for HIV/AIDS, Viral Hepatitis, STD, and TB Prevention, Division of STD Prevention. Chancroid. Available from: https://www.cdc.gov/std/tg2015/chancroid.htm.
61. Sternberg SS, Mills SE, Carter D. Sternberg's diagnostic surgical pathology, 2 vol., 5th ed. Philadelphia, PA: Wolters Kluwer Health/Lippincott Williams & Wilkins; 2010 (xv, 418 pages, 83 unnumbered pages).
62. Weedon D, Strutton G, Rubin AI, Weedon D. Weedon's skin pathology. 3rd ed. Oxford: Churchill Livingstone; 2010. 1041 p.
63. Joseph AK, Rosen T. Laboratory techniques used in the diagnosis of chancroid, granuloma inguinale, and lymphogranuloma venereum. Dermatol Clin. 1994;12(1):1–8.
64. Romero L, Huerfano C, Grillo-Ardila CF. Macrolides for treatment of Haemophilus ducreyi infection in sexually active adults. Cochrane Database Syst Rev. 2017;12:CD012492.
65. Centers for Disease Control and Prevention, National Center for HIV/AIDS, Viral Hepatitis, STD, and TB Prevention, Division of STD Prevention Donovanosis. Available from: https://www.cdc.gov/std/tg2015/donovanosis.htm.
66. O'Farrell N, Moi H. 2016 European guideline on donovanosis. Int J STD AIDS. 2016;27(8):605–7.
67. Centers for Disease Control and Prevention, National Center for HIV/AIDS, Viral Hepatitis, STD, and TB Prevention, Division of STD Prevention LGV. Available from: https://www.cdc.gov/std/tg2015/lgv.htm.
68. Isaksson J, Carlsson O, Airell A, Stromdahl S, Bratt G, Herrmann B. Lymphogranuloma venereum rates increased and Chlamydia trachomatis genotypes changed among men who have sex with men in Sweden 2004–2016. J Med Microbiol. 2017;66(11):1684–7.
69. Peuchant O, Touati A, Sperandio C, Henin N, Laurier-Nadalie C, Bebear C, et al. Changing pattern of Chlamydia trachomatis strains in lymphogranuloma venereum outbreak, France, 2010–2015. Emerg Infect Dis. 2016;22(11):1945–7.
70. Scieux C, Barnes R, Bianchi A, Casin I, Morel P, Perol Y. Lymphogranuloma venereum: 27 cases in Paris. J Infect Dis. 1989;160(4):662–8.
71. Collins L, White JA, Bradbeer C. Lymphogranuloma venereum. BMJ. 2006;332(7533):66.
72. Centers for Disease Control and Prevention. Recommendations for the laboratory-based detection of Chlamydia trachomatis and Neisseria gonorrhoeae—2014. MMWR Recomm Rep. 2014;63(RR-02):1–19.
73. Centers for Disease Control and Prevention, National Center for HIV/AIDS, Viral Hepatitis, STD, and TB Prevention, Division of STD Prevention. Chlamydia. Available from: https://www.cdc.gov/std/tg2015/chlamydia.htm.
74. Faro S. Chlamydia trachomatis infection in women. J Reprod Med. 1985;30(3 Suppl):273–8.
75. Haggerty CL, Gottlieb SL, Taylor BD, Low N, Xu F, Ness RB. Risk of sequelae after Chlamydia trachomatis genital infection in women. J Infect Dis. 2010;201(Suppl 2):S134–55.
76. O'Connell CM, Ferone ME. Chlamydia trachomatis genital infections. Microb Cell. 2016;3(9):390–403.
77. Edwards JM, Campbell AR, Tait A, Lusher M. Demonstration of Chlamydia trachomatis in colposcopic cervical biopsy specimens by an immunoperoxidase method. J Clin Pathol. 1991;44(12):1027–9.
78. Centers for Disease Control and Prevention, National Center for HIV/AIDS, Viral Hepatitis, STD, and TB Prevention, Division of STD Prevention. Warts. Available from: https://www.cdc.gov/std/tg2015/warts.htm.
79. Kurman RJ, International Agency for Research on Cancer, World Health Organization. WHO classification of tumours of female reproductive organs. 4th ed. Lyon: International Agency for Research on Cancer; 2014. 307 p.
80. Clavero O, McCloskey J, Molina VM, Quiros B, Bravo IG, de Sanjose S, et al. Squamous intraepithelial lesions of the anal squamocolumnar junction: histopathological classification and HPV genotyping. Papillomavirus Res. 2017;3:11–7.
81. Roberts JM, Cornall AM, Ekman D, Law C, Poynten IM, Jin F, et al. Papillary immature metaplasia of the anal canal: a low-grade lesion that can mimic a high-grade lesion. Am J Surg Pathol. 2016;40(3):348–53.
82. Anderson J, Clark RA, Watts DH, Till M, Arrastia C, Schuman P, et al. Idiopathic genital ulcers in women infected with human immunodeficiency virus. J Acquir Immune Defic Syndr Hum Retrovirol. 1996;13(4):343–7.
83. Burgener A, McGowan I, Klatt NR. HIV and mucosal barrier interactions: consequences for transmission and pathogenesis. Curr Opin Immunol. 2015;36:22–30.
84. Farcasanu M, Kwon DS. The influence of cervicovaginal microbiota on mucosal immunity and prophylaxis in the Battle against HIV. Curr HIV/AIDS Rep. 2018;15(1):30–8.
85. Nazli A, Chan O, Dobson-Belaire WN, Ouellet M, Tremblay MJ, Gray-Owen SD, et al. Exposure to HIV-1 directly impairs mucosal epithelial barrier integrity allowing microbial translocation. PLoS Pathog. 2010;6(4):e1000852.
86. Peters BM, Yano J, Noverr MC, Fidel PL Jr. Candida vaginitis: when opportunism knocks, the host responds. PLoS Pathog. 2014;10(4):e1003965.
87. Sobel JD. Vaginitis. N Engl J Med. 1997;337(26):1896–903.
88. Sobel JD. Vulvovaginal candidosis. Lancet. 2007;369(9577):1961–71.
89. Foxman B. The epidemiology of vulvovaginal candidiasis: risk factors. Am J Public Health. 1990;80(3):329–31.
90. Hoffmann JN, You HM, Hedberg EC, Jordan JA, McClintock MK. Prevalence of bacterial vaginosis and Candida among postmenopausal women in the United States. J Gerontol B Psychol Sci Soc Sci. 2014;69(Suppl 2):S205–14.
91. Mendling W, Friese K, Mylonas I, Weissenbacher ER, Brasch J, Schaller M, et al. Vulvovaginal Candidosis (excluding chronic mucocutaneous candidosis). Guideline of the German Society of Gynecology and Obstetrics (AWMF registry no. 015/072, S2k level, December 2013). Geburtshilfe Frauenheilkd. 2015;75(4):342–54.
92. Blostein F, Levin-Sparenberg E, Wagner J, Foxman B. Recurrent vulvovaginal candidiasis. Ann Epidemiol. 2017;27(9):575–82, e3.
93. Foster KW, Ghannoum MA, Elewski BE. Epidemiologic surveillance of cutaneous fungal infection in the United States from 1999 to 2002. J Am Acad Dermatol. 2004;50(5):748–52.
94. Ely JW, Rosenfeld S, Seabury Stone M. Diagnosis and management of tinea infections. Am Fam Physician. 2014;90(10):702–10.
95. Otero L, Palacio V, Vazquez F. Tinea cruris in female prostitutes. Mycopathologia. 2002;153(1):29–31.
96. Chang SE, Lee DK, Choi JH, Moon KC, Koh JK. Majocchi's granuloma of the vulva caused by Trichophyton mentagrophytes. Mycoses. 2005;48(6):382–4.
97. Luchsinger I, Bosshard PP, Kasper RS, Reinhardt D, Lautenschlager S. Tinea genitalis: a new entity of sexually transmitted infection? Case series and review of the literature. Sex Transm Infect. 2015;91(7):493–6.

98. Sand FL, Thomsen SF. Skin diseases of the vulva: infectious diseases. J Obstet Gynaecol. 2017;37(7):840–8.
99. Koumans EH, Sternberg M, Bruce C, McQuillan G, Kendrick J, Sutton M, et al. The prevalence of bacterial vaginosis in the United States, 2001–2004; associations with symptoms, sexual behaviors, and reproductive health. Sex Transm Dis. 2007;34(11):864–9.
100. Malaguti N, Bahls LD, Uchimura NS, Gimenes F, Consolaro ME. Sensitive detection of thirteen bacterial vaginosis-associated agents using multiplex polymerase chain reaction. Biomed Res Int. 2015;2015:645853.
101. Schwebke JR, Muzny CA, Josey WE. Role of Gardnerella vaginalis in the pathogenesis of bacterial vaginosis: a conceptual model. J Infect Dis. 2014;210(3):338–43.
102. Kenyon C, Colebunders R, Crucitti T. The global epidemiology of bacterial vaginosis: a systematic review. Am J Obstet Gynecol. 2013;209(6):505–23.
103. Eade CR, Diaz C, Chen S, Cole AL, Cole AM. HIV-enhancing factors are secreted by reproductive epithelia upon inoculation with bacterial vaginosis-associated bacteria. Protein Pept Lett. 2015;22(8):672–80.
104. Mitchell C, Marrazzo J. Bacterial vaginosis and the cervicovaginal immune response. Am J Reprod Immunol. 2014;71(6):555–63.
105. Fredricks DN, Fiedler TL, Thomas KK, Oakley BB, Marrazzo JM. Targeted PCR for detection of vaginal bacteria associated with bacterial vaginosis. J Clin Microbiol. 2007;45(10):3270–6.
106. Bakardzhiev I, Chokoeva A, Tchernev G, Wollina U, Lotti T. Tinea profunda of the genital area. Successful treatment of a rare skin disease. Dermatol Ther. 2016;29(3):181–3.
107. Ramsey ML. Pseudomonas folliculitis associated with use of hot tubs and spas. Phys Sportsmed. 1989;17(5):150–62.
108. Zisova LG, Dobrev HP, Tchernev G, Semkova K, Aliman AA, Chorleva KI, et al. Tinea atypica: report of nine cases. Wien Med Wochenschr. 2013;163(23–24):549–55.
109. Bhide A, Nama V, Patel S, Kalu E. Microbiology of cysts/abscesses of Bartholin's gland: review of empirical antibiotic therapy against microbial culture. J Obstet Gynaecol. 2010;30(7):701–3.
110. Cabrera H, Skoczdopole L, Marini M, Della Giovanna P, Saponaro A, Echeverria C. Necrotizing gangrene of the genitalia and perineum. Int J Dermatol. 2002;41(12):847–51.
111. Kilpatrick CC, Alagkiozidis I, Orejuela FJ, Chohan L, Hollier LM. Factors complicating surgical management of the vulvar abscess. J Reprod Med. 2010;55(3–4):139–42.
112. Kim TH, Seap B, Kim SA, Heo GE. Vulvar abscess caused by methicillin-resistant Staphylococcus aureus (MRSA) in a postmenopausal woman. J Menopausal Med. 2016;22(2):118–21.
113. Thurman AR, Satterfield TM, Soper DE. Methicillin-resistant Staphylococcus aureus as a common cause of vulvar abscesses. Obstet Gynecol. 2008;112(3):538–44.
114. Wood SC. Clinical manifestations and therapeutic management of vulvar cellulitis and abscess: methicillin-resistant Staphylococcus aureus, necrotizing fasciitis, Bartholin abscess, Crohn disease of the vulva, hidradenitis suppurativa. Clin Obstet Gynecol. 2015;58(3):503–11.
115. Dave AJ, Sethi A, Morrone A. Female genital mutilation: what every American dermatologist needs to know. Dermatol Clin. 2011;29(1):103–9.
116. Koussidis GA. Gynecologic rarities: a case of periclitoral abscess and review of the literature. Am J Obstet Gynecol. 2012;207(5):e3–5.
117. Rouzi AA. Epidermal clitoral inclusion cysts: not a rare complication of female genital mutilation. Hum Reprod. 2010;25(7):1672–4.
118. Gupta M, Saini V, Poddar A, Kumari S, Maitra A. Acquired clitoromegaly: a gynaecological problem or an obstetric complication? J Clin Diagn Res. 2016;10(12):QD10–1.
119. Markle W, Conti T, Kad M. Sexually transmitted diseases. Prim Care. 2013;40(3):557–87.
120. Ko CJ, Elston DM. Pediculosis. J Am Acad Dermatol. 2004;50(1):1–12; quiz 3–4.
121. Sangare AK, Doumbo OK, Raoult D. Management and treatment of human lice. Biomed Res Int. 2016;2016:8962685.
122. Chosidow O. Scabies and pediculosis. Lancet. 2000;355(9206):819–26.
123. Stamm AW, Kobashi KC, Stefanovic KB. Urologic dermatology: a review. Curr Urol Rep. 2017;18(8):62.
124. Bakos L, Reusch MC, D'Elia P, Aquino V, Bakos RM. Crusted scabies of the vulva. J Eur Acad Dermatol Venereol. 2007;21(5):682–4.
125. Hall LD, Eminger LA, Hesterman KS, Heymann WR. Epstein-Barr virus: dermatologic associations and implications: part I Mucocutaneous manifestations of Epstein-Barr virus and nonmalignant disorders. J Am Acad Dermatol. 2015;72(1):1–19; quiz 19–20.
126. Halvorsen JA, Brevig T, Aas T, Skar AG, Slevolden EM, Moi H. Genital ulcers as initial manifestation of Epstein-Barr virus infection: two new cases and a review of the literature. Acta Derm Venereol. 2006;86(5):439–42.
127. Haidari G, MacMahon E, Tong CY, White JA. Genital ulcers: it is not always simplex. Int J STD AIDS. 2015;26(1):72–3.
128. Griffiths P, Baraniak I, Reeves M. The pathogenesis of human cytomegalovirus. J Pathol. 2015;235(2):288–97.
129. McGalie CE, McBride HA, McCluggage WG. Cytomegalovirus infection of the cervix: morphological observations in five cases of a possibly under-recognised condition. J Clin Pathol. 2004;57(7):691–4.
130. Slyker J, Farquhar C, Atkinson C, Asbjornsdottir K, Roxby A, Drake A, et al. Compartmentalized cytomegalovirus replication and transmission in the setting of maternal HIV-1 infection. Clin Infect Dis. 2014;58(4):564–72.
131. Abou M, Dällenbach P. Acute cervicitis and vulvovaginitis may be associated with Cytomegalovirus. BMJ Case Rep. 2013;2013:bcr2013008884. https://doi.org/10.1136/bcr-2013-008884.
132. Choi YL, Kim JA, Jang KT, Kim DS, Kim WS, Lee JH, et al. Characteristics of cutaneous cytomegalovirus infection in non-acquired immune deficiency syndrome, immunocompromised patients. Br J Dermatol. 2006;155(5):977–82.
133. Centers for Disease Control and Prevention, National Center for HIV/AIDS, Viral Hepatitis, STD, and TB Prevention, Division of STD Prevention. Schistosomiasis. Available from: https://www.cdc.gov/parasites/schistosomiasis/index.html.
134. Christinet V, Lazdins-Helds JK, Stothard JR, Reinhard-Rupp J. Female genital schistosomiasis (FGS): from case reports to a call for concerted action against this neglected gynaecological disease. Int J Parasitol. 2016;46(7):395–404.
135. Richens J. Genital manifestations of tropical diseases. Sex Transm Infect. 2004;80(1):12–7.
136. Ricosse JH, Emeric R, Courbil LJ. [Anatomopathological aspects of schistosomiasis. A study of 286 pathological specimens (author's transl)]. Med Trop (Mars). 1980;40(1):77–94.
137. Hegertun IE, Sulheim Gundersen KM, Kleppa E, Zulu SG, Gundersen SG, Taylor M, et al. S. haematobium as a common cause of genital morbidity in girls: a cross-sectional study of children in South Africa. PLoS Negl Trop Dis. 2013;7(3):e2104.
138. Kjetland EF, Ndhlovu PD, Mduluza T, Gomo E, Gwanzura L, Mason PR, et al. Simple clinical manifestations of genital Schistosoma haematobium infection in rural Zimbabwean women. Am J Trop Med Hyg. 2005;72(3):311–9.
139. Kleppa E, Klinge KF, Galaphaththi-Arachchige HN, Holmen SD, Lillebo K, Onsrud M, et al. Schistosoma haematobium infection and CD4+ T-cell levels: a cross-sectional study of young South African women. PLoS One. 2015;10(3):e0119326.
140. Poggensee G, Kiwelu I, Weger V, Goppner D, Diedrich T, Krantz I, et al. Female genital schistosomiasis of the lower genital tract:

prevalence and disease-associated morbidity in northern Tanzania. J Infect Dis. 2000;181(3):1210–3.
141. John AR, Canaday DH. Herpes zoster in the older adult. Infect Dis Clin N Am. 2017;31(4):811–26.
142. Warren-Gash C, Forbes H, Breuer J. Varicella and herpes zoster vaccine development: lessons learned. Expert Rev Vaccines. 2017;16(12):1191–201.
143. Brown D. Herpes zoster of the vulva. Clin Obstet Gynecol. 1972;15(4):1010–4.
144. Philip KE, Goodman A, Pallawela SN, Sathia L, Webster DP. A not so simplex case of genital herpes. BMJ Case Rep. 2013;2013:bcr2013009993. https://doi.org/10.1136/bcr-2013-009993.
145. Cymerman RM, Kaplan Hoffmann R, Rouhani Schaffer P, Pomeranz MK. Vulvar infections: beyond sexually transmitted infections. Int J Dermatol. 2017;56(4):361–9.
146. Fishman A, Ortega E, Girtanner RE, Kaplan AL. Malacoplakia of the vagina presenting as a pelvic mass. Gynecol Oncol. 1993;49(3):380–2.
147. Chalvardjian A, Picard L, Shaw R, Davey R, Cairns JD. Malacoplakia of the female genital tract. Am J Obstet Gynecol. 1980;138(4):391–4.
148. Bhaijee F, Sebastian S, Lewin J. Vaginal malakoplakia: a benign mimic of pelvic malignancy in a postmenopausal female. Am J Clin Pathol. 2015;140:A171.
149. Yousef GM, Naghibi B, Hamodat MM. Malakoplakia outside the urinary tract. Arch Pathol Lab Med. 2007;131(2):297–300.
150. Yong M, Parkinson K, Goenka N, O'Mahony C. Diabetes and genital warts: an unhappy coalition. Int J STD AIDS. 2010;21(7):457–9.
151. Radja N, Lau R. Extensive genital warts associated with HTLV-I infection. Int J STD AIDS. 2004;15(3):202–3.
152. Gormley RH, Kovarik CL. Human papillomavirus-related genital disease in the immunocompromised host: part I. J Am Acad Dermatol. 2012;66(6):867.e1–14; quiz 81–2.
153. Werner RN, Westfechtel L, Dressler C, Nast A. Anogenital warts and other HPV-associated anogenital lesions in the HIV-positive patient: a systematic review and meta-analysis of the efficacy and safety of interventions assessed in controlled clinical trials. Sex Transm Infect. 2017;93(8):543–50.
154. Centers for Disease Control and Prevention, National Center for HIV/AIDS, Viral Hepatitis, STD, and TB Prevention, Division of STD Prevention. Available from: https://www.cdc.gov/tb/publications/guidelines/default.htm.
155. Centers for Disease Control and Prevention, National Center for HIV/AIDS, Viral Hepatitis, STD, and TB Prevention, Division of STD Prevention. Bartonella. Available from: https://www.cdc.gov/bartonella/clinicians/index.html.
156. Long SR, Whitfeld MJ, Eades C, Koehler JE, Korn AP, Zaloudek CJ. Bacillary angiomatosis of the cervix and vulva in a patient with AIDS. Obstet Gynecol. 1996;88(4 Pt 2):709–11.
157. Ramdial PK, Sing Y, Ramburan A, Dlova NC, Bagratee JS, Calonje E. Bartonella quintana-induced vulval bacillary angiomatosis. Int J Gynecol Pathol. 2012;31(4):390–4.

4 Vulvar Ectopic Tissues, Cysts, and Benign Adnexal Tumors

Anastasia M. Konstantinova, Michal Michal, and Dmitry V. Kazakov

Abstract

The vulva represents the female external genitalia external to the hymen, extending anteriorly to the mons pubis, posteriorly to the anus, and laterally to the inguinal-gluteal folds. It contains various histological structures including hair follicles, sebaceous, sweat, anogenital mammary-like, vestibular, and periurethral glands, which can give rise to various benign adnexal tumors. This chapter addresses the recent literature and our personal experience on benign cystic lesions, ectopic tissues, lesions of major and minor vestibular glands, benign lesions of anogenital mammary-like glands, and benign adnexal tumors of the vulva. Discussed are the normal anatomy and histology of the vulva as well as the clinical presentation, histopathological and immunohistochemical features and the differential diagnosis of paraurethral and Bartholin's gland cyst, mesonephric-like and mesothelial cyst, prostatic-type tissue of the vulva, endometriosis, hidradenoma papilliferum, fibroadenoma and benign phyllodes tumor, lactating adenoma, adenosis tumor, mammary-type fibrocystic disease and hamartoma, syringoma, cylindroma, spiradenoma, spiradenocylindroma, apocrine and eccrine mixed tumors and others.

Keywords

Vulva · Histology · Benign · Adnexal · Anogeniltal mammary-like glands

A. M. Konstantinova
Department of Pathology, Clinical Research and Practical Center for Specialized Oncological Care, Saint-Petersburg, Russia

Medical Faculty, Department of Pathology, Saint-Petersburg State University, Saint-Petersburg, Russia

Department of Pathology, Saint-Petersburg Medico-Social Institute, Saint-Petersburg, Russia

M. Michal · D. V. Kazakov (✉)
Medical Faculty in Pilsen, Sikl's Department of Pathology, Charles University in Prague, Pilsen, Czech Republic

Bioptical Laboratory, Pilsen, Czech Republic
e-mail: kazakov@biopticka.cz

4.1 Anatomy and Histology

The vulva represents the female external genitalia external to the hymen, extending anteriorly to the mons pubis, posteriorly to the anus, and laterally to the inguinal-gluteal folds. The main anatomic structures comprising of the vulva include the mons pubis, labia majora, labia minora, clitoris, vulvar vestibule and vestibulovaginal bulbs, urinary meatus, vaginal opening and hymen. Apart from the epidermis and adnexa, major and minor vestibular glands and anogenital mammary-like glands are histological constituents of the vulva [1, 2].

The mons pubis is a rounded prominence of fatty tissue located over the pubic symphysis of the pubic bones. It is covered by the skin with a stratified squamous keratinized epithelium, hair follicles, eccrine glands, and sensory receptors [2]. Hair follicle depth within the vulva is greatest in the mons pubis, with the depth up to 2.72 mm [3].

The labia majora are two large longitudinal folds of the skin that extend from the mons pubis, merge with the inguinal-gluteal folds laterally and with the perineal body posteriorly. The labia majora lie laterally and parallel to the labia minora, separated from the latter by the intralabial sulcus. Each labium majus has two surfaces, an outer one, pigmented and covered with pubic hair, containing apocrine and eccrine sweat glands, and an inner one, containing an abundance of sebaceous glands. These glands are not associated with hair follicles and open directly onto the epithelial surface. Sebaceous glands within the labia majora may have a depth of up to 2.03 mm [3]. The labia majora are covered with a squamous epithelium (Fig. 4.1) and contain a thin layer of smooth muscle that vaguely resemble the dartos muscle of the scrotum and a large amount of subcutaneous adipose tissue fat [1, 2, 4].

Medial to the labia majora, mainly within the sulcus between the labia majora and minora, *anogenital mammary-like glands* (AGMLG) are present (Fig. 4.1). Long regarded as ectopic or supernumerary breast tissue, anogenital mammary-like glands are now considered a

W. Zheng et al. (eds.), *Gynecologic and Obstetric Pathology, Volume 1*, https://doi.org/10.1007/978-981-13-3016-2_4

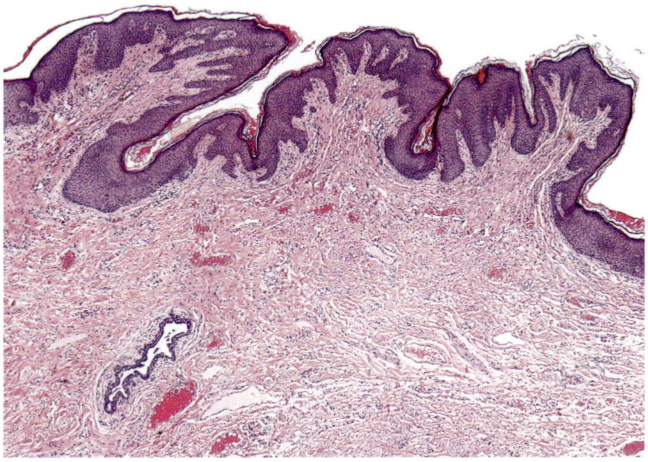

Fig. 4.1 The medial part of labia majora is covered by the squamous pigmented epithelium with a thin keratin layer. Note an anogenital mammary-like gland in the dermis

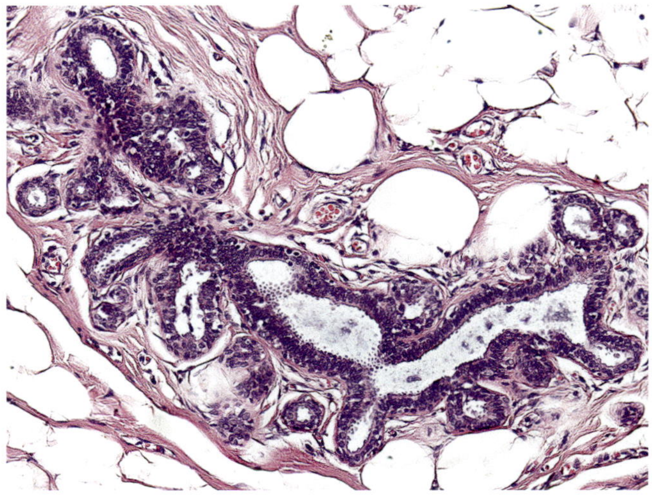

Fig. 4.2 An anogenital mammary-like gland with more complex structures showing outpouchings

normal constituent of the anogenital area [5–9]. Normal AGMLG exhibit a varying cytoarchitectural complexity and lined by a simple cuboidal to columnar epithelium surrounded by an outer myoepithelial layer. These glands vary from simple glandular structures with round lumina surrounded by a loose or dense fibrotic stroma, to more complex units closely imitating breast tissue (Fig. 4.2) [5, 7, 10]. Elastic fibers around anogenital glands can be found. The maximal depth of AGMLG is 3.9 mm, with a range of 0.64–3.9 mm [11]. Immunohistochemically, luminal cells show intermediate to strong expression of low molecular weight CKs ("luminal" keratins), ER (nuclear), PR (nuclear), AR (nuclear), and intermediate to strong expression of EMA (membranous, cytoplasmic), GCDFP-15 (cytoplasmic), mammaglobin (cytoplasmic), MUC1 (membranous, cytoplasmic), and GATA3 (nuclear). Furthermore, some cells in the luminal layer were positive for the high molecular weight CKs (cytoplasmic), CK5 (cytoplasmic), CK5/6 (cytoplasmic), CK14 (cytoplasmic), and CK17 (cytoplasmic), and p16 (nuclear, cytoplasmic). The outer cells of AGMLG are positive for myoepithelial markers and mostly for high molecular weight CKs ("basal" keratins"). The positivity for E-cadherin (membranous), CD138 (membranous), and MSH2 (nuclear) is seen in both layers of cells [12].

The excretory system of AGMLG opens to the epidermal surface and lined with columnar epithelium surrounded by myoepithelial cell layer which merges into a squamous epithelium. In some cases, elastic fibers surrounding excretory ducts of AGMLG can be found. Vulvar small clear cells (Toker cells), similar to Toker cells of the nipple, are arranged as single cells, in small clusters, or rarely form gland-like structures, can be detected in the lower epidermis around the openings of AGMLG ducts (Fig. 4.3a). Toker cells can be highlighted by using immunohistochemical staining with CK7 (membranous, cytoplasmic) (Fig. 4.3b) [10, 11, 13].

The labia minora are paired flaps of skin medial to the labia majora that bordered the vulvar vestibule. Anteriorly, each labium minus divides into two portions surrounding the clitoris: the upper part of each lip passes above the clitoris forming a prepuce and the lower part passes beneath the glans clitoridis and becomes the frenulum. Hart's line seen on the inner aspect of the labia minora represents the sides of the vestibule and marks the change from the vulvar skin covered by the epithelium of the stratified squamous type with thin keratin layer to the smoother transitional skin of the vulva covered by a not keratinized, generally highly glycogenated epithelium. Most of the epithelium of the labia minora is pigmented and the dermis does not contain skin appendages [1, 2].

4.1.1 Clitoris

The clitoris is a complex erectile structure located at the front of the vulva, containing attached root and free body and covered by protective fold of skin—preputium clitoridis. The visible portion of the clitoris is the clitoral glans. The clitoral crura are composed of erectile tissue similar to that seen in the penile corpora cavernosa (Fig. 4.4). They consist of cavernous veins surrounded by longitudinal smooth muscle as well as small centrally placed muscular arteries enveloped by the tunica albuginea. The glans clitoridis is highly sensitive, containing many nerve endings with abundant numbed of Pacinian corpuscles and covered by a squamous mucosa without glands (Fig. 4.4) [1, 2, 4].

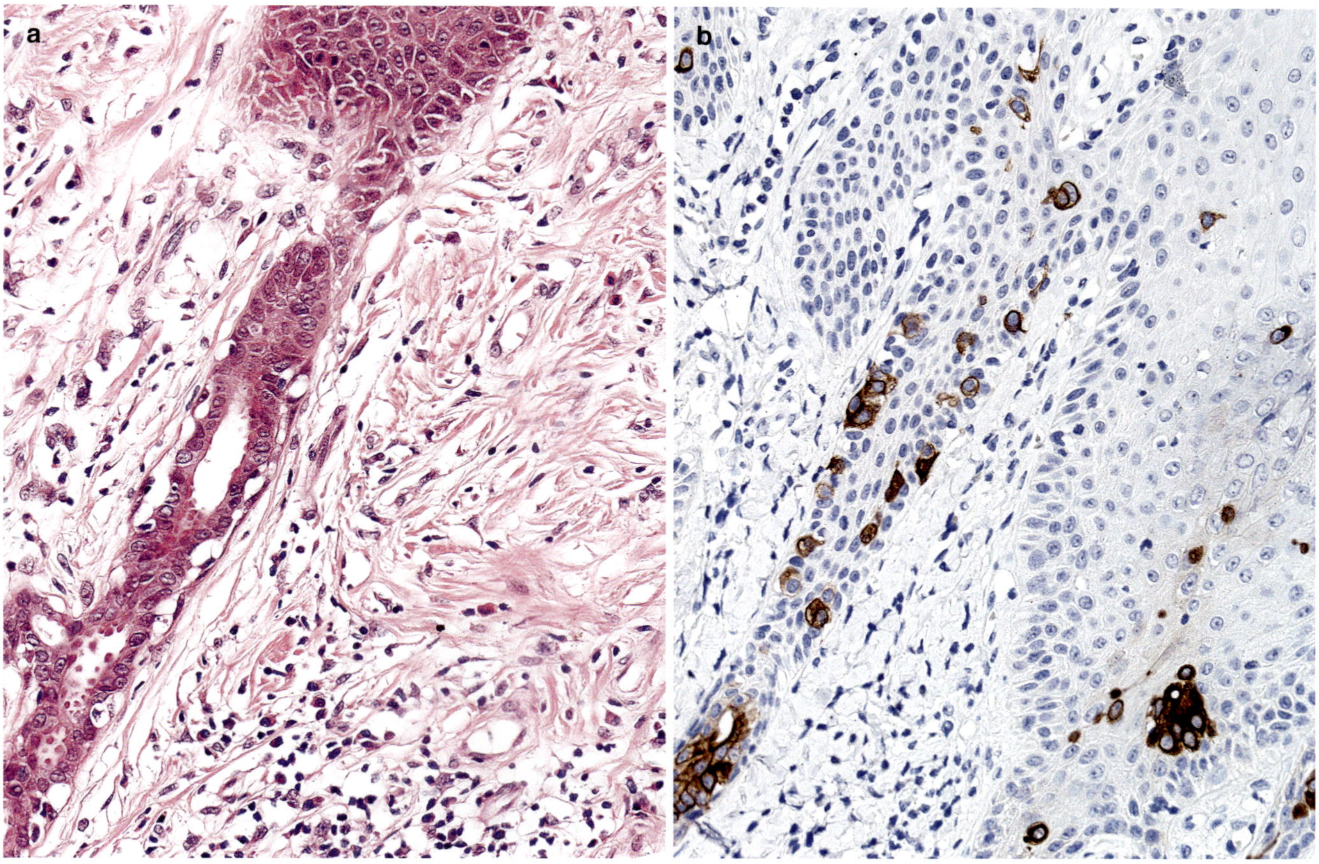

Fig. 4.3 Vulvar Toker cells in the lower epidermis around the openings of AGMLG duct (**a**). Positive immunohistochemical staining with CK7 (**b**)

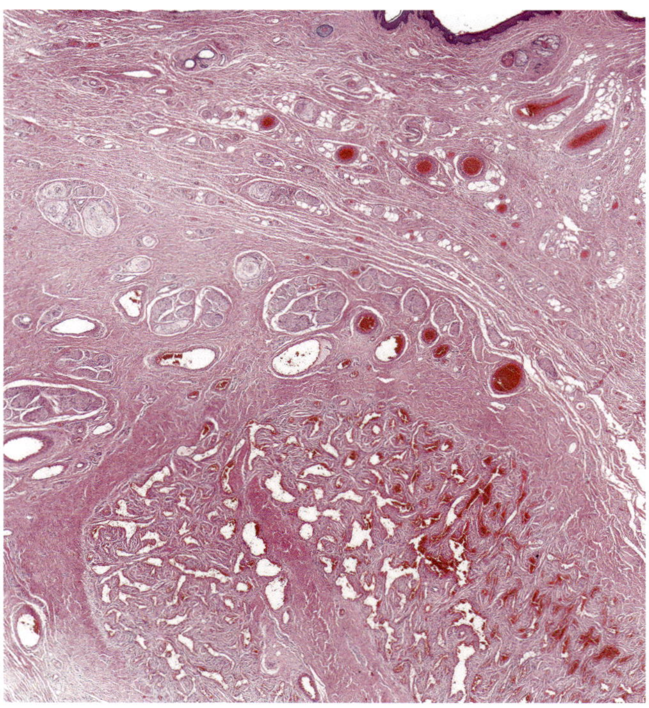

Fig. 4.4 The clitoris is covered by the squamous epithelium and contains erectile tissue, Pacinian corpuscles, and nerve bundles

4.1.2 Vulvar Vestibule

The vulvar vestibule is part of the vulva between the Hart's line inside the labia minora and the hymen. Both the vaginal opening and urethral orifice are within the vestibule. Additionally, within the vulvar vestibule are gland openings from both the major and minor vestibular glands, as well as the paired opening of the periurethral Skene's ducts. The external urethral orifice is placed behind the clitoris and in front of the vagina. Urethral meatus is lined by a transitional epithelium that merges with the stratified squamous epithelium of the vestibule. The vaginal orifice, the most proximal boundary of the vulvar vestibule, is a median slit below and behind the opening of the urethra. The vaginal introitus is lined by a nonkeratinized and glycogen-rich stratified squamous epithelium [1, 2].

4.1.2.1 Vestibular Glands

The major vestibular glands (Bartholin's glands) are paired glands which correspond to the male bulbourethral glands (Cowper's glands). They are located in the posterolateral area of the vulva and open into the vestibule. Bartholin's gland is composed of acini lined by mucus-secreting columnar cells surrounded by a peripheral layer of myoepithelial cells

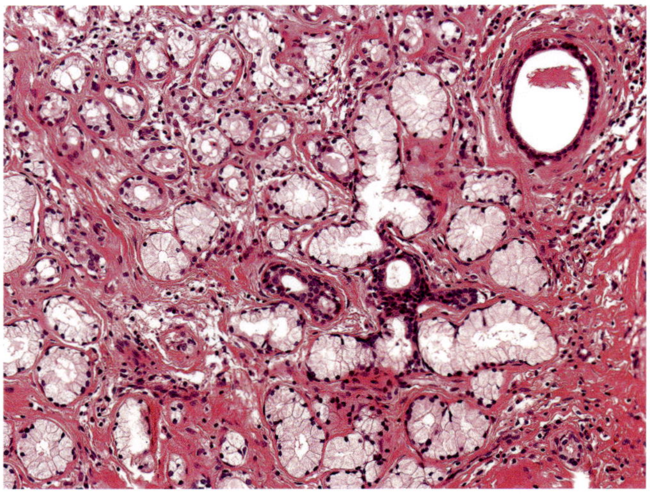

Fig. 4.5 Normal major (Bartholin's) vestibular glands acini lined by columnar mucin-producing cells with an adjacent duct

(Fig. 4.5). The secretion of these acini empties into Bartholin's duct, which is lined by a transitional-like epithelium. At the vestibular surface the distal part of the duct is lining by a non-keratinized squamous epithelium [1, 14, 15].

Minor vestibular glands, the analogue to the glands of Littre of the male urethra, are small simple glands that enter directly to the mucosal surface of the posterior vestibule. Majority of women have from 2 to 10 glands with a maximum depth of 2.27 mm. These glands have a mucus-secreting epithelium which changes to a stratified squamous epithelium near their exit at the vestibular surface [1, 15, 16].

4.1.2.2 Periurethral Glands

The major periurethral (Skene) glands are a paired organ located on either side of the urethral meatus and represent the female homologue of the male prostate. The glands are lined by mucinous pseudostratified columnar epithelial cells, whereas ducts are lined by a transitional epithelium that merges with the vestibular squamous epithelium [17].

Immediately adjacent to most of urethra are the periurethral glands of Huffman (minor periurethral glands) composed of a columnar mucinous epithelium [1, 2, 17].

Blood supply to the vulva is via the femoral artery and the internal iliac artery. Nerve supply to the vulva is via the pudendal nerve, iliohypogastric, ilioinguinal, and genitofemoral nerves. Parasympathetic innervation of erectile tissue occurs via pelvic splanchnic nerves [1, 2].

4.2 Benign Cystic Lesions

4.2.1 Paraurethral (Skene's) Gland Cyst

Skene's gland cyst results from dilatation of the duct of the paraurethral gland. The infection or inflammation is thought to be the cause of the ductal occlusion. The lesion is usually asymptomatic, measuring 1–2 cm, and involves the upper lateral introitus. Skene's duct cysts are a rare cause of an interlabial mass, especially in newborns [18, 19].

4.2.1.1 Histopathology

The Skene's gland cysts are lined by either a stratified squamous or transitional epithelium with rare mucinous cells [2, 15, 20].

4.2.2 Mesonephric-like (Gartner) Cyst

Mesonephric-like cysts are derived from the Wolffian ducts and involve the lateral aspect of the vulva. Clinically, the cyst presents as a thin-walled, translucent cyst containing clear fluid [21].

4.2.2.1 Histopathology

The cyst is lined by a cuboidal to columnar non-ciliated epithelium [2, 15, 20].

4.2.3 Cyst of the Canal of Nuck (Mesothelial Cyst)

The Canal of Nuck is a cystic remnant of the processus vaginalis, the rudimentary sac of peritoneal mesothelium that accompanies the round ligament as it traverses the inguinal canal, ending in the labium majus. Failure of closure of this structure results in blockage and cystic dilatation (female hydrocele) [22]. Clinically, patients present with an asymptomatic, nontender swelling in the groin, rarely in the labium majus or mons pubis. The condition is seen mainly in girls and young female patients.

4.2.3.1 Histopathology

The wall of the cyst is lined by low cuboidal cells of the mesothelial origin, which can be confirmed immunohistochemically with calretinin (nuclear and cytoplasmic staining) and D2–40 (membranous and cytoplasmic staining). The wall is surrounded by a loose fibrous tissue. Trauma may result in rupture; stromal fibrosis and hemosiderin deposition can be observed [2, 15, 20].

4.2.4 Epidermal Inclusion Cyst

Epidermoid (infundibular) cysts are usually solitary, asymptomatic, slow-growing lesions that are commonly present on the scalp, neck, and face; rarely they are located in the clitoris and labium majus. It is thought that the formation of the cysts results from the embedding and invagination of a squamous epithelium in the line of the scar. Then the epithelium desquamates and produces a cystic mass. These cysts could develop many years after the initial injury, e.g., surgical excision, circumcision, and genital piercing.

4.2.4.1 Histopathology

The wall of the cyst is formed by a keratinizing epithelium with the presence of a granular layer and the lumen contains abundant laminated keratin [20, 23, 24]. In some cases, the lumina are filled with calcium deposits and show hair shafts, suggesting that some of the lesions represent true infundibular cysts rather than epidermal invaginations [15].

4.3 Ectopic Tissues

4.3.1 Prostatic-Type Tissue of the Vulva

Skene's glands are thought to represent the female homologue of the male prostate. Occurrence of prostatic-type tissue in the lower female genital tract is rare and probably derived from the Skene's glands misplaced during embryologic development. Only isolated cases of prostatic-type tissue of the vulva have been reported in the literature [25, 26]. The ages of these three patients ranged from 43 to 58 years. In one case, the lesion presented with intermittent pea-sized swellings on the labia majora, whereas in other two cases the prostatic tissue was an incidental microscopic finding [25, 26].

4.3.1.1 Histopathology

Microscopically, small lobular clusters of benign glands and nests of epithelial cells were seen in the superficial dermis (Fig. 4.6). In two cases, these small glands were lined by a double-layered epithelium and there were bright, eosinophilic cytoplasmic granules in some of the luminal cells, resembling Paneth cell-like change reported in the male prostate. In the remaining case, the epithelial elements were predominantly squamous with tubules located around the periphery. In all three cases, the glands were positive for PSA (cytoplasmic) and in two cases they were positive for prostatic acid phosphatase (PrAP) (cytoplasmic) [25, 26].

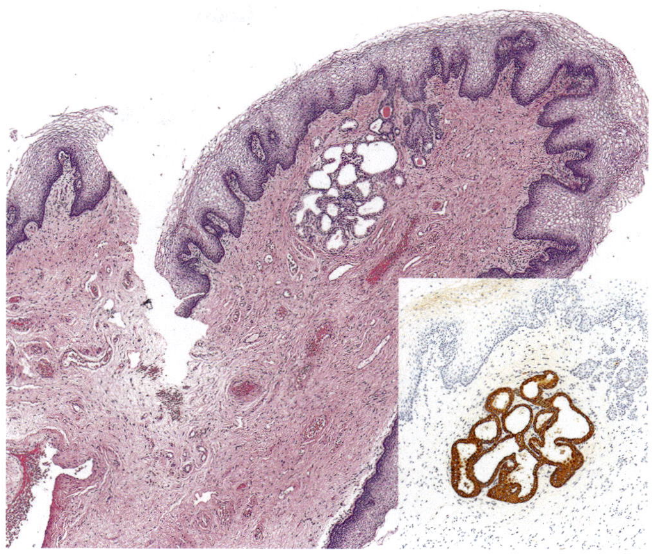

Fig. 4.6 Prostatic-type tissue in the vulva presented as small lobular cluster of benign glands within the superficial dermis. Insets: the glands manifest positivity for prostatic acid phosphatase (Courtesy of Colin J.R. Stewart, FRCPA, Perth, Western Australia, Australia)

4.3.2 Endometriosis

Endometriosis of the vulva is rare condition wherein endometrial-type glands and stroma occur within the vulva. It can be seen at sites of trauma, cutaneous scars after episiotomy, Bartholin's gland cyst removal, etc., supporting the implantation theory of origin (Fig. 4.7). Endometriosis of the vulva may present as a mass lesion, or may bleed or swell with the menstrual cycle [27–29].

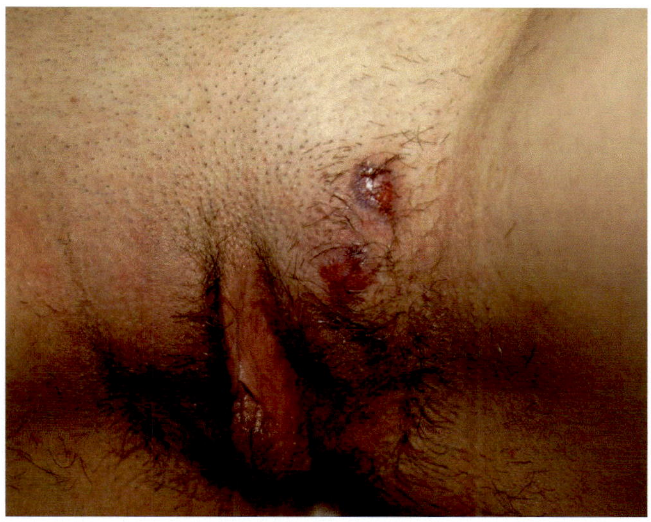

Fig. 4.7 Vulvar endometriosis in the cutaneous scar (Courtesy of Dr. Jiří Bouda, Pilsen, Czech Republic)

4.3.2.1 Histopathology

Histologically, both the endometrial glandular epithelium and the endometrial stroma with hemosiderin-laden macrophages are present (Fig. 4.8). In women under progesterone treatment and pregnancy the decidualization can be observed. A wide spectrum of microscopic changes, including hyperplasia and many types of metaplastic alterations of the Müllerian epithelium can be found [2, 15].

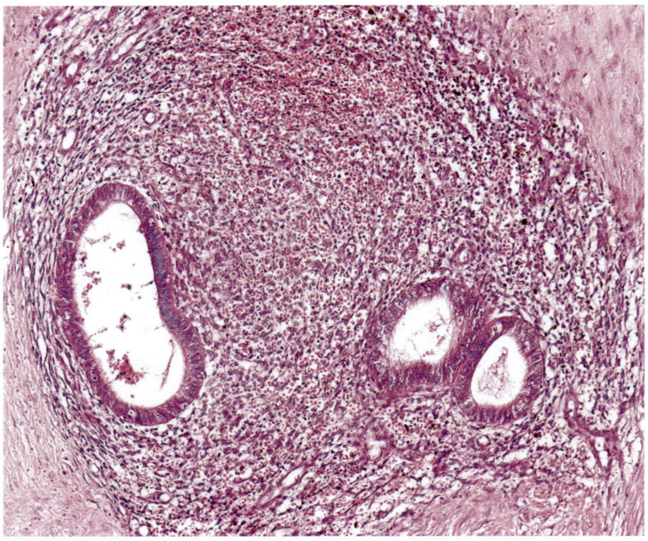

Fig. 4.8 Vulvar endometriosis. Both the endometrial glands and stroma are evident

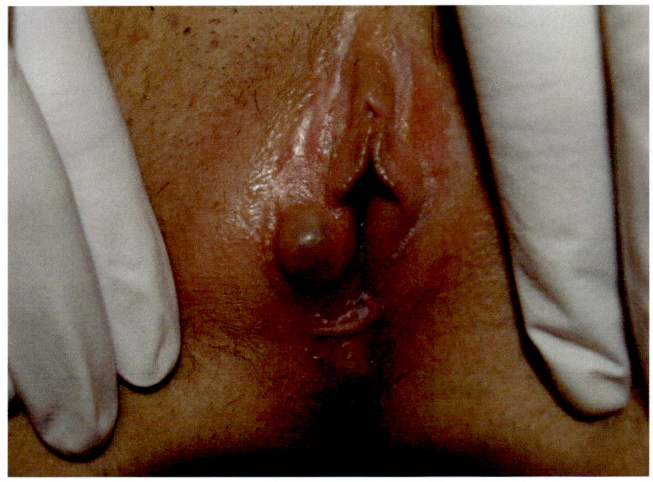

Fig. 4.9 Bartholin's gland cyst. Translucent nodular-cystic lesion in the vulva (Courtesy of Dr. Jiří Bouda, Pilsen, Czech Republic)

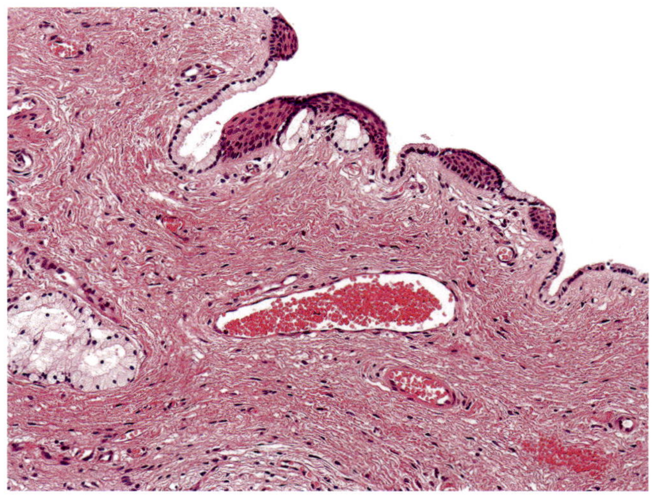

Fig. 4.10 Bartholin's gland cyst is lined by a squamous and mucinous epithelium

4.4 Lesions of Major and Minor Vestibular Glands

4.4.1 Bartholin's Gland Cyst

Bartholin's gland (duct) cyst results from dilatation of Bartholin's duct due to obstruction of its vestibular orifice. It occurs in 3% of adult women and usually asymptomatic. Patients present with cystic or nodular lesion of variable size located in the posterolateral introitus (Fig. 4.9) [15, 30, 31].

4.4.1.1 Histopathology

Bartholin's gland cysts are lined by a transitional, squamous, ciliated, or mucinous epithelium or by any combination of these epithelial types (Fig. 4.10). Rarely, areas resembling the fallopian tube epithelium or apocrine-type secretion can be noticed. A portion of Bartholin's glands tissue is almost always present near the cyst or attached to the cystic wall. Inflammation is common and can result in the destruction of the cyst.

4.4.1.2 Differential Diagnosis

Mucous cysts are smaller than Bartholin's gland cyst. Also, Bartholin's gland cysts are distinguished from cysts of mesonephric origin by staining for mucin, which is negative in mesonephric lesions. Epidermoid cyst most frequently located in the labia majora and clitoris is lined by a stratified squamous epithelium. Cyst of the canal of Nuck can be differentiated from Bartholin's gland cyst by its position in the superolateral position of the labia majora and lining by flattened mesothelial cells [2, 15].

4.4.2 Mucous Cyst

Mucous cysts probably result from occlusion of a minor vestibular gland. It is mostly observed in adult women. The majority of these cysts are small and present no symptoms, while some may grow larger causing discomfort.

4.4.2.1 Histopathology

Mucous cysts appear as smaller cysts lined by columnar mucinous cells resting on the basement membrane and filled with mucin. Squamous cells may also be seen [2, 15].

4.4.3 Nodular Vestibular Gland Hyperplasia

Nodular hyperplasia is a rare benign lesion of major vestibular gland. It is probably the most common solid lesion of Bartholin's glands [32]. Nodular hyperplasia presents as an asymptomatic or slightly painful small nodular lesion.

4.4.3.1 Histopathology

Nodular hyperplasia displays a lobular architecture with an increased number of secretory acini with preservation of the normal duct structures (Fig. 4.11). Areas with a diffuse growth of acini can be seen. The acinar cells are cuboidal or columnar, with mucin-filled cytoplasm and bland nuclei. Duct dilatations, squamous metaplasia of the ductal epithelium, mild lymphohistiocytic infiltrate, and duct rupture with extravasated stromal mucin have been reported in nodular hyperplasia [15, 31–33].

4.5 Benign Lesions of Anogenital Mammary-Like Glands

Benign and malignant lesions affecting anogenital mammary-like glands, including authentic neoplasms and various epithelial or stromal changes, are histopathologically very similar or identical to their mammary counterparts [5, 7, 11, 34–42]. Some lesions involving AGMLG demonstrate a stromal change identical to that known in mammary pathology as pseudoangiomatous stromal hyperplasia (PASH) [35]. It appeared as slit-like, open anastomosing channels devoid of erythrocytes and lined by discontinuous, inconspicuous cells without atypia or mitotic activity (Fig. 4.12) [35]. Areas of PASH have been described in anogenital fibroadenomas, phyllodes tumors, in complex neoplastic lesions and in one case of mild hyperplasia of anogenital mammary-like glands, stromal sclerosis and substantial lipomatous metaplasia [35, 41, 43–45]. Multinucleated cells associated with PASH were detected in one patient who suffered from neurofibromatosis [43]. PASH is distinguished from low-grade angiosarcoma by the lack of cytologic atypia, mitotic activity, intraluminal erythrocytes, and negativity for CD31 [35, 41].

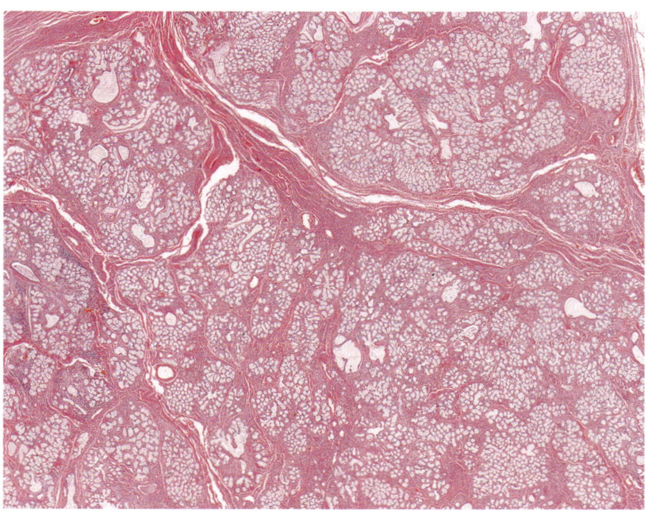

Fig. 4.11 Nodular hyperplasia of Bartholin's glands displays an increased number of acini with preservation of normal duct-acinar relationship

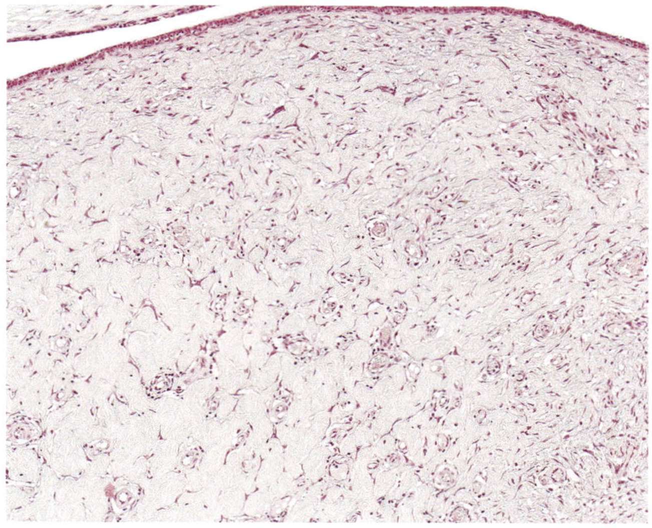

Fig. 4.12 Pseudoangiomatous stromal hyperplasia in the fibroepithelial lesion of anogenital mammary-like glands characterized by slit-like, open anastomosing channels devoid of erythrocytes and lined by discontinuous, inconspicuous cells without atypia or mitotic activity

4.5.1 Hidradenoma Papilliferum

Hidradenoma papilliferum (HP), also known as papillary hidradenoma, is the most common benign glandular neoplasm of the vulva which can be compared conceptually as the cutaneous counterpart of mammary intraductal papilloma [40, 46–49]. The lesion often presents as a small (from 0.5 to 2 cm) solitary asymptomatic nodule or cyst-like lesion on the labia minora and labia majora. The age of the patients ranges from 29 to 90 years. This is a benign tumor, but it may recur if incompletely excised [31].

4.5.1.1 Histopathology

HP is characterized by a cytoarchitectural variability, sometimes within the same tumor: some tumors are solid and composed of papillary and tubular areas, whereas others are predominantly cystic [10, 40, 46, 47, 49, 50]. Some HP have a connection to the epidermis or follicular infundibulum [51–53]. The neoplasm exhibits a complex pattern of branching and anastomosing tubules interconnected in a labyrinthine manner, with bands of fibrous tissue between them, focally forming papillae (Fig. 4.13a). A luminal layer of the tubules and papillae is formed by epithelial cells surrounded by a layer of myoepithelial cells. Decapitation secretion is a common feature. Epithelial metaplastic changes (oxyphilic (Fig. 4.13a, b), mucinous and squamous metaplasia, clear cell change), morphological features analogous to those occurring in benign breast disease (sclerosing adenosis-like

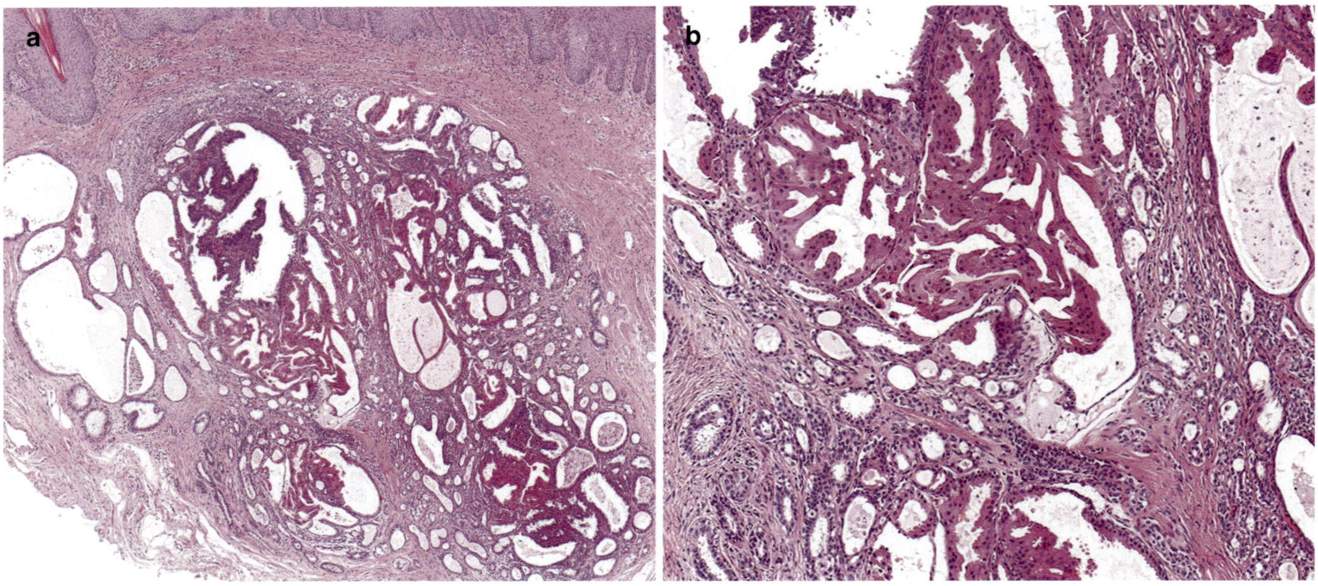

Fig. 4.13 Hidradenoma papilliferum. Intradermal solid-cystic neoplasm with a complex pattern of branching and anastomosing tubules and papillae (**a**). Prominent oxyphilic metaplasia (**b**)

changes, atypical and usual ductal hyperplasia and solid and "streaming" growth patterns can be seen [15, 40]. The mitotic index in HP can be up to 13/10 HPF, but it does not predict a more aggressive outcome [48]. Several cases of ductal carcinoma in situ arising in HP have been reported [42, 54]. In some cases, remnants of AGMLGs may be seen adjacent to the HP [40]. Two cases with mixed histopathological features of fibroadenoma and hidradenoma papilliferum and PASH have been reported [41, 44]. In addition, HP can rarely be seen in association with various benign and malignant lesions, including Bartholin's gland abscess, squamous cell carcinoma, and extramammary Paget disease [40, 55–57].

4.5.1.2 Differential Diagnosis

Prominent oxyphilic metaplasia, accompanied by nuclear enlargement, especially in areas with solid growth, may bear a resemblance to adenocarcinoma. In fact, such changes are analogous to atypical apocrine adenosis of the breast [47]. In cases with a connection to the overlying epidermis with reactive epidermal hyperplasia and prominent plasma cell infiltrate, HP may simulate syringocystadenoma papilliferum. Prominent, yet focal hyperplasia of stromal myofibroblast-like cells (HP) should not be confused with sarcomatoid carcinoma [15].

4.5.2 Fibroadenoma and Benign Phyllodes Tumor

Fibroadenoma and benign phyllodes tumor arising in AGMLGs are biphasic, circumscribed, epithelial-stromal neoplasms identical to homonymous mammary neoplasms. These lesions are rare, with approximately 40 cases of vulvar fibroadenoma and 11 cases of vulvar benign phyllodes tumor and reported to date [58] and affect predominately women of reproductive age, but they may be found in postmenopausal women and rarely in prepubertal girls [59]. These fibroepithelial neoplasms present as solitary, firm, asymptomatic nodules with an average size of 3 cm [43]. Multiple cases of fibroadenoma [60–62] and phyllodes tumors [63–65] have been reported. Enlargement may occur during pregnancy [66, 67]. Local recurrence after surgical excision can occur in phyllodes tumors [63, 68].

4.5.2.1 Histopathology

Fibroadenomas are well-circumscribed neoplasms composed of branching and anastomosing glandular structures surrounded by a paucicellular stroma showing low or no mitotic activity (Fig. 4.14). The pericanalicular growth pattern is typified by retention of round or oval duct lumina, whereas the intracanalicular growth pattern is characterized by stromal compression of the lumina sometimes producing slit-like structures. Cystic dilatation of duct lumina, apocrine secretion, and intraluminal papillary projections may be seen [10, 15, 43]. A case of mammary-type juvenile fibroadenoma has been reported [43].

Phyllodes tumor shows a growth pattern with leaf-like projections (Fig. 4.15a). The stroma is usually hypercellular, with periglandular condensation; cellularity commonly varies within a neoplasm (Fig. 4.15a, b). Three categories of the phyllodes tumor are recognized: benign, low grade, and high grade. The grade is defined by the atypia in the stroma. Except for a single case of high-grade neoplasm showing a rhabdomyosarcomatous stroma [69], the reported examples of vulvar phyllodes tumor were either benign or low grade [10, 43].

Columnar cell change, usual and florid ductal hyperplasia, pseudoangiomatous stromal hyperplasia, metaplastic changes in epithelial and stromal changes and lactation-like changes are rare features occurring in fibroadenoma and benign phyllodes tumor involving AGMLGs [15].

These neoplasms show overlapping features and in some cases the differentiation between fibroadenoma and benign or low-grade malignant phyllodes tumor may be very difficult. The stroma in phyllodes tumor is more cellular than fibroadenomas and variable in different foci of the lesion. Additionally, phyllodes tumor has less regular outlines than fibroadenoma which is usually a sharply demarcated lesion [15].

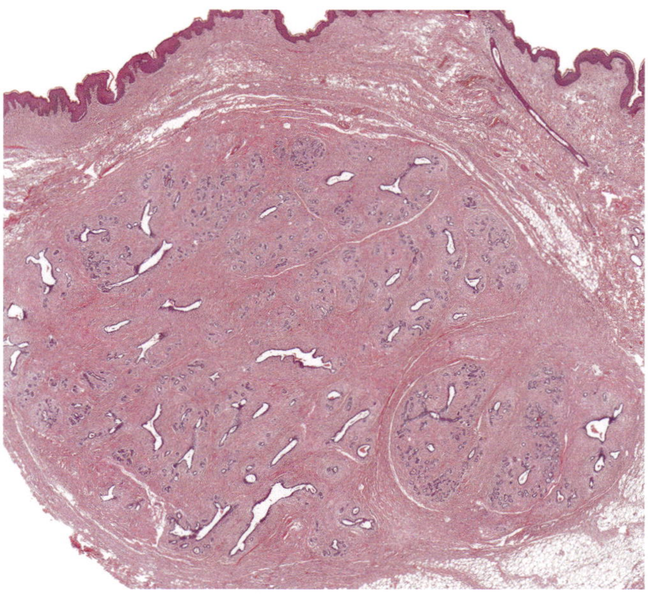

Fig. 4.14 Whole mount histological section evidencing a fibroadenoma arising in anogenital mammary-like glands

Fibroepithelial foci resembling fibroadenoma may rarely be found in other "complex" lesions of AGMLGs [41, 44].

4.5.2.2 Differential Diagnosis

Focal lactation-like change in a lesion of AGMLGs can be confused with malignancy. The clue to the diagnosis is the presence of intracytoplasmic vacuoles and intraluminal secretion. In lactating adenoma, the whole lesion manifests this feature.

Areas of PASH should be distinguished with low-grade angiosarcoma, which shows at least mild nuclear pleomorphism and immunopositivity for vascular markers [2, 15].

4.5.3 Lactating Adenoma

Lactating adenoma arising from AGMLGs is extremely rare and associated with pregnancy. The lesion can be solitary or multiple presenting as masses [70–73].

4.5.3.1 Histopathology

The lesion is well circumscribed and composed of densely packed round tubules lined by large cells with hyperchromatic nuclei and containing intracytoplasmic vacuoles and intraluminal secretion. Additionally, cystic changes, duct ectasia, and apocrine metaplasia have been described [71].

4.5.3.2 Differential Diagnosis

Lactating adenoma can be misdiagnosed as adenocarcinoma [15]. Rarely, lactation-like changes may occur in other lesions of AGMLGs, such as fibroadenoma [10, 66].

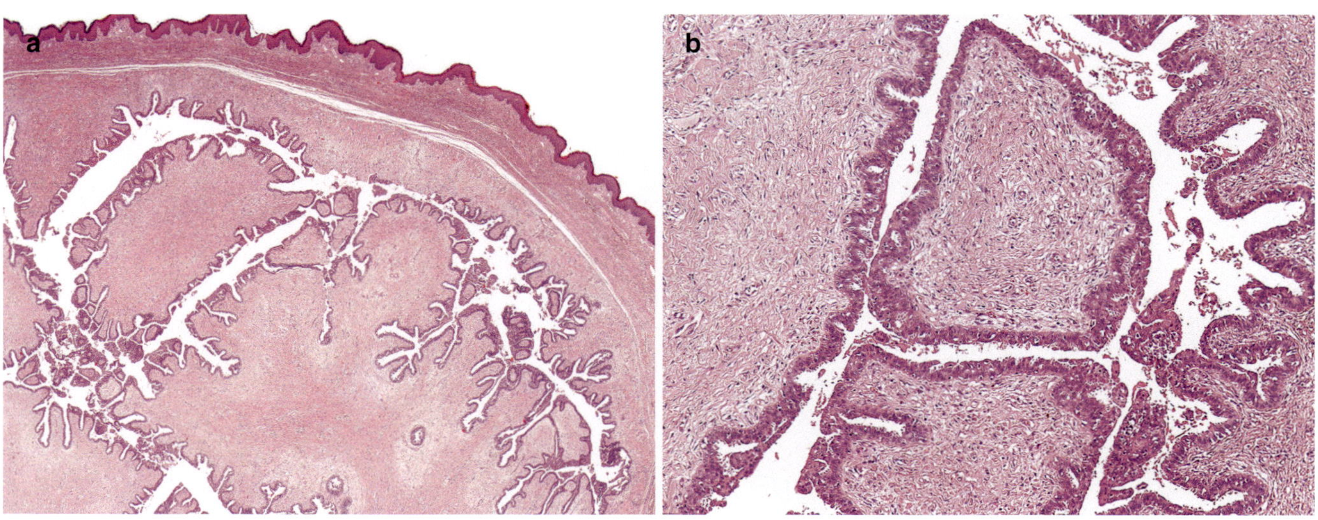

Fig. 4.15 Benign phyllodes tumors of the vulva with a leaf-like intracanalicular growth pattern and stromal hypercellularity (**a**, **b**)

4.5.4 Adenosis Tumor

Sclerosing adenosis may occur as a component of different lesions of AGMLG, including hidradenoma papilliferum, phyllodes tumor, and fibroadenoma [10, 40]. In addition, sclerosing adenosis can itself produce a clinically detectable lesion, the adenosis tumor. It is a very rare condition, with two reported lesions located in the perianal area and one in the vulva, ranging in size from 7 to 20 mm. The ages of these three patients were from 46 to 60 years [36, 74].

4.5.4.1 Histopathology

Sclerosing adenosis is a compact proliferation of small ductal structures with luminal epithelial cells which are often atrophic and attenuated with the preservation of the peripheral myoepithelial cell layer in a sclerotic stroma. Lesions are well demarcated, unencapsulated with irregular distribution of the glands (Fig. 4.16a). The luminal cells showed no cytological and nuclear atypia and visible is only minimal regular mitotic activity. Decapitation secretion is seen (Fig. 4.16b). Different patterns, including variably sized microcysts and cysts, some with papillary projections having hyalinized cores, areas reminiscent of usual ductal hyperplasia, various metaplastic changes in the epithelial and myoepithelial components can be noted. Isolated, typical AGMLG can be found in the periphery of the lesion.

4.5.4.2 Differential Diagnosis

Vulvar sclerosing adenosis can be confused with an invasive adenocarcinoma, but in the adenosis the myoepithelial cells at the periphery of the glands is a constant feature and can be highlighted by myoepithelial markers (actin S (membranous, cytoplasmic), calponin (cytoplasmic), CD10 (cytoplasmic, membranous), and others) [36, 74].

4.5.5 Mammary-Type Fibrocystic Disease

Mammary-type fibrocystic disease is rare condition clinically presenting as a cutaneous nodule simulating a tumor.

4.5.5.1 Histopathology

The changes are identical to those seen in the homonymous lesions in the breast and include cysts, oxyphilic (apocrine) metaplasia, fibrosis, calcification, chronic inflammation, and epithelial hyperplasia which are the basic morphological changes seen in fibrocystic disease (Fig. 4.17) [39].

4.5.6 Mammary-Type Hamartoma

A single case of mammary-type hamartoma in the anogenital area had been reported. It was a well-circumscribed 4.5-cm nodule in a patient with bilateral gigantomastia and nodular pseudoangiomatous stromal hyperplasia in the axilla [38]. The cutaneous lesion was located in the perianal area, but it presumably can be found in the vulva where AGMLG are more numerous.

4.5.6.1 Histopathology

Microscopically, the lesion demonstrated circumscribed margins, dense stromal fibrosis, islands of adipose tissue, cystic dilatation of ducts, scattered benign breast-type lobules, and a sparse focal infiltrate of lymphocytes (Fig. 4.18). In addition, adjacent intact AGMLGs were found [38].

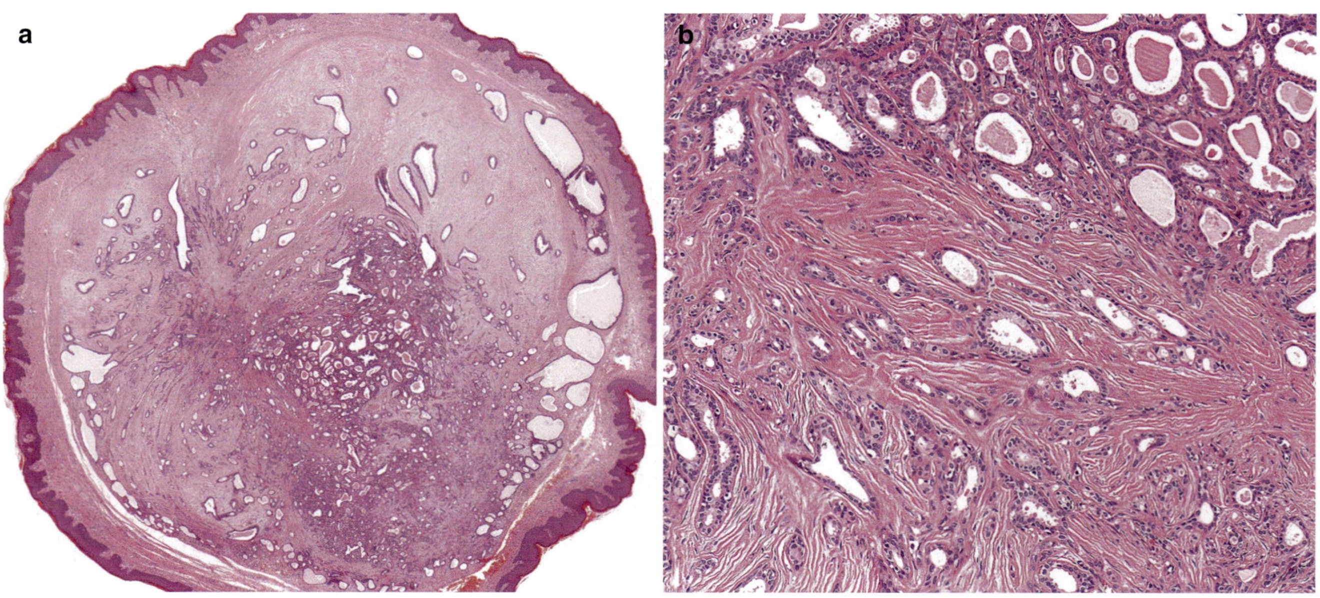

Fig. 4.16 Adenosis tumor. A well-demarcated, unencapsulated lesion (**a**). Areas of sclerosing adenosis composed of compressed tubular structures with a preserved myoepithelial layer in a sclerotic stroma (**b**)

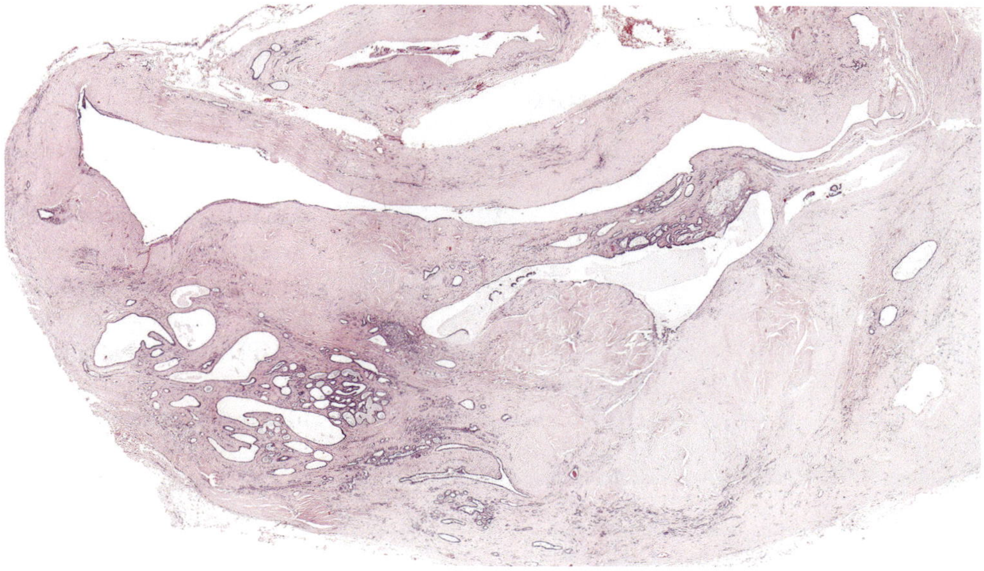

Fig. 4.17 Mammary-type fibrocystic disease. The lesion is well circumscribed but not encapsulated and displays marked stromal sclerosis and variably sized cysts

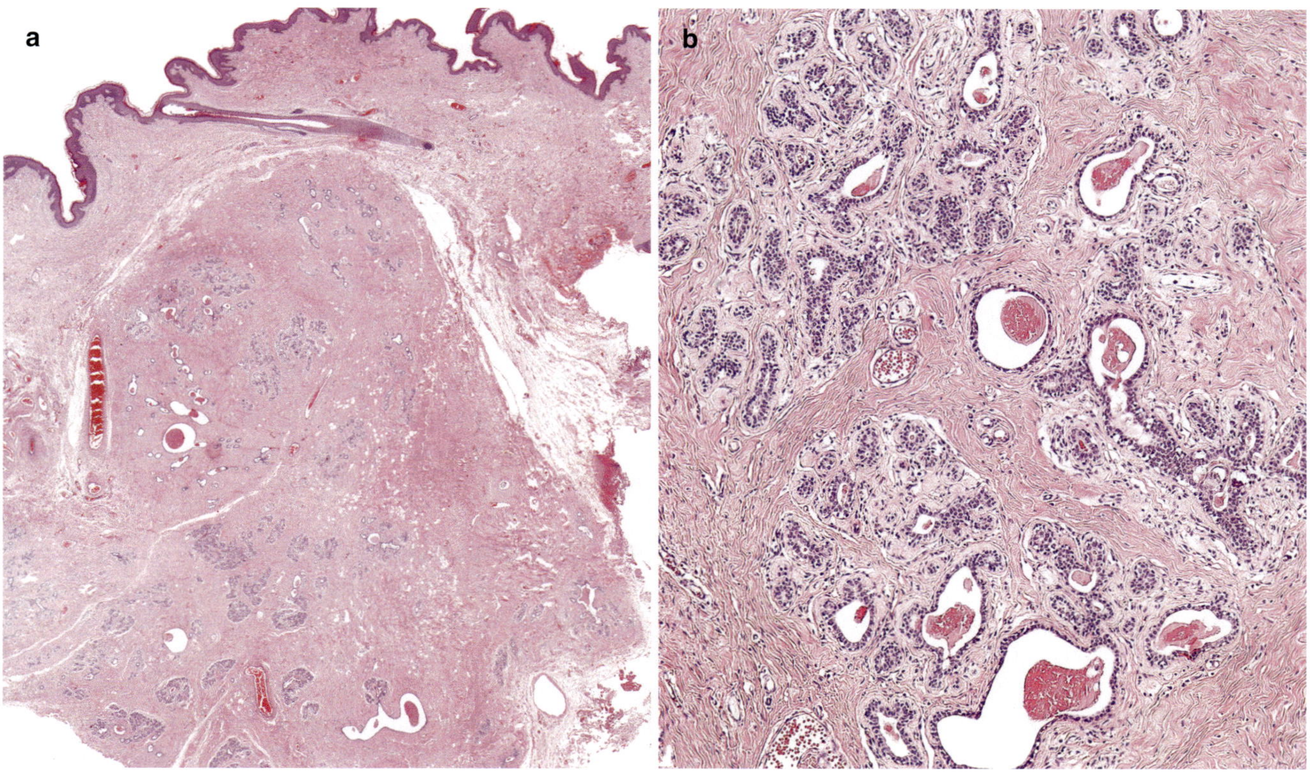

Fig. 4.18 Mammary-type hamartoma. The lesion is a sharply demarcated mass composed predominantly of dense sclerotic collagen, containing numerous well-developed mammary-type lobules, some of which ducts exhibit cystic dilatation (**a**, **b**)

4.6 Benign Adnexal Tumors

4.6.1 Syringoma

Syringoma is a small benign adnexal neoplasm usually presenting in the vulva as multiple, asymptomatic, small, smooth-surfaced, skin-colored, pink or brownish papules (Fig. 4.19). Adolescents and young adults are mostly affected. Familial cases of syringoma and coexistence with Down's syndrome have been reported [31]. The most common sites of involvement are the lower eyelids. Vulva is also a common site wherein syringomas present with symptom of pruritis and occur on an erythematous background. Vulvar

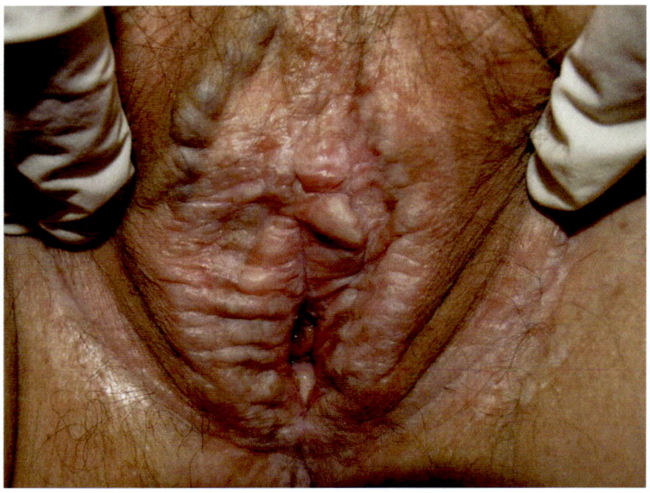

Fig. 4.19 Vulvar syringomas. Multiple small papules in the vulva (Courtesy of Dr. Jiří Bouda, Pilsen, Czech Republic)

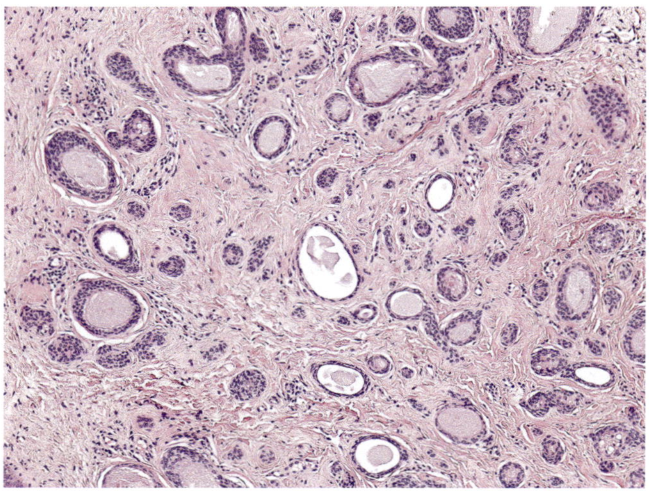

Fig. 4.20 Vulvar syringoma. The lesion consists of small solid and ductal structures in sclerotic collagenous stroma. "Comma-like" or "tadpole-like" elements can be seen

syringomas have commonly been described in association with extragenital lesions [75, 76].

4.6.1.1 Histopathology

Histopathologically, syringoma is usually a small, well-circumscribed neoplasm confined to the upper part of the dermis consisting of small solid and ductal structures that have peculiar geometric shapes (comma-like or tadpole-like) and are relatively evenly distributed in sclerotic collagenous stroma (Fig. 4.20). The cords, nests, and tubules of syringomas branch and anastomose. The epithelial aggregates are composed of monomorphous cuboidal cells with small nuclei and inconspicuous nucleoli. In most conventional syringomas most epithelial cells are eosinophilic and some cells have pale cytoplasm. The deep location of vulvar syringoma is unusual [77]. Clear cell change, prominent keratinization (squamous metaplasia), extension into the deeper dermis or subcutis, and presence of numerous mast cells in the stroma can be seen in syringoma. A clear cell variant has been associated with diabetes mellitus in many instances [31].

4.6.1.2 Differential Diagnosis

Syringomatous ductal proliferations and syringoma-like structures can be associated with several inflammatory and neoplastic conditions including extramammary Paget's disease (EMPD), basal cell carcinoma, reexcision specimens, prurigo nodularis, and others. A particular pitfall in the vulva are syringomatoid structures occurring in EMPD [78]. Microcystic adnexal carcinoma (MAC) and syringoma can have a morphological overlap but have different clinical presentation. MAC is extremely rare in the vulva. Moreover, microcystic adnexal carcinomas is usually a deeply infiltrative neoplasm with perineural extension which is larger, asymmetric, and less circumscribed than syringoma, although exceptionally rare vulva syringoma may show deep extension [2, 15, 20, 31, 77].

4.6.2 Spiradenoma, Cylindroma, and Spiradenocylindroma

Spiradenoma, cylindroma, and spiradenocylindroma are closely related entities comprising of a morphological spectrum. All three neoplasms occur either sporadically or may be part of Brooke-Spiegler syndrome with the head and neck area is the predilection side, but rare lesion has been reported in the vulva [79]. Clinically, sporadic tumors are solitary asymptomatic nodules affecting adult or elderly patients. In patients with Brooke-Spiegler syndrome lesions are multiple in various combinations with other adnexal neoplasms, mostly trichoepitheliomas [80–84].

4.6.2.1 Histopathology

Tumors are well circumscribed, sometimes encapsulated, and may be multi- or uninodular. Histologically, spiradenoma presents as a nodule composed of pale large cells and lymphocytes intermixed with small basaloid cells. Within the nodules the epithelial cells are arranged in a trabecular, reticular, or solid fashion (Fig. 4.21a). Focal ductal differentiation can be evident.

Cylindroma represents multinodular lesions composed of a basaloid cells surrounded by eosinophilic basement membrane material arranged in a jigsaw puzzle (mosaic-like). The peripheral cells are often darker than those cells located in the center and show palisading (Fig. 4.21b).

Spiradenocylindroma demonstrate areas typical of both spiradenoma and cylindroma, with at least 10% of its volume conforming to either of the two patterns. The elements of these two tumors are either closely intermingled or sharply demarcated [15].

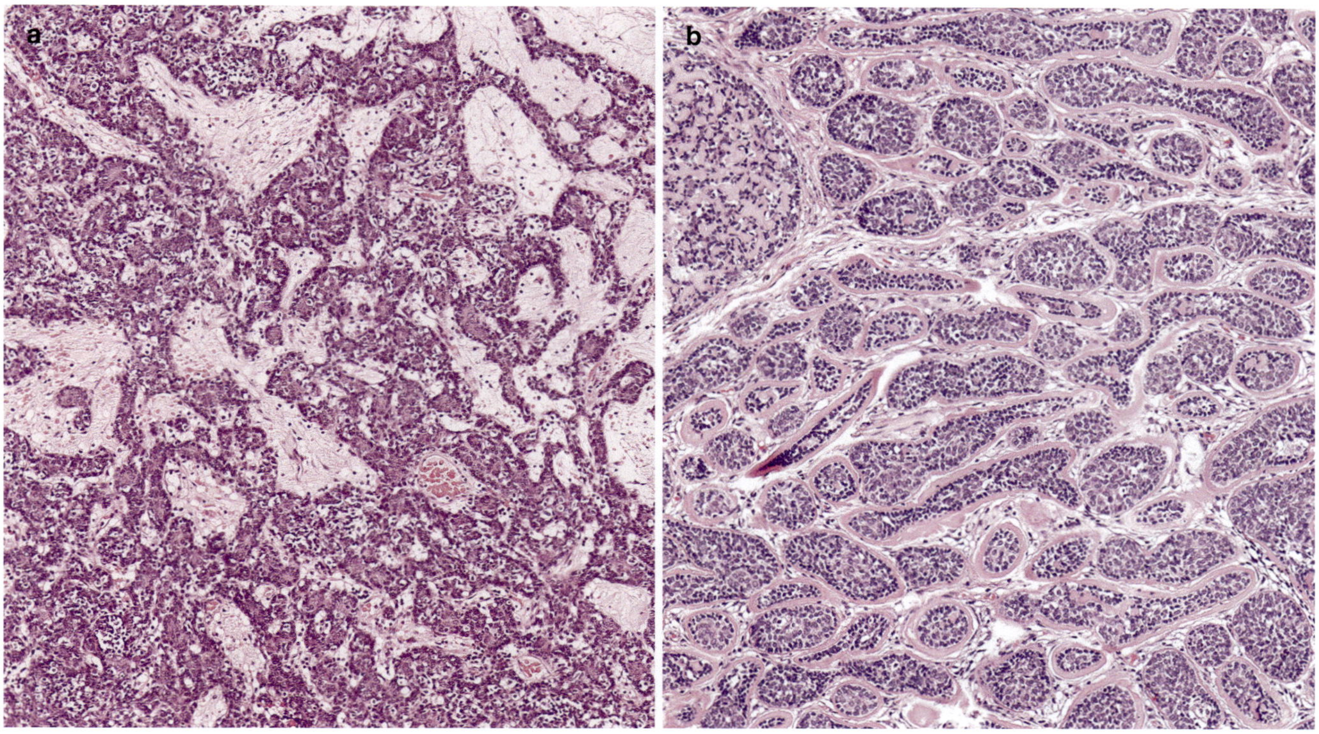

Fig. 4.21 Spiradenoma. Small basaloid neoplastic cells are arranged in a trabecular pattern. Note intratumoral lymphocytes (**a**). Cylindroma. A neoplasm manifesting jigsaw puzzle arrangement of islands of basaloid cells surrounded by eosinophilic basement membrane material (**b**)

Marked cystic changes, a poorly developed jigsaw puzzle pattern in cylindroma, other lines of adnexal differentiation, adenomatous component, adenoid cystic carcinoma-like pattern, metaplastic changes in the epithelial component, prominence of lymphocytes, and others can be seen [2, 15, 20, 31].

4.6.2.2 Differential Diagnosis

Spiradenoma with a prominent trabecular pattern can be confused with sebaceous neoplasms with a carcinoid-like or labyrinthine/sinusoidal pattern but the clue to the diagnosis is the presence of intratumoral lymphocytes.

Cylindroma and spiradenocylindroma may resemble basaloid (cloacogenic) carcinoma of the anus, but carcinoma have cellular atypia, in situ component, and common positivity for p16 [2, 15, 31].

4.6.3 Apocrine and Eccrine Mixed Tumors (Chondroid Syringoma)

Mixed tumors of the skin (pleomorphic adenoma) are usually classified into the more common apocrine type and the rare eccrine type. Usually they are slowly growing solitary nodules on the head or extremities of the middle-aged and elderly persons [2, 85]. Only a few vulvar cases of chondroid syringoma of both types have been reported in the literature [86–90]. The tumor may recur if not completely excised [31].

4.6.3.1 Histopathology

Apocrine mixed tumors show considerable variation in their epithelial, myoepithelial, and stromal components and usually characterized by branching tubular structures, often manifesting apocrine secretion, embedded in a chondromyxoid cartilaginous or osseous stroma (Fig. 4.22a). In contrast to its apocrine counterpart, eccrine mixed tumors do not display signs of decapitation secretion, sebaceous or follicular differentiation. The epithelial component of eccrine mixed tumors is composed of simple monolayered tubular elements, small epithelial nests, strands and cords, or singe cell units set in myxohyaline and cartilaginous stroma (Fig. 4.22b) [85].

4.6.3.2 Differential Diagnosis

Rare cases of chondroid syringoma with predominance of stromal component can be confused with mesenchymal neoplasms. In such cases it is important to recognize a minor epithelial component which can by highlighted by cytokeratin immunostaining.

Prominent myoepithelial differentiation may require distinction from myoepithelioma, but myoepithelioma is composed entirely of myoepithelial cells without any glandular or ductal differentiation.

So-called vulvar microglandular adenosis-like neoplasm described by Raiguru et al. represents an example of eccrine mixed tumor [91].

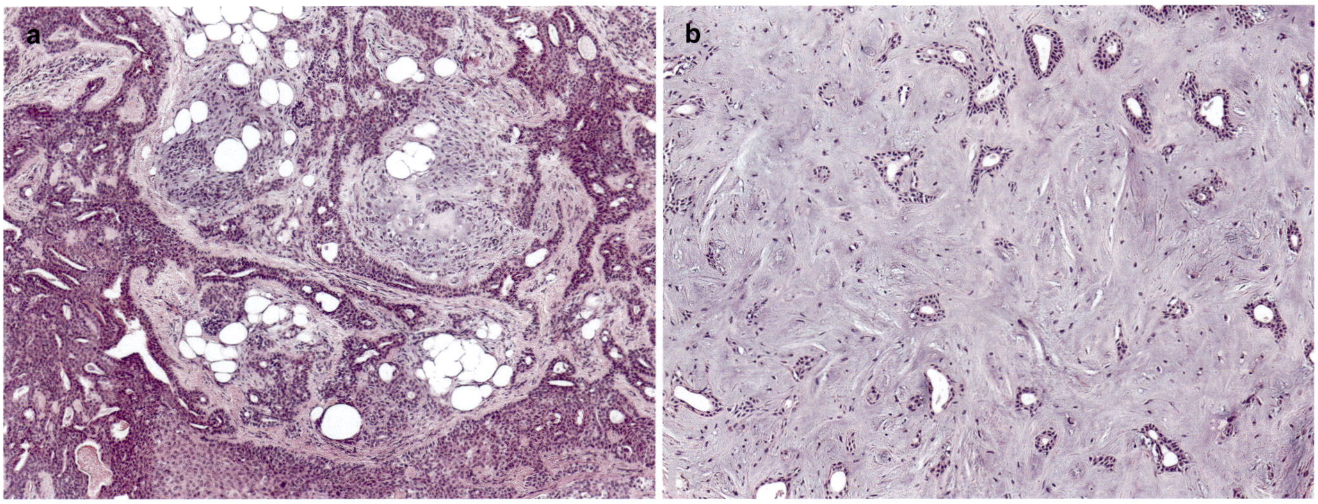

Fig. 4.22 Apocrine mixed tumor. Interconnected, double-layered ductal structures and myoepithelial cells set in fibromyxoid stroma (**a**) Eccrine mixed tumor. Ductal elements are monolayered and are surrounded by myxoid and hyalinized stroma (**b**)

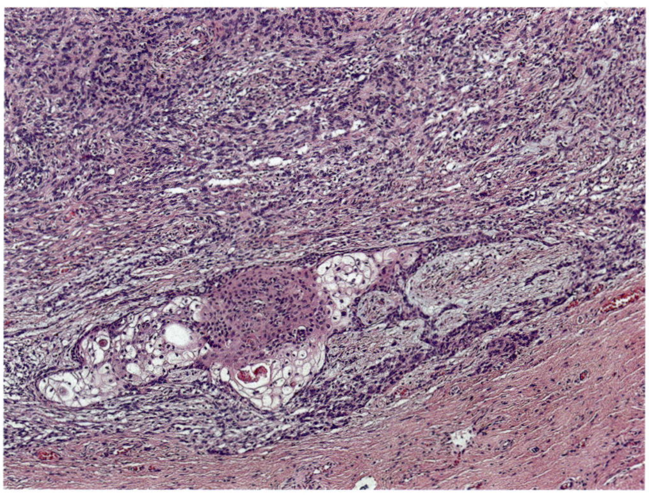

Fig. 4.23 Mixed tumor of the vagina. The neoplasm is composed of epithelial elements and stromal-type spindled cells

The malignant counterpart of chondroid syringoma, the malignant chondroid syringoma is characterized by infiltrative growth, nuclear pleomorphism, mitotic activity, and necrosis [2, 15].

One should keep in mind a distinctive neoplasm occurring in or near the hymen or its remnants, the mixed tumor of the vagina. Microscopically, it is composed of benign epithelial (islands of mature squamous, mucinous glands, or clear cell epithelium) and stromal-type spindled elements (Fig. 4.23) [92, 93].

4.6.4 Other Benign Adnexal Neoplasms

Other benign adnexal neoplasms, including poroma, pilomatricoma, hidradenoma, sebaceoma, and trichoepithelioma have been identified in the vulva [83]. Rare cases of vulvar myoepithelioma and trichofolliculoma have been reported [94–97]. Yoshida et al. described nine cases of "myoepithelioma-like tumors of the vulvar region" with the deficiency of SMARCB1 expression in all cases [98].

References

1. Mills SE. Histology for pathologists. Philadelphia, PA: Lippincott Williams & Wilkins; 2012.
2. Hoang MP, Selim MA. Vulvar pathology. New York: Springer; 2015.
3. Shatz P, Bergeron C, Wilkinson EJ, et al. Vulvar intraepithelial neoplasia and skin appendage involvement. Obstet Gynecol. 1989;74:769–74.
4. Ross MH, Kaye GI, Pawlina W. Histology: a text and atlas. Philadelphia, PA: Lippincott Williams & Wilkins; 2003.
5. van der Putte S. Anogenital "sweat" glands. Histology and pathology of a gland that may mimic mammary glands. Am J Dermatopathol. 1991;13:557–67.
6. van der Putte SC. Ultrastructure of the human anogenital "sweat" gland. Anat Rec. 1993;235:583–90.
7. van der Putte S. Mammary-like glands of the vulva and their disorders. Int J Gynecol Pathol. 1994;13:150–60.
8. van der Putte SC, van Gorp LH. Cysts of mammarylike glands in the vulva. Int J Gynecol Pathol. 1995;14:184–8.
9. van der Putte SC. Clear cells of Toker in the developing anogenital region of male and female fetuses. Am J Dermatopathol. 2011;33:811–8. https://doi.org/10.1097/DAD.0b013e31820fdc7d.
10. Kazakov DV, Spagnolo DV, Kacerovska D, et al. Lesions of anogenital mammary-like glands: an update. Adv Anat Pathol. 2011;18:1–28. https://doi.org/10.1097/PAP.0b013e318202eba5.
11. Konstantinova AM, Kyrpychova L, Belousova IE, et al. Anogenital mammary-like glands: a study of their Normal histology with emphasis on glandular depth, presence of columnar epithelial cells, and distribution of elastic fibers. Am J Dermatopathol. 2017;39:663–7. https://doi.org/10.1097/DAD.0000000000000744.
12. Konstantinova AM, Stewart CJ, Kyrpychova L, et al. An immunohistochemical study of anogenital mammary-like glands. Am

J Dermatopathol. 2017;39:599–605. https://doi.org/10.1097/DAD.0000000000000724.
13. Willman J, Golitz L, Fitzpatrick J. Vulvar clear cells of Toker: precursors of extramammary Paget's disease. Am J Dermatopathol. 2005;27(3):185–8.
14. Rorat E, Ferenczy A, Richart RM. Human Bartholin gland, duct, and duct cyst. Histochemical and ultrastructural study. Arch Pathol. 1975;99:367–74.
15. Kazakov DV, Michal M, Kacerovska D, et al. Cutaneous adnexal tumors. Philadelphia, PA: Lippincott Williams & Wilkins; 2012.
16. Pyka RE, Wilkinson EJ, Friedrich EG Jr, et al. The histopathology of vulvar vestibulitis syndrome. Int J Gynecol Pathol. 1988;7:249–57.
17. Wilkinson EJ, Stone IK. Atlas of vulvar disease. Philadelphia, PA: Lippincott Williams & Wilkins; 2012.
18. Costantino E, Ganesan GS. Skene's gland cyst as an interlabial mass in a newborn girl. BMJ Case Rep. 2016;2016. https://doi.org/10.1136/bcr-2016-215042.
19. Moralioglu S, Bosnali O, Celayir AC, et al. Paraurethral Skene's duct cyst in a newborn. Urol Ann. 2013;5:204–5. https://doi.org/10.4103/0974-7796.115754.
20. Heller DS. Benign tumors and tumor-like lesions of the vulva. Clin Obstet Gynecol. 2015;58:526–35. https://doi.org/10.1097/GRF.0000000000000133.
21. Junaid TA, Thomas SM. Cysts of the vulva and vagina: a comparative study. Int J Gynaecol Obstet. 1981;19:239–43.
22. Schneider CA, Festa S, Spillert CR, et al. Hydrocele of the canal of Nuck. N J Med. 1994;91:37–8.
23. Al-Ojaimi EH, Abdulla MM. Giant epidermoid inclusion cyst of the clitoris mimicking clitoromegaly. J Low Genit Tract Dis. 2013;17:58–60. https://doi.org/10.1097/LGT.0b013e318259a410.
24. Kroll GL, Miller L. Vulvar epithelial inclusion cyst as a late complication of childhood female traditional genital surgery. Am J Obstet Gynecol. 2000;183:509–10. https://doi.org/10.1067/mob.2000.105963.
25. Kazakov DV, Stewart CJ, Kacerovska D, et al. Prostatic-type tissue in the lower female genital tract: a morphologic spectrum, including vaginal tubulosquamous polyp, adenomyomatous hyperplasia of paraurethral Skene glands (female prostate), and ectopic lesion in the vulva. Am J Surg Pathol. 2010;34:950–5. https://doi.org/10.1097/PAS.0b013e3181e0f371.
26. Kelly P, McBride HA, Kennedy K, et al. Misplaced Skene's glands: glandular elements in the lower female genital tract that are variably immunoreactive with prostate markers and that encompass vaginal tubulosquamous polyp and cervical ectopic prostatic tissue. Int J Gynecol Pathol. 2011;30:605–12. https://doi.org/10.1097/PGP.0b013e31821713b6.
27. Katz Z, Goldchmit R, Blickstein I. Post-traumatic vulvar endometriosis. Eur J Pediatr Surg. 1996;6:241–2. https://doi.org/10.1055/s-2008-1066519.
28. Kazakov DV, Ondic O, Zamecnik M, et al. Morphological variations of scar-related and spontaneous endometriosis of the skin and superficial soft tissue: a study of 71 cases with emphasis on atypical features and types of mullerian differentiations. J Am Acad Dermatol. 2007;57:134–46. https://doi.org/10.1016/j.jaad.2006.11.036.
29. Mihmanli V, Ozkan T, Genc S, et al. Endometriosis of episiotomy scar: a case report. Clin Exp Obstet Gynecol. 2015;42:543–4.
30. Berger MB, Betschart C, Khandwala N, et al. Incidental Bartholin gland cysts identified on pelvic magnetic resonance imaging. Obstet Gynecol. 2012;120:798–802. https://doi.org/10.1097/AOG.0b013e3182699259.
31. Kurman RJ, Carcangiu ML, Herrington CS, et al. WHO classification of tumours of female reproductive organs. Lyon: IARC; 2014.
32. Koenig C, Tavassoli FA. Nodular hyperplasia, adenoma, and adenomyoma of Bartholin's gland. Int J Gynecol Pathol. 1998;17:289–94.
33. Kazakov DV, Curik R, Vanecek T, et al. Nodular hyperplasia of the Bartholin gland: a clinicopathological study of two cases, including detection of clonality by HUMARA. Am J Dermatopathol. 2007;29:385–7. https://doi.org/10.1097/DAD.0b013e31806f54b3.
34. Belousova IE, Kazakov DV, Michal M, et al. Vulvar toker cells: the long-awaited missing link: a proposal for an origin-based histogenetic classification of extramammary Paget disease. Am J Dermatopathol. 2006;28:84–6. https://doi.org/10.1097/01.dad.0000194052.65695.f1.
35. Kazakov DV, Bisceglia M, Mukensnabl P, et al. Pseudoangiomatous stromal hyperplasia in lesions involving anogenital mammary-like glands. Am J Surg Pathol. 2005;29:1243–6.
36. Kazakov DV, Bisceglia M, Sima R, et al. Adenosis tumor of anogenital mammary-like glands: a case report and demonstration of clonality by HUMARA assay. J Cutan Pathol. 2006;33:43–6. https://doi.org/10.1111/j.0303-6987.2006.00391.x.
37. Kazakov DV, Hugel H, Vanecek T, et al. Unusual hyperplasia of anogenital mammary-like glands. Am J Dermatopathol. 2006;28:134–7. https://doi.org/10.1097/01.dad.0000183890.09480.d9.
38. Hayes MM, Konstantinova AM, Kacerovska D, et al. Bilateral gigantomastia, multiple synchronous nodular pseudoangiomatous stromal hyperplasia involving breast and bilateral axillary accessory breast tissue, and perianal mammary-type hamartoma of anogenital mammary-like glands: a case report. Am J Dermatopathol. 2016;38:374–83. https://doi.org/10.1097/DAD.0000000000000498.
39. Konstantinova AM, Kacerovska D, Michal M, et al. A tumoriform lesion of the vulva with features of mammary-type fibrocystic disease. Am J Dermatopathol. 2013;35:e124–7. https://doi.org/10.1097/DAD.0b013e318284860c.
40. Konstantinova AM, Michal M, Kacerovska D, et al. Hidradenoma papilliferum: a clinicopathologic study of 264 tumors from 261 patients, with emphasis on mammary-type alterations. Am J Dermatopathol. 2016;38:598–607. https://doi.org/10.1097/DAD.0000000000000495.
41. Vazmitel M, Pavlovsky M, Kacerovska D, et al. Pseudoangiomatous stromal hyperplasia in a complex neoplastic lesion involving anogenital mammary-like glands. J Cutan Pathol. 2009;36:1117–20. https://doi.org/10.1111/j.1600-0560.2009.01250.x.
42. Vazmitel M, Spagnolo DV, Nemcova J, et al. Hidradenoma papilliferum with a ductal carcinoma in situ component: case report and review of the literature. Am J Dermatopathol. 2008;30:392–4. https://doi.org/10.1097/DAD.0b013e31817c6a7d.
43. Kazakov DV, Spagnolo DV, Stewart CJ, et al. Fibroadenoma and phyllodes tumors of anogenital mammary-like glands: a series of 13 neoplasms in 12 cases, including mammary-type juvenile fibroadenoma, fibroadenoma with lactation changes, and neurofibromatosis-associated pseudoangiomatous stromal hyperplasia with multinucleated giant cells. Am J Surg Pathol. 2010;34:95–103. https://doi.org/10.1097/PAS.0b013e3181c6e5c5.
44. Konstantinova AM, Kacerovska D, Michal M, et al. A composite neoplastic lesion of the vulva with mixed features of fibroadenoma and hidradenoma papilliferum combined with pseudoangiomatous stromal hyperplasia containing multinucleated giant cells. Am J Dermatopathol. 2014;36:e171–4. https://doi.org/10.1097/DAD.0b013e31828742e4.
45. Vella JE, Taibjee SM, Sanders DS, et al. Fibroadenoma of the anogenital region. J Clin Pathol. 2008;61:871–2. https://doi.org/10.1136/jcp.2007.052290.
46. Meeker JH, Neubecker RD, Helwig EB. Hidradenoma papilliferum. Am J Clin Pathol. 1962;37:182–95.
47. Kazakov DV, Mikyskova I, Kutzner H, et al. Hidradenoma papilliferum with oxyphilic metaplasia: a clinicopathological study of 18 cases, including detection of human papillomavirus. Am J Dermatopathol. 2005;27:102–10.

48. Sington J, Chandrapala R, Manek S, et al. Mitotic count is not predictive of clinical behavior in hidradenoma papilliferum of the vulva: a clinicopathologic study of 19 cases. Am J Dermatopathol. 2006;28:322–6.
49. Scurry J, van der Putte SC, Pyman J, et al. Mammary-like gland adenoma of the vulva: review of 46 cases. Pathology. 2009;41:372–8. https://doi.org/10.1080/00313020902884493.
50. Woodworth H Jr, Dockerty MB, Wilson RB, et al. Papillary hidradenoma of the vulva: a clinicopathologic study of 69 cases. Am J Obstet Gynecol. 1971;110:501–8.
51. Nishie W, Sawamura D, Mayuzumi M, et al. Hidradenoma papilliferum with mixed histopathologic features of syringocystadenoma papilliferum and anogenital mammary-like glands. J Cutan Pathol. 2004;31:561–4. https://doi.org/10.1111/j.0303-6987.2004.00176.x.
52. Parks A, Branch KD, Metcalf J, et al. Hidradenoma papilliferum with mixed histopathologic features of syringocystadenoma papilliferum and anogenital mammary-like glands: report of a case and review of the literature. Am J Dermatopathol. 2012;34:104–9. https://doi.org/10.1097/DAD.0b013e31820e63e8.
53. Stewart CJ. Syringocystadenoma papilliferum-like lesion of the vulva. Pathology. 2008;40:638–9. https://doi.org/10.1080/00313020802320770.
54. Pelosi G, Martignoni G, Bonetti F. Intraductal carcinoma of mammary-type apocrine epithelium arising within a papillary hydradenoma of the vulva. Report of a case and review of the literature. Arch Pathol Lab Med. 1991;115:1249–54.
55. Docimo S Jr, Shon W, Elkowitz DE. Bartholin's abscess arising within hidradenoma papilliferum of the vulva: a case report. Cases J. 2008;1:282. https://doi.org/10.1186/1757-1626-1-282.
56. Simpson WA, Burke M, Frappell J, et al. Paget's disease, melanocytic neoplasia and hidradenoma papilliferum of the vulva. Histopathology. 1988;12:675–9.
57. Stefanato CM, Finn R, Bhawan J. Extramammary Paget disease with underlying hidradenoma papilliferum: guilt by association? Am J Dermatopathol. 2000;22:439–42.
58. Konstantinova AM, Shelekhova KV. [Fibroepithelial neoplasms of anogenital mammary-like glands: a case report and review of the literature]. Arkh Patol. 2017;79: 40–47.
59. Zhang J, Chen Y, Wang K, et al. Prepubertal vulval fibroma with a coincidental ectopic breast fibroadenoma: report of an unusual case with literature review. J Obstet Gynaecol Res. 2011;37:1720–5. https://doi.org/10.1111/j.1447-0756.2011.01580.x.
60. Hassim AM. Bilateral fibroadenoma in supernumerary breasts of the vulva. J Obstet Gynaecol Br Commonw. 1969;76:275–7.
61. Assor D, Davis JB. Multiple apocrine fibroadenomas of the anal skin. Am J Clin Pathol. 1977;68:397–9.
62. Audisio T, Crespo-Roca F, Giraudo P, et al. Fibroadenoma of the vulva—simultaneous with breast fibroadenomas and uterine myoma. J Low Genit Tract Dis. 2011;15:75–9. https://doi.org/10.1097/LGT.0b013e3181de72e5.
63. Tbakhi A, Cowan DF, Kumar D, et al. Recurring phyllodes tumor in aberrant breast tissue of the vulva. Am J Surg Pathol. 1993;17:946–50.
64. Tresserra F, Grases PJ, Izquierdo M, et al. Fibroadenoma phyllodes arising in vulvar supernumerary breast tissue: report of two cases. Int J Gynecol Pathol. 1998;17:171–3.
65. Ozbudak IH, Akkaya H, Akkaya B, et al. Phyllodes tumor of the vulva: report of two cases. Turk Patoloji Derg. 2013;29:73–6. https://doi.org/10.5146/tjpath.2013.01153.
66. Lev-Cohain N, Kapur P, Pedrosa I. Vulvar fibroadenoma with lactational changes in ectopic breast tissue. Case Rep Obstet Gynecol. 2013;2013:924902. https://doi.org/10.1155/2013/924902.
67. Xanos ET, Kennedy DA, Grosen EA. Pregnancy-related fibroadenoma of ectopic breast tissue in the vulva. J Low Genit Tract Dis. 1997;1:182–4.
68. Heffernan TP, Sarode VR, Hoffman B, et al. Recurrent phyllodes tumor of the vulva: a case report with review of diagnostic criteria and differential diagnosis. Int J Gynecol Pathol. 2010;29:294–7. https://doi.org/10.1097/PGP.0b013e3181c14a8c.
69. Fu L, Lau S, Roy I, et al. Phyllodes tumor with malignant stromal morphology of the vulva: a case report and review of the literature. Int J Gynecol Pathol. 2011;30:198–202. https://doi.org/10.1097/PGP.0b013e3181f45f58.
70. Gugliotta P, Fibbi ML, Fessia L, et al. Lactating supernumerary mammary gland tissue in the vulva. Appl Pathol. 1983;1:61–5.
71. O'Hara MF, Page DL. Adenomas of the breast and ectopic breast under lactational influences. Hum Pathol. 1985;16:707–12.
72. Scarabin C, Koskas M, Bornes M, et al. Gigantomastia and vulvar lactating adenoma in a patient with myasthenia during pregnancy. Am J Obstet Gynecol. 2010;203:e5–8. https://doi.org/10.1016/j.ajog.2010.07.001.
73. Lee ES, Kim I. Multiple vulvar lactating adenomas. Obstet Gynecol. 2011;118:478–80. https://doi.org/10.1097/AOG.0b013e31821ecaa2.
74. Kinkor Z, Michal M. [Anogenital mammary type sclerosing adenosis—two case reports and the review of literature]. Ceska Gynekol. 2004;69:292–7.
75. Young AW Jr, Herman EW, Tovell HM. Syringoma of the vulva: incidence, diagnosis, and cause of pruritus. Obstet Gynecol. 1980;55:515–8.
76. Scherbenske JM, Lupton GP, James WD, et al. Vulvar syringomas occurring in a 9-year-old child. J Am Acad Dermatol. 1988;19:575–7.
77. Kazakov DV, Bouda J Jr, Kacerovska D, et al. Vulvar syringomas with deep extension: a potential histopathologic mimic of microcystic adnexal carcinoma. Int J Gynecol Pathol. 2011;30:92–4. https://doi.org/10.1097/PGP.0b013e3181ee5c9e.
78. Konstantinova AM, Hayes MM, Stewart CJ, et al. Syringomatous structures in extramammary Paget disease: a potential diagnostic pitfall. Am J Dermatopathol. 2016;38:653–7. https://doi.org/10.1097/DAD.0000000000000497.
79. Kazakov DV, Zelger B, Rutten A, et al. Morphologic diversity of malignant neoplasms arising in preexisting spiradenoma, cylindroma, and spiradenocylindroma based on the study of 24 cases, sporadic or occurring in the setting of Brooke-Spiegler syndrome. Am J Surg Pathol. 2009;33:705–19.
80. Grossmann P, Vanecek T, Steiner P, et al. Novel and recurrent germline and somatic mutations in a cohort of 67 patients from 48 families with Brooke-Spiegler syndrome including the phenotypic variant of multiple familial trichoepitheliomas and correlation with the histopathologic findings in 379 biopsy specimens. Am J Dermatopathol. 2013;35:34–44. https://doi.org/10.1097/DAD.0b013e31824e7658.
81. Michal M, Lamovec J, Mukensnabl P, et al. Spiradenocylindromas of the skin: tumors with morphological features of spiradenoma and cylindroma in the same lesion: report of 12 cases. Pathol Int. 1999;49:419–25.
82. Kazakov DV. Brooke-Spiegler syndrome and phenotypic variants: an update. Head Neck Pathol. 2016;10:125–30. https://doi.org/10.1007/s12105-016-0705-x.
83. Baker GM, Selim MA, Hoang MP. Vulvar adnexal lesions: a 32-year, single-institution review from Massachusetts General Hospital. Arch Pathol Lab Med. 2013;137:1237–46. https://doi.org/10.5858/arpa.2012-0434-OA.
84. Young AL, Kellermayer R, Szigeti R, et al. CYLD mutations underlie Brooke-Spiegler, familial cylindromatosis, and multiple familial trichoepithelioma syndromes. Clin Genet. 2006;70:246–9. https://doi.org/10.1111/j.1399-0004.2006.00667.x.
85. Kazakov DV, Kacerovska D, Hantschke M, et al. Cutaneous mixed tumor, eccrine variant: a clinicopathologic and immunohistochemical study of 50 cases, with emphasis on unusual histopatho-

logic features. Am J Dermatopathol. 2011;33:557–68. https://doi.org/10.1097/DAD.0b013e318206c1a3.
86. Chome J, Giard R. [Case report of an unusual tumor of the vulva; epithelioma of rearranged stroma or so-called mixed tumor]. Bull Fed Soc Gynecol Obstet Lang Fr. 1956;8:562–5.
87. Dykgraaf RH, van Veen MM, van Bekkum-de Jonge EE, et al. Pleomorphic adenoma of the vulva: a review illustrated by a clinical case. Int J Gynecol Cancer. 2006;16:920–3. https://doi.org/10.1111/j.1525-1438.2006.00423.x.
88. Ordonez NG, Manning JT, Luna MA. Mixed tumor of the vulva: a report of two cases probably arising in Bartholin's gland. Cancer. 1981;48:181–6.
89. Rorat E, Wallach RC. Mixed tumors of the vulva: clinical outcome and pathology. Int J Gynecol Pathol. 1984;3:323–8.
90. Wilson D, Woodger BA. Pleomorphic adenoma of the vulva. J Obstet Gynaecol Br Commonw. 1974;81:1000–2.
91. Rajguru A, Moulla A, Ogunremi A, et al. Vulval microglandular adenosis-like neoplasm with chondromyxoid stroma: report of a unique case. Int J Gynecol Pathol. 2016;35:123–6. https://doi.org/10.1097/PGP.0000000000000230.
92. Branton PA, Tavassoli FA. Spindle cell epithelioma, the so-called mixed tumor of the vagina. A clinicopathologic, immunohistochemical, and ultrastructural analysis of 28 cases. Am J Surg Pathol. 1993;17:509–15.
93. Fukunaga M, Endo Y, Ishikawa E, et al. Mixed tumour of the vagina. Histopathology. 1996;28:457–61.
94. Fukunaga M. Myoepithelioma of the vulva. APMIS. 2003;111:416–20.
95. Peterdy GA, Huettner PC, Rajaram V, et al. Trichofolliculoma of the vulva associated with vulvar intraepithelial neoplasia: report of three cases and review of the literature. Int J Gynecol Pathol. 2002;21:224–30.
96. Georgantopoulou C, Aird I. Management of myoepithelioma of the vulva—case report and review of the literature. Eur J Gynaecol Oncol. 2009;30:203–5.
97. Meenakshi M, McCluggage WG. Myoepithelial neoplasms involving the vulva and vagina: report of 4 cases. Hum Pathol. 2009;40:1747–53. https://doi.org/10.1016/j.humpath.2009.04.025.
98. Yoshida A, Yoshida H, Yoshida M, et al. Myoepithelioma-like tumors of the vulvar region: a distinctive group of SMARCB1-deficient neoplasms. Am J Surg Pathol. 2015;39:1102–13. https://doi.org/10.1097/PAS.0000000000000466.

5 Vulvar Squamous Neoplasia

Susanne K. Jeffus

Abstract

Vulvar cancer affects 2.5 per 100,000 women per year and represents 0.4% of all new cancer cases in the USA. It is primarily a disease of elderly women with those between the ages of 75 and 84 most commonly affected. The majority of vulvar cancers (90%) are squamous cell carcinomas. In contrast to the cervix, where virtually all squamous neoplasia is driven by human papillomavirus (HPV) infection, two distinct pathways to invasive squamous cell carcinoma are recognized in the vulva: the HPV-dependent and the HPV-independent pathway. While exceptions occur and rare overlap exists, these two pathways differ with respect to epidemiologic, clinical, histopathologic, and molecular characteristics. Recently, a third pathway has been proposed but requires further investigation.

Keywords

Vulva · Vulvar intraepithelial neoplasia · VIN · LSIL · HSIL · Differentiated VIN · Squamous cell carcinoma

5.1 Introduction

Vulvar cancer affects 2.5 per 100,000 women per year and represents 0.4% of all new cancer cases in the USA [1]. It is primarily a disease of elderly women with those between the ages of 75 and 84 most commonly affected. The majority of vulvar cancers (90%) are squamous cell carcinomas. In contrast to the cervix, where virtually all squamous neoplasia is driven by human papillomavirus (HPV) infection, two distinct pathways to invasive squamous cell carcinoma are recognized in the vulva: the HPV-dependent and the HPV-independent pathway [2]. While exceptions occur and rare overlap exists, these two pathways differ with respect to epidemiologic, clinical, histopathologic, and molecular characteristics. Recently, a third pathway has been proposed but requires further investigation [3].

The precursor lesion in the HPV-dependent pathway is usual vulvar intraepithelial neoplasia (uVIN). It presents in younger women, is clinically distinct, frequently multifocal, associated with smoking, and less likely to progress to invasive cancer. It typically gives rise to basaloid or warty squamous cell carcinoma. In contrast, the HPV-independent pathway is characterized by *Tp53* mutations. The precursor is differentiated VIN (dVIN), which is more subtle clinically and rapidly evolves into well- to moderately differentiated keratinizing squamous cell carcinoma. This pathway has a proclivity for older women (seventh and eighth decade). Risk factors include vulvar dermatoses such as lichen sclerosus or lichen simplex chronicus. A potential third pathway has recently been proposed in which *PIK3CA* and *ARID2* mutations drive the development of atypical verruciform vulvar lesions collectively referred to as differentiated exophytic vulvar intraepithelial lesion (DE-VIL). These may play a risk factor in the development of a small subset of HPV-independent well-differentiated squamous cell carcinomas of the vulva but require further investigation (Fig. 5.1) [2–4].

5.2 Vulvar Intraepithelial Neoplasia

5.2.1 Current Nomenclature

Over the last century, the nomenclature of intraepithelial lesions of the vulva has steadily evolved [5, 6]. In 2012, a consensus document referred to as the LAST (Lower Anogenital Standardization Terminology) Project was published by the College of American Pathologists (CAP) and the American Society for Colposcopy and Cervical Pathology (ASCCP) [7]. LAST recommends a two-tiered nomenclature for HPV-associated squamous intraepithelial lesions across

S. K. Jeffus (✉)
Department of Pathology, University of Arkansas for Medical Sciences, Little Rock, AR, USA
e-mail: skjeffus@uams.edu

W. Zheng et al. (eds.), *Gynecologic and Obstetric Pathology, Volume 1*, https://doi.org/10.1007/978-981-13-3016-2_5

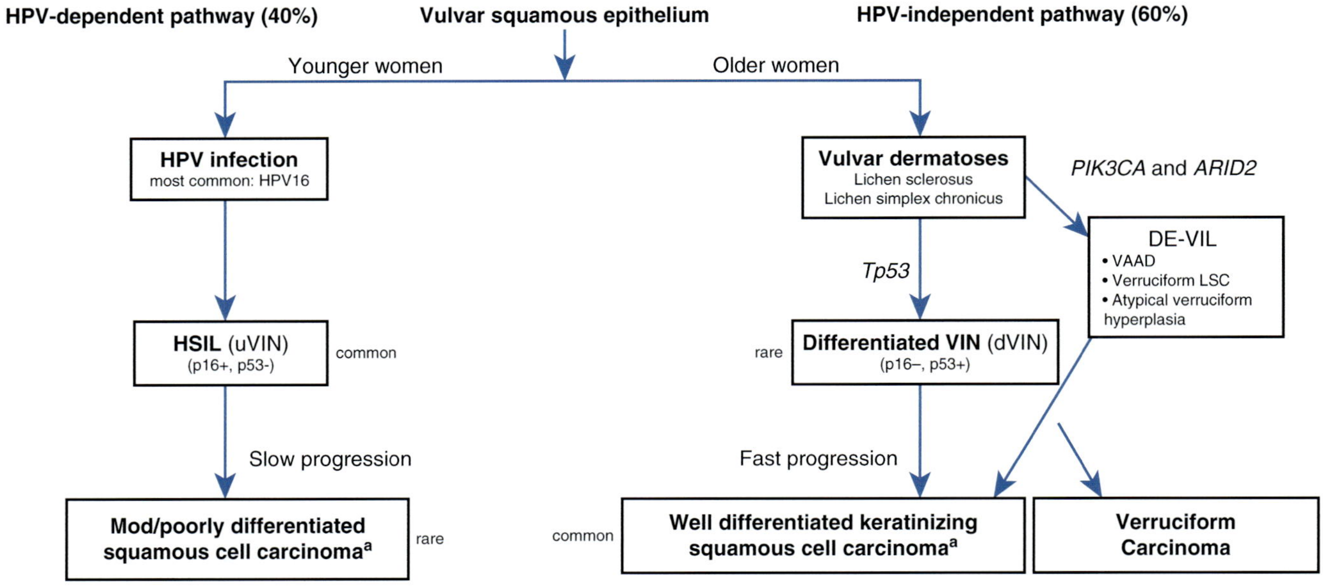

Fig. 5.1 Summary of current pathways to squamous cell carcinoma of the vulva (adopted and modified via Refs. [2–4]). [a]Morphologic overlap occurs; some p16+/HPV+ squamous cell carcinomas are of the keratinizing type, while some non-keratinizing tumors are p16−/HPV−

the entire anogenital tract: low-grade squamous intraepithelial lesion (LSIL) and high-grade squamous intraepithelial lesion (HSIL). This new classification has effectively replaced the previous three-tiered intraepithelial neoplasia (IN-1,2,3) scheme. Aside from better reproducibility, the designations of LSIL and HSIL reflect the underlying HPV biology more accurately. HSIL has a potential risk of progression to invasive cancer requiring conservative excision. LSIL on the other hand has a negligible risk and is managed expectantly. The simplified LAST nomenclature also unifies the varied language of preinvasive anogenital lesions, improving communication between pathologists and clinicians. The LAST recommendations were subsequently endorsed by the World Health Organization (WHO) in its 2014 Classification of Tumours of Female Reproductive Organs and by the International Society for the Study of Vulvovaginal Disease (ISSVD) in 2015 [6–8]. Hence, HPV-related vulvar lesions are currently classified in keeping with the two-tiered SIL nomenclature.

According to LAST, the designation of LSIL encompasses both exophytic (condyloma acuminatum) and flat lesions (VIN 1/flat condyloma). Whether LSIL of the vulva is precancerous is a matter of debate in the literature [6, 9–14]. Both WHO and ISSVD classify condyloma acuminatum under benign squamous lesions and reserve the "LSIL" designation for VIN 1/flat condyloma/HPV effect [6, 8]. If LAST terminology is consistently utilized in daily practice, clarification of LSIL with "condyloma acuminatum" or "VIN 1/flat condyloma/HPV effect" in parentheses is of value for the clinician who must navigate the ever changing landscape of nomenclature designations. Similarly, older and more established vulvar terminology for HSIL (e.g., VIN 2/3, VIN usual type) can be included in parentheses to further improve communication [7].

In addition to LSIL and HSIL, vulvar intraepithelial neoplasia also includes differentiated type VIN (dVIN), a high-grade intraepithelial squamous neoplasia not related to infection by HPV. First described by Abell and Gosling in 1961 and referred to as "intraepithelial carcinoma simplex type," dVIN remained a relatively under-recognized intraepithelial precursor until the landmark paper by Yang and Hart in 2000 [15, 16]. Because of its lack of association with HPV, dVIN was not addressed by LAST. The most recent WHO and ISSVD nomenclature recommend "VIN, differentiated type" over older terms such as "VIN 3, differentiated type" or "simplex type VIN" [6, 8]. Table 5.1 summarizes the current vulvar nomenclature for intraepithelial lesions.

5.2.2 Low-Grade Squamous Intraepithelial Lesion

5.2.2.1 Clinical Features

Low-grade squamous intraepithelial lesions of the vulva can be broadly subdivided based on appearance into exophytic and flat lesions. Condylomata (venereal warts) are common exophytic growths that affect approximately 1 million women each year and are typically associated with low-risk HPV types 6 and 11. Clinically, they can range from small excrescences to bulky cauliflower-like growths, frequently in a multifocal distribution (Fig. 5.2). In contrast to the classic genital wart, flat vulvar LSIL (VIN 1, flat condyloma, HPV effect) is rare and represents an active infection by low- or high-risk HPV types.

Table 5.1 Overview of current terminology (LAST, WHO, ISSVD) for vulvar intraepithelial neoplasia

HPV status	Nomenclature[a] (2012, LAST)	Nomenclature (2014, WHO)	Nomenclature (2015, ISSVD)	Synonyms (older terminology)
HPV-related vulvar intraepithelial lesions	LSIL	LSIL[b]	LSIL[b] (flat condyloma, HPV effect)	Condyloma acuminatum Flat condyloma/HPV effect VIN 1, VIN I Mild dysplasia
	HSIL	HSIL	HSIL (VIN usual type)	VIN, usual type VIN 2, VIN II, moderate dysplasia VIN 3, VIN III, severe dysplasia, carcinoma in situ Bowen disease
HPV-unrelated vulvar intraepithelial lesions	–	VIN, differentiated type	VIN, differentiated type	VIN 3, differentiated type VIN, simplex type Intraepithelial carcinoma, simplex type

[a]LSIL and HSIL can be further clarified by including synonyms or older terminology (e.g., VIN) in parentheses. Of note, LSIL includes exophytic and flat condyloma in the LAST classification

[b]Exophytic condyloma (condyloma acuminatum) is not included in the LSIL designation but is grouped with benign squamous lesions

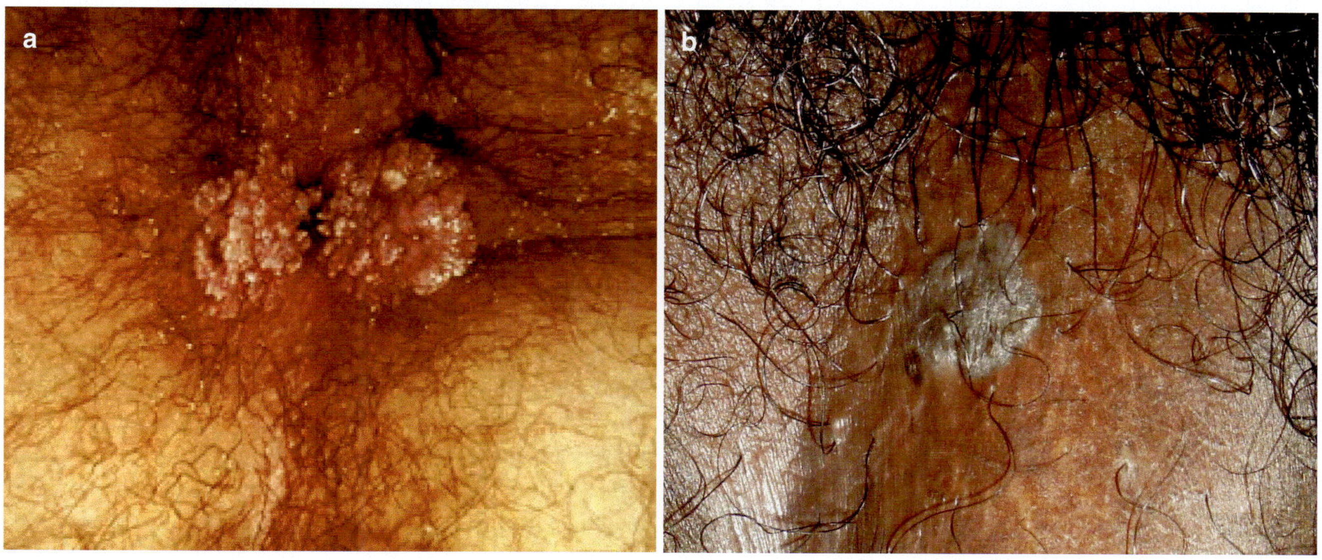

Fig. 5.2 Vulvar condyloma accuminata. The surface of lesions can be verrucous (**a**) or flat (**b**). The color of lesions can range from flesh-colored (**a**) to darker or lighter (**b**). (Courtesy of Dr. Kenneth Hatch, University of Arizona)

5.2.2.2 Histopathologic Features

Microscopically, the architectural changes of a condyloma are best appreciated on low-power examination. On scanning magnification, the acanthotic squamous epithelium shows a papillary configuration with a rounded, undulating surface (sometimes referred to as resembling knuckles) and prominent fibrovascular cores. Hyperkeratosis, parakeratosis, and hypergranulosis can be present. Nuclear atypia is mild and characterized by nuclear enlargement, hyperchromasia, chromatin condensation, and irregular nuclear membranes. Classic cytologic features of binucleation with perinuclear clearing (koilocytosis) are frequently observed but on occasion more difficult to find or even absent. Mitotic figures are confined to the lower third of the epithelium (Fig. 5.3). In contrast, flat lesions demonstrate an acanthotic squamous epithelium with a smooth, flat-topped surface. Koilocytic atypia and distribution of mitotic figures mirror its exophytic counterpart (Fig. 5.4).

5.2.2.3 Ancillary Studies

As in other anogenital sites, the diagnosis of a low-grade squamous intraepithelial lesion should be based on morphologic criteria rather than ancillary studies such as immunohistochemistry (IHC). According to LAST, p16^{INK4a} (p16) is neither recommended nor required as an adjunct stain in classic cases of LSIL and does not resolve the diagnostic dilemma of reactive atypia versus LSIL (see Sect. 5.4 for full discussion) [7]. Of note, vulvar lesions with unequivocal features of condyloma or flat LSIL/VIN 1 demonstrate either negative or rarely positive staining with p16 [14, 17].

Genital warts in infants and children can occur as a consequence of vertical transmission (childbirth) and through non-

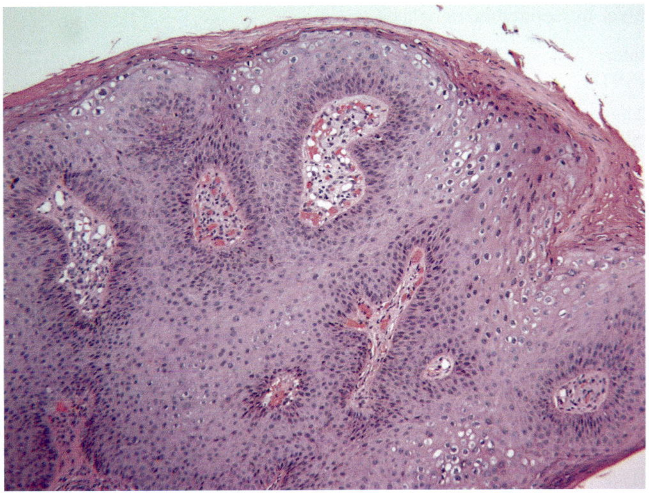

Fig. 5.3 LSIL (condyloma acuminatum). Low-power view shows a papillary configuration of acanthotic squamous epithelium with an undulating, rounded surface and fibrovascular cores. Koilocytic atypia is prominent in the upper layers of the epithelium (H&E 100×)

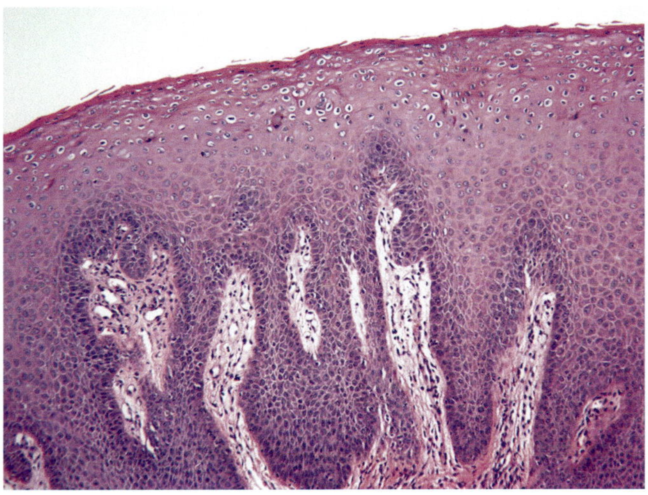

Fig. 5.4 LSIL (VIN 1, flat condyloma, HPV effect). The acanthotic squamous epithelium demonstrates a smooth, flat-topped surface. Koilocytic atypia is prominent in the upper layers of the epithelium (H&E 100×)

sexual transmission (skin to skin contact) but can also raise the concern for sexual abuse. Histologic examination may be required in select cases (e.g., uncertain clinical picture). HPV testing by PCR or hybridization is not recommended in a routine investigation of potential sexual abuse. For a detailed review on this topic, the reader is referred to the excellent review by Bussen et al. [18].

5.2.2.4 Differential Diagnosis

Fibroepithelial/Squamous Papilloma

Some exophytic lesions of the vulva closely resemble condylomata architecturally but lack koilocytosis. In this instance, several practical approaches for the diagnosis are acceptable including "fibroepithelial papilloma," "condyloma without cytopathic effect," "squamous papilloma, possibly condyloma," or "verrucous keratosis." A comment should be included in the report to explain the differential diagnosis and that HPV effect cannot be excluded.

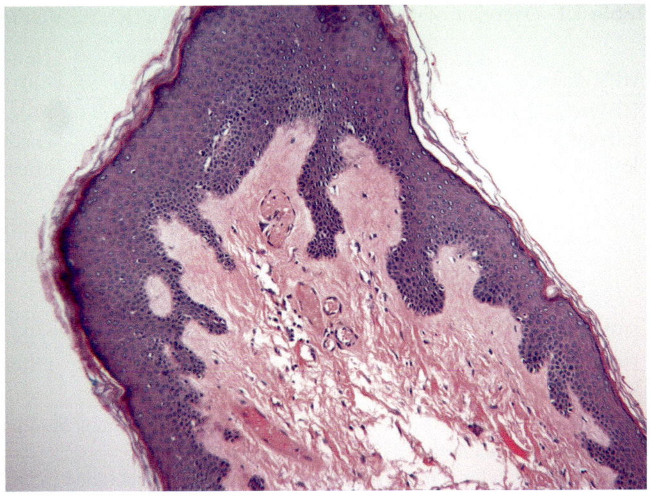

Fig. 5.5 Fibroepithelial polyp (skin tag). Unremarkable squamous epithelium overlies a fibrous stroma with delicate small vessels (H&E 100×)

Vestibular (Squamous) Papilloma

Vestibular (squamous) papillomas are delicate exophytic growths exclusively found in the area of the vestibule. These lesions are either solitary or multifocal and are not related to HPV. A fibrovascular core is covered by bland squamous epithelium. Glycogenated cells can mimic HPV effect. However, nuclear atypia (enlargement, chromatic clumping, irregular nuclear membranes) or bone fide koilocytosis is absent [19].

Fibroepithelial Polyp (Skin Tag, Acrochordon)

Fibroepithelial polyps are benign sessile to pedunculated lesions of the hair-bearing skin of the vulva. No relation to HPV has been identified. Microscopically, a keratinized squamous epithelium covers a stroma with a thick fibrovascular core. The squamous epithelium can vary in thickness but remains cytologically bland, lacking koilocytic changes (Fig. 5.5).

Fibroepithelial Stromal Polyp

Fibroepithelial stromal polyps are benign exophytic growths. The squamous epithelium lacks papillary features and nuclear atypia but may show mild acanthosis. The cellularity of the stroma can range from hypocellular to hypercellular and is remarkable for stellate and multinucleated stromal cells, which are concentrated around vessels and at the epithelial-stromal interface. Edema and myxoid change can be seen. Particularly in pregnancy, these polyps can mimic a

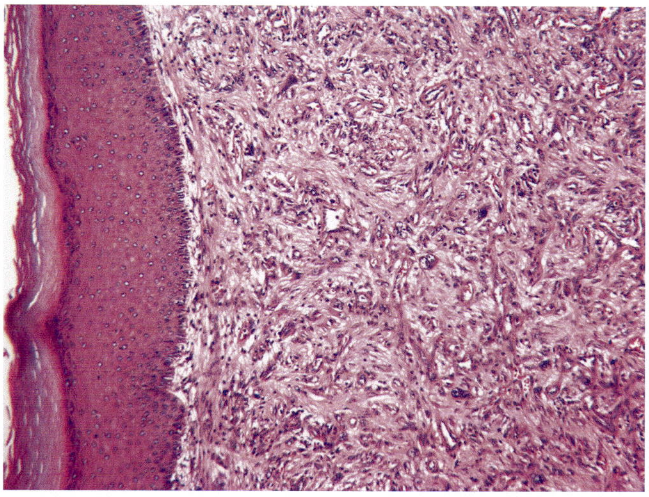

Fig. 5.6 Fibroepithelial stromal polyp from a pregnant woman. The stromal compartment is markedly hypercellular and exhibits nuclear pleomorphism and multinucleation. Mitotic figures (not shown) were present. This lesion has a pseudosarcomatous appearance but is benign (H&E 100×)

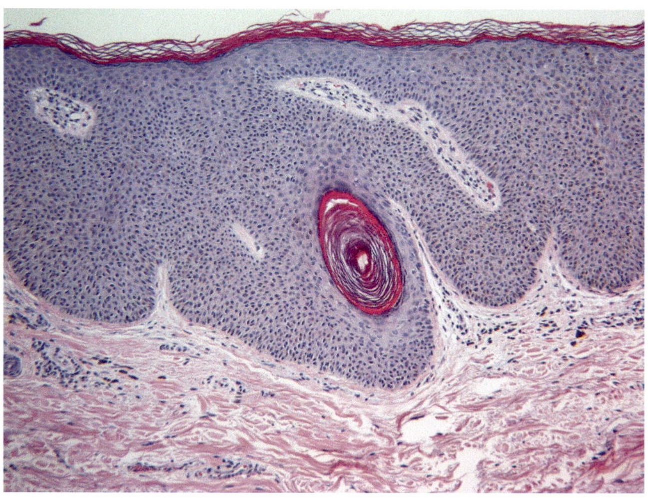

Fig. 5.7 Seborrheic keratosis. Cytologically bland basaloid cells and intraepithelial keratin-filled pseudo-horn cysts (H&E, 100×)

sarcoma due to the hypercellularity, pleomorphism, and mitotic activity in the stromal compartment (Fig. 5.6) [20].

Seborrheic Keratosis

Vulvar seborrheic keratosis (SK) is morphologically similar to cutaneous SK and is characterized by a proliferation of cytologically bland basaloid cells. Intraepithelial keratin-filled pseudo-horn cysts may be seen (Fig. 5.7). In contrast to extragenital seborrheic keratoses, a substantial subset of vulvar seborrheic keratoses have been documented to harbor low-risk HPV subtypes, leading to a proposed designation of "seborrheic keratosis-like condyloma" by some authors [21–23].

Condyloma Lata

Condyloma lata are genital papules that are seen in the second stage of syphilis, which is caused by *Treponema pallidum*, a sexually transmitted spirochete. Papillomatosis and acanthosis are accompanied by a brisk inflammatory infiltrate, which may obscure the dermal-epidermal junction. The inflammatory infiltrate is rich in plasma cells, which are centered on stromal vessels. A positive Warthin-Starry stain or spirochete immunohistochemistry supports the diagnosis (Fig. 5.8) [24].

Angiokeratoma

Angiokeratoma is a benign vascular lesion that can resemble a genital wart clinically. Of the five subtypes, two can affect the vulva: angiokeratoma corporis diffusum and the idiopathic type. The former is characterized by clustered papules in a bathing suit distribution and is classically associated with Anderson-Fabry disease, an X-linked recessive lysosomal storage disease. Lesions are solitary or multiple red to brown with a verrucous surface. Microscopically, an acanthotic and hyperkeratotic squamous epithelium overlies a dermis with vascular ectasia. Thrombosis of the vascular spaces is a common finding (Fig. 5.9) [25].

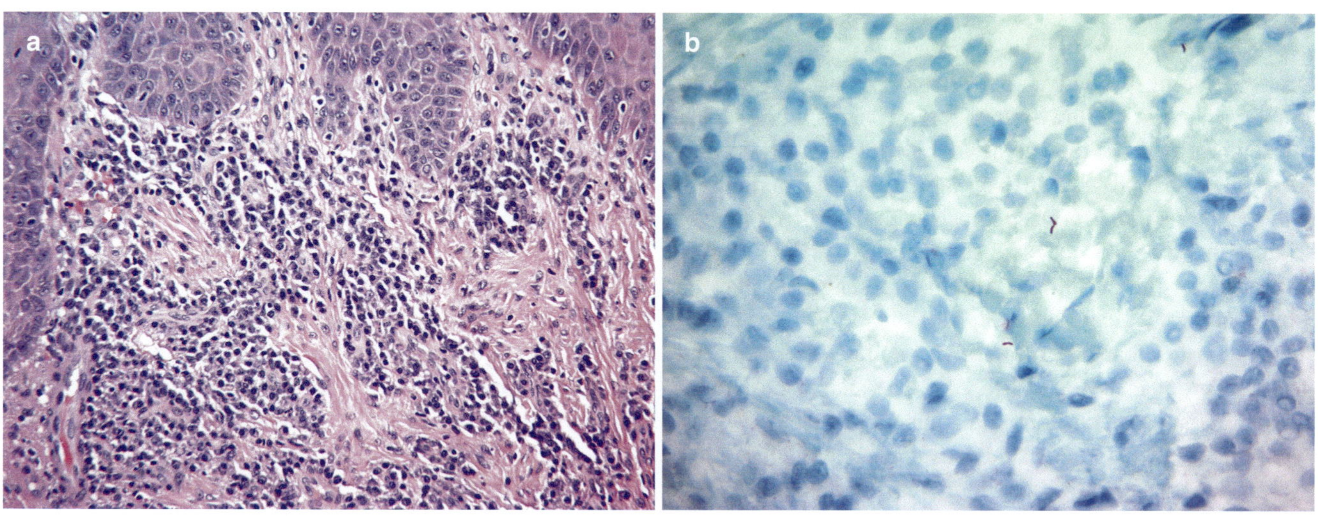

Fig. 5.8 Condyloma lata. Brisk plasma cell infiltrate in the dermis (H&E, 200×). Inset: Spirochete immunohistochemical stain is positive supporting the diagnosis (600×)

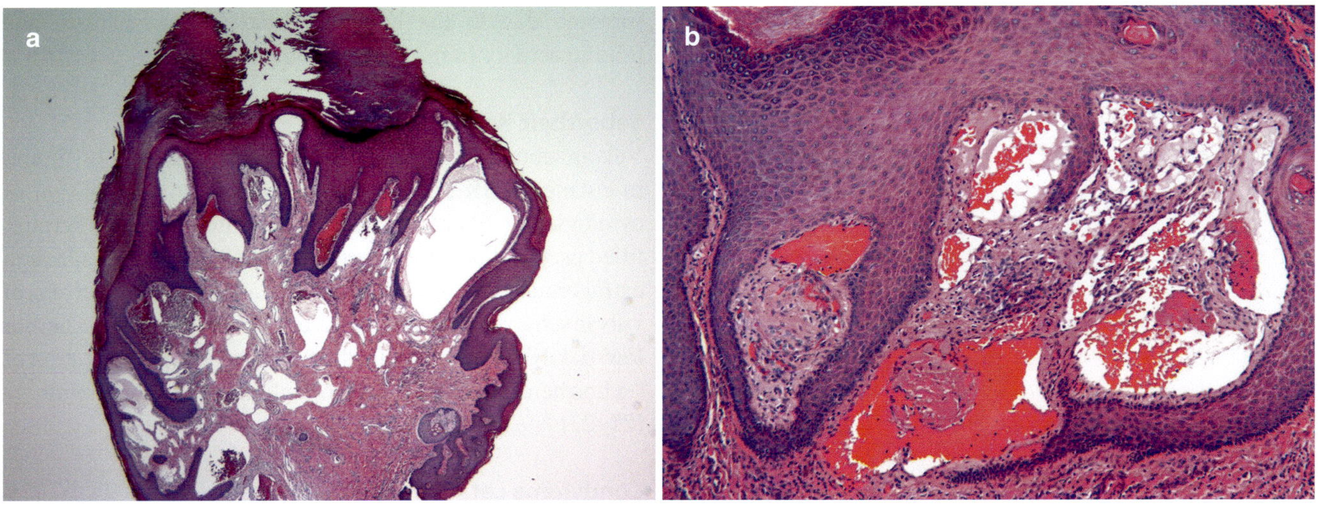

Fig. 5.9 Angiokeratoma. (**a**) Squamous epithelium with hyperkeratosis overlying dilated vascular spaces in the dermis (H&E, 20×), (**b**) some demonstrating vascular thrombosis (H&E, 100×)

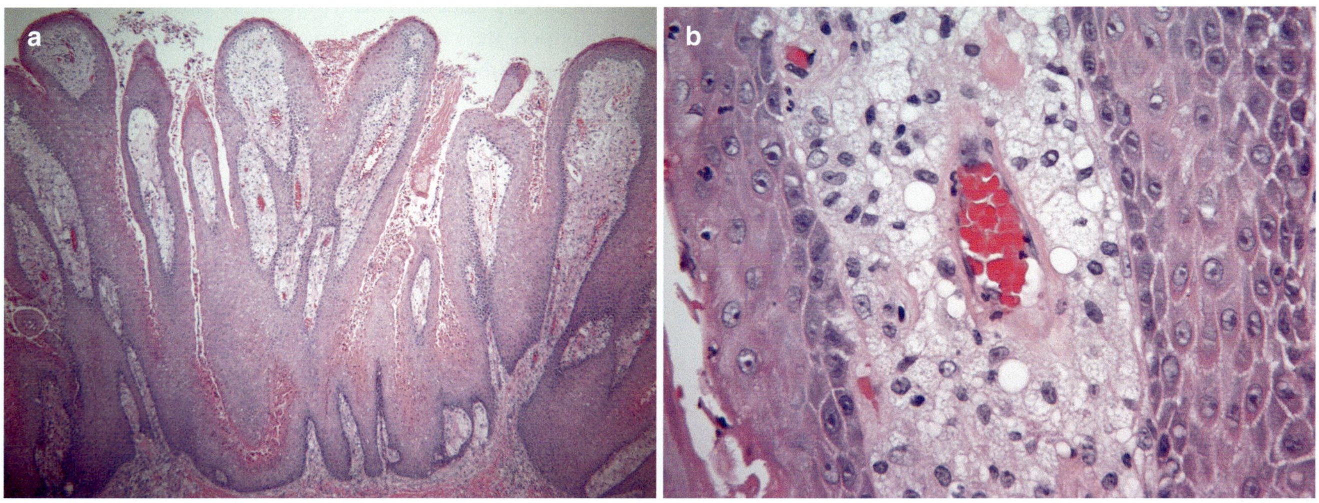

Fig. 5.10 Verruciform xanthoma. (**a**) Exophytic and papillary squamous epithelium with regular psoriasiform acanthosis (H&E, 40×) and (**b**) papillae distended by foamy macrophages (H&E, 400×)

Verruciform Xanthoma

Verruciform xanthoma (VX) is a rare benign entity, which can occur at any site, but has a propensity for mucosal surfaces, including the vulva. VX lesions are usually asymptomatic, have a yellow-orange color, and mimic other verrucous growths of the vulva. Microscopically, VX is composed of an exophytic and papillary squamous epithelium with regular psoriasiform acanthosis with rete ridge plugs of brightly eosinophilic stacked parakeratosis (Fig. 5.10a). Awareness of this histologic pattern is essential so that the astute pathologist can then search for the sometimes subtle but diagnostic features of dermal papillae distended by foamy macrophages (Fig. 5.10b). A CD68 stain is positive in the xanthoma cells. Of note, VX patients often have vulvar dystrophies such as lichen sclerosus and lichen planus [26–28]. In contrast to other xanthomatous lesions, VX is not associated with serum lipid abnormalities.

Acantholytic and Epidermolytic Acanthoma

Occasionally discrete and localized abnormalities in keratinocyte biology may lead to a clinically apparent verrucoid papule on the vulva resembling condyloma acuminatum or HSIL. Histologically, a lesion may show disassociation of keratinocytes (acantholysis) or dissolution of the intracellular keratin framework (epidermolysis). Acantholysis is due to defective cell-cell adhesion between keratinocytes; a solitary papule demonstrating only acantholysis may be referred to as an acantholytic acanthoma. The phenomenon of epidermolytic hyperkeratosis (EHK) is due to mutations in keratin proteins, resulting in histologically visible keratin filament clumping and intracellular eosinophilic globules with overlying hyperkeratosis. A solitary lesion showing EHK, likely representing a focal mosaic gene defect, may be referred to as epidermolytic acanthoma [29, 30].

Reactive Changes and Infection

The distinction between reactive changes or a subtle LSIL (VIN 1/flat condyloma) can be challenging at times. Just like in the cervix, no ancillary test can aid in this distinction; it is a histopathologic diagnosis. Strict adherence to diagnostic criteria (nuclear features) with assessment at low to intermediate power (4× and 10× rather than 40×) is advised to avoid overinterpretation of reactive changes as HPV effect. The nuclear atypia in reactive and inflammatory conditions is usually mild with uniform nuclear enlargement and prominent nucleoli while nuclear membranes remain smooth. In inflamed or ulcerated specimens, exclusion of viral cytopathic effect and vulvar fungal infection with special stains (e.g., PAS, GMS, HSV) is essential (Fig. 5.11).

Multinucleated Atypia of the Vulva

Multinucleation of vulvar epithelium is of uncertain etiology and can be seen particularly in young, reproductive age women [31]. It is not associated with HPV infection. Clustering of multiple nuclei in the lower to mid layers of the epithelium is a key feature. Nuclear atypia is at most mild and nucleoli can be present.

Squamous Cell Hyperplasia and Lichen Simplex Chronicus

Squamous cell hyperplasia is a relatively nonspecific morphologic pattern characterized by acanthosis with hyperkeratosis or parakeratosis. Nuclear atypia and inflammation are notably absent. Lichen simplex chronicus (LSC) is a pattern of vulvar dystrophy characterized by acanthosis with hypergranulosis, hyperkeratosis, or parakeratosis and scattered (chronic) inflammation in the dermis (Fig. 5.12). On occasion, LSC can be verruciform but lacks nuclear atypia. Performance of special stains for fungal organisms (PAS, GMS) should be included in the routine work up of cases with squamous cell hyperplasia or LSC.

HSIL

HSIL (particularly the warty subtype) can architecturally resemble a condyloma on low power examination. However, close attention to severity of nuclear atypia and distribution of mitotic activity with extension above the lower one-third of the epithelium aids in the diagnostic distinction. In small or tangentially sectioned biopsies, when the differential of LSIL versus HSIL cannot be resolved on H&E alone, adjunct immunohistochemical staining with p16 is of value. Block positive p16 staining in this setting supports the diagnosis of HSIL (see Sect. 5.4). The distinction between LSIL and HSIL is crucial because LSIL is in general managed expectantly while HSIL is conservatively excised.

Verrucous Carcinoma

Verrucous carcinoma is an extremely well-differentiated squamous cell carcinoma of older women characterized by marked acanthosis. Verrucous carcinoma is not associated with HPV. Notably, by definition, minimal to no epithelial atypia is present. A small and superficial biopsy sample may be misleading and interpreted as benign. Key features for the diagnosis center on the constellation of clinical impression, size of the lesion, and presence of invasion. The invasive front is broad, bulbous, and pushing rather than ragged and infiltrative (see Sect. 5.3).

5.2.2.5 Prognosis and Management

Condyloma acuminatum is considered a benign squamous lesion due to its strong association with low-risk HPV subtypes. However, many patients experience a protracted clinical

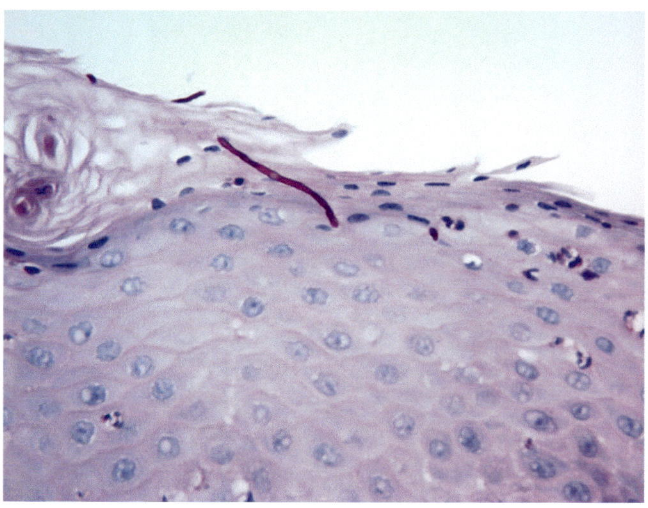

Fig. 5.11 Vulvovaginal candidiasis. PAS-D stain highlights pseudohyphae (H&E, 400×)

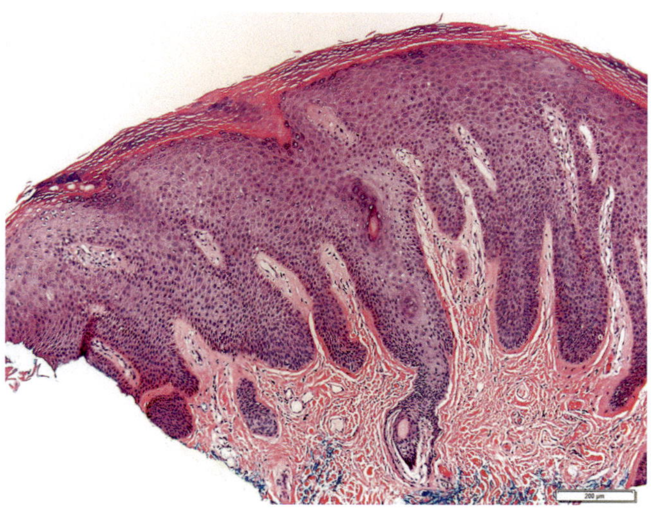

Fig. 5.12 Lichen simplex chronicus. Acanthotic squamous epithelium with hypergranulosis and sparse chronic inflammatory infiltrate (H&E, 100×)

course, particularly if smoking, immunocompromised, or pregnant. Rarely, transformation due to infection with hr-HPV can lead to HSIL or even invasive cancer arising in a condyloma. LSIL/VIN 1 (flat condyloma) is rare and its premalignant potential is debatable but infection with hr-HPV subtypes has been documented. The LSIL cohort is in general managed expectantly, unless the patient is symptomatic or desires removal of the lesion(s) due to cosmetic reasons. Resection, laser ablation, 5-fluorouracil (5-FU), imiquimod, podophyllin, and cryotherapy are all acceptable treatment methods. Risk-reducing measures for the development of LSIL include smoking cessation and immunization with the HPV vaccine. The latter is available as a quadrivalent (HPV genotype 6, 11, 16, 18) and 9-valent (HPV genotypes 6, 11, 16, 18, 31, 33, 45, 52, 58) vaccine and can be given up to age 26 [32].

5.2.3 High-Grade Squamous Intraepithelial Lesion

5.2.3.1 Clinical Features

Vulvar HSIL (former VIN 2/3, VIN usual type or uVIN) is frequently encountered in daily practice. It most commonly occurs in younger (reproductive age) patients, is almost exclusively associated with hr-HPV (particularly HPV 16), and has a proclivity for multifocal distribution. Aside from hr-HPV, other risk factors include smoking, SIL at other anogenital sites, and immunosuppression. On gross examination, vulvar HSIL presents as a macule, papule, or exophytic growth with discoloration ranging from white, gray to red. Pigmented lesions are not infrequent. Patients complain of burning or itching; however, some lesions are asymptomatic (Fig. 5.13) [15, 33–41].

5.2.3.2 Histopathologic Features

Microscopically, on low power examination an acanthotic epithelium with loss of orderly maturation is noted. The frequent association with parakeratosis and/or hyperkeratosis should prompt the pathologist to evaluate for features of HSIL, which include cell crowding with high nuclear to cytoplasmic ratios, nuclear pleomorphism, hyperchromasia, and chromatin clumping (Fig. 5.14). Mitotic figures, including atypical ones, are usually readily identified and visible above the basal layer with a tendency to involve all levels of the epithelium. Dyskeratotic cells (corp ronds or apoptotic bodies) may be present. Of note, nuclear abnormalities must extend above the lower one-third of the epithelium to qualify for the diagnosis of HSIL; most lesions however show near to full thickness atypia. On the labia majora, HSIL has a tendency to involve the adnexal structures; this feature should not be interpreted as invasive carcinoma (see Sect. 5.3.2.4) (Fig. 5.15).

HSIL is further subclassified into warty, basaloid, or mixed subtypes; however, this distinction lacks clinical significance. The basaloid, or undifferentiated, type mimics cervical HSIL; it exhibits a smooth surface and is com-

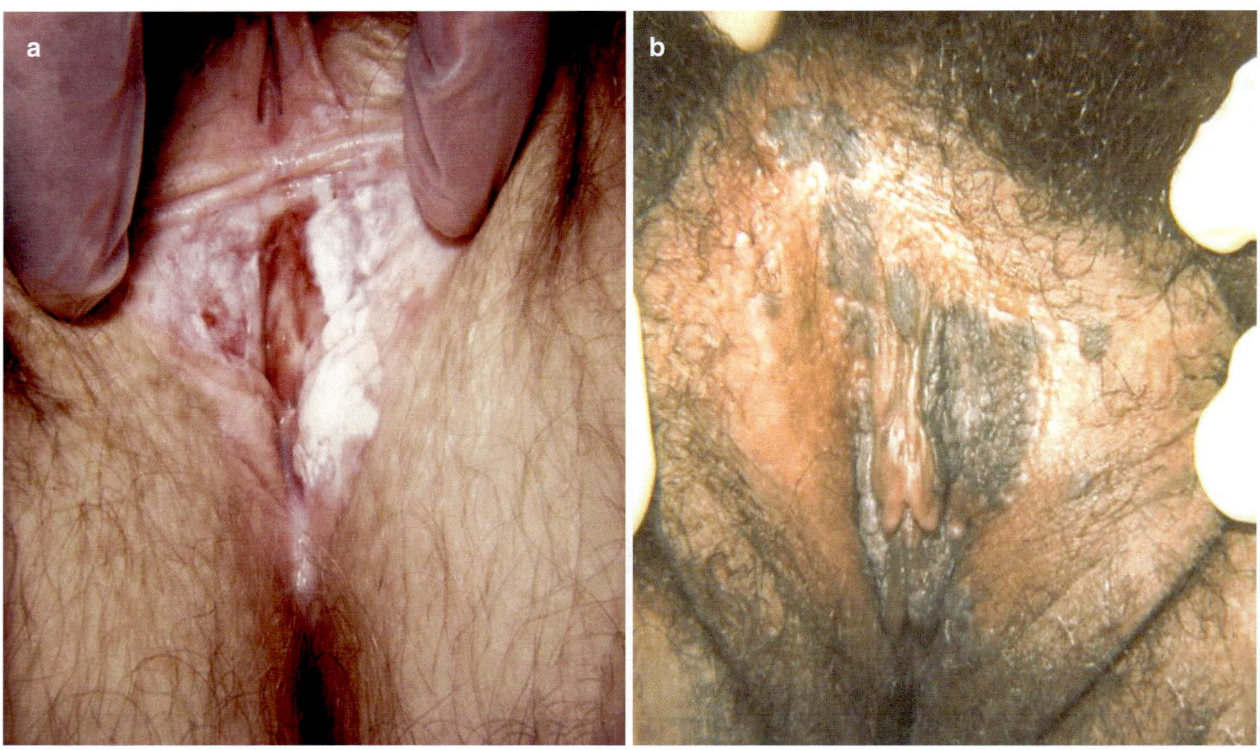

Fig. 5.13 Vulvar HSIL. The lesions present as a macule, papule, or exophytic growth with discoloration ranging from white (**a**), gray to red or pigmented (**b**). (Courtesy of Dr. Kenneth Hatch, University of Arizona)

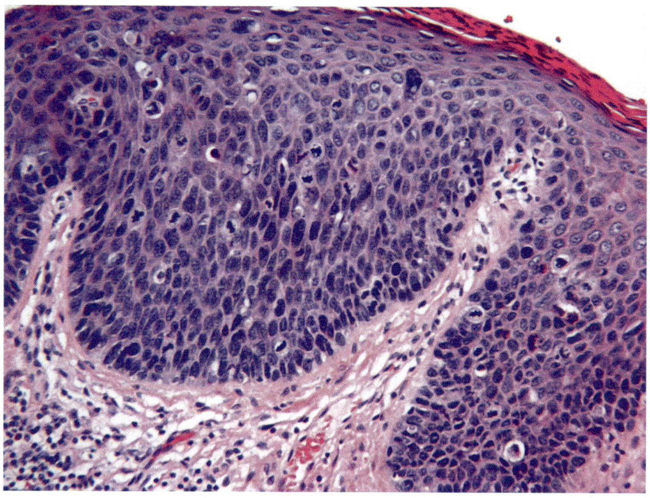

Fig. 5.14 HSIL, basaloid subtype. The basaloid, or undifferentiated, type mimics cervical HSIL; it exhibits a smooth (often keratotic) surface and is composed of a homogenous population of small, hyperchromatic cells filling the epidermis resulting in a striking blue appearance. Nuclear abnormalities exceed the bottom one-third of the epithelium and include cell crowding with high nuclear-to-cytoplasmic ratios, nuclear pleomorphism, hyperchromasia, and chromatin clumping. Mitotic figures and apoptotic bodies are usually readily identified and visible above the basal layer with a tendency to involve all levels of the epithelium (H&E, 200 ×)

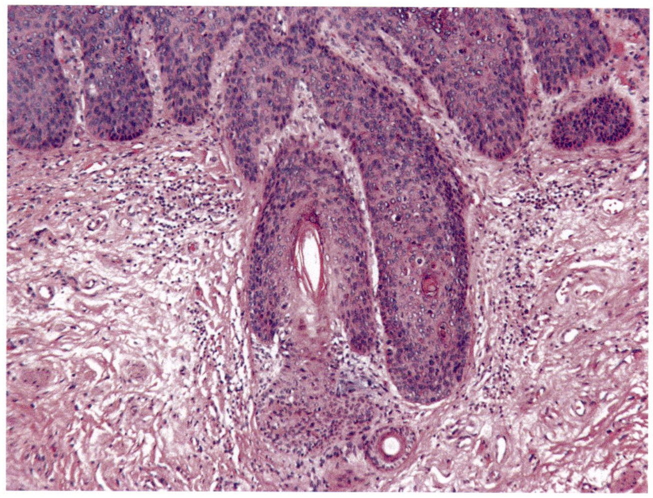

Fig. 5.15 HSIL involving adnexal structures of the labia majora (H&E, 100×)

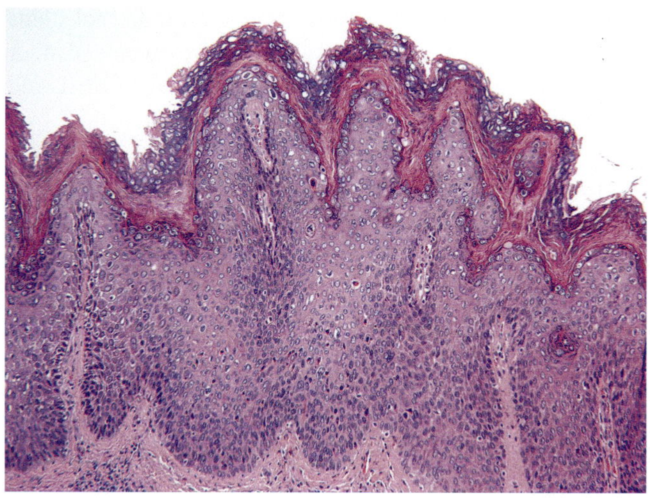

Fig. 5.16 HSIL, warty subtype. The warty type has a spiked (condylomatous) surface and dysplastic cells with more eosinophilic cytoplasm. Nuclear atypia, mitotic figures, and dyskeratotic cells are easily recognized and exceed the bottom one-third of the epithelium (H&E, 100×)

posed of a homogenous population of small, hyperchromatic cells filling the epidermis resulting in a striking blue appearance on low power (Fig. 5.14). In contrast, warty HSIL shows an undulating (condylomatous or spiked) surface with prominent parakeratosis and/or hyperkeratosis and is characterized by cells with eosinophilic cytoplasm and conspicuous nuclear pleomorphism (Fig. 5.16). Frequently, HSIL exhibits both warty and basaloid features. Rare variants of vulvar HSIL include pagetoid VIN and VIN with mucinous differentiation [42–44] (Fig. 5.17). Awareness of these rare variants of HSIL is needed and careful exclusion of extramammary Paget disease and its mimics should be undertaken (see Sect. 5.3.2.4).

5.2.3.3 Ancillary Studies

The diagnosis of vulvar HSIL is usually rendered on H&E without need for ancillary studies. Foremost, appropriate grossing and embedding are essential to yield well-oriented sections in vulvar specimens. In suboptimal scenarios, liberal ordering of deeper levels to achieve full face sections or to clarify tangential sectioning is advised. Strict adherence to diagnostic criteria and judicious utilization of the immunohistochemical stain p16 resolve most diagnostic dilemmas. In the lower female anogenital tract, p16 is recommended by LAST as the (only) biomarker of choice to support a diagnosis of HSIL [7]. p16 is recommended in cases for which the diagnosis of HSIL is considered but not unequivocally diagnostic on H&E impression alone. In this setting, a lesion with strong and diffuse (block) p16 positivity is considered diagnostic of vulvar HSIL while mimics will be negative (see Sect. 5.3.2.4 and Sect. 5.4 for full discussion). Other IHC stains (e.g., ProEx C and Ki-67/MIB-1) have been studied as alternatives to or in combination with p16 but do not improve performance characteristics [7].

5.2.3.4 Differential Diagnosis

Reactive Changes and Infection

A hyperplastic and markedly inflamed squamous epithelium can result in atypical changes that mimic HSIL in small biopsy specimens. An infectious etiology must be considered first. Viral cytopathic effect should be excluded on H&E or

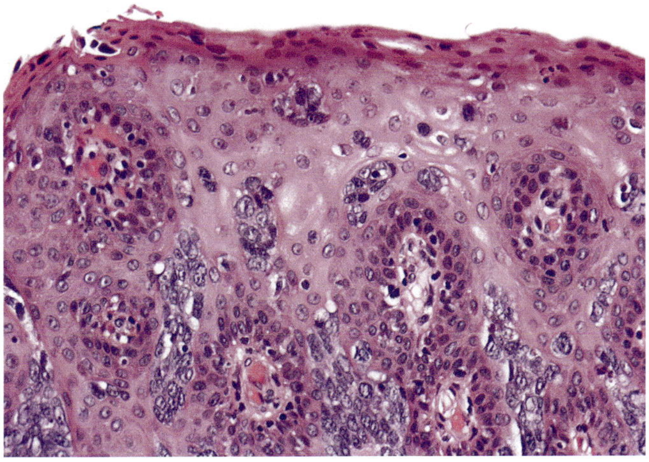

Fig. 5.17 HSIL, pagetoid variant. Dysplastic cells are distributed singly or in small clusters throughout the epithelium (H&E, 100×)

with help of ancillary stains (e.g., HSV stain). Special stains for fungal organisms (PAS or GMS) are recommended. A p16 immunohistochemical stain will be positive in HSIL and negative in reactive epithelial atypia.

Multinucleated Atypia of the Vulva

Multinucleation of vulvar epithelium is of uncertain etiology and can be seen particularly in young, reproductive age women. Clustering of multiple nuclei in the lower to mid layers of the epithelium is a key feature. Nuclear atypia is at most mild and nucleoli can be present.

Radiation Atypia

The patient's clinical history of radiation is essential. Interpretation of vulvar specimens in this setting is approached with much more caution. Morphologic features to support radiation atypia include multinucleation, bizarre cells with preserved N/C ratios, cytoplasmic vacuolization as well as stromal fibrosis and/or homogenization and atypia of endothelial cells.

Seborrheic Keratosis

Vulvar seborrheic keratosis (SK) is morphologically similar to cutaneous SK and is characterized by a proliferation of cytologically bland basaloid cells. Intraepithelial keratin-filled pseudo-horn cysts may be seen. In contrast to extragenital seborrheic keratoses, a substantial subset of vulvar seborrheic keratoses have been documented to harbor low-risk HPV subtypes, leading to a proposed designation of "seborrheic keratosis-like condyloma" by some authors [21–23]. Nuclear atypia, numerous mitotic figures, and dyskeratotic cells as seen in HSIL are notably absent (compare Figs. 5.7 and 5.14).

LSIL

Occasionally, small and tangentially sectioned biopsies raise the diagnostic dilemma of LSIL (VIN 1) or HSIL (VIN 2/3) with an equivocal initial H&E impression. Deeper levels and p16 staining are indicated in this scenario, with the latter supporting HSIL if block positivity is identified. The distinction between LSIL and HSIL is crucial because LSIL is in general managed expectantly and HSIL is conservatively excised.

Differentiated-Type VIN

Differentiated-type VIN (dVIN) (see full discussion in Sect. 5.2.4) can enter the differential diagnosis with HSIL (uVIN) in several scenarios. The (rare) basaloid variant of dVIN is morphologically indistinguishable from the (common) basaloid subtype of HSIL. Ordi et al. described four postmenopausal women with HPV negative precursor lesions characterized by a proliferation of basaloid cells filling the epithelium, resembling basaloid HSIL [45]. Nevertheless, by immunohistochemistry, these intraepithelial lesions were negative for p16 and strongly positive for p53, supporting a diagnosis of a dVIN variant. The warty subtype of HSIL can be mistaken for dVIN on low-power examination of a small biopsy because of its striking eosinophilic appearance. However, close examination shows near to full thickness atypia, which can be further supported by block positivity for p16. Similarly, HPV-associated lesions with superimposed LSC changes may impart a blander and "differentiated" look. But on high-power review, nuclear atypia extends above the lower third of the epithelium and a p16 stain is positive. Tandem p16 and p53 staining is therefore of value in select, challenging cases. Table 5.2 compares and contrasts key clinicopathologic features of HSIL (uVIN) and dVIN.

Condyloma with Treatment Effect

Condyloma with podophyllin effect can mimic HSIL. Podophyllin is a resin mixture from plants and has medicinal properties, including the treatment of genital warts [46]. The treatment effect is histologically most striking after 48 h and disappears by day 7. Key features are abundant necrotic keratinocytes and mitotic figures within the lower layers of the squamous epithelium. However, nuclear atypia is absent and an orderly maturation is maintained. Knowledge of recent treatment aids in the diagnostic distinction [47].

Pseudobowenoid Papulosis

Pseudobowenoid papulosis refers to condylomata, which exhibit degenerative cellular changes and prominent apoptosis in the upper layers of the epithelium while lacking nuclear atypia, apoptosis, or atypical mitoses in the lower layers.

The latter distinguishes it from HSIL or condyloma with podophyllin effect [48].

Extramammary Paget Disease of the Vulva and Mimics

Paget disease of the vulva is a glandular intraepithelial neoplasm, which predominantly affects postmenopausal Caucasian women. In contrast to Paget disease of the breast, an underlying malignancy is only rarely identified. Morphologically, the neoplastic glandular cells are distributed singly or in small aggregates throughout the squamous epithelium. The lesional cells are large and consist of eosinophilic to pale cytoplasm and nuclei with prominent nucleoli (Fig. 5.18). Intracytoplasmic mucin and/or lumens can be focally appreciated on high-power magnification. Involvement of adnexal structures and resection margins is common while true invasion into the dermis is rare [49]. On initial diagnosis, performance of ancillary stains (Table 5.3) is recommended to distinguish vulvar Paget disease from its mimics including pagetoid VIN, melanoma (in situ), or secondary Paget disease due to spread from a colorectal or urothelial primary [17, 42, 43, 50, 51].

Table 5.2 Comparison of key clinicopathologic features of HSIL (uVIN) and dVIN

Key features	HSIL (uVIN)	Differentiated-type VIN (dVIN)
Age	Younger cohort (fourth to seventh decade)	Older cohort (seventh to ninth decade)
Gross appearance	Well demarcated, synchronous or metachronous lesions	Poorly demarcated, solitary
Risk factors	Smoking SIL at other anogenital sites Immunosuppression	Vulvar dermatoses (LS, LSC)
Histopathology	Warty and/or basaloid Conspicuous full thickness atypia	Atypia confined to basal layer with abrupt maturation of upper layers
HPV status	Positive	Negative
Tp53 mutation	No	Yes
Immunophenotype	p16 positive p53 negative	p16 negative p53 positive
Treatment	Conservative excision	Conservative excision
Risk of disease progression to invasive carcinoma	Low	High

LS lichen sclerosus, *LSC* lichen simplex chronicus

Invasive Squamous Cell Carcinoma

Tangential sectioning of vulvar specimens can represent a diagnostic challenge in the distinction of HSIL from an (superficially) invasive squamous cell carcinoma. Moreover, adnexal structures on the labia majora are readily colonized by HSIL (as deep as several millimeters). Awareness of these phenomena is key to avoid misclassification as invasive squamous cell carcinoma. In these scenarios, adherence to strict criteria for invasion is essential. Histopathologic features of bone fide invasion include architectural complexity (irregular borders, lack of basement membrane), paradoxical maturation (budding of nests or individual tumor cells with striking eosinophilia compared to the adjacent in situ component), and stromal response (desmoplasia or brisk chronic inflammation). Comparison of involved to adjacent uninvolved adnexal structures is of value. Adnexal structures colonized by

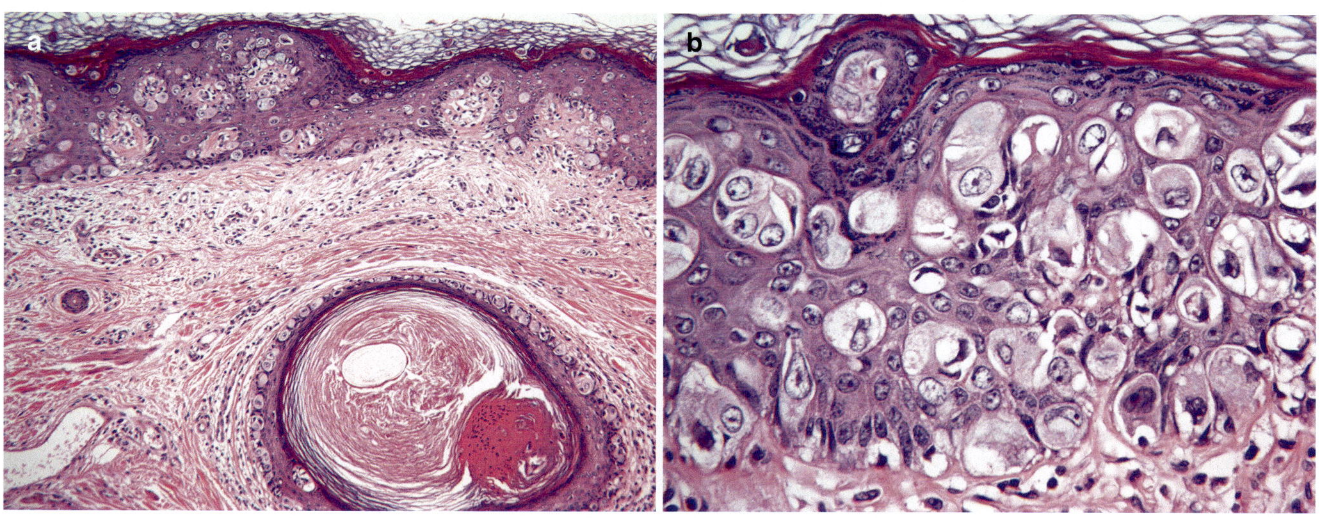

Fig. 5.18 Paget disease of the vulva. (**a**) Intraepithelial neoplastic glandular cells are distributed singly or in small clusters throughout the squamous epithelium. Note the extension into underlying adnexal structures, a frequent finding (H&E, 100×). (**b**) The lesional glandular cells are large and exhibit prominent nucleoli and abundant eosinophilic to pale cytoplasm (H&E, 400×)

Table 5.3 Extramammary Paget disease of the vulva and its mimics—summary of ancillary stains

	p16	p40 (or p63)	CK7	CK20	CDX-2	CEA	GCDFP	GATA-3	S-100	HMB45	Melan-A
Extramammary Paget disease	−/+	−	+	−/+	−	+	+	+	+/−	−	−
Secondary Paget disease due to colorectal primary	−	−	+/−	+	+	+/−	−	−	−	−	−
Secondary Paget disease due to urothelial primary	+/−	+	+	+	−	−	−	+	−	−	−
Melanoma (in situ)	−	−	−	−	−	−	−	−	+	+	+
Pagetoid HSIL	+	+	−	−	−	−	−	−	−	−	−

+ positive, − negative, *CEA* carcinoembryonic antigen, *GCDFP* gross cystic disease fluid protein

HSIL show an orderly, parallel arrangement, are well circumscribed, and lack a stromal response or budding nests with paradoxical maturation. If true invasion is present, accurate determination of depth of invasion is crucial and should follow established guidelines for measurement (see Sect. 3). However, despite established histologic criteria, Abdel-Mesih et al. noted that interobserver agreement among gynecologic pathologists is only fair in the determination of in situ or superficially invasive disease [52].

5.2.3.5 Prognosis and Management

Vulvar HSIL is a premalignant condition. Spontaneous regression is rare and has been described as a constellation of clinical features referred to as bowenoid papulosis, which presents as multifocal papular lesions in young adults typically in association with pregnancy [53–56]. Bowenoid papulosis is not a distinct pathologic entity and demonstrates morphologic features indistinguishable from HSIL.

HSIL's progression risk to invasive squamous cell carcinoma is much less common in comparison to women with dVIN (see below), ranging from 5 to 6% (treated) and 10 to 15% (untreated) [57]. Older women, immunocompromised states, or patients with large lesions are at much higher risk of progression or concurrent squamous cell carcinoma [58]. Risk-reducing measures for the development of HSIL include smoking cessation and immunization with the HPV vaccine.

Wide local excision (WLE) is the initial, preferred treatment of choice for vulvar HSIL, particularly when occult invasion cannot be excluded clinically [32]. Lesions are ideally excised with 0.5–1.0 cm margins. If there is no clinical concern for an occult squamous cell carcinoma, then alternative management options to WLE include local excision, laser ablation, and off-label use of topical imiquimod. Regardless of procedure, patients with a history of treated HSIL are not only at risk for recurrence but also vulvar cancer throughout life. Self-examination and close clinical monitoring with annual examinations of the vulva are essential. Recurrence rates after treatment range from 9% to 50%. Factors associated with an increased recurrence risk include smoking, multifocal distribution, positive margin status, and nonsurgical treatment [32].

5.2.4 Differentiated Vulvar Intraepithelial Neoplasia

5.2.4.1 Clinical Features

In contrast to HSIL, dVIN is the intraepithelial precursor lesion in the HPV-independent pathway and typically occurs in postmenopausal women as a subtle, solitary lesion. It can arise in and is clinically difficult to distinguish from vulvar dermatoses (e.g., lichen sclerosus, lichen simplex chronicus). dVIN is a high-grade intraepithelial lesion but represents only 2–10% of all VIN. While a prospective diagnosis of dVIN is rare, 80% of invasive squamous cell carcinomas contain an adjacent dVIN component. Possible explanations for this discrepancy are multifactorial and include its more subtle clinical appearance, a much more rapid disease progression (5–64 months) to invasive squamous cell carcinoma, misdiagnosis as a reactive condition, and poor interobserver agreement [16, 59]. Hence, recognition and accurate classification of a lesion as dVIN is essential.

5.2.4.2 Histopathologic Features

As described by Yang and Hart, dVIN is defined by a constellation of histopathologic features in the correct clinical setting (Table 5.4) [16]. The low power impression is that of an acanthotic and mature squamous epithelium which can be easily misclassified as a reactive lesion. Parakeratosis as well as elongated and anastomosing rete ridges are frequently observed. The atypia in dVIN is strictly confined to the (para) basal layer with abrupt maturation of the mid to upper layers of the squamous epithelium. Basal layer keratinocytes demonstrate architectural disarray and enlargement. Nuclei contain prominent nucleoli and abundant eosinophilic cytoplasm. Dyskeratosis, if present, includes premature maturation of basal layer keratinocytes or keratin pearl formation within the elongated rete ridges. Mitotic figures including atypical mitotic figures are present in the basal layer (Fig. 5.19). Van den Einden et al. listed the following five histomorphologic features (in order of diagnostic relevance) as strong indicators of a diagnosis of dVIN: (1) atypical mitotic figures in basal layer, (2) basal cellular atypia, (3) dyskeratosis, (4) prominent nucleoli, and (5) elongated and/or anastomosing

Table 5.4 Histologic features of differentiated VIN

Constellation of histologic features for a diagnosis of differentiated VIN
• Basal cellular atypia with maturation of upper layers of the epithelium
• Atypical mitoses in basal layer
• Dyskeratosis (premature maturation of keratinocytes or keratin pearl formation in rete)
• Prominent nucleoli
• Elongated and/or anastomosing rete ridges
• Epidermal thickening/hyperplasia
• Parakeratosis

rete ridges [59]. In addition, a survey of expert gynecologic and dermatopathologists found that basal layer atypia was (by consensus) the single histologic feature imperative for the diagnosis of dVIN [60]. Deemed equally important was the correct clinical setting (visible lesion, history of vulvar dermatoses or cancer, age (older than 40), or a persistent lesion unresponsive to steroids). This study also emphasized that ancillary immunohistochemical staining (e.g., p53) was not considered essential for the diagnosis.

Noteworthy is a recent description of a basaloid variant of dVIN. Ordi et al. described four cases, which on gross appearance and histomorphology alone were indistinguishable from HPV-associated HSIL/uVIN (full thickness proliferation of basaloid cells) [45]. However, these lesions were identified in older women, lacked detectable HPV, demonstrated a p53 positive/p16 negative immunophenotype, and predominantly evolved into well-differentiated keratinizing squamous cell carcinomas, all features in keeping with a dVIN variant.

Despite established criteria for the diagnosis of dVIN, poor interobserver agreement is readily acknowledged in the literature compounding the vexing nature of this entity. Van de Nieuwenhof et al. reviewed cases diagnosed as lichen sclerosus in women with and without progression to invasive squamous cell carcinoma; in women with progression 42% of lichen sclerosus cases were retrospectively reclassified as dVIN [61]. Van den Einden et al. showed the agreement among pathologists in training, general surgical pathologists, and gynecologic pathologists to range from poor to moderate with increased agreement following an educational session of the diagnostic criteria for dVIN [59]. However, only pathologists with gynecologic subspecialty training were shown to have substantial agreement and only after completion of the educational session. These studies underscore the challenge of this diagnosis. The pathologist is encouraged to study the histologic features of dVIN in the more commonly encountered resection specimens of well-differentiated keratinizing squamous cell carcinomas of older women. Intradepartmental or inter-institutional consultation with a gynecologic pathologist or dermatopathologist before sign out of a biopsy with dVIN is also encouraged. If no consensus is achieved or the histologic features fall short of dVIN, a diagnosis of "squamous cell hyperplasia with atypia, see comment" is certainly prudent. Particularly in the elderly, vulvar lesions with abnormal maturation, no matter how cytologically bland, warrant close clinical follow-up. Given the rapid progression of dVIN to invasive squamous cell carcinoma, it is imperative that the pathologist not only conveys to the clinician the meaning of this rare diagnosis (a high-grade intraepithelial lesion requiring excision) but also the importance of close clinical monitoring with biopsy of any new or evolving lesions.

5.2.4.3 Ancillary Studies

An increase in research-based publications and review articles over the last decade has contributed to the increased recognition of dVIN [2, 17, 23, 33, 59–65]. Differentiated VIN must be distinguished from HSIL/uVIN and vulvar inflammatory dermatoses [66]. No single biomarker reliably establishes a diagnosis of dVIN; it remains a histologic diagnosis. This concept was underscored by a survey of expert vulvar pathologists, in which no immunohistochemical stain emerged as a consensus biomarker for the diagnosis of dVIN [60]. However, the published literature to date supports the use of few select ancillary stains. By immunohistochemistry, dVIN demonstrates a p53 positive/p16 negative immunophenotype. A positive p53 stain is defined as strong and diffuse nuclear reactivity limited to the basal and suprabasilar layers or complete absence of nuclear staining (null pattern) compared to wild-type p53 labeling of nonlesional tissue. Ki-67 (MIB-1) will show an elevated proliferation index, also in a (supra)basilar rather than full thickness staining pattern. In challenging cases, tandem application of these ancillary stains can be informative but the pathologist must be aware of interpretative pitfalls (see Sect. 5.3.2.4 and Sect. 5.4 for full discussion).

5.2.4.4 Differential Diagnosis

HSIL

HPV-associated VIN (HSIL/uVIN) enters in the differential diagnosis with dVIN, particularly when the warty subtype or superimposed changes of LSC are present. While these lesions demonstrate more eosinophilia and may mimic dVIN on low power, pleomorphism is present throughout the entire lesion (full thickness atypia), albeit less striking in the upper layers. In addition, p16 staining is positive while p53 is either negative or accentuated (see Sect. 5.4). Therefore, tandem p16 and p53 staining is of value to avoid misdiagnosis of dVIN, particularly in small biopsies [62].

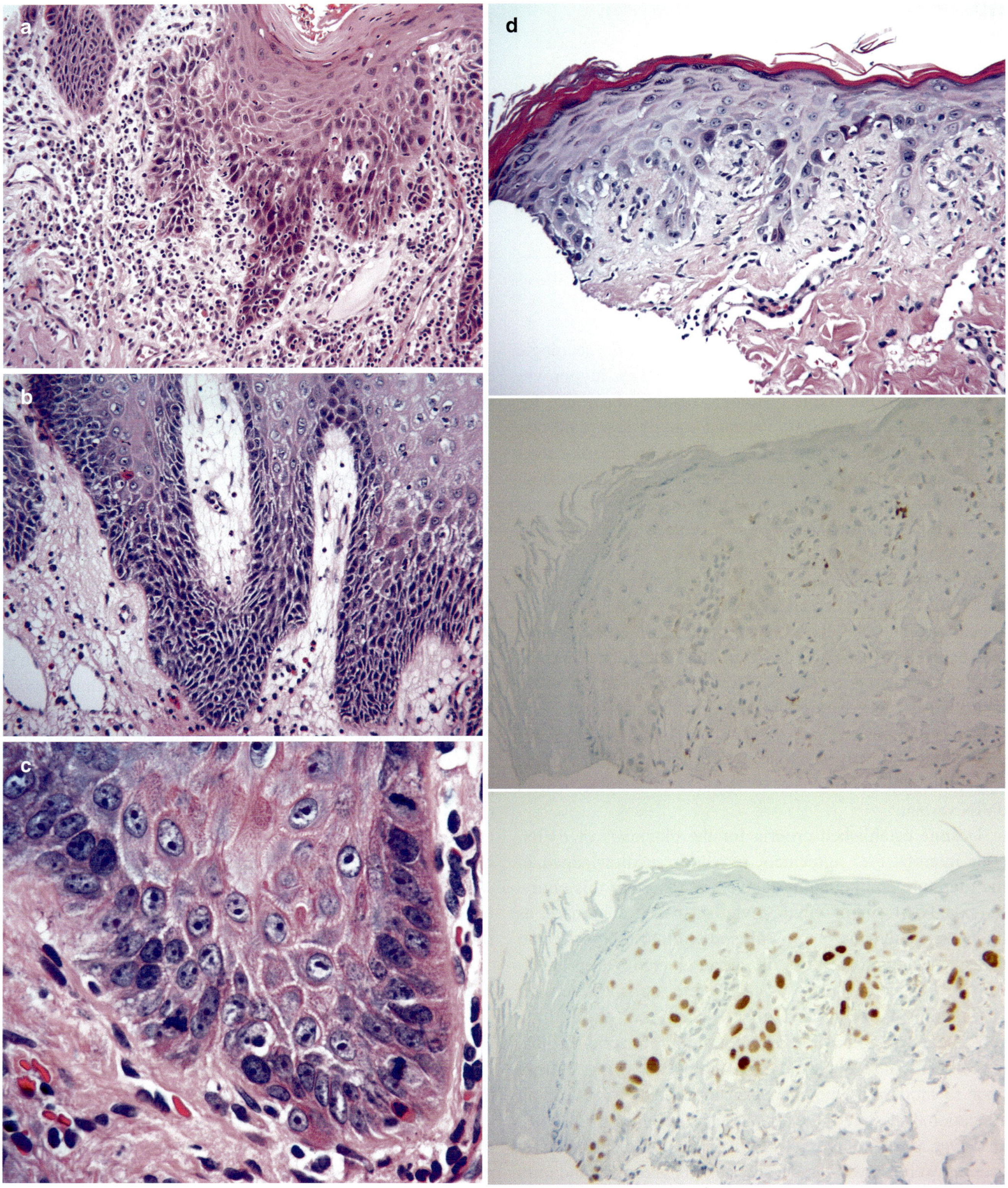

Fig. 5.19 Differentiated VIN. (**a**) Acanthotic and mature squamous epithelium with overlying parakeratosis. As the atypia is restricted to the (para)basal layer, dVIN can readily be mistaken for reactive lesion on low power (H&E, 200×). (**b**) Elongated and anastomosing rete in dVIN. The basal layer is characterized by nuclear atypia, mitotic figures, and frequent dyskeratotic cells (H&E, 200×). (**c**) (Inset) High-power examination of the basal layer further supports the constellation of histologic features for dVIN including marked nuclear atypia, prominent nucleoli, mitotic figures, dyskeratotic cells, and premature maturation of keratinocytes (H&E, 600×). (**d**) Another example of dVIN. The diagnosis is supported by the constellation of histologic features (note the marked basilar atypia) and the p53+/p16− immunophenotype (inset) (H&E and IHC, 200×)

Lichen Simplex Chronicus

LSC is a histologic pattern of vulvar dystrophy characterized by variably elongated rete, hypergranulosis, hyperkeratosis and/or parakeratosis, and scattered chronic inflammatory cells within the dermis (Fig. 5.12). It lacks the conspicuous basilar atypia of dVIN. p53 by immunohistochemistry can demonstrate an increased staining but the staining intensity is weak and the labeling index within the basal cells is low. Special stains (PAS or GMS) are recommended to exclude a fungal infection. Of note, LSC can be a secondary histologic pattern superimposed onto dVIN, lichen sclerosus, or other neoplastic or inflammatory disorders due to rubbing or scratching of the lesion (Fig. 5.20).

Lichen Sclerosus

Lichen sclerosus (LS) is an inflammatory dermatosis of the vulva that presents in a bimodal distribution (prepubertal or postmenopausal women). Clinically, early LS presents as vulvar erythema and thinning of the mucosa starting around the clitoris and spreading in a figure eight configuration. Over time, the affected skin becomes atrophic, porcelain white, and is accompanied by scarring and stenosis of the introitus.

"Early" changes of LS are histologically subtle and are characterized by a lichenoid chronic inflammatory infiltrate at the epidermal-dermal junction (Fig. 5.21) [67]. Sclerosis is either absent or focal and the morphologic pattern overlaps with other lichenoid dermatoses, such as lichen planus (LP). Well-developed (classic) LS is characterized by an atrophic epidermis, loss of rete ridges, a subepithelial band of homogenized and hyalinized eosinophilic collagen bundles with entrapped, delicate, small vessels, and a lichenoid inflammatory (lymphocyte predominant) infiltrate below the sclerosis (Fig. 5.22). No basal atypia is present. Scratching and rubbing of the lesion results in LS with superimposed changes of LSC [68]. LS is treated with topical steroids.

Women with lichen sclerosus have a very low (2–5%) risk of progression to invasive squamous cell carcinoma of the vulva [61, 69–73]. In resection specimens of such cancers, lichen sclerosus and dVIN are frequently seen adjacent to the invasive component and are touted to represent a continuum in the HPV-independent pathway to squamous cell carcinoma. While classic LS is a relatively straightforward diagnosis in daily practice, some cases of LS display "atypical" features (parakeratosis, conspicuous dyskeratosis, hyperplasia, or basal atypia). Both LS and atypical LS can demonstrate increased labeling with p53. Whether atypical LS represents a distinct histopathologic entity with an increased progression risk compared to classic LS is controversial. The histomorphologic overlap between LS with superimposed "reactive" changes, atypical LS or a "relaxed" interpretation of dVIN underscores the vexing nature of this disease spectrum which is plagued by interobserver variability and few, albeit polarizing, publications [61, 71, 74, 75]. Certainly, LS (with or without atypia) should be closely monitored clinically, re-biopsied upon evolution, or conservatively excised if unresponsive to steroids [72].

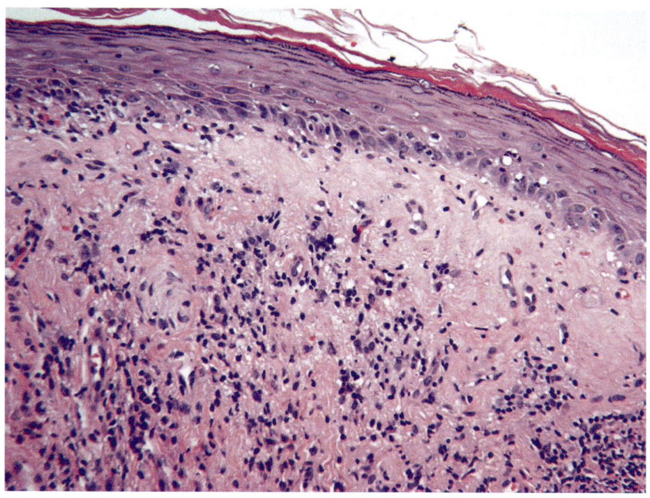

Fig. 5.21 Early lichen sclerosus. A lichenoid chronic inflammatory infiltrate is present at the epidermal-dermal junction and in the dermis. Sclerosis is scant (H&E, 200×)

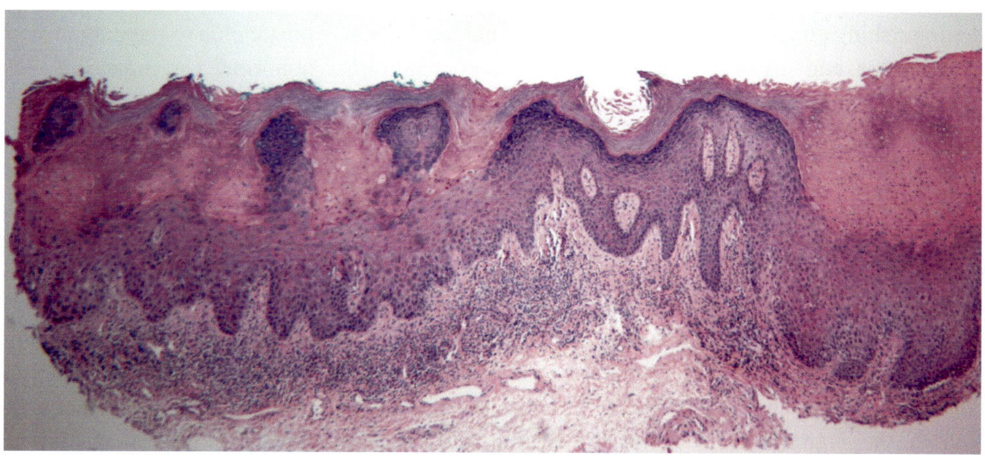

Fig. 5.20 Differentiated VIN with superimposed changes of lichen simplex chronicus (H&E, 20×)

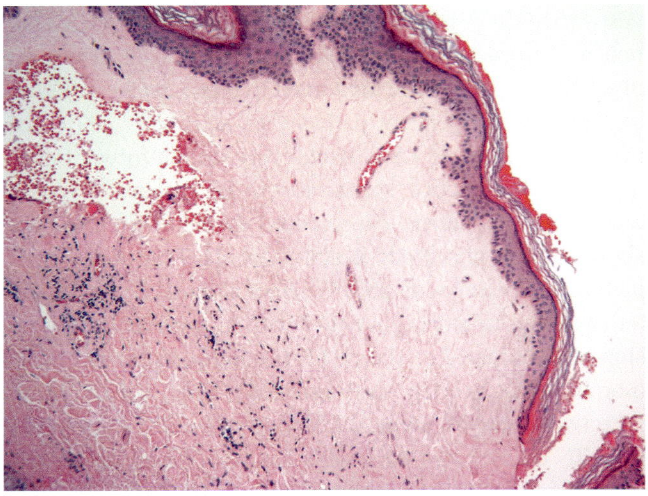

Fig. 5.22 Lichen sclerosus. An atrophic epidermis, loss of rete ridges, a subepithelial band of sclerosis with entrapped, delicate, small vessels, and a lichenoid inflammatory infiltrate below the sclerosis are all classic features of well-developed lichen sclerosus. No basal atypia is present (H&E, 200×)

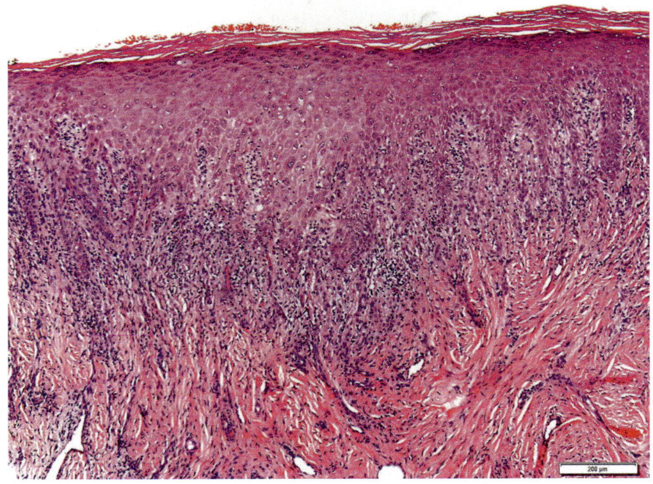

Fig. 5.23 Lichen planus. LP is characterized by compact orthokeratosis, hypergranulosis, saw tooth rete ridges, dyskeratotic cells at epidermal-dermal junction (Civatte bodies), basal vacuolar change, and a band-like lymphocyte predominant inflammatory infiltrate in the dermis, which obscures the basal epithelial layer (H&E, 100×)

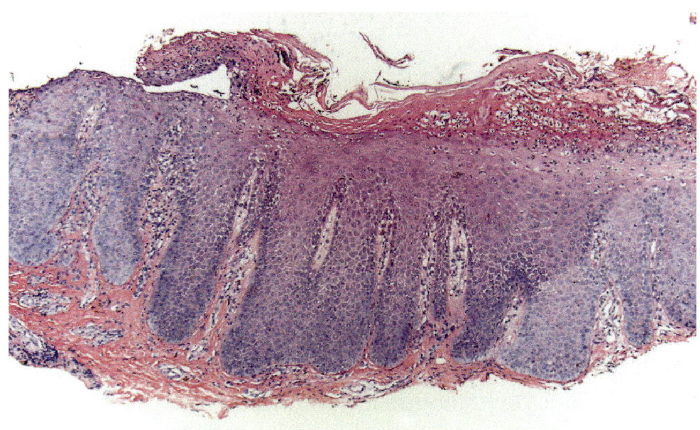

Fig. 5.24 Psoriasis. Microscopically, psoriasis is characterized by uniformly elongated rete (regular acanthosis) with loss of the granular layer. Parakeratotic plaques with neutrophils (Munro microabscesses) are a diagnostic clue to the diagnosis (H&E, 100×)

Lichen Planus

Lichen planus (LP) is a chronic cell-mediated immune reaction resulting in cytotoxicity to keratinocytes. Vulvovaginal LP is commonly associated with oral lesions. It presents as erosive, papulosquamous, or rarely hypertrophic lesions. Erosive LP is most common and consists of erythematous eroded epithelium with lacy reticulated plaques. The lesions are symmetric and improve with steroids. Microscopically, the classic features of papulosquamous LP include wedge-shaped hypergranulosis, compact orthokeratosis, saw tooth rete ridges, dyskeratotic cells at the epidermal-dermal junction (Civatte bodies), basal vacuolar change, and a band-like lymphocyte predominant inflammatory infiltrate in the dermis which obscures the basal epithelial layer (Fig. 5.23). Histologically, erosive LP may show ulceration and erosion, but careful inspection of any intact epithelium should show some of the aforementioned criteria; it can also demonstrate overlapping features with dVIN [76]. Moreover, LP can show strong confluent positive staining with p53 [76]. Key distinguishing characteristics from dVIN include the clinical presentation and improvement with topical corticosteroids [66, 76].

Psoriasis

Psoriasis is a chronic, relapsing disease that can involve the vulva. In its classic form, it is clinically easily recognized due to well-circumscribed, scaly, plaque-like lesions. In contrast, the inverse form of psoriasis is poorly demarcated. Lesions exhibit erythema, lack overt scales, and have a proclivity for skin folds. Microscopically, psoriasis is characterized by uniformly elongated rete (regular acanthosis) with loss of the granular layer (Fig. 5.24) [66]. Parakeratotic plaques with neutrophils (Munro microabscesses) are a diagnostic clue to the diagnosis. Absence of basal layer atypia or abnormal keratinization excludes dVIN. A negative PAS or GMS stain excludes a fungal infection.

Reactive Changes and Infection

Patients with vulvovaginal candidiasis present with pruritus, vaginal soreness, dyspareunia, and abnormal vaginal discharge. Microscopically, variable spongiosis, parakeratosis, hyperplasia, and inflammation (neutrophil dominant) are present. While reactive changes can produce cytologic atypia including nucleoli, reactive cells should be uniformly enlarged, display smooth nuclear membranes, and lack the tinctorial differences and basal atypia of dVIN. A PAS or

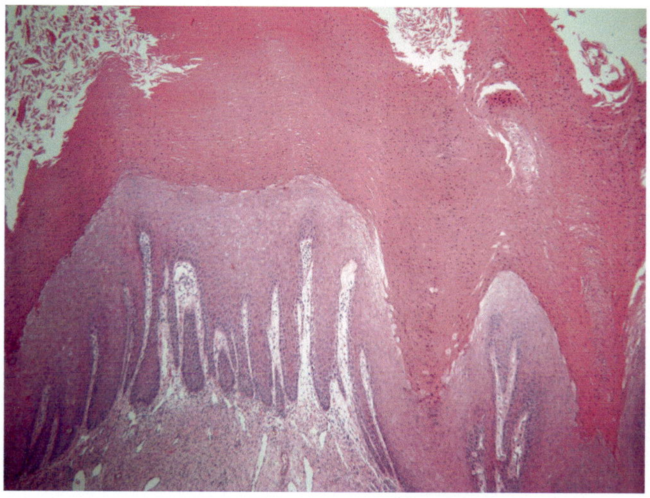

Fig. 5.25 Vulvar acanthosis with altered differentiation. VAAD is characterized by marked acanthosis with a variable verruciform growth pattern, pallor of the superficial squamous epithelium with loss of the granular layer, and stacked parakeratosis. It is a risk factor for the development of vulvar cancer and requires close clinical follow-up (H&E, 40×)

GMS stain is a helpful adjunct stain to highlight fungal elements in support of the diagnosis (Fig. 5.11) [66].

Differentiated Exophytic Vulvar Intraepithelial Lesions (DE-VIL)

In 2004, Nasciemento et al. coined the term vulvar acanthosis with altered differentiation (VAAD) to describe vulvar lesions with the following histologic triad: (1) marked acanthosis with a variable verruciform growth pattern, (2) pallor of the superficial squamous epithelium with loss of the granular layer, and (3) stacked parakeratosis (Fig. 5.25) [4]. These lesions are HPV-independent, occur in older women (seventh to ninth decade), and are closely associated with LS and verruciform LSC. More importantly, they represent a risk factor for the development of well-differentiated squamous cell carcinomas of the vulva and are a candidate precursor to verrucous carcinoma. Key distinguishing characteristics from dVIN include lack of nuclear atypia and presence of epithelial cell pallor in the upper layers. VAAD requires close clinical follow-up with biopsy of any new or evolving lesions.

In 2017, Watkins et al. studied verruciform lesions of the vulva including VAAD, verruciform LSC, and atypical verruciform hyperplasias [3]. These lesions presented in predominantly postmenopausal women and were associated with progression to HPV negative, well- to moderately differentiated keratinizing squamous cell carcinomas. Based on their results, Watkins et al. proposed the umbrella term "differentiated exophytic vulvar intraepithelial lesion" (DE-VIL) for this unique cohort which is characterized by: (1) verruciform morphology, (2) abnormalities in keratinocyte differentiation, (3) absence of conspicuous basal atypia, (4) absence of *Tp53* mutations, and (5) a high frequency of *PIK3CA* mutations. These criteria set it apart from verruciform presentations of HSIL/uVIN and dVIN. Of utmost interest is the identification of a high frequency of *PIK3CA* and *ARID2* mutations and a striking absence of *Tp53* mutations in this cohort. Watkins et al. theorized that the PI3K/AKT/mTOR pathway may potentially be a third (less common) pathway to squamous cell carcinomas of the vulva (Fig. 5.1). Currently DE-VIL is considered a risk factor for the development of vulvar cancer and requires close clinical follow-up. Whether DE-VIL represents an immediate precursor (akin to HSIL/uVIN or dVIN) in a third pathway to invasive vulvar cancer requires further studies.

Verrucous Carcinoma

Verrucous carcinoma is an extremely well-differentiated squamous cell carcinoma of older women. It is not associated with HPV infection. Notably, by definition, minimal to no epithelial atypia is present. The invasive front is broad, bulbous, and pushing rather than infiltrative. Verrucous carcinoma can be a challenging biopsy interpretation, particularly in a superficial sample, and bone fide invasion is essential for the diagnosis. Correlation with clinical impression and size of the lesion is also of value (see Sect. 3).

5.2.4.5 Prognosis and Management

Like HSIL, dVIN is a high-grade intraepithelial lesion requiring wide local excision [32]. In contrast to HPV-related SIL, 85% of patients diagnosed with dVIN have prior, concurrent or subsequent invasive squamous cell carcinoma [77]. Furthermore, disease progression to vulvar cancer is relatively rapid (ranging from 5 to 64 months) [77, 78], recurrence rates are higher [79], and survival from associated squamous cell carcinoma is lower [80]. Hence, accurate classification of dVIN on a vulvar biopsy is essential. Risk factors for development of dVIN include a history of inflammatory vulvar dermatoses; in particular, women with lichen sclerosus have a small risk of progression to invasive squamous cell carcinoma and require close clinical monitoring [81, 82].

5.3 Squamous Cell Carcinoma

5.3.1 Clinical Features

Squamous cell carcinoma of the vulva is an uncommon gynecologic cancer. It is an invasive epithelial malignancy with varying degrees of squamous differentiation. The majority of vulvar cancers (>90%) are squamous cell carcinomas (vSCC). Depending on the size and location of the lesion, patients can be either asymptomatic or present with pruritus, pain, bleeding, dysuria/

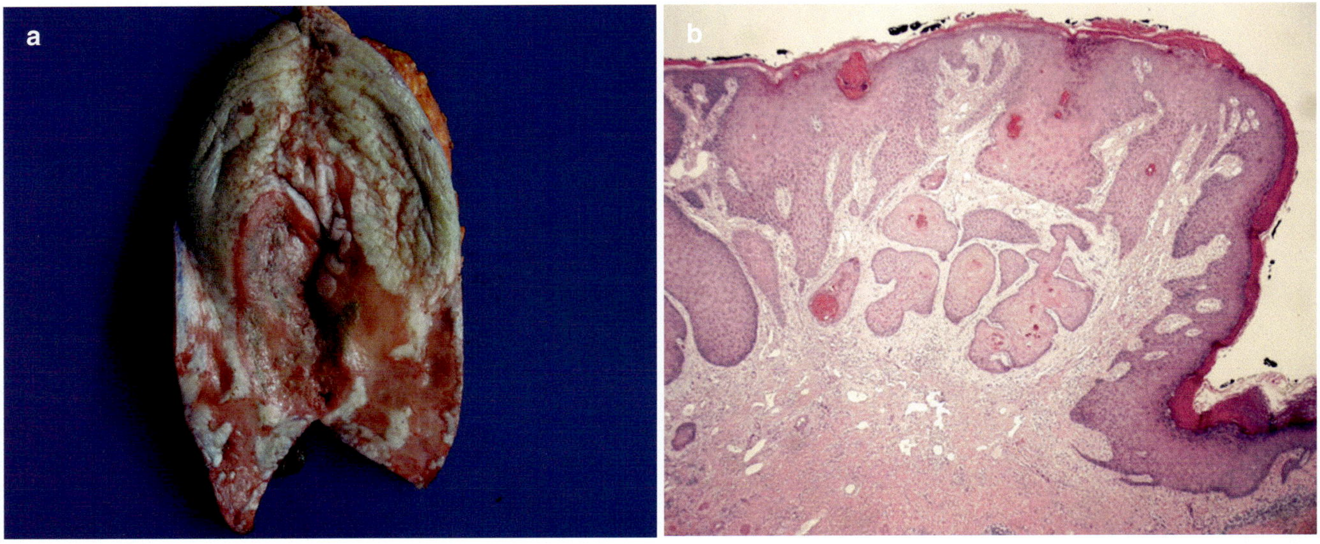

Fig. 5.26 Squamous cell carcinoma. (**a**) Clinical and (**b**) microscopic image of an invasive vulvar squamous cell carcinoma (H&E, 40×)

dyspareunia, or a malodorous discharge. vSCC varies in gross appearance from plaque-like, nodular, verruciform to ulcerated (Fig. 5.26). Clinical presentation and histopathology of vSCC is also influenced by HPV status. Squamous cell carcinoma arising through the HPV-dependent pathway affects younger women with a history of smoking, immunosuppression, HPV-driven VIN, or dysplasia at other anogenital sites. In contrast, HPV-independent vSCC has a predilection for older women and often co-exists with chronic vulvar inflammatory conditions (e.g., lichen sclerosus) and differentiated VIN (Fig. 5.1) [8].

5.3.2 Histopathologic Features

5.3.2.1 Superficially Invasive Squamous Cell Carcinoma

According to LAST, a superficially invasive squamous cell carcinoma (SISCCA) of the vulva fulfills the American Joint Committee on Cancer (AJCC)/International Union against Cancer (UICC) and International Federation of Gynecology and Obstetrics (FIGO) criteria for a pT1a/stage IA tumor (Table 5.5) [7, 83]. SISCCA is defined as ≤2 cm in size, confined to the vulva or perineum with an invasive component of ≤1 mm. No clinically suspicious regional lymph nodes or metastatic disease should be present. Patients with SISCCA have an excellent prognosis and are treated with conservative surgical excision without lymphadenectomy [84]. Before making a diagnosis of SISCCA, the pathologist should ask the following questions:

- Is invasion in fact established?
- Is the measurement of tumor size and depth of invasion accurate?
- Is the tumor completely excised?
- Is lymph-vascular invasion present?

Is Invasion in Fact Established?

Histopathologic features of bone fide invasion include architectural complexity (irregular borders, lack of basement membrane), paradoxical maturation (budding of nests or individual tumor cells with striking eosinophilia compared to the adjacent in situ component), and stromal response (desmoplasia or brisk chronic inflammation) (Fig. 5.27). However, invasion can at times be difficult to establish in vulvar specimens. Despite histologic criteria for invasion, Abdel-Mesih et al. noted that interobserver agreement among gynecologic pathologists is only fair in the determination of in situ or superficially invasive disease [52]. Limiting factors in the evaluation include tangential sectioning, VIN involvement of adnexal structures, and prominent inflammation obscuring the epithelial-stromal interface. Mimics (pseudoinvasion) such as pseudoepitheliomatous hyperplasia or artifactual displacement of squamous epithelium due to previous biopsy should also be excluded.

Tangential Sectioning of VIN

Tangentially sectioned VIN appears as nests of cells within the superficial portions of the stroma (Fig. 5.28). The nests of VIN are well circumscribed with round borders. Frequently, a thin eosinophilic band of basement membrane material can be seen enveloping each individual nest. The cells remain homogeneous and mirror their overlying in situ component. No overt features of invasion (as described above) are present. Performance of deeper levels is helpful; frequently connection with the overlying epithelium can be established.

Table 5.5 Summary of current FIGO and TNM staging of vulvar carcinoma [69]

FIGO stage	pT	pN	pM	Definition
Stage I	pT1	N0	M0	Tumor confined to vulva and/or perineum
IA	pT1a	N0	M0	≤2 cm in size with DOI of ≤1 mm
IB	pT1b	N0	M0	>2 cm in size or any size with DOI >1 mm
Stage II	pT2	N0	M0	Tumor of any size with extension to adjacent perineal structures: lower/distal third of urethra or vagina, anal involvement
Stage III	pT1 or T2	N1 or N2	M0	Tumor of any size with inguinofemoral lymph node involvement
Stage IIIA	pT1 or T2	N1a or N1b	M0	N1a: 1–2 LN metastasis <5 mm N1b: 1 LN metastasis ≥5 mm
Stage IIIB	pT1 or T2	N2a or b	M0	N2a: ≥3 LN metastasis, each <5 mm N2b: ≥2 LN metastasis, ≥5 mm
Stage IIIC	pT1 or T2	N2c	M0	N2c: extracapsular spread
Stage IV	pT1, T2, or T3	N3 or any N	M0 or M1	Tumor extends to other regional or distant sites
Stage IVA	pT1, T2	N3	M0	Tumor of any size with fixed or ulcerated lymph node metastasis
Stage IVA	pT3	Any N	M0	Tumor of any size with extension to: upper/proximal two-thirds of urethra or vagina, bladder or rectal mucosa or fixed to pelvic bone ± nodal disease
Stage IVB	Any T	Any N	M1	Distant metastasis (includes pelvic lymph nodes)

T primary tumor, *N* regional lymph node, *M* distant metastasis, *LN* lymph node

VIN Involvement of Adnexal Structures

Adnexal structures on the labia majora are readily colonized by VIN (as deep as several millimeters) (Fig. 5.15). Adnexal structures colonized by VIN show an orderly, parallel arrangement, are well circumscribed, and lack a stromal response or budding tumor cells with paradoxical maturation. The cells colonizing the adnexal structures are cytologically similar to the overlying in situ component. Comparison to adjacent uninvolved adnexal structures is of value.

Pseudoepitheliomatous Hyperplasia

Pseudoepitheliomatous hyperplasia (PEH) is a histologic pattern characterized by an acanthotic squamous epithelium with associated dermal fibrosis. However, no to minimal cytologic atypia is present and mitotic figures, if present, are rare. Perineural and lymph-vascular invasion are notably absent. In the vulva, PEH has been associated with granular cell tumor, lichen sclerosus, immunocompromised status, and infection [85–88].

Artifactual Displacement of Squamous Epithelium

On occasion, displaced fragments of squamous epithelium are identified in the stroma. Displacement is favored if the cytologic appearance of the epithelium is bland (non-neoplastic) and/or biopsy site changes are present. Deeper levels are also of value. Some seemingly displaced fragments connect readily to the overlying squamous epithelium in deeper sections.

Is the Measurement of Tumor Size and Depth of Invasion Accurate?

For tumors confined to the vulva and/or perineum (pT1), both tumor size (≤2 or >2 cm) and depth of invasion (≤1

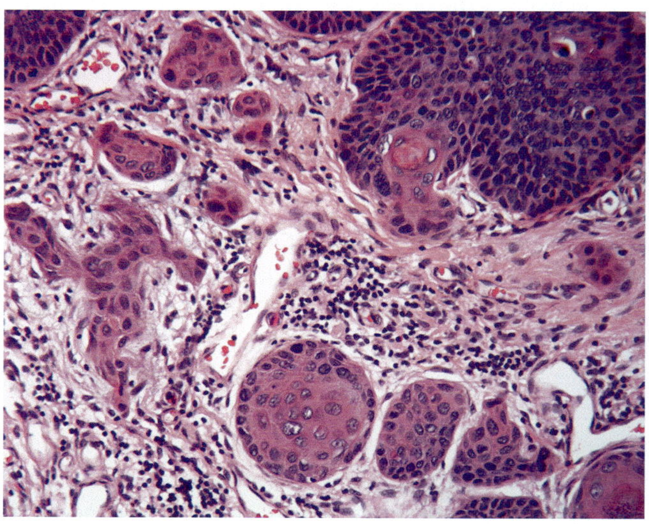

Fig. 5.27 Superficial invasion from overlying HSIL (uVIN). Invasive nests are characterized by paradoxical maturation and a focal stromal desmoplastic response (H&E, 200×)

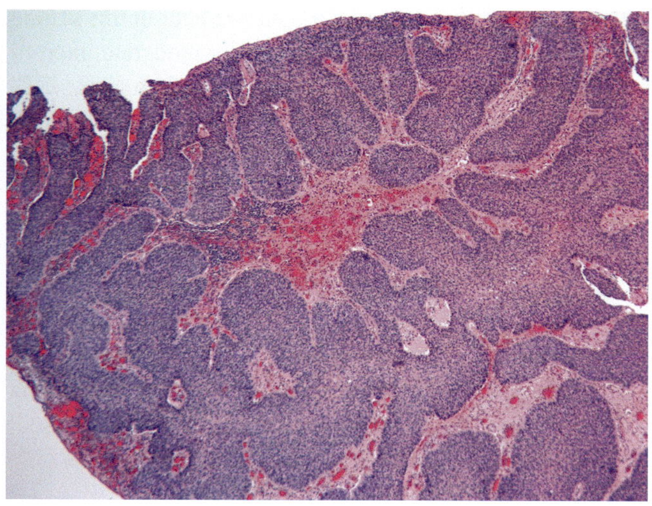

Fig. 5.28 HSIL (uVIN), tangentially sectioned. The nests connect and resemble the overlying in situ component. Note the lack of paradoxical maturation or stromal response (H&E, 100×)

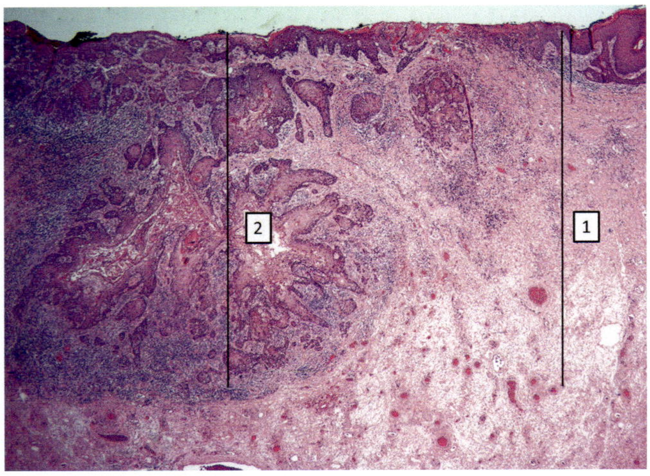

Fig. 5.29 Measurement of invasion in vulvar squamous cell carcinoma. Depth of invasion [1] is measured from the adjacent most superficial dermal papillae (epithelial-stromal interface) to the deepest point of invasion. Tumor thickness [2] is measured from the surface (even if ulcerated) of the tumor to the deepest point of invasion. If the surface is extensively keratinized, the bottom of the granular layer is used as a starting point. Tumor thickness can be reported in addition to DOI or in lieu of DOI (in difficult cases) (H&E, 20×)

or >1 mm) are important (Table 5.5). Accurate measurements are crucial because pT1a tumors are excised conservatively while pT1b tumors are treated with more extensive surgery and regional (femoral and inguinal) lymph node dissection. The latter therapeutic strategy carries significant morbidity, including wound dehiscence, infection, and lymphedema. Measurement of depth of invasion (DOI) should be given in millimeters and follow established guidelines. For vSCC, the tumor is measured from the adjacent most superficial dermal papillae (epithelial-stromal interface) to the deepest point of invasion (Fig. 5.29). If DOI appears superficial, an ocular micrometer should be utilized. Reproducibility studies for DOI measurement in this setting are sparse with one publication reporting moderate interobserver agreement among gynecologic pathologists [52]. Tumor thickness can be provided in lieu of DOI in difficult cases but is not a staging parameter [89–91]. Tumor thickness is measured from the surface of the tumor to the deepest point of invasion (Fig. 5.29). If the tumor surface displays keratinization, tumor thickness is measured from the bottom of the granular layer [92].

Is the Tumor Completely Excised?

The term superficially invasive squamous cell carcinoma should only be used if the lesion has been completely excised.

Is Lymph-Vascular Space Invasion Present?

The pathology report should include the presence or absence of lymph-vascular invasion (LVI) (Table 5.6). While LVI does not factor into the determination of stage, it predicts the risk of nodal spread [93–95]. In SISCCA without LVI, the risk of nodal disease is essentially zero [84]. Sentinel node excision may be utilized in cases with clinically suspicious lymph nodes or LVI [95].

Table 5.6 Reporting of vulvar squamous cell carcinoma [69]

Pathology report: squamous cell carcinoma of the vulva	
Essential elements	Optional (but informative) elements
• Histologic type and grade • Tumor size (in cm)[a] • Depth of invasion (in mm)[b] • LVI • Margin status (distance in mm) • Lymph nodes (if applicable) – Number, size, extranodal extension of metastasis	• Background VIN, vulvar dystrophy • Pattern of invasion (infiltrative or pushing) • Stromal response (fibromyxoid) • Perineural invasion

[a]Tumor size should also be correlated clinically
[b]DOI should be measured from the adjacent most superficial dermal papillae to the deepest point of invasion. Tumor thickness can be provided in addition to or in lieu of DOI but is not a staging parameter

5.3.2.2 Histologic Types

Keratinizing Squamous Cell Carcinoma

Keratinizing squamous cell carcinoma of the vulva is the most common histologic subtype (65–80%). It is a well- to moderately differentiated malignancy characterized by tumor cells with abundant eosinophilic cytoplasm, abnormal keratinization, and keratin pearl formation (Fig. 5.30). In resection specimens, differentiated VIN and lichen sclerosus are frequently identified adjacent to the invasive component (Fig. 5.31).

Non-keratinizing Squamous Cell Carcinoma

This subtype of squamous cell carcinoma lacks overt keratinization or keratin pearl formation and arises predominantly in a background of HPV-driven vulvar dysplasia. Due to its poorly differentiated appearance, adjunct immunohistochemical stains are sometimes required to support the diagnosis.

Basaloid and Warty Squamous Cell Carcinoma

Basaloid and warty SCC resemble their in-situ counterparts (basaloid and warty HSIL) [96]. These tumors typically arise in association with hr-HPV infection (e.g., HPV 16) in patients with a history of or concurrent anogenital HSIL. Basaloid SCC is characterized by small, uniform, immature tumor cells with high N/C ratios growing in sheets, nests, and cords. Keratinization can be focal. Larger tumor islands may show central comedo-type necrosis (Fig. 5.32). The tumor nests tend to invade in a pushing manner and are frequently surrounded by a brisk lymphoplasmacytic response. In contrast to basaloid SCC, warty (condylomatous) SCC has a spiked/papillary and hyperkeratotic surface. It exhibits conspicuous nuclear pleomorphism, koilocytosis, and keratin pearl formation (Fig. 5.33).

Verrucous Carcinoma

Verrucous carcinoma (VC) is an extremely well-differentiated squamous cell carcinoma in older women [97–99]. It presents as an exophytic, slow-growing mass and can be readily misclassified as a benign lesion on a superficial biopsy. As its name implies, it has a verrucous architecture. Broad bulbous rete pegs invade the underlying stroma in a pushing rather than infiltrative manner (Fig. 5.34). Cytologic atypia is absent to minimal and mitotic figures are confined to the basal layer. Conspicuous nuclear pleomorphism, koilocytosis, an infiltrative pattern of invasion, or metastatic disease all argue against a diagnosis of VC and should prompt the exclusion of a (co-existing) conventional keratinizing squamous cell carcinoma. VC is frequently seen in association with lichen sclerosus, lichen simplex chronicus, and vulvar acanthosis with altered differentiation (De-VIL) [3]. HPV status of VC has been inconsistent in the literature. Most recent studies have concluded that VC is likely unrelated to either HPV infection or *Tp53* mutations unless associated with other subtypes of vSCC [100]. VC may be the result of a third, yet to be fully explored, pathway (Fig. 5.1) [3]. Conservative surgical

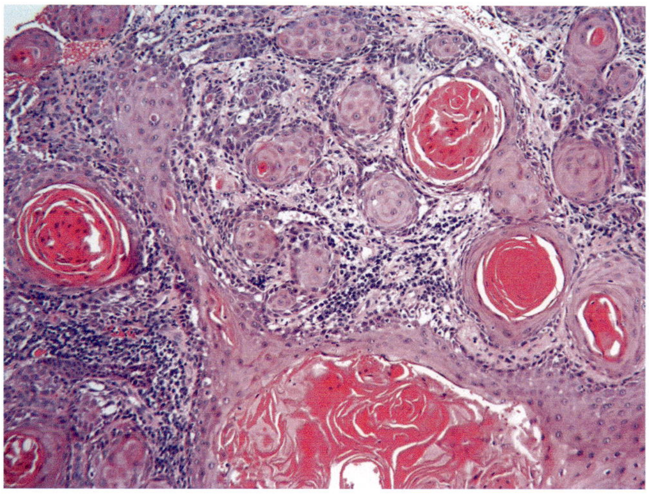

Fig. 5.30 Squamous cell carcinoma, keratinizing type. Tumor cells demonstrate abundant eosinophilic cytoplasm, abnormal keratinization, and keratin pearl formation (H&E, 100×)

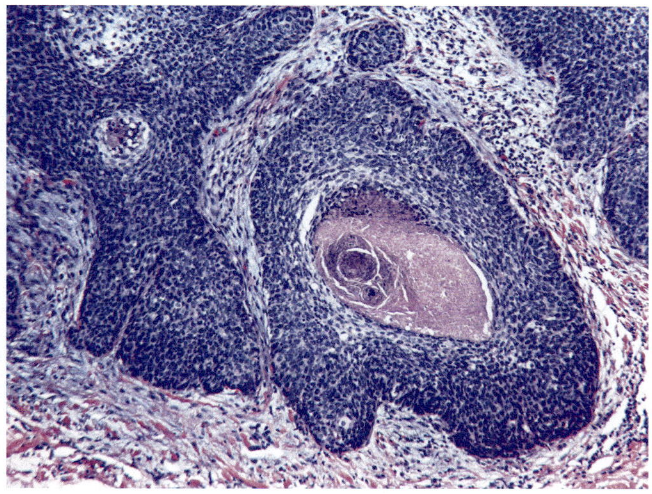

Fig. 5.32 Squamous cell carcinoma, basaloid type. Basaloid SCC is characterized by small, uniform, immature tumor cells with high N/C ratios growing in sheets, nests, and cords. Keratinization (not shown) is usually present but can be focal. Larger tumor islands may show central comedo-type necrosis (H&E, 100×)

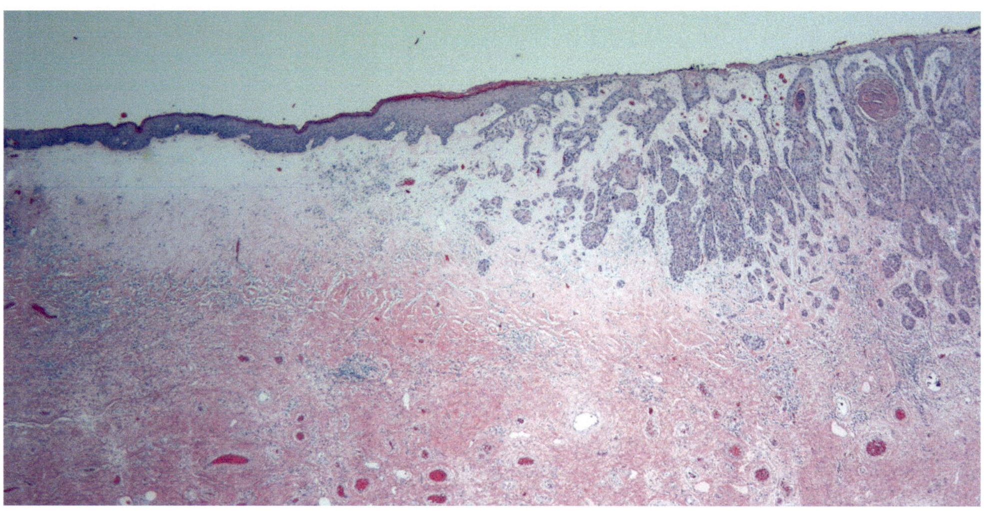

Fig. 5.31 Squamous cell carcinoma, keratinizing type, arising in a background of lichen sclerosus and differentiated VIN (H&E, 20×)

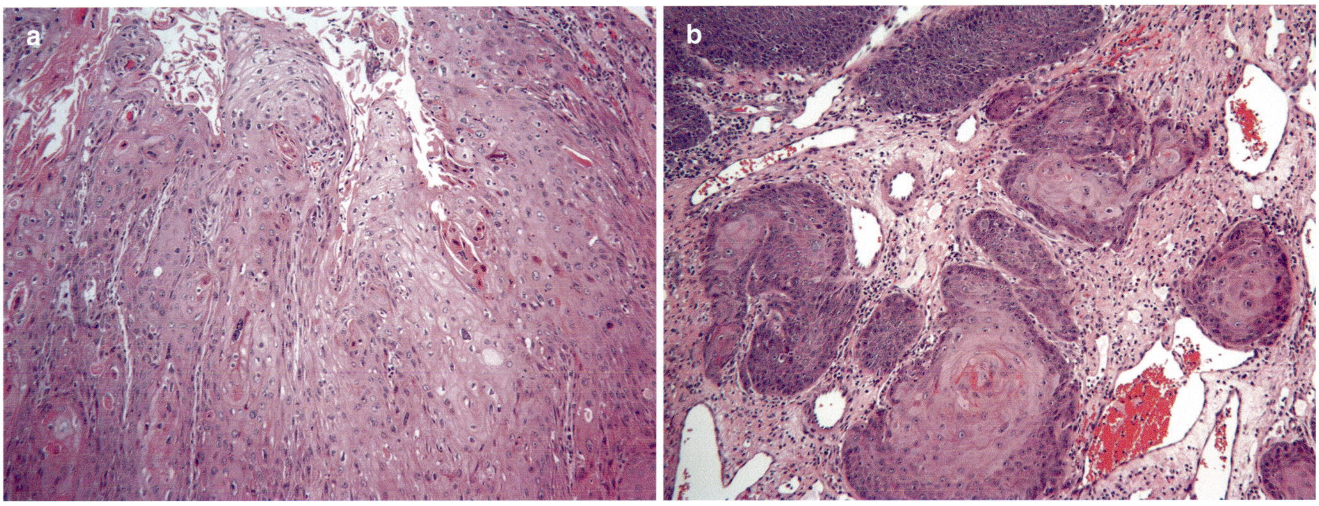

Fig. 5.33 Squamous cell carcinoma, warty (condylomatous) type. (**a**) The surface of this large and exophytic mass is "condylomatous" and shows multinucleated and koilocytic atypia. (**b**) Conspicuous pleomorphism is present within the invasive tumor front (H&E, 100×)

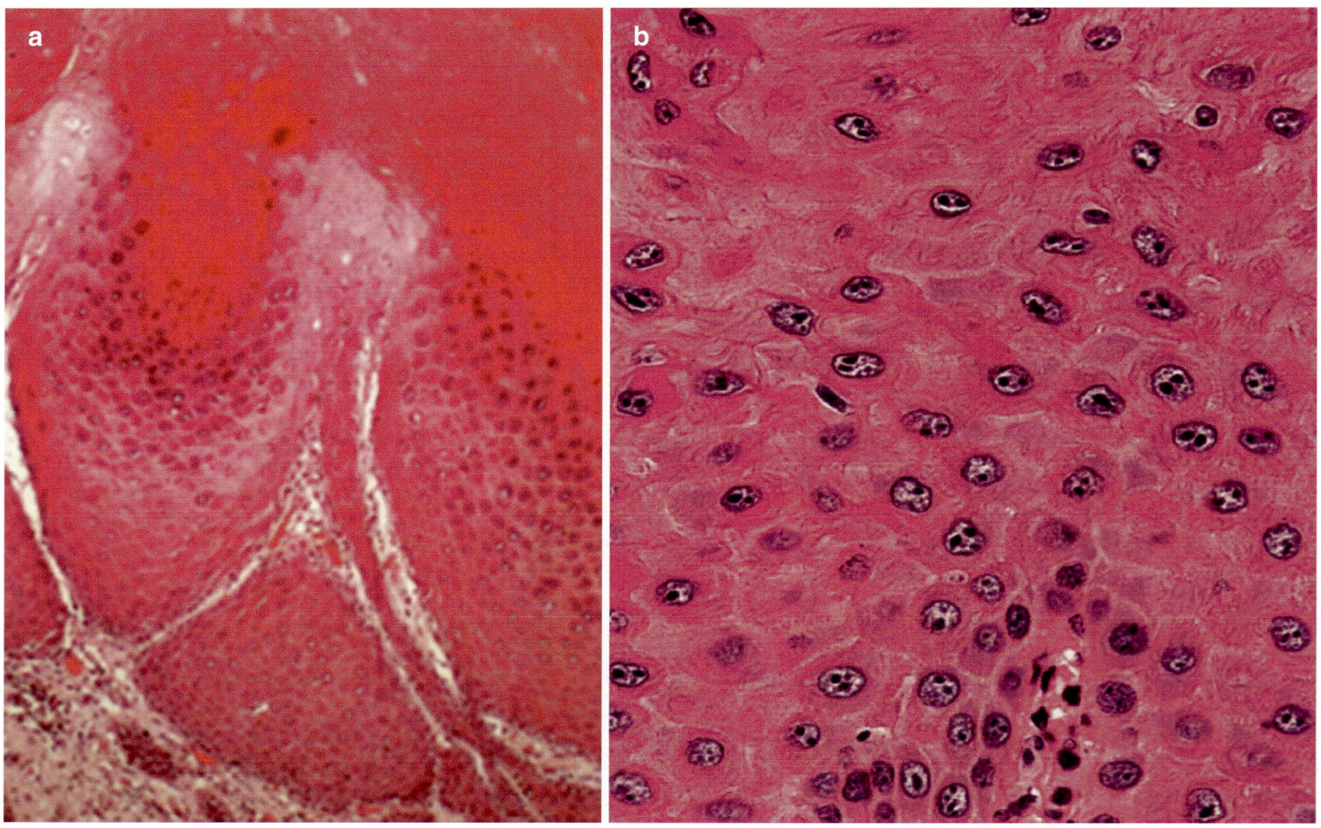

Fig. 5.34 Verrucous carcinoma. (**a**) The tumor front consists of broad bulbous rete pegs that invade the underlying stroma in a pushing manner. (**b**) The tumor is extremely well differentiated with minimal to no cytologic atypia (H&E, 100× and 400×)

excision is the treatment of choice due to minimal to no risk of metastatic spread. Recurrence is related to inadequate resection.

Other Rare Types of Vulvar Squamous Cell Carcinoma

Rare reported variants include vSCC with tumor giant cells as well as sarcomatoid (spindle cell), acantholytic (pseudoangiosarcomatoid or adenoid), plasmacytoid, and lymphoepithelioma-like SCC [101–108].

Grading of Squamous Cell Carcinoma

There is no universally accepted grading system for vSCC. Two proposed schemes exist and are summarized in Table 5.7 [83, 109].

Table 5.7 Grading schemes for vulvar squamous cell carcinoma

Grade	AJCC grading scheme [69]	GOG grading scheme[a] [96]
Gx	Grade cannot be assessed	Grade cannot be assessed
G1	Well differentiated	No undifferentiated cells
G2	Moderately differentiated	<50% Undifferentiated cells
G3	Poorly differentiated	>50% Undifferentiated cells
G4	Undifferentiated	All undifferentiated cells

[a]Gynecologic Oncology Group (GOG) grading is based on the percentage of undifferentiated tumor cells, which are defined as: small poorly differentiated to undifferentiated tumor cells with scant cytoplasm infiltrating the stroma as clusters or cords

5.3.2.3 Ancillary Studies

In the absence of bone fide histologic features of squamous differentiation (keratin pearl formation, intercellular bridges), ancillary studies may be required. Particularly in a small biopsy with a poorly differentiated (non-keratinizing) squamous cell carcinoma, biomarkers p40 or p63 are a valuable tool to support the diagnosis and exclude other poorly differentiated malignancies of the vulva.

While HPV status is not yet utilized for management decisions in vSCC, this information may prove of value in the future. In general, the majority of keratinizing squamous cell carcinomas are strongly positive for p53, while the basaloid, warty, and otherwise non-keratinizing subtypes of vSCC are immunoreactive with antibodies to p16 and negative (wild-type) for p53, reflecting the underlying pathophysiology. However, exceptions occur. Recently, several studies have shown that p16 is a reliable biomarker for the classification of vSCC based on HPV infection, and is superior to histomorphology alone (see Sect. 5.3.2.4 and Sect. 5.4 for full discussion) [110–113].

5.3.2.4 Differential Diagnosis

Keratoacanthoma or Well-Differentiated (Keratinizing) Squamous Cell Carcinoma?

Keratoacanthoma (KA) is a cutaneous neoplasm, which commonly occurs on sun-exposed skin. KA is well known clinically for its rapid growth and tendency to spontaneously regress. In the vulva, KA is an exceedingly rare diagnosis [114]. Microscopically, keratoacanthomas exhibit an inverted (endophytic) growth pattern with a central keratin-filled crater. The keratinocytes are well differentiated with minimal to no cytologic atypia and a low mitotic index. Although some features have been noted to be more common in KA, no single histologic feature can differentiate a KA from a well-differentiated SCC. In fact, many pathologists regard KA as a variant of well-differentiated SCC rather than a strictly distinct entity. The unique clinical presentation in conjunction with the histomorphology aids in the diagnosis. Conservative excision is the management of choice for vulvar KA.

Inverted Follicular Keratosis or Squamous Cell Carcinoma?

Inverted follicular keratosis (IFK) is commonly encountered on the head and facial region. It is exceedingly rare in the vulva [115]. It is considered a type of irritated seborrheic keratosis with an endophytic (pseudoinfiltrative) growth pattern, generally growing down along hair follicle epithelium. It exhibits uniform basaloid cells with varying degrees of squamous differentiation in the form of squamous eddies and pearls. In contrast to squamous cell carcinoma, IFK is symmetrical and lacks conspicuous pleomorphism, desmoplastic stromal reaction, or background dysplasia.

Basal Cell Carcinoma or Basaloid Squamous Cell Carcinoma?

Basal cell carcinoma (BCC) is rare but can occur in the vulva [116, 117]. BCC is characterized by a uniform proliferation of basaloid cells with low-grade atypia. Conspicuous palisading of nuclei occurs at the periphery of the tumor nests and clefts with the surrounding stroma are a clue to the diagnosis (Fig. 5.35). Of note, squamous differentiation can occur in the center of the tumor islands and is still in keeping with a diagnosis of BCC. A background of VIN is notably absent, so is the nuclear pleomorphism typical of a basaloid SCC. Immunohistochemistry can further aid in the distinction. BCC is immunoreactive with antibodies to BerEp4 which distinguishes it from basaloid SCC [118]. Of note, p63 and p16 can both be positive in BCC and (if positive) have limited value in the differential diagnosis with basaloid SCC [111]. Basal cell carcinoma of the vulva is managed by local excision without lymphadenectomy.

Warty Squamous Cell Carcinoma or Keratinizing Squamous Cell Carcinoma?

Warty SCC exhibits conspicuous koilocytosis, multinucleation, and nuclear pleomorphism, features that set it apart from the conventional vSCC.

Warty Squamous Cell Carcinoma or Verrucous Carcinoma?

While architecturally similar to VC on low power, warty SCC demonstrates conspicuous koilocytosis, nuclear pleomorphism, and an infiltrative pattern of invasion, all features not seen in verrucous carcinoma.

VAAD or Verrucous Carcinoma?

VAAD and verrucous carcinoma share overlapping histomorphologic features. VAAD has been identified as a risk factor in the development of VC. The presence of a large mass lesion and histologic evidence of invasion support a diagnosis of VC.

Giant Condyloma of Buschke and Lowenstein or Verrucous Carcinoma?

Similar to verrucous carcinoma, giant condyloma is a slow-growing, exophytic and expansile tumor. In contrast to VC, it

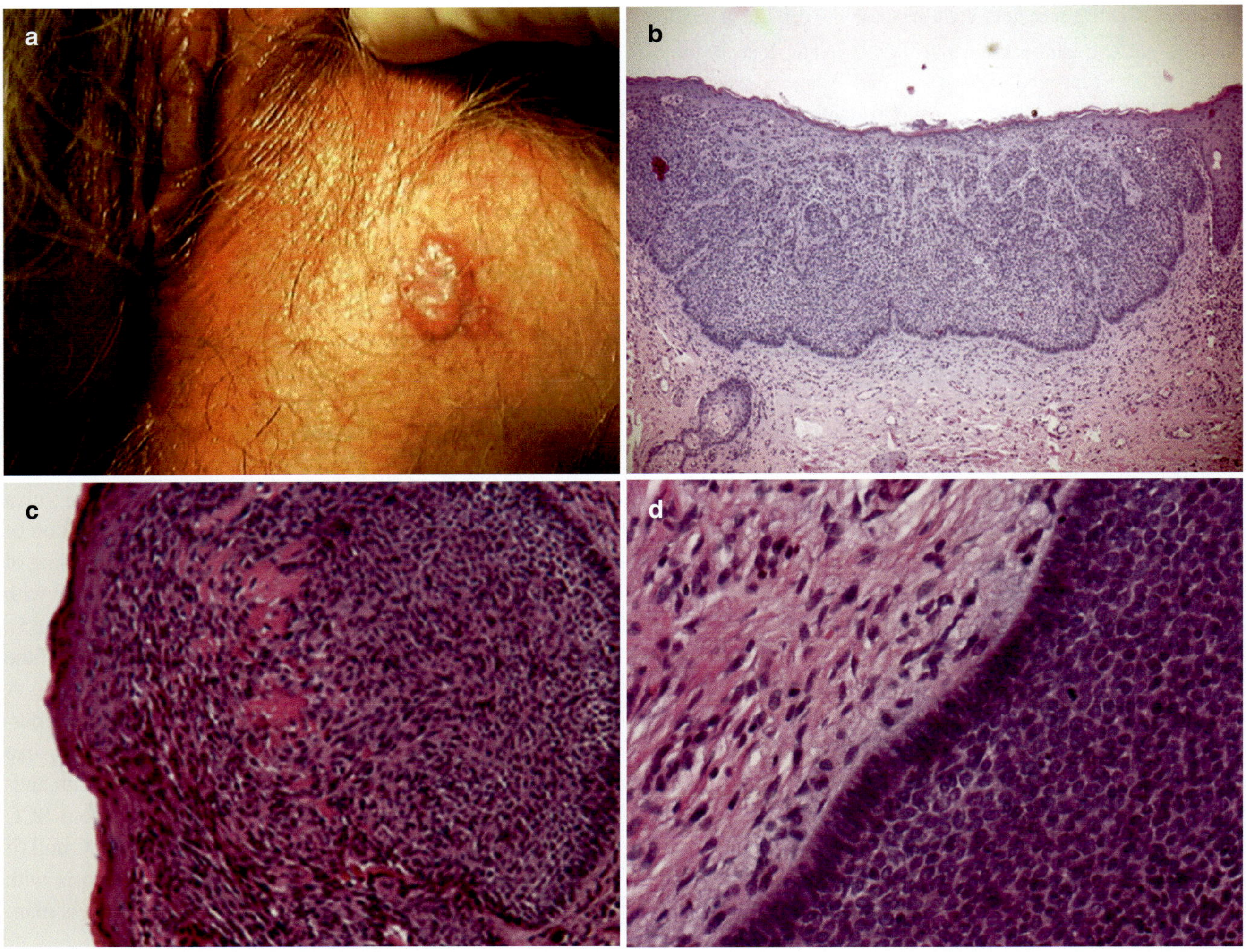

Fig. 5.35 Basal cell carcinoma. (**a**) Clinical image of a BCC. (**b**) Low power shows a proliferation of uniform basaloid cells. (**c**, **d**) High-power evaluation shows cytologically bland basaloid cells with peripheral palisading (H&E, 10× and 400×)

is associated with low-risk HPV and morphologically demonstrates papillomatosis and koilocytosis.

Malignant Melanoma or Squamous Cell Carcinoma?

Particularly if amelanotic, malignant melanoma of the vulva can enter in the differential diagnosis with vSCC. Immunohistochemical stains aid in the distinction. Melanoma is immunoreactive with antibodies to S-100, SOX-10, Melan-A, or HMB-45. Focal reactivity with cytokeratins can occasionally be observed. p40/p63 is negative in melanoma. In addition, background in situ components can be a valuable clue to the diagnosis.

Merkel Cell Carcinoma, Small Cell Carcinoma, or Poorly Differentiated, Non-keratinizing Squamous Cell Carcinoma?

Merkel and small cell carcinoma are both aggressive, high-grade neuroendocrine carcinomas, which rarely involve the vulva. Both have a similar morphology demonstrating a "neuroendocrine" architectural growth pattern (organoid, trabecular, nested, corded) and tumor cells composed of high N/C ratios, nuclear molding, and fine "salt and pepper" chromatin. Necrosis, mitotic figures, and apoptosis are readily identified. Performance of ancillary stains, particularly in small biopsy specimens, is of value. Markers of squamous differentiation (p40/p63) are usually (but not always) negative and help exclude a poorly differentiated non-keratinizing squamous cell carcinoma. Both small cell and Merkel cell carcinoma express markers of neuroendocrine differentiation (synaptophysin, chromogranin) and cytokeratins (AE1/AE3, Cam 5.2, etc.). The latter may demonstrate a unique para-nuclear dot pattern of reactivity. TTF-1 is expressed in the majority of small cell carcinomas (regardless of primary site) while Merkel cell carcinoma is characteristically positive for CK20.

5.3.2.5 Prognosis and Management

Regardless of pathogenesis, current prognostic factors are applicable to all vulvar SCC. Vulvar squamous cell carcinoma spreads by direct extension into adjacent structures and metastasizes to regional (inguino-femoral) lymph nodes. Distant metastasis is rare and encompasses involvement of pelvic lymph nodes. Prognosis in vulvar SCC depends on stage. Stage is determined by tumor size, depth of invasion, extension into adjacent structures, and lymph node status (Table 5.5). Depth of invasion determines risk of spread to groin lymph nodes. Tumors with DOI ≤1 mm have an almost negligible risk while this risk approaches 20% when the DOI increases to 5 mm [89]. Lymph node involvement is one of the most powerful prognostic factors and patient outcome significantly worsens with increasing number of nodes involved, larger size of deposits, and presence of extracapsular extension [119–122]. Patients with groin node involvement have a 5-year survival of 20–40% compared to those without lymph node metastasis (70–90%) [123]. Overall, 5-year survival rates are 85–98% for stage I and drop to 10–30% in stage IV patients [109]. While vSCC carries a high overall morbidity and mortality, superficially invasive squamous cell carcinoma of the vulva (stage IA) is the exception. It has an excellent prognosis. Five- and ten-year survival is 100% and 94%, respectively [84]. Lymph node sampling is not routinely performed in these superficially invasive tumors due to the overall negligible risk of nodal metastasis.

Recurrence rates vary from 12 to 37% with a reported 5-year survival of 25–50% [123–125]. Recurrences (local, groin, and distant) usually occur within the first 2 years after initial diagnosis [123–125]. Some consider a "local recurrence" beyond 2 years as a de novo tumor due to field cancerization effect [125]. Patient age, tumor size, focality, grade, depth of invasion, lymph-vascular space invasion, lymph node status, precursor lesions, and margin status all impact recurrence rates [125–131]. The desired width of tumor-free margin for resections is not well defined in the literature, with some citing no local recurrence if >8 mm is achieved [129], while other studies differ [132–136]. Recently, tumor growth pattern and the stromal response have been investigated and found to represent informative elements [137–139]. Tumors with an infiltrative (finger-like) pattern of invasion frequently demonstrate a fibromyxoid stromal response. Such tumors are associated with an increased risk of nodal metastasis and recurrence compared to tumors with a pushing invasive front. In addition, these tumors are more likely to demonstrate perineural invasion, which has been identified as an independent prognostic factor of recurrence [140]. The concept of epithelial-mesenchymal transition has been proposed as the underlying mechanism for these more aggressive vSCC [141]. Hence, growth pattern, stromal response, and perineural invasion represent optional but informative elements in the pathology report (Table 5.6). Of note, both groin recurrence (any lymph node metastasis in the groin with or without the presence of a local recurrence after treatment of vSCC) and distant metastasis are associated with high mortality (85–100%) [142].

The prognostic value of HPV status in vSCC is not yet fully elucidated due to conflicting data in the literature. While this area requires further study, some publications have shown that HPV-independent vSCCs have higher rates of recurrence and decreased overall survival compared to HPV-dependent vSCC [143–146]. Recently, Lee et al. investigated the value of p16 as a potential prognostic biomarker and found higher progression-free survival, overall survival, and lower rates of local recurrence in women with p16 positive tumors [147].

Surgery is the main treatment modality for vSCC [148]. Stage IA tumors are excised conservatively (with 1 cm margin) without lymphadenectomy, while all other surgically resectable tumors are excised with uni- or bilateral groin lymph node dissection [149]. Sentinel lymph node biopsy represents an alternative in patients with a tumor <4 cm without clinically suspicious lymph nodes [150–152]. Neoadjuvant chemotherapy or chemoradiation is an option for patients who would benefit from reduction of bulky locally advanced disease prior to surgery. Adjuvant radiation is considered in patients with close (<8 mm) or involved surgical margins and nodal metastasis [153, 154]. Recurrence is managed surgically with re-excision or local radiation. Groin recurrence is treated with surgery and/or adjuvant (chemo) radiation while palliative chemotherapy is the last resort for patients with distant (including pelvic) recurrence. Currently, HPV status of the primary tumor does not determine therapy. For a detailed discussion on surgical management, the reader is referred to an excellent review by Deppe et al. [149].

5.4 Select Biomarkers

5.4.1 p16^{INK4a}

p16^{INK4a} (p16) is a surrogate biomarker for infection with hr-HPV. p16 is recommended by LAST as the (only) biomarker of choice to support a diagnosis of HSIL in the lower female anogenital tract [7]. A positive p16 stain should follow the "block positivity" concept: strong nuclear or nuclear and cytoplasmic staining in contiguous lesional cells involving the basal layer with extension upward to include at least 1/3 of the epithelium (Fig. 5.36b). Full thickness staining is frequently observed but not required. Sole cytoplasmic positivity, noncontiguous patchy positivity (checkerboard-like pattern), and basal layer only staining are considered negative. Before ordering a p16 stain, the pathologist should adhere to the LAST criteria for p16 utilization to avoid over- or mis-use [7]. p16 is helpful in resolving the following diagnostic dilemmas in vulvar specimens:

1. HSIL or mimic (reactive, atrophic epithelium)
2. LSIL (VIN 1) or HSIL (VIN 2/3) if the H&E impression is equivocal
3. Discordance between two pathologists over diagnosis of HSIL

Just like in the cervix and other anogenital sites, the H&E impression dictates the diagnosis in bone fide cases of no SIL, LSIL, or HSIL; p16 staining is not a requirement in these settings. Of note, vulvar lesions with classic features of flat LSIL/VIN 1 are rarely positive with p16 [14, 17]. Furthermore, p16 does not resolve the diagnostic dilemma of reactive atypia versus LSIL/VIN 1. p16 is consistently negative in dVIN, including the basaloid variant [45, 155]. Therefore, p16 block positivity strongly argues against a diagnosis of dVIN (Figs. 5.19, 5.36, and 5.37).

In squamous cell carcinoma of the vulva, morphology typically correlates well with p16 and HPV status: basaloid and warty carcinomas are more likely to be p16+/HPV+ while p16−/HPV− tumors are of the well-differentiated keratinizing type or verrucous carcinoma. However, exceptions occur. In a recent study of 1594 vSCCs, histologic criteria alone did not reliably predict p16 and HPV status (e.g., 36.5% of p16+HPV+ tumors were keratinizing and 5.2% of p16−HPV− tumors were basaloid/warty) [110]. In addition, several studies have shown that p16 is a reliable biomarker for the classification of vSCC based on HPV infection, and is superior to histomorphology alone [110–113]. In a study by Santos et al., p16 demonstrated 100% sensitivity and 98.7% specificity in the detection of HPV-associated vSCC [112]. While p16 and HPV status are not yet utilized for management decisions in vSCC, this may prove of value in the future. Of note, p16 staining can be observed in basal cell carcinoma of the vulva and if positive is not a distinguishing stain in the differential with basaloid SCC.

5.4.2 p53

Mutations in *Tp53* are the hallmark of the non-HPV-related pathway to invasive squamous cell carcinoma. Hence, the most commonly described biomarker for dVIN is p53 [16, 64, 75, 111, 156–160]. By immunohistochemistry (IHC), two patterns of p53 positivity are recognized which support a diagnosis of dVIN (Fig. 5.36f, i):

1. Strong and diffuse nuclear staining of consecutive basal layer keratinocytes with suprabasilar extension, or
2. Lack of nuclear staining (null pattern)

Full thickness p53 positivity is usually not observed because mutant p53 is degraded as a function of cellular maturation. The labeling index (p53 positivity in 200 consecutive basal layer cells) in dVIN typically approaches or exceeds 90% [16]. The null pattern of p53 has been reported in 25–30% of dVIN [75]. Comparison to patchy and weak p53 positivity in less than 10% of basal cells (wild-type staining) of adjacent, nonlesional squamous epithelium aids in the evaluation. Pitfalls of p53 interpretation include overexpression of p53 in the setting of vulvar dermatoses (e.g., LS and LP) and squamous cell hyperplasia because inflammation and cell stress upregulate and stabilize wild-type p53 [161–163]. Strong confluent p53 staining in basal layer keratinocytes can therefore be seen in these settings in a significant subset of cases. An accentuated pattern of p53 wild-type positivity (increased intensity, frequency 5–50%, throughout the epithelium, with patchy, noncontiguous basal cell staining) has recently been described by Jeffreys et al. [62]. This pattern of reactivity was encountered in cases for which the differential diagnosis was dVIN versus HSIL (uVIN), particularly the warty subtype. All accentuated p53 cases also demonstrated block p16 staining, in keeping with HSIL (uVIN) (Fig. 5.37). Hence, tandem p53/p16 staining is of particular value in small biopsies with ambiguous histologic features and avoids inadvertent misclassification.

In squamous cell carcinoma, most (50–70%) of HPV-independent tumors demonstrate p53 expression by immunohistochemistry. In contrast, p53 is consistently negative in HPV-driven vSCC [111, 112].

5.4.3 MIB-1 (Ki-67)

MIB-1 (Ki-67) is a marker of cellular proliferation. It is a nuclear stain. It is increased and involves most layers of the epithelium in HPV-related VIN but restricted to the basal and parabasal layers in dVIN. However, it is also increased in reactive and inflammatory conditions and in isolation is neither sensitive nor specific for dVIN [64, 155, 163, 164]. MIB-1 may be reserved as an adjunct marker in a panel of stains. It is not routinely used in the diagnosis of squamous cell carcinoma.

5.4.4 CK17

Cytokeratin 17 (CK17) is a cytoskeletal intermediate protein which has been utilized in the evaluation of squamous neoplasia in the oral cavity, cervix, and anus [165–168]. In a study by Podoll et al., dVIN showed a moderate to strong diffuse cytoplasmic expression with antibodies to

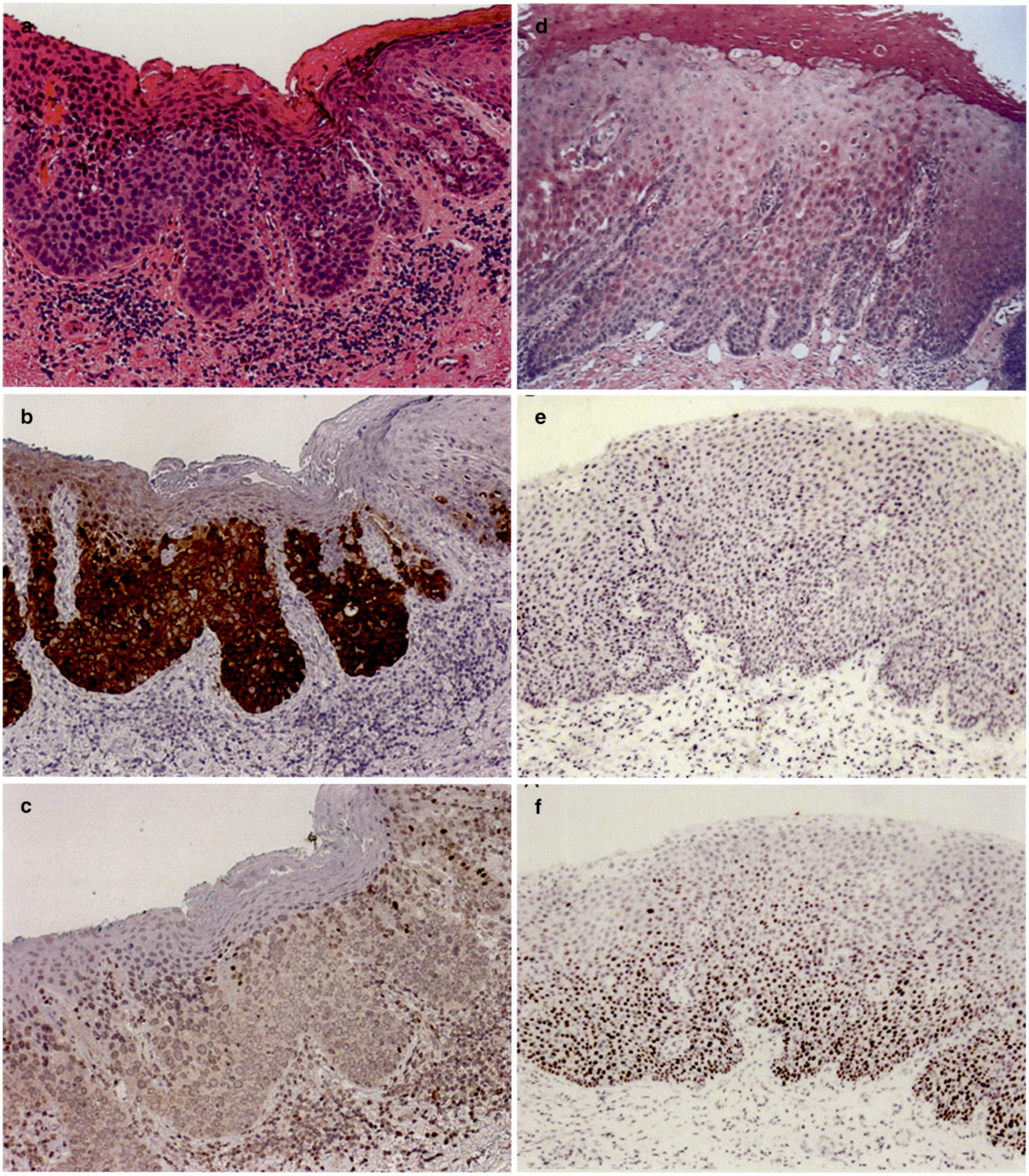

Fig. 5.36 Comparison of immunophenotype of HSIL/uVIN and dVIN. (**a**) HSIL. (**b**) p16 block positive staining. (**c**) p53 wild type (negative). (**d**) dVIN. (**e**) p16 (negative). (**f**) Contiguous basal and parabasal p53 reactivity (positive). (**g**) dVIN. (**h**) p16 (negative). (**i**) p53 null (positive) (200×)

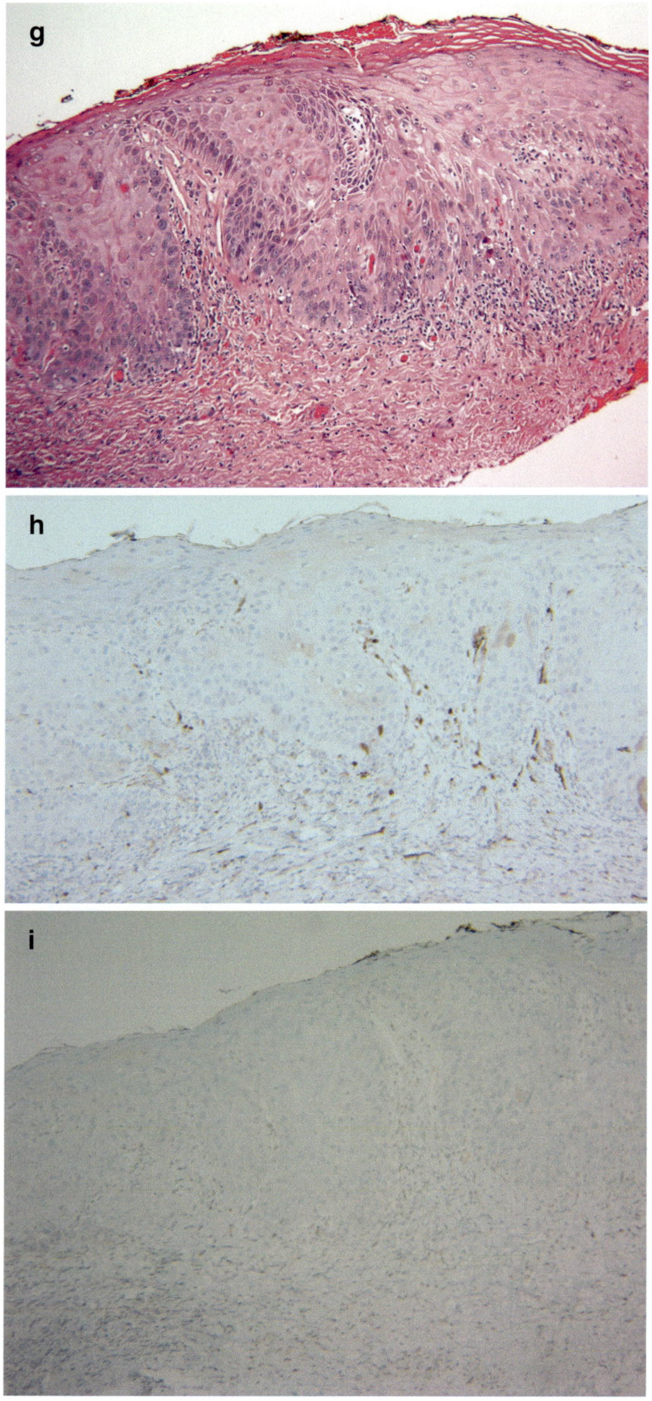

Fig. 5.36 (continued)

CK17 in a full thickness or suprabasal distribution [168]. In contrast, CK17 reactivity in HSIL/uVIN and LSC was weak and restricted to the superficial portions of the epithelium. However, CK17 failed to differentially stain LS which exhibited the same pattern of reactivity as dVIN. Therefore, reliance on CK17 in the diagnosis of dVIN should be avoided. CK17 may be reserved as an

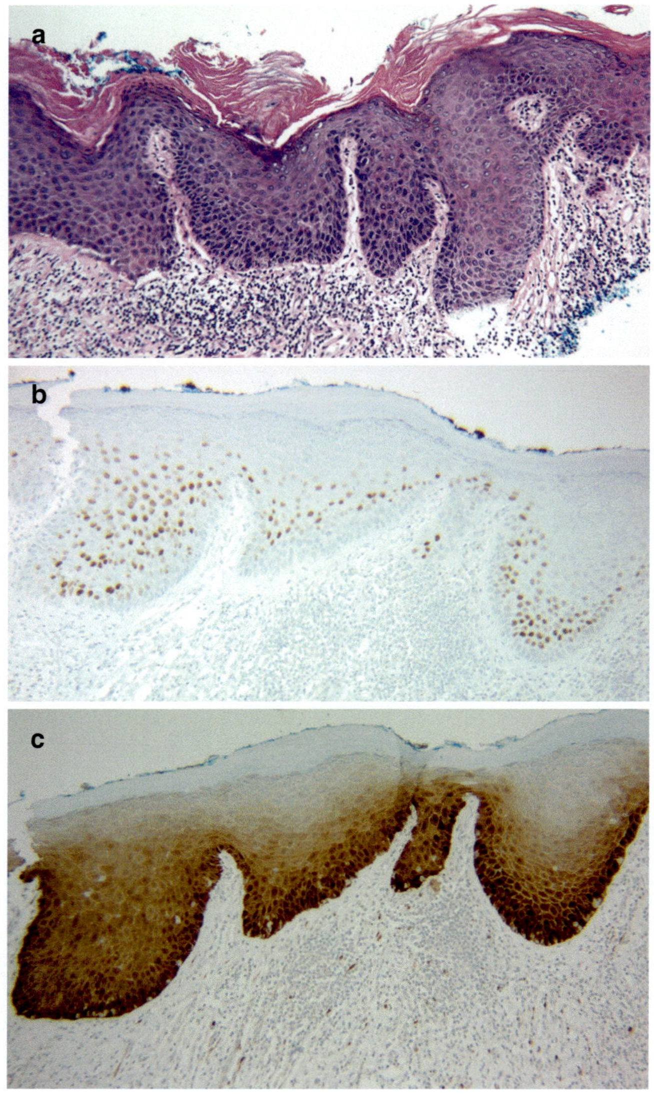

Fig. 5.37 HSIL (uVIN/VIN 2/3). (**a**) HSIL. Distinguishing features from dVIN include more striking pleomorphism and full thickness atypia. In some cases of HSIL (particularly the warty subtype), the nuclear atypia is less striking in the upper layers of the epithelium (H&E, 200×). (**b**) p16 shows block positivity (200×). (**c**) p53 staining is negative (not shown) in HSIL or can be accentuated (increased intensity, frequency 5–50%, throughout the epithelium, with patchy, noncontiguous basal cell staining) (200×)

adjunct marker in a panel of stains. CK17 is not routinely used in the diagnosis of squamous cell carcinoma.

5.4.5 p63/p40

p63 and p40 are both biomarkers of squamous differentiation. p40 is an isoform of p63 and a more specific marker for squamous cell carcinoma. Both are robust nuclear stains and utilized when the differential diagnosis includes a poorly differentiated squamous cell carcinoma.

5.5 Molecular Pathogenesis

5.5.1 HPV-Dependent Pathway

Whether vulvar LSIL is in fact a precancer or just a reactive change or human papillomavirus effect is a debate in the literature. It is associated with both low- and high-risk HPV subtypes.

HSIL of the vulva is a clonal premalignant condition that exhibits loss of heterozygosity and X-chromosome inactivation [169–172]. Chromosomal gains and losses in HPV-associated vSCC are similar to those in the cervix, with gains in 3q most commonly identified [173]. HSIL and its associated vSCC show a strong association with hr-HPV infection, particularly HPV 16 [174, 175]. In a large meta-analysis by Faber et al., 76% of VIN and 40% of vSCC tested positive for HPV [41]. The pathogenesis of HPV-driven carcinogenesis is well documented. In short, HPV protein E6 causes the degradation of tumor suppressor p53 resulting in rare to no p53 expression. p16 is a prototypic INK4 protein whose function is to inhibit cyclin-dependent kinase-mediated phosphorylation of the retinoblastoma (Rb) gene product leading to downregulation of cell proliferation. In the setting of persistent infection with hr-HPV, the E7 oncoprotein binds to the host Rb protein, which results in the inactivation of Rb as well as release and subsequent activation of the transcription factor E2F. These actions commit the cell to division. Simultaneously, E2F causes a marked increase in the production of p16; however, its inhibitory effect on cell proliferation is lost. This paradoxical overexpression makes p16 a sensitive surrogate biomarker for hr-HPV-associated SIL and vSCC.

5.5.2 HPV-Independent Pathway

Genetic mutations in *Tp53* mutations are the hallmark of dVIN and evolution to vSCC unrelated to HPV infection [156–159, 176–178]. Mutant p53 (due to a missense mutation) is more stable than wild-type p53 protein; therefore, accumulation of p53 in the nucleus can be detected by immunohistochemistry. But p53 expression does not always indicate the presence of a *Tp53* mutation (e.g., inflammation can prolong the p53 half-life), and not all mutations produce immunodetectable p53 protein. The latter (p53 null pattern) is due to deletions or nonsense mutations resulting in no detectable p53 protein by IHC. Other genetic events in this pathway include allelic imbalance, microsatellite instability, *PTEN and CDKN2A* mutations, DNA aneuploidy and tetraploidy, and hypermethylation of the *RASSF2A*, *MGMT*, and *TSP1* gene promoters [169, 178–180]. HPV has reportedly been detected in dVIN but is rare [16, 177, 181]. Not all HPV-independent squamous cell carcinomas of the vulva develop in the setting of *Tp53* mutations. *PIK3CA* and *ARID2* mutations drive the development of atypical verruciform vulvar lesions collectively referred to as differentiated exophytic vulvar intraepithelial lesion (DE-VIL) [3]. These may play a risk factor in the development of a small subset of *Tp53* and HPV-independent squamous cell carcinomas of the vulva. This potential third pathway requires further investigation.

Acknowledgment The author thanks Dr. Sara Shalin for her review and editorial comments during the preparation of this chapter.

References

1. SEER cancer statistics factsheets: vulvar cancer. Surveillance, epidemiology, and end results program. National Cancer Institute, 2017. Available at: http://seer.cancer.gov/statfacts/html/vulva.html. Accessed on 29 Nov 2017
2. Del Pino M, Rodriguez-Carunchio L, Ordi J. Pathways of vulvar intraepithelial neoplasia and squamous cell carcinoma. Histopathology. 2013;62:161–75.
3. Watkins J, Howitt BE, Horowitz N, et al. Differentiated exophytic vulvar intraepithelial lesions are genetically distinct from keratinizing squamous cell carcinomas and contain mutations in PIK3CA. Mod Pathol. 2017;30:448–58.
4. Nasciemento AF, Granter SR, Cviko A, et al. Vulvar acanthosis with altered differentiation. A precursor to verrucous carcinoma? Am J Surg Pathol. 2004;28(5):638–43.
5. Wilkinson EJ, Cox JT, Selim MA, et al. Evolution of terminology for human-papillomavirus-infection-related vulvar squamous intraepithelial lesions. J Lower Gen Tract Dis. 2015;19(1):81–7.
6. Bornstein J, Bogliatto F, Haefner H, et al. The 2015 International Society for the Study of Vulvovaginal Disease (ISSVD) terminology of vulvar squamous intraepithelial lesions. J Lower Gen Tract Dis. 2016;20:11–4.
7. Darragh TM, Colgan TJ, Cox JT, et al. The lower anogenital squamous terminology standardization project for HPV-associated lesions: background and consensus recommendations from the College of American Pathologists and the American Society for Colposcopy and Cervical Pathology. J Low Genit Tract Dis. 2012;16:205–42.
8. Crum C, Herrington CS, McCluggage WG, et al. Tumours of the vulva; epithelial tumours. In: Kleihues P, editor. WHO classification of tumours of the female genital reproductive organs, WHO Blue Book Series. 4th ed. Lyon: IRAC Press; 2014. p. 232–40.
9. Srodon M, Stoler MH, Baber GB, et al. The distribution of low and high-risk HPV types in vulvar and vaginal intraepithelial neoplasia (VIN and VaIN). Am J Surg Pathol. 2006;30(12):1513–8.
10. Sideri M, Jones RW, Heller DS, et al. Comment on the article: Srodon M, Stoler MH, Baber GB, et al. The distribution of low and high-risk HPV types in vulvar and vaginal intraepithelial neoplasia (VIN and VaIN). Am J Surg Pathol. 2007;31(9):1452.
11. Gasco M, Sullivan A, Repellin C, et al. Coincident inactivation of 14-3-3s and p16^{INK4a} is an early event in vulvar squamous neoplasia. Oncogene. 2002;21:1876–81.
12. Hillemanns P, Wang X. Integration of HPV-16 and HPV-18 DNA in vulvar intraepithelial neoplasia. Gynecol Oncol. 2006;100:276–82.

13. Logani S, Lu D, Quint WGV, et al. Low-grade vulvar and vaginal intraepithelial neoplasia: correlation of histologic features with human papillomavirus DNA detection and MIB-1 immunostaining. Mod Pathol. 2003;16:735–41.
14. Lewis N, Blanco LZ Jr, Maniar KP. p16 expression and biological behavior of flat vulvar low-grade squamous intraepithelial lesions (LSIL). Int J Gynecol Pathol. 2016;36:486–92.
15. Abell MR, Gosling JRG. Intraepithelial and infiltrative carcinoma of vulva: Bowen's type. Cancer. 1961;2:318–29.
16. Yang B, Hart WR. Vulvar intraepithelial neoplasia of the simplex (differentiated) type: a clinicopathologic study including analysis of HPV and p53 expression. Am J Surg Pathol. 2000;24:429–41.
17. Yang EJ, Kong CS, Longacre TA. Vulvar and anal intraepithelial neoplasia: terminology, diagnosis, and ancillary studies. Adv Anat Pathol. 2017;24(3):136–50.
18. Bussen S, Sutterlin M, Schmidt U, et al. Anogenital warts in childhood—always a marker of sexual abuse? Geburtshilfe Frauenheilkd. 2012;72(10):43–8.
19. Bergeron C, Ferenczy A, Richart RM, et al. Micropapillomatosis labialis appears unrelated to human papillomavirus. Obstet Gynecol. 1990;76:281–6.
20. Nucci MR, Young RH, Fletcher CD. Cellular pseudosarcomatous fibroepithelial stromal polyps of the lower female genital tract: an underrecognized lesion often misdiagnosed as sarcoma. Am J Surg Pathol. 2000;24(2):231–40.
21. Bai H, Cviko A, Granter S, et al. Immunophenotypic and viral (human papillomavirus) correlates of vulvar seborrheic keratosis. Hum Pathol. 2003;34(6):559–64.
22. Li J, Ackerman AB. "Seborrheic keratosis" that contain human papillomavirus are condyloma acuminatum. Am J Dermatopathol. 1994;16(4):559–64.
23. Medeiros F, Nascimento AF, Crum CP. Early vulvar squamous neoplasia. Advances in classification, diagnosis and differential diagnosis. Adv Anat Pathol. 2005;12:20–6.
24. Bruins FG, van Deudekom FJ, deVries HJ. Syphilitic condylomata lata mimicking anogenital warts. BMJ. 2015;17:350:h1259.
25. Terzakis E, Androutsopoulos G, Zygouris D, et al. Angiokeratoma of the vulva. Eur J Gynaecol Oncol. 2011;32(5):597–8.
26. Reich O, Regauer S. Recurrent verruciform xanthoma of the vulva. Int J Gynecol Pathol. 2003;23:75–7.
27. Santa Cruz DJ, Martin SA. Verruciform xanthoma of the vulva. Report of two cases. Am J Clin Pathol. 1979;71(2):224–8.
28. Fite C, Plantier F, Dupin N, et al. Vulvar verruciform xanthoma: ten cases associated with lichen sclerosus, lichen planus, or other conditions. Arch Dermatol. 2011;147(9):1087–92.
29. Quinn TR, Young RH. Epidermolytic hyperkeratosis in the lower female genital tract: an uncommon simulant of mucocutaneous papillomavirus infection—a report of two cases. Int J Gynecol Pathol. 1997;16(2):163–8.
30. Swann MH, Pujals JS, Pillow J, et al. Localized epidermolytic hyperkeratosis of the female external genitalia. J Cutan Pathol. 2003;30(6):379–81.
31. McLachlin CM, Mutter GL, Crum CP. Multinucleate atypia of the vulva. Report of a distinct entity not associated with human papillomavirus. Am J Surg Pathol. 1994;18(12):1233–9.
32. Committee on Gynecologic Practice and the American Society for Colposcopy and Cervical Pathology. Committee opinion: management of vulvar intraepithelial neoplasia. Obstet Gynecol. 2016;128(4):e178–82.
33. Fox H, Wells M. Recent advances in the pathology of the vulva. Histopathology. 2003;42(3):209–16.
34. Baandrup L, Varbo A, Munk C, et al. In situ and invasive squamous cell carcinoma of the vulva in Denmark 1978–2007—a nationwide population-based study. Gynecol Oncol. 2011;122:45–9.
35. Dittmer C, Katalinic A, Mundhenke C, et al. Epidemiology of vulvar and vaginal cancer in Germany. Arch Gynecol Obstet. 2011;284:169–74.
36. Jakobsson M, Pukkala E, Pavavonen J, et al. Cancer Incidence among Finnish women with surgical treatment for cervical intraepithelial neoplasia, 1987–2006. Int J Cancer. 2011;128: 1187–91.
37. Santoso JT, Long M, Crigger M, et al. Anal intraepithelial neoplasia in women with genital intraepithelial neoplasia. Obstet Gynecol. 2010;116:578–82.
38. Gormley RH, Kovarik CL. Human papillomavirus-related genital disease in the immunocompromised host. Part I. J Am Acad Dermatol. 2012;66:867–14.
39. Massad LS, Xie X, Darragh T, et al. Genital warts and vulvar intraepithelial neoplasia: natural history and effects of treatment and human immunodeficiency virus infection. Obstet Gynecol. 2011;118:831–9.
40. Chafe W, Richards A, Morgan L, et al. Unrecognized invasive carcinoma in vulvar intraepithelial neoplasia (VIN). Gynecol Oncol. 1988;31:154–65.
41. Faber MT, Sand FL, Albieri V, et al. Prevalence and type distribution of human papillomavirus in squamous cell carcinoma and intraepithelial neoplasia of the vulva. Int J Cancer. 2017;141:1161–9.
42. Armes JE, Lourie R, Bowlay G, et al. Pagetoid squamous cell carcinoma in situ of the vulva: comparison with extramammary Paget disease and nonpagetoid squamous cell neoplasia. Int J Gynecol Pathol. 2008;27(1):118–24.
43. Raju RR, Goldblum JR, Hart WR. Pagetoid squamous cell carcinoma in situ (pagetoid Bowen's disease) of the external genitalia. Int J Gynecol Pathol. 2003;22(2):127–35.
44. McCluggage WG, Jamison J, Boyde A, et al. Vulval intraepithelial neoplasia with mucinous differentiation: report of 2 cases of a hitherto undescribed phenomenon. Am J Surg Pathol. 2009;33(6):945–9.
45. Ordi J, Alejo M, Fuste V, et al. HPV-negative vulvar intraepithelial neoplasia (VIN) with basaloid histologic pattern. An unrecognized variant of simplex (differentiated) VIN. Am J Surg Pathol. 2009;33(11):1659–65.
46. Marcus J, Carnisa C. Podophyllin therapy for condyloma acuminatum. Int J Dermatol. 1990;29(10):693–8.
47. Wade TR, Ackerman AB. The effects of resin podophyllin on condyloma acuminatum. Am J Dermatopathol. 1984;6(2):109–22.
48. Nucci MR, Genest DR, Tate JE, et al. Pseudobowenoid change of the vulva: a histologic variant of untreated condylata acuminatum. Mod Pathol. 1996;9(4):375–9.
49. Hart WR, Millman JB. Progression of intraepithelial Paget's disease of the vulva to invasive carcinoma. Cancer. 1977;40:2333–7.
50. Morbeck D, Tregnago AC, Baiocchi G, et al. GATA3 expression in primary vulvar Paget disease: a potential pitfall leading to misdiagnosis of pagetoid urothelial intraepithelial neoplasia. Histopathology. 2017;70(3):435–41.
51. Sah SP, McCluggage WG. Florid vulval Paget disease exhibiting p16 immunoreactivity and mimicking classic VIN. Int J Gynecol Pathol. 2013;32(2):221–7.
52. Abdel-Mesih A, Daya D, Onuma K, et al. Interobserver agreement for assessing invasion in stage 1A vulvar squamous cell carcinoma. Am J Surg Pathol. 2013;37:1336–41.
53. Friedrich EG Jr. Reversible vulvar atypia: a case report. Obstet Gynecol. 1972;42:40–6.
54. Wade TR, Kopf AW, Ackerman AB. Bowenoid papulosis of the genitalia. Arch Dermatol. 1979;115:306–8.
55. Fleury FJ. Letter to the editor: Bowenoid papulosis of the genitalia, in reply. Arch Dermatol. 1980;116:274.
56. Patterson JW, Kao GF, Graham JH, et al. Bowenoid papulosis. A clinicopathologic study with ultrastructural observations. Cancer. 1986;57:823–36.
57. Jones RW, Rowan DW, Stewart AW. Vulvar intraepithelial neoplasia: aspects of the natural history and outcome in 405 women. Obstet Gynecol. 2005;106:1319–26.

58. Nugent EK, Brooks RA, Barr CD, et al. Clinical and pathologic features of vulvar intraepithelial neoplasia in premenopausal and postmenopausal women. J Low Genit Tract Dis. 2011;15(1): 15–9.
59. Van den Einden LCG, de Hullu JA, Massuger LFAG, et al. Interobserver variability and the effect of education in the histopathologic diagnosis of differentiated vulvar intraepithelial neoplasia. Mod Pathol. 2013;26:874–80.
60. Reutter JC, Walters RA, Selim A. Differentiated vulvar intraepithelial neoplasia: what criteria do we use in practice? J Low Genit Tract Dis. 2016;20:261–6.
61. van de Nieuwenhof HP, Bulten J, Hollema H, et al. Differentiated vulvar intraepithelial neoplasia is often found in lesions, previously diagnosed as lichen sclerosus, which have progressed to vulvar squamous cell carcinoma. Mod Pathol. 2011;24(2):297–305.
62. Jeffreys M, Jeffus SK, Herfs M, et al. Accentuated p53 staining in usual type vulvar dysplasia—a potential diagnostic pitfall. Pathol Res Pract. 2018;214:76–79 [Epub ahead of print].
63. Bigby DM, Eva LJ, Fong KL, et al. The natural history of vulvar intraepithelial neoplasia, differentiated type: evidence for progression and diagnostic challenges. Int J Gynecol Pathol. 2016;35(6):574–84.
64. Mulvaney NJ, Allen DG. Differentiated intraepithelial neoplasia of the vulva. Int J Gynecol Pathol. 2007;27:125–35.
65. Hoang LN, Park KJ, Soslow RA, et al. Squamous precursor lesions of the vulva: current classification and diagnostic challenges. Pathology. 2016;48(4):291–302.
66. Hoang MP, Reuter J, Papalas J, et al. Vulvar inflammatory dermatoses: an update and review. Am J Dermatopathol. 2014;36(9):689–704.
67. Regauer S, Liegl B, Reich O. Early vulvar lichen sclerosus: a histopathologic challenge. Histopathology. 2005;47:340–7.
68. Carlson JA, Lamb P, Malfetano J, et al. Clinicopathologic comparison of vulvar and extragenital lichen sclerosus: histologic variants, evolving lesions, and etiology of 141 cases. Mod Pathol. 1998;11(9):844–54.
69. Rodke G, Friedrich EG Jr, Wilkinson WJ. Malignant potential of mixed vulvar dystrophy (lichen sclerosus associated with squamous cell hyperplasia). J Reprod Med. 1988;33:545–50.
70. Micheletti L, Preti M, Radici G, et al. Vulvar lichen sclerosus and neoplastic transformation: a retrospective study of 976 cases. J Low Genit Tract Dis. 2016;20(2):180–3.
71. Chiesa-Vottero A, Dvoretsky PM, Hart WR. Histopathologic study of thin vulvar squamous cell carcinomas and associated cutaneous lesions: a correlative study of 48 tumors in 44 patients with analysis of adjacent vulvar intraepithelial neoplasia types and lichen sclerosus. Am J Surg Pathol. 2006;30:310–8.
72. Jones RW, Sadler L, Grant S, et al. Clinically identifying women with vulvar lichen sclerosus at increased risk of squamous cell carcinoma: a case control study. J Reprod Med. 2004;49: 808–11.
73. Carlson JA, Ambros R, Malfetano J, et al. Vulvar lichen sclerosus and squamous cell carcinoma: a cohort, case control, and investigational study with historical perspective; implications for chronic inflammation and sclerosis in the development of neoplasia. Hum Pathol. 1998;29(9):932–48.
74. Weyers W. (2013) Hypertrophic lichen sclerosus with dyskeratosis and parakeratosis—a common presentation of vulvar lichen sclerosus not associated with a significant risk of malignancy. Am J Dermatopathol. 2013;35:713–21.
75. Singh N, Leen SL, Han G, et al. Expanding the morphologic spectrum of differentiated VIN (dVIN) through detailed mapping of cases with p53 loss. Am J Surg Pathol. 2015;39:52–60.
76. Day T, Bowden N, Jaaback K, et al. Distinguishing erosive lichen planus from differentiated vulvar intraepithelial neoplasia. J Lower Gen Tract. 2016;20(2):174–9.
77. Eva LJ, Ganesan R, Chan KK, et al. Differentiated-type vulvar intraepithelial neoplasia has a high risk association with vulvar squamous cell carcinoma. Int J Gynecol Cancer. 2009;19:741–4.
78. van de Nieuwenhof HP, Massuger LF, van der Avoort IA, et al. Vulvar squamous cell carcinoma development after diagnosis of VIN increases with age. Eur J Cancer. 2009;45:851–6.
79. Eva LJ, Ganesan R, Chan KK, et al. Vulval squamous cell carcinoma occurring in a background of differentiated vulval intraepithelial neoplasia is more likely to recur: a review of 154 cases. J Reprod Med. 2008;53:397–401.
80. Van de Nieuwenhof HP, van Kempen LC, de Hullu JA, et al. The etiologic role of HPV in vulvar squamous cell carcinoma fine tuned. Cancer Epidemiol Biomark Prev. 2009;18:2061–7.
81. Leibowitch M, Neill S, Pelisse M, et al. The epithelial changes associated with squamous cell carcinoma of the vulva: a review of the clinical and histological and viral findings in 78 women. Br J Obstet Gynaecol. 1990;97:1135–9.
82. Carli P, Cattaneo A, De Magnis A, et al. Squamous cell carcinoma arising in vulval lichen sclerosus: a longitudinal cohort study. Eur J Cancer Prev. 1995;4:491–5.
83. Gibb RK, Olawaiye AB, Chen L-M, et al. Vulva. In: Amin MB, Edge SB, Greene FL, et al., editors. AJCC cancer staging manual. 8th ed. New York, NY: Springer; 2017. p. 633–40.
84. Magrina JF, Gonzalez-Bosquet J, Weaver AL, et al. Squamous cell carcinoma of the vulva stage IA: long-term results. Gynecol Oncol. 2000;76(1):24–7.
85. Lee ES, Allen D, Scurry J. Pseudoepitheliomatous hyperplasia in lichen sclerosus of the vulva. Int J Gynecol Pathol. 2003;22(1):57–62.
86. Lack EE, Worsham GF, Callihan MD, et al. Granular cell tumor: a clinicopathologic study of 110 patients. J Surg Oncol. 1980;13(4):301–16.
87. Frimer M, Chudnoff S, Hebert T, et al. Pseudoepitheliomatous hyperplasia mimicking vulvar cancer in a patient with AIDS. J Low Genit Tract Dis. 2011;15(1):66–8.
88. Tangjitgamol S, Loharamtaweethong K, Thawaramara T, et al. Vulvar pseudoepitheliomatous hyperplasia associated with herpes simplex virus type II mimicking cancer in an immunocompromised patient. J Obstet Gynaecol Res. 2014;40(1):255–8.
89. Yoder BJ, Rufforny I, Massoll NA, et al. Stage IA vulvar squamous cell carcinoma: an analysis of tumor invasive characteristics and risk. Am J Surg Pathol. 2008;32:765–72.
90. Kurzl R, Messerer D, Baltzer J, et al. Comparative morphometric study on the depth of invasion in vulvar carcinoma. Gynecol Oncol. 1988;29:12–25.
91. Dvoretsky PM, Bonfiglio TA, Helmkamp BF, et al. The pathology of superficially invasive, thin vulvar squamous cell carcinoma. Int J Gynecol Pathol. 1984;3:331–42.
92. Wilkinson E. Premalignant and malignant tumors of the vulva. In: Kurman RJ, Ellenson L, Ronnett BM, editors. Blaustein's pathology of the female genital tract. 6th ed. Boston, MA: Springer; 2011. p. 55–103.
93. Chan JK, Sugiyama V, Pham H, et al. Margin distance and other clinic-pathologic prognostic factors in vulvar carcinoma; a multivariate analysis. Gynecol Oncol. 2007;104:636–41.
94. Raspagliesi F, Hanozet F, Ditto A, et al. Clinical and pathologic prognostic factors in squamous cell carcinoma of the vulva. Gynecol Oncol. 2006;102:333–7.
95. Hauspy J, Beiner M, Harley I, et al. Sentinel lymph node in vulvar cancer. Cancer. 2007;110:1015–22.
96. Kurman RJ, Toki T, Schiffman MH. Basaloid and warty carcinomas of the vulva. Distinctive types of squamous cell carcinoma frequently associated with human papillomaviruses. Am J Surg Pathol. 1993;17:133–45.
97. Liu G, Li Q, Shang X, et al. Verrucous carcinoma of the vulva: a 20 year retrospective study and literature review. J Low Genit Tract Dis. 2016;20(1):114–8.

98. Gualco M, Bonini S, Foglia G, et al. Morphologic and biologic studies of ten cases of verrucous carcinoma of the vulva supporting the theory of a discrete clinic-pathologic entity. Int J Gynecol Cancer. 2003;13:317–24.
99. Japaze H, Van Dinh T, Woodruff JD. Verrucous carcinoma of the vulva: study of 24 cases. Obstet Gynecol. 1982;60:462–6.
100. del Pino M, Bleeker MC, Quint WG, et al. Comprehensive analysis of human papillomavirus prevalence and the potential role of low-risk types in verrucous carcinoma. Mod Pathol. 2012;25(10):1354–63.
101. Horn L, Liebert UG, Edelmann J, et al. Adenoid squamous carcinoma (pseudoangiosarcomatous carcinoma) of the vulva: a rare but highly aggressive variant of squamous cell carcinoma—report of a case and review of the literature. Int J Gynecol Pathol. 2008;27:288–91.
102. Santos LD, Krivanek MJ, Chan F, et al. Pseudoangiosarcomatous squamous cell carcinoma of the vulva. Pathology. 2006;38:581–3.
103. Niu W, Heller DS, D'Cruz C. Lymphoepithelioma-like carcinoma of the vulva: a case report. J Lower Gen Tract Dis. 2003;7:136–9.
104. Wilkinson EJ, Croker BP, Friedrich EG Jr, et al. Two distinct pathologic types of giant cell carcinoma of the vulva. A report of two cases. Reprod Med. 1988;33:519–22.
105. Choi D, Lee J, Lee S, et al. Squamous cell carcinoma with sarcomatoid features of the vulva: a case report and review of the literature. Gynecol Oncol. 2006;103:363–7.
106. Bigby SM, Eva LJ, Jones RW. Spindle cell carcinoma of the vulva: a series of 4 cases and review of the literature. Int J Gynecol Pathol. 2014;33(2):203–12.
107. Lasser A, Cornog JL, Morris JM. Adenoid squamous cell carcinoma of the vulva. Cancer. 1974;33:224–7.
108. Tran TA, Carlso JA. Plasmacytoid squamous cell carcinoma of the vulva. Int J Gynecol Pathol. 2008;27(4):601–5.
109. Homesley HD, Bundy BN, Sedlis A, et al. Assessment of current International Federation of Gynecology and Obstetrics staging of vulvar carcinoma relative to prognostic factors for survival (a Gynecologic Oncology Group study). Am J Obstet Gynecol. 1991;164(4):997–1004.
110. Rakislova N, Clavero O, Alemany L, et al. Histological characteristics of HPV-associated and -independent squamous cell carcinomas of the vulva: a study of 1,594 cases. Int J Cancer. 2017;141:2517–27.
111. Santos M, Montagut C, Mellado B. Immunohistochemical staining for p16 and p53 in premalignant and malignant epithelial lesions of the vulva. Int J Gynecol Pathol. 2004;23(3):206–14.
112. Santos M, Landolfi S, Olivella A. p16 overexpression identified HPV-positive vulvar squamous cell carcinomas. Am J Surg Pathol. 2006;30(11):1347–56.
113. Cheng AS, Karnezis AN, Jordan S. p16 immunostaining allows for accurate subclassification of vulvar squamous cell carcinoma into HPV-associated and HPV-independent cases. Int J Gynecol Pathol. 2015;35:385–93.
114. Chen W, Koenig C. Vulvar keratoacanthoma: a report of two cases. Int J Gynecol Pathol. 2004;23:284–6.
115. Roth LM, Look KY. Inverted follicular keratosis of the vulvar skin: a lesion that can be confused with squamous cell carcinoma. Int J Gynecol Pathol. 2000;19:369–73.
116. Gibson GE, Ahmed I. Perianal and genital basal cell carcinoma: a clinicopathologic review of 51 cases. J Am Acad Dermatol. 2001;45:68–71.
117. Takahashi H. Non-ulcerative basal cell carcinoma arising on the genitalia. J Dermatol. 2000;27:798–801.
118. Tellechea O, Reis JP, Domingues JC, et al. Monoclonal antibody BerEp4 distinguishes basal cell carcinoma from squamous cell carcinoma of the skin. Am J Dermatopathol. 1993;15:452–5.
119. van der Steen S, de Nieuwenhof HP, Massuger L. New FIGO staging system of vulvar cancer indeed provides a better reflection of prognosis. Gynecol Oncol. 2010;119(3):520–5.
120. Hoffman JS, Kumar NB, Morley GW. Prognostic significance of groin lymph node metastases in squamous cell carcinoma of the vulva. Obstet Gynecol. 1985;66:402–5.
121. Pinto AP, Schlecht NF, Pintos J, et al. Prognostic significance of lymph node variables and human papillomavirus DNA in invasive vulvar carcinoma. Gynecol Oncol. 2004;92:856–65.
122. Luchini C, Nottegar A, Solmi M. Prognostic implications of extranodal extension in node-positive squamous cell carcinoma of the vulva: a systematic review and meta-analysis. Surg Oncol. 2016;25(1):60–5.
123. Gadducci A, Cionini L, Romanini A, et al. Old and new perspectives in the management of high-risk, locally advanced or recurrent, and metastatic vulvar cancer. Crit Rev Oncol Hematol. 2006;60(3):227–41.
124. Coulter J, Gleeson N. Local and regional recurrence of vulval cancer: management dilemmas. Best Pract Res Clin Obstet Gynaecol. 2003;17(4):663–81.
125. Nooij LS, Brand FA, Gaarenstroom KN, et al. Risk factors and treatment for recurrent vulvar squamous cell carcinoma. Crit Rev Oncol Hematol. 2016;106:1–13.
126. Podratz KC, Symmonds RE, Taylor WF. Carcinoma of the vulva: analysis of treatment failures. Am J Obstet Gynecol. 1982;143:340–51.
127. Boyce J, Fruchter RG, Kasambilides E, et al. Prognostic factors in carcinoma of the vulva. Gynecol Oncol. 1985;20:364–77.
128. Binder SW, Huang I, Fu YS. Risk factors for the development of lymph node metastasis in vulvar squamous cell carcinoma. Gynecol Oncol. 1990;37:9–16.
129. Heaps JM, Fu YS, Montz FJ. Surgical-pathologic variables predictive of local recurrence in squamous cell carcinoma of the vulva. Gynecol Oncol. 1990;38:309–14.
130. Burger MP, Hollema H, Emanuels AG, et al. The importance of the groin node status for the survival of T1 and T2 vulvar carcinoma patients. Gynecol Oncol. 1995;57:327–34.
131. Woelber L, Mahner S, Voelker K, et al. Clinicopathological prognostic factors and patterns of recurrence in vulvar cancer. Anticancer Res. 2009;29:545–52.
132. de Hullu JA, Hollema H, Lolkema S, et al. Vulvar carcinoma. The price of less radical surgery. Cancer. 2002;95(11):2331–8.
133. Chan JK, Sugiyama V, Pham H, Gu M, et al. Margin distance and other clinico-pathologic prognostic factors in vulvar carcinoma: a multivariate analysis. Gynecol Oncol. 2007;104(3):636–41.
134. Woelber L, Choschzick M, Eulenburg C, et al. Prognostic value of pathological resection margin distance in squamous cell cancer of the vulva. Ann Surg Oncol. 2011;18(13):3811–8.
135. Groenen SM, Timmers PJ, Burger CW. Recurrence rate in vulvar carcinoma in relation to pathological margin distance. Int J Gynecol Cancer. 2010;20(5):869–73.
136. Viswanathan AN, Pinto AP, Schultz D, et al. Relationship of margin status and radiation dose to recurrence in post-operative vulvar carcinoma. Gynecol Oncol. 2013;130(3):545–9.
137. Drew PA, Al-Abbadi MA, Orlando CA, et al. Prognostic factors in carcinoma of the vulva: a clinicopathologic and DNA flow cytometric study. Int J Gynecol Pathol. 1996;15:235–41.
138. Ambros RA, Malfetano JH, Mihm MC Jr. Clinicopathologic features of vulvar squamous cell carcinomas exhibiting prominent fibromyxoid stromal response. Int J Gynecol Pathol. 1996;15(2):137–45.
139. Jeffus SK, Gehlot A, Holthoff E, et al. A fibromyxoid stromal response is associated with an infiltrative tumor morphology, perineural invasion, and lymph node metastasis in squamous cell carcinoma of the vulva. Am J Surg Pathol. 2015;39(9):1226–33.

140. Holthoff ER, Jeffus SK, Gehlot A, et al. Perineural invasion is an independent pathologic indicator of recurrence in vulvar squamous cell carcinoma. Am J Surg Pathol. 2015;39(8):1070–4.
141. Holthoff ER, Spencer H, Kelly T, et al. Pathologic features of aggressive vulvar carcinoma are associated with epithelial-mesenchymal transition. Hum Pathol. 2016;56:22–30.
142. Gonzalez Bosquet J, Magrina JF, Gaffey TA, et al. Long-term survival and disease recurrence in patients with primary squamous cell carcinoma of the vulva. Gynecol Oncol. 2005;97(3):828–33.
143. Lindell G, Nasman A, Jonsson C, et al. Presence of human papillomavirus (HPV) in vulvar squamous cell carcinoma (VSCC) and sentinel node. Gynecol Oncol. 2010;117(2):312–6.
144. Monk BJ, Burger RA, Lin F, et al. Prognostic significance of human papillomavirus DNA in vulvar carcinoma. Obstet Gynecol. 1995;85(Pt 1):709–15.
145. Ansink A, van der Velden J. Surgical interventions for early squamous cell carcinoma of the vulva. Cochrane Database Syst Rev. 2000;(2):CD002036.
146. Larsson GL, Helenius G, Andersson S, et al. Human papillomavirus (HPV) and HPV 16-variant distribution in vulvar squamous cell carcinoma in Sweden. Int J Gynecol Cancer. 2012;22(8):1413–9.
147. Lee LJ, Howitt B, Catalano P, et al. Prognostic importance of human papillomavirus (HPV) and p16 positivity in squamous cell carcinoma of the vulva treated with radiotherapy. Gynecol Oncol. 2016;142(2):293–8.
148. Rouzier R, Haddad B, Atallah D, et al. Surgery for vulvar cancer. Clin Obstet Gynecol. 2005;48:869–78.
149. Deppe G, Mert I, Winer IS. Management of squamous cell vulvar cancer: a review. J Obstet Gynaecol Res. 2014;40(5):1217–25.
150. van der Zee AG, Oonk MH, de Hullu JA, et al. Sentinel node dissection is safe in the treatment of early stage vulvar cancer. J Clin Oncol. 2008;26(6):884–9.
151. Farias-Eisner R, Cirisano FD, Grouse D, et al. Conservative and individualized surgery for early squamous carcinoma of the vulva: the treatment of choice for stage I and II (T1-2N0-1M0) disease. Gynecol Oncol. 1994;53(1):55–8.
152. Te Grootenhuis NC, van der Zee AG, van Doorn HC, et al. Sentinel nodes in vulvar cancer: long-term follow-up of the Groningen International Study on sentinel nodes in vulvar cancer (GROINSS-V) I. Gynecol Oncol. 2016;140(1):8–14.
153. Faul CM, Mirmow D, Huang Q, et al. Adjuvant radiation for vulvar carcinoma: improved local control. Int J Radiat Oncol Biol Phys. 1997;38:381–9.
154. Hacker NF, Eifel PJ, van der Velden J. Cancer of the vulva. Int J Gynaecol Obstet. 2012;119(Suppl 2):S90–6.
155. Hoevenaars BM, van der Avoort IA, de Wilde PC, et al. A panel of p16(INK4A), MIB1 and p53 proteins can distinguish between the 2 pathways leading to vulvar squamous cell carcinoma. Int J Cancer. 2008;123(12):2767–73.
156. Choschzik M, Hantaredja W, Tennstedt P, et al. Role of TP53 mutations in vulvar carcinomas. Int J Gynecol Pathol. 2011;30:497–504.
157. Rosenthal AN, Hopster D, Ryan A, et al. Immunohistochemical analysis of p53 in vulval intraepithelial neoplasia and vulval squamous cell carcinoma. Br J Cancer. 2003;88:251–6.
158. Soufir N, Queille S, Liboutet M, et al. Inactivation of the CDKN2A and the p53 tumour suppressor genes in external genital carcinomas and their precursors. Br J Dermatol. 2007;156:448–53.
159. Pinto AP, Miron A, Yassin Y, et al. Differentiated vulvar intraepithelial neoplasia contain tp53 mutations and is genetically linked to vulvar squamous cell carcinoma. Mod Pathol. 2010;23:404–12.
160. Hantschmann P, Sterzer S, Jeschke U, et al. P53 expression in vulvar carcinoma, vulvar intraepithelial neoplasia, squamous cell hyperplasia and lichen sclerosus. Anticancer Res. 2005;25:1739–45.
161. Liegl B, Regauer S. p53 immunostaining in lichen sclerosus is related to ischaemic stress and is not a marker of differentiated vulvar intraepithelial neoplasia (d-VIN). Histopathology. 2006;48:268–74.
162. Rolfe KJ, MacLean AB, Crow JC, et al. TP53 mutations in vulval lichen sclerosus adjacent to squamous cell carcinoma of the vulva. Br J Cancer. 2003;89:2249–53.
163. Rolfe KJ, Eva LJ, MacLean AB, et al. Cell cycle proteins as molecular markers of malignant change in vulvar lichen sclerosus. Int J Gynecol Cancer. 2001;11:113–8.
164. Stewart CJR, Crook ML. Fascin and cyclin D1 immunoreactivity in non-neoplastic vulvar squamous epithelium, vulvar intraepithelial neoplasia and invasive squamous carcinoma: correlation with Ki67 and p16 protein expression. J Clin Pathol. 2014;67:319–25.
165. Ikeda K, Tate G, Suzuki T, et al. Coordinate expression of cytokeratin 8 and cytokeratin 17 immunohistochemical staining in cervical intraepithelial neoplasia and cervical squamous cell carcinoma: an immunohistochemical analysis and review of the literature. Gynecol Oncol. 2008;108:598–602.
166. Nazarian RM, Primiani A, Doyle LA, et al. Cytokeratin 17: an adjunctive marker of invasion in squamous neoplastic lesions of the anus. Am J Surg Pathol. 2014;38:78–85.
167. Nobusawa A, Sano T, Negishi A, et al. Immunohistochemical staining patterns of cytokeratins 13, 14, and 17 in oral epithelial dysplasia including orthokeratotic dysplasia. Pathol Int. 2014;64:20–7.
168. Podoll MB, Singh N, Gilks CB, et al. Assessment of CK17 as a marker for the diagnosis of differentiated vulvar intraepithelial neoplasia. Int J Gynecol Pathol. 2017;36(3):273–80.
169. Pinto AP, Lin MC, Sheets EE, et al. Allelic imbalance in lichen sclerosus, hyperplasia, and intraepithelial neoplasia of the vulva. Gynecol Oncol. 2000;77:171–6.
170. Rosenthal AN, Ryan A, Hopster D, et al. Molecular evidence of a common clonal origin and subsequent divergent clonal evolution in vulval intraepithelial neoplasia, vulval squamous cell carcinoma and lymph node metastases. Int J Cancer. 2002;99:549–54.
171. Tate JE, Mutter GL, Boynton KA, et al. Monoclonal origin of vulvar intraepithelial neoplasia and some vulvar hyperplasias. Am J Pathol. 1997;150:315–22.
172. Ueda Y, Enomoto T, Miyatake T, et al. Analysis of clonality and HPV infection in benign, hyperplastic, premalignant, and malignant lesions of the vulvar mucosa. Am J Clin Pathol. 2004;122:266–74.
173. Thomas LK, Bermejo JL, Vinokurova S, et al. Chromosomal gains and losses in human papillomavirus-associated neoplasia of the lower genital tract—a systematic review and meta-analysis. Eur J Cancer. 2014;50(1):85–98.
174. Crum CP, Braun LA, Shah KV, et al. Vulvar intraepithelial neoplasia: correlation of nuclear DNA content and the presence of a human papillomavirus (HPV) structural antigen. Cancer. 1982;49:468–71.
175. Hampl M, Sarajuuri H, Wentzensen N, et al. Effect of human papillomavirus vaccines on vulvar, vaginal and anal intraepithelial lesions and vulvar cancer. Obset Gynecol. 2006;108:1361–8.
176. Hording U, Junge J, Daugaard S, et al. Vulvar squamous cell carcinoma and papillomaviruses: indications for two different etiologies. Gynecol Oncol. 1994;52:241–6.
177. Haefner HK, Tate JE, MacLachlin CM, et al. Vulvar intraepithelial neoplasia: age, morphologic phenotype, papillomavirus DNA and coexisting invasive carcinoma. Hum Pathol. 1995;26:147–54.
178. Trietsch MD, Nooji LS, Gaarenstroom KN, et al. Genetic and epigenetic changes in vulvar squamous cell carcinoma and its precursor lesions: a review of the current literature. Gynecol Oncol. 2015;136:143–57.

179. Van der Avoort IAM, van de Nieuwenhof HP, Otte-Holler I, et al. High levels of p53 expression correlate with DNA aneuploidy in (pre) malignancies of the vulva. Hum Pathol. 2010;41:1475–85.
180. Guerrero D, Guarch R, Ojer A, et al. Differential hypermethylation of genes in vulvar cancer and lichen sclerosus coexisting or not with vulvar cancer. Int J Cancer. 2011;128:2853–64.
181. Van der Avoort IA, Shirango H, Hovenaars BM, et al. Vulvar squamous cell carcinoma is a multifactorial disease following two separate and independent pathways. Int J Gynecol Pathol. 2006;25:22–9.

6 Vulvar Glandular and Other Neoplasms

Andrew Dunn, Michael DeWall, and Jennifer Kaley

Abstract

This chapter will address vulvar neoplasms with glandular differentiation as well as neuroendocrine carcinoma and metastatic tumors. These entities are rare, as the vast majority of malignancies of the vulva are squamous in origin. Careful consideration of the differential diagnosis, as well as knowledge of any pertinent clinical history, is essential when evaluating these lesions.

Keywords

Adenosquamous carcinoma · Adenocarcinoma · Bartholin Merkel · Cloacogenic · Metastasis

6.1 Adenosquamous Carcinoma of the Vulva

6.1.1 Clinical Features

Adenosquamous carcinoma of the vulva is uncommon, comprising just 18 of 135 cases of vulvar cancer in one large study [1]. The mean age of diagnosis is 65–70 years, and this entity may be associated with chronic vulvar inflammatory disease [2]. Adenosquamous carcinoma of the vulva is not associated with human papilloma virus (HPV), though this is based on the study of relatively few cases [2, 3]. In a study by Carson et al., only one of 16 cases was positive for an undetermined type of HPV DNA [3]. This tumor involves the labium majus, and many also involve the labium minus [1]. Adenosquamous carcinoma has been proposed to arise from mucin-secreting glands of the hair shaft [4], Bartholin glands [5], and, in one report, a hidradenoma papilliferum [6].

A. Dunn · M. DeWall · J. Kaley (✉)
Department of Pathology, University of Arkansas for Medical Sciences, Little Rock, AR, USA
e-mail: ALdunn2@uams.edu; mrdewall@uams.edu; Jrkaley2@uams.edu

6.1.2 Microscopic Findings

Adenosquamous carcinoma is characterized by a blend of tumor cells showing squamous and glandular differentiation. The glandular areas are usually lined by a single layer of cells, while multilayering results in a squamoid appearance with frequent areas of keratinization, dyskeratosis, and acantholysis (Fig. 6.1). Solid areas within the tumor frequently consist of spindled squamoid cells. The tumor is deeply invasive in many cases and may involve the vagina and other adjacent perineal structures.

6.1.3 Immunohistochemistry

The lesional cells are diffusely positive for a high-molecular-weight keratin stain, and carcinoembryonic antigen (CEA) stain can be used to highlight glandular differentiation.

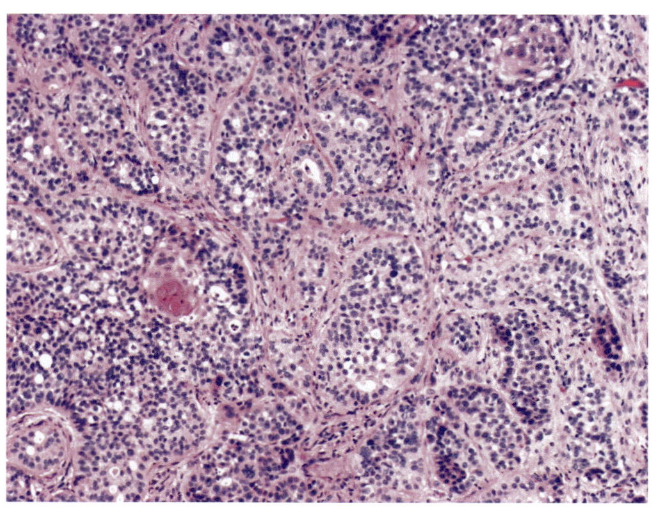

Fig. 6.1 Adenosquamous carcinoma, showing areas of dyskeratosis adjacent to gland formation (original magnification, 100×)

W. Zheng et al. (eds.), *Gynecologic and Obstetric Pathology, Volume 1*, https://doi.org/10.1007/978-981-13-3016-2_6

6.1.4 Differential Diagnosis

The growth pattern of the acantholytic, or pseudoglandular, variant of *squamous cell carcinoma* can mimic that of adenosquamous carcinoma (Fig. 6.2). Careful examination for the presence of true glandular differentiation is necessary for the latter diagnosis [2]. *Invasive Paget disease* and *amelanotic melanoma* are also considerations on the differential diagnosis. This differential can be narrowed down through the use of appropriate immunohistochemistry, if necessary. These entities as well as their immunohistochemical profiles are discussed separately in this chapter.

6.1.5 Prognosis and Treatment

Vulvar adenosquamous carcinoma has a worse prognosis than squamous cell carcinoma of a comparable stage [1] and is associated with a higher rate of metastasis [7]. Patients with adenosquamous carcinoma typically present at a clinically more advanced stage of disease than those with conventional squamous cell carcinoma; Underwood et al. observed that 2/3 of the patients in their study were T3 or higher when diagnosed [1]. Treatment varies depending on the extent of disease. Surgical treatment includes wide local excision or partial radical vulvectomy with lymphadenectomy; however, advanced- or late-stage disease may require the combination of surgery and chemoradiation.

6.1.6 Adenocarcinoma

This section discusses extramammary Paget disease, carcinoma arising in ectopic breast tissue, skin appendage adenocarcinoma, and carcinoma of the Bartholin gland.

6.2 Extramammary Paget Disease

6.2.1 Clinical Features

Extramammary Paget disease (EMPD) is a rare intraepithelial adenocarcinoma that may arise from primary or secondary spread of malignant cells. EMPD comprises 1–2% of all vulvar malignancies [8], but in terms of EMPD sites, the vulva is the most common. Other less common areas of involvement include the perianal region, eyelids, groin, and scrotum [9]. Secondary EMPD represents spread of an internal malignancy, often a genitourinary or gastrointestinal source, and may represent up to 30% of EMPD cases [10]. Ruling out internal malignancy is vital as this portends different prognostic and therapeutic implications.

Women affected by EMPD of the vulva are usually between 50 and 80 years old [11]. Clinically, lesions present as multicentric moist, red pruritic plaques with or without ulceration. Erythema with hyperkeratotic scale may lead to a clinical differential diagnosis of more common conditions such as eczema, *Candida albicans* infection, or vulvar intraepithelial neoplasia. While pruritus is the most common symptom, up to 10% of patients may be asymptomatic, and diagnosis may not occur until 2 years after symptom onset [12].

6.2.2 Microscopic Findings

EMPD is characterized by large, atypical cells with pale cytoplasm, namely, Paget cells, arranged singly or in nests, occupying the lower level of the epidermis (Fig. 6.3). Cytologically, Paget cells display pale cytoplasm and enlarged vesicular nuclei with prominent nucleoli.

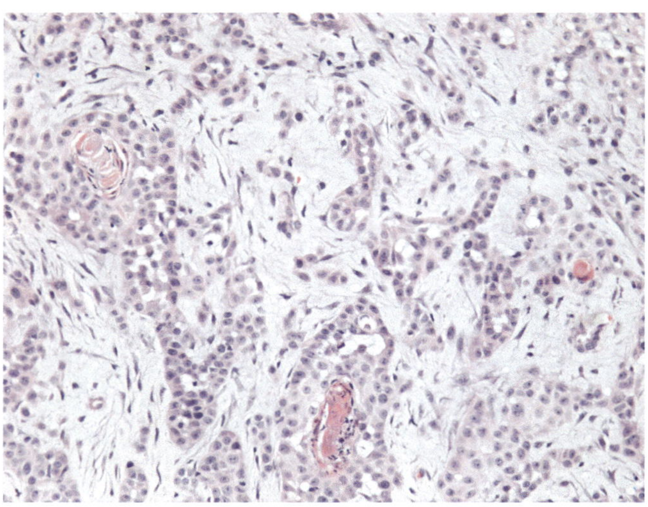

Fig. 6.2 Squamous cell carcinoma with acantholytic features (original magnification, 200×)

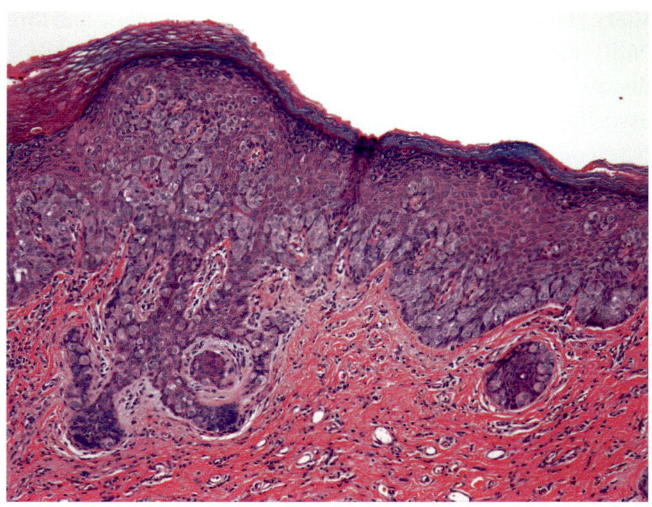

Fig. 6.3 Extramammary Paget disease, lower third of the epidermis is involved by small clusters or single cells with noticeably fainter cytoplasm staining (original magnification, 100×)

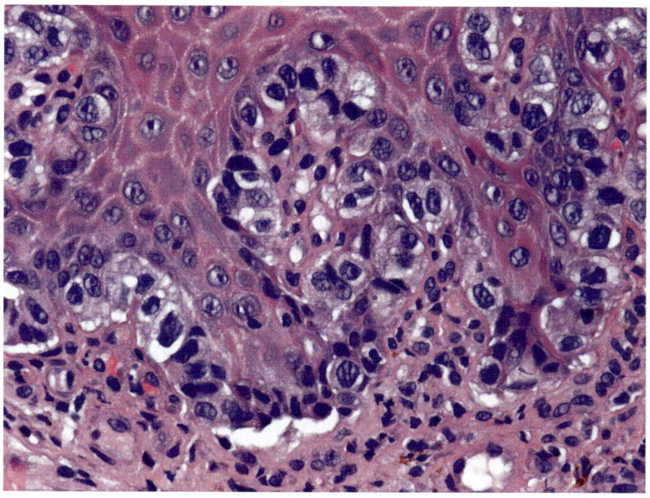

Fig. 6.4 Extramammary Paget disease, the presence of cytoplasmic vacuoles aids in the diagnosis of an adenocarcinoma (original magnification, 400×)

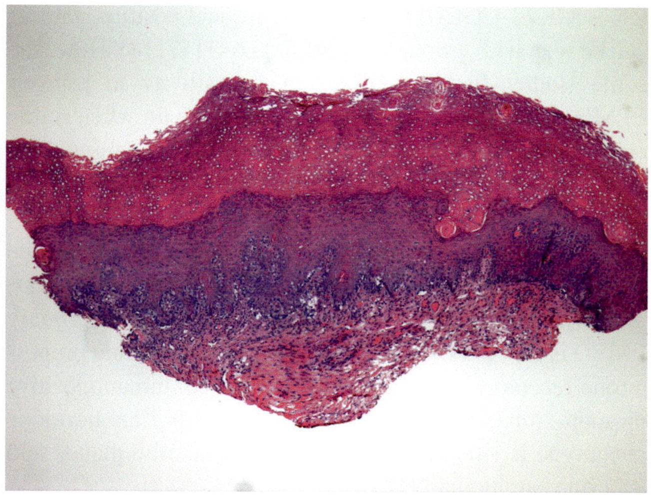

Fig. 6.5 Extramammary Paget disease. Overlying epidermal changes, including squamous hyperplasia as seen here, are often encountered in EMPD (original magnification, 40×)

Cytoplasmic vacuoles may be seen (Fig. 6.4). Occasionally, Paget cells may be found in the upper layers of the epidermis or extending along adnexal structures. Similar to other cutaneous tumors, adnexal extension does not equate invasive disease, and preservation of the basal keratinocytes is a key clue to ruling out invasion [11]. Direct stromal invasion may be difficult to find given the multicentric nature of EMPD, but its incidence may be as high as 47% [13].

Other histologic patterns can be observed in EMPD and include glandular and acantholysis-like patterns [14]. The glandular pattern is uncommon but shows intraepidermal glands with polarization of tumor cells around a central lumen. The acantholytic pattern demonstrates tumor cells falling apart within the epidermis and creating spaces; this lack of cohesion between tumor cells and neighboring keratinocytes imparts a pseudoglandular appearance. Invasion is characterized by malignant cells located in the dermis as nests or single cells with clear delineation from the basement membrane. Rare reports have described invasion presenting as mucinous carcinoma [10]. Some studies have found correlation between the presence of invasion and the histologic pattern of EMPD, but these studies are limited in sample size and not restricted to vulvar EMPD [14].

Epidermal changes are commonly encountered in association with EMPD. Hyperplasia and anastomosis of the epidermal rete ridges have been described in EMPD of the perianal region [15]. Other epidermal proliferations include papillomatous hyperplasia, fibroepithelioma-like hyperplasia, and squamous hyperplasia (Fig. 6.5). Concurrent in situ and invasive squamous cell carcinoma have also been observed in cases of vulvar EMPD [16]. One must be aware of these benign and malignant epidermal changes as they may obscure or distract from a diagnosis of EMPD.

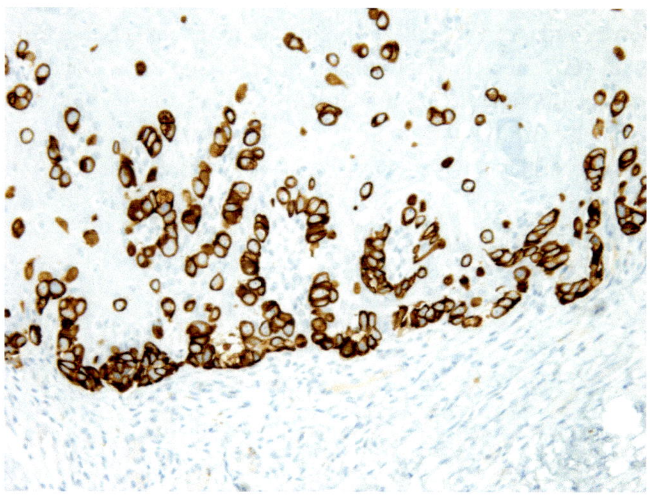

Fig. 6.6 Extramammary Paget disease. Immunohistochemical staining for cytokeratin 7 shows positivity in the EMPD cells that are predominantly found in the lower epidermis. Note the negativity for CK7 in the normal keratinocytes (original magnification, 200×)

6.2.3 Immunohistochemistry

Immunohistochemical staining patterns are useful when attempting to differentiate between primary and secondary EMPD. EMPD tumor cells typically express low molecular weight cytokeratin, epithelial membrane antigen (EMA), gross cystic disease fluid protein 15 (GCDFP-15), and carcinoembryonic antigen (CEA). Primary EMPD has an immunoprofile of CK7+/CK20-/GCDFP15+ (Fig. 6.6). Positivity for Her2/neu may be seen in 30–50% of primary EMPD. Secondary EMPD immunophenotypes depend upon the primary site. Secondary EMPD from an anorectal primary will be CK7-/CK20+/GCDFP15- as well as MUC2+ and CDX2+. EMPD from a urothelial primary is usually

CK7+/CK20 +/GCDFP-15-, and additional positive staining can be seen with uroplakin-3 and GATA-3 [17, 18]. However, some studies have found GATA-3 positivity in primary EPMD, which may make it a less reliable stain when ruling out a urothelial primary [19]. A summary of an immunohistochemical panel which may be useful in distinguishing primary from secondary EMPD is provided in (Table 6.1).

Intracellular mucin is highlighted by the use of special stains such as periodic acid Schiff, Alcian blue, or mucicarmine [20]. In terms of hormone receptor status, primary EMPD is characteristically negative for estrogen and progesterone receptors; androgen receptor can be immunopositive in approximately half of cases. Interestingly, this hormone phenotype is similar to that of benign apocrine glands and apocrine carcinoma [21].

6.2.4 Differential Diagnosis

Superficial spreading melanoma and *melanoma in situ* may have similar cytological and architectural features. Large cells with prominent nucleoli can form nests and show pagetoid spread throughout the epidermis; however, melanoma will typically involve the basal layer, whereas EMPD shows an intact basal layer with displacement of keratinocytes (Fig. 6.7). Melanin pigment may be more prominent in variants of melanoma, but occasional melanin may be seen in Paget cells [11]. Paget cells are usually negative for melanocytes markers such as S-100, HMB45, Melan-A, and SOX10 [20]. In addition, melanoma is negative for mucins by various special stains.

Squamous cell carcinoma (SCC), in situ or invasive, is a much more common entity that may show pagetoid spread of neoplastic cells (Fig. 6.8). A histologic clue is full-thickness atypia with effacement of the basal layer in squamous lesions. SCC will lack glandular formation and intracellular mucin and is usually negative for CK7 and GCDFP-15 and positive for CK5/CK6, p63, and p16 [22]. *Usual-type vulvar intraepithelial neoplasia* (uVIN) falls on the premalignant spectrum of SCC, and, like SCC, pagetoid spread has been described. Diffuse, full-thickness positivity with p16 aids in the diagnosis of uVIN.

Sebaceous carcinoma, which typically involves the head and neck, is another rare malignancy which may show cytologic and architectural overlap with EMPD. Sebaceous carcinoma is cytologically characterized by atypical basaloid cells showing foci of sebocytic differentiation in the form of multiple lipid-filled vacuoles with nuclear indentation. Architecturally, the intraepidermal portion often shows pagetoid spread, and dermal invasion is apparent (Fig. 6.9). Immunohistochemistry is a useful tool in cases of superfi-

Table 6.1 Immunophenotypes of EMPD

		Secondary EMPD		
	Primary EMPD	Anorectal	Urothelial	Cervical
Cytokeratin 7	+	–	+	+
Cytokeratin 20	–	+	+	–
GCDFP-15	+	–	–	–
Additional positive stains	Her-2/neu	MUC-2 CDX-2	GATA-3 Uroplakin-3	p63 p16

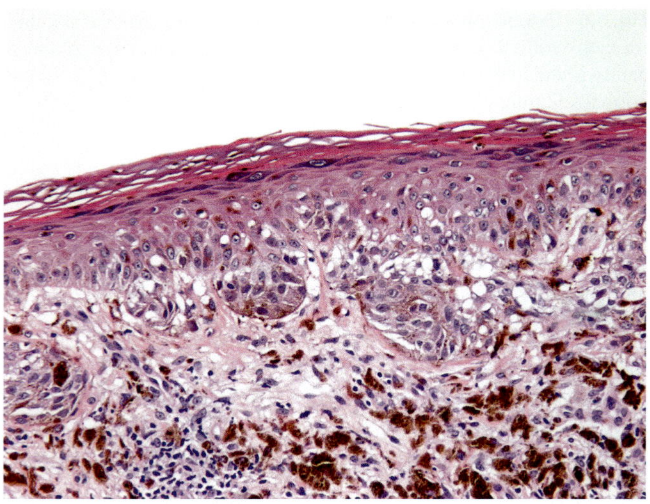

Fig. 6.7 Superficial spreading melanoma with basally located melanocytes. Note the grayish cytoplasm, lack of mucin vacuoles, and presence of melanin (original magnification, 200×)

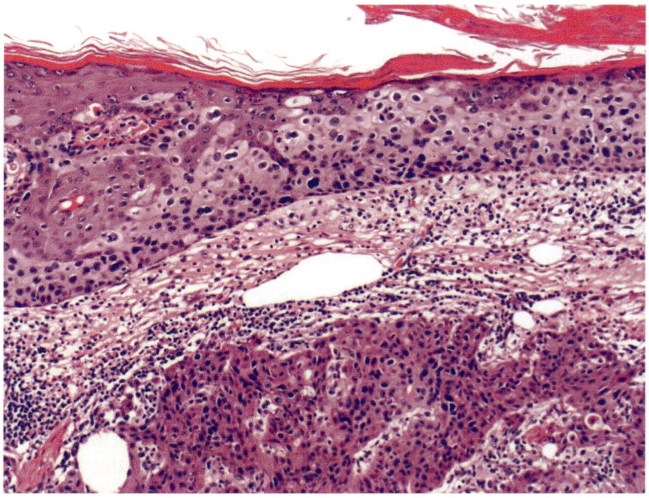

Fig. 6.8 Squamous cell carcinoma with pagetoid spread (original magnification, 100×)

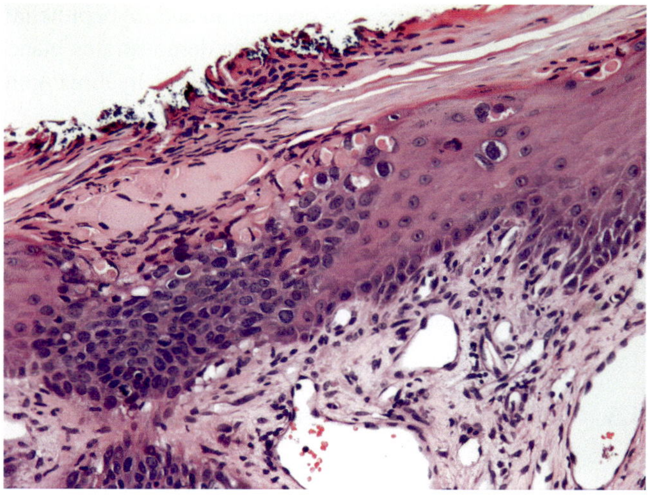

Fig. 6.9 Sebaceous carcinoma with intraepidermal spread (original magnification, 200×)

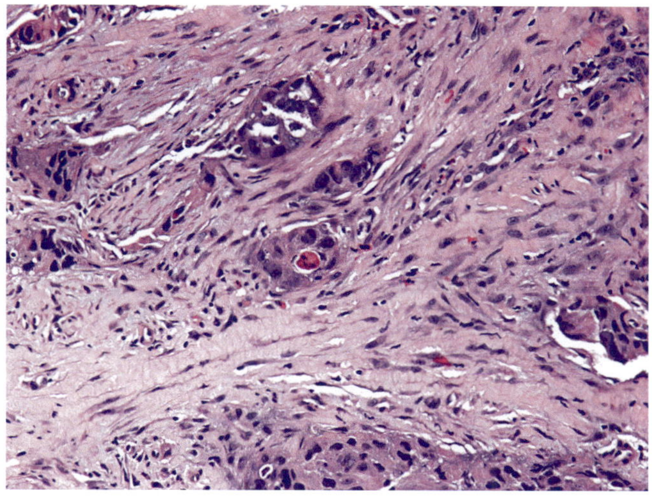

Fig. 6.10 Ductal adenocarcinoma showing high-grade nuclear features with surrounding desmoplastic stroma (original magnification, 200×)

cially sampled sebaceous carcinoma in which the dermal component is not readily visualized. Sebaceous carcinoma shows membranous positivity for adipophilin around lipid vesicles, and staining for nuclear factor XIIIa has been proposed as a sensitive marker of sebaceous differentiation [23, 24]. Sebaceous tumor cells will be negative for GCDFP-15 and CEA.

6.3 Carcinoma Arising in Ectopic Breast Tissue

6.3.1 Clinical Features

Ectopic breast tissue is the result of incomplete ectodermal involution and may be found anywhere from the axilla to the vulva [25]. Clinically, palpable ectopic breast tissue may be mistaken as a lipoma due to a predominance of adipose tissue. As with other ectopic tissue, there remains a small but present risk for malignancy. Only a few dozen cases of carcinoma arising from ectopic breast tissue have been reported. Patients tend to be in their late 60s, but patients as young as 44 years old have been reported [26]. Lesions may be slightly tender and average 3 cm in size. As with any vulvar mass in a postmenopausal woman, vulvar lesions should be approached with a high suspicion for malignancy.

6.3.2 Microscopic Findings

Breast carcinoma arising from ectopic breast tissue has the same morphologic variants as seen in breast primaries. *Ductal carcinoma* is characterized by infiltrating angulated glands with varying degrees of nuclear atypia (Fig. 6.10).

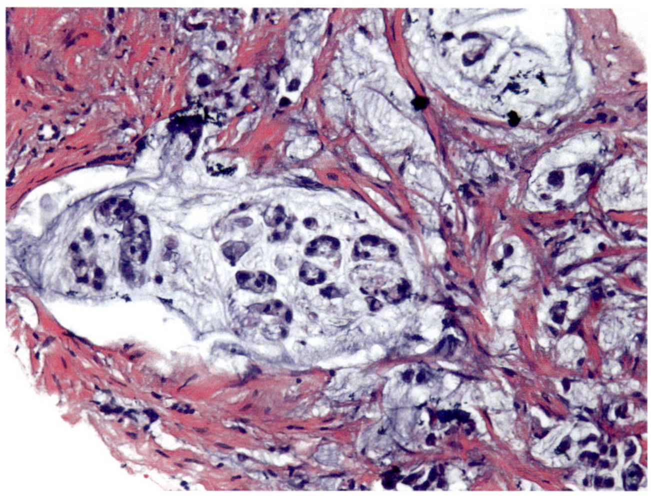

Fig. 6.11 Mucinous carcinoma is comprised of islands of low-grade neoplastic cells floating in mucin (original magnification, 200×)

Tumors can range from well-formed glands (low-grade) to sheets of tumor cells with high mitotic activity (high-grade). Ductal carcinoma in situ may be identified by distended glands filled with a monotonous population of cells with or without comedonecrosis.

Mucinous carcinoma is another variant of breast carcinoma that may be seen in the vulva. This variant features an abundance of extracellular mucin with floating islands of tumor cells (Fig. 6.11). Tumor cells are typically well-differentiated with low-grade nuclear features. Thin fibrous septa traverse the mucin pools and form compartments.

Lobular carcinoma is typically low-grade and shows invasion as single cells arranged in cords.

It is essential to assess lymphovascular invasion and subsequent lymph node metastasis in cases of breast carcinoma arising from ectopic tissue. Previous reviews of the literature have reported lymph node metastasis in up to 66% of cases [26].

Normal benign changes of the breast may also be found in ectopic breast tissue [27]. An example is lactational change, which features closely packed glands with cytoplasmic blebs and vacuoles. Relative increases in cellularity and prominent nucleoli raise the suspicion for malignancy, but overall well-circumscribed architecture and clinical awareness are key in recognizing benign mimics.

6.3.3 Immunohistochemistry

Similar to primary breast carcinoma, carcinoma arising out of ectopic breast tissue will stain positively for pancytokeratin, CK7, mammoglobin, and gross cystic disease fluid protein (GCDFP-15) [26]. Over half of cases will stain estrogen receptor (ER) and progesterone receptor (PR) positive. Her2/neu, human epidermal growth factor receptor 2, is typically negative in these carcinomas. Given the infrequency of Her2/neu positivity, many authors only require positivity in ER or PR as part of their diagnostic criteria for breast carcinoma arising from the vulva [28].

6.3.4 Differential Diagnosis

Other patterns of primary breast carcinoma are less likely but should be considered in the differential diagnosis.

6.3.5 Prognosis and Therapy

Given the rarity of breast carcinoma arising from ectopic breast tissue, there are no widely accepted treatment guidelines at this time. In the event of a positive sentinel node, lymph node mapping with subsequent lymphadenectomy has been researched and strongly supported by some authors [29]. Treatment plans for vulvar primaries may mirror those of breast primaries: personalization of surgical, chemotherapeutic, and hormonal therapies [26].

6.4 Phyllodes Tumor

The lesional transformation of mammary-like tissue is not restricted solely to the ductal epithelium as stromal lesions, while rare, can also occur. Typically, lesions present as solitary, mobile, and painless nodules involving the labia majora [30]. Prior literature review of vulvar phyllodes tumor characterized the gross findings as a well-circumscribed white lesion with a pushing margin and papillary-like fronds [30]. The histologic features are similar to that of a primary breast phyllodes tumor and include leaflike fronds of stromal overgrowth covered by a bilayer of epithelium and myoepithelial cells. Higher power view of the stroma demonstrates bland spindle cells in a collagenized background; hyalinization may be focal when present [31].

Immunohistochemical staining shows the ductal epithelial cells are positive for ER and PR, which in contrast, are negative in the stromal spindle cells [30]. The myoepithelial cells are positive for SMA and S-100. The stromal spindle cells are also positive for CD34, vimentin, and SMA; ER and PR are usually negative.

6.5 Skene's Gland Adenocarcinoma

While the periurethral Skene's gland is part of the genitourinary system, it is important to recognize that the exceedingly rare Skene's gland adenocarcinoma may be encountered as a vulvar lesion. This tumor typically affects women in their 60s, and median tumor size has been reported to be 3.0 cm. Pain may be elicited by the perineural invasion of the tumor.

Gross features include poor circumscription with invasive borders; the surface is usually solid, although necrosis may be present [32]. Histologic features may vary widely as the tumor may show features similar to prostatic, intestinal, or adenoid cystic carcinomas. Prostatic differentiation will show highly atypical cells with cribiforming or tubular formation, and immunostaining may show positivity for PSA, CA-125, and P504S [33]. Intestinal differentiation will show cribiforming with glandular areas and signet rings. Similar to other tumor that show intestinal features, immunostaining will show positivity for CDX2 and MUC2 [32].

6.6 Skin Appendage Adenocarcinoma

Due to the presence of hair, apocrine glands, and sebaceous glands found throughout the vulvar skin, the malignant counterparts of these cell lines have been reported in the vulva. Approximately half of malignant vulvar adnexal tumors are some form of EMPD, and the other less frequent malignant tumors include sebaceous carcinoma, apocrine carcinoma, and microcystic adnexal carcinoma [34]. Adenoid cystic carcinoma is discussed later in this chapter as a carcinoma of the Bartholin gland.

6.6.1 Clinical Features

Due to a higher density of skin appendages, cutaneous adnexal malignancies are much more common on the head and neck of patients in their 50s and 60s. However, there are multiple case reports of such lesions affecting the vulva. Typically, these lesions present as a slowly growing papule

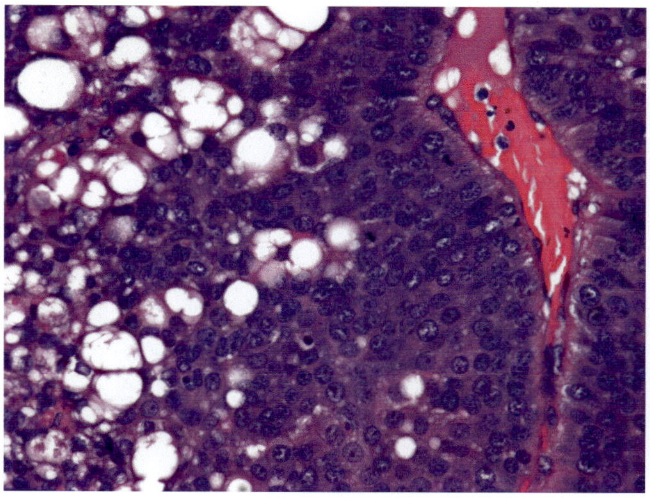

Fig. 6.12 Sebaceous carcinoma. Oftentimes focal, the presence of lipid vacuoles that indent the nucleus is useful in identifying sebaceous carcinoma and differentiating it from basal cell carcinoma (original magnification, 400×)

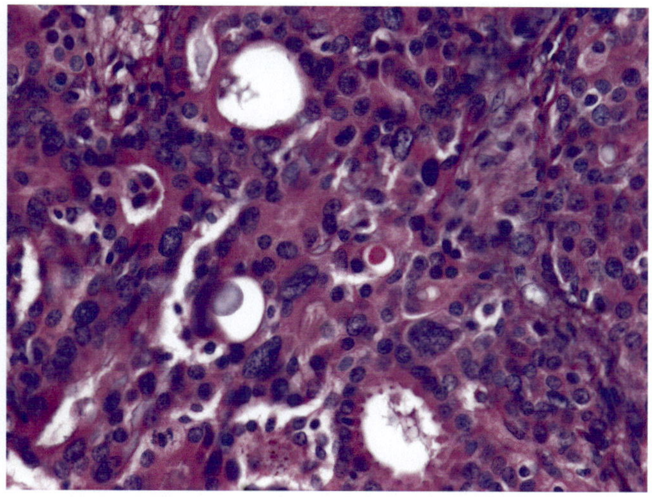

Fig. 6.13 Apocrine carcinoma showing marked nuclear atypia with areas of gland formation and apical snouting (original magnification, 400×)

with various degrees of pain or paresthesia, which is likely secondary to nerve involvement [35]. Ulceration and pain are variable, and lesions average 3.0 cm in size [35, 36].

Coloration varies from flesh-colored to slightly yellow as is the case for *sebaceous carcinoma* due to its increased lipid content [37].

6.6.2 Microscopic Findings

Sebaceous carcinoma is characterized by lobules of basaloid cells with marked atypia and mitoses. Well-differentiated tumors will display clear cell change in the center of the tumor nodules, and tumor cells will have multiple lipid vacuoles that indent the nucleus (Fig. 6.12). Within the tumor nodules, central comedonecrosis is a common finding. With poorly differentiated tumors, there are less obvious malignant sebocytes and more basaloid cells with prominent atypia. Occasionally, these cells may have a squamous appearance, which may lead to confusion with much more common entities such as squamous cell carcinoma.

Apocrine carcinoma features large eosinophilic cells arranged in cords and nests within the dermis. At scanning magnification, these tumors can appear benign as there may be an overall nodular growth of tightly packed glands. Higher power viewing reveals these glands dissecting through collagen fibers with various degrees of cribiforming. Tumor cells may showed marked atypia and have characteristic decapitation secretion and apical snouting (Fig. 6.13) [38].

Microcystic adnexal carcinoma (MAC) is a slow growing but locally aggressive sweat gland tumor that may be confused with benign syringoma, desmoplastic trichoepithelioma, or infiltrative basal cell carcinoma, especially when interpreting a superficial biopsy. At low power, MAC is asymmetric and poorly circumscribed and usually extends into the deep dermis and subcutis. The superficial aspect of the tumor shows keratinous cysts and basaloid strands with variable ductal differentiation. The stroma displays a desmoplastic response. MAC may also grow as nests and cords, and there is a characteristic "tadpole-like" trailing of the ductal component, which is architecturally similar to syringoma (Fig. 6.14) [35]. Key histologic features to distinguish MAC from syringoma are the presence of perineural invasion and extension of the low-grade ductal structures into the subcutaneous tissue or muscle (Fig. 6.15). As opposed to MAC, syringomas and desmoplastic trichoepitheliomas are sharply demarcated laterally at the base of the lesion. As such, a sufficiently deep biopsy is required for accurate diagnosis.

6.6.3 Immunohistochemistry

Sebaceous carcinoma can be readily identified on routine staining in well-differentiated cases. For cases with poor differentiation, immunohistochemistry has more utility. Epithelial membrane antigen (EMA) positivity is helpful in well-differentiated sebaceous carcinomas, as positivity helps rule out basal cell carcinoma, which is EMA negative [39]. Adipophilin, which is a protein found within lipid droplets in cells, is a highly sensitive and specific immunostain for sebaceous neoplasms [40]. Nuclear positivity for androgen receptor can be seen even in poorly differentiated sebaceous carcinomas, but this does not rule out basal cell carcinoma as over half of BCC may be androgen receptor positive [41]. Positivity for nuclear factor XIIIa may be helpful in supporting sebaceous differentiation [24].

Apocrine carcinoma expresses gross cystic disease fluid protein-15 (GCDFP-15), estrogen receptor, and androgen

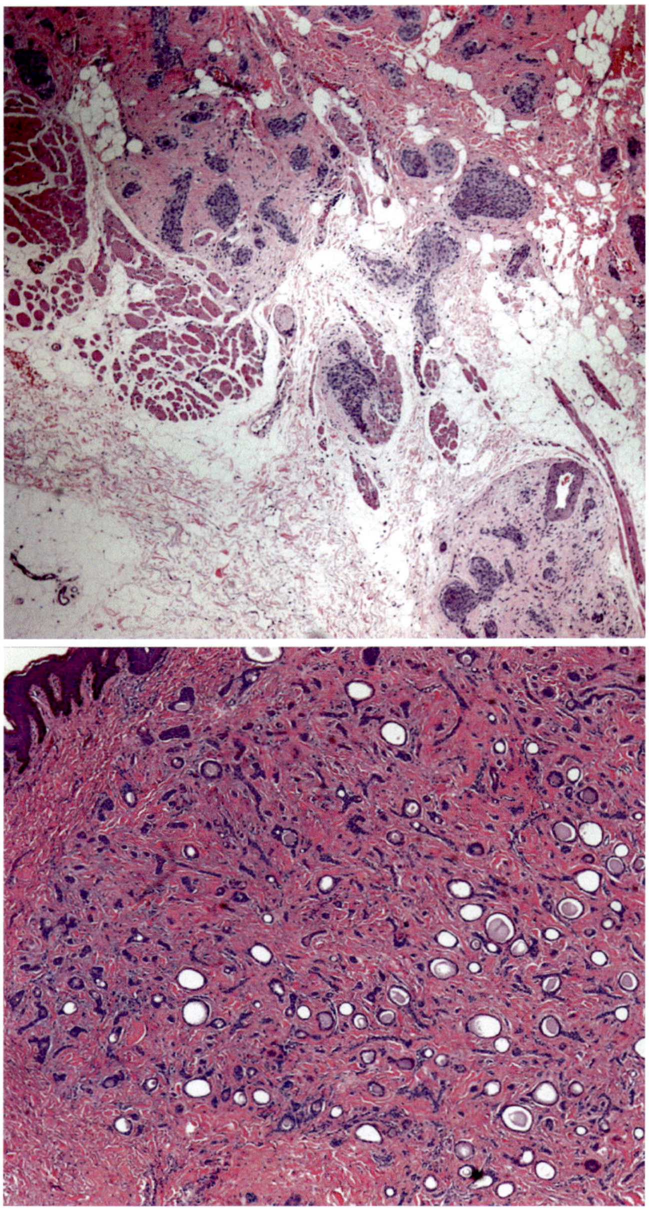

Fig. 6.14 Microcystic adnexal carcinoma (top) is composed of low-grade cells forming nests and cords with occasional lumen formation. Invasion into the subcutis and perineural invasion are key to the diagnosis. Syringoma (bottom) has the same nested and corded architecture, but involvement is limited to the dermis and usually well-circumscribed (original magnification, 40×)

receptor [42]. One must be careful when relying on histology or immunohistochemistry for the diagnosis of cutaneous apocrine carcinoma versus breast carcinoma. Hormone receptors and GCDFP-15 are positive in both entities, and immunostaining patterns with mammoglobin may not fully elucidate tumor origin. Thorough review of clinical history and searching for neighboring mammary-like glands are helpful in making this rare diagnosis.

Pancytokeratin may be useful to highlight the extent of tumor spread in *MAC*. BerEP4 negativity may be useful to differentiate MAC from an infiltrative or morpheaform basal cell carcinoma, which shows intense BerEP4 positivity [43]. Cytokeratin 15 negativity and cytokeratin 19 positivity helps distinguish MAC from desmoplastic trichoepithelioma; although, some studies have found various degrees of CK15 positivity in MAC [43, 44]. CK20-positive Merkel cells are present as colonizing desmoplastic trichoepitheliomas but are absent in basal cell carcinomas and microcystic adnexal carcinomas [45].

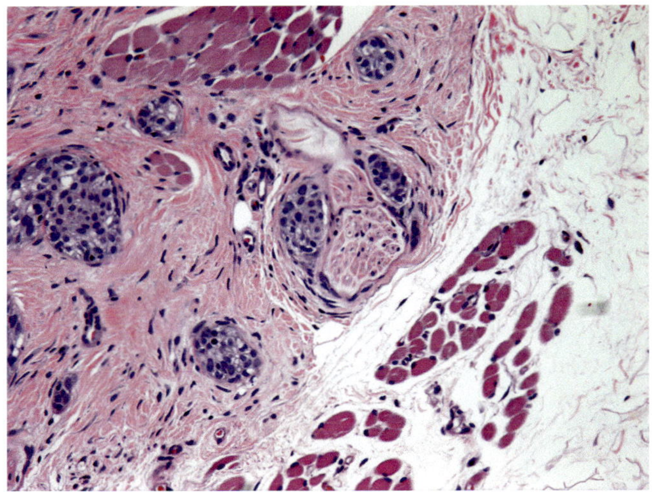

Fig. 6.15 Microcystic adnexal carcinoma. The presence of subcutaneous or, in this case, perineural invasion is essential feature to make the diagnosis of MAC (original magnification, 200×)

6.7 Carcinoma of the Bartholin Gland

6.7.1 Clinical Features

Carcinomas of the Bartholin gland comprise less than 5% of vulvar carcinomas and less than 1% of all gynecologic cancers. The most common histologic subtype is squamous cell carcinoma, followed by adenocarcinoma and less common tumors such as adenoid cystic carcinoma and small cell neuroendocrine carcinoma [46, 47]. Such tumors typically present as a painless mass of the posterolateral vulva in postmenopausal females. Patients may complain of pruritus, vulvodynia, or abnormal bleeding. One should be cautious when diagnosing any Bartholin gland "cyst" reported in a postmenopausal female and approach such lesions with a high suspicion for malignancy [48]. The biopsy should provide appropriate depth, and one must exclude more common diagnoses such as metastasis.

6.7.2 Pathologic Features

6.7.2.1 Gross Findings

Bartholin gland carcinoma is usually an ill-defined mass that has an average size of 4.0 cm [49]. The lesion may be cystic or firm, and focal areas of necrosis may be identified on the cut surface.

6.7.2.2 Microscopic Findings

Squamous Cell Carcinoma

The most common histologic subtype of Bartholin gland carcinoma is squamous cell carcinoma (SCC). Similar to SCC of other organs, various degrees of differentiation and keratinization can be seen. Identification of carcinoma in situ within the Bartholin gland duct is a histologic clue to tumor origin.

Adenocarcinoma

The second most common histologic subtype, adenocarcinoma, may show papillary or solid patterns. Intraductal adenocarcinoma features markedly atypical cells tracking along the Bartholin gland duct extending to the squamous-lined surface. Other features include cribiforming and intraductal necrosis similar to that seen in intraductal carcinoma in situ of breast origin. Invasion is noted by angulated glands with adjacent desmoplastic stroma. Cytologically, tumor cells are hyperchromatic with irregular nuclear borders and increased N:C ratio.

Adenoid Cystic Carcinoma

Morphologic features of adenoid cystic carcinoma of the Bartholin gland are identical to those seen in the salivary gland and other sites. The tumor is composed of infiltrating glands with a characteristic cribiforming pattern, commonly described as "cookie-cutter" (Fig. 6.16). Morphology is commonly a mixture of tubuloglandular and nested patterns [50]. Eosinophilic basement membrane-like material is found within these cribiforming neoplastic glands. Similar to a primary salivary gland malignancy, perineural invasion is commonly found in adenoid cystic carcinoma [51].

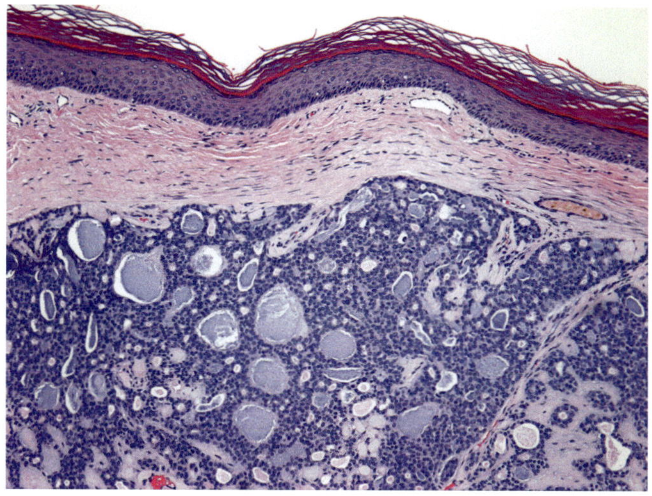

Fig. 6.16 Adenoid cystic carcinoma showing punched out luminal spaces characteristic of adenoid cystic carcinoma (original magnification, 100×)

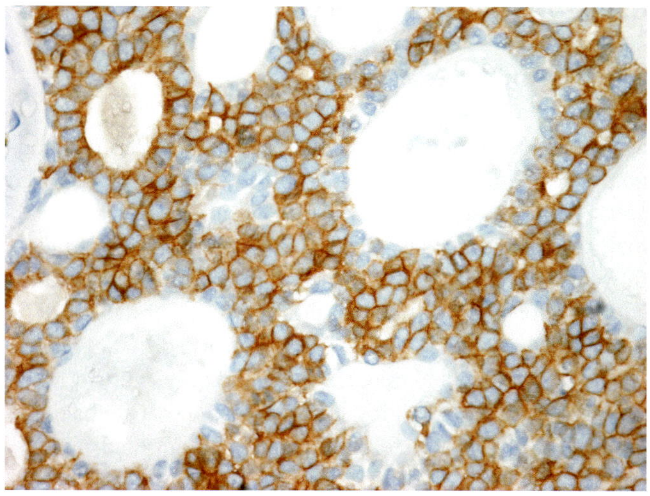

Fig. 6.17 Adenoid cystic carcinoma. Membranous and cytoplasmic immunopositivity for CD117 (c-kit) may be restricted to luminal cells or involve all tumor cells (original magnification, 400×)

Small Cell Carcinoma

Small cell carcinoma is a poorly differentiated neuroendocrine carcinoma that shows "small blue cells" at low power. Architectural features include tumor cells arranged in nests or trabeculae. Tumor cells show enlarged nuclei with a thin rim of cytoplasm, and nuclear molding is abundant. Extensive crush artifact is present, which may raise suspicion for lymphoma.

6.7.2.3 Immunohistochemistry

In cases of poorly differentiated neoplasms, immunohistochemistry may play a vital role (Table 6.1). SCC will stain positively for p63, high molecular weight cytokeratin, CEA, and EMA. Infection with HPV type 16 in cases of Bartholin gland SCC makes diffuse p16 positivity a surrogate marker for HPV infection [47, 52].

Adenoid cystic carcinoma shows membrane and cytoplasmic positivity for c-kit (CD117) in the luminal cells; although, the pattern of immunopositivity may differ by tumor pattern (Fig. 6.17) [53]. Peripheral myoepithelial cells show p63 nuclear positivity (Fig. 6.18) and variable nuclear and cytoplasmic S-100 positivity, which demonstrates the myoepithelial component of this tumor [54]. Luminal tumor cells are also positive for CK 8/18, AE1/AE3, and EMA [52].

Small cell carcinoma shows variable membrane and cytoplasmic positivity, if any, for keratins. Nuclear TTF-1 positivity is not site-specific, and positivity has been described to vary by tumor origin [55]. Oftentimes, cytoplasmic positivity for neuroendocrine markers, such as synaptophysin and chromogranin, is essential to determine neuroendocrine origin.

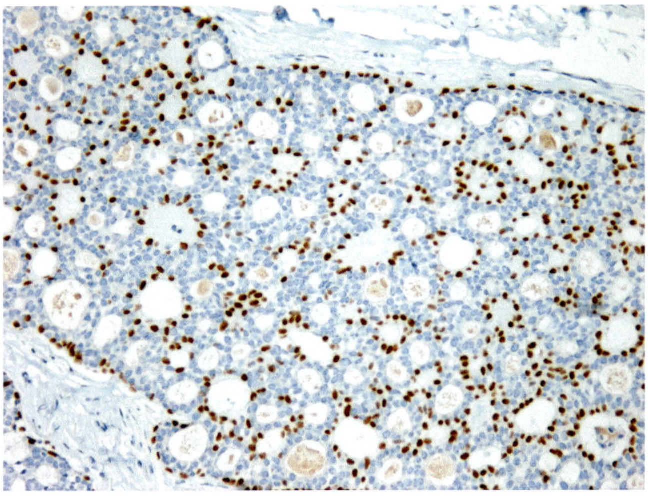

Fig. 6.18 Adenoid cystic carcinoma. Nuclear positivity for p63 highlights myoepithelial cells within adenoid cystic carcinoma (original magnification, 200×)

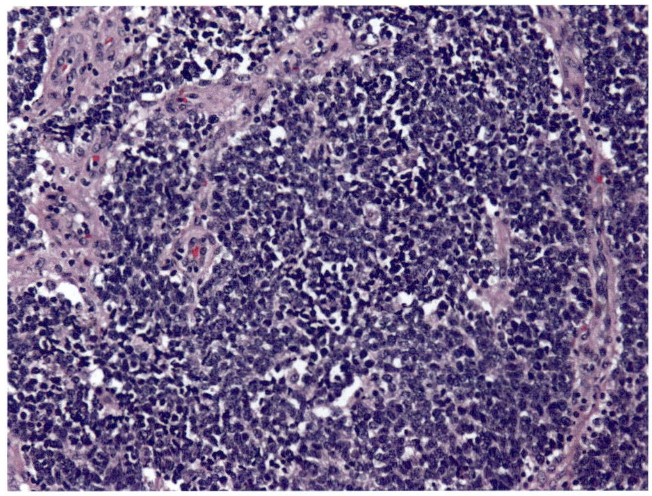

Fig. 6.19 Merkel cell carcinoma consists of sheets of tumor cells that give a "blue" appearance due to high N:C ratio (original magnification, 200×)

6.8 Merkel Cell Carcinoma

6.8.1 Clinical Features

Merkel cell carcinoma (MCC) is an aggressive cutaneous neuroendocrine carcinoma that typically affects sun-exposed areas with over half located on the head and neck. A vast majority of patients are Caucasians with an average age of 69 years [56]. Vulvar MCC is quite rare, which makes clinical behavior more difficult to predict [57]. Similar to MCC of the head and neck, vulvar MCC is marked by aggressive clinical behavior and recurrence. Clinically, vulvar MCC presents as a rapidly growing red-blue mass at the labia majora [58]. Tumor size can average 7.5 cm, and patients commonly complain of tenderness, pruritus, and ulceration. Time to presentation can be delayed, and overall disease duration can range from 1 to 18 months [58]. Similar to other mass lesions of the vulva, MCC may be clinically mistaken for a Bartholin gland cyst or abscess. As mentioned earlier in this chapter, one should have a high index of suspicion for malignancy when encountering a suspected Bartholin gland cyst in a postmenopausal patient.

6.8.2 Microscopic Findings

MCC is characterized by nests and trabeculae of cells with high nuclear to cytoplasmic ratio (Fig. 6.19) [59]. The tumor may show areas of invasion with adjacent mucinous and mucin-filled spaces similar to that seen in basal cell carcinoma [60]. Larger tumors tend to display geographic necrosis. Increased mitoses and apoptotic debris can be found throughout the tumor [61]. Lymphovascular invasion is commonly present and usually best appreciated at the tumor periphery. MCC tumor cells have been reported to display pagetoid spread in up to 20% of cases [60, 62].

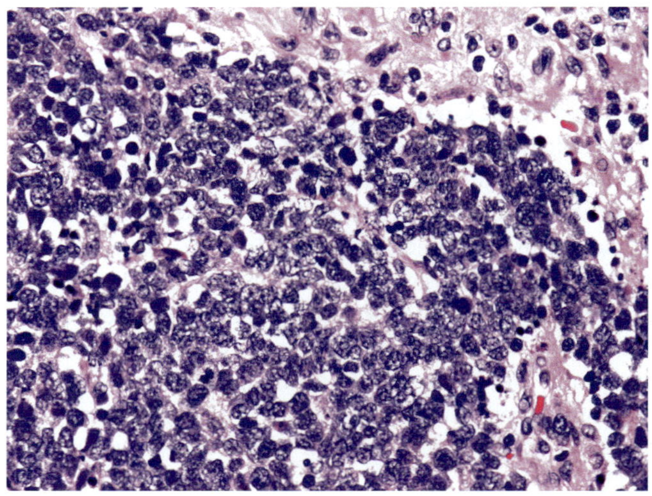

Fig. 6.20 High nuclear/cytoplasm ratio with "salt and pepper" chromatin and nuclear molding are characteristic features of Merkel cell carcinoma (original magnification, 400×)

Similar to neuroendocrine carcinomas arising from other locations, nuclear features of MCC exhibit homogeneous "salt and pepper" chromatin, nuclear molding, and inconspicuous nucleoli (Fig. 6.20) [60]. These nuclear features are key factors to distinguish from basal cell carcinoma, which would show well-developed peripheral palisading of tumor cells. Crush artifact is typically present, and the extent of crush may raise suspicion for a hematolymphoid neoplasm.

6.8.3 Immunohistochemistry

Given the histologic overlap of MCC with other entities, immunohistochemistry plays a vital role in excluding other

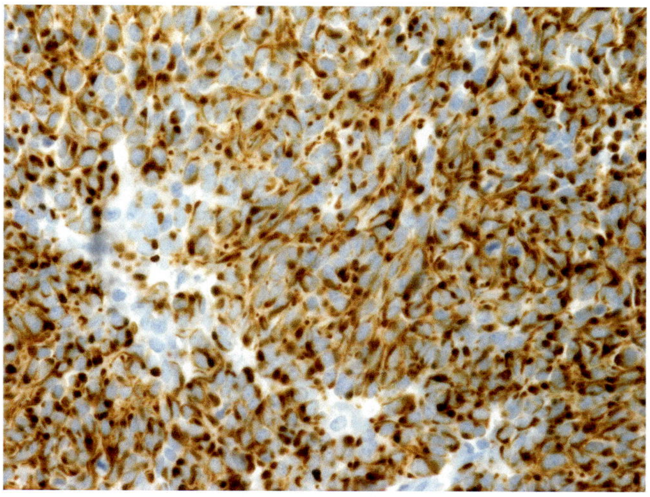

Fig. 6.21 Immunohistochemical staining for cytokeratin 20 shows perinuclear “dot-like” staining (original magnification, 400×)

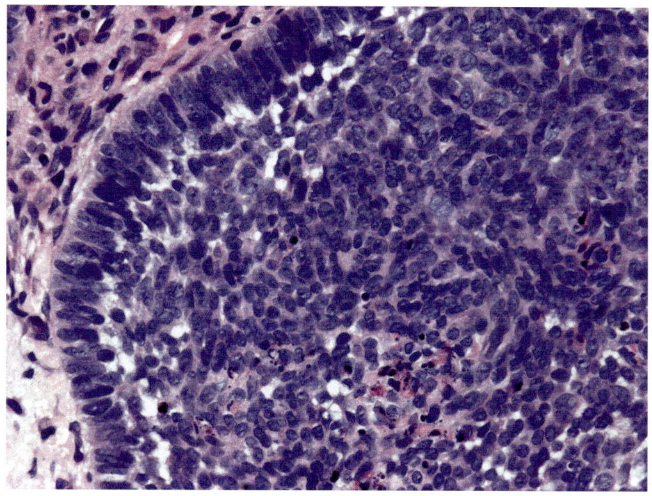

Fig. 6.22 Basal cell carcinoma has characteristic palisading of tumor cells at the tumor-stroma interface (original magnification, 400×)

high-grade tumors. Pancytokeratin is positive in approximately half of cases of vulvar MCC, and low molecular weight keratin can be positive in as few as 20% of cases [58]. Typically, MCC stains negative for CK7 and positive for CK20, but a subset of MCC with CK20-/CK7+ has been reported [63, 64]. In the setting of CK20 positivity, MCC has a classic perinuclear dot-like positivity (Fig. 6.21) [58]. Like other neuroendocrine tumors, there must be some degree of positivity for chromogranin, synaptophysin, or neuron-specific enolase. As with all immunostains, caution must be used when dealing with areas of crush artifact.

6.8.4 Differential Diagnosis

Basal cell carcinoma, when considering overall cutaneous distribution, is the most common cutaneous malignancy [65]. The correlation between basal cell carcinoma and cumulative UV exposure is well established, and the majority is found at the head and neck [66]. Once thought to be rare as a vulvar neoplasm, approximately 2% of basal cell carcinomas arise in the vulva [67]. The average age of affected patient is 70 years old, and lesions typically average 2.0 cm with ulceration a common finding. Clinical symptoms are non-specific and include bleeding, pruritus, and pain [67]. Histologically, basal cell carcinoma is characterized by peripheral palisading of basaloid cells with high nuclear/chromatin ratio (Fig. 6.22). Common morphologic patterns include superficial invasion, nodular, and infiltrative. Similar to MCC, basal cell carcinoma has mucinous stroma, but basal cell carcinoma exhibits artifactual retraction of the tumor-stroma interface. Mitotic activity is less frequent than in MCC. Immunostaining for basal cell carcinoma will show positivity for Ber-EP4 and negativity for CK20, synaptophysin, and chromogranin-A.

Lymphoma can rarely affect the gynecologic tract, and the most common type affecting the vulva is diffuse large B-cell lymphoma [68]. Lymphomas may be histologically distinguished from MCC in various ways. Unlike the trabecular and nested patterns of invasion seen in MCC, lymphomas tend to form sheets of dyscohesive cells. Similar to MCC, crush artifact and necrosis may be common, but lymphomas will not have the “salt and pepper” chromatin pattern seen in neuroendocrine tumors. A broad stain such as CD45 will stain positively in lymphomas, while cytokeratins and neuroendocrine markers will be negative. Lymphoblastic lymphoma, which may lack CD45, is a notable exception.

Extrapulmonary small cell carcinoma is rare and occurs in approximately 2% of all cases of small cell carcinoma [69]. Small cell carcinoma arising from the gynecologic tract commonly involves the cervix, but areas of less frequent involvement include the ovary, fallopian tube, and vulva. Histologically, small cell carcinoma of the gynecologic tract is identical to that of other sites, including lung primaries. Tumor cells are arranged in sheets or trabeculae, and there is frequently necrosis with increased mitotic rate [69]. A thorough clinical and radiologic history is essential when determining primary versus secondary small cell carcinoma. It should be noted that TTF-1 expression is not specific for small cell carcinoma of pulmonary origin and should not be used to distinguish primary from metastatic small cell carcinomas involving extrapulmonary sites. However, TTF-1 expression may be useful in distinguishing TTF-1 negative Merkel cell carcinomas from cutaneous metastasis of small cell carcinomas, which are TTF-1 positive [55, 70]. Small cell carcinoma is usually negative for CK20, which aids in distinguishing it from MCC.

6.9 Cloacogenic Neoplasms

6.9.1 Clinical Features

Cloacogenic carcinoma of the vulva is an extremely rare variant of primary adenocarcinoma of the vulva with as few as 20 cases reported in the literature [71]. The average age of presentation is 51 years old with a range of 35 to 67 years old [71, 72]. Anatomically, primary adenocarcinomas of the vulva are thought to arise from the Bartholin glands that are normally present in the vulvar area [73–76]. Other possible origins are sweat glands, Skene's glands, minor vestibular glands, or endometriotic implants. Cloacogenic carcinoma is thought to arise from embryonic or ectopic rests of cloacogenic tissue [77]. Rare multicentric cases have been described [78].

6.9.2 Microscopic Findings

Histologically, these lesions resemble colonic adenocarcinoma. A feature found in the majority cases is direct continuity of the tumor with the epidermis [71, 73–77, 79]. The neoplastic cells form glands, and the cells lining the acini are columnar and often stratified. Proliferation into gland-in-gland patterns, varying numbers of goblet cells, and a prominent brush border may be observed [77, 80].

6.9.3 Immunohistochemistry and Histochemistry

Reported cases have shown positive staining with CEA, broad-spectrum cytokeratin, CDX-2, and p53 antigen [72, 73] and variable staining for CK7 and CK20 [79]. A recent case report described diffuse positivity for p53 and only focal positivity for p16INK4a [81]. Neuroendocrine markers such as synaptophysin may highlight endocrine cells [77]. Alcian blue, mucicarmine, and PAS with diastase decorate goblet cells, indicating the presence of enteric-type sialomucins [77].

6.9.4 Differential Diagnosis

As the morphology and potentially the immunophenotype of the tumor are essentially identical to that of colonic adenocarcinoma, a thorough clinical workup is necessary to exclude metastasis from a colonic origin [71, 72, 80].

6.9.5 Prognosis and Treatment

Treatment typically includes wide local excision or, less often, radical vulvectomy with or without local lymph node excision. Most of these tumors are indolent in nature with excision seemingly curative [71, 75, 76, 79]; however, local recurrence has been reported [77] as well as rare more aggressive forms with distant metastasis [72, 74].

6.10 Metastatic Tumors

6.10.1 Clinical Features

Metastatic tumors of the vulva are rare, accounting for 5–8% of vulvar malignancies [2]. These lesions present in females with a median age of 55 years old and are most common in perimenopausal or postmenopausal women; however, the age range of presentation is wide, with patients presenting anywhere from 18 to 84 years of age [82]. In a study of 66 cases of metastatic tumors to the vulva, Neto et al. found that in roughly half of cases, the tumor was of gynecologic origin; 43.9% were from nongynecologic origin, and the remaining had unknown primaries [82]. Primary sites reported in the literature include the anogenital squamous lesions, anal adenocarcinoma, endometrium, lung, and breast [83–87]. Clinical presentation varies from multiple nodules to a single mass. Some less frequent presentations include bleeding, pruritus, swelling, local discomfort, or a cystic lesion [82]. Anatomically, the labium majus is the most commonly involved site [82].

6.10.2 Microscopic Findings

Histologically, metastatic disease resembles the primary tumor.

6.10.3 Immunohistochemistry

Immunohistochemistry varies by the tumor origin; therefore, a wide panel may be necessary to evaluate these lesions depending on the histologic appearance, especially in the absence of a known primary tumor (Table 6.2). CK7 and CK20 are widely used markers in this setting, and PAX-8 (nuclear), which has a moderate to high sensitivity and high specificity for diagnosing carcinomas of Mullerian origin, may also be useful [88]. Table 6.3 provides a summary of immunohistochemical stains which are useful in pinpointing the origin of a metastatic tumor.

Table 6.2 Positive immunohistochemical staining patterns of Bartholin gland carcinoma subtypes [52]

Squamous cell carcinoma	p16 (HPV positive), p63, CEA, CK19
Adenocarcinoma	CAM 5.2, CA 19–9, CEA, EMA
Adenoid cystic carcinoma	Epithelial cells: AE1/AE3, CK 8/18, EMA Myoepithelial cells: CD117, p63, S-100
Small cell carcinoma	CAM 5.2, CD56, neuron-specific enolase, chromogranin, synaptophysin

Table 6.3 Useful immunohistochemical stains for working up metastatic tumors to the vulva [2, 18]

	CK7	CK20	TTF-1	GCDFP-15	ER	PR	Vimentin	p16	CEA
Endometrium	+	–			+		+	Patchy +	–
Lung	+	–	+						
Breast	+	–	–	+	+/–	+/–			
Primary EMPD	+	–		+					
Urothelial	+	+		–					

6.10.4 Differential Diagnosis

Primary Paget Disease must be distinguished from metastasis or direct extension of urothelial carcinoma [89]. Immunohistochemistry is necessary in this circumstance – the immunoprofile of vulvar Paget disease is GCDFP+/CK7+/CK20-, while urothelial neoplasia is GCDFP-/CK7+/CK20+ (Table 6.1).

Primary breast carcinoma arising in ectopic breast tissue versus metastatic breast carcinoma is a particularly challenging differential diagnosis and usually cannot be made on histologic and immunohistochemical grounds alone. Metastatic breast carcinoma to the vulva has been described only 20 times in the literature [86, 87, 90–97], and one case of synchronous vulvar metastasis arising from a low-grade ductal carcinoma has been reported [95]. The diagnosis of metastatic disease is supported by a known history of breast malignancy, with the vulvar tumor demonstrating identical histological, immunohistochemical, and hormone receptor status – with the exception that in some cases the hormone receptor status may change due to spontaneous mutations [91, 93]. On the other hand, the presence of normal ectopic breast tissue in the vulvar specimen would suggest a primary lesion.

The knowledge of a preexisting malignancy and the absence of intraepithelial involvement aid in the diagnosis of metastasis. Thorough clinical history, relevant imaging, and physical examination are often necessary to determine the tumor of origin (Table 6.3).

6.10.5 Prognosis and Treatment

A variety of therapeutic methods have been used including any combination of surgery, chemotherapy, and/or radiation, depending on the extent of disease and tumor of origin. Prognosis is usually poor as distant metastases often suggest late-stage disease.

References

1. Underwood JW, Adcock LL, Okagaki T. Adenosquamous carcinoma of skin appendages (adenoid squamous cell carcinoma, pseudoglandular squamous cell carcinoma, adenoacanthoma of sweat gland of lever) of the vulva: a clinical and ultrastructural study. Cancer. 1978;42(4):1851.
2. Crum CP, Haefner HK, Peters WA. Diagnostic gynecologic and obstetric pathology. 3rd ed. Philadelphia, PA: Elsevier, Inc.; 2018.
3. Carson LF, Twiggs LB, Okagaki T, Clark BA, Ostrow RS, Faras AJ. Human papillomavirus DNA in adenosquamous carcinoma and squamous cell carcinoma of the vulva. Obstet Gynecol. 1988;72(1):63.
4. Johnson WC, Helwig EB. Adenoid squamous cell carcinoma (adenoacanthoma). A clinicopathologic study of 155 patients. Cancer. 1966;19(11):1639.
5. Rhatigan RM, Mojadidi Q. Adenosquamous carcinomas of the vulva and vagina. Am J Clin Pathol. 1973;60(2):208.
6. Bannatyne P, Elliott P, Russell P. Vulvar adenosquamous carcinoma arising in a hidradenoma papilliferum, with rapidly fatal outcome: case report. Gynecol Oncol. 1989;35(3):395.
7. Lasser A, Cornog JL, Morris JM. Adenoid squamous cell carcinoma of the vulva. Cancer. 1974;33(1):224.
8. Curtin JP, Rubin SC, Jones WB, Hoskins WJ, Lewis JL Jr. Paget's disease of the vulva. Gynecol Oncol. 1990;39(3):374.
9. Jones IS, Crandon A, Sanday K. Paget's disease of the vulva: diagnosis and follow-up key to management; a retrospective study of 50 cases from Queensland. Gynecol Oncol. 2011;122(1):42.
10. Asaka S, Yoshizawa A, Sano K, Uhara H, Honda T, Ota H. A case of vulval extramammary paget disease with dermal invasion showing mucinous carcinoma. Int J Gynecol Pathol. 2015;34(4):396.
11. Shaco-Levy R, Bean SM, Vollmer RT, et al. Paget disease of the vulva: a histologic study of 56 cases correlating pathologic features and disease course. Int J Gynecol Pathol. 2010;29(1):69.
12. Tebes S, Cardosi R, Hoffman M. Paget's disease of the vulva. Am J Obstet Gynecol. 2002;187(2):281.
13. Zhang C, Zhang P, Sung CJ, Lawrence WD. Overexpression of p53 is correlated with stromal invasion in extramammary Paget's disease of the vulva. Hum Pathol. 2003;34(9):880.
14. Shiomi T, Yoshida Y, Shomori K, Yamamoto O, Ito H. Extramammary Paget's disease: evaluation of the histopathological patterns of Paget cell proliferation in the epidermis. J Dermatol. 2011;38(11):1054.
15. Goldblum JR, Hart WR. Perianal Paget's disease: a histologic and immunohistochemical study of 11 cases with and without associated rectal adenocarcinoma. Am J Surg Pathol. 1998;22(2):170.
16. Brainard JA, Hart WR. Proliferative epidermal lesions associated with anogenital Paget's disease. Am J Surg Pathol. 2000;24(4):543.
17. Brown HM, Wilkinson EJ. Uroplakin-III to distinguish primary vulvar Paget disease from Paget disease secondary to urothelial carcinoma. Hum Pathol. 2002;33(5):545.
18. Zhao M, Zhou L, Sun L, et al. GATA3 is a sensitive marker for primary genital extramammary Paget disease: an immunohistochemical study of 72 cases with comparison to gross cystic disease fluid protein 15. Diagn Pathol. 2017;12(1):51.
19. Morbeck D, Tregnago AC, Netto GB, et al. GATA3 expression in primary vulvar Paget disease: a potential pitfall leading to misdiagnosis of pagetoid urothelial intraepithelial neoplasia. Histopathology. 2017;70(3):435.
20. Goncalves Amorim A, Batista Fraga Mendes B, Neves Ferreira R, Chambo Filho A. Paget disease of the vulva: diagnosis by immunohistochemistry. Case Rep Dermatol Med. 2015;2015:162483.

21. Diaz de Leon E, Carcangiu ML, Prieto VG, et al. Extramammary Paget disease is characterized by the consistent lack of estrogen and progesterone receptors but frequently expresses androgen receptor. Am J Clin Pathol. 2000;113(4):572.
22. Fox H, Wells M. Recent advances in the pathology of the vulva. Histopathology. 2003;42(3):209.
23. Ostler DA, Prieto VG, Reed JA, Deavers MT, Lazar AJ, Ivan D. Adipophilin expression in sebaceous tumors and other cutaneous lesions with clear cell histology: an immunohistochemical study of 117 cases. Mod Pathol. 2010;23(4):567.
24. Clark LN, Elwood HR, Uhlenhake EE, Smoller BR, Shalin SC, Gardner JM. Nuclear factor XIIIa staining (clone AC-1A1 mouse monoclonal) is a highly sensitive marker of sebaceous differentiation in normal and neoplastic sebocytes. J Cutan Pathol. 2016;43(8):657.
25. Dordevic M, Jovanovic B, Mitrovic S, Dordevic G. Ectopic mammary tissue in vulva. Vojnosanit Pregl. 2008;65(5):407.
26. Ishigaki T, Toriumi Y, Nosaka R, et al. Primary ectopic breast cancer of the vulva, treated with local excision of the vulva and sentinel lymph node biopsy: a case report. Surg Case Rep. 2017;3(1):69.
27. Pieh-Holder KL. Lactational ectopic breast tissue of the vulva: case report and brief historical review. Breastfeed Med. 2013;8:223.
28. Intra M, Maggioni A, Sonzogni A, et al. A rare association of synchronous intraductal carcinoma of the breast and invasive carcinoma of ectopic breast tissue of the vulva: case report and literature review. Int J Gynecol Cancer. 2006;16(Suppl 1):428.
29. Cripe J, Eskander R, Tewari K. Sentinel lymph node mapping of a breast cancer of the vulva: case report and literature review. World J Clin Oncol. 2015;6(2):16.
30. Lee S, Nodit L. Phyllodes tumor of vulva: a brief diagnostic review. Arch Pathol Lab Med. 2014;138(11):1546.
31. Heffernan TP, Sarode VR, Hoffman B, Lea J. Recurrent phyllodes tumor of the vulva: a case report with review of diagnostic criteria and differential diagnosis. Int J Gynecol Pathol. 2010;29(3):294.
32. Muto M, Inamura K, Ozawa N, et al. Skene's gland adenocarcinoma with intestinal differentiation: a case report and literature review. Pathol Int. 2017;67(11):575.
33. Tsutsumi S, Kawahara T, Hattori Y, et al. Skene duct adenocarcinoma in a patient with an elevated serum prostate-specific antigen level: a case report. J Med Case Rep. 2018;12(1):32.
34. Baker GM, Selim MA, Hoang MP. Vulvar adnexal lesions: a 32-year, single-institution review from Massachusetts General Hospital. Arch Pathol Lab Med. 2013;137(9):1237.
35. Buhl A, Landow S, Lee YC, Holcomb K, Heilman E, Abulafia O. Microcystic adnexal carcinoma of the vulva. Gynecol Oncol. 2001;82(3):571.
36. Jacobs DM, Sandles LG, Leboit PE. Sebaceous carcinoma arising from Bowen's disease of the vulva. Arch Dermatol. 1986;122(10):1191.
37. Sullivan SA, Tran AQ, O'Connor S, Gehrig PA. Sebaceous carcinoma of the vulva: a case report and review of the literature. Gynecol Oncol Rep. 2016;18:40.
38. Rutten A, Kutzner H, Mentzel T, et al. Primary cutaneous cribriform apocrine carcinoma: a clinicopathologic and immunohistochemical study of 26 cases of an under-recognized cutaneous adnexal neoplasm. J Am Acad Dermatol. 2009;61(4):644.
39. Kyllo RL, Brady KL, Hurst EA. Sebaceous carcinoma: review of the literature. Dermatol Surg. 2015;41(1):1.
40. Izumi M, Mukai K, Nagai T, et al. Sebaceous carcinoma of the eyelids: thirty cases from Japan. Pathol Int. 2008;58(8):483.
41. Evangelista MT, North JP. Comparative analysis of cytokeratin 15, TDAG51, cytokeratin 20 and androgen receptor in sclerosing adnexal neoplasms and variants of basal cell carcinoma. J Cutan Pathol. 2015;42(11):824.
42. Robson A, Lazar AJ, Ben Nagi J, et al. Primary cutaneous apocrine carcinoma: a clinico-pathologic analysis of 24 cases. Am J Surg Pathol. 2008;32(5):682.
43. Aslam A. Microcystic adnexal carcinoma and a summary of other rare malignant adnexal tumours. Curr Treat Options in Oncol. 2017;18(8):49.
44. Sellheyer K, Nelson P, Kutzner H, Patel RM. The immunohistochemical differential diagnosis of microcystic adnexal carcinoma, desmoplastic trichoepithelioma and morpheaform basal cell carcinoma using BerEP4 and stem cell markers. J Cutan Pathol. 2013;40(4):363.
45. Ferringer T. Immunohistochemistry in dermatopathology. Arch Pathol Lab Med. 2015;139(1):83.
46. Jones MA, Mann EW, Caldwell CL, Tarraza HM, Dickersin GR, Young RH. Small cell neuroendocrine carcinoma of Bartholin's gland. Am J Clin Pathol. 1990;94(4):439.
47. Felix JC, Cote RJ, Kramer EE, Saigo P, Goldman GH. Carcinomas of Bartholin's gland. Histogenesis and the etiological role of human papillomavirus. Am J Pathol. 1993;142(3):925.
48. Finan MA, Barre G. Bartholin's gland carcinoma, malignant melanoma and other rare tumours of the vulva. Best Pract Res Clin Obstet Gynaecol. 2003;17(4):609.
49. Bhalwal AB, Nick AM, Dos Reis R, et al. Carcinoma of the Bartholin gland: a review of 33 cases. Int J Gynecol Cancer. 2016;26(4):785.
50. Heller DS. Benign tumors and tumor-like lesions of the vulva. Clin Obstet Gynecol. 2015;58(3):526.
51. Yoon G, Kim HS, Lee YY, et al. Analysis of clinical outcomes of patients with adenoid cystic carcinoma of Bartholin glands. Int J Clin Exp Pathol. 2015;8(5):5688.
52. Di Donato V, Casorelli A, Bardhi E, et al. Bartholin gland cancer. Crit Rev Oncol Hematol. 2017;117:1.
53. Penner CR, Folpe AL, Budnick SD. C-kit expression distinguishes salivary gland adenoid cystic carcinoma from polymorphous low-grade adenocarcinoma. Mod Pathol. 2002;15(7):687.
54. Rabban JT, Swain RS, Zaloudek CJ, Chase DR, Chen YY. Immunophenotypic overlap between adenoid cystic carcinoma and collagenous spherulosis of the breast: potential diagnostic pitfalls using myoepithelial markers. Mod Pathol. 2006;19(10):1351.
55. Kaufmann O, Dietel M. Expression of thyroid transcription factor-1 in pulmonary and extrapulmonary small cell carcinomas and other neuroendocrine carcinomas of various primary sites. Histopathology. 2000;36(5):415.
56. Dancey AL, Rayatt SS, Soon C, Ilchshyn A, Brown I, Srivastava S. Merkel cell carcinoma: a report of 34 cases and literature review. J Plast Reconstr Aesthet Surg. 2006;59(12):1294.
57. Gil-Moreno A, Garcia-Jimenez A, Gonzalez-Bosquet J, et al. Merkel cell carcinoma of the vulva. Gynecol Oncol. 1997;64(3):526.
58. Nguyen AH, Tahseen AI, Vaudreuil AM, Caponetti GC, Huerter CJ. Clinical features and treatment of vulvar Merkel cell carcinoma: a systematic review. Gynecol Oncol Res Pract. 2017;4:2.
59. Khoury-Collado F, Elliott KS, Lee YC, Chen PC, Abulafia O. Merkel cell carcinoma of the Bartholin's gland. Gynecol Oncol. 2005;97(3):928.
60. Ball NJ, Tanhuanco-Kho G. Merkel cell carcinoma frequently shows histologic features of basal cell carcinoma: a study of 30 cases. J Cutan Pathol. 2007;34(8):612.
61. Iavazzo C, Terzi M, Arapantoni-Dadioti P, Dertimas V, Vorgias G. Vulvar merkel carcinoma: a case report. Case Rep Med. 2011;2011:546972.
62. Winer IS, Lonardo F, Johnson SC, Deppe G. Merkel cell carcinoma in a patient with noninvasive vulvar Paget's disease. Am J Obstet Gynecol. 2012;207(1):e9.
63. Jensen K, Kohler S, Rouse RV. Cytokeratin staining in Merkel cell carcinoma: an immunohistochemical study of cytokeratins 5/6, 7, 17, and 20. Appl Immunohistochem Mol Morphol. 2000;8(4):310.
64. Calder KB, Coplowitz S, Schlauder S, Morgan MB. A case series and immunophenotypic analysis of CK20-/CK7+ primary neuroendocrine carcinoma of the skin. J Cutan Pathol. 2007;34(12):918.

65. Miller DL, Weinstock MA. Nonmelanoma skin cancer in the United States: incidence. J Am Acad Dermatol. 1994;30(5 Pt 1):774.
66. Gilchrest BA, Eller MS, Geller AC, Yaar M. The pathogenesis of melanoma induced by ultraviolet radiation. N Engl J Med. 1999;340(17):1341.
67. de Giorgi V, Salvini C, Massi D, Raspollini MR, Carli P. Vulvar basal cell carcinoma: retrospective study and review of literature. Gynecol Oncol. 2005;97(1):192.
68. Kosari F, Daneshbod Y, Parwaresch R, Krams M, Wacker HH. Lymphomas of the female genital tract: a study of 186 cases and review of the literature. Am J Surg Pathol. 2005;29(11):1512.
69. Crowder S, Tuller E. Small cell carcinoma of the female genital tract. Semin Oncol. 2007;34(1):57.
70. Agoff SN, Lamps LW, Philip AT, et al. Thyroid transcription factor-1 is expressed in extrapulmonary small cell carcinomas but not in other extrapulmonary neuroendocrine tumors. Mod Pathol. 2000;13(3):238.
71. Liu SH, Ho CM, Huang SH, Shih BY, Lee FK. Cloacogenic adenocarcinoma of the vulva presenting as recurrent Bartholin's gland infection. J Formos Med Assoc. 2003;102(1):49.
72. Chibbar R, Wood KA, Giede CK, Agrawal A. Unusually aggressive primary cloacogenic carcinoma of the vulva: a case report and literature review. Case Rep Clinical Med. 2013;02(05):4.
73. Zaidi SN, Conner MG. Primary vulvar adenocarcinoma of cloacogenic origin. South Med J. 2001;94(7):744.
74. Tiltman AJ, Knutzen VK. Primary adenocarcinoma of the vulva originating in misplaced cloacal tissue. Obstet Gynecol. 1978;51(1 Suppl):30s.
75. Ghamande SA, Kasznica J, Griffiths CT, Finkler NJ, Hamid AM. Mucinous adenocarcinomas of the vulva. Gynecol Oncol. 1995;57(1):117.
76. Kennedy JC, Majmudar B. Primary adenocarcinoma of the vulva, possibly cloacogenic. A report of two cases. J Reprod Med. 1993;38(2):113.
77. Willen R, Bekassy CB, Bozoky B, Cajander S. Cloacogenic adenocarcinoma of the vulva. Gynecol Oncol. 1999;74(2):298.
78. Lee KC, Su WP, Muller SA. Multicentric cloacogenic carcinoma: report of a case with anogenital pruritus at presentation. J Am Acad Dermatol. 1990;23(5 Pt 2):1005.
79. Dube V, Veilleux C, Plante M, Tetu B. Primary villoglandular adenocarcinoma of cloacogenic origin of the vulva. Hum Pathol. 2004;35(3):377.
80. Crum CP, Nucci MR, Lee KR. Diagnostic gynecologic and obstetric pathology. 2nd ed. Philadelphia, PA: Saunders/Elsevier; 2011.
81. Lee IH, Kim MK, Lee YK, Hong SR, Lee KH. Primary mucinous adenocarcinoma of the vulva, intestinal type. Obstet Gynecol Sci. 2017;60(4):369.
82. Neto AG, Deavers MT, Silva EG, Malpica A. Metastatic tumors of the vulva: a clinicopathologic study of 66 cases. Am J Surg Pathol. 2003;27(6):799.
83. Matsuo K, Hew KE, Im DD, Rosenshein NB. Clitoral metastasis of anal adenocarcinoma associated with rectovaginal fistula in long standing Crohn's disease. Eur J Obstet Gynecol Reprod Biol. 2009;144(2):182.
84. Sheen-Chen SM, Eng HL, Huang CC. Breast cancer metastatic to the vulva. Gynecol Oncol. 2004;94(3):858.
85. Rocconi RP, Leath CA 3rd, Johnson WM 3rd, Barnes MN 3rd, Conner MG. Primary lung large cell carcinoma metastatic to the vulva: a case report and review of the literature. Gynecol Oncol. 2004;94(3):829.
86. Curtin WM, Murthy B. Vulvar metastasis of breast carcinoma. A case report. J Reprod Med. 1997;42(1):61.
87. Alligood-Percoco NR, Kessler MS, Willis G. Breast cancer metastasis to the vulva 20 years remote from initial diagnosis: a case report and literature review. Gynecol Oncol Rep. 2015;13:33.
88. Heidarpour M, Tavanafar Z. Diagnostic utility of PAX8 in differentiation of mullerian from non-mullerian tumors. Adv Biomed Res. 2014;3:96.
89. Wilkinson EJ, Brown HM. Vulvar Paget disease of urothelial origin: a report of three cases and a proposed classification of vulvar Paget disease. Hum Pathol. 2002;33(5):549.
90. Miliaras D. Breast-like cancer of the vulva: primary or metastatic? A case report and review of the literature. Eur J Gynaecol Oncol. 2002;23(4):350.
91. Porzio G, Ficorella C, Calvisi G, Paris I, Ricevuto E, Marchetti P. Ductal breast carcinoma metastatic to the vulva: a case report. Eur J Gynaecol Oncol. 2001;22(2):147.
92. Julien V, Labadie M, Gauthier G, Ronger-Savle S. Clitoral metastasis from ductal breast cancer revealing metastases in multiple sites and review of the literature. J Low Genit Tract Dis. 2012;16(1):66.
93. Menzin AW, De Risi D, Smilari TF, Kalish PE, Vinciguerra V. Lobular breast carcinoma metastatic to the vulva: a case report and literature review. Gynecol Oncol. 1998;69(1):84.
94. Papaioannou N, Zervoudis S, Grammatikakis I, Peitsidis P, Palvakis K, Youssef TF. Metastatic lobular carcinoma of the breast to the vulva: a case report and review of the literature. J Egypt Natl Canc Inst. 2010;22(1):57.
95. Perrone G, Altomare V, Zagami M, et al. Breast-like vulvar lesion with concurrent breast cancer: a case report and critical literature review. In Vivo. 2009;23(4):629.
96. Sindico R, Mariani L, Atlante M, Vincenzoni C, Tulini R, Benevolo M. Vulvar metastasis from breast carcinoma: a case report and review of the literature. Eur J Gynaecol Oncol. 1998;19(4):386.
97. Valenzano Menada M, Papadia A, Lorenzi P, Fulcheri E, Ragni N. Breast cancer metastatic to the vulva after local recurrence occurring on a rectus abdominis myocutaneous flap: a case report and review of the literature. Eur J Gynaecol Oncol. 2003;24(6):577.

Vulvar Melanocytic Lesions

7

Katelynn Campbell and Sara C. Shalin

Abstract

Pigmented lesions arising in the lower female genital tract most commonly are found on the vulva and rarely in the vagina. Perigenital and genital pigmented lesions are identified in up to 10–12% of women in a primary care setting. Pigmented lesions do not always correspond to a melanocytic neoplasm; inflammatory processes, squamous lesions, and vascular lesions may all mimic melanocytic proliferations. This chapter seeks to provide an overview of the salient clinical and histologic features of various pigmented melanocytic lesions of the vulva.

Melanocytes normally reside in the basal layer of the epidermis of vulvar skin and mucosa, and the normal density of melanocytes in the peri-genital region is higher than in other cutaneous sun-protected sites. While the majority of pigmented lesions encountered in the lower genital tract are benign, the clinical appearance can be worrisome, and the presence of such lesions may be concerning to patients. The most common benign lesions include lentigines (melanotic macules), vulvar melanosis, and common acquired nevi. Melanocytic nevi arising in the peri-genital region may sometimes show architectural and cytologic irregularities which may be a frequent source of consternation for pathologists. These atypical nevi—encompassing atypical melanocytic nevus of the genital type, nevi arising in the setting of lichen sclerosus, and dysplastic nevi—may mimic melanoma clinically and histologically. Much less frequently, the presence of a pigmented lesion on the vulva reflects malignant melanoma. Vulvar melanoma, although rare, is the second most common malignancy of the vulva after squamous cell carcinoma. Overall, vulvar melanoma generally presents at an advanced stage and therefore has a poor prognosis. Prognostic features of importance and molecular signatures of vulvar melanoma will also be discussed. In general, familiarity with clinical features of malignancy and having a low threshold for biopsy of suspicious lesions is important for clinicians to increase the chances of early detection, which will significantly improve prognosis. Likewise, it is important for pathologists to recognize common and uncommon melanocytic lesions and to distinguish melanoma from its mimickers. This chapter seeks to address these issues and give pathologists a framework with which to handle these challenging specimens.

Keywords

Nevus · Nevi · Melanoma · Lentigo · Melanosis · Melanotic macule · Blue nevus · Spitz nevus · Special site nevus Atypical nevus

7.1 Melanotic Macule and Vulvar Melanosis

7.1.1 Clinical Features

Lentigo is the term applied by dermatopathologists for benign pigmented lesions arising on skin due to an increase in melanin pigment rather than a true significant proliferation in melanocytes. When occurring on nonkeratinized genital skin such as the labia minora, which is the preferred location for these lesions in the vulvar region, the term "melanotic macule" is commonly employed. As such, lentigo and melanotic macule are referring to similar benign pigmented lesions conceptually, although the pathogenesis of these two entities may be technically somewhat different [1]. For the purposes of this chapter, these entities can be viewed as

K. Campbell
Department of Pathology, University of Arkansas for Medical Sciences, Little Rock, AR, USA

S. C. Shalin (✉)
Department of Pathology, University of Arkansas for Medical Sciences, Little Rock, AR, USA

Department of Dermatology, University of Arkansas for Medical Sciences, Little Rock, AR, USA
e-mail: SCShalin@uams.edu

W. Zheng et al. (eds.), *Gynecologic and Obstetric Pathology, Volume 1*, https://doi.org/10.1007/978-981-13-3016-2_7

loosely synonymous terms. Vulvar melanosis (or genital melanosis) is often reserved for larger (>0.5 cm), more irregular, or multifocal pigmented patches with similar histologic features, although it should be noted that some authors consider all of these terms interchangeable. The pathogenesis of melanotic macules is not well understood, with theories suggesting defects in melanin transport to keratinocytes [2] and chronic irritation [3]. Human papillomavirus has been investigated as a cause but has not been detected in vulvar melanosis and thus is unlikely to be causative [4].

Melanotic macules are relatively common and have been estimated to comprise approximately 17% of pigmented vulvar lesions [5], with other sources estimating that they may be found on the vulva of about 10% of women [1]. In general, melanotic macules are uniform, evenly pigmented, and small in size. However, melanotic macules may also be multifocal and large, and both of these attributes may lead to clinical concern for vulvar melanoma [1]; some classify larger and multifocal melanotic macules under the terminology of vulvar melanosis (see below). Regardless of terminology, macules larger than 6 mm are worth sampling to exclude the possibility of melanoma [5].

Multiple melanotic macules (involving other mucosal sites such as orolabial mucosa) can alert the astute clinician to the possibility of a genetic syndrome. Melanotic macules are part of the constellation of features in genetic syndromes such as Carney complex or LAMB (showing a constellation of lentigines, atrial myxoma, mucocutaneous myxomas, and blue nevi), Peutz-Jeghers, LEOPARD (showing a combination of lentigines, electrocardiogram abnormalities, ocular hypertelorism, pulmonary stenosis, abnormalities of genitalia, retardation of growth, and deafness), Ruvalcaba-Myhre, and Laugier-Hunziker syndromes [6, 7]. Patients of any age, but particularly children presenting with multiple mucosal or genital melanotic macules, should have a complete and careful skin exam for other cutaneous syndromic findings and if appropriate, should be referred for genetic evaluation.

Vulvar melanosis (as defined above) is a rare phenomenon with an estimated incidence of 0.01% in dermatologic patients [6, 8, 9]. Lesions of vulvar melanosis may be multifocal, asymmetric, variably pigmented, and considerably larger than a solitary melanotic macule. As such, the clinical appearance of vulvar melanosis can be indistinguishable from vulvar melanoma. Importantly, the age of presentation differs between vulvar melanosis and melanoma, and this can be a helpful clue in differentiating the two entities. Patients with vulvar melanosis typically present at a younger age than those with vulvar melanoma, with most women presenting with vulvar melanosis in the second to fourth decades of life [1, 5, 9]. Vulvar melanosis can be seen in conjunction with lichen sclerosus, and the presence of superimposed lichen sclerosus can further amplify the clinical perception of atypia. Dermatoscopic evaluation of vulvar melanosis has most often demonstrated a "parallel" pattern of pigment, resembling a fingerprint of curved lines and streaks [10]. This pattern has also been referred to as "ringlike" [11]. This pattern likely correlates histologically with epithelial (rather than melanocytic) hyperplasia, as nevi uncommonly and melanoma never demonstrated this dermatoscopic pattern in one study [10].

7.1.2 Histological Features

The histologic features of melanotic macules and melanosis are identical, with both of these lesions demonstrating hyperpigmentation of basal keratinocytes (Fig. 7.1). Mild epithelial acanthosis and pigment incontinence with free papillary dermal melanin pigment and melanophages may be seen [4, 6, 12]. Slight melanocyte hyperplasia may be seen, with one study estimating a twofold increase of basilar melanocytes compared to normal skin (with a mean of one melanocyte for every 6.7 basal keratinocytes) [4]. However, confluence, cytologic atypia or pagetoid spread of melanocytes is not observed [9, 13] (Fig. 7.2). Ultrastructural examination has shown that genital melanotic macules harbor increased melanosomes, but the number and morphology of melanocytes are normal [6].

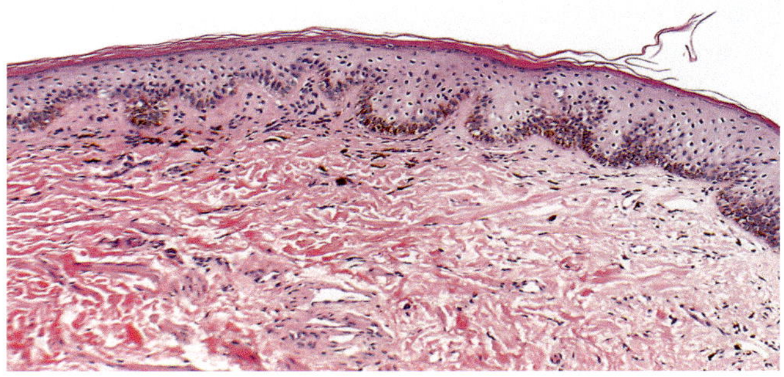

Fig. 7.1 Vulvar melanosis with evenly distributed hyperpigmentation within basal keratinocytes and pigment incontinence in the papillary dermis. Mild epidermal acanthosis can be seen

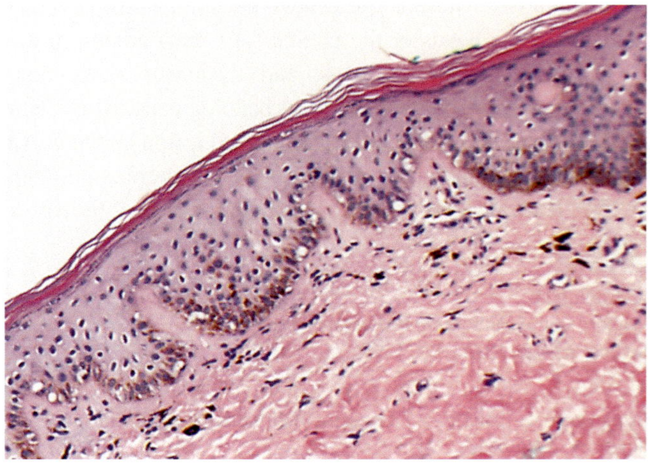

Fig. 7.2 Vulvar melanosis, demonstrating even distribution and regular number of melanocytes at the dermal-epidermal junction. No confluence or pagetoid spread of melanocytes is observed

7.1.3 Immunohistochemical Features

Ancillary testing is not routinely required in the diagnosis of melanotic macule or vulvar melanosis. Immunohistochemical stains to identify the number and location of melanocytes may be useful, particularly when there is a strong clinical impression of melanoma. Immunohistochemical stains such as MART-1 (Melan-A), Sox10, or MITF may be useful to delineate well-spaced, junctional melanocytes limited to the basal layer of the epidermis (Fig. 7.3). S100 protein will stain Langerhans cells within the suprabasilar epidermis that could be mistaken for pagetoid melanocytes, so the use of this stain is not advised.

7.1.4 Differential Diagnosis

The histopathologic differential diagnosis of a melanotic macule or vulvar melanosis includes true melanocytic proliferations. The identification of any nesting of melanocytes signifies the presence of a true melanocytic proliferation and excludes the diagnosis of melanotic macule or melanosis. Benign junctional or compound nevi show nests of melanocytes confined to the basilar epidermis and lack cytologic atypia of melanocytes or upward spread of melanocytes. Melanoma is characterized by single cell and nested growth in a confluent manner along the dermal-epidermal junction. Melanoma generally shows cytologic atypia, haphazard spread of melanocytes at all levels of the epidermis, and mitotic activity of any dermal component.

Another histologic mimic of melanotic macule is post-inflammatory hyperpigmentation. The histologic features of melanotic macule/vulvar melanosis may be indistinguishable from post-inflammatory hyperpigmentation, although pigmentation of keratinocytes may be less and dermal melanophages may be more in post-inflammatory hyperpigmentation. At best, this is a qualitative difference, and thus correlation with the clinical impression and any known previously existing inflammatory processes involving the area is imperative.

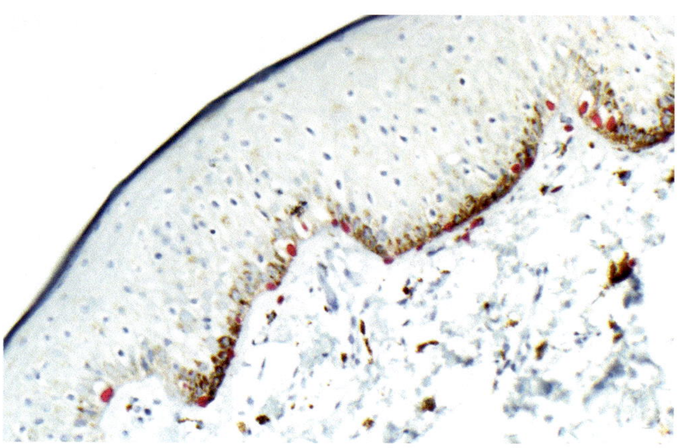

Fig. 7.3 Vulvar melanosis. SOX-10 stain demonstrates even distribution and regular number of melanocytes at the dermal-epidermal junction. No confluence or pagetoid spread of melanocytes is observed

7.1.5 Prognosis and Management

The relationship between vulvar melanosis and melanoma is still being investigated. Vulvar melanosis itself does not seem to confer a greater risk for melanoma, with one study showing no progression to genital melanoma with an average follow-up time of 30 months [9]. Most melanotic macules and vulvar melanosis persist over time but do not change or grow [6]. Any history of growth or change should prompt additional sampling or biopsy. Otherwise, clinical surveillance is the recommended management strategy. A recent study revealed a slightly increased incidence of genital melanosis in patients with a personal history of melanoma (including in non-genital locations), suggesting that diagnosis of melanosis should prompt complete body skin evaluation for other suspicious pigmented lesions [9].

7.2 Melanocytic Nevi of the Vulva

7.2.1 Common Melanocytic Nevus (Junctional Melanocytic Nevus, Compound Melanocytic Nevus, and Intradermal Melanocytic Nevus)

7.2.1.1 Clinical Features

Benign melanocytic nevi are common melanocytic lesions of the lower genital tract, with some sources estimating a prevalence of detection in 2.3% of women on routine gynecologic examination [14]. Nevi most commonly occur on the vulva and perineum, but rarely nevi may be found in the vagina. Vulvar nevi arise most commonly on the labia majora, and less frequently on the labia minora and clitoral hood [15]. Clinically, nevi present in childhood or young adulthood. On exam, they will be found to have uniform pigmentation and regular, well-demarcated borders (Fig. 7.4). Nevi may be completely flat, or they may be elevated from the skin, with domed or flat-topped surfaces [16]. The degree of pigmentation may vary considerably, with flat/macular lesions often showing darker pigmentation than the raised, papular lesions. Some nevi may even be polypoid and fleshy, resembling a skin tag and may lack clinical evidence of pigmentation.

The proposed clinical "ABCDE" guide for examining pigmented lesions can be applied to lesions in the vulvar region as well. The ABCDE mnemonic reminds clinicians (and patients!) to look for *a*symmetry, *b*order irregularities, *c*olor variegation, large *d*iameter, and a history of *e*volution

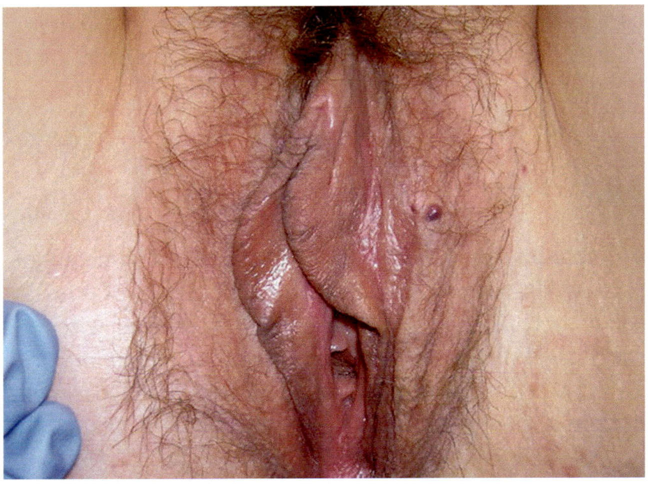

Fig. 7.4 Clinical image of a benign melanocytic nevus. Photo provided courtesy of previous edition in Chinese (Science Press, Beijing, China)

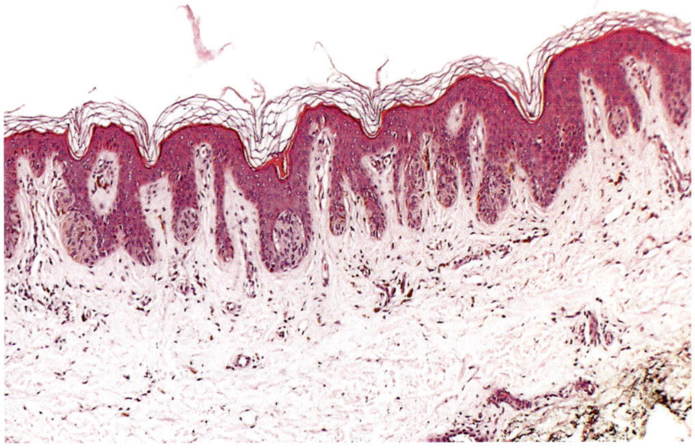

Fig. 7.5 Junctional melanocytic nevus. Nests of mature melanocytes are present only at the dermal-epidermal junction and generally located at the tips of rete ridges

or change as features to raise concern for melanoma. The converse of these parameters, namely, symmetry, well-demarcated borders, single, uniform coloration, small size, and stable growth history, are all features of benign nevi. Dermatoscopic evaluation of vulvar nevi often shows a homogenous or globular pigment pattern [10].

The clinical differential diagnosis of vulvar nevi includes other melanocytic neoplasms as well as vascular and squamous proliferations. Angiokeratomas or hemangiomas may appear as small, well-circumscribed dark brown to black lesions on the vulva. Vulvar intraepithelial neoplasia may be pigmented, as may seborrheic keratoses. These lesions are easily distinguished by biopsy.

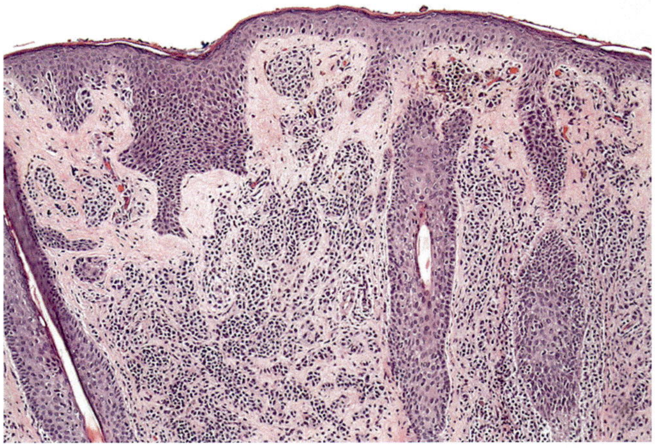

Fig. 7.6 Compound melanocytic nevus. Nests of mature melanocytes are present at the dermal-epidermal junction as well as within the dermis

7.2.1.2 Histologic Features

Histologically, vulvar nevi show similar features to nevi removed from other cutaneous sites. By definition, a melanocytic nevus is composed of small aggregates or nests of melanocytes that lack cytologic atypia. Melanocytic nests are present in the basilar epidermis in a junctional nevus (Fig. 7.5) and in both the dermis and basilar epidermis in a compound nevus [16] (Fig. 7.6). Junctional nests in both junctional and compound nevi should be located predominantly at the tips of the rete ridges, which may be elongated. Melanocytic nests are located solely in the dermis in an intradermal nevus (Fig. 7.7). In most series, intradermal nevi and compound nevi outnumber junctional nevi in the vulvar region [12, 17]. Corresponding with their clinical appearance, benign nevi show a circumscribed, symmetric proliferation of melanocytes on low-power examination. In any of these subsets of nevi, melanocytes should be relatively small in size and lack nucleoli. For nevi with a dermal component, the melanocytes show the phenomenon often referred to as "maturation," whereby the melanocytic nests, as well as the individual melanocytes, become smaller with dispersion

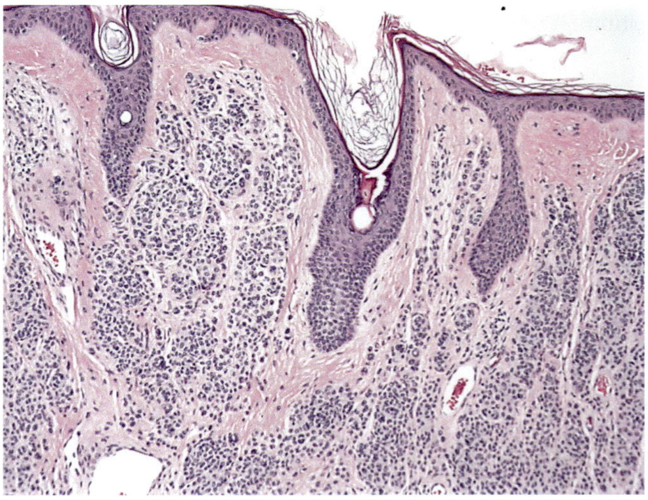

Fig. 7.7 Intradermal nevus. Nests of mature melanocytes are present within the dermis only

deeper into the dermis. Likewise, any cytoplasmic pigment that may be seen in junctional or superficial dermal melanocytes diminishes with further descent into the dermis. Mitotic figures should not be routinely encountered, but the presence of one or two in the absence of any other concerning architectural or cytologic features should not exclude the diagnosis. When mitotic figures are seen, they should be non-atypical and located in the superficial aspect of lesions only.

7.2.1.3 Immunohistochemical Features

Immunohistochemical stains are not required to diagnosis a vulvar melanocytic nevus and are generally only useful to confirm melanocytic derivation.

7.2.1.4 Differential Diagnosis

The histologic differential diagnosis of benign nevi generally includes other melanocytic lesions (Table 7.1). Junctional melanocytic nevi need to be distinguished from vulvar melanosis. The presence of any nesting of melanocytes excludes the diagnosis of melanotic macule/melanosis. Junctional nevi should show a predominantly nested pattern of growth. Single-cell proliferation of melanocytes along the dermal-epidermal junction and/or suprabasilar scatter of melanocytes should raise consideration for a melanoma in situ. Compound melanocytic nevi may share features with dysplastic nevi and atypical nevi of the genital type. These distinctions will be discussed further in the sections below.

Table 7.1 Melanocytic neoplasms arising in the vulva

	Conventional nevus	Blue nevus	Spitz nevus	Atypical nevus of genital type (AGN)	Nevus arising in lichen sclerosus (see text)	Dysplastic nevus	Melanoma
Clinical parameter							
Age at presentation	Any but generally younger, mean age mid-30s	Any but generally younger	Young (children and adolescents)	Generally younger, mean age early to mid-20s	Young (often prepuberal)	Any but generally younger	Older, generally postmenopausal
Preferential site	Labia majora> labia minora> clitoral hood	Unknown due to rarity	Hair-bearing skin (labia majora)	Mons pubis and labia majora> labia minora Hair-bearing skin> mucosa	Labia minora and clitoris Mucosa > hair-bearing skin	Hair-bearing skin (labia majora)	Labia majora> labia minora> clitoris
"ABCDE" rules Asymmetry Border irregularity Color variation Diameter Evolution (changing)	Absent Absent Uniform-1 color Small (<7 mm) No, stable	Absent Absent Uniform blue to black Small (<10 mm) No, stable	Absent Absent Uniform Small (<10 mm) Initial growth, then stable	Generally absent Generally absent 1–2 colors but uniform Usually <10 mm No, stable	Often present Often present May be present Small (mean = 6 mm) May be present	Often present Often present May be present Usually >5 mm May be present	Present Present Present Large Present
Frequency of diagnosis	Common	Rare	Rare	Rare	Rare	Rare	Rare
Histologic parameter							
Architectural symmetry	Present	Present	Present	Present	May be absent	May be absent	Absent
Maturation of dermal component	Present	Absent (see text)	Present	Present	Usually present	Usually present	Absent
Lentiginous junctional component	Absent	Absent (no junctional component)	Absent	Unusual	Present	Present	Often present with confluence
Large and dyshesive junctional nests	Absent	Absent (no junctional component)	Present	Present	Absent	Absent	May be present

(continued)

Table 7.1 (continued)

	Conventional nevus	Blue nevus	Spitz nevus	Atypical nevus of genital type (AGN)	Nevus arising in lichen sclerosus (see text)	Dysplastic nevus	Melanoma
Pagetoid spread of melanocytes	Absent	Absent (no junctional component)	May be present, confined to central zone Nests> single cells	Minimal, focal, and only in central portion	Maybe present, confined to zones of underlying lichen sclerosus	Minimal, focal, and only in central portion	Often present
Shouldering of junctional component	Absent	Absent (no junctional component)	Absent	+/– (see text)	Absent	Present	May be present as melanoma in situ
Melanocyte cytologic atypia	Absent	Absent (spindled, pigmented morphology	Present	Present, usually mild to moderate (uniform and superficial)	Usually absent	Present, usually random	Present, may be severe, diffuse and deep
Dermal mitotic figures	Exceedingly rare to absent	Absent	Rare, superficially located	Rare to absent, no atypical forms if seen	Absent	Absent	Present
Dermal fibrosis	Absent	May be present	May be present ("desmoplastic" Spitz)	Often present	Present (homogenous sclerosis)	Present (eosinophilic fibroplasia or lamellar fibrosis	Present if there is regression

Melanoma should be considered in the setting of asymmetric, large melanocytic proliferations. Nests may coalesce into zones of confluence in the intraepidermal component and the dermal component may lack the gradient of maturation, either overtly or subtly. The presence of abundant, atypical, or deep mitoses should prompt consideration of an aggressive melanocytic neoplasm.

7.2.1.5 Prognosis and Management

Vulvar melanocytic nevi are benign and do not require further management. They do not indicate a propensity for development of other, more aggressive melanocytic neoplasms.

7.2.2 Blue Nevus

7.2.2.1 Clinical Features

The term "blue nevus" describes darkly pigmented (generally blue to black) skin lesions whose histologic correlate is a dermal-based, spindled benign melanocytic proliferation. Although first described in the literatures by Dr. Tièche in 1906, the original use of the term is attributed to German dermatologist Josef Jadassohn [18, 19]. Several clinically and pathologically distinct variants of the original blue nevus described by Tièche and Jadassohn have since been described, including cellular blue nevus, sclerosing/desmoplastic blue nevus, hypomelanotic or amelonotic blue nevus, epithelioid blue nevus, and the controversial "malignant" blue nevus [20]. Blue nevi are not unique to the vulva and may occur on any mucocutaneous surfaces from the conjunctiva to the endocervix [21, 22]. Blue nevi of any variant are rarely reported to occur in the vulva, and only the prototypical classic blue nevus will be discussed in this chapter.

Blue nevi may present at any age and in either gender but are more common in children, young adults, and females [20, 23, 24]. Lesions typically present as single, small, (usually less than 1 cm) well-circumscribed macules or dome-shaped papules with a uniform coloration within a spectrum of reported colors from blue to gray to blue-black to simply black [23]. Often, the strikingly dark coloration of these lesions raises clinical suspicion for melanoma, especially if the blue nevus is part of a combined nevus, creating a heterogeneous pigment pattern. The distinct bluish-gray color that typifies these lesions is due to the presence of melanin deeper in the dermis, causing an optical phenomenon involving melanin's absorption of longer wavelengths of light and reflection of shorter wavelengths (blue color spectrum) known as the "Tyndall effect" [23, 25]. As mentioned previously, blue nevi can occur virtually anywhere on the body and are not limited to skin. The most common cutaneous locations include the dorsal extremities, face, scalp, and buttocks [20, 23]. Blue nevi have been reported in different locations along the gynecologic tract such as vagina [26], uterus [27], cervix [22], and vulva [28].

Occasionally, multiple blue nevi may indicate a genetic syndrome. LAMB syndrome (lentigines, atrial myxomas, mucocutaneous myxomas, and blue nevi) [29] has also been termed NAME syndrome (blue nevi, atrial myxomas, myxoid neurofibromas, and ephelides), and both are generally considered synonymous with the Carney complex, which may show a specific association with epithelioid blue nevi. Rare case reports describe benign blue nevi developing satellite nodules, which can either clinically mimic multiple blue nevi and raise suspicion for a syndrome or, more alarmingly, may resemble metastatic melanoma [30].

7.2.2.2 Histologic Features

On scanning magnification, blue nevi are symmetrical spindle cell lesions located in the dermis or submucosa, without a junctional component. Lesions sometimes have a V-shaped configuration with the base of the lesion parallel to the epidermis and the peak reaching deep within the dermis; sometimes lesions are more subtle with an increase in dermal cellularity and pigment. Blue nevi can track down adnexal structures and neurovascular bundles. Most blue nevi are associated with increased stromal fibrosis, as melanocytes grow between interspersed collagen bundles. The melanocytes themselves are elongated, spindled, or dendritic-type melanocytes with subtle cytoplasmic melanin pigment. These spindled melanocytes intersect between collagen to create a mesh-like appearance that is distinct from the typical nested appearance of a conventional nevus (Fig. 7.8). Nuclei are generally small and hyperchromatic and lack atypia. The pigmented cells persist into the deepest aspect of the lesion, which contributes to their characteristic blue-gray clinical appearance. Mitotic figures should be scarce to absent with no atypical forms present. Melanin-laden macrophages are commonly a component of classic blue nevi.

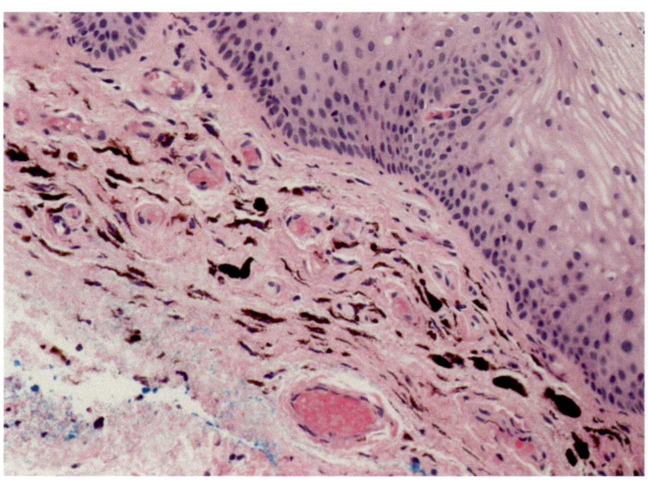

Fig. 7.8 Blue nevus of the vulva. Deeply pigmented dendritic melanocytes are seen in the submucosa. Image credit: Wenxin Zheng, MD

7.2.2.3 Immunohistochemical Features

Ancillary immunohistochemical stains are generally not required in the diagnosis of a blue nevus. Blue nevi express melanocytic markers (MART-1, HMB-45, SOX10, S100 protein) if confirmation of melanocytic origin is required.

7.2.2.4 Differential Diagnosis

The differential diagnosis of blue nevi includes hyperpigmented conventional nevi, as well as other benign spindle cell proliferations such as dermatofibroma or dermal scar. Conventional nevi may occasionally have abundant associated melanin pigment, particularly in patients with darker skin pigmentation. Conventional nevi, however, generally have epidermal and dermal components, a nested rather than spindled morphology of melanocytes, and nests of melanocytes generally show decreasing pigmentation with descent into the dermis.

Spindle cell lesions may mimic blue nevi. Dermatofibroma is a spindle cell proliferation of fibrohistiocytic origin whereby spindle cells entrap normal dermal collagen. Occasionally hemosiderin pigment may be part of a dermatofibroma, thus further mimicking a blue nevus. Similarly, dermal scar shows a spindle cell myofibroblastic proliferation and may occasionally have associated dermal pigment. Spindle cells of scar tend to be arranged horizontally with vertically oriented vessels and an attenuated epidermis and loss of associated appendages. If in doubt, immunohistochemistry for melanocytic markers will be negative in dermatofibroma and scar.

Blue nevi with marked sclerosis may resemble desmoplastic melanoma in rare cases, particularly at sites on the head and neck. As desmoplastic melanoma essentially never arises on the vulva, this should not enter the differential diagnosis at this site. However, sclerotic blue nevus can be distinguished from desmoplastic melanoma by the absence of cytologic atypia, characteristic preservation of HMB-45 or MART-1 immunoreactivity in spindle cells, and melanin pigment associated with the cells. In contrast, desmoplastic melanoma usually shows at least focal nuclear hyperchromasia with atypia, rare mitotic figures, loss of common and specific melanocytic antigens [31], and no associated pigment.

Other endogenous pigment deposition may mimic blue nevus as well. Hemosiderin deposition can sometimes mimic the marked pigmentation of blue nevi and may require an iron stain to distinguish it from melanin pigment, which, in contrast, is Fontana-Masson positive. Other nonneoplastic pigment depositional disorders may mimic blue nevi including post-inflammatory hyperpigmentation, iatrogenic pigmentation by drugs such as minocycline, and tattoo pigment. Pigmented cells in these conditions are exclusively macrophages and not melanocytes, so any melanocytic immunohistochemical stains should be negative. Additionally, in post-inflammatory hyperpigmentation, the pigmented macrophages preferentially precipitate around blood vessels, rather than creating a visible spindle cell "lesion" as in a blue nevus.

7.2.3 Spitz Nevus

7.2.3.1 Clinical Features

The Spitz nevus was first described by Sophie Spitz in 1948 and was considered at that time to represent a diagnosis of "juvenile melanoma" [32]. While this terminology is no longer used today, it nonetheless conveys the worrisome cytologic features of these benign melanocytic lesions.

Spitz nevi are benign acquired melanocytic neoplasms that may present at any age, but typically develop in children and adolescents. The average age at which a patient is diagnosed with Spitz nevus ranges in the literature from 21 years [33] to 26 years [34]. Generally, the comfort level among dermatopathologists associated with the diagnosis of Spitz nevus is inversely proportional to the age of the patient. A melanocytic neoplasm with Spitzoid cytologic features presenting in middle age or older should be carefully examined to exclude melanoma.

In infants and children, Spitz nevi arise on the lower extremities, trunk, and head/neck region most commonly. In older patients, these lesions present on the extremities and trunk and spare the face [33, 35, 36]. Spitz nevi of the vulva are rare (or at least under-reported!), and only a single case report of an intradermal Spitz nevus has been recorded in the English literature to date [37]. Spitz nevi typically present as single lesions; however, multiple Spitz nevi may occur (sometimes following the excision of a solitary lesion), and rare cases of eruptive Spitz nevi are reported in the literature [38]. Spitz nevi are usually nonpigmented (i.e., flesh-colored), pink-red, or reddish-brown, often with associated erythema secondary to vasodilation and vascular prominence. Spitz nevus may present as a polypoid, dome-shaped, flat, or papillomatous lesion. The textural characteristics of these nevi range from soft and fleshy (more common in children) to firm and immobile (more common in adults). Regardless of the described appearance, Spitz nevi should be symmetric and relatively small (~1 cm in greatest dimension) with even, regular borders [35]. Patients (or parents) may report an initial rapid growth phase, followed by stability of the lesion [35]. The clinical differential diagnosis for Spitz nevi is diverse and includes entities such as hemangioma, dermatofibroma, non-Spitz melanocytic nevus, seborrheic keratosis, viral wart, sebaceous nevus, epidermal nevus, and xanthogranuloma [33, 35].

7.2.3.2 Microscopic Findings

Just as blue nevi may simulate melanoma clinically with their dark blue to black appearance, Spitz nevi may simulate melanoma due to their cytologic features. Spitz nevi may be junctional, compound, or intradermal proliferations of large melanocytes with specific, uniformly atypical cytologic attributes. At low power, the architecture of Spitz nevi shows well-defined lateral demarcation with epidermal and dermal symmetry (Fig. 7.9). When a junctional component is prominent, there is usually acanthosis of the epidermis, often accompanied by hypergranulosis and hyperkeratosis. Junctional nests are often large, oval, and vertically oriented, but horizontal orientation of nests can also be present. Confluence of nests and dyshesion of melanocytes within the nests may also be seen (Fig. 7.10). Kamino bodies are small, extracellular aggregates of eosinophilic basement membrane material that can be seen within the epidermis near the dermal-epidermal junction [39]. Pagetoid spread of melanocytes, a feature more commonly associated with melanoma,

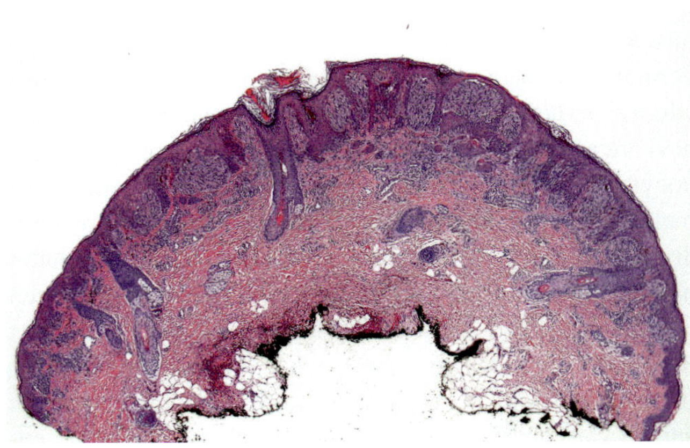

Fig. 7.9 Spitz nevus. Scanning magnification demonstrates a circumscribed melanocytic neoplasm with epithelial hyperplasia and large junctional nests

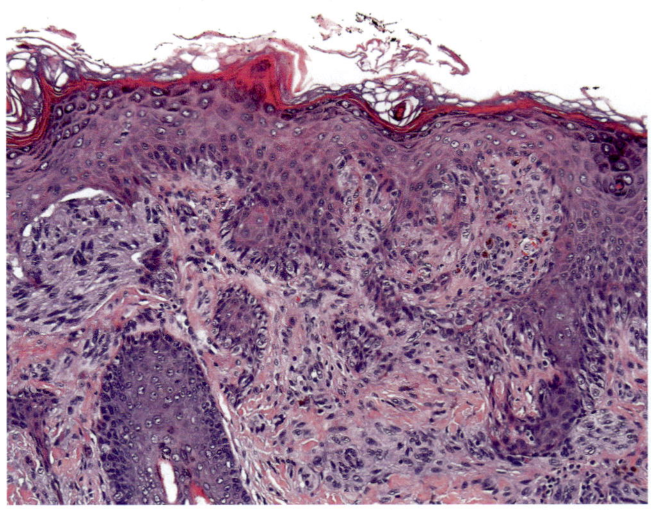

Fig. 7.10 Spitz nevus. Higher-power magnification shows clefting around junctional nests of spindled and epithelioid melanocytes. A Kamino body is present

may be seen in Spitz nevi. This upward ascent of melanocytes should be confined to the center of the lesion and is often seen as pagetoid spread of melanocytic *nests*, although individual single melanocytes may be seen as well. Epidermal attenuation or compression by melanocytes (so-called "consumption of the epidermis") should be absent; this feature should raise suspicion for melanoma [35].

Cytologic features of Spitz nevi are reproducible. Individual cell morphology can range from epithelioid and polygonal to spindle shape. Epithelioid morphology is considered by some to predominate in infancy and early childhood, whereas spindled morphology may be more common in adolescence and adulthood [35]. In the author's opinion, however, most Spitz nevi will have both spindled and epithelioid melanocytes. The nuclei of Spitz nevi are regular, round to oval shape, with smooth nuclear borders, marginated chromatin, and a distinct central punctate pink nucleolus (Fig. 7.11). Some deviation from this appearance, with more nuclear atypia, has been noted to occur in lesions presenting in infancy [35].

Spitz nevi should exhibit maturation where cells are largest in the central and superficial aspects of the nevus and gradually decrease in size toward the deep border. When pigment is present, it is generally coarse and granular and tends to be restricted to the superficial aspect of the nevus. The quality of the pigment has been described as a discriminating feature between Spitz nevus and melanoma: brown, granular melanin predominates in Spitz nevi, while gray, dust-like pigment should raise suspicion for melanoma [35]. Mitotic figures are not uncommonly detected in Spitz nevi. They should be restricted to the junctional and superficial dermal melanocytes. They should not be found in the deeper aspects of the lesion, and there should not be atypical forms. The dermis may have prominent vascularity. Additionally, a perivascular and/or interstitial lymphocytic infiltrate may be seen in association with the nevus [33, 37].

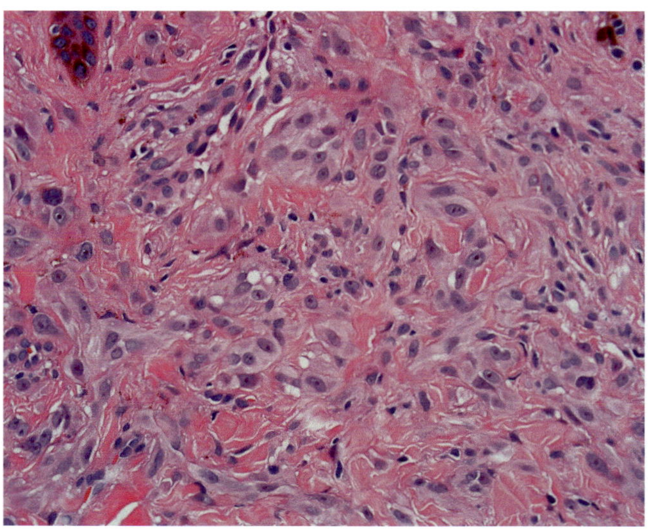

Fig. 7.11 Spitz nevus. The cytologic features of Spitz nevus are appreciated on high-power view, showing large, epithelioid melanocytes with ample eosinophilic cytoplasm, nuclei with distinct nucleoli, and smooth nuclear rims

While the overall architectural and cytologic features of Spitz may appear atypical when viewed in isolation or when compared to traditional nevi, these distinct morphologic features, when present uniformly throughout a lesion and arising in a young individual, can be confidently recognized as a Spitz nevus.

7.2.3.3 Immunohistochemical Features

Ancillary immunohistochemical stains are not always required in the diagnosis of Spitz nevus; however, familiarity with their usage may sometimes assist in avoiding a diagnostic pitfall. Spitz nevi express conventional melanocytic markers (MART-1, HMB-45, SOX10, S100 protein) if confirmation of melanocytic origin is required. These immunohistochemical stains will also accentuate the overall symmetry of a benign Spitz nevus.

HMB-45, as with other benign nevi, often shows a gradient of positivity. The stain tends to be positive in the superficial dermal aspect of Spitz nevi with diminished staining toward the base. Ki-67 (MIB1) may be useful in cases with a large dermal component. An overall low proliferative index (<2% in the series by Al Dhaybi et al. [40]) should be present in Spitz nevi, although there may be some staining superficially within the lesion. The presence of a low proliferative index in Spitz nevus contrasts with melanoma, in which the proliferative index is elevated, with one study documenting a range between 18 and 75% of dermal melanocytes [40]. Of note, this stain may be difficult to evaluate in inflamed lesions, as lymphocytes are frequently in the cell cycle and mark with Ki-67. Care must be taken to only evaluate melanocytes.

Some studies have noted p16 to have some diagnostic utility in distinguishing between Spitz nevus and Spitzoid melanoma. P16 nuclear and cytoplasmic staining, either in a diffuse or "checkerboard" pattern, was present in all 18 cases of Spitz nevi examined in one series, whereas loss of p16 was seen in all 6 cases of childhood Spitzoid melanoma [40]. This finding has been replicated by other groups [41]; however, it should be noted that p16 expression is less useful when atypical Spitz tumor is being considered in the differential diagnosis. Complete loss of p16 immunohistochemical expression may be seen in atypical Spitz tumors with homozygous deletion of 9p21 (the CDKN2A locus where p16 resides), whereas expression is retained in atypical Spitz tumors with heterozygous loss of this locus [41, 42].

7.2.3.4 Molecular Features

Spitzoid neoplasms encompass benign, atypical, and malignant counterparts. A full discussion of the nuances between each of these entities (benign Spitz nevus, atypical Spitz nevus/atypical Spitzoid neoplasm, and Spitzoid melanoma) is beyond the scope of this book, as the pathology of Spitzoid tumors is regarded as diagnostically challenging. Part of this is because the morphology of a Spitzoid neoplasm does not always predict clinical behavior or biologic potential. Advances in understanding of the molecular events present in Spitzoid neoplasms has allowed for creation of a molecular taxonomy, and it has been determined that some of these reproducible molecular aberrations correspond with clinical behavior better than simply histopathologic microscopic evaluation. For this reason, molecular testing is becoming increasingly common, particularly in the work-up of large or atypical spitzoid neoplasms. A thorough recent review of the subject by Tetzlaff and colleagues is recommended to interested readers [43].

One of the first described reproducible molecular signatures was the presence of copy number gains of chromosome 11p in a small subset of Spitz nevi [44]. Initially detected by comparative genomic hybridization (CGH), 11p amplification is usually detected by fluorescent in situ hybridization (FISH) in current routine practice and is estimated to be present in about 12–15% of Spitz nevi [43, 45]. The short arm of chromosome 11 encompasses the *HRAS* gene, and subsequent studies have documented frequent activating mutations in *HRAS* in the setting of 11p copy number increase (as well as in a smaller subset of cases without 11p amplification) [45]. Specific histologic features have been linked to the presence of 11p gain, including predominantly intradermal location with an infiltrative growth pattern within a fibrotic to sclerotic dermis, leading to the terminology of "desmoplastic Spitz nevus" [45, 46]. Importantly, *HRAS* mutations and 11p copy number gains have not been routinely detected in melanoma, so identification of these changes in isolation is generally reassuring of a benign and indolent clinical course [44, 46].

Kinase translocations are a frequent event in Spitzoid neoplasms, occurring in approximately 50% of cases [47]. The list of kinase genes that may be translocated is growing and includes *ALK*, *ROS1*, *NTRK1*, *BRAF*, *RET*, and *MET*, and translocation partners are equally varied [47–50]. Current research is focusing on histologic attributes of specific kinase fusion in Spitzoid neoplasms, with early reports suggesting that the involved kinase often results in predictable histopathologic features [43]. The detection of a kinase fusion does not necessarily assist with the diagnosis, as these fusions may occur in benign Spitz nevi, atypical Spitz tumors, and Spitzoid melanoma. Thus, while not able to predict biologic potential, the identification of a kinase fusion in a Spitz tumor has potential to guide treatment with targeted therapies (kinase inhibitors) if the lesion should result in an aggressive clinical course [43].

In contrast to conventional benign nevi and melanoma, Spitz nevi are unlikely to demonstrate mutations in the gene encoding *BRAF* kinase. However, a subset of atypical nevi with cytologic features resembling Spitz nevi have been detected in several families and sporadically; these Spitzoid neoplasms have documented loss of BAP1 expression in concert with frequent *BRAF* mutation. BAP-omas (or Wiesner's nevi) usually lack the junctional features seen in Spitz nevi, but demonstrate predominantly intradermal cellular nodules of epithelioid melanocytes with abundant cytoplasm, well-defined cytoplasmic borders, distinct nucleoli, and a lymphocytic host response [51–53]. *BAP1* mutation may occur sporadically or may be inherited in an autosomal dominant fashion; families with this mutation have a risk of cutaneous and uveal melanoma. BAP1 protein loss may be detected by immunohistochemistry, and detection of multiple BAP1-deficient melanocytic neoplasms should prompt genetic evaluation for germline mutation. *BAP1*-mutated Spitzoid neoplasms generally seem to have an indolent course; however, *BAP1* mutations may also be detected in a subset of melanomas, so identification of this molecular signature in isolation does not confer a diagnosis [43].

The presence of multiple chromosomal copy number aberrations (gains and/or losses) is at odds with a benign diagnosis. FISH panels or array CGH that detect multiple abnormal signals in a Spitzoid lesion would be more in keeping with melanoma than with Spitz nevus. In particular, 9p21 homozygous deletions have a higher risk of metastasis beyond the sentinel lymph nodes and death from melanoma and thus signify a risk factor for aggressive behavior [54, 55]. *TERT* promoter mutations have also been detected in a subset of atypical and malignant Spitzoid neoplasms and have been noted to have an aggressive course [56].

It should be noted that Spitzoid lesions exhibiting classically benign or malignant features should not be routinely submitted for molecular evaluation. Molecular testing, however, is beginning to have a role in assisting in the classification and anticipating the behavior of morphologically ambiguous lesions.

7.2.3.5 Differential Diagnosis

The diagnosis of Spitz nevi is historically difficult, and most pathologists agree that these lesions exist on a spectrum with the benign Spitz nevus as described in detail above at one end of the spectrum, and Spitzoid melanoma at the other end. In the middle of the spectrum is the so-called "atypical Spitz tumor," which has intermediate features between typical Spitz nevus and overt melanoma. The final diagnosis of these morphologically equivocal lesions often involves a constellation of clinical, pathologic, and, increasingly, molecular features [43, 57]. The absence of symmetric architecture, Kamino bodies, or "maturation" with descent into the dermis or the presence of numerous/atypical mitotic figures, ulceration, sheet-like dermal tumor cells, or a single-cell growth pattern within the junction should raise concern for an atypical Spitz tumor or Spitzoid melanoma and prompt careful evaluation.

Occasionally, other non-melanocytic lesions can enter the differential diagnosis, including keratinocytic neoplasms such as clonal seborrheic keratosis, dermal-based lesions such as epithelioid fibrous histiocytoma, and metastatic carcinoma. For each of these lesions, immunohistochemical markers for melanocytic derivation will be negative. Seborrheic keratosis is a benign keratinocytic neoplasm occurring most often in adults. The clonal variant has uniform intraepidermal nests of keratinocytes, often arranged in a whirling pattern. Epithelioid fibrous histiocytoma (EFH) is a dermal-based neoplasm in which cellular elements often have a Spitzoid cytomorphology, thus mimicking an intradermal Spitz nevus. Historically thought to be a variant of dermatofibroma, the relative recent description of *ALK* rearrangements (and ALK immunohistochemical reactivity) in the majority of these lesions has led to a revised theory that they are a unique fibrohistiocytic neoplasm [58]. Carcinoma, whether native or metastatic, may occasionally mimic the epithelioid tumor cells of Spitz nevi but will express a variety of keratins by immunohistochemistry.

7.2.3.6 Prognosis and Treatment

If clinicians are considering a Spitz nevus before biopsy, an excisional biopsy is preferred in order to examine the entire lesion. Partial biopsies decrease the likelihood of a definitive diagnosis being rendered.

Benign Spitz nevi will behave indolently and do not absolutely require additional treatment. However, some clinicians and dermatopathologists advocate for the narrow but complete re-excision of any partially sampled Spitz nevus for two reasons: (1) to ensure that the entire lesion has been evaluated histopathologically and (2) to decrease the likelihood of persistence or recurrent growth. Molecular profiles, as described in the previous section, may provide additional prognostic information in lesions with ambiguous histologic features and unclear diagnosis. The management of atypical Spitz tumors is beyond the scope of this chapter but is managed on a case by case approach, sometimes employing wider excisions and sentinel lymph node sampling [59]. Spitzoid melanoma would be treated as other melanomas and is discussed in the subsequent section.

7.2.4 Atypical Genital Nevus and Nevi Arising Association with Lichen Sclerosus

7.2.4.1 Clinical Features

The vulva is often considered a "special site" for nevi. In part this is because vulvar nevi may arise in the "milk line" that extends from the axillae and breasts to the vulva, and nevi arising along this trajectory often exhibit clinical and histological atypia. These nevi have been variably termed atypical genital nevi (AGN), atypical melanocytic nevi of the genital type (AMNGT) or nevi with special site features [15, 16]. Estimated to comprise between 5 and 10% of pigmented lesions from the vulvar region [15, 17], AGN possess atypical histologic features that may mimic melanoma, so familiarity with the features and the distinction from melanoma is paramount. AGN are diagnosed primarily in young women. These nevi variants often have a papillomatous surface, are larger in size than conventional nevi, and can have irregular borders [16, 17] (Fig. 7.12). In one large study, the median age of diagnosis of AGN was 26 years old (with a range of 6–54) [60], and another study found the median age of diagnosis to be 21 years [17]. This suggests that these lesions are detected and diagnosed in general at an earlier age than vulvar melanoma. The most common site of occurrence is mons pubis and labia majora, with fewer AGN being diagnosed from the labia minora, and estimates suggest that about one half to two-thirds of lesions arise on hair-bearing skin and the remaining one third to one half on mucosal surfaces [60, 61]. AGN in children, however, may be detected more commonly on mucosal epithelium [60]. Clinical sizes are often less than 1 cm; however, larger lesions up to 2 cm have been reported [60, 62]. Ideally, the clinician should notify the pathologist about the specific location (e.g., vulva, milk line) of a nevus being biopsied in order to allow the pathologist to accurately assess the histologic features and prevent overdiagnosis [16].

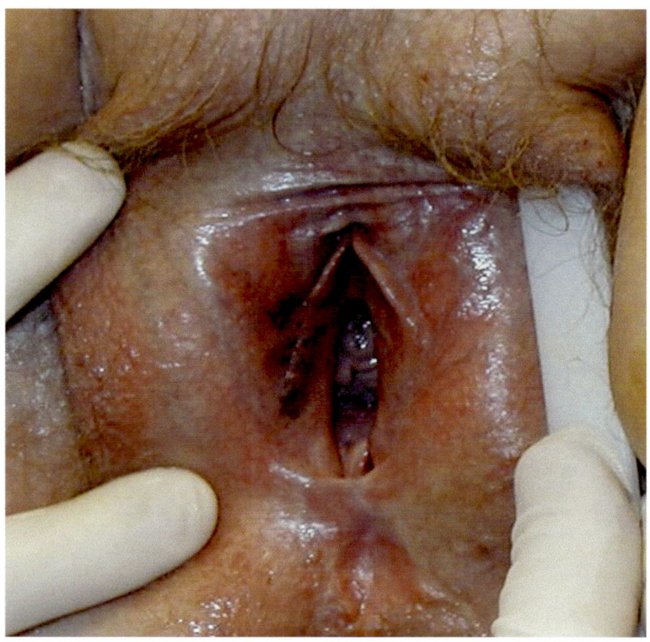

Fig. 7.12 Atypical melanocytic nevus of the genital type of the labia minorum demonstrates variable pigmentation, large size, and irregular borders. Photo provided courtesy of previous edition in Chinese (Science Press, Beijing, China)

The concomitant presence of lichen sclerosus can complicate the diagnosis of AGN or other genital nevi. Such combined lesions may show exaggerated clinical and histologic atypia due to the dermal sclerosis [63–65]. Nevi with superimposed lichen sclerosus are more likely to arise on the mucosal aspects of the vulva (labia minora and clitoris) in young females (often prepubertal) and have a mean diameter of 0.6 mm [65]. Treatment of the lichen sclerosus may lead to resolution of some of the concerning clinical and dermatoscopic features [63].

7.2.4.2 Histologic Features

Both architectural and cytologic features may be atypical in AGN. The low-power impression of an AGN is that of a symmetric and cellular lesion (Fig. 7.13). Coarse brown-gray cytoplasmic melanin pigment is often prominent in the superficial aspect of the lesion [61]. AGN are usually compound nevi that show variable size and shape of junctional nests. Junctional nests tend to be large and dyshesive and may arise at both the tips and sides of rete ridges, rather than exclusively at the tips [17, 62] (Fig. 7.14). Junctional nests may also be located in a horizontal alignment, creating an appearance of confluence [61, 62]. The dyshesive nature of junctional nests may create clefting artifact between melanocytes, and bridging between nests (a feature of dysplastic nevi) may be seen [60]. The presence of a lentiginous, single-cell growth pattern of melanocytes is unusual in these lesions but may be seen more at the periphery of the nevus [60]. Pagetoid extension of melanocytes above the basal layer should be minimal, focal, and confined to the center of the lesion [17, 60, 61] (Fig. 7.15). Some authors exclude lesions with a prominent "shoulder" (the presence of a junctional component persisting peripherally beyond the limits of a dermal component) as being AGN [62]; other authors note a shoulder phenomenon in a substantial percentage of nevi classified as AGN [60]. The dermal component of an AGN should be symmetric and show maturation of the individual cells and nests [17, 62]. Melanocytes may grow within adnexal epithelium. Dermal mitotic figures should not be abundant and should not be atypical and are found only in a minority of AGN [60]. Superficial bands of dermal fibrosis, distinct from the lamellar fibroplasia seen in dysplastic nevi, are noted to be present in at least half of AGN [17, 60, 61].

Some degree of cytologic atypia is permitted in AGN. Although most AGN have mild to moderate junctional cytologic atypia, occasionally atypia may be classified as severe [60]. In contrast to the random atypia seen in dysplas-

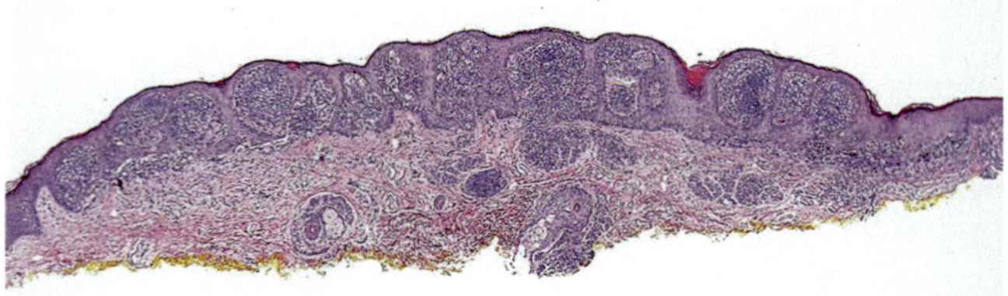

Fig. 7.13 Atypical melanocytic nevus of the genital type. Low-power assessment demonstrates a symmetric, cellular, and nodular compound nevus. Junctional melanocytic nests are variably sized

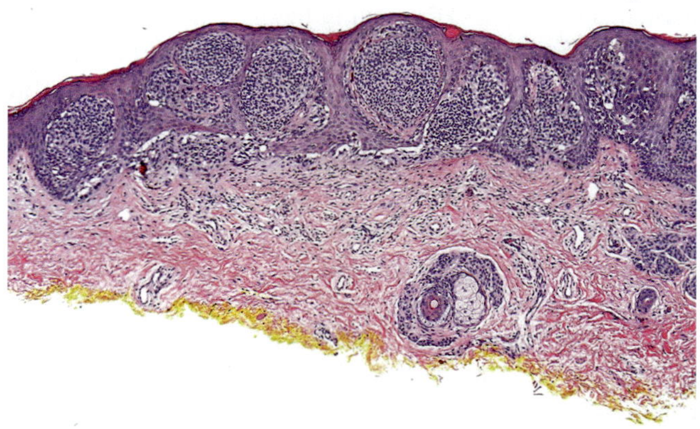

Fig. 7.14 Atypical melanocytic nevus of the genital type. Large junctional nests with some dyscohesive cells. Junctional nests arise from the sides as well as the tips of the rete ridges. Variable size of nests can give the illusion of confluence

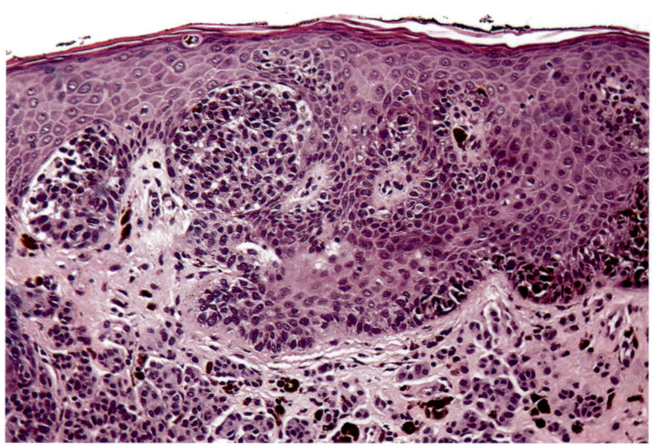

Fig. 7.15 Atypical melanocytic nevus of the genital type. Coarse brown-gray cytoplasmic melanin granules are often seen as well as mild cytologic atypia and focal pagetoid spread of junctional melanocytes. Photo provided courtesy of previous edition in Chinese (Science Press, Beijing, China)

tic nevi, the atypia of AGN tends to be uniform and diffusely present in the superficial aspect of the lesion [61]. Melanocytes in the epidermis and superficial dermis are typically larger with abundant eosinophilic cytoplasm and may show pink to red, variably distinct nucleoli [60, 62]. Cytoplasmic pigment may be dusty or coarse [60], and pigment dropout may be prominent [61]. Although these are atypical nevi, there does not appear to be an increased risk of malignant transformation [16, 17].

One particular pitfall of which to be aware when evaluating AGN and conventional vulvar nevi is the tendency for overdiagnosis when a nevus arises in the setting of lichen sclerosus. Several papers in the literature have explored the clinical and histologic overlap with malignancy of nevi biopsied in the setting of lichen sclerosus [63–65]. Such nevi will demonstrate atypical histopathologic features, although there is no agreement as to whether these lesions should be diagnosed specifically as AGN. Vulvar nevi with superimposed lichen sclerosus will demonstrate features seen in AGN, dysplastic nevi, recurrent (or persistent) nevi, and melanoma. Most literature suggests that nevi with superimposed lichen sclerosus most closely resemble recurrent nevi, a known mimic of melanoma in situ on cutaneous sites. The junctional component of nevi arising in lichen sclerosus generally assumes a lentiginous, single-cell growth pattern along an attenuated epidermis and may approach confluence [64, 65]. There may be central focal suprabasilar extension of melanocytes, both singly and in nests [66]. The presence of dermal sclerosis can be mistaken for dermal regression in a melanoma and may entrap melanocytic nests. Importantly, just as in recurrent nevi, any atypical junctional features should be strictly limited to the areas overlying the dermal sclerosis. Atypia extending beyond the dermal sclerosis should prompt consideration of a more aggressive neoplasm. The dermal melanocytes may show increased proliferation indices compared to conventional nevi uninvolved by lichen sclerosus but still lower than proliferation rates seen in melanoma [65].

7.2.4.3 Immunohistochemical and Molecular Features

The diagnosis of atypical nevus in the vulvar region—whether AGN, dysplastic, or nevus associated with lichen sclerosus—typically is made through examination of H&E sections alone. Ancillary testing with immunohistochemistry is not required, although in some cases may provide support for or against a significant pagetoid component. Molecular studies have noted a high incidence of BRAF V600E mutations in AGN and other non-overlapping mutational events compared to vulvar melanoma [67], so ultimately, mutational analysis may be useful in markedly atypical nevi where a melanoma diagnosis is being considered.

7.2.4.4 Differential Diagnosis

The differential diagnosis of AGN includes conventional and dysplastic nevi as well as vulvar melanoma (Table 7.1). The large dyshesive junctional nests of AGN generally are not seen in conventional acquired vulvar nevi. Conventional melanocytic nevi in the vulvar region tend to be papular, raised lesions that show a prominent dermal component with minimal epidermal component.

There is admitted overlap in the histology of dysplastic nevi and AGN. Dysplastic nevi are rare in the vulvar region, display a more lentiginous growth along the dermal-epidermal junction, and show random rather than uniform cytologic atypia [61]. Whether a shoulder favors a dysplastic nevus [62] or is permitted in AGN [60] remains debated in the literature.

Vulvar melanoma tends to be larger, arises in an older population, and lacks the symmetry of AGN. Severe cytologic atypia, expansile dermal growth with mitotic activity, and prominent lentiginous growth in the junction with pagetoid spread of melanocytes also favor a diagnosis of melanoma.

7.2.4.5 Prognosis and Management

The relationship between AGN and dysplastic nevi and familial melanoma risk is not completely clear. Most authors suggest that despite some of the overlapping clinical and histologic features of AGN with dysplastic nevi, the diagnosis of AGN does not seem to indicate a predisposition for growing atypical nevi and melanoma [62]. However, a subset of patients diagnosed with AGN may document a history of dysplastic nevi or melanoma [60, 61]; it is unclear whether this relationship may be due to the increased surveillance and lower threshold for biopsy that patients with such a history typically experience. Most AGN have a benign clinical course and do not recur, and none have progressed to melanoma [17, 60, 61]. No recurrence was seen in completely excised lesions, and recurrence was rare even in incompletely excised AGN [60]. Nevertheless, given the atypical histologic features, re-excision to ensure that the lesion has been appropriately sampled and to ensure complete removal is generally the method of treatment for these rare lesions [62].

Nevi arising in the setting of lichen sclerosus should be similarly excised if clinically feasible. However, it should be noted that treatment of the lichen sclerosus may lead to resolution of some of the concerning clinical and dermatoscopic features [63].

7.2.5 Dysplastic Nevus

Despite the word "dysplastic" within the name, there is no evidence that dysplastic nevi transform into more aggressive lesions over time. For this reason, terminology to describe these architecturally disordered and cytologically atypical lesions is not always uniform and the subject of much debate within dermatopathology circles. As this debate is beyond the scope of this chapter, we will use the term "dysplastic nevus" to encompass a spectrum of nevi that appear atypical both clinically and histologically and show fairly well agreed upon architectural features. Some pathologists tend to eschew the diagnosis of dysplastic nevus in genital sites such as the vulva, preferring to attribute the atypical features to the anatomic site, as discussed above in the section on atypical genital nevi. That said, verifiable accounts of dysplastic nevi on vulvar sites are present in the literature and many consider it an acceptable diagnosis to make on vulvar skin [62].

7.2.5.1 Clinical Features

By definition, dysplastic nevus is an acquired benign melanocytic proliferation. Dysplastic nevi have no predilection for the lower genital tract but occur incidentally in this area [16]. These nevi are usually large, show irregular borders, and range in color from pink to tan to brown, sometimes displaying two tones of color (Fig. 7.16) [16]. Lesions tend to exceed 0.5 cm in size and may be completely flat or flat with a raised center. A flat, tan brown or erythematous border is not uncommon and corresponds to the "shoulder" seen microscopically [13, 68]. Patients with many atypical nevi will often have nevi in sites such as the scalp and anogenital skin [16]. Dysplastic nevi of the vulva arise on the hair-bearing skin of the labia but do not occur on mucosal-type epithelium [62]. Despite the irregular appearance of these nevi, their behavior is benign [13]. Although dysplastic nevi themselves do not seem to progress to melanoma, patients with many dysplastic nevi are at an increased risk of developing melanoma. As such, the presence of numerous dysplastic nevi should prompt routine surveillance of the patient to ensure timely diagnosis of the melanoma he or she is likely to develop over time. Therefore, diagnosis of dysplastic nevus is not without consequence.

7.2.5.2 Histologic Features

The histologic features of dysplastic nevi in the lower genital tract are identical to dysplastic nevi on other cutaneous sites [13]. Dysplastic nevi show elongation of rete ridges, with junctional nests bridging between the rete ridges. There is usually also a lentiginous component typified by an increased density of junctional melanocytes interspersed by nesting of melanocytes (Fig. 7.17). Dysplastic nevi also demonstrate a "shoulder" phenomenon, which is defined by the peripheral/radial extension of the junctional component beyond any dermal component (Fig. 7.18). The dermis is characterized by concentric eosinophilic fibroplasia or lamellar fibrosis underneath the bridged junctional nests of melanocytes, a variable chronic inflammatory infiltrate, and prominent vasculature [13, 16, 68]. Cytologic atypia of melanocytes is requisite but is generally random rather than uniform [61, 68]. Some dysplastic nevi will have a dermal component, but melanocytic nests usually are limited to the papillary dermis and/or the superficial aspect of the reticular dermis.

7.2.5.3 Immunohistochemical and Molecular Features

Ancillary immunohistochemical studies are generally not required in the diagnosis of dysplastic nevi. The use of melanocytic markers to aid in the assessment of the degree of lentigi-

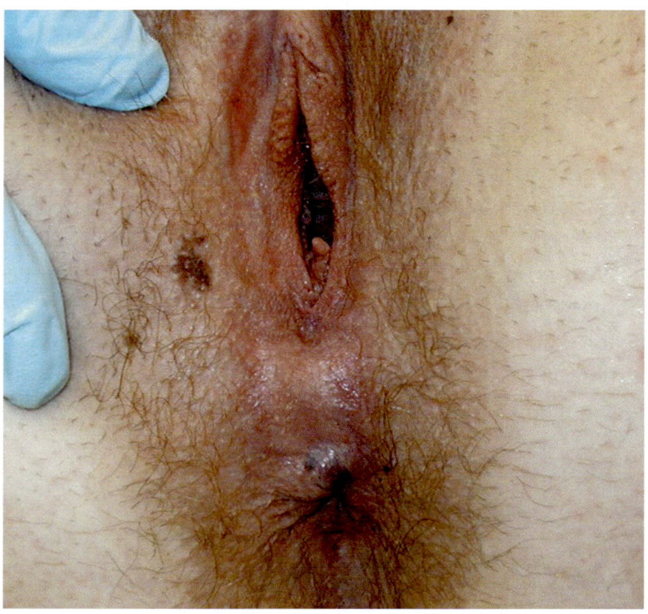

Fig. 7.16 Dysplastic nevus. Clinical image. Photo provided courtesy of previous edition in Chinese (Science Press, Beijing, China)

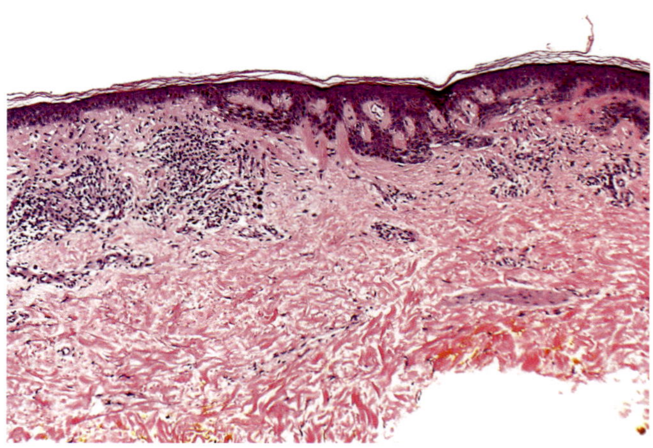

Fig. 7.17 Junctional dysplastic nevus that demonstrates elongated rete ridges, bridging of junctional nests and slight cytologic atypia. Eosinophilic fibroplasia is seen within the dermis beneath the bridged junctional nests

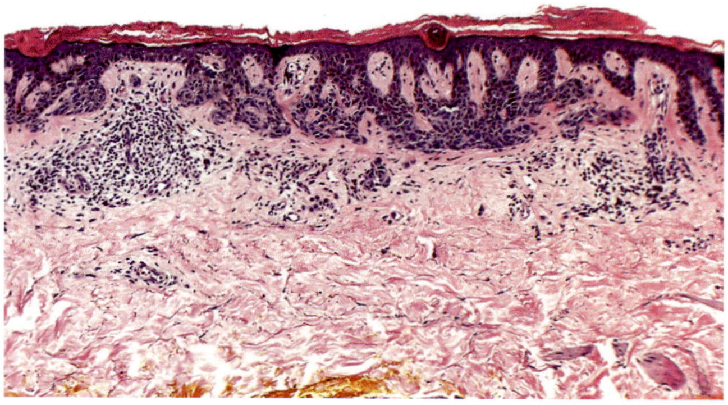

Fig. 7.18 Dysplastic nevus with the "shoulder" phenomenon whereby the junctional melanocytic component extends beyond the dermal component

nous spread may be helpful; it should be remembered that nuclear stains such as Sox10 and MITF may best estimate the number of junctional melanocytes, while cytoplasmic stains such as MART-1/Melan-A may overrepresent this number [69]. Occasionally, melanoma enters the differential diagnosis of a dysplastic nevus. In such cases, increasingly, molecular techniques are being introduced to provide ancillary information in the diagnosis of difficult melanocytic lesions. Techniques such as fluorescent in situ hybridization, gene expression profiling, and next-generation sequencing can be utilized to help distinguish between benign and malignant lesions [70–72].

7.2.5.4 Differential Diagnosis

The differential diagnosis of dysplastic nevi includes conventional nevi and atypical genital nevi as well as vulvar melanoma (Table 7.1). The junctional predominance and bridging junctional nests of dysplastic nevi generally are not seen in conventional acquired vulvar nevi. Conventional melanocytic nevi in the vulvar region tend to be papular, raised lesions that show a prominent dermal component with minimal epidermal component.

There is admitted overlap in the histology of dysplastic nevi and AGN. Dysplastic nevi are rare in the vulvar region, display a more lentiginous growth along the dermal-epidermal junction, and show random rather than uniform cytologic atypia [61]. Whether a shoulder favors a dysplastic nevus [62] or is permitted in AGN [60] remains debated in the literature.

Vulvar melanoma tends to be larger, arises in an older population, and lacks the nested architecture of dysplastic nevi. Severe cytologic atypia, expansile dermal growth with mitotic activity, and prominent lentiginous growth in the junction with pagetoid spread of melanocytes also favor a diagnosis of melanoma.

7.2.5.5 Prognosis and Management

Treatment of dysplastic nevi involves continued clinical surveillance or surgical excision. If pigmented lesions are biopsied with the clinical intent to remove the lesion completely, further treatment is generally not required after diagnosis [73]. There is general agreement that any lesion with considerable cytologic atypia should be completely excised [74].

7.3 Malignant Melanoma of the Vulva

7.3.1 Overview and Epidemiology

Malignant melanoma is a skin cancer with one of (if not the) highest mortality rates and is the malignant counterpart of a benign melanocytic nevus. Melanoma arising at gynecologic sites, including the vulva, vagina, and cervix, is rare and accounts for only 1–3% of melanoma in female patients [75, 76]. Despite its rarity, melanoma is the second most common skin cancer of the vulva after the more prevalent squamous cell carcinoma. Vulvar melanoma generally shows an aggressive clinical course, as many patients present at an advanced stage with thick primary tumors [13, 75]. Factors associated with a particularly poor prognosis include advanced age and black race [77]. Many studies of melanoma in the female reproductive tract combine data on vulvar, vaginal, and cervical melanoma, so separating out features unique to vulvar melanoma is sometimes challenging. Of gynecologic melanomas, approximately 70–80% arise in the vulva [75, 78]. Overall, vulvar melanomas have a 5-year survival rate ranging from 10 to 50% depending on the study [75–77, 79–81]. However, patients with vulvar melanomas generally seem to have better 5-year overall and disease-free survival than patients with melanoma arising in the vagina [79, 82].

7.3.2 Clinical Features

Vulvar melanoma is generally a disease of older (postmenopausal) women. Most patients present in their sixth or seventh decade of life [75, 76, 79–81]. Presenting symptoms may include bleeding, mass/swelling, discharge, pruritus, and pain [76, 80, 82, 83]. Anatomically speaking, vulvar melanoma arises most commonly on the labia majora, followed by labia minora, both labia majora and minora and finally within the clitoral/periclitoral area [76, 80, 83]. However, one study noted that any pigmented lesion arising on mucosal tissue of a postmenopausal woman was more likely to be melanoma than a nevus, so a mucosal location should not preclude consideration of the diagnosis [67]. Although any ethnic group may be affected by vulvar melanoma, Caucasian women have a higher incidence of diagnosis, just as with cutaneous melanoma [80]. The lesions themselves may be flat macules, raised papules, or nodular tumors of variable size. Most lesions are greater than 7 mm in diameter on average by the time of diagnosis [13, 84] (Figs. 7.19 and 7.20). Advanced lesions are often ulcerated, have irregular contours and

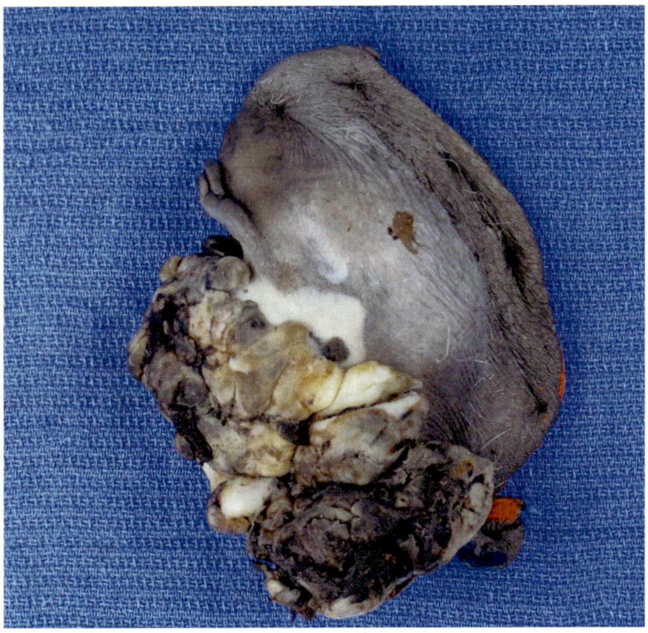

Fig. 7.19 Melanoma of labia minora. Initial presentation revealed this destructive, nodular mass, obliterating most of the vulvar structures in this partial vulvectomy specimen

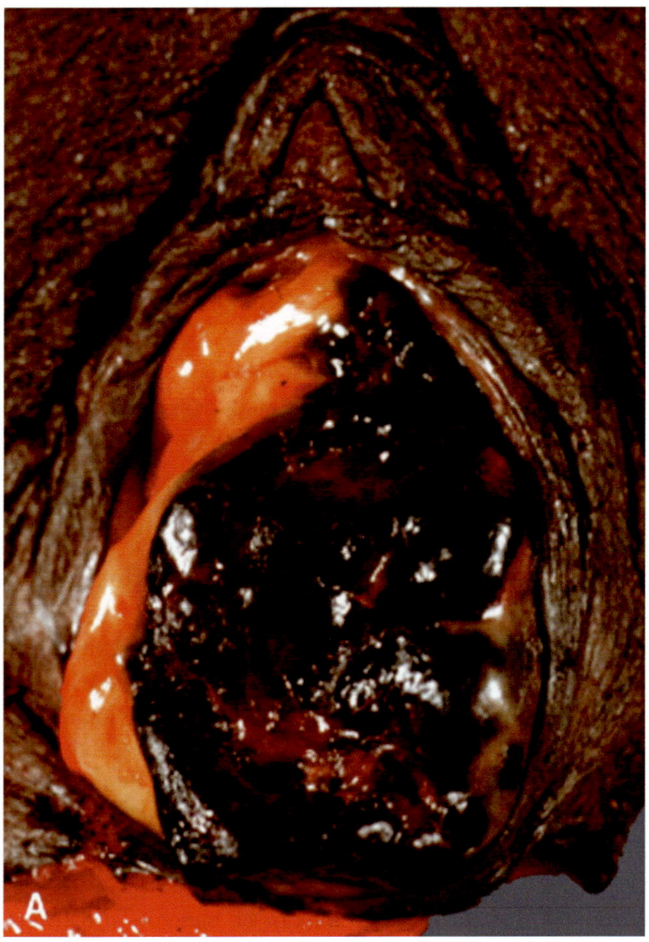

Fig. 7.20 Melanoma of the female reproductive tract, likely originating in vagina. Photo provided courtesy of previous edition in Chinese (Science Press, Beijing, China)

variable pigmentation, and may be accompanied by satellite nodules at the time of presentation [36]. Amelanotic presentation was reported in up to 27% of patients in a Swedish case series [83]. Amelanotic lesions can be erythematous and may demonstrate an ulcerated and friable red to pink nodule, resembling a pyogenic granuloma clinically [84].

Dermatoscopic evaluation of vulvar melanoma will show multiple patterns within the single lesion, including reticular, globular, and homogenous patterns [10]; multiple patterns within one lesion should prompt biopsy.

7.3.3 Histologic Features

Just as the clinical presentation of vulvar melanoma is varied, vulvar melanoma also displays a considerable morphologic spectrum histologically. There are differing reports in the literature regarding the most common histologic subtype. Among melanomas in the female reproductive tract, mucosal and nodular subtypes appear overrepresented compared to cutaneous melanomas [82, 85]. However, studies separating vulvar from non-vulvar (i.e., vaginal and cervical) gynecologic melanomas generally observe that subtypes and other parameters differ significantly in these two groups of tumors. Melanoma in situ (Figs. 7.21, 7.22, and 7.23) and superficial spreading type melanoma were most commonly represented in vulvar melanomas, together comprising over 60% of cases in one series [75] and a substantial subset in another series [85]. Mucosal lentiginous melanoma comprises 17–25% of vulvar melanoma [75, 85]. Nodular melanoma was rare in the vulva in one series but comprised 64% of non-vulvar (vaginal and cervical) melanomas [75], while this subtype was common in the vulva in another series [85]. Desmoplastic melanoma of the

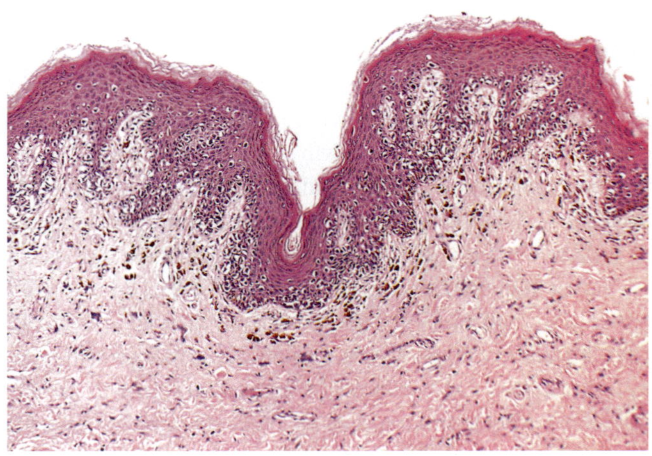

Fig. 7.21 Melanoma in situ. There is an increased density and confluence of melanocytes at the dermal-epidermal junction as well as cytologic atypia and pagetoid spread of melanocytes throughout the epidermis. There is no invasion of malignant melanocytes into the dermis

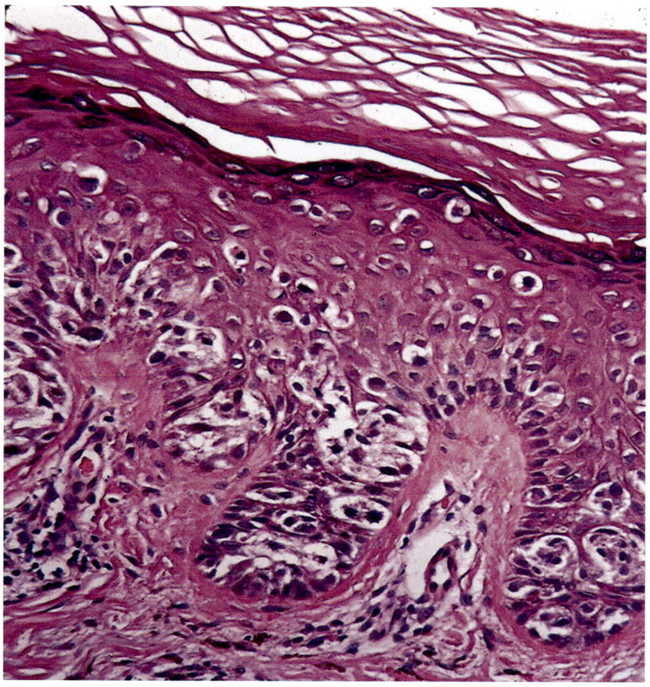

Fig. 7.22 Melanoma in situ. There is an increased density and confluence of atypical melanocytes at the dermal-epidermal junction with pagetoid spread. Photo provided courtesy of previous edition in Chinese (Science Press, Beijing, China)

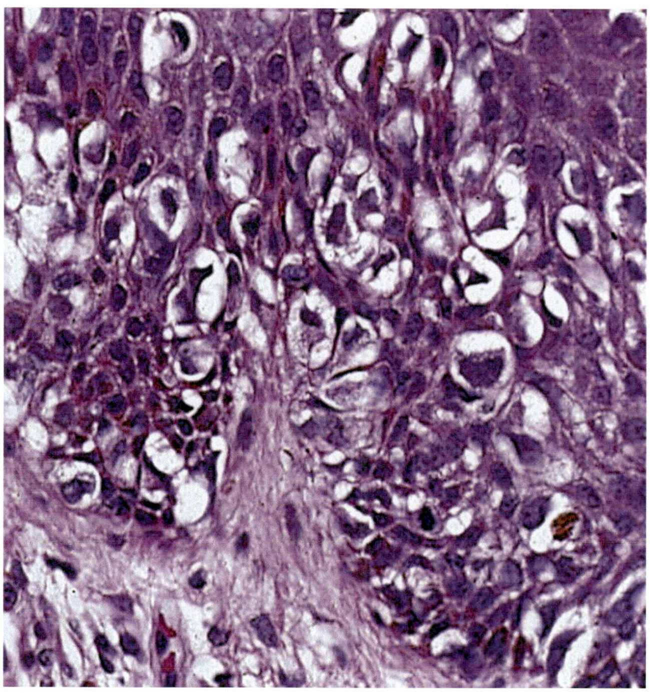

Fig. 7.23 Melanoma in situ. Cells demonstrate pagetoid spread with ample blue-gray cytoplasm, mimicking the histologic differential diagnosis of extramammary Paget's disease. Photo provided courtesy of previous edition in Chinese (Science Press, Beijing, China)

vulva has been reported but is exceptionally rare [86]. Independent of subtype, melanoma in the vulvar region is characterized by increased tumor thickness at initial presentation compared to other cutaneous melanomas, with reported median thicknesses ranging between 1.1 and 4.4 mm [75, 82, 83]. However, vulvar melanomas typically present with a thinner Breslow depth than tumors arising in the vagina or cervix [75]. Advanced tumors frequently show ulceration of the epidermis, and the dermal component is often expansile, cellular, and deeply invasive. Cytologically, melanoma tumor cells are generally large with pleomorphic nuclei (Fig. 7.24). Epithelioid morphology is more common than spindled morphology [85]. Mitotic activity is readily identified, and the cytologic and architectural maturation gradient that is appreciated in nevi is absent in melanoma. Tumors may also show a variety of other features including clear cell (or balloon cell) change, extensive melanin pigmentation or an absence of histologic pigment, and rhabdoid or spindled morphology. The mucosal lentiginous subtype is characterized by a broad, poorly defined junctional component that often extends well beyond any dermal invasion; this junctional pattern of growth can mimic the architecture of a dysplastic nevus on a partial biopsy. The histologic features of superficial spreading and nodular melanomas of the vulva are identical to those seen in other anatomic locations, with asymmetry prominent on scanning magnification and cytologic atypia on high magnification. Superficial spreading melanoma demonstrates a prominent intraepidermal component, with melanocytes observed at all layers of the epidermis. Single cell spread through the epidermis (pagetoid extension) predominates over nesting. Nodular melanoma is defined as an invasive melanoma that lacks a well-defined in situ component (Figs. 7.25 and 7.26). By definition, an intraepidermal component should not extend beyond three rete ridges in order to be classified as a nodular melanoma. This means that even if a superficial spreading type melanoma demonstrates deep invasion with an expansile nodule of tumor, it is still classified as superficial spreading rather than nodular

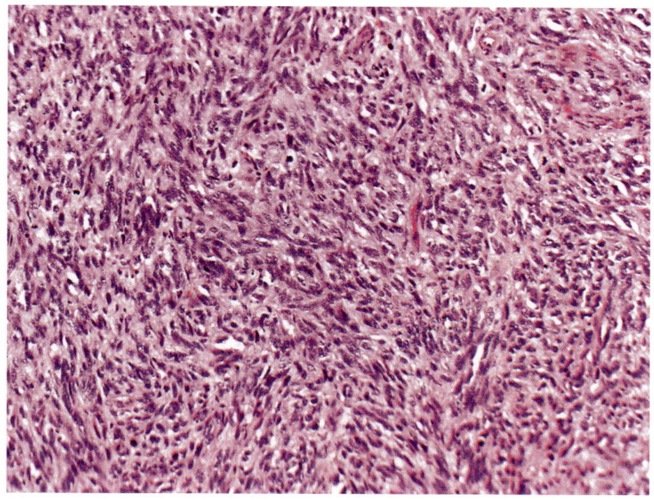

Fig. 7.24 Melanoma with prominent spindled morphology

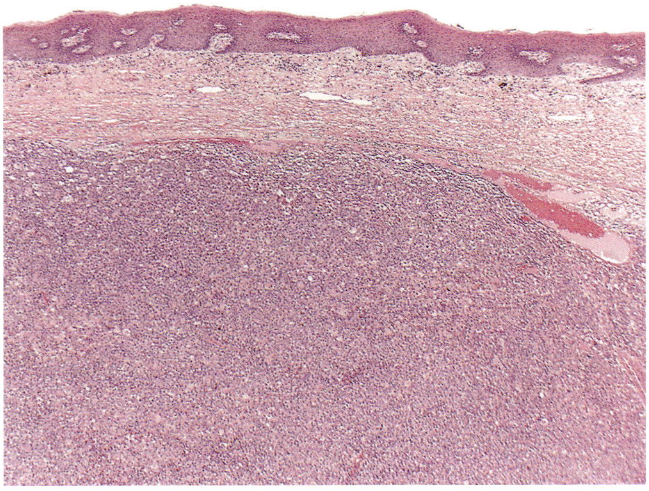

Fig. 7.25 Nodular melanoma. A dermal proliferation of atypical, epithelioid melanocytes is seen within the dermis and sparing the overlying epidermis

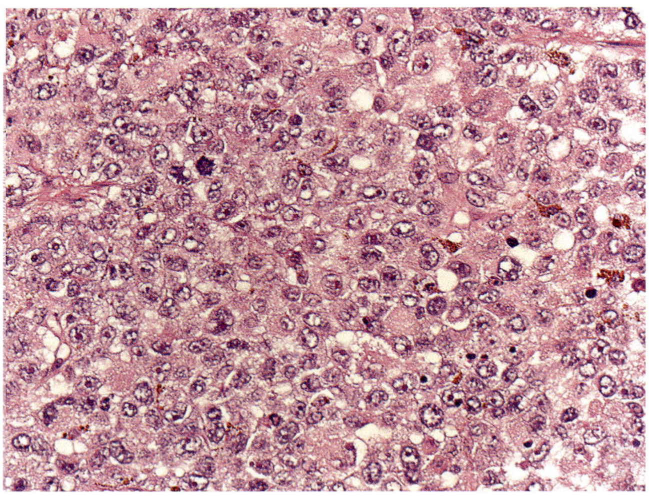

Fig. 7.26 Nodular melanoma. Tumor cells have prominent, pink-red nucleoli and open chromatin with a high mitotic index

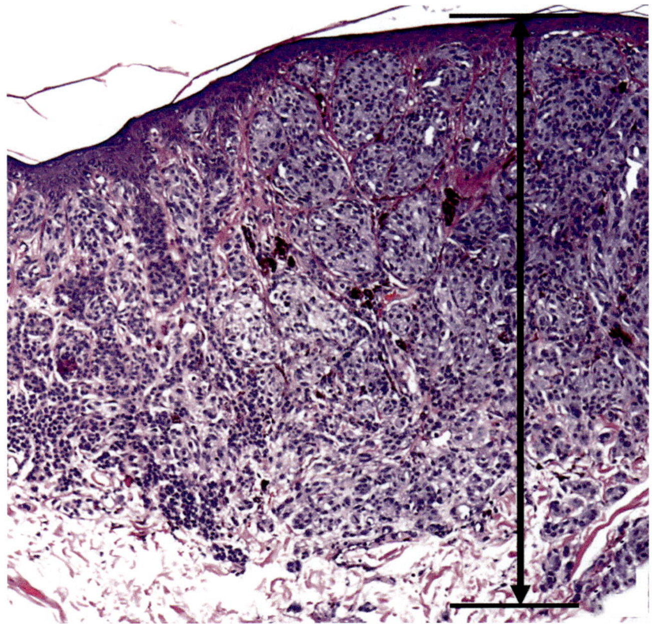

Fig. 7.27 Breslow's thickness measurement. In cases with no ulceration, measurement is from the granular layer of overlying epidermis to deepest invasive tumor cells. Photo provided courtesy of previous edition in Chinese (Science Press, Beijing, China)

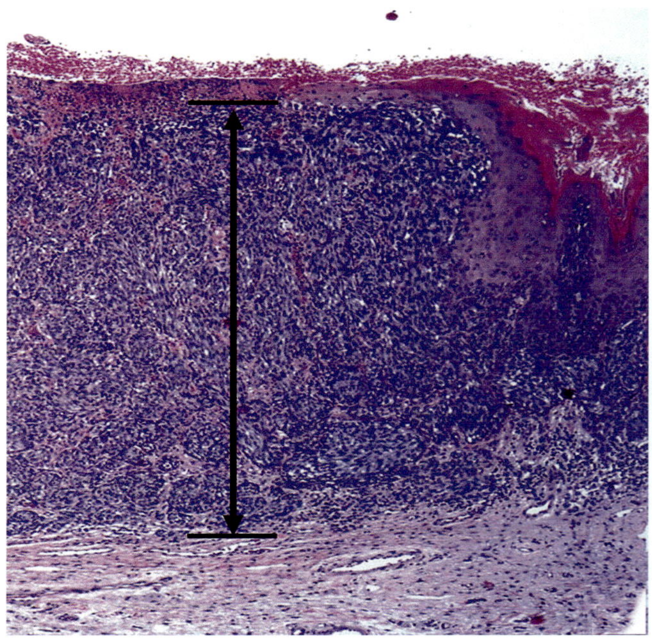

Fig. 7.28 In cases with ulceration, measurement is from base of overlying ulcer to deepest invasive tumor cells. Photo provided courtesy of previous edition in Chinese (Science Press, Beijing, China)

subtype. It should be remembered that while the pathogenesis of the different subtypes of melanoma likely differs in regard to common mutational events, histologic distinction between subtypes actually has no prognostic import at this point. However, familiarity with each of the patterns is important to prevent misdiagnosis.

Similar to the diagnosis of cutaneous melanoma, pathology reports for vulvar melanoma should include staging information at minimum about tumor thickness (Breslow depth), ulceration status, and mitotic rate as recommended by the American Joint Committee on Cancer (AJCC) [82]. Breslow depth is a measurement of the vertical thickness of the tumor measured histopathologically from the epidermal granular layer or from the base of the ulcer (if ulceration is present) , to the deepest dermal invasive melanoma cell [87] (Figs. 7.27 and 7.28). The most recent edition of the AJCC staging manual (8th edition) has removed the detection of mitotic figures as a criteria to upstage a thin melanoma [87]. Many dermatopathologists will provide synoptic reporting of melanomas with comprehensive evaluation of additional prognostic factors, including the presence or absence of lymphovascular invasion, neurotropism, regression, and tumor infiltrating lymphocytes.

7.3.4 Immunohistochemical Features

The use of immunohistochemistry in the work-up of vulvar melanoma is sometimes employed. If there is any doubt as to the derivation of the tumor cells, immunohistochemistry for melanocytic specific markers would be recommended. Melanocytic derivation of the tumor cells can be determined with relatively specific immunohistochemical stains HMB-45 and Melan-A/Mart-1 or with less specific but more sensitive stains such as Sox10 or S100 protein. These latter immunohistochemical stains are very sensitive in the detection of melanocytic cells, including spindle/desmoplastic subtypes [88]; however, both antibodies have additional immunoreactivities, including neural neoplasms and myoepithelial cells (among others). In general, tumor immunoreactivity with any one of these markers in the setting of morphologic features compatible with melanoma should be sufficient to confirm the diagnosis. Dual stains such as MART-1 combined with a proliferation marker (MIB-1/Ki-67) may be useful if there is a large dermal component and the pathologist wishes to evaluate for the proportion of dermal cells in the cell cycle. High numbers of co-labeled cells would indicate a high proliferative index in dermal melanocytes and be supportive of melanoma. Of note, this immunohistochemical technique has limited value in thin melanomas with a minimal dermal component. The use of Ki-67 alone can estimate the number of melanocytes undergoing cell division but will indiscriminately mark all such cells (including admixed lymphocytes) and therefore is difficult to interpret, particularly in very inflamed tumors. Lymphatic markers such as D2–40 (podoplanin) may be used to confirm lymphovascular invasion. Dual stains that utilize a lymphatic and melanocytic marker can confirm this impression with even more specificity [89].

Currently immunohistochemical stains are not routinely employed for prognostic purposes in vulvar melanoma. However, CD117 (CKIT) expression by immunohistochemistry has been shown in some studies to correlate with higher progression-free and/or disease-free survival [90, 91]. Other studies have noted that CD117 expression in melanoma may correlate with *KIT* copy number alterations [85, 92], but not necessarily mutations, and CD117 expression alone does not predict response to the tyrosine kinase inhibitor imatinib [85]. Thus, immunohistochemistry for CD117 as a screening tool is not currently routine practice.

7.3.5 Molecular and Genetic Features

Melanoma arising in the female genital tract has a high level of chromosomal instability and is characterized by many mutational events. Vulvar melanoma has documented mutational events similar to what is seen at other cutaneous sites but with differing frequencies, thereby emphasizing its unique yet shared pathogenesis. In vulvar melanoma, mutations and copy number alterations involving *KIT* are some of the most common genetic aberrations, being found in 20–44% of cohorts, depending on the study [67, 75, 78, 91]. *KIT* encodes the receptor tyrosine kinase KIT expressed on the surface of cells, which, when activated, links to signaling cascades important for cellular proliferation and growth. *KIT* mutations in melanoma are most commonly localized in exon 11 (L576P), leading to constitutive kinase activation; however, mutational events occur within other exons with some frequency [91, 93]. *KIT* copy number alterations (generally amplifications) have also been detected in a smaller subset of vulvar melanomas [85, 91]. The detection of *KIT* alterations within a vulvar melanoma will often allow patients with advanced disease to undergo treatment with tyrosine kinase inhibitors (imatinib, dasatinib, and sorafenib), although ultimate disease progression while on these therapies is to be expected [93].

BRAF mutation is one of the most commonly detected mutational events in melanoma, particularly associated with melanomas developing on the trunk and extremities and associated with intermittent rather than continuous UV exposure. *BRAF* mutations usually result in constitutive activation of signaling pathways involved in cell proliferation, differentiation, and survival [93]. In general, rates of *BRAF* mutation are lower in vulvar melanomas compared to other body sites, and varying percentages of *BRAF* mutation in vulvar melanoma have been reported in the literature, ranging from 0 to 36% [75, 78, 85, 94]. More recent series have been identifying higher rates of *BRAF* mutations [78, 94], speculated to be due to more sensitive detection methods. The activating V600E mutation most commonly identified in *BRAF*-mutated melanomas of cutaneous skin is found in a lower percentage of vulvar melanoma, and vulvar melanomas seem to demonstrate an increased incidence of other mutational events in *BRAF*, including inactivating mutations [78]. Those patients with an activating mutation (including the most common V600E) will be eligible for treatment with FDA-approved BRAF inhibitor therapy (vemurafenib and dabrafenib); patients with inactivating mutations in *BRAF* would not be expected to benefit from these treatments. A recent study by Dias-Santagata et al. identified three rare *BRAF* mutations—G469R, L597Q, and N581S—not previously reported in vulvar melanoma, which are currently undergoing investigation in clinical trials for therapeutic options [91]. *BRAF* mutations in vulva melanomas, overall, are associated with poor survival outcomes.

NRAS mutation can be seen in 12–28% of vulvar melanomas, depending on the series [75, 85, 91]. This frequency is similar to mutation rates in *NRAS* in melanoma from other cutaneous sites. *NRAS* mutations generally correlate with aggressive histologic features and poor survival [93]. Patients with *NRAS*-mutated melanomas might benefit from treatment with a MEK inhibitor [95], as the MAP kinase pathways are activated by NRAS, similar to BRAF. *NRAS* and *BRAF* mutations in melanomas are generally mutually exclusive [93].

NF1 mutations have been recently identified in 20% of vulvovaginal melanomas [91, 96, 97]. Targeted therapeutic strategies are not currently available to patients with *NF1* loss of function mutations, but immunotherapeutic agents are being investigated as potential treatment strategies for these tumors [98].

Other less commonly identified mutational events include mutations in *TP53* [67, 91], the TERT promoter [91], and genes involved in β-catenin signaling [75, 78].

Ancillary molecular techniques are increasingly employed in the diagnosis and prognosis of melanoma and include fluorescent in situ hybridization (FISH), gene expression profiling, array comparative genomic hybridization (CGH), mutational analysis, and next-generation sequencing. FISH employs a set of specific probes to genes known to be commonly mutated in melanoma. CGH identifies large-scale mutational aberrations across the genome in a melanocytic lesion but may miss small mutational events or translocations. Gene expression profiling assays exist both to help determine whether a melanocytic lesion is benign or malignant and to provide risk assessment in lesions already diagnosed as melanoma [70, 72]. Next-generation sequencing and mutational analysis identify potential druggable targets in an individual's melanoma, many of them being the specific mutations discussed above. Full description of each of these techniques is beyond the scope of this chapter, but the reader is referred to a recent review of such techniques [72].

7.3.6 Differential Diagnosis

As discussed earlier in this chapter, vulvar melanomas must be distinguished from melanosis, benign melanocytic nevi, especially those with atypical features such as atypical genital nevi and dysplastic nevi (Table 7.1). Non-melanocytic tumors may also enter the differential diagnosis and most notably include extramammary Paget disease, poorly differentiated squamous cell carcinoma, and vascular neoplasms.

Paget disease is an intraepidermal adenocarcinoma characterized by single cells and nests of tumor cells scattered at all layers of the epidermis (thus tumors that mimic this pattern of growth are said to have a "pagetoid" pattern of growth). Morphologically, these cells can resemble melanoma in situ with pleomorphic, enlarged nuclei and amphophilic blue-gray cytoplasm. Focal areas of dermal invasion may also occasionally be observed in Paget disease. Clues to distinguish Paget disease from melanoma include the presence of intracytoplasmic mucin or intraepidermal glandular formation, features not seen in melanoma. Moreover, the nests of Paget cells tend to preserve the basal layer of the epidermis whereas confluent junctional growth (both singly and in nests) in melanoma tends to replace the basal layer of keratinocytes. The diagnosis of Paget disease can easily be confirmed with positive staining for cytokeratin 7 and CEA, which typify the most common immunophenotype; these markers should be negative in melanoma.

In poorly differentiated squamous cell carcinomas, identification of a more well-differentiated area of the tumor is helpful. Areas of keratinization and intracellular bridges are seen in squamous cell carcinoma but not in melanoma. In difficult cases, the diagnosis can be made with immunohistochemistry with squamous cell carcinoma exhibiting positivity for markers such as p63, p40, and high molecular weight cytokeratins.

Vascular tumors may be more of a clinical mimic of melanoma than a histologic mimic. Thrombosis of dermal vascular channels can result in a dark brown to black clinical appearance. Vascular neoplasms are generally readily identified as such on histologic examination.

7.3.7 Staging, Prognosis, and Management

The 5-year overall and disease-free survival rates that have been reported for vulvar melanoma are generally low and range from 10 to 50% in different series [75, 76, 79–81]. The overall prognosis is generally poor, with a range of clinical outcomes [82]. Comparable to cutaneous melanoma, better outcome is associated with younger age at diagnosis, localized disease, lack of lymph node involvement, and histologically confirmed clear margins of excision [79–81, 83, 84, 87, 99]. Similar to cutaneous melanoma on other body sites, parameters predicting poorer prognosis include thick tumors (>1 mm), high mitotic rate, perineural invasion, and ulceration (Figs. 7.29 and 7.30). Molecular profiles are being increasingly investigated with relation to prognostic import. Some recent studies have shown *KIT* mutations and overexpression of CD117 to be associated with a more favorable prognosis [90, 91], although in Asian populations *KIT* mutations are correlated with a poorer prognosis [92, 100]. The presence of increased peritumoral regulatory T-cells (FoxP3-expressing) in vulvar melanoma was shown to correlate with improved survival, suggesting an important role for an intact adaptive immune response [101].

Management of vulvar melanoma depends on the extent of disease. Localized disease is managed through surgery with or without lymph node sampling. Radical procedures

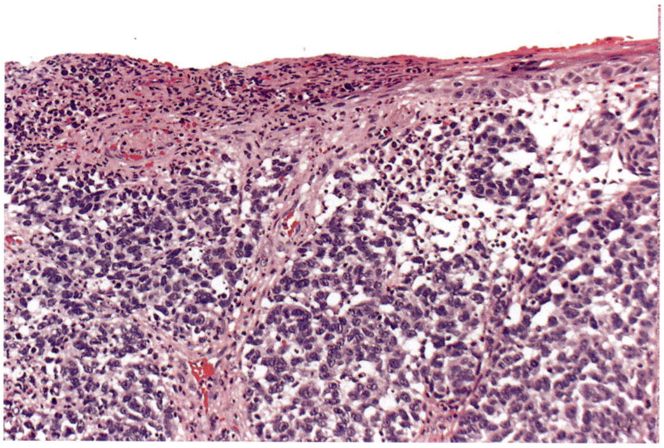

Fig. 7.29 Melanoma with ulceration of the epidermis, a poor prognostic indicator

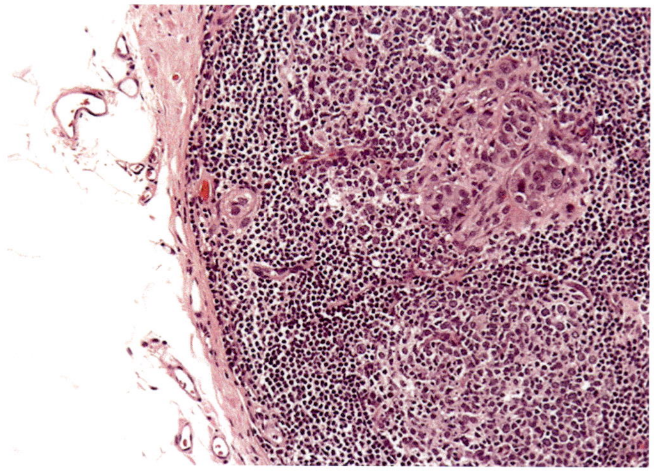

Fig. 7.31 Sentinel lymph node with metastatic melanoma seen on H&E. Photo provided courtesy of previous edition in Chinese (Science Press, Beijing, China)

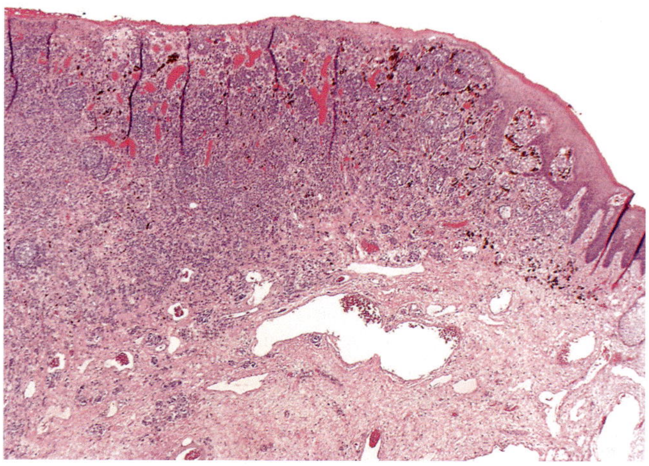

Fig. 7.30 Melanoma with ulceration of the epidermis, a poor prognostic indicator

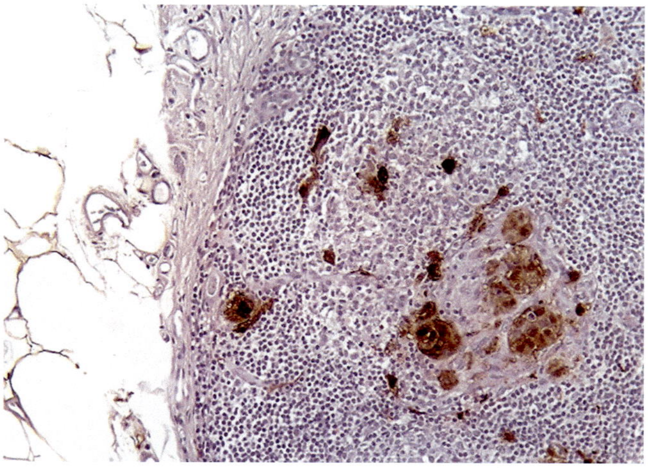

Fig. 7.32 Sentinel lymph node with metastatic melanoma confirmed with S-100 immunohistochemistry. Photo provided courtesy of previous edition in Chinese (Science Press, Beijing, China)

have shown no survival benefit over wide local excisions in vulvar melanoma [79], and treatment is shifting to more conservative partial vulvectomies. The recommended clinical excision margins for melanoma in situ, melanomas with Breslow's thickness 2.0 mm or less, and thickness greater than 2.0 mm are 0.5 cm, 1 cm, and 2 cm, respectively [102]. These surgical margins may sometimes be difficult to obtain in the vulvar region with its complex anatomy, and margins are often narrower [82]. One series noted that 20% of vulvar melanomas excised had a positive final margin, and vaginal melanomas had an even higher rate of incomplete excision (64%) [75]. An increased emphasis on early detection has stressed consistent and thorough physical examination at routine visits [79, 103–105].

Sentinel lymph node (SLN) mapping is recommended for all cutaneous melanomas staged pT2 and higher and can be considered in thinner melanomas with adverse prognostic features such as ulceration (pT1b lesions). SLN biopsy is less invasive and results in lower morbidity than elective lymph node dissection which used to be utilized. However, while SLN biopsy provides definite prognostic benefit, the therapeutic benefits of SLN biopsy remains debated. Some studies suggest therapeutic in addition to prognostic benefit such as the Multicenter Selective Lymphadenectomy Trial I (MSLT-I), which noted a disease-free survival advantage of SLN mapping with completion lymphadenectomy for node-positive cases compared with observation alone [106–108].

Patients diagnosed with metastatic melanoma either in regional lymph nodes (Figs. 7.31 and 7.32) or at distant sites historically have been treated with radiation and/or chemotherapy, neither of which is particularly effective. Advances in the understanding of the molecular pathogenesis and mutational events that contribute to melanomagenesis have increased the arsenal of effective therapeutics for patients. Targeted therapies based on molecular profile (such as BRAF inhibitors targeting activated BRAF mutations or tyrosine kinase inhibitors targeting KIT mutations) offer a higher rate of response but require documentation of an actionable mutation. Immunotherapy aimed to prime the patient's immune system to fight the tumor offers the promise of longer lasting, durable responses but is still only seen in a subset of patients. Combination therapies targeting multiple mutational drivers and the immune system are currently in trials and showing promising results [109].

References

1. Massi G, Leboit PE. Histological diagnosis of nevi and melanoma. 2nd ed. Berlin: Springer-Verlag; 2014.
2. Chapel TA, Taylor RM, Pinkus H. Volar melanotic macules. Int J Dermatol. 1979;18:222–5.
3. Veraldi S, Cavicchini S, Benelli C, et al. Laugier-Hunziker syndrome: a clinical, histopathologic, and ultrastructural study of four cases and review of the literature. J Am Acad Dermatol. 1991;25:632–6.
4. Jih DM, Elder DE, Elenitsas R. A histopathologic evaluation of vulvar melanosis. Arch Dermatol. 1999;135:857–8.
5. Allbritton JI. Vulvar neoplasms, benign and malignant. Obstet Gynecol Clin N Am. 2017;44:339–52.
6. Lenane P, Keane CO, Connell BO, et al. Genital melanotic macules: clinical, histologic, immunohistochemical, and ultrastructural features. J Am Acad Dermatol. 2000;42:640–4.
7. Pandolfino TL, Cotell S, Katta R. Pigmented vulvar macules as a presenting feature of the carney complex. Int J Dermatol. 2001;40:728–30.
8. Barnhill RL, Albert LS, Shama SK, et al. Genital lentiginosis: a clinical and histopathologic study. J Am Acad Dermatol. 1990;22:453–60.
9. Haugh AM, Merkel EA, Zhang B, et al. A clinical, histologic, and follow-up study of genital melanosis in men and women. J Am Acad Dermatol. 2017;76:836–40.
10. Ronger-Savle S, Julien V, Duru G, et al. Features of pigmented vulval lesions on dermoscopy. Br J Dermatol. 2011;164:54–61.
11. Ferrari A, Buccini P, Covello R, et al. The ringlike pattern in vulvar melanosis: a new dermoscopic clue for diagnosis. Arch Dermatol. 2008;144:1030–4.
12. Hoang MP, Selim MA. Vulvar pathology. 1st ed. New York: Springer; 2015.
13. Brown LMG, Singh N. Pathology of the vulva and vagina. New York: Springer; 2012.
14. Rock B, Hood AF, Rock JA. Prospective study of vulvar nevi. J Am Acad Dermatol. 1990;22:104–6.
15. Murzaku EC, Penn LA, Hale CS, et al. Vulvar nevi, melanosis, and melanoma: an epidemiologic, clinical, and histopathologic review. J Am Acad Dermatol. 2014;71:1241–9.
16. Edwards L. Pigmented vulvar lesions. Dermatol Ther. 2010;23:449–57.
17. Ribe A. Melanocytic lesions of the genital area with attention given to atypical genital nevi. J Cutan Pathol. 2008;35(Suppl 2):24–7.
18. Tieche M. Uber benigne melanome ("Chromatophorome") der haut- "Blaue Naevi". Virchows Arch Pathol Anat. 1906;186:212–29.
19. Niedelman ML. Blue nevus of Jadassohn and Tieche; report of a case. Arch Dermatol Syphilol. 1946;53:285–7.
20. Zembowicz A, Phadke PA. Blue nevi and variants: an update. Arch Pathol Lab Med. 2011;135:327–36.
21. Tucker SM, Linberg JV, Doshi HM. Conjunctival blue nevus associated with pyogenic granuloma. Can J Ophthalmol. 1994;29:95–6.
22. Diaz De Molnar AM, Guralnick M, Ferenczy A. Blue nevus of the endocervix: report of two cases and ultrastructure. Gynecol Oncol. 1978;6:373–82.
23. Murali R, McCarthy SW, Scolyer RA. Blue nevi and related lesions: a review highlighting atypical and newly described variants, distinguishing features and diagnostic pitfalls. Adv Anat Pathol. 2009;16:365–82.
24. Rodriguez HA, Ackerman LV. Cellular blue nevus. Clinicopathologic study of forty-five cases. Cancer. 1968;21:393–405.
25. Edwards EA, Duntley SQ. The pigments and color of living human skin. Am J Anat. 1939;65:1–33.
26. Tobon H, Murphy AI. Benign blue nevus of the vagina. Cancer. 1977;40:3174–6.
27. Eskue K, Prieto VG, Malpica A. Cellular blue nevus of the uterus: a case report and review of the literature. Int J Gynecol Pathol. 2010;29:583–6.
28. Yamazhan M, Ertas IE, Kandiloglu G, et al. Cellular blue nevus of the vulva mimicking Bartholin's gland abscess in a 15-year-old girl: a case report. Arch Gynecol Obstet. 2012;285:1009–11.
29. Rhodes AR, Silverman RA, Harrist TJ, et al. Mucocutaneous lentigines, cardiomucocutaneous myxomas, and multiple blue nevi: the "LAMB" syndrome. J Am Acad Dermatol. 1984;10:72–82.
30. Kang DS, Chung KY. Common blue naevus with satellite lesions: possible perivascular dissemination resulting in a clinical resemblance to malignant melanoma. Br J Dermatol. 1999;141:922–5.
31. Palla B, Su A, Binder S, et al. SOX10 expression distinguishes desmoplastic melanoma from its histologic mimics. Am J Dermatopathol. 2013;35:576–81.
32. Spitz S. Melanomas of childhood. Am J Pathol. 1948;24:591–609.
33. Requena C, Requena L, Kutzner H, et al. Spitz nevus: a clinicopathological study of 349 cases. Am J Dermatopathol. 2009;31:107–16.
34. Sepehr A, Chao E, Trefrey B, et al. Long-term outcome of Spitz-type melanocytic tumors. Arch Dermatol. 2011;147:1173–9.
35. Menezes FD, Mooi WJ. Spitz tumors of the skin. Surg Pathol Clin. 2017;10:281–98.
36. Lott JP, Wititsuwannakul J, Lee JJ, et al. Clinical characteristics associated with Spitz nevi and Spitzoid malignant melanomas: the Yale University Spitzoid neoplasm repository experience, 1991 to 2008. J Am Acad Dermatol. 2014;71:1077–82.
37. Plaza JA, De Stefano D, Suster S, et al. Intradermal spitz nevi: a rare subtype of spitz nevi analyzed in a clinicopathologic study of 74 cases. Am J Dermatopathol. 2014;36:283–94. quiz 295–287
38. Levy RM, Ming ME, Shapiro M, et al. Eruptive disseminated Spitz nevi. J Am Acad Dermatol. 2007;57:519–23.
39. Kamino H, Flotte TJ, Misheloff E, et al. Eosinophilic globules in Spitz's nevi. New findings and a diagnostic sign. Am J Dermatopathol. 1979;1:319–24.
40. Al Dhaybi R, Agoumi M, Gagne I, et al. p16 expression: a marker of differentiation between childhood malignant melanomas and Spitz nevi. J Am Acad Dermatol. 2011;65:357–63.
41. Harms PW, Hocker TL, Zhao L, et al. Loss of p16 expression and copy number changes of CDKN2A in a spectrum of spitzoid melanocytic lesions. Hum Pathol. 2016;58:152–60.
42. Yazdan P, Cooper C, Sholl LM, et al. Comparative analysis of atypical spitz tumors with heterozygous versus homozygous 9p21 deletions for clinical outcomes, histomorphology, BRAF mutation, and p16 expression. Am J Surg Pathol. 2014;38:638–45.

43. Tetzlaff MT, Reuben A, Billings SD, et al. Toward a molecular-genetic classification of Spitzoid neoplasms. Clin Lab Med. 2017;37:431–48.
44. Bastian BC, Wesselmann U, Pinkel D, et al. Molecular cytogenetic analysis of Spitz nevi shows clear differences to melanoma. J Invest Dermatol. 1999;113:1065–9.
45. Bastian BC, LeBoit PE, Pinkel D. Mutations and copy number increase of HRAS in Spitz nevi with distinctive histopathological features. Am J Pathol. 2000;157:967–72.
46. van Engen-van Grunsven AC, van Dijk MC, Ruiter DJ, et al. HRAS-mutated Spitz tumors: a subtype of Spitz tumors with distinct features. Am J Surg Pathol. 2010;34:1436–41.
47. Wiesner T, He J, Yelensky R, et al. Kinase fusions are frequent in Spitz tumours and spitzoid melanomas. Nat Commun. 2014;5:3116.
48. Yeh I, Tee MK, Botton T, et al. NTRK3 kinase fusions in Spitz tumours. J Pathol. 2016;240:282–90.
49. Yeh I, Botton T, Talevich E, et al. Activating MET kinase rearrangements in melanoma and Spitz tumours. Nat Commun. 2015;6:7174.
50. Shalin SC. A review of kinase fusions in melanocytic tumors. Lab Investig. 2017;97:158–65.
51. Wiesner T, Murali R, Fried I, et al. A distinct subset of atypical Spitz tumors is characterized by BRAF mutation and loss of BAP1 expression. Am J Surg Pathol. 2012;36:818–30.
52. Wiesner T, Obenauf AC, Murali R, et al. Germline mutations in BAP1 predispose to melanocytic tumors. Nat Genet. 2011;43:1018–21.
53. Busam KJ, Sung J, Wiesner T, et al. Combined BRAF(V600E)-positive melanocytic lesions with large epithelioid cells lacking BAP1 expression and conventional nevomelanocytes. Am J Surg Pathol. 2013;37:193–9.
54. Gerami P, Cooper C, Bajaj S, et al. Outcomes of atypical spitz tumors with chromosomal copy number aberrations and conventional melanomas in children. Am J Surg Pathol. 2013;37:1387–94.
55. Gerami P, Scolyer RA, Xu X, et al. Risk assessment for atypical spitzoid melanocytic neoplasms using FISH to identify chromosomal copy number aberrations. Am J Surg Pathol. 2013;37:676–84.
56. Lee S, Barnhill RL, Dummer R, et al. TERT promoter mutations are predictive of aggressive clinical behavior in patients with Spitzoid melanocytic neoplasms. Sci Rep. 2015;5:11200.
57. Abboud J, Stein M, Ramien M, et al. The diagnosis and management of the Spitz nevus in the pediatric population: a systematic review and meta-analysis protocol. Syst Rev. 2017;6:81.
58. Doyle LA, Marino-Enriquez A, Fletcher CD, et al. ALK rearrangement and overexpression in epithelioid fibrous histiocytoma. Mod Pathol. 2015;28:904–12.
59. Cerroni L, Barnhill R, Elder D, et al. Melanocytic tumors of uncertain malignant potential: results of a tutorial held at the XXIX symposium of the International Society of Dermatopathology in Graz, October 2008. Am J Surg Pathol. 2010;34:314–26.
60. Gleason BC, Hirsch MS, Nucci MR, et al. Atypical genital nevi. A clinicopathologic analysis of 56 cases. Am J Surg Pathol. 2008;32:51–7.
61. Brenn T. Atypical genital nevus. Arch Pathol Lab Med. 2011;135:317–20.
62. Elder DE. Precursors to melanoma and their mimics: nevi of special sites. Mod Pathol. 2006;19(Suppl 2):S4–20.
63. Neri I, Dika E, Fanti PA, et al. Genital melanocytic naevus on lichen sclerosus: an uncommon occurrence and a management proposal. J Eur Acad Dermatol Venereol. 2016;30:794–7.
64. Pinto A, McLaren SH, Poppas DP, et al. Genital melanocytic nevus arising in a background of lichen sclerosus in a 7-year-old female: the diagnostic pitfall with malignant melanoma. A literature review. Am J Dermatopathol. 2012;34:838–43.
65. Carlson JA, Mu XC, Slominski A, et al. Melanocytic proliferations associated with lichen sclerosus. Arch Dermatol. 2002;138:77–87.
66. El Shabrawi-Caelen L, Soyer HP, Schaeppi H, et al. Genital lentigines and melanocytic nevi with superimposed lichen sclerosus: a diagnostic challenge. J Am Acad Dermatol. 2004;50:690–4.
67. Yelamos O, Merkel EA, Sholl LM, et al. Nonoverlapping clinical and mutational patterns in melanomas from the female genital tract and atypical genital nevi. J Invest Dermatol. 2016;136:1858–65.
68. Clark WH Jr, Tucker MA. Problems with lesions related to the development of malignant melanoma: common nevi, dysplastic nevi, malignant melanoma in situ, and radial growth phase malignant melanoma. Hum Pathol. 1998;29:8–14.
69. Kim J, Taube JM, McCalmont TH, et al. Quantitative comparison of MiTF, Melan-a, HMB-45 and Mel-5 in solar lentigines and melanoma in situ. J Cutan Pathol. 2011;38:775–9.
70. Minca EC, Al-Rohil RN, Wang M, et al. Comparison between melanoma gene expression score and fluorescence in situ hybridization for the classification of melanocytic lesions. Mod Pathol. 2016;29:832–43.
71. Clarke LE, Flake DD 2nd, Busam K, et al. An independent validation of a gene expression signature to differentiate malignant melanoma from benign melanocytic nevi. Cancer. 2017;123:617–28.
72. Lee CY, Gerami P. Molecular techniques for predicting behaviour in melanocytic neoplasms. Pathology. 2016;48:142–6.
73. Maghari A. Dysplastic (or atypical) nevi showing moderate or severe Atypia with clear margins on the shave removal specimens are Most likely completely excised. J Cutan Med Surg. 2017;21:42–7.
74. Reddy KK, Farber MJ, Bhawan J, et al. Atypical (dysplastic) nevi: outcomes of surgical excision and association with melanoma. JAMA Dermatol. 2013;149:928–34.
75. Udager AM, Frisch NK, Hong LJ, et al. Gynecologic melanomas: a clinicopathologic and molecular analysis. Gynecol Oncol. 2017;147:351–7.
76. Wechter ME, Gruber SB, Haefner HK, et al. Vulvar melanoma: a report of 20 cases and review of the literature. J Am Acad Dermatol. 2004;50:554–62.
77. Vyas R, Thompson CL, Zargar H, et al. Epidemiology of genitourinary melanoma in the United States: 1992 through 2012. J Am Acad Dermatol. 2016;75:144–50.
78. Hou JY, Baptiste C, Hombalegowda RB, et al. Vulvar and vaginal melanoma: a unique subclass of mucosal melanoma based on a comprehensive molecular analysis of 51 cases compared with 2253 cases of nongynecologic melanoma. Cancer. 2017;123:1333–44.
79. Skovsted S, Nielsen K, Blaakaer J. Melanomas of the vulva and vagina. Dan Med J. 2017;64:A5336.
80. Weinstock MA. Malignant melanoma of the vulva and vagina in the United States: patterns of incidence and population-based estimates of survival. Am J Obstet Gynecol. 1994;171:1225–30.
81. Chang AE, Karnell LH, Menck HR. The National Cancer Data Base report on cutaneous and noncutaneous melanoma: a summary of 84,836 cases from the past decade. The American College of Surgeons Commission on Cancer and the American Cancer Society. Cancer. 1998;83:1664–78.
82. Seifried S, Haydu LE, Quinn MJ, et al. Melanoma of the vulva and vagina: principles of staging and their relevance to management based on a clinicopathologic analysis of 85 cases. Ann Surg Oncol. 2015;22:1959–66.
83. Ragnarsson-Olding BK, Kanter-Lewensohn LR, Lagerlof B, et al. Malignant melanoma of the vulva in a nationwide, 25-year study of 219 Swedish females: clinical observations and histopathologic features. Cancer. 1999;86:1273–84.
84. Raber G, Mempel V, Jackisch C, et al. Malignant melanoma of the vulva. Report of 89 patients. Cancer. 1996;78:2353–8.

85. Aulmann S, Sinn HP, Penzel R, et al. Comparison of molecular abnormalities in vulvar and vaginal melanomas. Mod Pathol. 2014;27:1386–93.
86. Mulvany NJ, Sykes P. Desmoplastic melanoma of the vulva. Pathology. 1997;29:241–5.
87. AJCC. AJCC cancer staging manual. 8th ed. New York: Springer; 2017.
88. Ramos-Herberth FI, Karamchandani J, Kim J, et al. SOX10 immunostaining distinguishes desmoplastic melanoma from excision scar. J Cutan Pathol. 2010;37:944–52.
89. Moy AP, Mochel MC, Muzikansky A, et al. Lymphatic invasion predicts sentinel lymph node metastasis and adverse outcome in primary cutaneous melanoma. J Cutan Pathol. 2017;44:734–9.
90. Heinzelmann-Schwarz VA, Nixdorf S, Valadan M, et al. A clinicopathological review of 33 patients with vulvar melanoma identifies c-KIT as a prognostic marker. Int J Mol Med. 2014;33:784–94.
91. Dias-Santagata D, Selim MA, Su Y, et al. KIT mutations and CD117 overexpression are markers of better progression-free survival in vulvar melanomas. Br J Dermatol. 2017;177:1376–84.
92. Kong Y, Si L, Zhu Y, et al. Large-scale analysis of KIT aberrations in Chinese patients with melanoma. Clin Cancer Res. 2011;17:1684–91.
93. Reddy BY, Miller DM, Tsao H. Somatic driver mutations in melanoma. Cancer. 2017;123:2104–17.
94. Wylomanski S, Denis MG, Theoleyre S, et al. BRAF mutations might be more common than supposed in vulvar melanomas. Exp Dermatol. 2018;27(2):210–3.
95. Dummer R, Schadendorf D, Ascierto PA, et al. Binimetinib versus dacarbazine in patients with advanced NRAS-mutant melanoma (NEMO): a multicentre, open-label, randomised, phase 3 trial. Lancet Oncol. 2017;18:435–45.
96. Hintzsche JD, Gorden NT, Amato CM, et al. Whole-exome sequencing identifies recurrent SF3B1 R625 mutation and comutation of NF1 and KIT in mucosal melanoma. Melanoma Res. 2017;27:189–99.
97. Yang HM, Hsiao SJ, Schaeffer DF, et al. Identification of recurrent mutational events in anorectal melanoma. Mod Pathol. 2017;30:286–96.
98. Johnpulle RA, Johnson DB, Sosman JA. Molecular targeted therapy approaches for BRAF wild-type melanoma. Curr Oncol Rep. 2016;18:6.
99. De Simone P, Silipo V, Buccini P, et al. Vulvar melanoma: a report of 10 cases and review of the literature. Melanoma Res. 2008;18:127–33.
100. Jin SA, Chun SM, Choi YD, et al. BRAF mutations and KIT aberrations and their clinicopathological correlation in 202 Korean melanomas. J Invest Dermatol. 2013;133:579–82.
101. Chlopik A, Selim MA, Peng Y, et al. Prognostic role of Tumoral PDL1 expression and Peritumoral FoxP3+ lymphocytes in vulvar melanomas. Hum Pathol. 2018;73:176–83.
102. Garbe C, Peris K, Hauschild A, et al. Diagnosis and treatment of melanoma. European consensus-based interdisciplinary guideline--update 2012. Eur J Cancer. 2012;48:2375–90.
103. Moxley KM, Fader AN, Rose PG, et al. Malignant melanoma of the vulva: an extension of cutaneous melanoma? Gynecol Oncol. 2011;122:612–7.
104. Suwandinata FS, Bohle RM, Omwandho CA, et al. Management of vulvar melanoma and review of the literature. Eur J Gynaecol Oncol. 2007;28:220–4.
105. Trimble EL, Lewis JL Jr, Williams LL, et al. Management of vulvar melanoma. Gynecol Oncol. 1992;45:254–8.
106. Leitao MM Jr. Management of vulvar and vaginal melanomas: current and future strategies. Am Soc Clin Oncol Educ Book. 2014:e277–81.
107. Wong SL, Balch CM, Hurley P, et al. Sentinel lymph node biopsy for melanoma: American Society of Clinical Oncology and Society of Surgical Oncology joint clinical practice guideline. J Clin Oncol. 2012;30:2912–8.
108. Morton DL, Thompson JF, Cochran AJ, et al. Sentinel-node biopsy or nodal observation in melanoma. N Engl J Med. 2006;355:1307–17.
109. Assi HI, Assi RE. Recent Progress in mutation-driven therapy, immunotherapy and combination therapy for the treatment of melanoma. Curr Cancer Drug Targets. 2017;17:137–57.

8 Soft Tissue Lesions of the Vulva and the Vagina

Carlos Parra-Herran

Abstract

With the exception of fibroepithelial stromal polyps, the entities covered in this section are uncommon. For this reason, a broad differential diagnosis must be considered when evaluating a soft tissue lesion in the vulvovaginal region. This differential can be narrowed by patient age (for instance, prepubertal vulvar fibroma and embryonal rhabdomyosarcoma in young women), clinical presentation (slow vs. rapidly growing mass, superficial vs. deep), and morphology (myxoid vs. fibromatous appearance; spindle vs. round tumor cells; obvious smooth muscle, adipocytic, fibroblastic/myofibroblastic, vascular, or Schwannian cell differentiation). Some lesions harbor characteristic genetic abnormalities (loss of the 13q14 locus in cellular angiofibroma and mammary-type myofibroblastoma or amplification of the 12q13-15 locus in atypical lipomatous tumor); in others, the diagnosis fully relies on histopathologic features. In any spindle cell proliferation of the vulva or vagina, *spindled invasive squamous cell carcinoma* and *desmoplastic malignant melanoma* should be considered and excluded through detailed examination and ancillary studies (immunohistochemistry, HPV testing). Entities included in this chapter are organized into benign, locally aggressive, and malignant categories (with the exception of smooth muscle tumors, which are covered together). The chapter emphasizes on lesions with anatomic predilection for the lower genital tract and likely derivation from specialized vulvovaginal stromal cells; while morphologic overlap exists among these lesions, their behavior and clinical management are indolent, with the exception of aggressive angiomyxoma. The latter, thus, should be always considered and excluded through careful assessment, radiologic correlation, and thorough margin assessment on excision material.

C. Parra-Herran (✉)
Department of Laboratory Medicine and Pathobiology, University of Toronto, Toronto, ON, Canada

Sunnybrook Health Sciences Centre, Toronto, ON, Canada
e-mail: carlos.parraherran@sunnybrook.ca

Keywords

Vulva · Vagina · Sarcoma · Mesenchymal · Angiomyxoma · Fibroepithelial polyp · Angiomyofibroblastoma · Myofibroblastoma · Angiofibroma · Hemangioma · Lymphangioma circumscriptum · Angiokeratoma · Rhabdomyoma · Lipoma · Dermatofibroma · Leiomyoma · Liposarcoma · Leiomyosarcoma · Rhabdomyosarcoma · Botryoides · Granular cell tumor · Schwannoma · Neurofibroma · Malignant peripheral nerve sheath tumor · Primitive neuroectodermal tumor · Angiosarcoma · Dermatofibrosarcoma · Myeloid sarcoma

8.1 Benign Lesions

8.1.1 Vulvovaginal Stromal Lesions

The lesions described in this section present preferentially in the vulvovaginal region. Tumors in this category are believed to originate in the specialized stroma of the vaginal and vulvar mucosa, since most express estrogen and progesterone receptors. There is significant morphologic and immunophenotypic overlap among these tumors. The following paragraphs aim to describe the most salient features of each entity and clues in their differential diagnosis. These are also presented schematically in Fig. 8.1.

8.1.1.1 Fibroepithelial Stromal Polyp

Clinical Features

Formerly known as "vulvovaginal polyp" [1], this lesion is common in the vagina [2, 3] and vulva [4] of women predominantly in their fourth decade; however, age rage is wide [1, 5, 6]. Associations with pregnancy and hormone therapy have been observed [2, 5, 7]. The lesion is typically asymptomatic and discovered incidentally on examination in most of cases, while in others it can present with bleeding or pain.

W. Zheng et al. (eds.), *Gynecologic and Obstetric Pathology, Volume 1*, https://doi.org/10.1007/978-981-13-3016-2_8

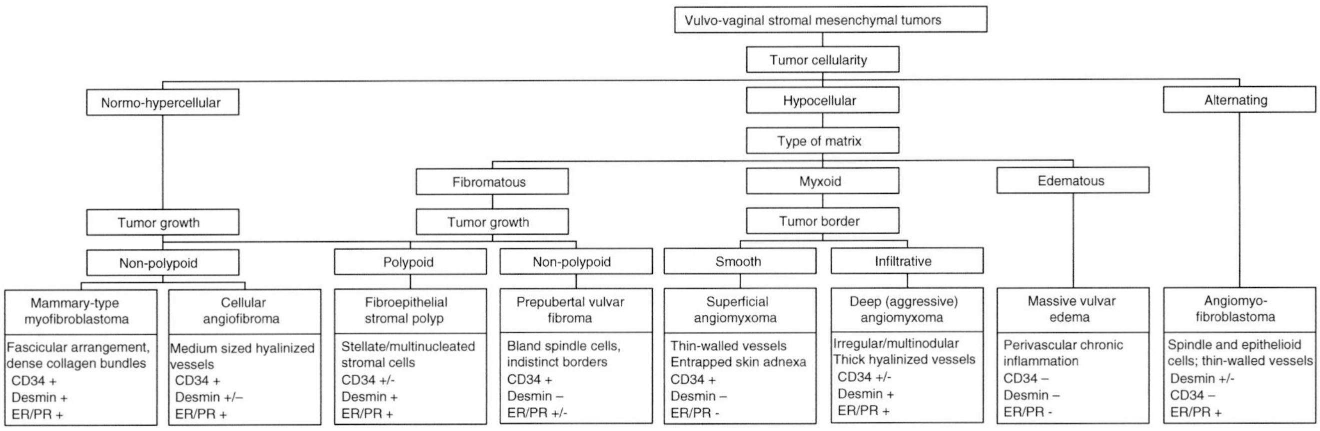

Fig. 8.1 Algorithmic approach to the diagnosis of vulvovaginal stromal tumors. Despite the significant morphologic and immunophenotypic overlap, the proposed features are relatively distinct for each entity and in combination can aid in the differential diagnosis

Pathologic Features

Macroscopically, the lesion is polypoid and pedunculated; when multiple and large, it may acquire a frond-like appearance. Size is variable, ranging from less than 1 to 18 cm [8]. On sectioning, the tissue is uniform white and soft to rubbery.

Microscopically, fibroepithelial stromal polyp is characterized by a uniformly collagenous stromal component containing bland myofibroblastic spindle cells. The lesion has variably sized blood vessels, which often are thick and large at the base of the polyp. Toward the superficial (subepithelial) aspect of the lesion, the stromal cells appear stellate and multinucleated with larger and more hyperchromatic nuclei (akin to the subepithelial stromal cells sometimes found in the normal vaginal mucosa, Fig. 8.2). Lesions are frequently bland, hypocellular, and may present significant atypia. Indeed, initial descriptions in the literature termed fibroepithelial polyps as “pseudosarcoma botryoides” and “cellular pseudosarcomatous fibroepithelial stromal polyp,” alluding to the frequent presence of large bizarre cells which could be mistaken for a malignant process [6, 9]. This scenario appears to be more common in cases presenting during pregnancy [4, 6].

Ancillary Studies

The stromal cells in fibroepithelial polyps are reported to express desmin, vimentin, estrogen, and progesterone receptors [1, 6, 10]. No recurrent molecular alterations have been reported to date.

Differential Diagnosis

Acrochordon (skin tag) is a term used for polyps outside of the genital area. While morphologically similar to skin tags, fibroepithelial polyp is the preferred term in the vulvovaginal region as it may have a different pathogenesis, given its association with sex hormone expression and the distinct presence of stellate stromal cells, native to the lower genital tract mucosa.

Fibroepithelial polyps exhibiting hypercellularity and stromal pleomorphism should be distinguished from malignant proliferations, importantly rhabdomyosarcoma. Unlike the latter, fibroepithelial stromal polyp lacks a cambium layer and has scattered bizarre stromal cells extending to the epithelial base. Embryonal rhabdomyosarcoma and genital rhabdomyoma both have cells with identifiable striations, which will be absent in cellular fibroepithelial polyp. Furthermore, embryonal rhabdomyosarcoma usually presents in prepubertal girls.

Fibroepithelial polyps may undergo torsion, which gives them an edematous, hypocellular, and congested appearance, potentially mimicking an angiomyxoma. Unlike fibroepithelial polyp, deep (aggressive) angiomyxoma involves deep connective tissue in an infiltrative fashion and is less likely polypoid. Superficial angiomyxoma is frequently lobulated, multinodular, and well demarcated from the underlying tissue. Lastly, vulvar hypertrophy is usually unilateral, and its stroma highly resembles fibroepithelial polyp microscopically; however, vulvar hypertrophy presents as non-polypoid enlargement of the labium minus. Some consider both entities part of a spectrum of stromal response to sex hormones [11].

Prognosis and Management

Fibroepithelial stromal polyps are benign, although they may recur if incompletely excised or during pregnancy [4, 6].

8.1.1.2 Angiomyofibroblastoma

Clinical Features

With few exceptions reported in the scrotum and upper female genital tract, angiomyofibroblastoma predominantly occurs in the vulva and vagina of reproductive-aged women,

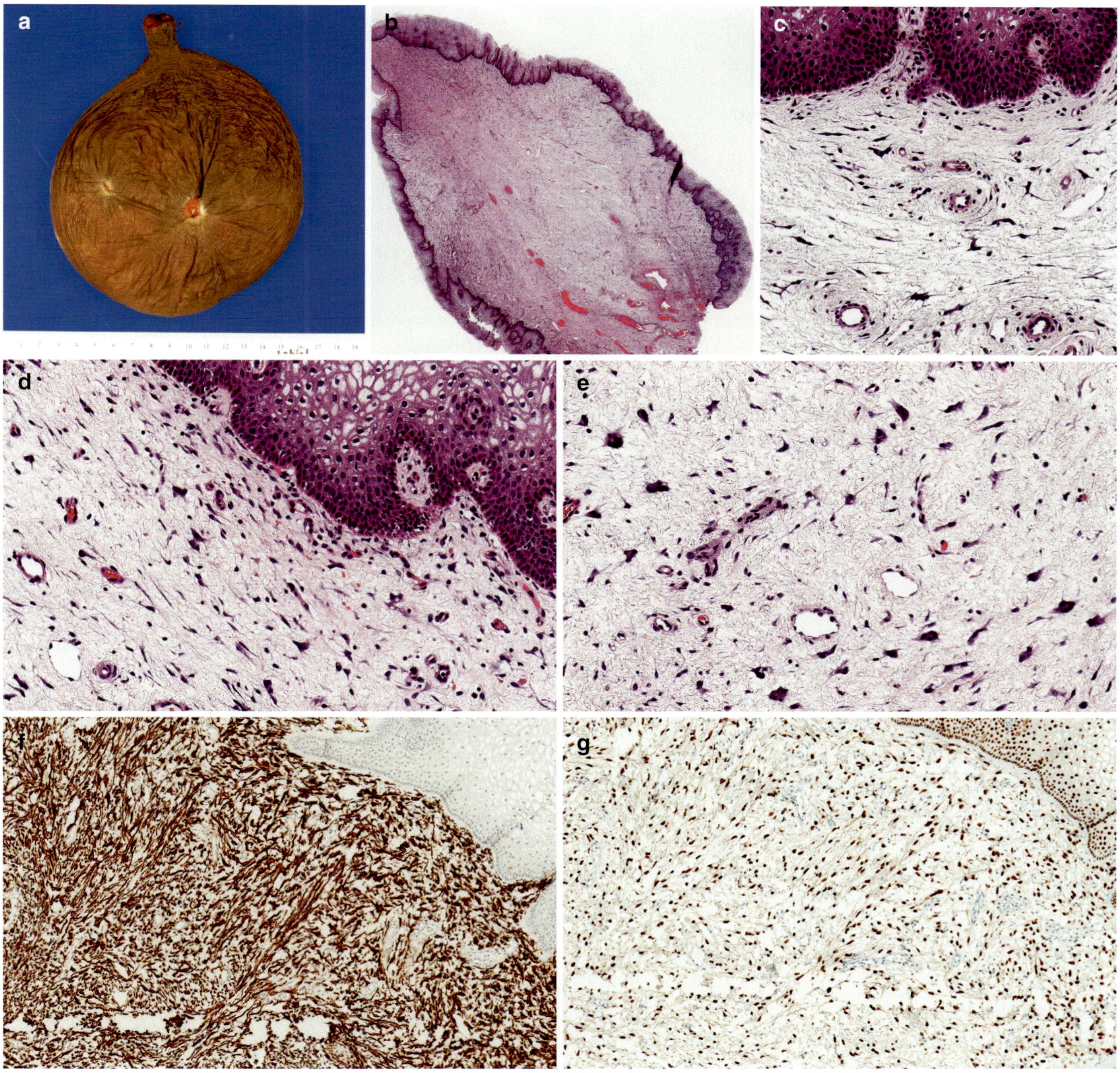

Fig. 8.2 Fibroepithelial stromal polyp. This lesion is usually exophytic and can be quite large (**a**, courtesy of Dr. C Matthew Quick); it contains uniform stromal cellularity and prominent vasculature toward the polyp base (**b**); stromal cells are characteristic with mildly enlarged multinucleated and stellate nuclei in a subepithelial location (**c**–**e**). They are usually positive for desmin (**f**) and ER (**g**)

presenting as a slow-growing painless mass [12–15]. The lesion is commonly excised under a clinical impression of lipoma or Bartholin gland cyst.

Pathologic Features

The tumor is soft and uniform under macroscopic examination. Size is ~5 cm on average but can be as large as 30 cm [15]. Histologically, the tumor is composed of mildly enlarged spindle and epithelioid stromal cells clustered around vessels, which are thin walled (capillary sized) and evenly distributed. Plasmacytoid and multinucleated forms can be observed. The lesion is well demarcated from the surrounding tissue. The lesion has heterogeneous cellularity under low-power magnification, given the presence of edema and perivascular stromal cell condensation (Fig. 8.3). In addition, adipose tissue is commonly present; indeed, a lipomatous variant has been proposed [16].

Ancillary Studies

Expression of smooth muscle markers is variable: 30–60% are positive for desmin, whereas 15–20% are positive for

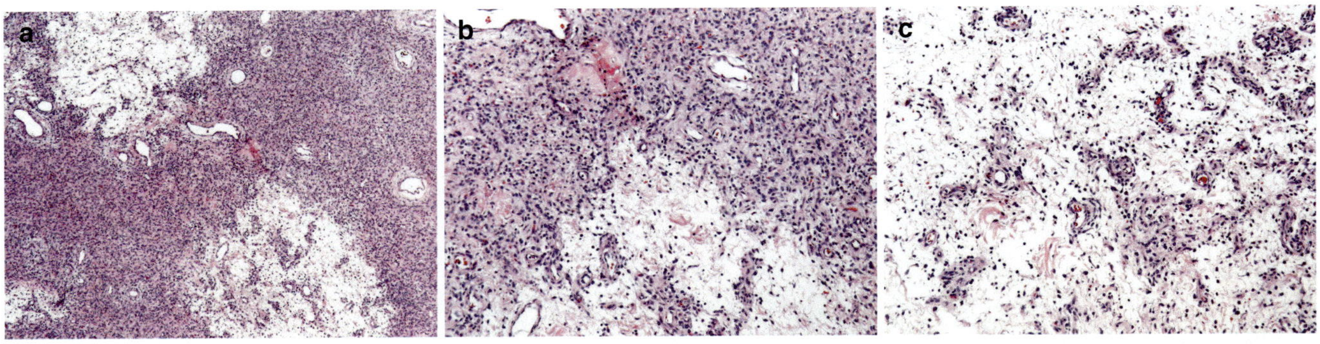

Fig. 8.3 Angiomyofibroblastoma. A biphasic pattern is noted in low power view (**a**), comprised of alternating hypercellular fascicular (**b**) and hypocellular edematous areas (**c**). Courtesy of Dr. C. Matthew Quick (University of Arkansas)

smooth muscle actin. CD34 tends to be negative (although expression is seen in up to 15% of cases) [17]. *HMGA2* rearrangements and monoallelic loss of *FOXO1* loci (13q14), characteristic of aggressive angiomyxoma, and cellular angiofibroma, respectively, are absent in angiomyofibroblastoma [17, 18].

Differential Diagnosis

The characteristic pattern of alternating hypocellular and hypercellular areas in angiomyofibroblastoma is an important clue in excluding other vulvovaginal mesenchymal lesions, importantly aggressive angiomyxoma which displays uniform hypocellularity. In addition, aggressive angiomyxoma contains thick-walled vessels, which are typically absent in angiomyofibroblastoma. Cellular angiofibroma tends to have larger (medium-sized) vessels with hyalinized walls, contrasting with the capillary-sized vasculature of angiomyofibroblastoma. In addition to having a more uniform cellular distribution, cellular angiofibroma, prepubertal vulvar fibroma, and mammary-type myofibroblastoma are all positive for CD34.

Prognosis and Management

Angiomyofibroblastoma is benign, and conservative local excision is curative. Sarcomatous transformation within angiomyofibroblastoma has been reported [19].

8.1.1.3 Cellular Angiofibroma

Clinical Features

Unlike other vulvovaginal mesenchymal proliferations, cellular angiofibroma presents at similar rates in the male inguinoscrotal region. Similar to angiomyofibroblastoma, vulvovaginal cellular angiofibroma preferentially occurs in adult women as a superficial, painless, slow-growing nodule [20, 21].

Pathologic Features

The lesion is usually less than 5 cm in size and grossly appears as non-polypoid and well circumscribed, although polypoid exceptions occur [22]. Histologically, cellular angiofibroma is composed of bland spindle-shaped cells arranged in a cellular distribution, intersected by short bundles of wispy collagen and small- to medium-sized hyalinized vessels (Fig. 8.4). Atypical features can be rarely seen, ranging from occasional atypical nuclei to focal frank sarcomatous transformation [23, 24]. The latter is identified as an abrupt transition to highly pleomorphic sarcoma with either liposarcoma or high-grade pleomorphic sarcoma appearance.

Ancillary Studies

By immunohistochemistry, the stromal cells have a "fibroblastic" phenotype with relatively high rates of CD34 (up to 60%) in addition to low rates of desmin and smooth muscle actin positivity (20%), as well as absence of H-Caldesmon expression [22]. As with other vulvovaginal stromal lesions, estrogen and progesterone receptor staining is positive in most cases. Cellular angiofibroma harbors monoallelic deletions of *RB1* and *FOXO1* at the 13q14 locus. These abnormalities are shared with spindle cell lipoma and mammary-type myofibroblastoma, which has led to an understanding of these three entities as a spectrum of the same biologic entity [25, 26].

Differential Diagnosis

The relative hypercellularity, overall absence of thick vessels, and positivity for CD34/desmin in cellular angiofibroma are helpful features in its distinction from aggressive angiomyxoma (thick vessels, hypocellular, CD34/desmin often negative) and angiomyofibroblastoma (thin vessels, alternating cellularity, CD34 negative). Of note, cellular angiofibroma shares significant morphologic, immunophenotypic, and molecular overlap with mammary-type myofibroblastoma, described below.

Prognosis and Management

Conservative local excision with negative margins is sufficient as these lesions behave in a benign fashion with no

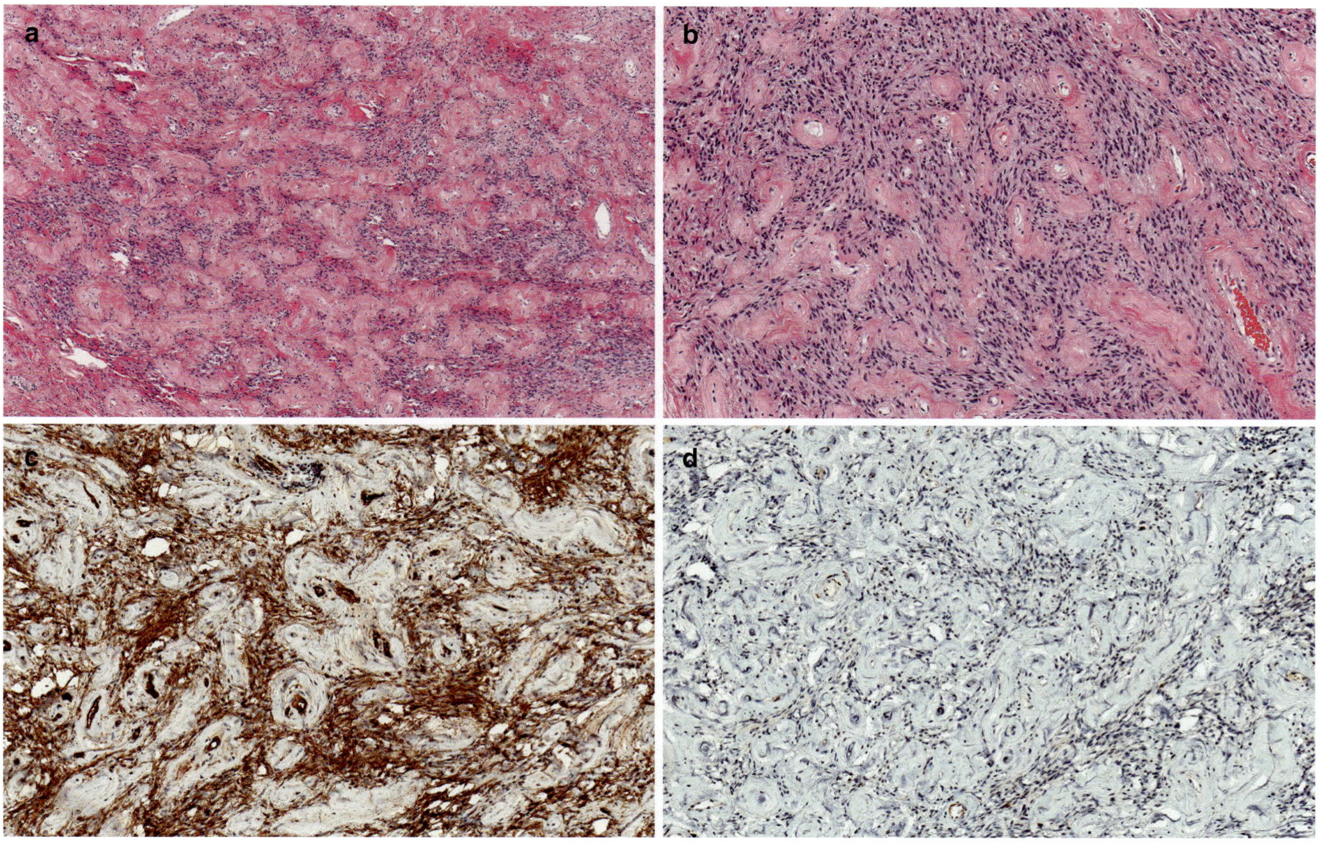

Fig. 8.4 Cellular angiofibroma. Stromal cells are densely packed imparting a hypercellular appearance (**a**); medium-sized vessels with hyalinized walls are uniformly dispersed (**b**). Stromal cells are positive for CD34 (**c**) and negative for desmin (**d**)

recurrences or metastatic potential. This seems to apply even to cases with atypia or sarcomatous transformation, although clinical follow-up is limited [23].

8.1.1.4 Mammary-Type Myofibroblastoma

Clinical Features

This tumor is not exclusive to the lower genital tract. As the name implies, mammary-type myofibroblastoma was first described in the breast, but its anatomic distribution is wide. It is, however, described in this section given its similarity with the other vulvovaginal lesions discussed [27]. Myofibroblastoma of the lower genital tract, also known as "superficial cervicovaginal myofibroblastoma," has a wide age of presentation (23–80 years); most cases arise in the vagina [28].

Pathologic Features

Myofibroblastoma grossly appears as a polypoid or superficial, soft to rubbery nodular mass, usually less than 10 cm in size [28]. Microscopically, the tumor features a sharp demarcation from the superficial dermis [29]. The neoplastic cells are bland and spindle in shape, arranged in fascicles, and separated by dense collagen (Fig. 8.5). Intratumoral adipose tissue and myxoid change have been described.

Ancillary Studies

Neoplastic cells in myofibroblastoma usually express estrogen and progesterone receptors (>95%), desmin (~90%), and CD34 (68%) [28, 29]. Monoallelic loss of *FOXO1* on 13q14 has been documented in lower genital myofibroblastoma [30], similar to its extragenital counterparts and related tumors (spindle cell lipoma and cellular angiofibroma).

Differential Diagnosis

Compared to mammary-type myofibroblastoma, aggressive angiomyxoma is less cellular and has an infiltrative interface. Cellular angiofibroma and mammary-type myofibroblastoma are related lesions, distinguishable only based on the more prominent vascular component and the absence of interspersed collagen bundles in the former. Angiomyofibroblastoma is different from myofibroblastoma in its alternating cellularity and delicate vasculature. Prepubertal vulvar fibroma presents in younger women, has an ill-demarcated interface, and lacks the fascicular architecture of myofibroblastoma.

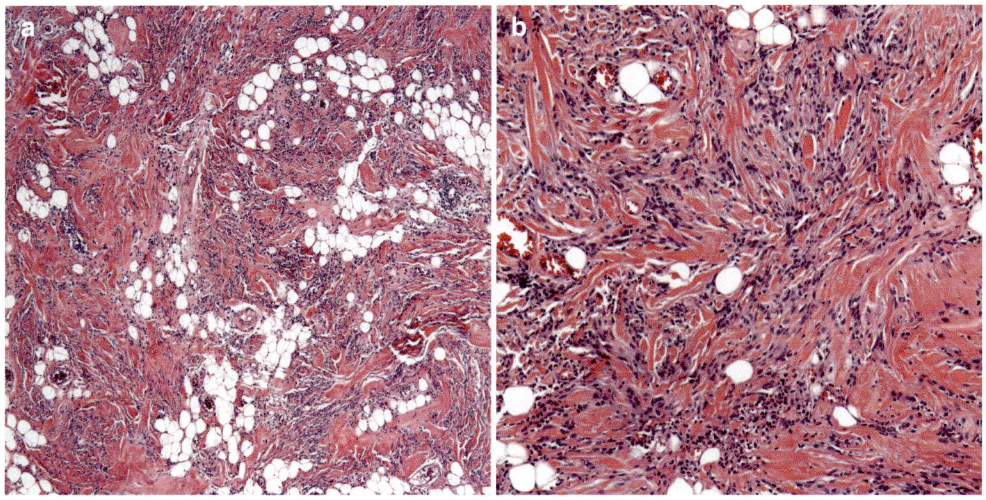

Fig. 8.5 Mammary-type myofibroblastoma. The lesion is composed of bland fusiform cells arranged in fascicles surrounding dense collagen bundles and with variable amounts of adipose tissue (**a**, **b**). Courtesy of Dr. C. Matthew Quick (University of Arkansas)

Prognosis and Management

Mammary type myofibroblastoma is a benign process with no recurrences or metastases documented to date.

8.1.1.5 Prepubertal Vulvar Fibroma

Clinical Features

With occasional exceptions seen in postmenopause [31], prepubertal vulvar fibroma affects premenarchal girls [32, 33]. The nature of prepubertal vulvar fibroma is uncertain; it may represent a response of the vulvar mesenchyme to the surge in sex hormones during puberty [33]. However, its unilaterality and potential for recurrence are features suggestive of a neoplastic process [32]. Patients present with slow-progressing, unilateral, painless vulvar enlargement, usually in the labium majus.

Pathologic Features

Prepubertal vulvar fibroma is characteristically superficial and small in size (median 4 cm). The microscopic borders tend to be indistinct, and extension to the resection margins is usually observed [32]. The lesion is comprised of bland fusiform cells individually dispersed in a fibrotic stroma, encasing adipose tissue and skin adnexa. The stroma can contain variable amounts of myxoid matrix, edema, and/or collagen.

Ancillary Studies

The spindle cell population is positive for estrogen receptor and CD34 but negative for desmin, smooth muscle actin, and S-100. Progesterone receptor expression is variable [33]. It is unknown if this lesion is associated with any recurrent genomic abnormality.

Differential Diagnosis

Prepubertal vulvar fibroma can simulate morphologically aggressive angiomyxoma, as both entities are hypocellular and have ill-defined margins. Aggressive angiomyxoma presents in reproductive-age and postmenopausal women and has a diffuse myxoid component. In challenging cases, CD34 can be of value (positive in vulvar fibroma, more often negative in aggressive angiomyxoma).

Prognosis and Management

Conservative surgical treatment is usually recommended. Prepubertal vulvar fibroma appears to be benign, although it may recur if margins are positive.

8.1.1.6 Superficial Angiomyxoma

Clinical Features

This lesion is not exclusive to the genital area. In fact, it is most frequent in the trunk and neck [34]. It is, nonetheless, closely related to the other tumors presented in this section. As its name implies, the tumor is typically superficial and frequently polypoid. An association between genital superficial angiomyxoma and Carney's complex has not been observed [35]. However, the occurrence of multiple angiomyxomas in other anatomic locations is highly associated with this condition.

Pathologic Features

Superficial angiomyxoma is usually small (less than 5 cm), multilobulated, and gelatinous. On microscopic examination, demarcation from the overlying superficial dermis can be appreciated. The neoplastic population is composed of bland spindle and stellate-shaped cells in a prominent myxoid background with a thin-walled vasculature (Fig. 8.6). Nests of benign epithelium (presumably entrapped adnexal structures) can be seen.

Ancillary Studies

Stromal cells are positive for CD34 and negative for desmin. Unlike most other vulvovaginal stromal tumors, superficial

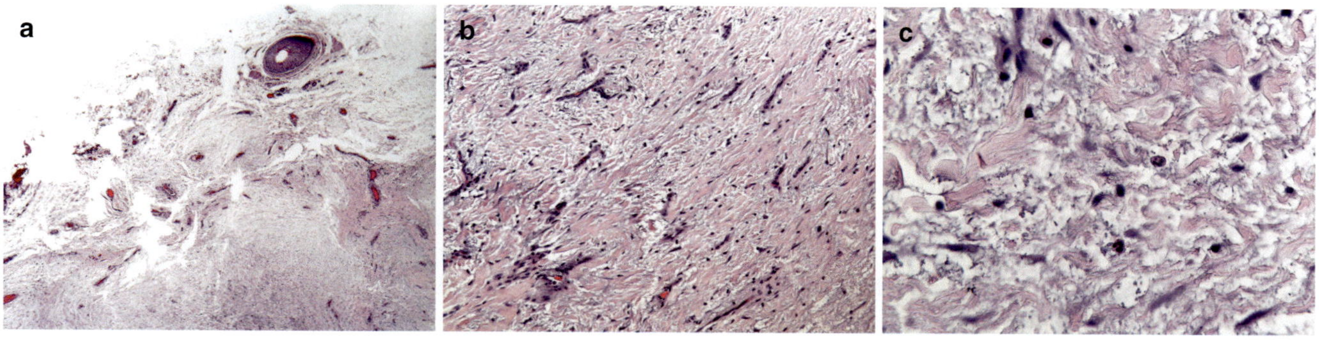

Fig. 8.6 Superficial angiomyxoma. Uniformly hypocellular lesion, commonly with intratumoral entrapped skin adnexal structures (**a**); stromal cells and thin-walled vessels are uniformly distributed (**b**); stromal cells are bland (**c**). Courtesy of Dr. Matt Quick (University of Arkansas)

angiomyxoma is negative for estrogen and progesterone receptors [36].

Differential Diagnosis

Outside of the vulvovaginal region, common mimickers of superficial angiomyxoma include sheath myxoma, trichodiscoma, trichofolliculoma, and low-grade myxofibrosarcoma [34]. In the female lower genital tract, the most important differential diagnosis is deep (aggressive) angiomyxoma. The latter tends to be large (>10 cm) and involves deep subcutaneous tissue, whereas superficial angiomyxoma is small and confined to the skin. Superficial angiomyxoma is multinodular, but the borders are smooth unlike deep angiomyxoma which is infiltrative. Positivity for desmin, estrogen receptor, and/or progesterone receptor argues against superficial angiomyxoma and should raise the possibility of aggressive angiomyxoma. Fibroepithelial stromal polyp is an important differential with superficial angiomyxoma, since both lesions are polypoid and when torsion and subsequent edema are present in the former. Superficial angiomyxoma is favored in the presence of a definitive myxoid stroma and when the lesion is well demarcated from the surrounding dermis.

Prognosis and Management

While regarded as a benign tumor, nondestructive recurrence has been reported, usually in the context of a positive margin [35]. Thus, excisional management should aim for a wide negative margin.

8.1.2 Other Benign Lesions

8.1.2.1 Genital Rhabdomyoma

Clinical Features

Extracardiac rhabdomyomas are rare and unrelated to tuberous sclerosis (unlike the more common cardiac rhabdomyoma). Rhabdomyoma of the genital type is very rare, accounting for 10% of all extracardial rhabdomyomas [37, 38]. They usually appear in the vagina of middle-aged women as a painless and slow-growing exophytic mass. The clinical impression is usually of a fibroepithelial polyp [39].

Pathologic Features

On gross examination, genital rhabdomyoma is polypoid and small, usually less than 3 cm. The lesion is comprised of fascicles of spindle and polygonal cells with abundant cytoplasm and striations identifiable under light microscopy. The nuclei are bland, round, and uniform with pale chromatin and conspicuous nucleoli. Mitotic activity, if present, is low. The striated cells are distributed throughout the lesion, predominantly in the subepithelial stroma.

Ancillary Studies

By immunohistochemistry, striated cells are positive for desmin, MyoD1, and myogenin (MYF4). No significant copy number alterations were identified in two cases recently tested [39]. Importantly, there was absence of heterozygosity in chromosomes 9q22.32 (*PTCH* gene) and 10q24.32 (*SUFU* gene), which has been reported in rhabdomyoma of cardiac, adult, and fetal types.

Differential Diagnosis

Genital rhabdomyoma is usually clinically mistaken for a fibroepithelial polyp. Microscopic identification of bland rhabdomyoblastic cells will point toward the right diagnosis. Immunohistochemistry is not generally needed, and it is key to bear in mind that fibroepithelial polyps can be positive for myogenin [40]. Another important differential diagnosis is embryonal rhabdomyosarcoma, which occurs in younger patients and displays conspicuous atypia, proliferation, and a characteristic cambium layer in the submucosa.

Prognosis and Management

Genital rhabdomyoma is benign with no recurrences or malignant transformation reported following local excision [39].

8.1.2.2 Lipoma

Clinical Features

Adipocytic neoplasms are exceedingly rare in the vulvovaginal region, presumably because of the scant amount of fat tissue in this anatomic location. Lipomas are typically described as single or multiple slow-growing, painless, mobile masses found in areas of swelling [41]. The diagnosis of lipoma is usually suspected clinically due to the characteristic soft consistency and mobility of the lesion. Interestingly, cases reported in children have a strong predilection for the right vulva [42, 43].

Pathologic Features

Vulvar lipoma appears grossly as a well circumscribed, soft, yellow, and tan mass. Microscopically, the lesion is composed of mature adipose tissue with variable amounts of collagenous septa (Fig. 8.7). A spindle cell/pleomorphic lipoma variant containing floret-like multinucleated cells has also been described in the vulva [44].

Differential Diagnosis

The principal differential diagnosis is with adipocytic malignancies, discussed later in this chapter. Lower genital angiomyofibroblastoma and mammary-type myofibroblastoma may contain significant amounts of adipose tissue, similar to lipoma. However, thorough examination and sampling will identify stromal areas diagnostic of these entities.

Prognosis and Management

Lipomas are benign. Observation is advisable unless symptoms persist, in which case excision is curative.

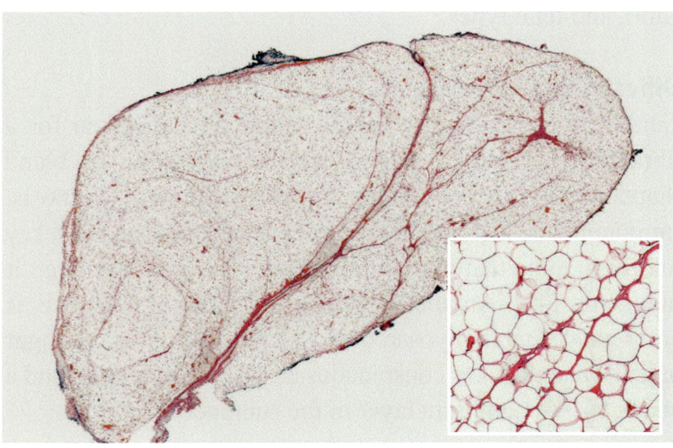

Fig. 8.7 Lipoma. Well-circumscribed lesion composed of mature adipose tissue and bands of collagen of variable thickness (insert)

8.1.2.3 Schwannoma and Neurofibroma

These benign lesions derived from peripheral nerve are occasionally seen in the vulvovaginal region and are described together given their benign nature and morphologic overlap.

Clinical Features

Vulvar schwannoma has been rarely described in this anatomic region [45–51]. Remarkably, of the few cases reported, the vast majority are located in the clitoris. It presents as a non-tender, soft mass, or as de novo clitoral enlargement [45, 46]. Age range widely varies, with predilection for middle-aged women.

Neurofibroma of the lower genital tract is similarly infrequent, occurring sporadically or in the context of neurofibromatosis type 1. The tumor frequently involves the clitoris causing clitoromegaly or a distinct mass [52–55]. Indeed, clitoromegaly can be a presenting sign of vulvar neurofibromatosis [56]. A case of a vaginal benign triton tumor (neurofibroma with rhabdomyomatous differentiation) has been reported [57].

Pathologic Features

Schwannomas are encapsulated lesions. Classic tumors display the characteristic alternating Antoni type A and Antoni type B areas. The former is composed of tightly packed sheaths of spindle cells with palisading and swirling patterns, while the latter is comprised of loosely packed spindle cells (Fig. 8.8). Cystic degeneration and Verocay body-like structures can be observed. A cellular variant, composed exclusively of Antoni A areas, has been described. Plexiform schwannoma, also reported in the vulva [46–48], is characterized by intraneural multinodular anastomosing growths (hence the term plexiform) with either conventional or cellular morphology. Ancient schwannoma is characterized by degenerative myxoid and hyalinized areas and bizarre hyperchromatic nuclei within Antoni B regions [50].

Neurofibroma arises within peripheral nerves and can be localized (single lesion within an otherwise preserved nerve), diffuse (large, obliterating the nerve, and involving surrounding fibroadipose tissue), or plexiform (mass of expanded nerves). Microscopically, neurofibroma is well circumscribed but not encapsulated. It is comprised of a mixture of spindle cells, small nerves, and mast cells embedded in a myxoid to collagenous stroma. Spindle cells have pointed ends, similar to schwannoma.

Ancillary Studies

Similar to extragenital sites, schwannomas are positive for S100 (stronger in Antoni A areas), GFAP, and CD57. Neurofibromas are also consistently positive for S100 but in a less diffuse fashion. Collagen type IV is positive in a pericellular fashion in both lesions. At the ultrastructural level,

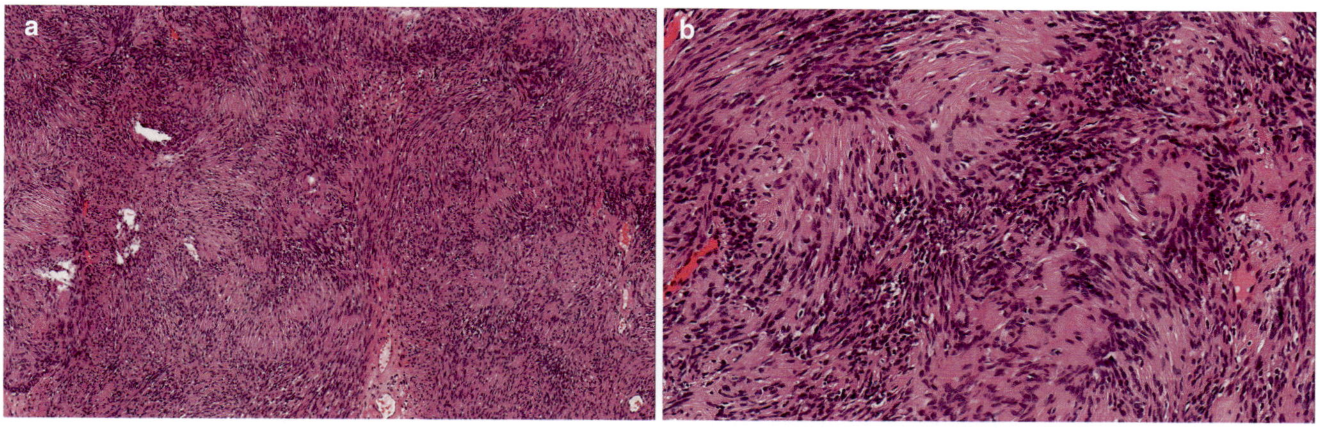

Fig. 8.8 Schwannoma. Lesion with alternating zones of hypercellularity (Antoni A) and hypocellularity (Antoni B) (**a**) and nuclear palisading on high-power magnification (**b**)

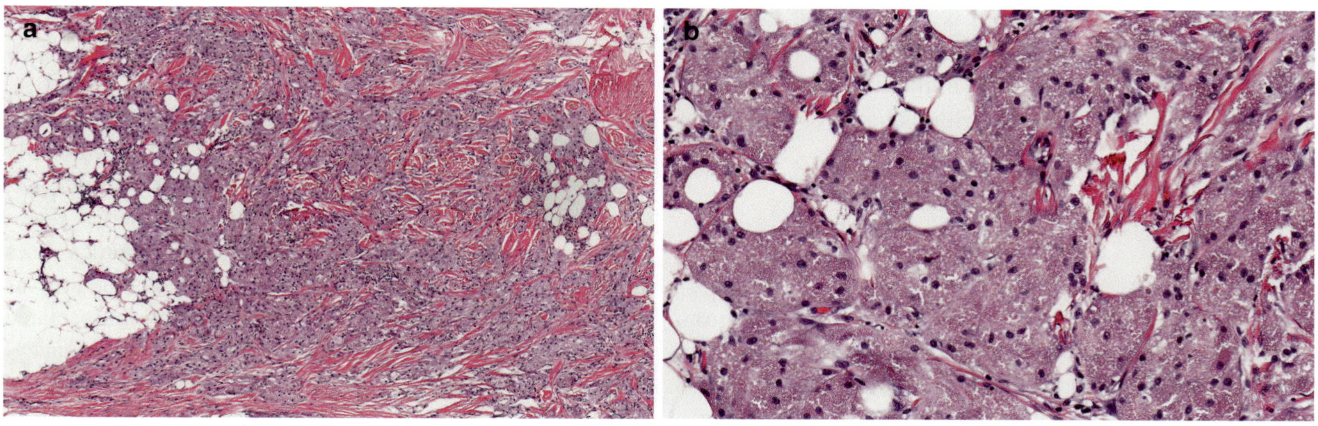

Fig. 8.9 Granular cell tumor. The tumor usually has an infiltrative interface with the surrounding tissue (**a**); it is composed of bland polygonal cells with abundant granular cytoplasm (**b**)

neurofibromas are composed of Schwann cells, perineurial cells, and fibroblasts.

Differential Diagnosis

Schwannoma and neurofibroma are clinically and morphologically similar. Distinguishing features of schwannoma include the presence of a true capsule, a biphasic cellular pattern, and diffuse positivity for S100. An important, and often difficult, distinction is between these two benign lesions and malignant peripheral nerve sheath tumor. The presence of the following features should suggest malignancy: prominent cellular atypia, hyperchromasia, necrosis, and proliferation (>1 mitosis in 10 HPFs).

Prognosis and Management

The treatment of choice for both schwannoma and neurofibroma is complete excision. Prognosis is favorable with no recurrences reported in the vulvar region [48].

8.1.2.4 Granular Cell Tumor

Clinical Features

Granular cell tumor is an uncommon neoplasm of neural sheath origin; 4–10% of cases arise in the vulva, usually the labium majus [58, 59]. It occurs more commonly in black and perimenopausal women (mean age 50 years) [60, 61]. The tumor is superficial and slow growing, often found incidentally.

Pathologic Features

Tumor size rarely exceeds 10 cm. Histologically, it consists of polygonal cells with abundant eosinophilic granular cytoplasm and round to ovoid central nuclei (Fig. 8.9). The interface with the surrounding tissue can be smooth or, less frequently, infiltrative. Perineural involvement is a common finding. The overlying epithelium usually displays reactive changes including pseudoepitheliomatous hyperplasia, which can be quite prominent [62].

Ancillary Studies

Tumor cells display ultrastructural evidence of neural (Schwannian) derivation and are positive for S100. The cells may also stain for NKI-C3, a nonspecific antibody against lysosomes. Intracytoplasmic granules (lysosomes) are periodic acid-Schiff (PAS)-positive, diastase-resistant.

Differential Diagnosis

The most relevant differential diagnosis, particularly in superficial biopsy specimens, is with squamous cell carcinoma, since the overlying epidermis of granular cell tumor is frequently hyperplastic. Upon close examination, a syncytial-like proliferation in the superficial dermis is characteristic of granular cell tumor.

Prognosis and Management

Conservative complete excision is the preferred treatment, since most lesions are indolent. Recurrence is uncommon, more likely seen in tumors with infiltrative edges and perineural invasion [58]. One case with malignant behavior has been reported [63].

8.1.2.5 Hemangioma

Clinical Features

Capillary hemangiomas are common in the vulvar region, seen as dome-shaped purple papules predominantly in elderly women [64]. Cavernous hemangiomas (also termed venous malformations) have a wider age of presentation including infants and adolescents (median age 44 years in a small series) [65]. Lesions tend to grow after puberty, at which point become symptomatic causing bleeding or mass effect. An association with pregnancy and postpartum complications has been reported [66, 67]. Cases mimicking clitoromegaly have also been described [68, 69].

Pathologic Features

Capillary hemangiomas are typically small (<2 cm). Cavernous hemangiomas, on the other hand, can be large and even efface the vaginal or vulvar surface macroscopically [65]. Like those in other anatomic locations, vulvovaginal hemangiomas contain irregularly dilated thin-walled venous channels lined by a monolayer of flat endothelial cells and surrounded by a thin muscular layer (Fig. 8.10). Intraluminal thrombosis can be observed.

Prognosis and Management

Capillary hemangiomas rarely require treatment; when symptomatic, electrocautery is a safe approach. Cavernous hemangiomas can be managed with simple excision or embolization. Prognosis is excellent after conservative treatment [65].

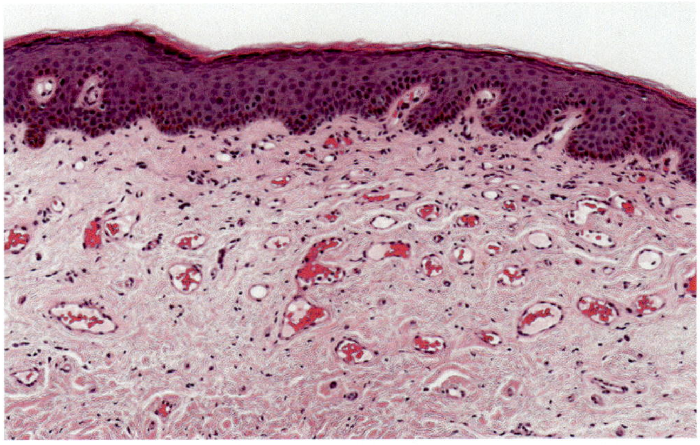

Fig. 8.10 Capillary hemangioma. Superficial proliferation of thin and small blood vessels lined by bland endothelium

8.1.2.6 Acquired Lymphangiectasia

Clinical Features

Acquired lymphangiectasia (lymphangioma circumscriptum) of the vulva is a reactive condition, most commonly secondary to lymphatic obstruction and distortion of the pelvic lymphatic vascular network. A recent case series, documenting cumulative evidence in the literature, grouped cases according to the cause of lymphatic obstruction as malignancy-associated (61%), Crohn's disease-associated (12%), and tuberculosis-associated (9%) [70]. Malignancy-related lymphangiectasia is due to lymphatic obstruction by a tumor and/or treatment (lymphadenectomy, radiation). In these patients, acquired lymphangiectasia can appear years after the initial cancer diagnosis. Patients usually complain of vulvar swelling, pain, discharge, and skin irritation, frequently leading to superimposed infection [71]. Median age at presentation is ~50 years [70].

Pathologic Features

Lesion size varies and can exceed 10 cm [72]. On gross examination, the overlying skin frequently appears irritated, and hyperplastic verrucoid changes can be exuberant. Histologically, the lesion is composed of markedly dilated intradermal lymphatics. Channels are lined by a single layer of flat endothelium and devoid of a muscular layer (Fig. 8.11).

Ancillary Studies

Endothelium lining the dilated channels is positive for CD31 and D2–40 by immunohistochemistry; CD34 is usually negative [72].

Prognosis and Management

Management depends on the clinical presentation and the condition of the locoregional lymphatic network. It includes laser therapy, cryotherapy, electrocautery, and surgical excision.

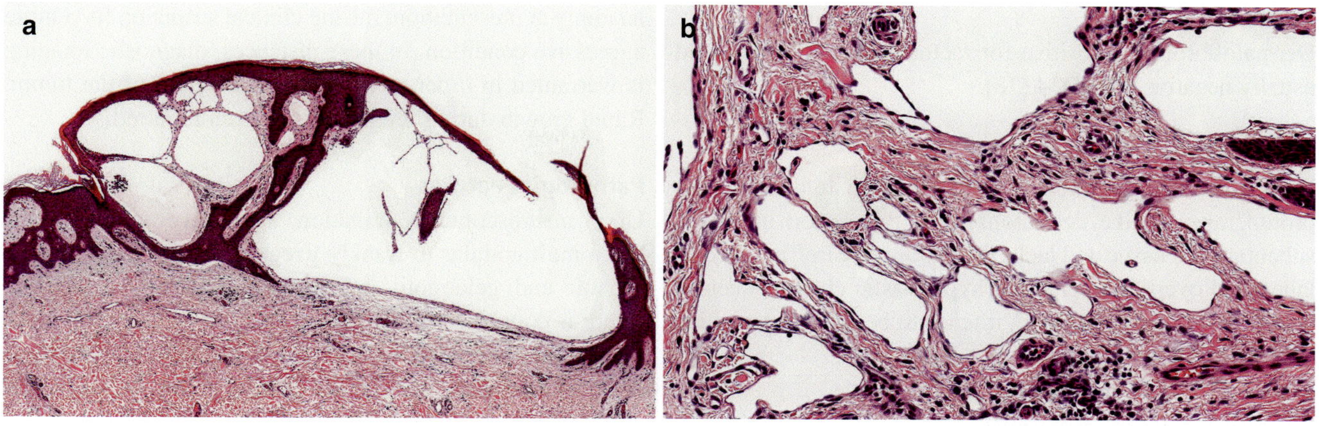

Fig. 8.11 Acquired lymphangiectasia. Markedly dilated lymphatic channels in the papillary dermis (**a**); vessels are lined by unremarkable endothelium and lack a muscular layer (**b**)

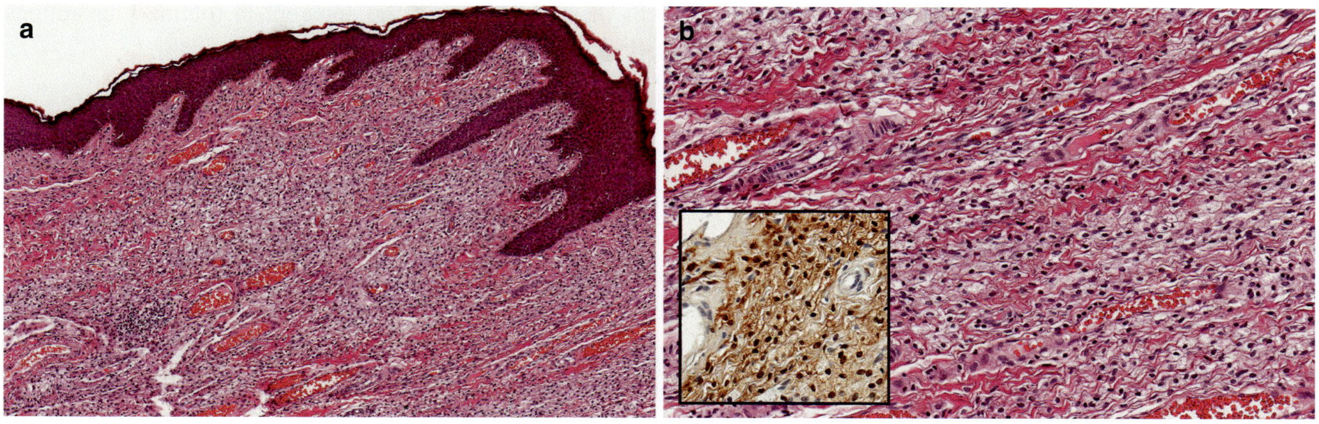

Fig. 8.12 Dermatofibroma. Subepithelial spindle cell proliferation with a storiform pattern (**a**). Cells dissect collagen bundles (**b**); they are positive for factor XIIIa (insert)

8.1.2.7 Angiokeratoma

Clinical Features

Angiokeratoma is a lesion that has a predilection for the vulvar region. Like other benign vascular proliferations discussed in this chapter, angiokeratoma is thought to represent a reactive ectatic process rather than true neoplasia. Vulvar angiokeratoma is also termed angiokeratoma of Fordyce (genital type), one of four types described in the literature [73]. Vulvar lesions are typical of perimenopausal women, although pediatric cases have been reported [73–75].

Pathologic Features

Vulvar angiokeratoma usually appears as a small (<1 cm) papule or warty nodule [76]. The lesion is comprised of dilated blood vessels in the papillary dermis, immediately surrounded by acanthotic and hyperkeratotic epidermis.

Prognosis and Management

In most cases, the lesion can be observed. If symptomatic, local excision is curative. In patients with multiple lesions, the possibility of Fabry's disease should be considered, especially if extending outside the genital area.

8.1.2.8 Dermatofibroma

Clinical Features

Dermatofibroma arises in the superficial dermal stroma. The vulva is an uncommon location, compared to more frequent locations like the extremities and trunk [77].

Pathologic Features

On gross examination, dermatofibroma appears as a flesh-colored or pigmented nodule or papule. On histologic examination, most vulvar dermatofibromas display a classic morphology: a relatively well-circumscribed spindle cell proliferation with a storiform pattern (Fig. 8.12). The spindle cells surround collagen bundles, more prominently at the lesion edges (polarized light can help visualized entrapped collagen within the lesion).

Ancillary Studies

Dermatofibroma is positive for factor XIIIa (diffusely) and usually negative for CD34 [78].

Differential Diagnosis

The principal diagnostic differential is dermatofibrosarcoma protuberans. Unlike dermatofibroma, this lesion infiltrates subcutaneous tissue and lacks the entrapped birefringent collagen and overlying epithelial hyperplastic changes seen in dermatofibroma. In addition, it tends to be diffusely positive for CD34 and negative for factor XIIIa.

Prognosis and Management

Classic dermatofibroma is considered benign; hence, observation or localized excision is appropriate. Other types (cellular, aneurysmal, atypical) have the potential for local recurrence; thus, initial sampling should be followed by re-excision if margins are positive [79, 80].

8.2 Locally Aggressive and Malignant Lesions

8.2.1 Vulvovaginal Stromal Lesions

8.2.1.1 Deep (Aggressive) Angiomyxoma

Clinical Features

Deep (aggressive) angiomyxoma is a locally infiltrative tumor predominantly described in the pelvis of women (vulva, vagina, and perineum) and men [81–84]. Sometimes the tumor is clinically mistaken for a Bartholin gland cyst; however, the lesion commonly reaches a large size (>10 cm), involves deep soft tissue structures, and distorts the pelvic anatomy at presentation, raising clinical suspicion for a more aggressive condition. In these instances, diagnostic imaging is warranted in order to determine the extent of the tumor. Rapid growth during pregnancy has been reported.

Pathologic Features

Upon macroscopic examination, aggressive angiomyxoma has a multinodular to frankly irregular outer aspect as well as soft and gelatinous cut surface. Microscopically, the tumor is composed of bland fusiform cells, individually dispersed in an abundant myxoid matrix. Although the vasculature pattern varies, large, thick, and hyalinized vessels tend to predominate. These large vessels are surrounded by stromal cells in a more dense fascicular distribution. The neoplasm dissects surrounding stroma in a frankly infiltrative fashion. Because of its low cellularity, the infiltrative nature of the tumor may not be apparent in routine preparations (Fig. 8.13).

Ancillary Studies

Aggressive angiomyxoma is positive for the estrogen receptor, desmin, and smooth muscle actin, particularly in the perivascular fascicles [85, 86]. Expression of CD34 is variable (up to 45%). Alterations of the *HMGA2* gene in the 12q15 locus have been documented in ~30% of aggressive angiomyxomas [18, 87]. Immunohistochemical expression of HMGA2 occurs in 37–83% of tumors, but does not correlate entirely with *HMGA2* gene rearrangement status [85, 88]. It is important to note that HMGA2 immunohistochemical expression has also been shown in leiomyomas, myxoid leiomyosarcoma, fibroepithelial polyps, and angiomyofibroblastomas [86, 88], limiting the specificity of this marker in the diagnosis of aggressive angiomyxoma. Nonetheless, when positive, HMGA2 can aid in determining the extent of

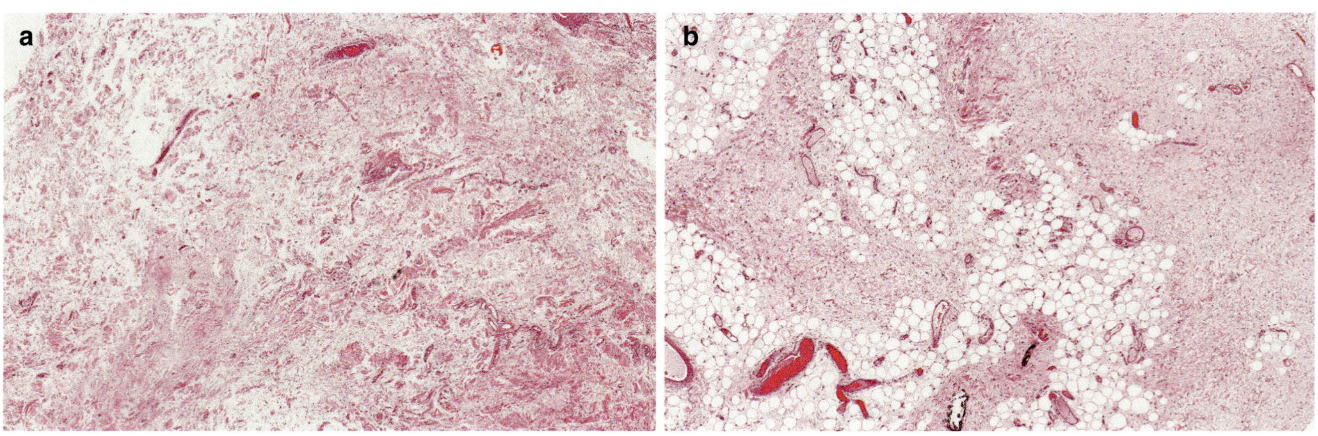

Fig. 8.13 Aggressive angiomyxoma. The lesion is uniformly hypocellular (**a**); given this deceptively bland appearance, the infiltrative tumor interface is difficult to distinguish from normal tissue (**b**); resection margins are frequently positive (**c**). Vasculature varies in size and distribution; however thick-walled vessels are consistently present (**d**). Neoplastic spindle cells are bland (**e**) and individually dispersed in a myxoid stroma (**f**, alcian blue stain pH 2.5). Tumor cells are positive for desmin (**g**), ER (**h**), and CD34 (**i**) and negative for smooth muscle actin (**j**)

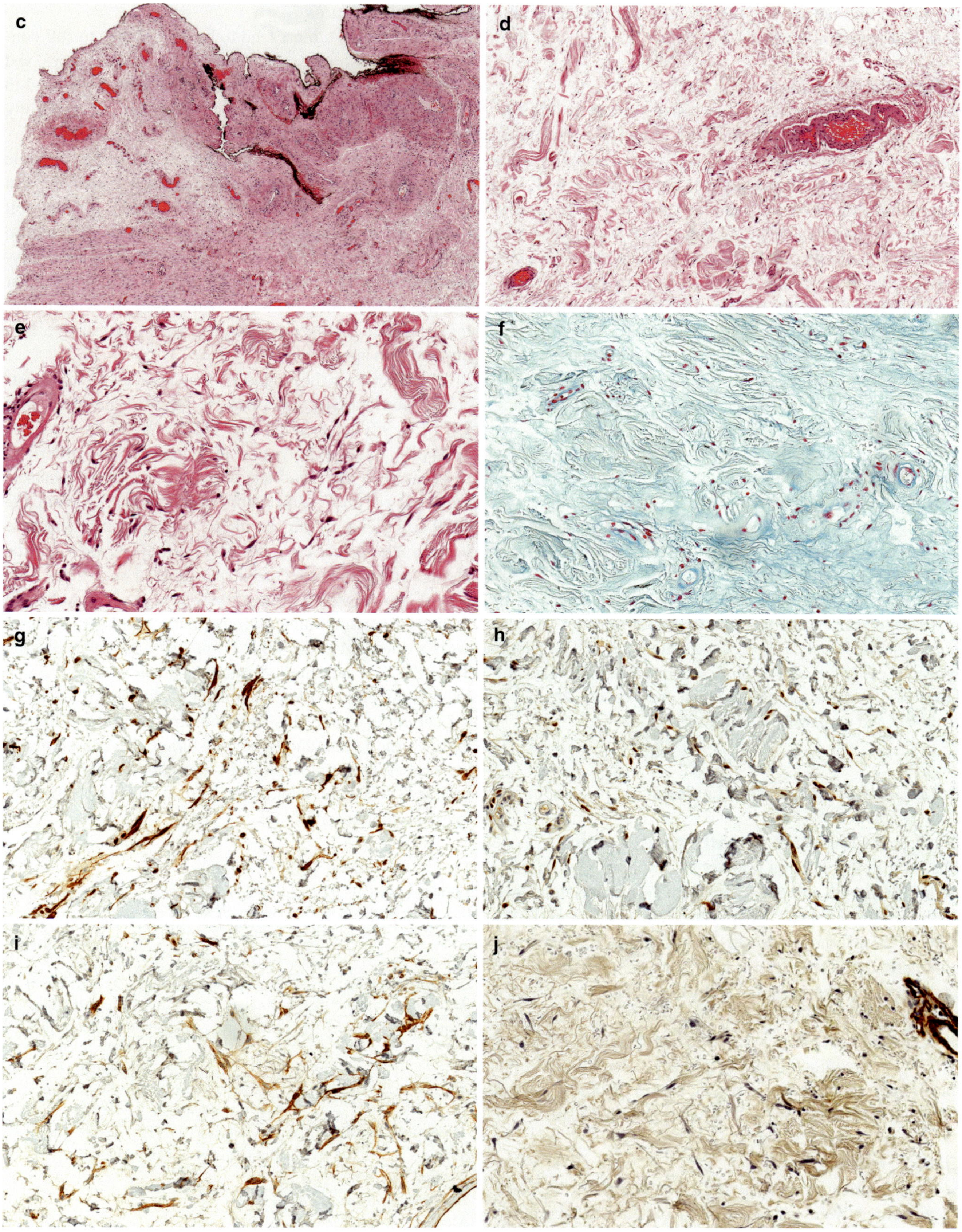

Fig. 8.13 (continued)

the tumor into adjacent tissues (which can be subtle) and assessing resection margins.

Differential Diagnosis

Virtually any of the other vulvovaginal stromal lesions discussed previously can overlap with aggressive angiomyxoma. Key distinguishing features of aggressive angiomyxoma are its large size, infiltrative nature, and involvement of deep soft tissues. Not discussed previously, *massive vulvar edema* can mimic aggressive angiomyxoma. Vulvar edema can be secondary to obesity, prolonged immobilization or previous pelvic lymphadenectomy. Unlike aggressive angiomyxoma, massive vulvar edema is characteristically bilateral and superficial. Microscopically, the presence of edematous fluid (instead of myxoid stroma) and the presence of perivascular chronic inflammation is in keeping with vulvar edema [89]. In two cases of vulvar edema reported, desmin, CD34, and hormone receptors were all negative [90].

Prognosis and Management

Local destructive recurrence occurs in 30–40% of aggressive angiomyxomas, sometimes years after the initial diagnosis. For this reason, long-term follow-up is necessary. A positive margin is a risk factor for recurrence [81, 82]; thus, a wide excision margin (at least 1 cm) is recommended after careful mapping of the lesion with preoperative imaging. Distant metastases and fatal cases are exceedingly rare [91]. There is sporadic evidence of response to gonadotrophin-releasing hormone (GnRH) agonists, which can be considered in recurrent and unresectable lesions [92].

8.2.2 Other Aggressive Lesions

8.2.2.1 Vulvovaginal Smooth Muscle Tumors

The English literature on primary vulvovaginal smooth muscle neoplasms has addressed benign, malignant, and unknown malignant potential (STUMP) categories together, given the rarity of these tumor types and the evolution of the diagnostic criteria used for their classification. These criteria differ from cutaneous and extragenital locations, since vulvovaginal smooth muscle neoplasms express hormone receptors and have clinical differences with their non-genital counterparts [93]. While traditionally the criteria have also differed from those used in the uterus, recent data supports a unified approach for both uterine and vulvovaginal neoplasms.

Clinical Features

Smooth muscle tumors involving the vagina and vulva occur more frequently in perimenopausal patients, although age range is wide. The lesions are usually superficial, non-tender, and commonly detected by the patient on self-examination.

Pathologic Features

Macroscopically, tumors tend to have a rubbery to soft consistency and whorled appearance. Tumor size varies and tends to be associated with behavior: benign tumors tend to be small (<3 cm), whereas malignant tumors are frequently larger than 5 cm.

Similar to uterine tumors, vulvovaginal smooth muscle neoplasms can be divided morphologically in conventional (spindle cell), epithelioid, and myxoid types. Spindle cell tumors are composed of intersecting fascicles of fusiform cells with tapered-end nuclei. Epithelioid tumors have varying proportions of round cells with eosinophilic to clear cytoplasm. Myxoid tumors are characterized by a prominent myxo-hyaline matrix dissecting fascicles and giving a lacy or plexiform appearance.

The criteria for the diagnosis of malignancy (leiomyosarcoma) were initially described by *Tavassoli and Norris* in 1979 [94, 95] and subsequently updated by *Nielsen* et al. in 1993 [96]. Recently, *Sayeed* et al. compared these criteria to those used in the classification of uterine smooth muscle tumors as per the World Health Organization [97]. While the 1979 criteria have high sensitivity, validation data and have been in use for decades, this recent study showed that the uterine smooth muscle criteria had superior specificity. This is by virtue of better classification of benign versus unknown malignant potential tumors. Importantly, coagulative necrosis is a criterion not included in the 1979 and 1996 criteria. Table 8.1 lists the criteria for the diagnosis of vulvovaginal leiomyosarcoma in these classification systems. In view of the current evidence, it is advisable to apply uterine smooth muscle criteria first and to include tumor size and border in the evaluation of equivocal cases (those that would be classified as STUMP or leiomyoma variant by uterine smooth muscle tumor criteria).

Table 8.1 Criteria for diagnosis of vulvovaginal leiomyosarcoma [97]

Vulvar [94, 95]	**Vulvar** [13, 96]	**Uterine smooth muscle** [97]
At least two of the following:	*At least three of the following:*	*At least two of the following:*
Tumor size ≥5 cm	Tumor size ≥5 cm	Moderate to severe nuclear atypia
≥5 mitoses/10 HPFs	Moderate to severe nuclear atypia	≥10 mitoses/10 HPFs
Infiltrative margins	≥5 mitoses/10 HPFs	Tumor cell necrosis
	Infiltrative margins	
Vaginal [94, 95]		
One of the following:		
Moderate to severe nuclear atypia AND ≥5 mitoses/10 HPFs		
Infiltrative margins		

In principle, the diagnosis of leiomyoma can be made when none of the listed features are identified after thorough sampling (Figs. 8.14 and 8.15). If features are present, but insufficient for leiomyosarcoma (either by uterine smooth muscle or by site specific criteria), the possibility of STUMP (also known as atypical smooth muscle tumor) should be considered [98].

Ancillary Studies

Vulvovaginal smooth muscle tumors express at least one smooth muscle marker [93], desmin and smooth muscle actin being the most sensitive and H-caldesmon the most specific. Cytogenetic abnormalities have been reported in sporadic cases of vulvar leiomyoma, including translocation (7;8)(p13:q11.2) [99] and inv.(12)(p12q13-q14) which is associated with *HMGA2* activation [100].

Prognosis and Management

Diagnostic criteria described above were based on patient outcomes, particularly local recurrence and distant metastases. Conservative complete excision usually suffices in tumors classified as leiomyoma. Conversely, leiomyosarcoma and tumors of unknown malignant potential should ideally have a wide (>1 cm) margin of excision, as well as close and long-term follow-up. Chemotherapy and radiation are usually considered for patients with tumor recurrence and/or metastases.

8.2.2.2 Rhabdomyosarcoma

Clinical Features

This tumor type is better characterized in the pediatric population, also known as "sarcoma botryoides," a subset of embryonal rhabdomyosarcoma involving the submucosa of the vagina and cervix. Mean age at presentation is ~6 years [101]. While most are sporadic, cases related to Li-Fraumeni syndrome and neurofibromatosis type 1 have been reported [102–104]. Genital rhabdomyosarcoma in adult women is very infrequent. The mass commonly manifests clinically with abnormal bleeding and/or pain.

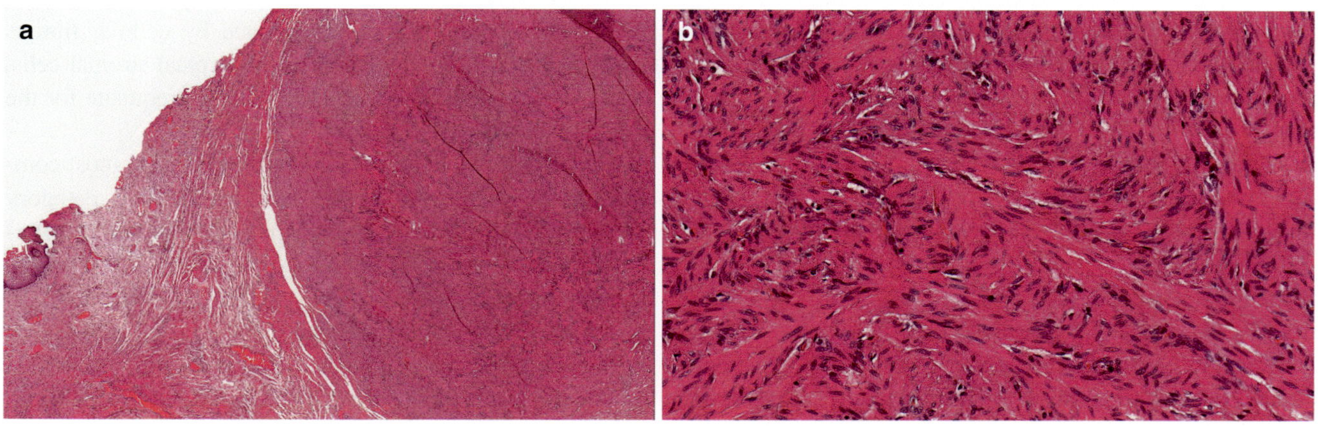

Fig. 8.14 Leiomyoma. Well-demarcated mass (**a**) composed of uniformly distributed fascicles of spindle cells; nuclei have tapered borders and uniform euchromatic nuclei (**b**)

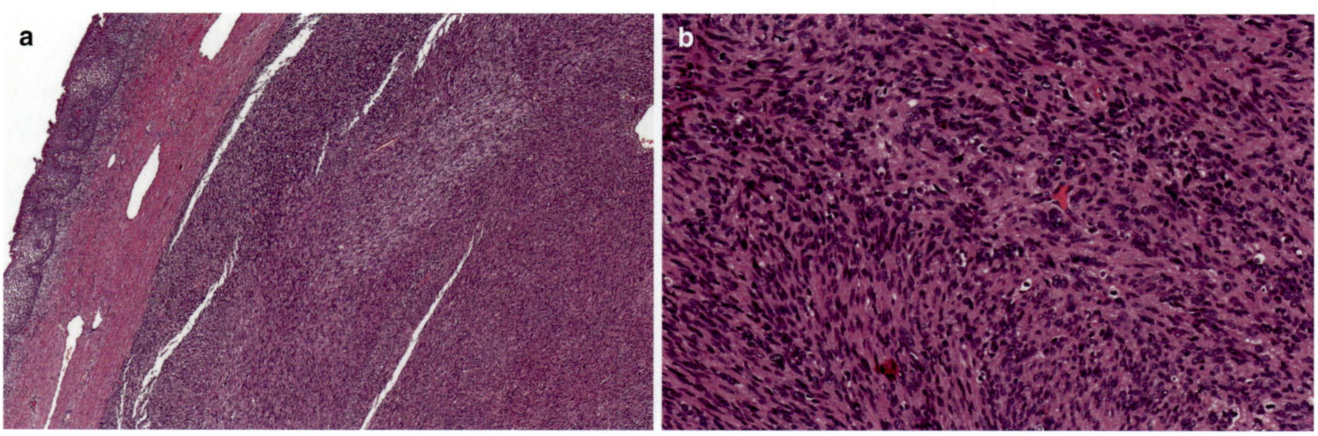

Fig. 8.15 Leiomyosarcoma. In contrast with the previous example, this lesion is hypercellular (**a**) and composed of markedly atypical and hyperchromatic nuclei with evident mitoses (**b**). Courtesy of Dr. Andre Pinto (University of Miami)

Pathologic Features

Median tumor size is 6 cm. In pediatric cases, tumors tend to grow as polypoid, frond-like masses (hence the name "*botryoides*"). The cut surface is typically homogeneous and soft; overlying mucosa can be ulcerated [102].

Most cases are of embryonal type (75% in one series) [105, 106]. Embryonal rhabdomyosarcoma is characterized by immature, round to spindle rhabdomyoblasts interspersed in a myxoid stroma. Cells contain oval nuclei and eccentric protrusions of eosinophilic cytoplasm resembling a tennis racket; striations can be seen. Chondroid differentiation can be observed. In the botryoid type, a layer of cells densely organized immediately beneath the vaginal epithelium is characteristic (cambium layer). The typical areas of hypercellularity can be subtle, since they are typically limited to the superficial stroma and absent in deeper portions of the tumor.

Non-embryonal types are mostly seen in postmenopausal women [105, 106]. Alveolar rhabdomyosarcoma is characterized by round blue cells forming sac (alveolar)-type spaces, interspersed with pleomorphic and giant cells. Pleomorphic rhabdomyosarcoma resembles other adult-type pleomorphic sarcomas with a storiform and fascicular appearance; definitive rhabdomyoblastic differentiation (cross-striations) is rare, and when present is only focal.

Ancillary Studies

The tumor cells are positive for desmin and specific skeletal muscle markers (myoglobin, MyoD1, and myogenin).

Differential Diagnosis

Cellular fibroepithelial stromal polyps can harbor atypical and pleomorphic cells mimicking botryoid rhabdomyosarcoma. However, they occur more frequently in adults, and the cellularity is concentrated toward the center of the lesion as opposed to the subepithelial cambium layer typical of botryoid embryonal rhabdomyosarcoma. Genital rhabdomyoma can also be polypoid; however, its population is bland, lacking the atypia and proliferation expected in genital rhabdomyosarcoma.

Prognosis and Management

The 5-year overall survival for lower genital rhabdomyosarcoma was 68% in one recent large series. Distant metastases are rare (~7% of cases) [105]. Younger age, early stage, and embryonal histology were associated with better prognosis. Indeed, outcome is favorable in most pediatric patients treated with surgery (local excision or radical resection), chemotherapy, and radiotherapy [101, 107]. In contrast, adult cases tend to be aggressive with high rates of advanced stage and nodal metastases, as well as low 5-year disease-specific survival (~30%) [105, 106]. The botryoid (exophytic) variant of embryonal rhabdomyosarcoma has an excellent prognosis (92% 10-year survival) in comparison with the usual (nonexophytic) type of embryonal rhabdomyosarcoma (68% 10-year survival) and other subtypes, particularly the alveolar subtype, which carries a much worse prognosis [108].

8.2.2.3 Atypical Lipomatous Tumor and Liposarcoma

Clinical Features

Atypical and malignant adipocytic tumors of the vulva are rare, with less than 20 cases in the English literature [109]. They typically occur in middle-aged women (median age 52) and have a mean size of 6 cm. Most are superficial and mobile and are often misdiagnosed as a benign tumor.

Pathologic Features

The most common histologic type is atypical lipomatous tumor (formerly well-differentiated liposarcoma) [109, 110]. Only the lipomatous variant has been described in the vulvovaginal region; other types (spindle cell, sclerosing, and inflammatory) have not been reported. Atypical lipomatous tumor is typically lobulated and is composed of mature adipocytes of different sizes separated by cellular fibrous septa, which contain hyperchromatic atypical stromal cells. Lipoblasts may be present but are not a prerequisite for the diagnosis.

Myxoid/round cell liposarcoma is the second most common tumor type seen in the vulva [109]. This category includes tumors with variable degrees of lipoblastic differentiation from the well (myxoid) to the poorly differentiated (round cell). This morphologic spectrum can sometimes be appreciated within the same tumor. Myxoid tumors consist of nodular growths of myxoid stroma containing vacuolated adipocytic and spindle non-lipomatous cells. Round cell tumors are comprised of sheets of large cells with scant cytoplasm, round nuclei, and prominent nucleoli. Pleomorphic liposarcoma has only been documented in one patient to date [111].

Ancillary Studies

Atypical lipomatous tumor is characterized by amplification of the 12q13–15 locus, which includes the *MDM2*, *TSPAN31*, *CDK4*, and *HMGA2* genes [112]. Myxoid/round cell liposarcoma is characterized by recurrent rearrangements of *DDIT3* (most commonly *FUS-DDIT3* fusion, *EWSR1-DDIT3* fusion in a minority of cases) [112]. *MDM2* amplification and *FUS-DDIT3* rearrangements have also been demonstrated in examples of vulvar atypical lipomatous tumor and vulvar myxoid leiomyosarcoma, respectively [109].

Differential Diagnosis

Malignant lesions can be subtle and mimic lipoma both clinically and pathologically. Atypical lipomatous tumor can be distinguished from lipoma by the presence of atypical cells

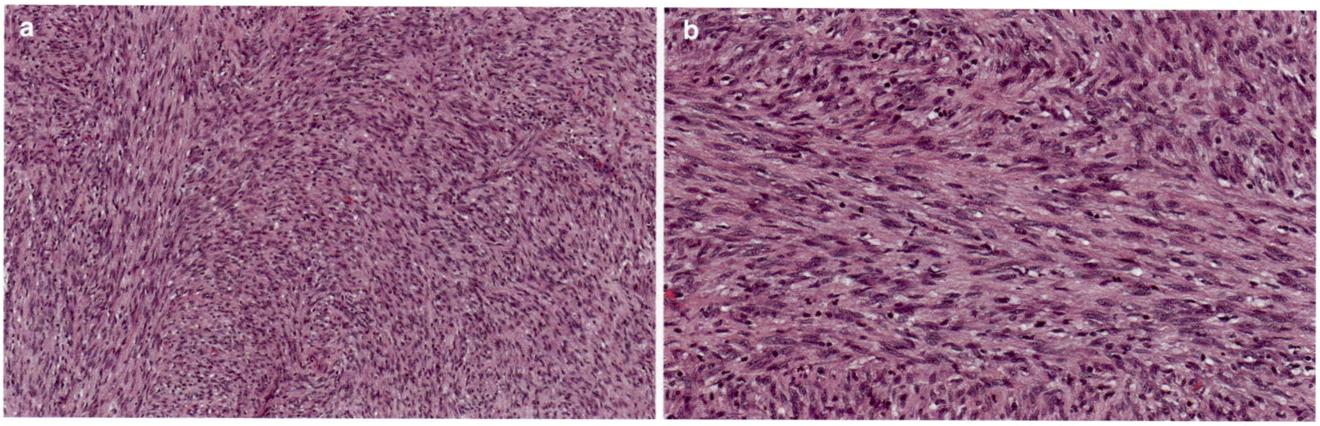

Fig. 8.16 Peripheral nerve sheath tumor. The picture depicts hypercellular areas of intersecting fascicles (**a**) composed of atypical spindle cells with pointed nuclei and conspicuous mitoses (**b**)

within fibrous septa and the variation in adipocyte size; if present, lipoblasts are also supportive of an atypical lipomatous tumor. In challenging cases, testing for 12q13–15 amplification can be of value. The differential diagnosis of myxoid liposarcoma of the vulva includes aggressive angiomyxoma, superficial angiomyxoma, and myxoid leiomyosarcoma. The presence of lipoblastic/adipocytic differentiation within the neoplastic/atypical population will argue against these possibilities and support liposarcoma. Testing for DDIT3 rearrangements should be considered in equivocal cases.

Prognosis and Management

Atypical lipomatous tumor is associated with local recurrence. Metastases have not been reported, except in tumors with a dedifferentiated component (a phenomenon not yet described in the vulvovaginal region). Myxoid liposarcomas tend to have an indolent outcome; conversely, round cell liposarcoma is an aggressive form [113]. Wide local excision with clear margins is the optimal treatment for vulvar liposarcoma, followed by close monitoring.

8.2.2.4 Malignant Peripheral Nerve Sheath Tumor

Clinical Features

This tumor is believed to originate in peripheral Schwann cells based on ultrastructural features indicative of Schwannian derivation. An association with neurofibromatosis type 1 is documented [114, 115]. Occurrence in the vulva and vagina is exceedingly rare [116–118]. The tumor appears predominantly in middle aged-women as a painful, rapid-growing mass which usually raises concern for malignancy.

Pathologic Features

The morphology of lower genital malignant peripheral nerve sheath tumor is identical to that described for extragenital sites. Alternating zones of hypercellularity and hypocellularity are characteristic, the latter being usually myxoid. The neoplastic population displays fusiform nuclei with pointed ends, hyperchromasia, pleomorphism, and conspicuous mitoses (>1 mitosis in 10 HPFs, Fig. 8.16). Peri- and intraneural invasion is common, sometimes with an evident plexiform pattern.

Ancillary Studies

S100 immunohistochemical expression is frequent (>80%) but usually focal; desmin and MDM2 expression is seen in a minority of tumors (~30%). The latter does not appear to correlate with *HMGA2* rearrangements [119]. Cytogenetic studies have revealed a complex tumor karyotype including structural abnormalities in chromosomes 17 and 22 [120].

Differential Diagnosis

Because the histologic appearance is usually nondescript, the differential diagnosis is wide, including benign (schwannoma) and malignant (fibrosarcoma, monophasic synovial sarcoma, leiomyosarcoma) conditions. The presence of cytologic atypia and mitotic activity should point against the possibility of schwannoma. In addition, S100 expression will be strong and diffuse in schwannoma and focal in peripheral nerve sheath tumor. Distinction from other types of sarcoma can be difficult; intimal tumor relationship with nerve structures and S100 expression in the absence of markers specific for other entities should raise the possibility of malignant peripheral nerve sheath tumor.

Prognosis and Management

Malignant peripheral nerve sheath tumors are aggressive neoplasms with high rates of recurrence and metastasis. Overall 5-year survival is ~40% [114]. Adverse prognostic features include high-grade morphology, personal diagnosis of neurofibromatosis type 1 syndrome, and positive margins on excision [115, 119].

8.2.2.5 Primitive Neuroectodermal Tumor

Clinical Features

Peripheral primitive neuroectodermal tumor is a round cell sarcoma of neuroectodermal derivation. Occurrence in the vulva and vagina is rare with small case series and single reports available in the English literature [121–123]. This tumor is more common in premenopausal women (median age 27 years).

Pathologic Features

Tumors tend to be small (mean size 5.8 cm) and superficial. The neoplasm is composed of large solid cellular aggregates of monomorphic round blue cells with hyperchromatic nuclei and scant cytoplasm (Fig. 8.17). Mitotic activity is usually high (over five mitoses per high-power field), and necrosis is frequent.

Ancillary Studies

Most cases show diffuse and strong membranous staining for CD99 and FLI-1 nuclear expression [123]. Synaptophysin and neuron-specific enolase are also positive [124]. The vast majority of tumors in the Ewing sarcoma/primitive neuroectodermal tumor family, including those in the vulvovaginal region, harbor a characteristic t(11;22)(q24;q12) translocation that results in a *EWS-FLI-1* fusion transcript [123].

Differential Diagnosis

The differential diagnosis is wide and includes other small round blue cell tumors (rhabdomyosarcoma, small cell carcinoma, melanoma). CD99 is highly sensitive for primitive neuroectodermal tumor but specific only when staining is strongly and diffusely membranous. In equivocal cases, detection of the *EWS-FLI1* translocation is keeping with primitive neuroectodermal tumor.

Prognosis and Management

Treatment involves wide surgical excision, chemotherapy, and/or radiation. The overall prognosis of lower genital primitive neuroectodermal tumor is largely dependent on the stage at presentation. Patients presenting with metastatic disease have a dismal prognosis [121, 122].

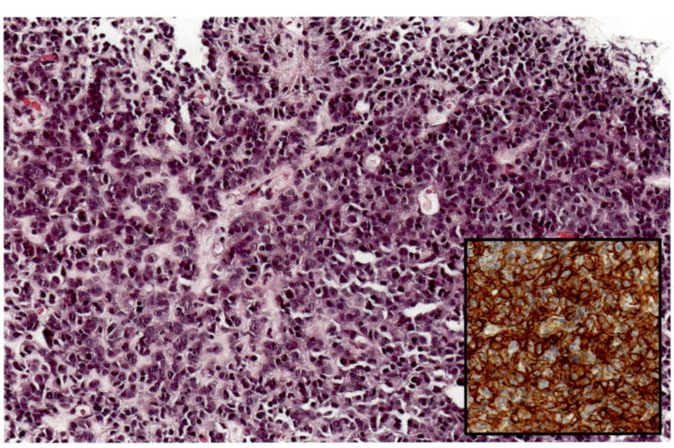

Fig. 8.17 Primitive neuroectodermal tumor. Monomorphic round blue cells with high nuclear-to-cytoplasmic ratio; CD99 expression is membranous, diffuse, and strong (insert)

8.2.2.6 Angiosarcoma

Only a few cases of angiosarcoma involving the vulvovaginal region are documented [125, 126]. Most are postmenopausal women presenting with a rapidly growing genital mass. Tumor size ranges from 1.5 to 8 cm (mean 3.5 cm). Microscopically, the tumor is composed of a deeply infiltrative malignant spindle and epithelioid cell population forming anastomosing vascular channels. Solid architecture and necrosis can be seen, particularly in poorly differentiated tumors (Fig. 8.18). Most patients reported had poor outcome with rapid recurrence and death of disease despite radical surgical treatment and radiation.

8.2.2.7 Dermatofibrosarcoma Protuberans

Clinical Features

Although this entity is commonly seen in the groin, cases restricted to the vulva are rare, with slightly over 50 cases reported in the English literature [127]. The lesion usually presents as a slow-growing nodule in the labium majus. Age at presentation is wide (mean 45 years).

Pathologic Features

The lesion is usually small (average 4 cm) [127]. Dermatofibrosarcoma protuberans can vary in appearance from a plaque or nodule to exophytic, multinodular growths which may be flesh colored or variably hypopigmented or hyperpigmented. Despite its name, the typical histologic appearance is bland, comprised of spindle cells with minimal to absent pleomorphism and low mitotic activity (less than 5 mitoses/10 PHFs), arranged in a storiform pattern (Fig. 8.19). Some cases contain areas of frank fibrosarcoma, characterized by pleomorphic and mitotically active spindle cells. The lesion is usually ill demarcated and infiltrates subcutaneous adipose tissue. The neoplasm is often separated from the normal-appearing epidermis by a rim of normal dermis.

Ancillary Studies

Immunohistochemically, tumors are diffusely and strongly positive for CD34 but negative for S100, C-KIT, factor XIII, smooth muscle, and epithelial markers, as well as hormone receptors. Positivity for PDGFR-α and β has been reported in vulvar lesions [128]. The tumor harbors a characteristic translocation t(17; 22)(q22; q13), generally in the form of a supernumerary ring chromosome, resulting in the formation of a chimeric fusion gene (*COL1A1/PDGFB*, i.e., collagen type I alpha I-platelet-derived growth factor beta) [129, 130].

Differential Diagnosis

An important distinction is with dermatofibroma (discussed above). Other benign entities frequently entertained in the

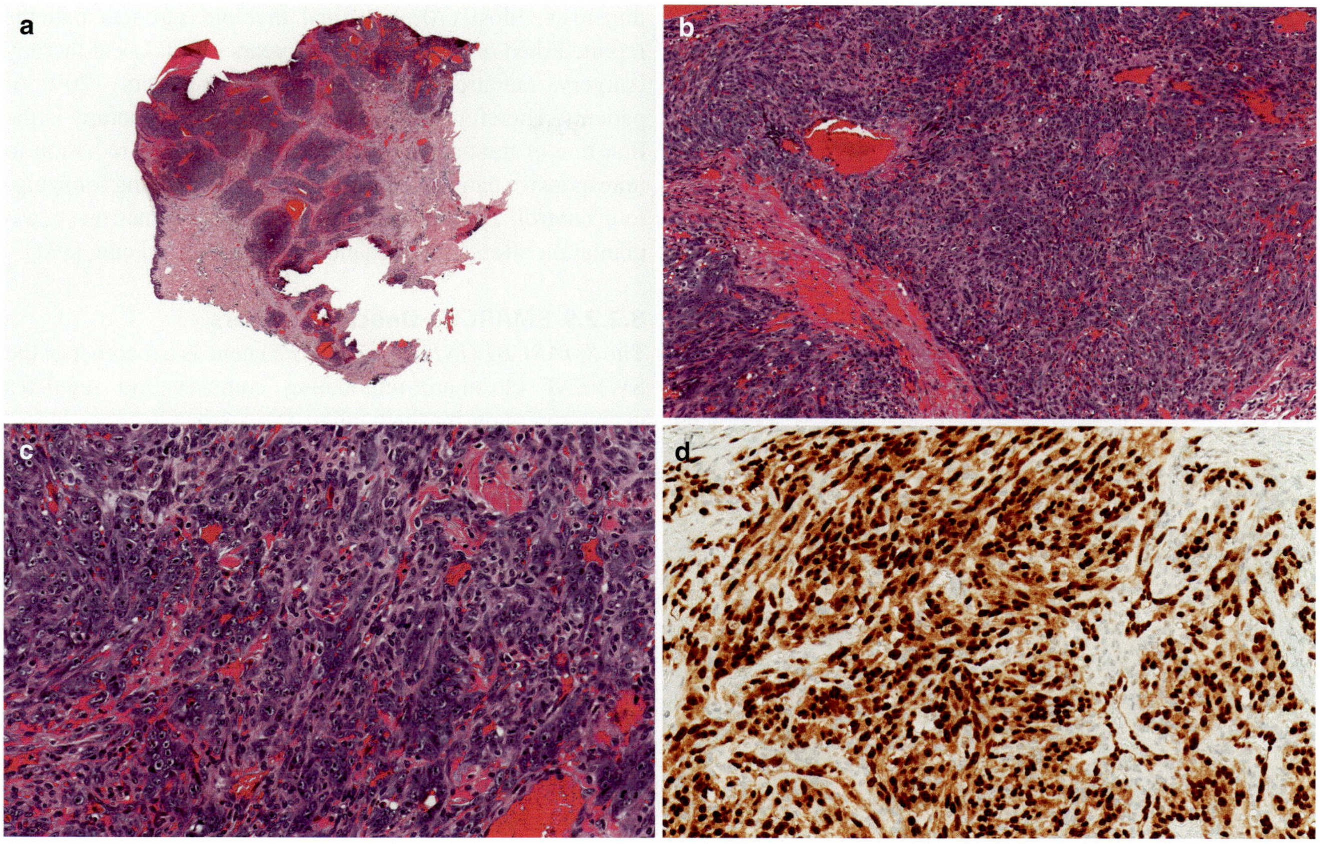

Fig. 8.18 Angiosarcoma. The lesion is infiltrative (**a**) and solid on low-power magnification (**b**). Poorly formed blood-filled channels and frankly atypical cells are noted on high-power magnification (**c**). Cells are diffusely positive for ERG (**d**)

differential are neurofibroma and schwannoma; S100 expression will be in favor of these and against dermatofibrosarcoma protuberans. Malignant peripheral nerve sheath tumor, another lesion of neural derivation, can also overlap with dermatofibrosarcoma and frequently express CD34; however, this tumor has a more peculiar appearance with alternating hypocellular and hypercellular areas [128].

Prognosis and Management

In contrast to dermatofibroma, dermatofibrosarcoma protuberans has significantly higher rates of local recurrence (50% of cases). Wide local excision is generally recommended. Since tumors frequently express PDGFR α and β, therapy with imatinib (Gleevec) is also a valid approach in recurrent or unresectable lesions, as evidenced in one case [128].

8.2.2.8 Myeloid Sarcoma

Clinical Features

Myeloid sarcoma (also known as granulocytic sarcoma, chloroma) is defined as immature myeloid cells forming a mass in an extramedullary location. Overall, most patients have a previous or concomitant history of a myeloid disorder in bone marrow and/or peripheral blood [131]. Interestingly, patients with female genital involvement frequently present only with the extramedullary mass and no evidence of leukemia [132, 133]. This represents a pitfall: in fact, up to 75% of non-leukemic cases are initially misdiagnosed as a lymphoma or non-hematopoietic malignancy [134]. Age ranges from 12 to 77 years (mean 39 years). Patients present with abnormal bleeding or a rapidly growing mass, most commonly centered in the vagina.

Pathologic Features

In most cases, the neoplastic population is composed of undifferentiated, large pleomorphic cells with a high nuclear-to-cytoplasmic ratio, apoptosis, and necrosis. When present, neutrophilic or eosinophilic precursors with lobulated nuclei and more abundant granular cytoplasm are helpful diagnostic clues. The proliferation is usually submucosal, seen as densely cellular aggregates that extend to the subepithelial stroma (but sparing the epithelium, Fig. 8.20).

Ancillary Studies

Immunohistochemistry is usually required to determine neoplastic lineage. Most lesions are granulocytic and express CD13, CD33, CD117, MPO, CD34, and/or CD38; they are either blastic (immature) or differentiated (promyelocytes and other mature forms). Monocytic/monoblastic (CD14, CD4, CD11b, CD64, lysozyme), erythroid (glycophorin A, blood group antigens), and megakaryoblastic (CD41, CD61, CD42) forms are less frequent [135].

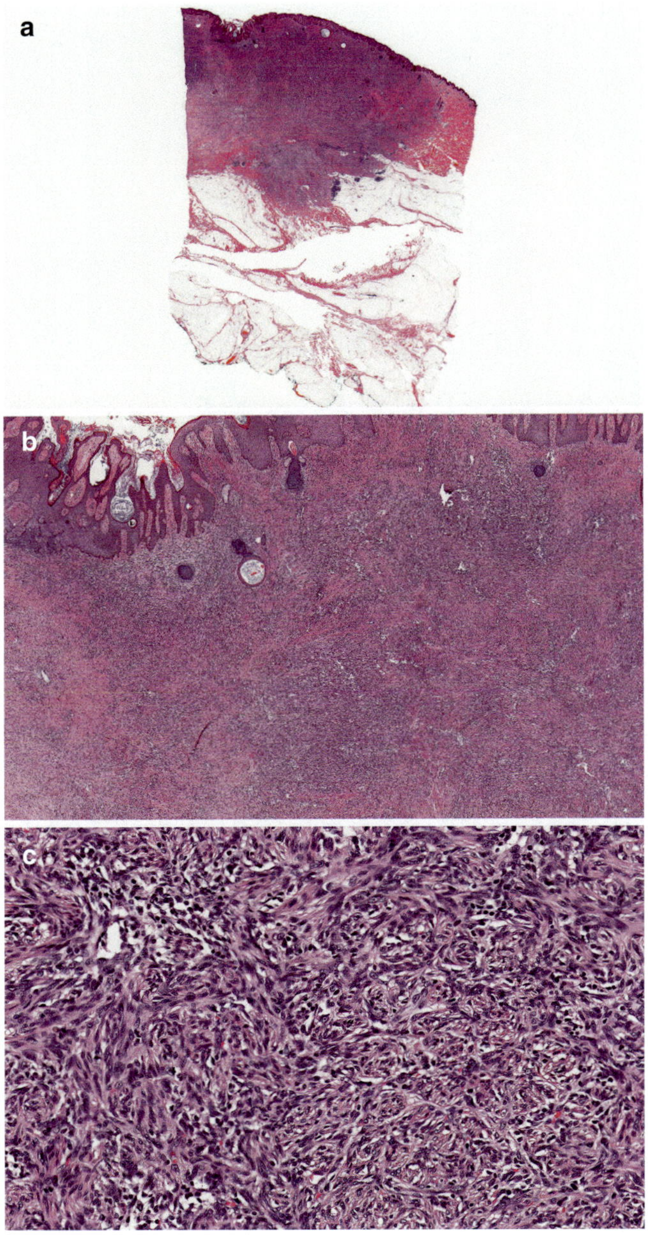

Fig. 8.19 Dermatofibrosarcoma protuberans. Multinodular and infiltrative growth (**a**) with uniform cellularity (**b**) and a storiform pattern on high power view; note the relative normocellularity of the neoplastic population (**c**)

Differential Diagnosis

The most important diagnostic considerations are poorly differentiated squamous cell carcinoma, rhabdomyosarcoma, primitive neuroectodermal tumor, melanoma, and lymphoma. Immunohistochemistry for myeloid, melanocytic, and epithelial markers is helpful in ascertaining the cell type and lineage.

Prognosis and Management

The prognosis of myeloid sarcoma is poor. 50% of non-leukemic patients will develop acute leukemia shortly after diagnosis. Most (70%) vaginal myeloid sarcoma patients reported died of disease within 3 years [135]. Local therapy (surgery, radiation) achieves remission in only 20% of patients. Therefore, systemic induction chemotherapy is the first line of treatment, followed by surgery and radiation in unresponsive patients or those requiring debulking for symptom control. Allogenic or autologous bone marrow transplantation offers higher chances of survival and cure [131].

8.2.2.9 SMARCB1-Deficient Tumors

The *SMARCB1* (*INI1/BAF47/SNF5*) gene is a member of the SWI/SNF chromatin-remodeling complex and regulates gene expression by uncoupling DNA from histones [136]. Alterations in this gene leading to loss of SMARCB1 expression were initially described in pediatric rhabdoid tumor and subsequently in proximal-type epithelioid sarcomas [137]. Other tumors found to harbor *SMARCB1* alterations include renal medullary carcinoma, epithelioid malignant peripheral nerve sheath tumor, myoepithelial carcinoma, and myxoid chondrosarcoma [138]. Lesions with myoepithelioma-like features have also been described within the spectrum of neoplasia with *SMARCB1* loss [139].

Clinical Features

Proximal-type epithelioid sarcoma is more frequent in the proximal extremities and pelvis. Primary vulvar involvement is rare with only 32 cases reported [140–142]. Similarly, there are 14 cases in the literature reported as malignant rhabdoid tumor of the vulva [143]. Both lesions present in young, premenopausal women (mean age at presentation 31–38 years).

Pathologic Features

Proximal-type epithelioid sarcoma and malignant rhabdoid tumor have strikingly similar pathologic features, and most authors consider them the same entity. Macroscopically, the tumor is firm to fleshy with frequent necrosis and hemorrhage. Microscopically, the tumor has a nodular arrangement. Rhabdoid differentiation, characterized by ovoid, polyhedral or spindle cell shape and eosinophilic cytoplasm, is seen in varying proportions (focal in epithelioid sarcoma, diffuse in rhabdoid tumor). Tumor cells have epithelioid to spindled shape, abundant cytoplasm and uniform nuclei with vesicular chromatin (Fig. 8.21). Conspicuous mitoses and necrosis are common. The tumor is variably myxoid (<5% to 95% of the tumor volume); non-myxoid areas have a diffuse fascicular or storiform architecture [136, 144].

Ancillary Studies

By immunohistochemistry, this family of lesions expresses epithelial membrane antigen and cytokeratins. Loss of SMARCB1/INI1 nuclear expression, which correlates with *SMARCB1* gene deletion at the 22q11.2 locus, is a

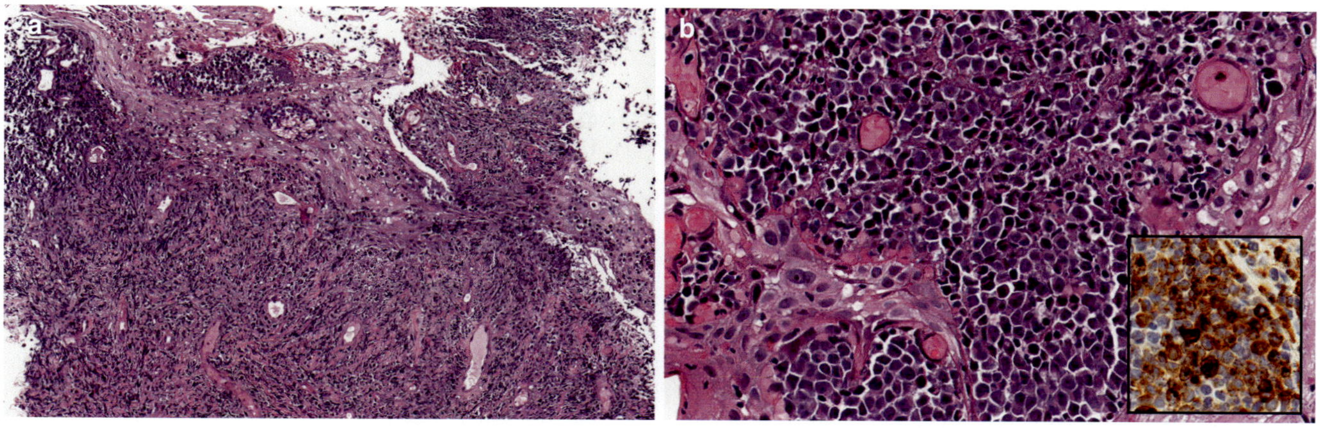

Fig. 8.20 Myeloid sarcoma. Dense proliferation of small, round blue cells in the subepithelial connective tissue (**a**). The population varies from immature (blastic) to maturing forms (**b**); strong expression of myeloperoxidase is in keeping with a myeloid lineage (insert)

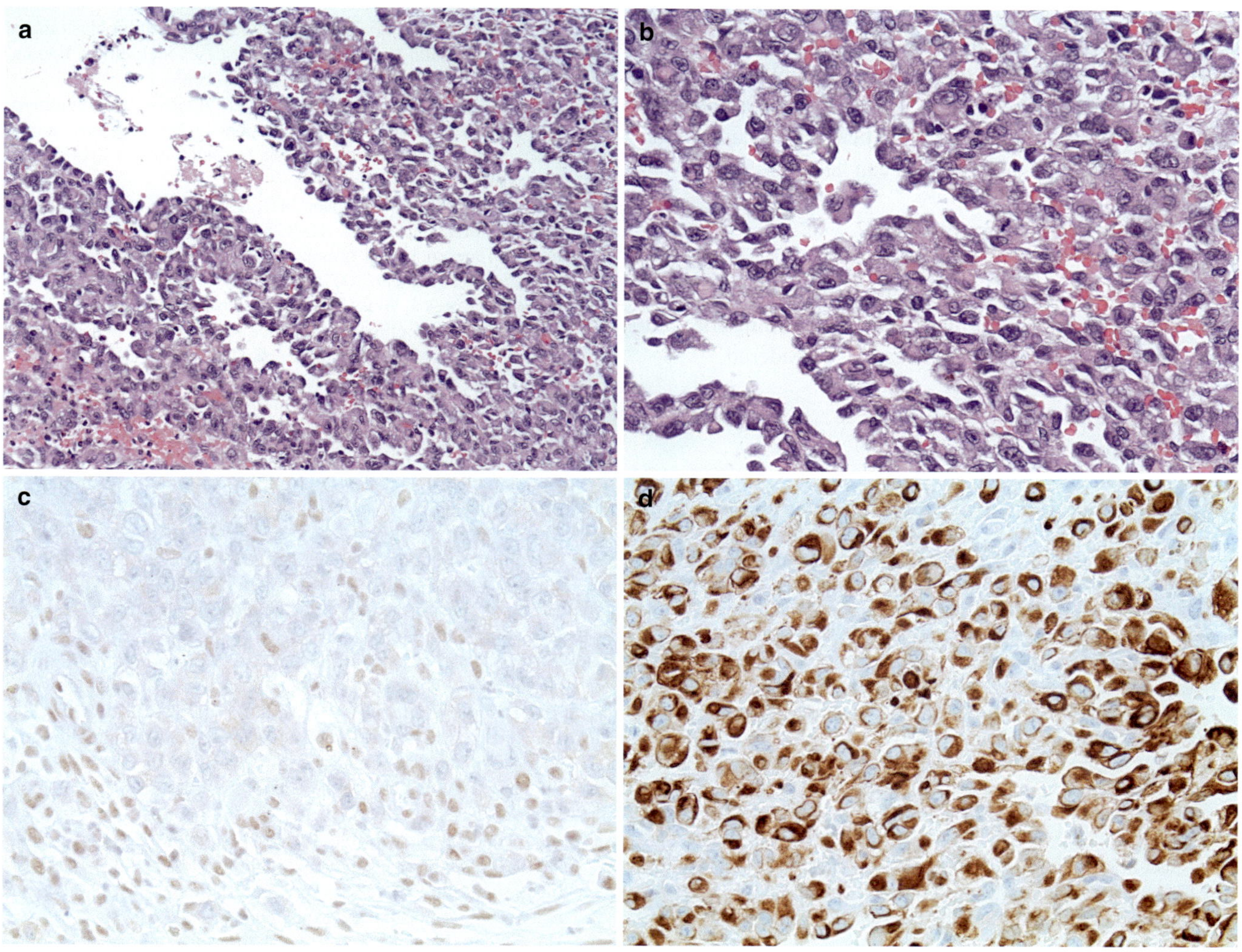

Fig. 8.21 *SMARCB1* deficient sarcoma. Tumor is usually multinodular and solid, sometimes with an "alveolar" pattern (**a**). Tumor cells display an epithelioid morphology with abundant eosinophilic cytoplasm and vesicular nuclei (**b**). Loss of nuclear INI1 expression, secondary to *SMARCB1* gene deletion, is characteristic (**c**). The tumor usually expresses cytokeratins (**d**). Courtesy of Dr. Oluwole Fadare (University of California, San Diego)

sensitive (>95% of cases) and specific finding in proximal-type epithelioid sarcoma [137, 145]. This characteristic feature has been also demonstrated, by immunohistochemistry and/or gene sequencing, in epithelioid sarcoma and myoepithelial neoplasms of the vulva [136, 139]. Myoepithelioma-like lesions also demonstrate negative S100 and CD34, as well as absence of *EWSR1*, *FUS*, and *NR4A3* rearrangements [139].

Differential Diagnosis

Given the epithelioid morphology and epithelial marker expression of this tumor type, it is important to distinguish it from a poorly differentiated squamous cell carcinoma. Identification of definitive epithelial features (cohesive nested areas, intercellular junctions), tumor connection with the surface, or an adjacent intraepithelial lesion should raise the possibility of carcinoma. INI1 immunohistochemistry must be considered in suspicious cases. The differential also includes other epithelioid mesenchymal neoplasms such as epithelioid smooth muscle tumors and angiomyofibroblastoma. Adequate sampling and identification of classic morphologic features for these entities can help.

Prognosis and Management

Tumors in this group demonstrate an aggressive behavior with 55% recurrence rate and fatality in 42–50% of patients [140, 143]. Treatment is primarily surgical aiming for complete resection; radiation therapy can be considered.

References

1. Mucitelli DR, Charles EZ, Kraus FT. Vulvovaginal polyps. Histologic appearance, ultrastructure, immunocytochemical characteristics, and clinicopathologic correlations. Int J Gynecol Pathol. 1990;9:20–40.
2. Chirayil SJ, Tobon H. Polyps of the vagina: a clinicopathologic study of 18 cases. Cancer. 1981;47:2904–7.
3. Burt RL, Prichard RW, Kim BS. Fibroepithelial polyp of the vagina. A report of five cases. Obstet Gynecol. 1976;47:52S–4S.
4. Ostör AG, Fortune DW, Riley CB. Fibroepithelial polyps with atypical stromal cells (pseudosarcoma botryoides) of vulva and vagina. A report of 13 cases. Int J Gynecol Pathol. 1988;7:351–60.
5. Halvorsen TB, Johannesen E. Fibroepithelial polyps of the vagina: are they old granulation tissue polyps? J Clin Pathol. 1992;45:235–40.
6. Nucci MR, Young RH, Fletcher CD. Cellular pseudosarcomatous fibroepithelial stromal polyps of the lower female genital tract: an underrecognized lesion often misdiagnosed as sarcoma. Am J Surg Pathol. 2000;24:231–40.
7. O'Quinn AG, Edwards CL, Gallager HS. Pseudosarcoma botryoides of the vagina in pregnancy. Gynecol Oncol. 1982;13:237–41.
8. Madueke-Laveaux OS, Gogoi R, Stoner G. Giant fibroepithelial stromal polyp of the vulva: largest case reported. Ann Surg Innov Res. 2013;7:8.
9. Miettinen M, Wahlström T, Vesterinen E, Saksela E. Vaginal polyps with pseudosarcomatous features. A clinicopathologic study of seven cases. Cancer. 1983;51:1148–51.
10. Hartmann CA, Sperling M, Stein H. So-called fibroepithelial polyps of the vagina exhibiting an unusual but uniform antigen profile characterized by expression of desmin and steroid hormone receptors but no muscle-specific actin or macrophage markers. Am J Clin Pathol. 1990;93:604–8.
11. Heller DS, Kuye OO. Recurrent hypertrophy of the labia minora: a hormonally related lesion possibly related to fibroepithelial stromal polyps of the vulva. J Low Genit Tract Dis. 2011;15:69–70.
12. Fletcher CD, Tsang WY, Fisher C, et al. Angiomyofibroblastoma of the vulva. A benign neoplasm distinct from aggressive angiomyxoma. Am J Surg Pathol. 1992;16:373–82.
13. Nielsen GP, Rosenberg AE, Young RH, et al. Angiomyofibroblastoma of the vulva and vagina. Mod Pathol. 1996;9:284–91.
14. Ockner DM, Sayadi H, Swanson PE, et al. Genital angiomyofibroblastoma. Comparison with aggressive angiomyxoma and other myxoid neoplasms of skin and soft tissue. Am J Clin Pathol. 1997;107:36–44.
15. Sims SM, Stinson K, McLean FW, et al. Angiomyofibroblastoma of the vulva: a case report of a pedunculated variant and review of the literature. J Low Genit Tract Dis. 2012;16:149–54.
16. Laskin WB, Fetsch JF, Tavassoli FA. Angiomyofibroblastoma of the female genital tract: analysis of 17 cases including a lipomatous variant. Hum Pathol. 1997;28:1046–55.
17. Magro G, Righi A, Caltabiano R, et al. Vulvovaginal angiomyofibroblastomas: morphologic, immunohistochemical, and fluorescence in situ hybridization analysis for deletion of 13q14 region. Hum Pathol. 2014;45:1647–55.
18. Medeiros F, Erickson-Johnson MR, Keeney GL, et al. Frequency and characterization of HMGA2 and HMGA1 rearrangements in mesenchymal tumors of the lower genital tract. Genes Chromosomes Cancer. 2007;46:981–90.
19. Folpe A, Tworek J, Weiss S. Sarcomatous transformation in angiofibroblastomas: a clinicopathological, histological and immunohistochemical study of eleven cases. Mod Pathol. 2001;14:12A.
20. Nucci MR, Granter SR, Fletcher CD. Cellular angiofibroma: a benign neoplasm distinct from angiomyofibroblastoma and spindle cell lipoma. Am J Surg Pathol. 1997;21:636–44.
21. Iwasa Y, Fletcher CDM. Cellular angiofibroma: clinicopathologic and immunohistochemical analysis of 51 cases. Am J Surg Pathol. 2004;28:1426–35.
22. Mandato VD, Santagni S, Cavazza A, et al. Cellular angiofibroma in women: a review of the literature. Diagn Pathol. 2015;10:114.
23. Chen E, Fletcher CDM. Cellular angiofibroma with atypia or sarcomatous transformation: clinicopathologic analysis of 13 cases. Am J Surg Pathol. 2010;34:707–14.
24. Ptaszyński K, Szumera-Ciećkiewicz A, Bartczak A. Cellular angiofibroma with atypia or sarcomatous transformation – case description with literature review. Pol J Pathol. 2012;63:207–11.
25. Flucke U, van Krieken JHJM, Mentzel T. Cellular angiofibroma: analysis of 25 cases emphasizing its relationship to spindle cell lipoma and mammary-type myofibroblastoma. Mod Pathol. 2011;24:82–9.
26. Maggiani F, Debiec-Rychter M, Vanbockrijck M, Sciot R. Cellular angiofibroma: another mesenchymal tumour with 13q14 involvement, suggesting a link with spindle cell lipoma and (extra)-mammary myofibroblastoma. Histopathology. 2007;51:410–2.
27. Howitt BE, Fletcher CDM. Mammary-type myofibroblastoma: clinicopathologic characterization in a series of 143 cases. Am J Surg Pathol. 2016;40:361–7.
28. Laskin WB, Fetsch JF, Tavassoli FA. Superficial cervicovaginal myofibroblastoma: fourteen cases of a distinctive mesenchymal tumor arising from the specialized subepithelial stroma of the lower female genital tract. Hum Pathol. 2001;32:715–25.
29. Ganesan R, McCluggage WG, Hirschowitz L, Rollason TP. Superficial myofibroblastoma of the lower female genital

tract: report of a series including tumours with a vulval location. Histopathology. 2005;46:137–43.
30. Magro G, Righi A, Casorzo L, et al. Mammary and vaginal myofibroblastomas are genetically related lesions: fluorescence in situ hybridization analysis shows deletion of 13q14 region. Hum Pathol. 2012;43:1887–93.
31. Ajibona OO, Richards CJ, Davies Q. A distinctive vulval fibroma of so-called prepubertal type in a postmenopausal patient. J Clin Pathol. 2007;60:437–8.
32. Iwasa Y, Fletcher CDM. Distinctive prepubertal vulval fibroma: a hitherto unrecognized mesenchymal tumor of prepubertal girls: analysis of 11 cases. Am J Surg Pathol. 2004;28:1601–8.
33. Vargas SO, Kozakewich HPW, Boyd TK, et al. Childhood asymmetric labium majus enlargement: mimicking a neoplasm. Am J Surg Pathol. 2005;29:1007–16.
34. Calonje E, Guerin D, McCormick D, Fletcher CD. Superficial angiomyxoma: clinicopathologic analysis of a series of distinctive but poorly recognized cutaneous tumors with tendency for recurrence. Am J Surg Pathol. 1999;23:910–7.
35. Fetsch JF, Laskin WB, Tavassoli FA. Superficial angiomyxoma (cutaneous myxoma): a clinicopathologic study of 17 cases arising in the genital region. Int J Gynecol Pathol. 1997;16:325–34.
36. McCluggage WG. A review and update of morphologically bland vulvovaginal mesenchymal lesions. Int J Gynecol Pathol. 2005;24:26–38.
37. Willis J, Abdul-Karim FW, di Sant'Agnese PA (1994) Extracardiac rhabdomyomas. Semin Diagn Pathol 11:15–25.
38. Iversen UM. Two cases of benign vaginal rhabdomyoma. Case reports. APMIS Acta Pathol Microbiol Immunol Scand. 1996;104:575–8.
39. Schoolmeester JK, Xing D, Keeney GL, Sukov WR. Genital Rhabdomyoma of the lower female genital tract: a study of 12 cases with molecular cytogenetic findings. Int J Gynecol Pathol. 2018;37(4):349–55.
40. McCluggage WG, Longacre TA, Fisher C. Myogenin expression in vulvovaginal spindle cell lesions: analysis of a series of cases with an emphasis on diagnostic pitfalls. Histopathology. 2013;63:545–50.
41. Odoi AT, Owusu-Bempah A, Dassah ET, et al. Vulvar lipoma: is it so rare. Ghana Med J. 2011;45:125–7.
42. Oh J-T, Choi SH, Ahn SG, et al. Vulvar lipomas in children: an analysis of 7 cases. J Pediatr Surg. 2009;44:1920–3.
43. Jóźwik M, Kołodziejczak M, Klonowska-Dziatkiewicz E, Jóźwik M. Giant vulvar lipoma in an adolescent girl: a case study and literature review. J Pediatr Adolesc Gynecol. 2014;27:e117–9.
44. Reis-Filho JS, Milanezi F, Soares MF, et al. Intradermal spindle cell/pleomorphic lipoma of the vulva: case report and review of the literature. J Cutan Pathol. 2002;29:59–62.
45. Park ST, Kim HM, Shin MK, Kim JW. An unusual case of vulvar schwannoma. World J Surg Oncol. 2015;13:139.
46. Sammarco AG, Abualnadi NM, Andraska EA, et al. Plexiform schwannoma: an unusual clitoral mass. Am J Obstet Gynecol. 2017;216:319.e1–2.
47. Azurah AGN, Grover S, McGregor D. Plexiform schwannoma of the clitoris in a young girl: a case report. J Reprod Med. 2013;58:365–8.
48. Chuang W-Y, Yeh C-J, Jung S-M, Hsueh S. Plexiform schwannoma of the clitoris. APMIS Acta Pathol Microbiol Immunol Scand. 2007;115:889–90.
49. Yegane RA, Alaee MS, Khanicheh E. Congenital plexiform schwannoma of the clitoris. Saudi Med J. 2008;29:600–2.
50. Fong KL, Bouwer H, Baranyai J, Jones RW. Ancient schwannoma of the vulva. Obstet Gynecol. 2009;113:510–2.
51. Hanafy A, Lee RM, Peterson CM. Schwannoma presenting as a Bartholin's gland abscess. Aust N Z J Obstet Gynaecol. 1997;37:483–4.
52. Nibhoria S, Kaur Tiwana K, Kaur M, Phutela R. Isolated vaginal neurofibroma presenting as vaginal wall cyst: a rare case report with review of literature. J Fam Reprod Health. 2016;10: 49–51.
53. Kidanto HL, Garrison J, Wangwe P. Large neurofibroma of the labia majora: a case report. Tanzan J Health Res. 2013;15:71–2.
54. Amita M, Darshit D, Rekha W, Hemant T. Giant neurofibroma of the vulva. Aust N Z J Obstet Gynaecol. 2005;45:84–5.
55. Wehmeijer LM, Hage JJ, Eberz B, van Beurden M. Partially plexiform neurofibroma of the labia minora and clitoral hood-a prognostic dilemma. J Low Genit Tract Dis. 2015;19:e55–7.
56. Sutphen R, Galán-Goméz E, Kousseff BG. Clitoromegaly in neurofibromatosis. Am J Med Genet. 1995;55:325–30.
57. Azzopardi JG, Eusebi V, Tison V, Betts CM. Neurofibroma with rhabdomyomatous differentiation: benign "triton" tumour of the vagina. Histopathology. 1983;7:561–72.
58. Lack EE, Worsham GF, Callihan MD, et al. Granular cell tumor: a clinicopathologic study of 110 patients. J Surg Oncol. 1980;13:301–16.
59. Hong SC, Lim YK, Chew SH, et al. Case report of granular cell tumor of the vulva and review of current literature. Gynecol Oncol Case Rep. 2012;3:20–2.
60. Horowitz IR, Copas P, Majmudar B. Granular cell tumors of the vulva. Am J Obstet Gynecol. 1995;173:1710–1713, 1714.
61. Levavi H, Sabah G, Kaplan B, et al. Granular cell tumor of the vulva: six new cases. Arch Gynecol Obstet. 2006;273:246–9.
62. Wolber RA, Talerman A, Wilkinson EJ, Clement PB. Vulvar granular cell tumors with pseudocarcinomatous hyperplasia: a comparative analysis with well-differentiated squamous carcinoma. Int J Gynecol Pathol. 1991;10:59–66.
63. Schmidt O, Fleckenstein GH, Gunawan B, et al. Recurrence and rapid metastasis formation of a granular cell tumor of the vulva. Eur J Obstet Gynecol Reprod Biol. 2003;106:219–21.
64. Heller DS. Benign Tumors and tumor-like lesions of the vulva. Clin Obstet Gynecol. 2015;58:526–35.
65. Wang S, Lang JH, Zhou HM. Venous malformations of the female lower genital tract. Eur J Obstet Gynecol Reprod Biol. 2009;145:205–8.
66. Celik F, Arioz DT, Köken GN, Yilmazer M. Very rare cause of vaginal mass in pregnancy: cavernous hemangioma. J Obstet Gynaecol Res. 2012;38:889–91.
67. Yu BR, Lee GE, Cho DH, et al. Genital tract cavernous hemangioma as a rare cause of postpartum hemorrhage. Obstet Gynecol Sci. 2017;60:473–6.
68. Bruni V, Pontello V, Dei M, et al. Hemangioma of the clitoris presenting as clitoromegaly: a case report. J Pediatr Adolesc Gynecol. 2009;22:e137–8.
69. Nayyar S, Liaqat N, Sultan N, Dar SH. Cavernous haemangioma mimicking as clitoral hypertrophy. Afr J Paediatr Surg AJPS. 2014;11:65–6.
70. Chang MB, Newman CC, Davis MDP, Lehman JS. Acquired lymphangiectasia (lymphangioma circumscriptum) of the vulva: clinicopathologic study of 11 patients from a single institution and 67 from the literature. Int J Dermatol. 2016;55:e482–7.
71. Vlastos A-T, Malpica A, Follen M. Lymphangioma circumscriptum of the vulva: a review of the literature. Obstet Gynecol. 2003;101:946–54.
72. Stewart CJR, Chan T, Platten M. Acquired lymphangiectasia ('lymphangioma circumscriptum') of the vulva: a report of eight cases. Pathology (Phila). 2009;41:448–53.
73. Doğan F, Bucak İH. Rare Giant Angiokeratoma of the vulva: a case report. Balk Med J. 2017;34:163–4.
74. Terzakis E, Androutsopoulos G, Zygouris D, et al. Angiokeratoma of the vulva. Eur J Gynaecol Oncol. 2011;32:597–8.
75. Yiğiter M, Arda IS, Tosun E, et al. Angiokeratoma of clitoris: a rare lesion in an adolescent girl. Urology. 2008;71:604–6.

76. Cohen PR, Young AW, Tovell HM. Angiokeratoma of the vulva: diagnosis and review of the literature. Obstet Gynecol Surv. 1989;44:339–46.
77. Gonzalez S, Duarte I. Benign fibrous histiocytoma of the skin. A morphologic study of 290 cases. Pathol Res Pract. 1982;174:379–91.
78. Abenoza P, Lillemoe T. CD34 and factor XIIIa in the differential diagnosis of dermatofibroma and dermatofibrosarcoma protuberans. Am J Dermatopathol. 1993;15:429–34.
79. Franquemont DW, Cooper PH, Shmookler BM, Wick MR. Benign fibrous histiocytoma of the skin with potential for local recurrence: a tumor to be distinguished from dermatofibroma. Mod Pathol. 1990;3:158–63.
80. Calonje E, Mentzel T, Fletcher CD. Cellular benign fibrous histiocytoma. Clinicopathologic analysis of 74 cases of a distinctive variant of cutaneous fibrous histiocytoma with frequent recurrence. Am J Surg Pathol. 1994;18:668–76.
81. Fetsch JF, Laskin WB, Lefkowitz M, et al. Aggressive angiomyxoma: a clinicopathologic study of 29 female patients. Cancer. 1996;78:79–90.
82. Granter SR, Nucci MR, Fletcher CD. Aggressive angiomyxoma: reappraisal of its relationship to angiomyofibroblastoma in a series of 16 cases. Histopathology. 1997;30:3–10.
83. Tsang WY, Chan JK, Lee KC, et al. Aggressive angiomyxoma. A report of four cases occurring in men. Am J Surg Pathol. 1992;16:1059–65.
84. Iezzoni JC, Fechner RE, Wong LS, Rosai J. Aggressive angiomyxoma in males. A report of four cases. Am J Clin Pathol. 1995;104:391–6.
85. Bigby SM, Symmans PJ, Miller MV, et al. Aggressive angiomyxoma [corrected] of the female genital tract and pelvis--clinicopathologic features with immunohistochemical analysis. Int J Gynecol Pathol. 2011;30:505–13.
86. van Roggen JFG, van Unnik JA, Briaire-de Bruijn IH, Hogendoorn PC. Aggressive angiomyxoma: a clinicopathological and immunohistochemical study of 11 cases with long-term follow-up. Virchows Arch Int J Pathol. 2005;446:157–63.
87. Rabban JT, Dal Cin P, Oliva E. HMGA2 rearrangement in a case of vulvar aggressive angiomyxoma. Int J Gynecol Pathol Off J Int Soc Gynecol Pathol. 2006;25:403–7.
88. McCluggage WG, Connolly L, McBride HA. HMGA2 is a sensitive but not specific immunohistochemical marker of vulvovaginal aggressive angiomyxoma. Am J Surg Pathol. 2010;34:1037–42.
89. McCluggage WG, Nielsen GP, Young RH. Massive vulval edema secondary to obesity and immobilization: a potential mimic of aggressive angiomyxoma. Int J Gynecol Pathol. 2008;27:447–52.
90. Fadare O, Brannan SM, Arin-Silasi D, Parkash V. Localized lymphedema of the vulva: a clinicopathologic study of 2 cases and a review of the literature. Int J Gynecol Pathol. 2011;30:306–13.
91. Blandamura S, Cruz J, Faure Vergara L, et al. Aggressive angiomyxoma: a second case of metastasis with patient's death. Hum Pathol. 2003;34:1072–4.
92. Fine BA, Munoz AK, Litz CE, Gershenson DM. Primary medical management of recurrent aggressive angiomyxoma of the vulva with a gonadotropin-releasing hormone agonist. Gynecol Oncol. 2001;81:120–2.
93. Newman PL, Fletcher CD. Smooth muscle tumours of the external genitalia: clinicopathological analysis of a series. Histopathology. 1991;18:523–9.
94. Tavassoli FA, Norris HJ. Smooth muscle tumors of the vulva. Obstet Gynecol. 1979;53:213–7.
95. Tavassoli FA, Norris HJ. Smooth muscle tumors of the vagina. Obstet Gynecol. 1979;53:689–93.
96. Nielsen GP, Rosenberg AE, Koerner FC, et al. Smooth-muscle tumors of the vulva. A clinicopathological study of 25 cases and review of the literature. Am J Surg Pathol. 1996;20:779–93.
97. Sayeed S, Xing D, Jenkins SM, et al. Criteria for risk stratification of vulvar and vaginal smooth muscle tumors: an evaluation of 71 cases comparing proposed classification systems. Am J Surg Pathol. 2018;42:84–94.
98. Nucci MR, Fletcher CD. Vulvovaginal soft tissue tumours: update and review. Histopathology. 2000;36:97–108.
99. Horton E, Dobin SM, Debiec-Rychter M, Donner LR. A clonal translocation (7;8)(p13;q11.2) in a leiomyoma of the vulva. Cancer Genet Cytogenet. 2006;170:58–60.
100. Guardiola MT, Dobin SM, Dal Cin P, Donner LR. Pericentric inversion (12)(p12q13-14) as the sole chromosomal abnormality in a leiomyoma of the vulva. Cancer Genet Cytogenet. 2010;199:21–3.
101. Yang J, Yang J, Yu M, et al. Clinical study on female genital tract Rhabdomyosarcoma in childhood: changes during 20 years in one Center. Int J Gynecol Cancer. 2017;27:311–4.
102. Dehner LP, Jarzembowski JA, Hill DA. Embryonal rhabdomyosarcoma of the uterine cervix: a report of 14 cases and a discussion of its unusual clinicopathological associations. Mod Pathol. 2012;25:602–14.
103. Diller L, Sexsmith E, Gottlieb A, et al. Germline p53 mutations are frequently detected in young children with rhabdomyosarcoma. J Clin Invest. 1995;95:1606–11.
104. Ferrari A, Bisogno G, Macaluso A, et al. Soft-tissue sarcomas in children and adolescents with neurofibromatosis type 1. Cancer. 2007;109:1406–12.
105. Nasioudis D, Alevizakos M, Chapman-Davis E, et al. Rhabdomyosarcoma of the lower female genital tract: an analysis of 144 cases. Arch Gynecol Obstet. 2017;296: 327–34.
106. Ferguson SE, Gerald W, Barakat RR, et al. Clinicopathologic features of rhabdomyosarcoma of gynecologic origin in adults. Am J Surg Pathol. 2007;31:382–9.
107. Andrassy RJ, Hays DM, Raney RB, et al. Conservative surgical management of vaginal and vulvar pediatric rhabdomyosarcoma: a report from the intergroup Rhabdomyosarcoma study III. J Pediatr Surg. 1995;30:1034–1036, 1037.
108. Leuschner I, Harms D, Mattke A, et al. Rhabdomyosarcoma of the urinary bladder and vagina: a clinicopathologic study with emphasis on recurrent disease: a report from the Kiel Pediatric Tumor Registry and the German CWS Study. Am J Surg Pathol. 2001;25:856–64.
109. Schoolmeester JK, Leifer AJ, Wang L, Hameed MR. Vulvar myxoid liposarcoma and well differentiated liposarcoma with molecular cytogenetic confirmation: case reports with review of malignant lipomatous tumors of the vulva. Int J Gynecol Pathol. 2015;34:390–5.
110. Nucci MR, Fletcher CD. Liposarcoma (atypical lipomatous tumors) of the vulva: a clinicopathologic study of six cases. Int J Gynecol Pathol. 1998;17:17–23.
111. Rogers RG, Thorp JM. Liposarcoma of the vulva: a case report. J Reprod Med. 1995;40:863–4.
112. Hameed M. Pathology and genetics of adipocytic tumors. Cytogenet Genome Res. 2007;118:138–47.
113. Brooks JJ, LiVolsi VA. Liposarcoma presenting on the vulva. Am J Obstet Gynecol. 1987;156:73–5.
114. Kolberg M, Høland M, Agesen TH, et al. Survival meta-analyses for >1800 malignant peripheral nerve sheath tumor patients with and without neurofibromatosis type 1. Neuro-Oncol. 2013;15:135–47.
115. Stucky C-CH, Johnson KN, Gray RJ, et al. Malignant peripheral nerve sheath tumors (MPNST): the Mayo Clinic experience. Ann Surg Oncol. 2012;19:878–85.
116. Lambrou NC, Mirhashemi R, Wolfson A, et al. Malignant peripheral nerve sheath tumor of the vulva: a multimodal treatment approach. Gynecol Oncol. 2002;85:365–71.

117. Maglione MA, Tricarico OD, Calandria L. Malignant peripheral nerve sheath tumor of the vulva. A case report. J Reprod Med. 2002;47:721–4.
118. Ozdal B, Oz M, Korkmaz E, et al. Malignant peripheral nerve sheath tumor of the vulva, an unusual differential diagnosis for vulvar mass. Int J Surg Case Rep. 2014;5:793–5.
119. Le Guellec S, Decouvelaere A-V, Filleron T, et al. Malignant peripheral nerve sheath tumor is a challenging diagnosis: a systematic pathology review, immunohistochemistry, and molecular analysis in 160 patients from the French sarcoma group database. Am J Surg Pathol. 2016;40:896–908.
120. Fletcher CD, Dal Cin P, de Wever I, et al. Correlation between clinicopathological features and karyotype in spindle cell sarcomas. A report of 130 cases from the CHAMP study group. Am J Pathol. 1999;154:1841–7.
121. Tunitsky-Bitton E, Uy-Kroh MJS, Michener C, Tarr ME. Primary Ewing sarcoma presenting as a vulvar mass in an adolescent: case report and review of literature. J Pediatr Adolesc Gynecol. 2015;28:e179–83.
122. Bancalari E, de Álava E, Tardío JC. Primary vaginal Ewing sarcoma: case report and review of the literature. Int J Surg Pathol. 2012;20:305–10.
123. McCluggage WG, Sumathi VP, Nucci MR, et al. Ewing family of tumours involving the vulva and vagina: report of a series of four cases. J Clin Pathol. 2007;60:674–80.
124. Xiao C, Zhao J, Guo P, et al. Clinical analysis of primary primitive neuroectodermal tumors in the female genital tract. Int J Gynecol Cancer. 2014;24:404–9.
125. Kruse A-J, Sep S, Slangen BFM, et al. Angiosarcomas of primary gynecologic origin: a clinicopathologic review and quantitative analysis of survival. Int J Gynecol Cancer. 2014;24:4–12.
126. Sheinis M, Cesari M, Selk A. Angiosarcoma of the vulva: a case report. J Low Genit Tract Dis. 2016;20:e6–7.
127. Nguyen AH, Detty SQ, Gonzaga MI, Huerter C. Clinical features and treatment of dermatofibrosarcoma protuberans affecting the vulva: a literature review. Dermatol Surg. 2017;43:771–4.
128. Edelweiss M, Malpica A. Dermatofibrosarcoma protuberans of the vulva: a clinicopathologic and immunohistochemical study of 13 cases. Am J Surg Pathol. 2010;34:393–400.
129. Vanni R, Faa G, Dettori T, et al. A case of dermatofibrosarcoma protuberans of the vulva with a COL1A1/PDGFB fusion identical to a case of giant cell fibroblastoma. Virchows Arch Int J Pathol. 2000;437:95–100.
130. Gökden N, Dehner LP, Zhu X, Pfeifer JD. Dermatofibrosarcoma protuberans of the vulva and groin: detection of COL1A1-PDGFB fusion transcripts by RT-PCR. J Cutan Pathol. 2003;30:190–5.
131. Pileri SA, Ascani S, Cox MC, et al. Myeloid sarcoma: clinicopathologic, phenotypic and cytogenetic analysis of 92 adult patients. Leukemia. 2007;21:340–50.
132. Oliva E, Ferry JA, Young RH, et al. Granulocytic sarcoma of the female genital tract: a clinicopathologic study of 11 cases. Am J Surg Pathol. 1997;21:1156–65.
133. Hu SC-S, Chen W-T, Chen G-S. Myeloid sarcoma of the vulva as the initial presentation of acute myeloid leukaemia. Br J Dermatol. 2016;174:234–6.
134. Meis JM, Butler JJ, Osborne BM, Manning JT. Granulocytic sarcoma in nonleukemic patients. Cancer. 1986;58:2697–709.
135. Skeete DH-A, Cesar-Rittenberg P, Jong R, et al. Myeloid sarcoma of the vagina: a report of 2 cases. J Low Genit Tract Dis. 2010;14:136–41.
136. Folpe AL, Schoolmeester JK, McCluggage WG, et al. SMARCB1-deficient vulvar neoplasms: a clinicopathologic, immunohistochemical, and molecular genetic study of 14 cases. Am J Surg Pathol. 2015;39:836–49.
137. Hornick JL, Dal Cin P, Fletcher CDM. Loss of INI1 expression is characteristic of both conventional and proximal-type epithelioid sarcoma. Am J Surg Pathol. 2009;33:542–50.
138. Hollmann TJ, Hornick JL. INI1-deficient tumors: diagnostic features and molecular genetics. Am J Surg Pathol. 2011;35:e47–63.
139. Yoshida A, Yoshida H, Yoshida M, et al. Myoepithelioma-like Tumors of the vulvar region: a distinctive group of SMARCB1-deficient neoplasms. Am J Surg Pathol. 2015;39:1102–13.
140. Patrizi L, Corrado G, Saltari M, et al. Vulvar "proximal-type" epithelioid sarcoma: report of a case and review of the literature. Diagn Pathol. 2013;8:122.
141. Rodrigues AI, Lopes HI, Lima O, Marta S. Proximal-type epithelioid sarcoma-unusual presentation: unilateral vulvar mass. BMJ Case Rep. 2015;2015:bcr2014208488. https://doi.org/10.1136/bcr-2014-208488.
142. Han CH, Li X, Khanna N. Epithelioid sarcoma of the vulva and its clinical implication: a case report and review of the literature. Gynecol Oncol Rep. 2016;15:31–3.
143. Dolanbay M, Kutuk MS, Uludag S, et al. Malignant rhabdoid tumor of the vulva: a case report and review of the literature. Taiwan J Obstet Gynecol. 2016;55:128–30.
144. Tajima S, Takahasi Y, Hikoaki M, Goto R. A SMARCB1-deficient vulvar neoplasm with prominent myxoid stroma: report of a case showing ERG and FLI1 expression. Int J Clin Exp Pathol. 2015;8:7526–32.
145. Kim H-J, Kim M-H, Kwon J, et al. Proximal-type epithelioid sarcoma of the vulva with INI1 diagnostic utility. Ann Diagn Pathol. 2012;16:411–5.

Benign Lesions of the Vagina

9

Pavel Dundr, Kristýna Němejcová, and Michaela Bártů

Abstract

This chapter describes the normal anatomy, histology and microflora of the vagina and a selection of benign vaginal diseases, including inflammatory and other disorders, with an emphasis on their etiopathogenesis and morphological features that may be necessary to achieve their correct diagnoses. Pathologic differential diagnosis is described in detail, especially in entities which can be confused with some premalignant or malignant diseases, such as malacoplakia, vaginal cysts and tumour-like lesions including fibroepithelial polyps, tubulosquamous polyps, postoperative spindle cell nodules and prolapsed fallopian tube. A discussion of vaginal adenosis is also included, including its historical perspective.

Keywords

Vagina · Benign diseases · Anatomy · Histology
Infectious diseases

9.1 Anatomy, Histology and Biostasis of the Vagina

9.1.1 Vaginal Anatomy and Histology

The vagina is an elastic, muscular, tubular structure which extends from the vestibule of the vulva to the uterus. It is located within the pelvis, posterior to the urinary bladder and anterior to the rectum. Its axis averages 30 degrees with the vertical and more than 90 degrees with the long axis of the uterus. The average length of the vagina in adults is about 9 cm; the anterior is shorter than the dorsal wall by about 3 cm, with the cervix filling the difference. During sexual arousal, the vagina expands in both length and width; its length and calibre are unrelated to symptoms of dyspareunia [1, 2]. It surrounds the exocervix and forms vault-like fornices between its cervical attachment and the lateral wall, which are deepest posteriorly. The anterior and posterior walls are in contact with each other, whereas the lateral walls remain fairly rigid and separated. This gives an H-shaped appearance to the vaginal canal in transverse sections.

Anteriorly, the vagina is in contact with the uterine cervix, the base of the bladder and the urethra. The urethra runs approximately one third of its length on the vagina, separated from the vagina by loose connective tissue, and then enters into the vaginal wall distally to become an inseparable part of vagina, with the fusion of their fasciae into a single dense layer.

Posteriorly, the upper fourth of the vagina is covered with peritoneum and forms the anterior part of the "cul-de-sac" or pouch of Douglas (rectouterine space). The adventitia of the middle half of the vagina is connected to the rectum by the rectovaginal septum. The lower fourth of the vagina is separated from the anal canal by the perineal body and anal and rectal sphincters. Laterally, the ureters run along both sides of the upper third of the vagina until entering the bladder wall. Distally, the vagina is partially surrounded by the levator ani and bulbocavernosus muscles and ultimately opens into the vestibule, situated beneath the urethra and between the inner margins of the labia minora.

The vasculature of the vagina is supplied by branches of the internal iliac artery: uterine, vaginal, middle rectal and internal pudendal arteries. Extensive arterial anastomoses provide an adequate blood supply, which minimizes the possibility of ischemic damage. The venous drainage forms a complex network, surrounds the vagina and communicates with the uterine, pudendal and rectal veins, which empty into the interior iliac veins.

The vaginal lymphatic system is complex and variable, with frequent crossovers between the left and right pelvis. The lymphatics of the upper anterior vagina and vaginal vault join those of the cervix and terminate in the medial chain of the external iliac lymph nodes, whereas the middle

P. Dundr (✉) · K. Němejcová · M. Bártů
First Faculty of Medicine, Institute of Pathology, Charles University and General University Hospital in Prague, Prague, Czech Republic
e-mail: pdundr@seznam.cz

W. Zheng et al. (eds.), *Gynecologic and Obstetric Pathology, Volume 1*, https://doi.org/10.1007/978-981-13-3016-2_9

drains into internal iliac lymph nodes. The posterior portion of the vagina drains into the inferior gluteal, sacral and anorectal lymph nodes. The lymphatics of the distal vagina as well as the vulva drain into the femoral lymph nodes. It is important to note that, as a consequence of extensive anastomotic channels, any pelvic, anorectal or femoral node may be involved in the lymphatic drainage of any part of the vagina. In a simplified way, the tumours in the upper vagina can spread in a similar way to cervical carcinomas, and tumours in the lower vagina tend to involve superficial iliac and deep pelvic nodes, like vulvar cancer.

The nerve supply to the vagina is primarily derived from the superior hypogastric plexus of the autonomic nervous system. This plexus bifurcates and is joined by branches of the second through to the fifth sacral nerves, forming the pelvic plexuses. The upper part of the vagina is innervated by the uterovaginal plexus, and the lower vagina through the fibres of the pudendal nerve.

Histologically, the vaginal wall consists of three principal layers: the mucosa, muscularis and adventitia. The mucosa, on gross examination, forms ill-defined laterally oriented folds or rugae of about 2–5 mm thickness, which vary according to location and hormonal stimulation. The rugal pattern of the vaginal mucosa contributes to the organ's elasticity, and rugae are more prominent in nulliparous than in multiparous women.

The mucosa is lined by a non-keratinized glycogenated squamous epithelium (Fig. 9.1). The mature stratified squamous epithelium can be subdivided into several layers; basal,

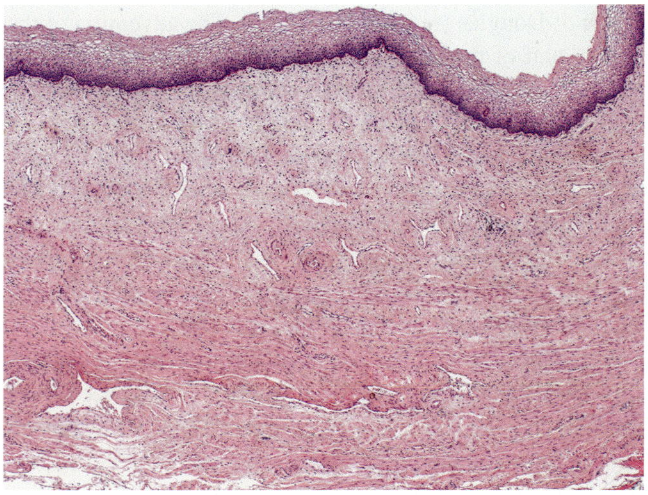

Fig. 9.1 Normal histology of the vagina. The mucosa is lined by non-keratinized squamous epithelium composed of basal layer, parabasal layers and glycogenated intermediate and superficial cells. Beneath the mucosa there is lamina propria, consisting of loose connective tissue with elastic fibres rich in venous and lymphatic vessels. In deeper part of the vaginal wall, there is muscularis, formed by loose bundles of smooth muscle cells

parabasal, intermediate and superficial. Mitoses are usually confined to the basal and parabasal layers, which are the active proliferative compartments. The basal layer consists of a single layer of columnar cells, with the long axis of the cells perpendicular to the basement membrane. The basal cells have scant cytoplasm and relatively large, oval and uniformly hyperchromatic nuclei. Occasional melanocytes are also found in about 3% of women. The parabasal layer usually consists of two to five layers of small cuboidal cells, with a centrally located, round and uniformly hyperchromatic nucleus. The intermediate layer is of variable thickness. The cells in this layer have moderate quantities of slightly flattened cytoplasm and oval nuclei with finely dispersed chromatin. The cells have variously prominent intercellular bridges, and the long cell axis of both nucleus and cytoplasm is parallel to the basement membrane. The superficial layer also varies in thickness. The cells are polygonal, contain abundant acidophilic cytoplasm and have an orientation similar to intermediate cells. Keratohyalin granules are sometimes seen in the cytoplasm. The nuclei are centrally located, small, round, hyperchromatic and pyknotic. In the intermediate and superficial cell layers, there may be present variable quantities of glycogen, which accumulates initially in a perinuclear location within intermediate cells, resulting in a clear zone around the nucleus. This appearance may resemble HPV changes with the perinuclear clearing (koilocytes), and the normal mucosal cells can be distinguished by having normal-sized nuclei and by their characteristic location in the middle rather than the superficial third of the epithelium. The normal vaginal mucosa lacks glands. The lamina propria (or submucosa) consists of a loose fibrovascular stroma with elastic fibres and nerves and a rich venous and lymphatic network. Superficially, beneath the squamous epithelium is a poorly defined zone containing atypical, large, stellate, polygonal or spindle stromal cells with scant cytoplasm. Some of these cells have multinucleated or multilobulated hyperchromatic nuclei. This band of stroma extends in an irregular fashion from the endocervix to the vulva, and these atypical stromal cells are thought to give rise to fibroepithelial polyps.

The muscularis consists of poorly delineated bundles of smooth muscle, forming the inner circular and outer longitudinal layers, continuous with the muscle layers of the uterus. Some of the outer longitudinal layers pass into the lateral pelvic wall and contribute to the inferior portion of the cardinal ligaments. The sphincter around the distal vagina is formed by the bulbospongiosus (bulbocavernosus) muscular fibres. The adventitia is a thin coat of dense connective tissue, containing the lymphatic and venous plexuses and nerve bundles. It joins with the loose connective tissue of the surrounding pelvis.

9.1.2 Steroid Hormone Effect on Vaginal Epithelia

Steroid hormones regulate the proliferation and differentiation of epithelial cells in the female genital tract. Their effect is primarily mediated through intranuclear steroid receptors. These receptors are present in all three layers of the vaginal wall, but the highest intensity of their expression is found in the squamous cells of the vaginal mucosa [3].

The thickness and maturation of the vaginal epithelium is mainly regulated by estrogen and varies throughout the menstrual cycle and throughout the various stages of the life cycle (birth, childhood, reproduction and the postmenopausal years). Vaginal epithelial receptors, particularly the estrogen nuclear receptor 1 (ESR1, formerly named ERα), integrate estrogen and growth factor signalling to mediate the switch between cell proliferation and differentiation [4]. Animal model investigations suggest that the proliferation and maturation of vaginal epithelium are mediated by the stromal estrogen receptors in a paracrine manner, whereas differentiation is promoted by epithelial estrogen receptors [4].

In the proliferative phase of the menstrual cycle, the epithelium progressively proliferates and matures fully in response to estrogens. This is reflected in a high expression of the proliferation marker Ki-67 coinciding with high serum estrogen levels [5]. During the secretory phase, higher levels of progesterone inhibit the maturation of the vaginal epithelium at the intermediate cell level, resulting in decreased thickness of the epithelium. Before puberty and after menopause, estrogenic activity is low or absent, and the vaginal epithelium fails to mature and hence remains thin. An exception to this can be seen in newborns where the vaginal epithelium is frequently mature because of the influence of placental estrogens, but it rapidly regresses to atrophy within about 4 weeks. Upon reaching puberty, in response to increased estrogen production by the maturing ovaries, the intermediate cell layer proliferates, and the superficial cells undergo maturation.

During the menopausal period, the changes in the vaginal mucosa are characterized by a gradual reduction in the thickness of the epithelium, loss of rugae and reduced tissue elasticity and lubrication. The decrease of estrogen hormones leads to the progressive loss of superficial cells, gradually followed by the decline and loss of intermediate cells, and finally the thinning of the epithelium leaves only six to eight layers of parabasal cells.

Vaginal atrophy could also be found in premenopausal women, where it is most commonly encountered either as a consequence of iatrogenic decrease of estrogen levels or during the postpartum period due to the loss of placental estrogen and the antagonistic action of prolactin on estrogen production during lactation [6].

Atrophy can cause some local symptoms of vaginal dryness, itch, discomfort, symptomatic prolapse, change in vaginal discharge or dyspareunia. Local or systemic exposure of the atrophic mucosa to estrogen leads to maturation of squamous cells, and thus the same level of maturation similar to the proliferative phase of the menstrual cycle could be achieved.

Estrogen also affects the maintenance of vaginal smooth muscle bundle density, growth and the functions of vascular and nonvascular smooth muscle in the subepithelial vaginal layers and nerve ending morphology as well as their density. In addition, estrogens have been shown to enhance genital sensation and play a role during sexual arousal. In the early phases of sexual response, the proximal two thirds of the vagina lengthen and increase in volume, followed by constriction of the distal third [2]. Estrogens also affect the genes involved in the immune response and many other factors involved in maintaining a healthy condition and moisture in the vaginal mucosa. Vaginal lubrication typically results from increased vascular pressure and genital engorgement caused by dilatation of the vaginal vasculature in response to excitatory stimuli (mediated by hormones, particularly estrogen, neurotransmitters and nitric oxide) [7]. The fluid is usually acidic (pH around 4.6) and contains a variable amount of antibodies, enzymes and their inhibitors, which may play a role in the liquefaction of coagulated semen and the capacitation of spermatocytes or have antimicrobial activity [8].

9.1.3 Biostasis of the Vagina

The vagina and its microbiota form a balanced ecosystem, which plays an important role in preventing colonization by pathogenic organisms, including those responsible for bacterial vaginosis, sexually transmitted and urinary tract infectious agents. The ecosystem reflects a delicate balance which includes the interplay of steroid hormones, vascularity, vaginal acidity and glycogen [8]. This can easily be disturbed by chemical, mechanical or hormonal manipulation. The vaginal flora is a dynamic and closely interrelated system comprised of a vast diversity of microorganism species (more than 200 bacterial species, dominated by *Lactobacillus* spp.), which varies and changes from birth through menarche to menopause [9]. Initial colonization at birth comes from the vaginal microbiota or from the skin or mouth microbiota of the mother. Before menarche the vagina is colonized by diverse assemblages of enteric and skin species of microorganisms, and the pH of the vagina is nearly neutral [10]. Around the start and during the reproductive phase of women's lives, hormonal changes trigger certain changes in the spectrum of bacterial species. The increased estrogen levels support the proliferation of the vaginal epithelium and the intraepithelial production of glycogen, whereas progesterone causes the cytolysis of epithelial cells and the release of glycogen. The glycogen and its breakdown products are metabolized by lactobacilli and other bacteria to lactic acid, leading to acidification of the vaginal microenvironment to pH of 3.8–4.4, which is defined as normal [9]. After menopause, the decreasing estrogen levels lead to the altered composition of the vaginal microbiota.

The importance of lactic acid-producing bacteria in the vagina was discovered by Albert Döderlein in 1892. *Lactobacillus* spp. are a group of Gram-positive, anaerobic bacteria that produce lactic acid as a by-product of glycogen fermentation and serve as a natural resistance factor against potentially pathogenic microorganisms. The production of lactic acid maintains the low vaginal pH and so creates an unsuitable environment for pathogenic microbial species such as *Trichomonas vaginalis* and *Candida* spp. [11]. Other defensive mechanisms include competitive adhesion to the vaginal epithelium, production of antibacterial substances (bacteriocins) and hydrogen peroxide and the interactions between the plasminogen-plasmin system and the local immune system [11]. Maintaining a high number of lactic acid bacteria is regarded as a hallmark of health. The disruption of the vaginal ecosystem may cause various diseases and is also associated with an increased risk of infection, including but not limited to human immunodeficiency virus infection [11].

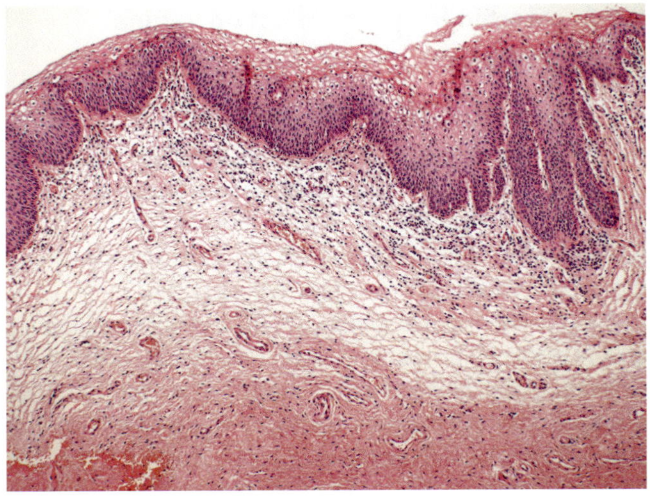

Fig. 9.2 Chronic nonspecific vaginitis. The mucosa is covered by normal stratified squamous epithelium. There is a mild inflammatory (predominantly lymphocytic) infiltrate in the lamina propria

9.2 Inflammatory Disorders of the Vagina

The normal vaginal flora is varied and constitutes a dynamic ecosystem known as the vaginal microbiota, which is delicately balanced and influenced by factors such as vaginal acidity, glycogen, vascularity and the interactions of steroid hormones [12]. Although the make-up of vaginal flora changes from birth throughout the reproductive life and menopause, the predominant microorganisms in a healthy vaginal environment are represented by *Lactobacillus* species. These species are not only able to colonize the vaginal mucosa but, more importantly, produce antimicrobial substances which act to prevent the growth of pathogenic microorganisms [13].

Urogenital infections, especially in premenopausal women, represent an important female health problem as they often require antibiotic treatment and their recurrence and relapse rates tend to be high.

Vaginitis

Vaginitis is an inflammation of the vagina characterized by the presence of inflammatory response consistent with alterations in the vaginal ecosystem (Fig. 9.2). In contrast, the term *vaginosis* is, strictly speaking, used to describe an altered vaginal ecosystem with reduced beneficial vaginal lactobacilli but a demonstrable absence of inflammatory response [14]. The three most prevalent diagnoses comprising 70% of all reported cases of vaginitis include bacterial vaginosis (BV), trichomoniasis and vulvovaginal candidiasis (VVC) [15]. Another significant condition is represented by a recently recognized entity called aerobic vaginitis.

Vaginitis is primarily a clinical diagnosis based on the presence of subjective symptoms of various kinds of discomfort (pruritus and pain being among the most frequent complaints) and the presence of a vaginal discharge, although building the diagnosis on discharge alone may at times lead to overdiagnosis [12]. What is commonly termed "vaginal discharge" often includes not only the pathological discharge caused by vaginitis but also simply the increased production of vaginal fluid, which can be frequently observed in the middle of the menstrual cycle when the cervical and uterine mucus become rather watery and profuse. It is therefore important to take into account the typical signs pointing to a vaginitis-associated discharge, such as the odour, colour, consistency and quantity of the discharge.

9.2.1 Bacterial Infections

9.2.1.1 Bacterial Vaginosis

Bacterial vaginosis (BV) is the most common cause of acute vaginitis. It is described as a polymicrobial disorder accompanied by an increase in the vaginal pH to over 4.5, reduced or absent lactobacillus colonization and overgrowth of several facultative and obligate anaerobic bacteria (Fig. 9.3) [16]. A large number of studies have demonstrated that despite its generally mild clinical presentation, bacterial vaginosis is associated with a variety of adverse pregnancy outcomes, such as miscarriage, preterm delivery of a low-birth-weight infant, premature rupture of the membranes,

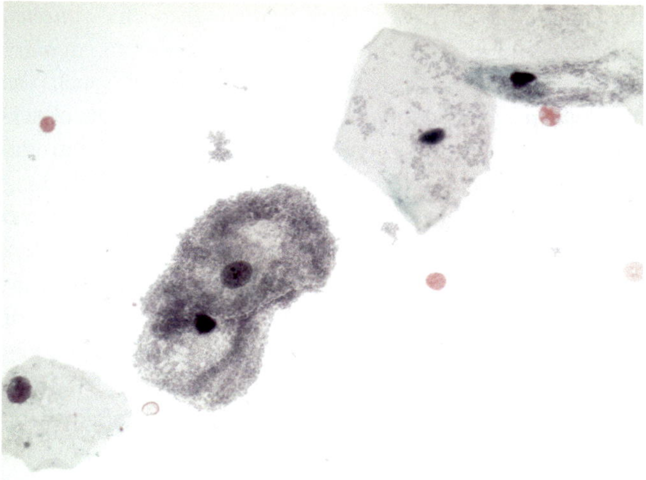

Fig. 9.3 Bacterial vaginosis. Typical clue cells can be seen, consisting of squamous cells covered by bacteria (in this case *Gardnerella vaginalis*)

chorioamnionitis, amniotic fluid infections and post-caesarean endometritis [17–20]. Bacterial vaginosis has also been reported to increase the risk of contracting a sexually transmitted disease, including an increased susceptibility to the human immunodeficiency virus [17, 20]. Other gynaecological complications include pelvic inflammatory disease, tubal infertility, postoperative infections and cervicitis [21].

Bacterial vaginosis is characterized by a thin, watery, fishy-smelling discharge, positive "amine" odour test (which can be easily demonstrated by adding 10% potassium hydroxide solution to a drop of vaginal discharge on a slide, with the resulting production of volatilized amines causing the distinctive odour) and a wet mount showing >20% clue cells (vaginal epithelial cells with a large number of attached bacteria) [22]. The underlying cause of bacterial vaginosis is described as a shift in the balance of the vaginal microflora with a reduction in lactobacilli and an increase in facultative and anaerobic bacteria (in either their number and/or type) [23]. This bacterial overgrowth can be caused by a number of anaerobic and other bacteria, primarily represented by *Gardnerella vaginalis*, *Mobiluncus* spp., *Prevotella* spp., *Bacteroides* spp., *Streptococcus* spp., *Megasphaera* spp., *Ureaplasma urealyticum*, *Atopobium vaginae* and *Mycoplasma* spp. [17, 21, 24].

Bacterial vaginosis can be diagnosed either based on the clinical Amsel's criteria or by the Nugent method, which has become the gold standard for histopathological diagnosis [25, 26]. Clinical diagnosis requires the fulfilment of at least three of the four main features described above (vaginal pH > 4.5, specific discharge, positive "amine" odour test and the presence of >20% clue cells on the wet mount). One of the shortcomings of using clinical criteria is that these cannot be applied to postmenopausal women, as the vaginal pH of these patients is constantly elevated above 4.5 due to the lack of hormonal stimulation and estrogenization of the vaginal mucosa (which lacks the glycogen deposits needed by the lactobacilli and these in turn cannot proliferate and produce lactic acid and hydrogen peroxide in the process). The amount of discharge in these women can also pose a problem, because vaginal discharge tends to be scarce, which makes judging its quality and quantity difficult [16].

The Nugent method was first suggested at the beginning of 1990s as a part of the Vaginal Infection and Prematurity Study [26]. The score is based on interpreting Gram-stained smears of the vaginal discharge, working under the assumption that the vaginal ecosystem of normal, healthy women is fully colonized by lactobacilli. The Nugent method quantitatively evaluates three different morphotypes: (1) lactobacilli, (2) *Gardnerella*-like species (*Gardnerella vaginalis*, *Bacteroides* spp., *Prevotella* spp., *Porphyromonas* spp.) and (3) *Mobiluncus* spp. in five different fields under oil immersion (magnification ×1000). The average number of lactobacilli morphotypes (large Gram-positive rods), *Gardnerella*-like morphotypes (small Gram-variable rods) and *Mobiluncus* spp. morphotypes (small, curved Gram-variable or Gram-negative rods) in five fields is established and then ranked. The points assigned to each morphotype are then combined, and the sum represents the patient's final Nugent score, which classifies the vaginal flora as normal (Nugent score 0–3), intermediate altered flora (Nugent score 4–6) and full-blown bacterial vaginosis (Nugent score 7–10) (Table 9.1).

However, given the differences between vaginal flora in fertile, perimenopausal and postmenopausal women, it has been suggested that the Nugent score system is inadequate for evaluating the normal and intermediate vaginal flora in women over the age of 40 years [16]. Due to the physiological decrease in lactobacillus colonization during the peri- and postmenopausal period, it is quite common for the vaginal flora of these patients to show an absence of lactoba-

Table 9.1 Nugent scoring system for Gram-stained vaginal smears for the diagnosis of bacterial vaginosis [26]

Score	*Lactobacillus* morphotype	*Gardnerella*-like spp. morphotypes	Curved Gram-variable rods
0	>30	0	0
1	5–30	<1	<1, 1–4
2	1–4	1–4	5–30, >30
3	<1	5–30	
4	0	>30	
Final Nugent Score (NS): the sum of the scores for the presence of *Lactobacillus*, *Gardnerella*-like morphotypes and curved Gram-variable rods			
NS 0–3: normal vaginal flora			
NS 4–6: intermediate altered flora			
*NS 4**: intermediate abnormal flora (acc. to Cauci et al.) [16]			
NS 7–10: bacterial vaginosis			

cilli morphotypes without an increase in bacterial vaginosis-associated microorganisms. It has therefore been proposed that, when dealing with this specific age group, the mere absence of lactobacilli morphotypes (without the accompanying limited overgrowth of *Gardnerella*-like and *Mobiluncus* spp.) should not be assigned the Nugent score of 4, but a score of 4*, and this special kind of mixed flora should be termed "intermediate abnormal flora".

Nevertheless, due to the high percentage of women with bacterial vaginosis who are asymptomatic, the Nugent scoring method cannot be always utilized. In such cases the use of a Pap smear was suggested as a suitable test for diagnosing bacterial vaginosis, with the sensitivity of 78% and specificity and positive predictive value of 86.9% [27]. Although the cervicovaginal smear is an effective tool, the Bethesda system for reporting the results only recognizes one category—"shift in vaginal flora suggestive of bacterial vaginosis"—and studies have therefore proposed utilizing the 1988 Dutch coding system (KOPAC), which differentiates between two categories: "dysbacteriosis O3" (clue cells with coccobacilli in the background) and "*Gardnerella vaginalis* O5" (blue mountain cells completely covered by a mountain of blue-staining round bacteria) [28]. Given the clinical significance of pure *Gardnerella* infection, the distinction between simple dysbacteriosis and *Gardnerella* infection is very desirable.

9.2.1.2 Aerobic Vaginitis

Aerobic vaginitis (AV) is an infectious entity which was first officially recognized by Donders et al. in 2002 as a condition characterized by abnormal (dysbiotic) vaginal microflora, which is different from bacterial vaginosis and thus represents an individual entity [29].

The diagnostic criteria of bacterial vaginosis have now been firmly established, with the Nugent score providing a clear definition of normal microflora (Nugent score of 3 or less) and a full-blown case of BV (Nugent score of 7–10). It is the category between these two marginal groups, called intermediate altered microflora, which has proved to be somewhat problematic in respect to establishing what exactly defines this altered state. This particular type of microflora, together with the varying degrees of associated vaginal atrophy and inflammation (unlike the suppressed immune response typical for bacterial vaginosis), was therefore called aerobic vaginitis [30]. The prevalence of aerobic vaginitis is reported to be between 8.3 and 10.8% of pregnant women and between 5.0 and 23.74% in symptomatic non-pregnant women [31]. The most severe presentation of aerobic vaginitis is comparative to desquamative inflammatory vaginitis [32].

Similarly to bacterial vaginosis, aerobic vaginitis also results from a shift in the balance of the vaginal microbiota. The altered microflora in aerobic vaginitis consists of commensal aerobic microorganisms of intestinal origin, comprised of *Escherichia coli*, *Staphylococcus aureus*, *Enterococcus faecalis*, group B *Streptococcus* (*S. agalactiae*) and coagulase-negative staphylococci such as *Staphylococcus epidermidis* [29]. Clinical symptoms of aerobic vaginitis include a typical vaginal discharge, introital and vaginal redness, dyspareunia in some (especially long standing) cases and subjective complaints of stinging and burning sensations. The discharge in aerobic vaginitis differs from the one typical for bacterial vaginosis—it shows a typically purulent character with high viscosity, yellowish or greenish colour, homogenous consistency and foul-smelling rotten odour (but no fishy smell). Due to the epithelial disruption, the vaginal mucosa appears red and inflamed on macroscopic examination, and in severe cases erosions, ulcerations and ecchymotic bleeding may be present. The severe cases may also involve cervix, which then exhibits similar superficial erosions and ulcerations, hyperemia and scattered ecchymotic bleeding [33].

The recommended diagnostic method is a wet mount microscopy of the vaginal fluid, using a scoring system similar to the one in bacterial vaginosis in order to categorize the vaginal microflora into normal microflora and light, moderate and severe case of aerobic vaginitis [29, 30]. The AV score is composite and consists of lactobacillary grade, number of leucocytes, proportion of toxic leucocytes (leucocytes with toxic granulation), background microflora and proportion of parabasal cells. Each of these criteria is assigned points: 0 for absent, 1 for moderate and 2 for severe. The final AV score is then calculated by adding these points. The score of 0–2 means no aerobic vaginitis, 3–4 means light aerobic vaginitis, 5–6 means moderate vaginitis and a score of 7–10 corresponds to severe aerobic vaginitis (Table 9.2).

The most important characteristics distinguishing aerobic vaginitis from bacterial vaginosis, from the view of a pathologist, include the presence of various degrees of mucosal inflammation (severe cases with scattered bleeding points or ulcers) and severely depressed lactobacilli on wet smears (with the presence of chains of cocci, numerous leucocytes, toxic leucocytes and parabasal cells). There are also specific findings in the Gram stain (deficiency of lactobacilli with increased levels of Gram-positive bacteria and Gram-negative small rods from *Enterobacteriaceae*) [33].

Aerobic vaginitis is associated with several significant clinical implications. Firstly, it is often found mixed with other vaginal infections, namely, vulvovaginal candidiasis, bacterial vaginosis and trichomonal vaginitis, resulting in atypical complaints and symptoms which may make the syndromic diagnosis problematic [34, 35]. Secondly, aerobic vaginitis has been associated with various adverse pregnancy outcomes such as increased risk of preterm delivery, premature rupture of fetal membranes, chorioamnionitis and funisitis of the fetus [30, 32].

Table 9.2 The scoring system for the diagnosis of aerobic vaginitis [29, 30]

Sub-score	LBG	No. of toxic leucocytes	Proportion of toxic leucocytes	Background flora	PBC
0	I, IIa	≤10/hpf	None or sporadic	Unremarkable or cytolysis	None or < 1%
1	IIb	>10/hpf and ≤ 10/epithelial cell	≤50% of all leucocytes	Small coliform bacilli	≤10%
2	III	>10/epithelial cell	>50% of all leucocytes	Chains or cocci	>10%
Sub-score: 0 points (criterion absent), 1 point (moderate), 2 points (severe)					
Final AV score: *0–2* means no signs of aerobic vaginitis, *3–4* light aerobic vaginitis, *5–6* moderate aerobic vaginitis and *7–10* severe vaginitis					
PBC—proportion of parabasal cells					
LBG—Lactobacillary grade					
I	Normal vaginal microflora, containing mostly lactobacillary cell types with no or very few coccoid bacteria				
II	Diminished numbers of lactobacilli mixed with other bacteria				
	IIa—slightly disturbed microflora				
	IIb—moderately disturbed microflora				
III	No lactobacilli, microflora is dominated by numerous other bacteria (cocci, anaerobic coccobacilli or small bacilli)				

9.2.1.3 Streptococcus Group B

Group B streptococci (GBS), or *Streptococcus agalactiae*, are considered to be a normal part of the vaginal microflora and as such non-pathogenic in the vagina [36]. Reports suggest that at least 25% of women are regularly colonized with GBS in the vagina and rectum [22]. So far no specific histopathologic changes descriptive of GBS vaginitis have been described.

Unlike the case of GBS vaginitis, GBS morbidity among the obstetrical population is well established. Cervicovaginal colonization with group B streptococci at 23–26 weeks' gestation is associated with an increased risk of preterm birth and delivery of a low-birth-weight infant, while colonization at delivery shows association with neonatal sepsis, although the exact factors determining the risk of developing such complications are still unknown [37]. Other reported complications include intraamniotic infection and endomyometritis [38]. *Streptococcus agalactiae* is also responsible for a number of serious infections in newborns of colonized mothers, including pneumonia, meningitis and septicaemia [39].

9.2.1.4 Streptococcus Group A

Group A beta-haemolytic streptococci (GAS), or *Streptococcus pyogenes*, are an established cause of cellulitis, necrotizing fasciitis, erysipelas, impetigo and puerperal infections. Aside from the well-known soft tissue and skin infections, *Streptococcus pyogenes* also represents one of the rarer causes of vaginitis.

Group A streptococcal vaginitis is usually encountered in prepubescent girls, although reports of findings in adult women are increasing [40, 41]. Clinical symptoms of GAS vulvovaginitis are usually acute and more severe than the signs caused by other types of vaginitis [42]. The most common complaints include vulvar and vaginal pain, often spreading to the perianal regions, pruritus and dyspareunia. The discharge associated with GAS infection is typically copious, malodorous (foul-smelling, with absence of the fishy smell characteristic of BV), yellow and seropurulent in consistency. Vaginal walls may display a marked oedema and erythema.

The diagnosis is usually made by correlating the clinical signs and symptoms with the results of a wet mount and Gram stain and can be confirmed by a culture with overgrowth of group A streptococci. Both wet mount and Gram stain of a vaginal smear usually show numerous polymorphonuclear leukocytes, singlets, doublets or chains of Gram-positive cocci and the absence of lactobacilli [41].

9.2.1.5 Toxic Shock Syndrome (TSS)

Toxic shock syndrome (TSS) is a potentially fatal, acute systemic illness caused by an infection with *Staphylococcus aureus* strains producing toxic shock syndrome toxins (TSST-1) or by *Streptococcus pyogenes* M types I and III (group A beta-haemolytic streptococcus, GABHS) capable of producing streptococcal pyrogenic exotoxin A (SPeA), streptococcal pyrogenic exotoxin C (SPeC), protein cysteine SPeB, mitogenic factor (MF, SPeF) and streptococcal superantigen (SSA) [43, 44]. The interaction of these toxins with the immune system of the host leads to a massive release of pro-inflammatory cytokines including TNF-α, TNF-β, IL-1, IL-2 and IL-6, which are responsible for the severe shock response and resulting organ failure.

Toxic shock syndrome can be divided into menstrual and nonmenstrual cases. The menstrual cases are typically found in the adolescent and fertile female population and are associated with vaginal colonization by *S. aureus*, while the nonmenstrual cases are common in postmenopausal women, men and children [44, 45]. Recently, a relationship between the vaginal microbiota and the risk of TSS has been proposed, suggesting that women with aerobic vaginitis (colonized by *Streptococcus agalactiae* and *Enterococcus* spp.) may be more susceptible to menstrual toxic shock syndrome as the presence of these bacteria significantly induces TSST-1 production [46]. Staphylococcal TSS was first described in the 1980s among young American women using superabsorbent tampons [47]. It is generally more common than streptococcal, which is however reportedly increasing in frequency and characterized by a poor outcome and mortality rate as high as 80% [43, 48, 49].

9.2.2 Fungal Infections

9.2.2.1 Vulvovaginal Candidiasis

Vulvovaginal candidiasis (VVC) is a fungal disease predominantly caused by *Candida albicans*, which is responsible for up to 65–90% of vaginal *Candida* spp. infections, with the non-albicans *Candida* species being responsible for up to 30% of infections [24]. The most common non-*Candida* species found in the vaginal isolates, in descending order, are *C. glabrata*, *C. tropicalis*, *C. parapsilosis* and *C. krusei*. Their clinical significance is given by the fact that while *C. albicans* remains sensitive to azole treatment, non-albicans *Candida* species have shown fluconazole resistance [50–52]. The emergence of *C. glabrata* has been a special cause for concern, as its incidence has been increasing continually since the first reports of a few rare cases in the 1990s [53].

Vulvovaginal candidiasis caused by *Candida* spp. is the second most common vaginal infection, and, according to statistics, up to 70–75% of women of a reproductive age will suffer from at least one clinical episode of VVC [15, 54, 55].

The development of a symptomatic infection first requires the colonization of the vagina with *Candida* spp., which usually occurs by a local introduction of the organism from the perineum and perianal areas through digital or sexual contact. Following the contact, *Candida* adheres to the vaginal epithelium and causes either asymptomatic colonization or, when it switches from its yeast cell morphology to its hyphal form, leads to VVC [56]. The literary prevalence of colonization in asymptomatic women varies, with positive vaginal cultures of *Candida* species being found in 15–37% of asymptomatic women [50]. In a healthy host, there is a balance between *Candida* spp. and the other microorganisms forming the vaginal microbiota, and *Candida* is therefore considered as a commensal organism, well tolerated in low numbers. This balance in the vaginal ecosystem can become disturbed in a number of situations. The predisposing factors include uncontrolled diabetes mellitus (and the role of glycosuria in promoting *Candida* colonization), frequent antibiotic use, high-estrogen oral contraception, hormone replacement therapy and immunosuppression [15, 57].

Typical clinical symptoms of acute VVC include mainly the characteristic vaginal discharge, which is non-malodorous and of a cheesy or curd-like consistency and colour [14]. The most common subjective complaints are of intense vulvar itching, soreness, superficial dyspareunia and dysuria. The gross macroscopic findings include oedema, reddened and erythematous mucosa with possible fissuring and satellite skin lesions.

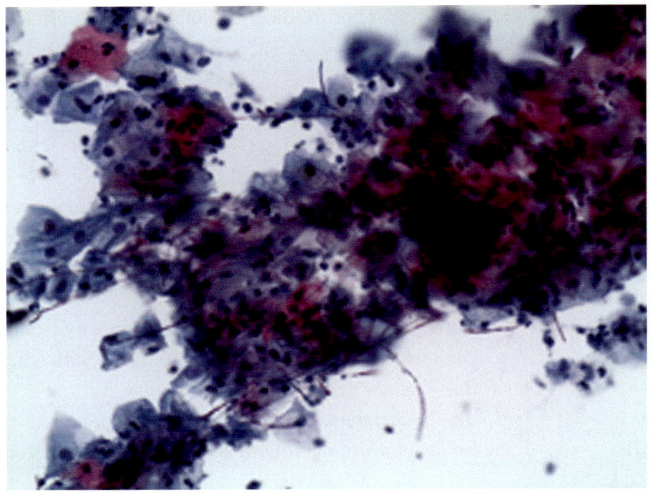

Fig. 9.4 Candida albicans. Numerous yeast and pseudohyphae are present, intermingled with superficial squamous cells (cytology specimen; Papanicolaou staining)

The microscopic diagnosis can be based on an examination of a cytology specimen or wet mount of the discharge or a Gram stain (Fig. 9.4). The presence of blastospores and pseudohyphae is diagnostic of VVC, although their morphologic appearance is not entirely specific and the reported sensitivity of the wet prep exam is only about 65% [12]. Biopsy samples are used rarely in diagnosing vulvovaginal candidosis, but if they are available the main microscopic findings include marked acute neutrophilic infiltration of the epithelium, predominantly mononuclear inflammation and congested blood vessels in the stroma and reactive changes of the squamous epithelium [12, 22]. The superficial layers of the squamous epithelium may show adhering desquamated epithelial cells, which can be intertwined with identifiable pseudohyphae (long, tube-like filaments arranged in parallel with constrictions between the individual cells).

9.2.2.2 Actinomycosis

Actinomyces is a Gram-positive, non-spore-forming, nonmotile and non-acid-fast anaerobic bacterium, which is found as a normal commensal organism in the oral cavity, respiratory tract and gastrointestinal tract. The vagina of up to 27% of healthy, asymptomatic women may also be colonized [22, 58]. The most commonly encountered member of the *Actinomyces* genus is *Actinomyces israelii*, with other relatively common species being *Actinomyces turicensis* (isolated in up to 18.5% of clinical cases of actinomycosis and recently reported as the cause of systemic bacteraemia in a patient with pyometra), *A. naeslundii*, *A. viscosus* and *A. bovis* [59, 60]. The colonization of the vaginal flora is considered to follow a transfer of the organism from the intestine, and infection is usually initiated if there is a local breach of the mucosal barrier. In the pathologic setting, *Actinomyces* has been associated with infections of mainly the female upper reproductive tract (cervicitis, endometritis, tuboovarian and pelvic abscesses); however there was also a reported case of a rare primary involvement of the vulva [58]. Actinomycosis of the female genital tract has a significantly higher prevalence in women with long-lasting intrauterine contraceptive devices [12]. The estimated prevalence of *Actinomyces israelii* infection among women with IUDs is reportedly between 1.6 and 11%, with a strong positive association with the duration of application and with plastic devices without a hormonal or metal load [61]. The length of time the device has spent in the uterine cavity before the development of an infection is variable, but up to 85% of cases reportedly occur after 3 or more years [62].

Actinomycosis of the vagina is uncommon, but it may be observed in women with intravaginal foreign bodies (such as IUDs or suture material). The presence of foreign bodies is considered to enable the overgrowth of actinomycetes and cause vaginitis. The infection is characteristic by its slow, but continuous, progress across anatomical sites leading to the formation of extensive granulomatous, suppurative abscesses which may cause perforations of the skin and drain via multiple sinus tracts. The abscesses are usually surrounded by copious granulation tissue and abundant dense, fibrous scar tissue [63]. If the perforation involves any of the surrounding abdominopelvic organs, fistulas may form between the affected organs. The draining pus contains multiple small, soft yellowish so-called sulphur granules which consist of branching aggregates of the organisms, but are not specific for actinomycosis as they can also be observed with *Nocardia* and fungal infections [64]. The presence of sulphur granules (also called Gupta bodies or actinomycotic drusen) indicates a local tissue reaction to the infection [58].

The clinical presentation associated with infection includes postcoital bleeding, malodorous vaginal discharge, pruritus and in case of abdominopelvic abscesses abdominal pain [22].

The diagnosis of genital actinomycosis may be a difficult one, as the clinical signs are often nonspecific and the use of Papanicolaou-stained cytologic slides reportedly lacks specificity and sensitivity and has a low positive predictive value—for example, in one study of women with actinomycotic abscesses, only half of those with an available Pap smear test were positive for *Actinomyces* [64].

Microscopically, Pap smears typically show the presence of inflammatory cells and characteristic collections of fine, filament-like blue bacterial structures radiating from a dense, basophilic central core [61]. Additional Gram stain and Gomori methenamine silver stain may be used to confirm the presence of *Actinomyces* and distinguish it from pseudoactinomycotic radiate granules that are noninfectious and a common finding in women with intrauterine devices [62]. Pseudoactinomycotic radiate granules (PAMRAGs) are composed of neutral glycoproteins, lipids and calcium, often showing lamination in the centre ("tidewater" marks) and club-like peripheral projections (Fig. 9.5) [65]. They are a specific form of a tissue response to the presence of an IUD and may be frequently found on their own in the absence of an *Actinomyces* infection or sometimes can be identified in the surroundings of actinomycotic sulphur granules.

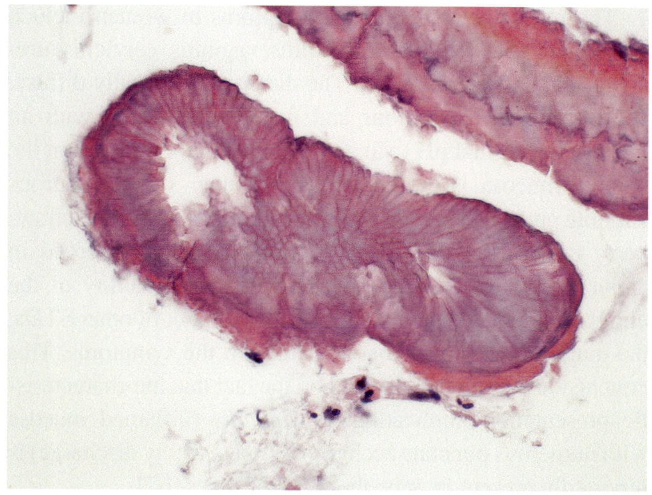

Fig. 9.5 Pseudoactinomycotic radiate granules (PAMRAGs). Note the club-like peripheral projections

Although the finding of sulphur granules surrounded by pus is highly suggestive of actinomycosis, the gold standard for diagnosis remains to be culture, which is unfortunately a lengthy procedure as *Actinomyces* are a fastidious and slow-growing species [66].

9.2.3 Protozoal Infections

9.2.3.1 Trichomoniasis

Trichomoniasis is the most common non-viral, curable sexually transmitted infection in the world [24]. It is caused by *Trichomonas vaginalis*, a flagellated protozoan parasite of the human reproductive system [67]. This extracellular, facultatively anaerobic and obligatory sexually transmitted microorganism is uniquely adapted to the epithelial lining of the human vagina, uterine cervix and both the male and female urethra [68]. In women, *Trichomonas vaginalis* infection may be relatively asymptomatic, but it usually presents as vaginitis and/or cervicitis, while in men it tends to be asymptomatic in the majority of cases.

The most common gynaecologic complications of trichomoniasis include endometritis, adnexitis, pyosalpinx and atypical pelvic inflammatory disease [69]. Trichomoniasis has also been linked to various adverse pregnancy outcomes including premature rupture of membranes, preterm birth and low birth weight [70].

The most common clinical symptoms in women include abnormal vaginal discharge, pruritus, vaginitis, cervicitis, urethritis and dyspareunia [71]. The discharge is usually diffuse, yellow to green in colour and malodorous, often with an increase in vaginal pH (>5). On macroscopic examination the vaginal mucosa is erythematous and may show numerous variable punctate haemorrhages, which led to the term "strawberry cervix" (*colpitis macularis*) and can be observed in about 5–50% of women [72]. Due to the variability of the clinical presentation and similarity to a number of other STDs, the diagnosis cannot be based purely on the symptoms. This conclusion is further supported by the fact that the characteristic presentation implicating *T. vaginalis* (inflamed mucosa with numerous punctate ecchymoses and a frothy discharge) is reportedly present in only about 2% of cases [67].

The gold standard for diagnosis of trichomoniasis is still considered to be the identification of trichomonads by culture in Diamonds medium. However, the cultures require an incubation time of 7 days (although some signs of growth can already be observed after 48 h), which is not desirable in a clinical setting where the proper treatment needs to be administered without unnecessary delay. The alternatives to cultures include the visualization of trichomonads on wet mount and microscopy, combined with a positive whiff test and a vaginal discharge pH of >4.5 [14].

The wet mount of a saline preparation of the vaginal (or cervical) discharge allows for identification of the motile organisms, which are visible as ovoid shapes about 10–20 μm in diameter, with polar flagella which provide the typical jerky swaying motion [12]. This method is simple, easy to access and very cost-effective. Unfortunately, studies show that the sensitivity of microscopic evaluation is rather low (around 60%) and further decreases in cases when there is a delay between the sample acquisition and evaluation, due to the reduction in parasite motility, making it harder to identify. A delay of as little as 10 min can decrease the sensitivity by further 20% [67]. It is also possible to use the Pap smear test, where the organisms appear as pear-shaped cells with a "lancet"-shaped nucleus and red cytoplasmic granules, but its sensitivity for diagnosis is also considered to be poor [22].

Biopsy specimens are uncommon, and if used the organisms are not directly detectable, although there is a variety of inflammatory and reactive changes which may point to their presence. The vaginal squamous epithelium may be spongiotic, with numerous neutrophils which can sometimes form intraepithelial abscesses. The epithelium may show irregular acanthosis with pseudoepitheliomatous hyperplasia. The submucosa often exhibits an inflammatory response, with hyperaemia and a dense, nonspecific chronic inflammatory infiltrate composed predominantly of lymphocytes and plasmocytes [12, 22].

With the wide range of emerging molecular technology methods, providing superior sensitivity and specificity when compared with wet mount examination, the preferred diagnostic methods are shifting towards PCR-based essays and commercially available nucleic acid amplification tests (NAATs). A standard PCR essay was reported to have a sensitivity of 97% and specificity of 98%, and the same authors also mention that the sensitivity of wet mount microscopy in their study reached only 36%, while the sensitivity of culture reached 70% [73].

Recently, immunocytochemistry (ICC) was suggested as another possible diagnostic method, which could be more accessible in the clinical setting of developing countries (where the trichomoniasis epidemic seems to be most pronounced) than the modern techniques of nucleic acid amplification tests (NAATs) and PCR-based essays [74].

9.2.4 Viral Infections

9.2.4.1 Herpes Simplex Virus

Herpes simplex virus (HSV) is one of the most prevalent sexually transmitted infections with an estimated more than 500 million adults globally infected with either HSV type 1 or 2 [75]. In the United States alone, there are approximately 750,000 new cases of genital herpes every year, with a prevalence of 20 million cases [76]. The majority of the genital tract infections have traditionally been caused by the type 2, although HSV-1 is becoming increasingly more common [77]. Most of the cases are clinically asymptomatic, and intermittent asymptomatic viral shedding can occur with genital HSV-2 infection [78].

The classical case of primary symptomatic infection begins with about 3 days to 2 weeks following the exposure. Malaise, fever, vulvar pain and painful reactive inguinal lymphadenopathy are usually the first to occur. Shortly afterwards the first multiple small vesicles begin to appear on the vulva or vaginal and perianal mucosa [76]. The vesicles quickly turn into pustules, and due to the maceration in the moist environment of the vagina, these are replaced by numerous painful ulcers with yellowish-white erythematous base, which can be accompanied by intermittent bleeding and vaginal discharge. The ulcerative phase typically lasts about 10 days. Then the ulcers crust over and begin to heal, leaving no scars. In rare cases, herpetic infection can become chronic and chronic hypertrophic herpetic vulvovaginitis may clinically resemble a neoplasm (or in fact harbour an invasive squamous cell carcinoma) [65].

The microscopic appearance is usually evaluated in cytological smears or biopsies from the base or edges of a fresh ulcer (Tzanck preparation), keeping in mind that in a tissue section the characteristic changes are more commonly present at the edge of the ulcer [22]. The characteristic findings include vesicles involving the entire thickness of the epithelium, with infected cells showing typical bi- or multinucleation and "ground-glass" nuclei (or the subsequent eosinophilic or basophilic intranuclear inclusions, best identified in viable epithelial cells or at the interface between the ulcer and viable epithelium). With the progression of the infection, the vesicles are transformed into ulcers, which are characterized by the presence of a diffuse, full-thickness epithelial necrosis consisting of dead and degenerating epithelial cells. In cases when the edges of the ulcer and the changes at their interface are not readily identifiable, HSV-targeted immunostaining can be of great help in highlighting the infected cells. The dermal stroma underlying herpetic ulcers may show a variable degree of inflammatory infiltrate, which may contain numerous neutrophils. It is also possible to use HSV-targeted in situ hybridization when in need of a diagnostic confirmation.

Although the histopathology of herpetic genital lesions is well described, in clinical settings the diagnosis usually does not require verification by a pathologist and is made based on the typical clinical presentation. Following the primary infection recurrent episodes (or a secondary infection) are fairly common and usually occur with the highest frequency during the first year after the initial infection.

9.2.4.2 Cytomegalovirus

In a healthy immunocompetent host, cytomegalovirus (CMV) infection is usually asymptomatic. If the infection does become clinically apparent, it is most commonly in the form of mononucleosis syndrome, and its association with vulvovaginitis (or cervicitis) is rare [79]. Cytomegalovirus infection, similarly to genital herpes, begins with the eruption of multiple small vesicles which turn into vaginal ulcers, which makes it easily confused with HSV infection, and the frequency of CMV vulvovaginitis is probably underestimated [79]. In HIV-positive patients, the ulcers can also involve the cervix and vulva, and in severe cases of immunosuppression, they can take on an aphthous appearance, often be very deep and even progress to fistulas.

Microscopically, vaginal swabs from the freshly unroofed vesicles show changes involving the entire epithelium. The infected epithelial cells characteristically display one enlarged nucleus, intracytoplasmic inclusions, and, similarly to HSV, intranuclear inclusions can also be observed. The nucleus has been described to have an "owl's eye" appearance due to a peripheral clearing of the chromatin [22]. The diagnosis can be further confirmed by immunohistochemical staining or PCR, especially in cases when the differentiation between HSV and CMV is problematic.

9.2.4.3 Epstein-Barr Virus

The Epstein-Barr virus is a rare cause of painful, ulcerative genital disease, found predominantly in teenage or young adult women [65]. Apart from genital ulcers, other symptoms of the disease include the typical features of mononucleosis (malaise, fever, sore throat) and lymphadenopathy, which may be distant from the site of the ulcers. The onset of genital ulcers may even precede the manifestation of mononucleosis and be the first sign of an active EBV infection. As the vulvar and vaginal pathology tends to be nonspecific, the final diagnosis can be confirmed serologically (by increased titres of antibodies against the viral capsid antigen, early antigen or nuclear antigen) or with the use of PCR. Microscopy of the ulcerated lesions shows infiltration with acute and mononuclear inflammatory cells, while the intact non-ulcerated lesions may display only mild, superficial chronic inflammatory perivascular infiltrate [76].

9.2.4.4 HIV

The prevalence of women among the HIV-infected population has been steadily increasing since the 1980s, when women made up 8% of all AIDS cases reported in the United States, to the 25% reported by the late 1990s. In 2000, women represented about 40% of the infected population worldwide, with almost 12 million female patients with HIV [80].

In women, the genital tract represents the most common acquisition and transmission site of the virus, as well as a reservoir for HIV once the infection has been contracted [81]. Although HIV/AIDS shows no gross or microscopic changes specific to the vagina, recently it has been discussed that in HIV-positive women, the genital tract may become a site of chronic inflammation causing a disruption of the epithelial barrier [82].

The significance of HIV when discussing vaginal infections lies in the synergistic relationship between HIV and other sexually transmitted diseases, as the presence of an STD is considered to increase the risk of both acquiring and transmitting HIV [80, 83]. The factors implicated in contracting the human immunodeficiency virus infection include the inflammation associated with STDs (which may increase the local concentration of immune cells in the vulvovaginal region, allowing for them to be targeted by HIV) and the presence of ulcers in some of the STDs, with the ulcers serving as a gateway for the virus [84].

9.2.5 Genital Manifestations of Other STDs

Sexually transmitted infections comprise a wide range of causative agents and clinical presentations, usually sharing a common feature of involving various parts of the lower genital tract with systemic symptoms and involvement. Many of the infections have been historically well-known and their pathogenesis, manifestation and symptoms well-established by the standards of modern medicine. For the purposes of this chapter, only the vagina-specific morphology and clinical manifestation will be discussed.

9.2.5.1 Genital Ulcer Disease

Syphilis

Syphilis is an ulcerative disease caused by the spirochete *Treponema pallidum*, which can cause significant complications in an untreated individual and has been associated with an increased risk of the acquisition and transmission of the HIV infection [75, 77]. In 2012, the estimated prevalence of syphilis was 18 million cases worldwide, with an estimated incidence of 5.6 million new cases in men and women ages 15–49 globally, making syphilis the least common of the four main curable STDs, the others being chlamydia, gonorrhoea and trichomoniasis [85].

The primary lesion of syphilis is the syphilitic chancre, which is most commonly seen on the skin of the vulva and perianal regions although the vaginal, cervical or oropharyngeal mucosa may also be affected. The presentation of the typically non-painful chancre is followed by a regional lymphadenopathy, fever and malaise, and if left untreated, the rapid systemic dissemination of the pathogen may progress to the secondary (characterized by mucocutaneous rash and papules—condylomata lata) and tertiary stage (leading to the formation of granulomatous lesions—gummas) of the disease [78].

The gross pathology of the chancre is characterized by an indurated ulcer with a typical "punched-out" appearance. Histologically, there is a marked dermal infiltrate of lymphocytes, macrophages and neutrophils, with a perivascular plasmacellular infiltrate accompanied by endothelial swelling and proliferation (also called plasma cell endarteritis) [65, 76]. The edges of the ulcers often show pseudoepitheliomatous epidermal thickening. For the demonstration of the organism within the lesion, silver stains (such as Warthin-Starry or Steiner stain) have traditionally been used, revealing the spirochetes in their typical perivascular distribution. Another method of detection is the dark field examination of secretions expressed from the lesions; however, the rather low sensitivity and often high background of these methods are not ideal, and in doubtful cases the application of immunohistochemical stains is preferable [76, 78].

Condylomata lata, the lesions of secondary syphilis, are typically found on various mucocutaneous surfaces, which in the genital tract may include the vagina although the involvement of the vulva is much more common. The lesions are characterized by a broad morphology with the macroscopic appearance of papules, pustules, macules and hyperkeratotic lesions. Histologically, the early changes are usually observed in the form of perivascular dermatitis with numerous plasma cells in the infiltrate, without any significant changes in the overlying epithelium. With the progression of the disease, the lesions can take on a lichenoid histomorphology with a psoriasiform epidermal hyperplasia, accompanied by a dense, band-like inflammatory infiltrate at the dermoepidermal junction, consisting predominantly of plasma cells, lymphocytes and macrophages. It is not uncommon for this infiltrate to spread and involve the deep vascular plexus. If the lesions are rich in spirochetes (which may be observed as slender, "left-handed" spirals with a length of 6–16 μm), the epidermis may show psoriasiform spongiform pustules containing neutrophils either in the epidermis or in the superficial crusts covering these lesions. The involved vessels may display variable endothelial swelling. The inflammatory infiltrate in late-stage lesions is often of a more granulomatous character, with the presence of epithelioid granulomas [22].

Tertiary lesions occurring in the genital tract are extremely rare, and, if present, they are characterized by gummas with central area of necrosis, surrounded by fibrous lymphohistiocytic infiltrate with numerous plasma cells [76].

Chancroid

Chancroid is a rare infection caused by *Haemophilus ducreyi*, a Gram-negative bacillus which is most prevalent in the tropical and subtropical areas. The typical clinical presentation is a combination of painful genital ulcers and tender suppurative inguinal lymphadenopathy. The gross pathology is characterized by single or multiple erythematous papules, which change into pustules, and following the rupture of the pustule's cover, a shallow ulcer is formed, releasing purulent exudate and revealing a friable, erythematous base with ragged undermined edges [78]. The individual lesions are usually small, measuring approximately 1–2 mm in diameter, and once the lesions become ulcerative, they may form larger confluent areas of up to 3 cm in diameter [12].

Biopsies are not usually required for the diagnosis, which (especially in the endemic regions of the disease) is often made based on the clinical symptoms alone. However, evaluation of the histopathology may be needed when other ulcerative conditions (such as herpes and syphilis) need to be excluded. The microscopic appearance of the chancroid ulcers shows a characteristic three-zone distribution: (1) a superficial zone with neutrophilic infiltrate, fibrin and erythrocytes, (2) a middle zone with vascular changes and a band of granulation tissue and (3) a deep zone with marked lymphoplasmacellular infiltrate [65, 76].

Lymphogranuloma Venereum

Lymphogranuloma venereum (LGV) is caused by the L1, L2 and L3 serotypes of the obligatory intracellular microorganism *Chlamydia trachomatis*. Traditionally, LGV was a disease endemic to tropical and subtropical areas, but in recent years a number of cases have been reported in Europe, North America and Australia [86]. LGV is an ulcerative disease where the first clinical manifestation is situated in the inoculation site, which is mostly the vulva, but an involvement of the vagina is also possible.

Similarly to syphilis, LGV infection progresses in three stages. The first stage occurs at the site of inoculation, beginning with the development of painless, small and shallow genital ulcers or papules [78]. In the vagina, these are most commonly found on the posterior vaginal wall and may be accompanied by a mucopurulent vaginal discharge. The accompanying infiltrate consists of mixed chronic inflammatory cells, with numerous plasma cells, lymphocytes and histiocytes including giant cells [65]. Granulomas can be present. The ulcers are self-resolving and heal without any residual scarring.

The second stage involves the regional lymph nodes and presents as painful lymphadenopathy. In men, inguinal adenopathy is the most common, while only about 20% of infected women present with lymphadenopathy at this site, and the most predominant lymphadenopathy is intra-abdominal or retroperitoneal (when the primary lesion is located on the posterior wall of the vagina), causing a clinically symptomatic anorectal syndrome [87]. The affected lymph nodes are usually matted in clusters (buboes) and frequently rupture spontaneously with the formation of fistulas and sinus tracts. If a biopsy of these lymph nodes is taken, it may reveal a characteristic stellate (or serpiginous) area of necrotizing inflammation, which may be surrounded by areas of acute inflammation with abscess formation, chronic inflammation or a granulomatous inflammation ("suppurating granulomas") [76].

The tertiary state of LGV is a result of untreated infection and comprises local complications due to extensive necrosis and scarring of the affected lymph nodes. The damage to the lymphatic drainage can lead to a local lymphoedema or even in extreme cases elephantiasis of the genitalia [62]. The reparatory process often leads to a fibrotic scarring of the vagina and rectum, resulting in genito-anorectal syndrome, chronic proctitis, rectal stenosis, scarring of the vulva and the formation of strictures and fistulae [87].

Due to the largely nonspecific histopathological findings, the diagnosis can be supported by immunohistochemical staining and is made in correlation with serology (complement fixation tests) and culture.

Granuloma Inguinale

Granuloma inguinale is an ulcerative genital disease otherwise known as donovanosis, caused by the intracellular Gram-negative bacteria *Klebsiella granulomatis*, previously known as *Calymmatobacterium granulomatis*. The primary lesions may be found in the vulva, vagina or cervix following the inoculation through sexual contact or faecal contamination [65].

Macroscopically, the lesions are made up of painless erythematous papules, nodules or progressive ulcers (the most common, ulcerovegetative form of the disease) [62]. The ulcers eventually merge together to form larger areas of hypertrophic, "beefy red" granulation-like tissue with rolled edges, which is highly vascular and frequently bleeds upon contact. In some cases the ulcers persist for a long time (months to years) and may resemble a squamous cell carcinoma in their appearance. Associated inguinal lymphadenopathy is not common with granuloma inguinale (unlike LGV), but it may be mimicked by the formation of subcutaneous, ulcerating abscesses termed pseudobuboes [78].

Smears or biopsy samples taken from the ulcerated lesions consist mostly of granulation tissue, rich in mixed inflammatory infiltrate consisting of neutrophils, macrophages, plasma cells and lymphocytes. The chronic inflammatory infiltrate may extend into the dermis, frequently associated with endarteritis of the dermal vessels. The cytoplasm of some of the macrophages contains the pathognomonic vacuoles with ingested coccoid to bacillary organisms displaying characteristic surrounding halos, called Donovan bodies. In some cases, these may also be observed extracellularly. The Donovan bodies are key to the microscopic diagnosis and can be best visualized on a Giemsa or Warthin-Starry (the appearance of small safety pins) stained slide, which is prepared by pressing the biopsy tissue from the edge of the ulcer between two slides and then staining the imprint. The ulcerated surface is often covered by a fibrinous exudate, with multiple necroses and microabscesses within the epidermis [12, 62, 65, 76]. If left untreated, the natural course of the disease is slow and progressive, and healing of the (often extensive) ulcerations leads to the formation of abundant, disfiguring fibrous tissue which can eventually result in genital mutilation.

9.2.5.2 Discharge-Causing Diseases

Gonorrhoea

Gonorrhoea, a disease caused by the organism *Neisseria gonorrhoeae*, is the second most commonly reported bacterial STD in the United States, with a total of 350,062 cases reported in the United States in 2014 and a national gonorrhoea rate of 110.7 cases per 100,000 population [77]. Literary data estimated the global prevalence of gonorrhoea in 2012 to be 27 million cases, with an estimated incidence of 78 million cases [85].

In the female genital tract, gonorrhoea is associated predominantly with infectious cervicitis and as such plays an important role in the development of pelvic inflammatory disease and also has been associated with various negative pregnancy outcomes [75]. The mucopurulent discharge, one of the main clinical symptoms of gonorrhoeal cervicitis, can sometimes be suggestive of a vaginal infection, but a simple colposcopy exam is usually sufficient to rule out this entity.

Chlamydia Trachomatis

Chlamydia is the most frequently reported bacterial sexual transmitted disease, with the estimated overall worldwide prevalence of 128 million cases and incidence of 131 million new cases a year [85]. In the United States alone, there was a total of 1,441,789 cases of chlamydial infection reported to the CDC in 2014, corresponding to a rate of 456.1 cases per 100,000 population [77]. The significant morbidity associated with this curable STD includes pelvic inflammatory disease, chronic pelvic pain, tubal infertility and increased risk of ectopic pregnancy [75].

The infection is most common in the adolescent population and often clinically asymptomatic. It is a frequent cause of cervicitis, causing a mucopurulent discharge which not unlike in the case of gonorrhoea may mimic bacterial or aerobic vaginitis. On closer inspection however, mucopurulent cervicitis is easily distinguishable from such entities. In some cases, the inflammation may show chronic inflammatory infiltrate, sometimes even leading to follicular cervicitis with multiple subepithelial and periglandular lymphoid follicles in the endocervical mucosa, often with germinal centres [65]. The causative *Chlamydia* microorganisms can be confirmed by immunohistochemical staining. If a biopsy specimen is not available, chlamydial infection can also be observed in a cervical smear. The typical (although not always present) signs include cytoplasmic vacuolization, squamous and glandular cells with a ragged cytoplasmic border (so-called moth-eaten appearance) and a coccal-like background with a few scattered neutrophils. In the case of follicular cervicitis, occasional streaks of lymphocytes and their immature forms may be distinguishable [62].

9.2.6 Parasitic Infections

Parasitic vaginitis has traditionally been a rare entity in developed countries, but the incidence is likely to increase as the global travel and migration increases as well. In the endemic regions of mostly tropical and subtropical climate of Africa, Central America, Middle East and Asia, these infections are encountered much more frequently and constitute an important source of reproductive morbidity in women.

9.2.6.1 Schistosomiasis

Schistosomiasis (or bilharzia) is an intravascular infection caused by the freshwater trematode worms *Schistosoma*, which are endemic especially to the tropical and subtropical regions of Africa, Asia and the Middle East. The transmission occurs when a person is in contact with freshwater contaminated by faeces or urine containing the parasite eggs, which first infect a specific freshwater snail (in case of *S. haematobium* the *Bulinus* snail) serving as an intermediate host from which the infection can be transmitted to humans [88]. Most commonly, female genital schistosomiasis (FGS) is caused by an infection with *S. haematobium* (also termed urinary schistosomiasis, or more recently urogenital schistosomiasis), but there are also reports of genital affliction with *S. mansoni* and *S. japonicum* [89]. The deposition of schistosomiasis eggs follows their transmission into the genital tract, which occurs via blood vessel anastomoses in the pelvic organs. It is assumed that in cases of pure *S. haematobium* genital infection (without the involvement of the urinary tract), the transmission probably occurred due to individual blood vessel patterns, blood flow and the localization of worms.

The lower female genital tract is a common site for the deposition of *Schistosoma haematobium* ova, and it is estimated that probably millions of women may suffer from an undiagnosed genital schistosomiasis. The reported prevalence of FGS in its endemic areas ranges from 33 to 75% [89]. The infection is a significant cause for morbidity, and it has been associated with infertility, preterm delivery, increased risk of extrauterine pregnancy, menstrual disorders and lower abdominal or back pain [90, 91].

The clinical presentation of genital schistosomiasis may be very mild or completely asymptomatic. The most commonly recorded subjective complaints are of a malodorous, bloody or yellow vaginal discharge, dysuria, low abdominal pain, dyspareunia and postcoital bleeding [90]. Other symptoms associated with FGS also include genital itching, stress incontinence and pollakisuria [92]. A serious and debilitating complication of chronic vaginal schistosomiasis is the formation of rectovaginal and vesicovaginal fistulas, often requiring surgical intervention [93].

Colposcopic examination reveals either the characteristic "sandy patches", which are typically located predominantly on the cervix, or polypoid/papillomatous tumour-like prominences and papulae with irregular surface, which are more common to the vaginal walls and vulva [94]. Sandy patches are described as slightly elevated lesions with a characteristic rough, sand-like surface which is gritty on section. The correlating histologic image shows marked areas of fibrosis with disintegrated eggs and only a minimal inflammatory infiltration. On the other hand, the polypoid or papillomatous lesions consist of large masses of mostly viable eggs, with a dense surrounding inflammatory reaction rich in eosinophils. Both sandy patches and polypoid/papillomatous lesions may show epithelial hyperplasia. Erosions and superficial ulcerations of the vagina and vulva have also been described. The infection is characterized by the deposition of eggs, either inside the epithelial layer or inside the connective tissue stroma. The eggs themselves are usually easy to identify due to their characteristic size, shape and a lateral or terminal spine, especially if there is a clinically expressed suspicion of this diagnosis [88]. Careful examination may demonstrate either viable eggs (with mature miracidia containing intact germinal cells) or calcified, non-viable ova. The surrounding tissue reaction ranges from an abundant granulation tissue with numerous newly formed blood vessels and immature fibroblasts to areas of fibrosis. Fibrosis is ultimately considered to be the end-stage pathology in schistosomiasis.

Until recently, the gold standard for diagnosis was considered to be the crushed biopsy of genital tissue (quantitative compressed biopsy technique, QCBT). The tissue is crushed between two glass slides, together with a drop of 0.5% tryptan blue in physiological saline (aiding in the microscopic differentiation between dead and viable eggs) and examined microscopically [90, 93]. However, ethical concerns have been raised about the performance of a diagnostic biopsy, seeing as the procedure is invasive, associated with bleeding and may lead to blood exposure during sexual intercourse between the female and her partner, raising the risk of HIV acquisition and transmission [95]. Also, the focal localization of the eggs means that they might be missed in a crushed biopsy. After the 2010 FGS consensus meeting in Copenhagen, it was established that in endemic areas the presence of at least one of the three defined visual clinical findings is sufficient to make the diagnosis. These findings are (1) aceto-negative single or clustered grains, (2) homogenous yellowish sandy patches and (3) rubbery tubercles or papules [96]. Wet smears and Pap smears may also help in identifying the parasite eggs, but with a reported value of 15%, their sensitivity is rather low [89].

9.2.6.2 Enterobiasis

Enterobiasis is an infection caused by the nematode *Enterobius vermicularis*, also known as pinworm, threadworm or seat-worm. It is the most common helminthic infection in humans, with a prevalence of about 209 million people infected worldwide [97].

Enterobius vermicularis (EV) is considered as a mainly intestinal parasite, living predominantly in the caecum and colon. The gravid females of the parasite migrate to the perianal region at night, where they emerge on the perianal and perineal skin and deposit their eggs [98].

Extraintestinal enterobiasis is a rare presentation of the infection caused by migration of the pinworms into other anatomical locations, most commonly to the female genital tract [99]. Both the upper and lower genital tract may be affected, with a suggested ascending course of pinworm migration which can even reach past the fallopian tubes and ovaries into the pelvic peritoneum or even infect the human embryo [100]. In some cases, EV was identified as the cause of extensive pelvic masses, pelvic pain mimicking endometriosis, pelvic inflammatory disease (necessitating hysterectomy with bilateral salpingo-oophorectomy) and ovarian cysts [97]. The most serious gynaecological complications of invasive female genital tract enterobiasis include bacterial co-infection, infertility, tuboovarian abscess formation, granulomata of the vulva, uterus and ovaries and generalized peritonitis [99, 100].

The proposed mechanism of female genital tract infection is a direct migration of the parasites from the anus and perianal region into the vagina. It has also been suggested that the vagina may serve as a potential reservoir for EV [98].

A variety of clinical symptoms have been reported, ranging from vaginal discharge, vulvar and vaginal itching and postcoital spotting to a severe, distressing nocturnal perineal or vaginal pain [97, 99, 101]. However, the majority of the cases represented an incidental finding in asymptomatic females (>70%).

The diagnosis of a classical *Enterobius vermicularis* infection is based predominantly on the clinical symptoms, typical patient history and the demonstration of the eggs, usually on a piece of a tape that is applied over the anus and left in place over night. In case of genital enterobiasis, live pinworms can sometimes be spotted in either the vaginal introitus or collected from vaginal swabs, usually from the anterior or posterior fornix [97, 102]. Tissue biopsies are not routinely performed for this diagnosis, but the presence of the nematode may be an incidental finding especially in cases of pelvic involvement mimicking malignancy.

The characteristic smear finding is of variable amounts of EV eggs. The inflammation may be mild or severe and is an important sign that the *Enterobius* parasite actually originated in the genital tract rather than contaminated the slide from its usual perianal distribution. The inflammatory infiltrate usually contains numerous neutrophils and cellular debris, and in some cases there are also eosinophils and macrophages present. The eggs have a typical appearance of small, ovoid, flattened objects resembling pumpkin seeds in shape, with dimensions between 20 and 60 μm [103]. The shell of these eggs is characteristically thick, double-contoured and birefringent. Inside the eggs there may be visible coarsely granular embryos or curved larvae in different stages of delivery (entirely inside the egg, partially expelled or completely delivered) [99]. The background may also frequently show reactive and reparative columnar cells, sometimes almost completely obscured by the inflammatory infiltrate. The differential diagnosis includes mainly other parasitic infections (especially *Trichuris trichiura*, *Strongyloides stercoralis*, *S. haematobium* and *Entamoeba histolytica*), but also contaminating materials such as pollen (brown, oval structures measuring approximately 10×2 μm, with refractile smooth walls, an absence of nuclei and internal structures, sometimes forming chains) [103, 104].

9.2.6.3 Other Rare Parasitic Vaginitides

Vaginal amoebiasis is a rarer presentation of *Entamoeba histolytica* infection. Classic amoebiasis affects the large intestine and leads to amoebic dysentery, colitis and development of liver abscesses [105]. *E. histolytica* has an infective cyst stage and a pathogenic, motile trophozoite stage. The trophozoites may form larger aggregates and behave as microemboli, being carried via the bloodstream to other organs (particularly portal circulation), which is considered to be one of the possible ways of extraintestinal spread. However, there are cases of female genital amoebiasis with no documented intestinal infection [106].

The main clinical findings are represented by ulcerative lesions with indurated base located on the vulva, vagina or cervix, the appearance of which may often mimic carcinoma (which in some cases was found together with the amoebiasis-caused ulcer) [105]. The ulcers may be covered by a fibrinopurulent exudate resembling "anchovy sauce", with numerous microscopic trophozoites [22]. Neglected cases of uncontrolled infection have been demonstrated to progress in a locally devastating manner, leading to necrotizing vulvitis requiring a surgical intervention or even a radical vulvectomy [105].

The microscopic diagnosis is most commonly done in cervical or cervicovaginal smear specimens or in a biopsy of the ulcerated lesion. The cytological appearance of the parasite is that of round or ovoid shapes with a diameter of 15–60 μm, with a basophilic staining and clearly defined ectoplasm and endoplasm. The endoplasm has a finely granular structure and shows one of the most typical characteristics of *E. histolytica*—the parasite frequently ingests erythrocytes, which can be visible as orange or pink spheres within the phagocytic vacuoles and greatly aid in establishing the diagnosis of amoebiasis [107]. The ectoplasm on the other hand is less basophilic and more homogenous and often shows a typical "helmet-like" placement covering only about half the surface of the trophozoite, taking on a crescent shape. In some cases the trophozoites might not be well preserved on the slide, and the ectoplasm becomes less distinguishable, giving the appearance of a clear halo around the endoplasm. The nuclei are often placed eccentrically, with a characteristic, central small karyosome, delicate peripheral chromatin and a single unidirected pseudopod [108]. The background of the smears has been described as "dirty", given by the presence of numerous leucocytes, red blood cells, histiocytes, bacteria (frequently with *Trichomonas vaginalis*) and intermixed cell detritus [107].

In tissue sections, the amoebic penetration through the vaginal mucosa causes extensive cell necrosis. The very commonly occurring secondary bacterial infection leads to frequently observed purulent sloughing of the mucosa and the dense inflammatory infiltrate in the submucosa [106].

9.3 Other Benign Disorders of the Vagina

9.3.1 Malacoplakia

The term "malacoplakia"is derived from the Greek "malakos" (soft) and "plakos" (plaque), first described in 1901 by von Hansemann. Malacoplakia is a rare granulomatous disease caused by impaired macrophage response, most commonly involving the urinary tract. The etiology and pathogenesis of malacoplakia is still not fully understood, but it is proposed that it is associated with immunosuppression, infection and systemic illnesses. An important role is played by some bacteria, such as *Escherichia coli*, *Proteus*, *Mycobacterium tuberculosis* and *Staphylococcus aureus*, but it is clear that other factors must contribute as well, since these infections are much more common than malacoplakia itself. Malacoplakia could therefore be the result of improperly functioning lysosomes, probably caused by a low level or deficit of cyclic guanosine monophosphate and/or β-glucuronidase (both essential to efficient lysosomal bactericidal activity), leading to the incomplete removal of bacteria and the persistence of bacterial residues within the phagolysosome [109].

9.3.1.1 Gross and Microscopic Features

In the vagina, malacoplakia typically forms yellow polypoid nodules arising from the vaginal mucosa, sometimes accompanied by a vaginal discharge [8]. They may also present as a mass lesion. Microscopically, the lesion is characterized by the accumulation of histiocytes with abundant granular to pale foamy cytoplasm (von Hansemann cells) (Fig. 9.6). There are also numerous interspersed plasma cells, lymphocytes and a variable numbers of intracellular and extracellular concentrically laminated basophilic masses (Michaelis-Gutmann bodies), scattered in a scant fibrous stroma, infiltrated with lymphoid cells. Michaelis-Gutmann bodies are supposed to arise from the mineralization of calcium and iron salts on residual microorganism glycolipids. They are pathognomonic of malacoplakia and their finding is fundamental for the diagnosis [109]. The

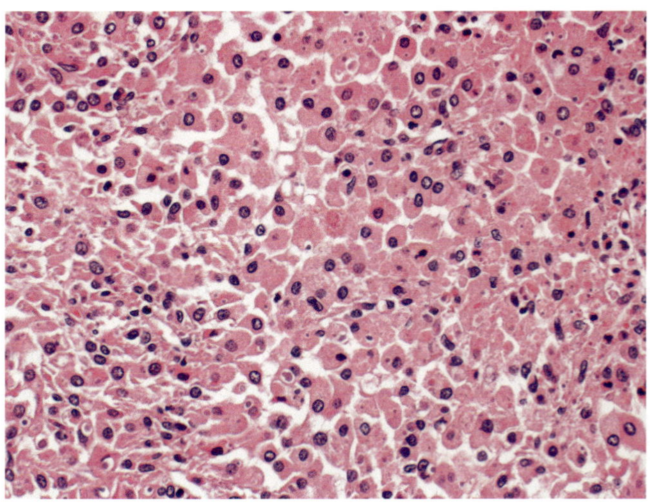

Fig. 9.6 Malacoplakia. The lesion is characterized by the accumulation of numerous histiocytes with abundant cytoplasm. Numerous amphophilic or basophilic laminated bodies (Michaelis-Gutmann bodies) can be seen

correct diagnosis may be supported by the finding of degenerating bacteria on tissue Gram stain, silver stain or by electron microscopy [8]. In a final "end-stage", malacoplakia may show significant scarring, making the aforementioned pathognomonic cells difficult to identify.

9.3.1.2 Differential Diagnosis

The differential diagnosis includes nonspecific granulomatous inflammation and haematopoietic neoplasms, with which malacoplakia may rarely coexist. As previously noted, the finding of Michaelis-Gutmann bodies establishes the diagnosis. Concurrent haematopoietic diseases can be excluded by careful analysis of the density, phenotype and distribution of the non-histiocytic populations.

9.3.2 Trauma and Iatrogenic Injury

9.3.2.1 Trauma

Vaginal lacerations can occur in association with an injury to the pelvic area (in particular in pelvic fractures), in penetrating injuries, and after vaginal delivery, especially with instrumental deliveries. An episiotomy, a surgical cut of the vagina and perineum, may prevent serious tears during childbirth, but on the other hand, an episiotomy guarantees perineal trauma and sutures. Patients with vaginal lacerations present with abnormal vaginal discharge or intermenstrual bleeding.

Tampon use may also cause ulcerations of the vaginal mucosa, and in rare cases toxic shock syndrome has been described. Tampon ulcer is typically a single ulcer with an irregular border of granulation tissue, mostly localized in one of the vaginal fornices [110]. Microscopically, the ulcers may contain fibrillar foreign bodies within the exudate, and the ulcers heal spontaneously within 2–3 months after ceasing tampon usage (Figs. 9.7 and 9.8) [110]. The pathogenic mechanism for the association of tampons with toxic shock syndrome is not well understood. Menstrual toxic shock syndrome is thought to be associated with colonization by toxic shock syndrome toxin-1 producing *Staphylococcus aureus* in women with insufficient antibody titres [111]. One of the proposed mechanisms is that tampon use further enables the production of toxic shock syndrome toxin-1 by exposing the vagina to more oxygen [112].

9.3.2.2 Fistula

Vesicovaginal and ureterovaginal fistulas are a rare complication of female pelvic surgery, most commonly the result of gynaecological surgery. Other causes include radiotherapy, injury during the healing process or severe pelvic pathology (such as pelvic tumour, trauma, congenital anomalies, foreign body and abscess). In developing countries genitourinary fistulas are most commonly related to childbirth [113].

Fistulas are usually painless and result in the leakage of urine from the vagina, which might be either intermittent or, more characteristically, continuous. They can cause vulvar irritation or more serious recurrent infections or pyelonephritis which can be the cause of renal insufficiency. Microscopically, little or no epithelial lining, variable amounts of granulation tissue, fibrosis and chronic inflammation can be seen. Infrequently, vaginal calculi which originate from the deposition of urinary salts in the vagina may be present.

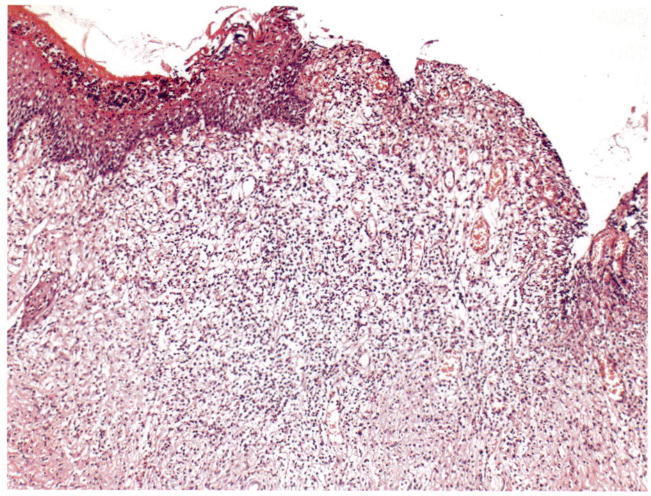

Fig. 9.7 Chronic tampon ulcer. The epidermis at the edge of the ulcer is irritated, with numerous mixed inflammatory cells. Granulation tissue is apparent in the area of ulceration, with numerous vessels and pronounced inflammation

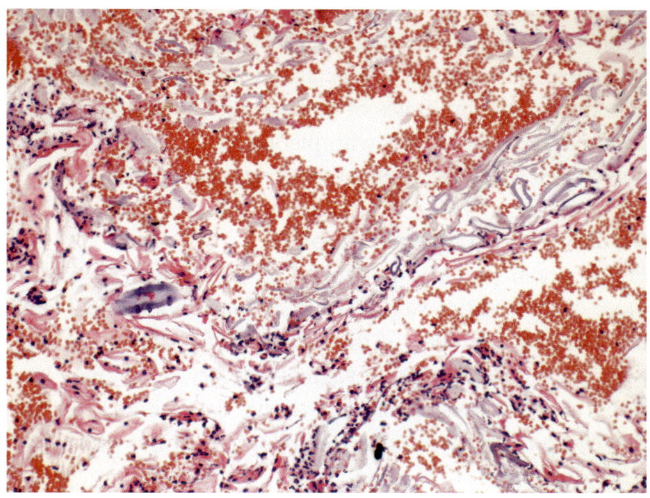

Fig. 9.8 Foreign (tampon) material. The fragments of tampon fibres intermingled with squamous cells, leucocytes and erythrocytes

9.3.2.3 Radiation

The vaginal alterations after radiotherapy may be divided into acute or chronic postradiotherapy reaction. The acute reaction occurs during or immediately after radiotherapy, and acute changes may include mucosal inflammation, hyperaemia, epithelial denudation leading to ulceration and endothelial injury causing small-vessel thrombosis, oedema and smooth muscle necrosis [114]. The chronic postradiotherapy changes largely follow the general principles of chronic treatment complications and occur later than 3 months post radiotherapy. These reactions include changes in the microvasculature, with the loss of capillaries and impaired microcirculation, and changes in the vaginal mucosa caused by increased collagen production in the submucosal fibromuscular connective tissue. This leads to secondary atrophic changes of the vaginal mucosa, obliteration of the muscle and vasculature resulting in hypoxia, tissue atrophy and fibrosis with a shortening and stenosis of the vagina [114]. Eventually, ulceration, necrosis and fistulae can develop. Pathological dilation of capillaries also results in telangiectasias, which are prone to bleeding. In addition to these more general changes, treatment-related loss of ovarian function and consequent hormonal insufficiencies can augment the mucosal alterations.

Microscopically, atrophic mucosa with thinned epithelium may be seen, along with fibrosis, vascular changes with obliteration and thrombosis. The dilation of small blood vessels lined with plump endothelial cells containing large nuclei with vesicular chromatin may also be observed. There may also be variable infiltrates of plasma cells, granulation tissue and bizarre stromal cells with pleomorphic, hyperchromatic nuclei which may be scattered within the stroma (Fig. 9.9).

9.3.2.4 Pelvic Organ Prolapse

Pelvic organ prolapse is defined as the descent of one or more of the anterior vaginal wall, the posterior vaginal wall, the uterus or the apex of the vagina [115]. The prolapse is principally associated with vaginal delivery, which may lead to pelvic floor muscle and connective tissue injury, but the cause of prolapse is multifactorial. Hysterectomy, pelvic surgery and conditions associated with increased intra-abdominal pressure (including obesity, chronic cough, constipation and repeated heavy lifting) also contribute to prolapse. Its prevalence increases with age, and it may occur in up to 50% of parous women.

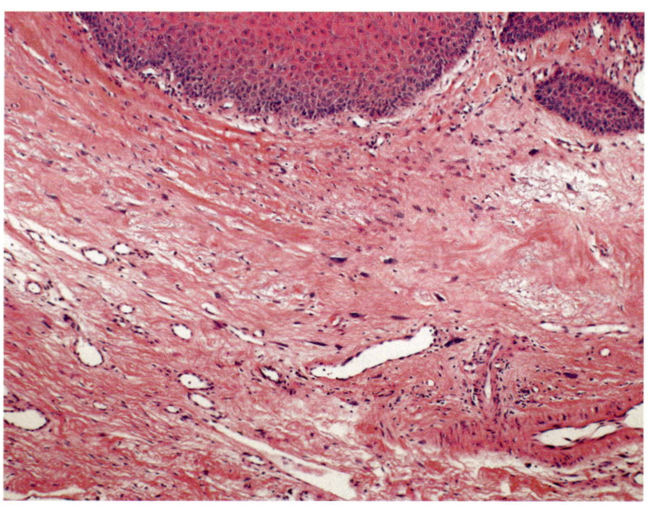

Fig. 9.9 Postradiotherapy changes. There is a fibrosis of lamina propria with increased amount of elastic fibres, dilatation of capillaries and mild chronic inflammatory infiltrate. Stromal cells with hyperchromatic atypical nuclei are scattered within the stroma

The prolapse is either asymptomatic or presents with various symptoms including vaginal bulge, pelvic pressure and incontinence. Microscopically, vaginal mucosa presents variable degrees of acanthosis, hyperkeratosis or parakeratosis; sometimes erosions or reparative changes can be seen. Treatment options include observation, surgery and the use of vaginal pessaries. The surgical options are reconstructive pelvic surgery with or without mesh augmentation and obliterative surgery [116].

9.3.3 Emphysematous Vaginitis

Emphysematous vaginitis is a rare condition, characterized by the presence of multiple, discrete, gas-filled cystic cavities in the vaginal mucosa and on the exocervix. It is a benign, self-limited disease with a benign clinical course. Its etiology is not completely understood, but it is proposed that it could be an unusual manifestation of a common vaginal infection in immunocompromised patients [117]. Although a number of microorganisms have been studied, a confirmed relationship with emphysematous vaginitis has only been found for *Trichomonas vaginalis* and *Gardnerella vaginalis* [118].

The lesions present as variably sized nodules (gas-filled bubbles), most commonly in the upper two thirds of the vagina and/or on the cervix, on occasion producing crepitus or a "popping sound" which relieves the pressure sensation. Chemical analyses of the gaseous content show a wide variety of gases, with high proportions of nitrogen and oxygen and smaller proportions of carbon dioxide, sulphur dioxide and argon [118]. The patients mostly present with symptoms of pruritus and vaginal discharge, although some are aware of popping sounds during sexual intercourse. Microscopically, the lesion is characterized by variably sized cysts in the stroma, which may be empty or contain pink, hyaline-like material. The cysts are mainly located in the outermost portion of the lamina propria in the subepithelial space and are lined by either multinucleated giant cells, squamous cells or both and accompanied by minimal chronic inflammatory cell infiltrate (Fig. 9.10a, b) [8].

9.3.4 Desquamative Vaginitis

Desquamative inflammatory vaginitis is a rare form of chronic vaginitis, characterized by yellow discharge, vaginal irritation and dyspareunia. The vaginal walls show signs of inflammation with increased erythema and petechiae, mainly

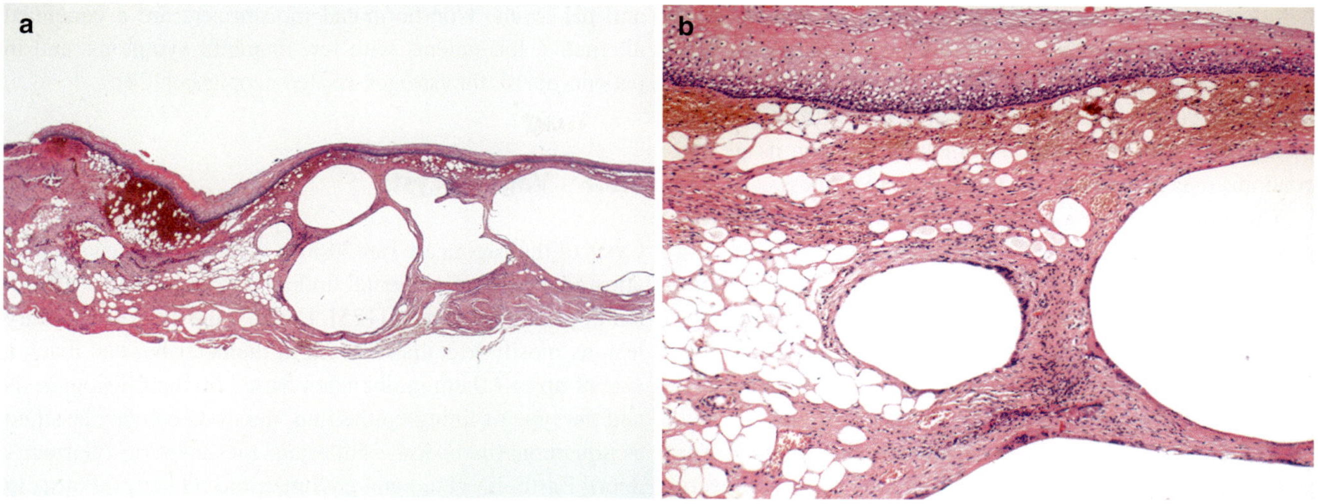

Fig. 9.10 Emphysematous vaginitis. Low-power view showing numerous variable-sized empty spaces located in the vaginal wall (**a**). Some of the cysts are lined by multinucleated giant cells. There is a mild focal chronic inflammatory infiltration in the stroma (**b**)

in the upper half of the vagina. Occasionally, erythematous papules with a pale centre or pseudomembranes are seen [119]. Symptoms and signs are nonspecific, and the diagnosis of desquamative vaginitis follows the exclusion of a wide range of all other disorders causing erosion (such as pemphigus vulgaris, lichen planus and pemphigoid). Infectious forms of inflammatory vaginitis also need to be carefully ruled out. Microscopically, the affected vaginal mucosa shows only a nonspecific inflammatory reaction. The vaginal discharge is usually copious, purulent to haemorrhagic with a high proportion of parabasal cells and numerous neutrophils. The vaginal flora is abnormal with lower levels or a loss of lactobacilli and their replacement by other organisms (mainly Gram-positive cocci and/or *Escherichia coli*) but is frequently negative for infectious pathogens [120]. The vaginal pH is always elevated above 4.5 [119]. Desquamative vaginitis usually affects premenopausal and perimenopausal women, with normal serum estrogen levels.

The etiology of the disease remains unknown, although a number of different etiologies have been suggested to play a key role in the pathogenesis. These include, for example, a bacterial infection, but no single bacterial or viral agent has been identified by culture. Kallikrein-related peptidases (serine proteases which play a crucial role in skin desquamation) have also been considered in the pathogenesis [121]. Due to the overlap of some of the symptoms and signs with other immune-mediated vaginal diseases (such as lichen planus and pemphigus), and the favourable response to anti-inflammatory agents, there is a suggestion that the etiology could be immune mediated, but the serologic studies needed to confirm an immune basis of the disease have not been forthcoming [119]. Desquamative vaginitis is commonly treated with vaginal clindamycin and local vaginal corticosteroids, with clinical improvement in more than 86% of patients [119].

9.3.5 Vaginal Calculus

Vaginal calculi are rare and can be classified as primary or secondary, depending on the presence or absence of a foreign body nidus. Primary vaginal calculi are more common than secondary calculi and originate from the deposition of urinary salts in the vagina without an obvious nidus. They can be caused by various etiological factors, such as vesicovaginal and urethrovaginal fistulas, congenital anomalies of the genitourinary tract or pelvis radiotherapy, vaginal outlet obstruction (acquired or congenital) and neurogenic bladder [122].

Primary vaginal calculi are usually associated with an infection with urease-producing bacteria, changing the normally acidic pH of the vagina to alkaline and therefore predisposing the precipitation of triple phosphate (struvite) calculi [123]. Secondary vaginal calculi result from the crystallization of urinary constituents around a foreign body in the vagina. In exceptionally rare cases, a preexisting bladder calculus may travel into the vagina through the vesicovaginal septum and become a secondary vaginal calculus [123]. Vaginal calculus can act as a foreign body, and it can reach such dimensions that it obstructs the whole vagina, with the resulting pressure on other organs causing obstruction of the bowel or urinary tract.

9.3.6 Atrophic Vaginitis

Atrophic vaginitis is a form of vaginitis caused by estrogen deficiency. It occurs in postmenopausal women as a physiologic event or in premenopausal women where it is caused by iatrogenic or otherwise mediated decrease of estrogen levels (administration of anti-estrogen medication as a part of the treatment for breast cancer, endometriosis, leiomyoma or infertility; chemotherapy- or radiotherapy-induced ovarian failure; premature ovarian failure; endocrine or immunologic disorders). Some women may develop atrophic vaginitis postpartum due to the loss of placental estrogen or while breastfeeding due to the antagonistic action of prolactin on estrogen production. Some medications, smoking, tampon usage and condoms may also cause or worsen vaginal dryness.

The atrophic mucosa is thin and dry, with a loss of glycogen and a lack of lactobacilli, thus leading to the increase of vaginal pH, followed by changes in the vaginal flora. Transudation through the vaginal epithelium is reduced. Due to these changes, the thin, atrophic vaginal mucosa is more susceptible to injuries and infection from pathogenic bacteria such as staphylococci, group B streptococci and *E. coli*. Simple atrophy can thus transform into atrophic vaginitis. The patients may be asymptomatic, or there may be symptoms of vaginal dryness, itching, irritation, mucosal bleeding, dyspareunia and sometimes watery discharge. The vaginal mucosa is macroscopically pale, shiny smooth with a loss of rugal folds and easily traumatized. Often, inflammation with patchy erythema and petechiae may be present. Microscopically, there is a reduction or a loss of the superficial and intermediate cell layers; the epithelium may be thinned to six to eight layers of parabasal cells that may also predominate in cytologic vaginal smears (Fig. 9.11). Sometimes the degenerative features of parabasal cells can mimic dysplasia, which has to be excluded. There may be small ulcerations with acute inflammation interspersed among regions of intact atrophic epithelium. The submucosa is infiltrated by variably dense infiltrates of mononuclear inflammatory cells. Both systemic and topical estrogen treatments are effective in the treatment for relieving the symptoms of atrophic vaginitis, but topical vaginal estrogen is preferred because of the low systemic absorption and reduced risk of adverse effects when compared with oral therapy. The response to estrogen therapy is usually good, with epithelial cell maturation and a return of premenopausal flora and pH levels. Non-hormonal moisturizers are a beneficial alternative for patients with few or minor symptoms and in patients at risk for estrogen-related neoplasia [124].

9.3.7 Vaginal Cysts

Cysts of the vagina are rare lesions which can be asymptomatic and represent incidental finding or can present as a vaginal or paravaginal mass [125]. Usually, the cysts are solitary lesions mostly less than 2.0 cm in diameter but can reach a size of up to 7.0 cm in diameter. Based on their histogenesis and the type of lining epithelium, the cysts can be classified as squamous inclusion, Müllerian, mesonephric (Gartner's duct), Bartholin gland and endometrioid. Other rare cysts in this area include the paravaginal/paraurethral cyst caused by an ectopic ureterocele and the paravaginal epidermoid cyst.

9.3.7.1 Squamous Inclusion Cyst

The squamous inclusion cyst is the most common vaginal cyst, which is usually secondary to episiotomy or surgical procedure. The size of these cysts varies from a few millimetres to several centimetres. Microscopically, the cyst is lined by stratified squamous epithelium. The cyst can be filled with keratin from desquamated squamous cells (Fig. 9.12).

9.3.7.2 Mesonephric (Gartner's Duct) Cyst

Mesonephric cyst is usually lateral or anterolateral and can be single or multiple. This cyst accounts for about 10% of vaginal cysts. It arises from a persistent, vestigial form of Wolffian ducts. The size varies from a few millimetres to several centimetres. Microscopically, the cyst is lined by bland-appearing cuboidal cells lacking cilia or intracellular mucin production (Fig. 9.13a, b). This feature is particularly helpful in the differential diagnosis against Müllerian cyst.

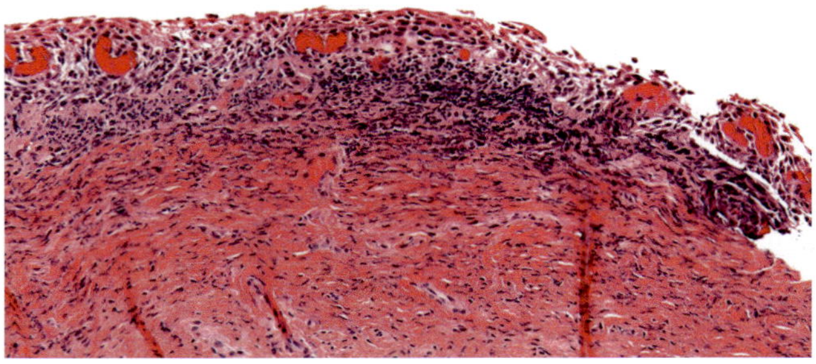

Fig. 9.11 Atrophic vaginitis

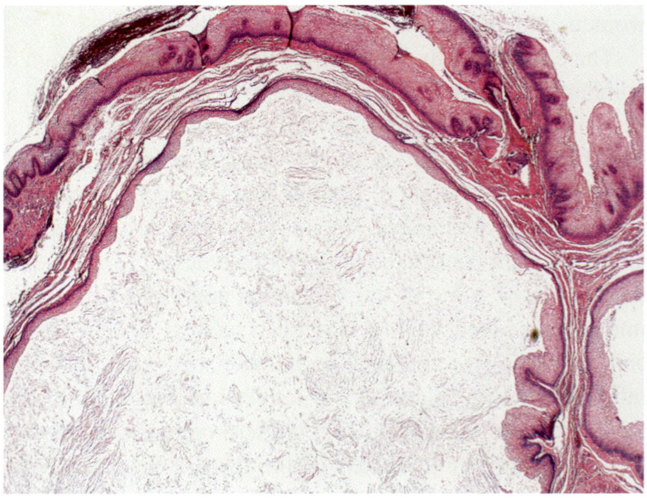

Fig. 9.12 Squamous inclusion cyst. The cyst is lined by a stratified squamous epithelium. Inside the cyst there is a keratin material

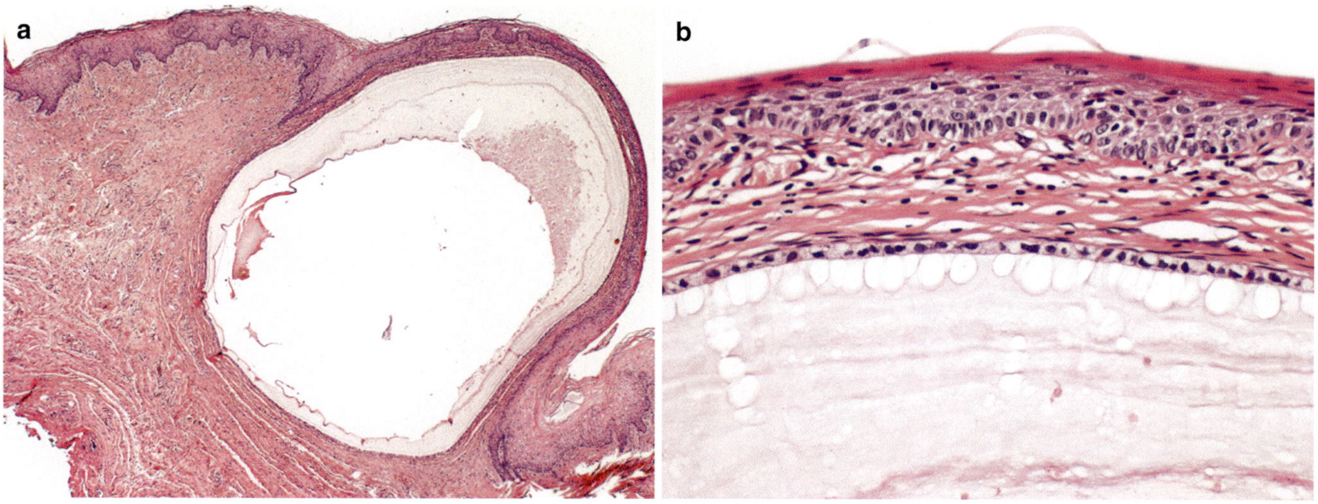

Fig. 9.13 Mesonephric (Gartner's duct) cyst. Unilocular cyst located directly beneath the superficial mucosal epithelium, containing eosinophilic material (**a**). The cyst is lined by a single row of cuboidal epithelium lacking cilia (**b**)

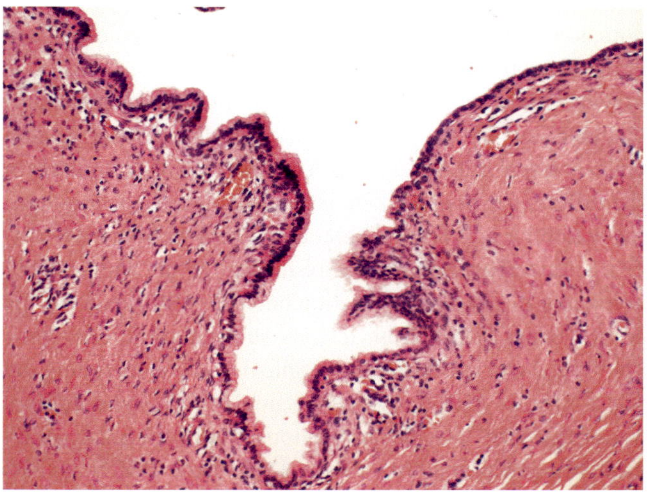

Fig. 9.14 Müllerian cyst. The cyst is lined by mucinous epithelium; however, any Müllerian type of epithelium can occur

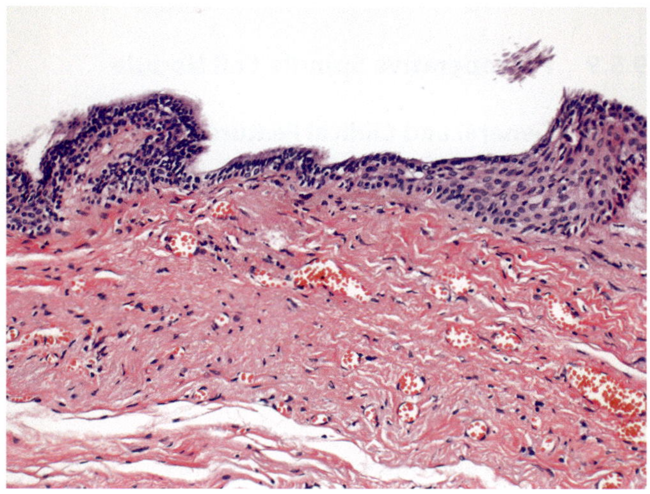

Fig. 9.15 Bartholin gland cyst. The cyst is partly lined by mucinous epithelium similar to the epithelium of normal Bartholin gland duct. On the right side metaplastic squamous epithelium is seen

9.3.7.3 Müllerian Cyst

Müllerian cysts usually present as small (up to 2 cm) midline cystic masses. Microscopically, the cysts may be lined by any type of Müllerian epithelium, including mucinous, ciliated tubal and endometrial (Fig. 9.14). Squamous metaplasia may occur.

9.3.7.4 Bartholin Gland Cyst

Bartholin gland cyst occurs in the distal part of vagina, near the opening of the Bartholin gland duct into the vestibule. This cyst is usually associated with occlusion of the duct, due to mucus retention, inflammation or trauma. Microscopically, the lining epithelium can be mucinous, squamous or transitional in type (Fig. 9.15). Commonly, all types of epithelium may be found within a single lesion. Inflammatory changes are not uncommon.

9.3.8 Vaginal Granulation Tissue

Granulation tissue occurring in the vagina is a common finding, especially after hysterectomy. It can, however, also be found in other settings such as mesh implants for uterine prolapse or can be associated with local trauma [126]. Grossly, granular or polypoid, single or multiple, reddish and sometimes haemorrhagic lesions are present. Clinically it may cause bleeding or discharge. Histologically, the lesion shows the typical features of nonspecific granulation tissue, which is highly vascular with pronounced inflammatory infiltrate including neutrophils, lymphocytes, plasma cells and macrophages (Fig. 9.16). It can contain scattered bizarre stromal cells that may lead to confusion with a malignant neoplasm, particularly if the previous hysterectomy has been performed due to a malignant tumour.

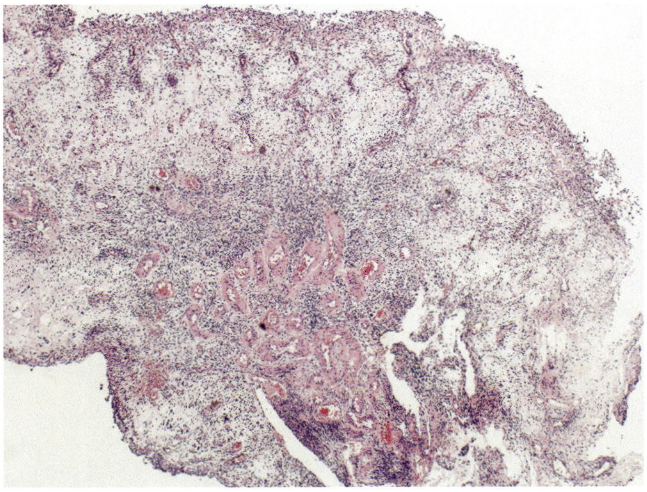

Fig. 9.16 Granulation tissue. Polypoid arrangement of granulation tissue with stromal oedema, pronounced vascularization and multiple mixed inflammatory cells

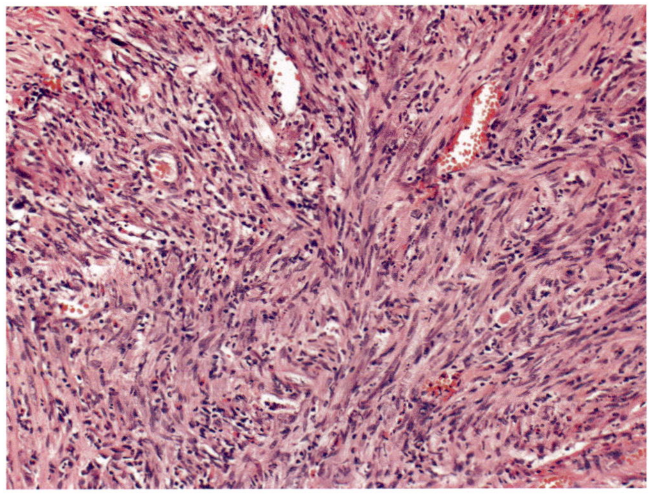

Fig. 9.17 Postoperative spindle cell nodule. The lesion consists of proliferation of spindle cells with bland nuclei, forming fascicles. Scattered inflammatory cells are present in the background

9.3.9 Postoperative Spindle Cell Nodule

9.3.9.1 General and Clinical Features

The postoperative spindle cell nodule (PSCN) is a rare benign lesion of the lower urogenital tract, mostly occurring in the urinary bladder [127]. The lesion is mostly preceded by instrumentation, usually a surgical procedure, and arises within 1–3 months after surgery (in the upper vagina it usually follows a vaginal hysterectomy, whereas in the lower vagina it usually follows an episiotomy). However, cases without such association may occur.

9.3.9.2 Gross and Microscopic Features

Grossly, they are soft sessile or polypoid masses that are typically less than 5 cm in greatest dimension. Microscopically, the lesion consists of the non-neoplastic proliferation of spindle cells forming intersecting fascicles, small blood vessels, myxoid stroma and scattered various inflammatory cells (Fig. 9.17) [127, 128]. The lesional cells show bland nuclei. Mitotic activity can be brisk (more than 25 mitoses/10 HPF); however, no atypical mitoses should be present. Immunohistochemically, the lesions express vimentin, actin and cytokeratins in most cases, in about 50% of cases desmin and rarely EMA. It is usually poorly circumscribed and may infiltrate the adjacent tissue to a limited degree. There may be superficial ulceration, acute superficial and deeper chronic inflammatory cells scattered within the lesion, along with foci of haemorrhage and oedema.

9.3.9.3 Differential Diagnosis

The most important differential diagnosis includes sarcomatoid carcinoma, sarcoma and inflammatory myofibroblastic tumour (IMT). The distinguishing between PSCN and sarcomatoid carcinoma can be difficult, as the lesions share some morphological and immunohistochemical features; however, in contrast to PSCN, sarcomatoid carcinoma is characterized by the presence of markedly atypical spindle cells, atypical mitoses and actin negativity. Other tumours in the differential diagnosis include sarcomas, especially leiomyosarcoma and Kaposi sarcoma. These tumours are also characterized by the presence of nuclear atypia and possibly atypical mitoses. The distinction between PSCN and IMT is controversial [129]. Both lesions showed significant morphological and immunohistochemical overlap, including the possibility of ALK-1 overexpression [130]. Some authors prefer the term "pseudosarcomatous myofibroblastic proliferation", encompassing both IMT and PSCN [130]. However, this is disputable as IMT is usually not associated with any previous surgery and in about 1/3 of cases can recur. Recurrence is not a feature characteristic of PSCN. Moreover, PSCN is usually small (<1 cm) and IMTs tend to be larger.

9.3.10 Prolapsed Fallopian Tube

Fallopian tube prolapse is an uncommon complication caused by either an abdominal or, more commonly, a transvaginal hysterectomy. The patients usually present with pain, vaginal discharge or bleeding. During colposcopy, a red haemorrhagic granular mass can be visible in the vaginal vault, resembling granulation tissue or a tumour [131]. Histologically, the tissue is composed of complex epithelial proliferation, which is commonly polypoid, with tubular and papillary pattern and inflammation in the fibrovascular stroma. The fimbriae are usually not apparent. The epithelial cells are typical of the fallopian tube, including the ciliary,

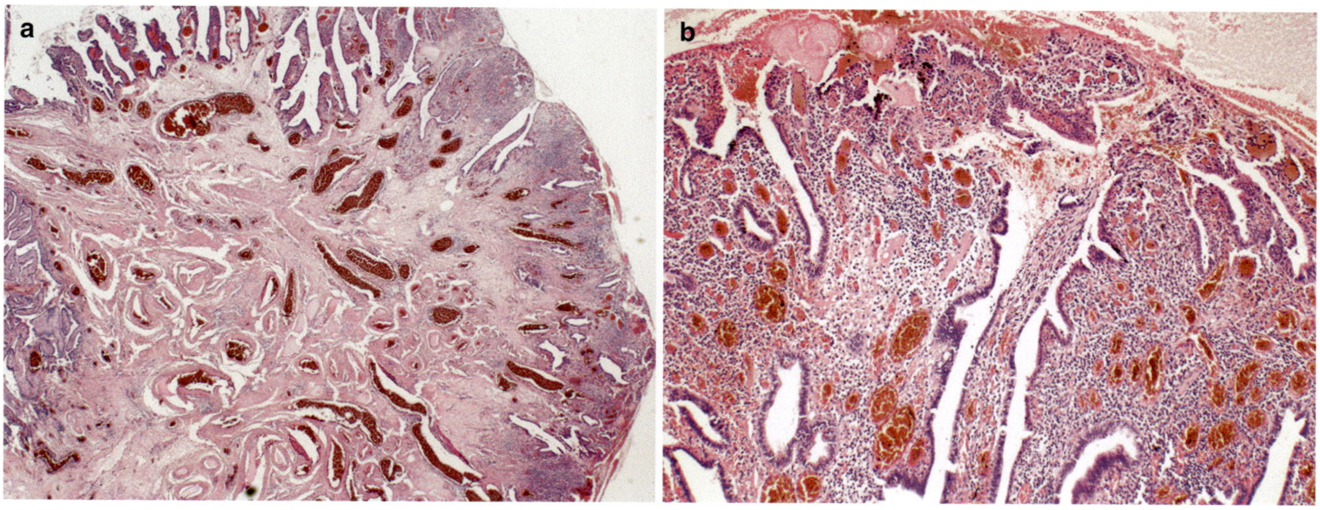

Fig. 9.18 Fallopian tube prolapse. Polypous arrangement of prolapsed Fallopian tube with partly blunted plicae (**a**). The architecture of normal tube is distorted; however, the epithelium is typical of Fallopian tube with the predominance of secretory- and ciliated-type cells (**b**)

secretory and intercalated cells. The differential diagnosis includes endometriosis, vaginal adenosis and primary or metastatic adenocarcinomas. The most important differential diagnosis is against the adenocarcinoma. In this context, the history of the hysterectomy is helpful. Microscopically, the presence of underlying smooth muscle bundles and typical fallopian tube epithelium is characteristic; however, distortion of the normal fallopian tube structure is usually present, including degenerative changes, nuclear crowding, atypia and epithelial hyperplasia due to chronic irritation and inflammation (Fig. 9.18a, b). In these cases, achieving a correct diagnosis can be more difficult [132, 133].

9.3.11 Vaginal Stromal Sclerosis

Vaginal stromal sclerosis represents a change which may be associated with vaginal atrophy [134]. Clinically, it is characterized by the presence of single or multiple plaques or nodules which are firm in consistency. Histologically, the characteristic feature is stromal sclerosis with prominent elastosis, merging imperceptibly with surrounding stroma without an apparent "grenz zone". This can be helpful in the differential diagnosis of some benign stromal tumours occurring in this area, such as myofibroblastoma. Other entities should be considered as well, including amyloidosis and ligneous vaginitis. Amyloidosis of the vagina is usually part of a generalized disease; however, it rarely can occur as a localized disease [135]. Special stains (Congo red, Sirius red) will rule out this possibility. Ligneous vaginitis can occur in patients with plasminogen deficiency [136]. Histologically, homogenous, eosinophilic, fibrin-rich deposits in subepithelial and/or perivascular location are present, associated with chronic inflammatory changes [137].

9.3.12 Fibroepithelial Polyps

9.3.12.1 General and Clinical Features

Fibroepithelial polyps (FP) of the vagina are benign, uncommon lesions that are cured by simple excisions [138, 139]. Approximately 20–25% of FP occurs in pregnant patients, and about 10% of patients have a history of hormonal therapy. The pathogenesis is not well understood, but these lesions probably represent a reactive hyperplastic process which can be hormonally dependent [140]. Most cases are hypocellular, and in these cases, the diagnosis is usually straightforward; however, there are some histologic features which can be suspicious of malignancy, including hypercellularity, increased mitotic activity, atypical mitoses and nuclear atypia.

9.3.12.2 Gross and Microscopic Features

Mostly, these lesions are solitary but may occasionally be multiple. Most lesions are less than 4 cm in greatest dimension, although occasional polyps may be as large as 10 cm. Microscopically, the lesions consist of stromal and epithelial component (Fig. 9.19a–d). The epithelial component, composed of stratified squamous epithelium, is usually intact but may be hyperplastic (i.e. with acanthosis and/or hyperkeratosis). The stromal component shows a much more potentially variable appearance. Typically, the stroma is hypocellular and oedematous, with prominent vessels. Rarely, the stroma can be myxoid. Stromal cells are spindle or stellated and commonly multinucleated. In some cases, nuclear atypia may be present including bizarre hyperchromatic or vesicular nuclei. Increased mitotic activity of more than ten mitoses per ten high-power fields can be found, including atypical mitoses. Cases associated with increased stromal cellularity are designated as "cellular pseudosarco-

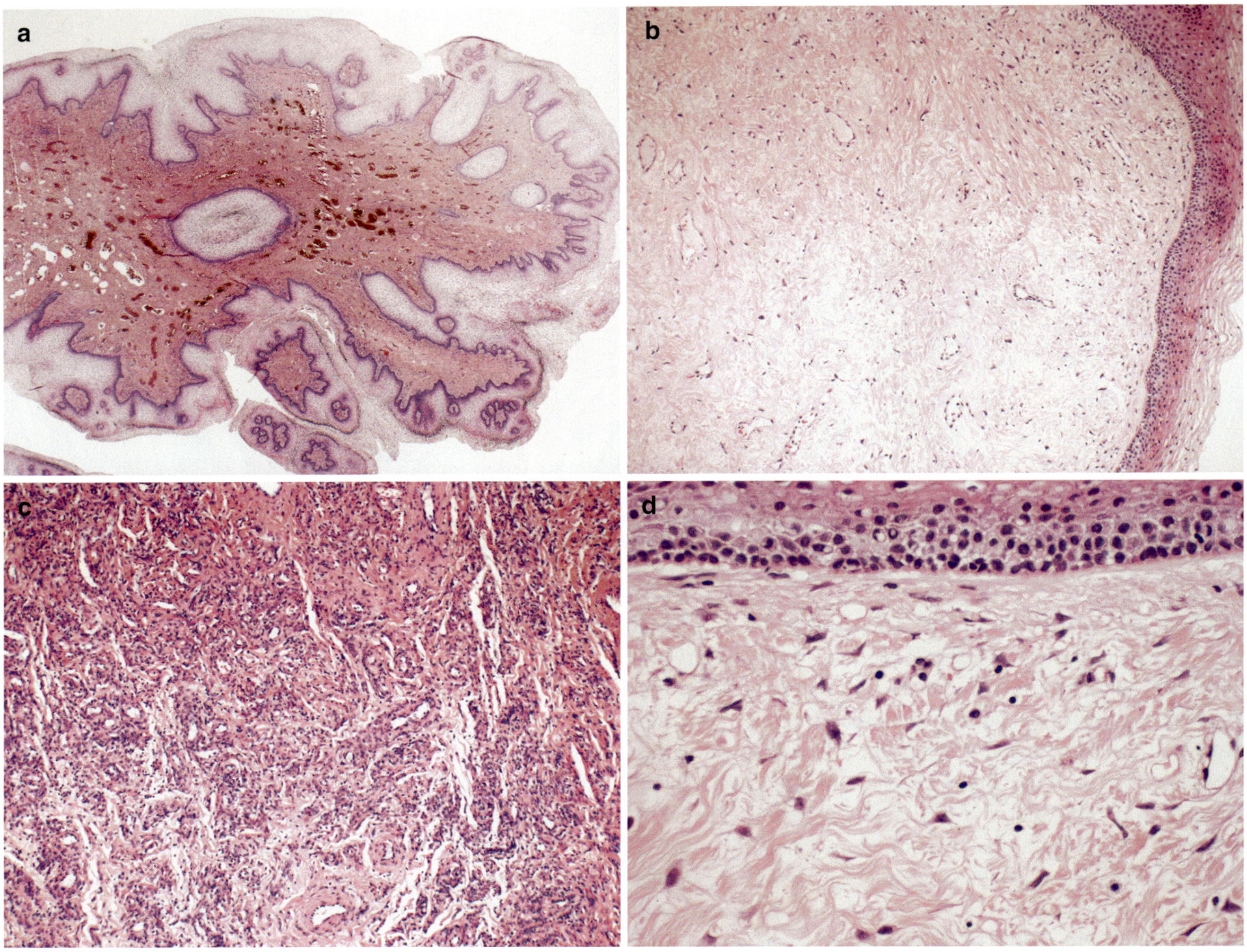

Fig. 9.19 Fibroepithelial polyp. The lesion consists of epithelial component of hyperplastic squamous epithelium and a stromal component (**a**). The stromal component can be variably cellular, ranging from hypocellular (commonly with stromal oedema (**b**)) to hypercellular with pronounced vascularity (**c**). The characteristic stromal cells are spindle or stellated and can be multinucleated (**d**). No grenz zone can be seen

matous fibroepithelial stromal polyps" and occur commonly, but not invariably, during pregnancy [140].

9.3.12.3 Differential Diagnosis

The differential diagnosis of FE with atypical cells and increased cellularity encompasses sarcomas, especially leiomyosarcoma, rhabdomyosarcoma, low-grade endometrial stromal sarcoma, malignant peripheral nerve sheath tumour and dermatofibrosarcoma protuberans. Other neoplasms in the differential diagnosis include tumours belonging to the category of benign stromal tumours of the lower female genital tract, such as aggressive angiomyxoma, cellular angiofibroma, superficial angiomyxoma and myofibroblastoma. Features which help us to achieve the correct diagnosis include (1) presence of multinucleated cells, which are rare in sarcomas; (2) absence of "cambium" layer, typical, for example, for rhabdomyosarcoma; (3) absence of sharp boundary (grenz zone) with the surrounding stroma; (4) exophytic polypous growth of FP; and (5) age of the patient (e.g. sarcoma botryoides usually occurs in children of up to 5 years of age). Immunohistochemistry is generally not very helpful, but in the above-mentioned differential diagnosis, it can be beneficial. The stromal cells of FE polyps are usually desmin and vimentin positive and only rarely smooth muscle actin positive. Expression of estrogen and progesterone receptors is common. Very rarely, the stromal cells of FP may express myogenin, but the pattern of expression is typically restricted, as compared with the diffuse expression that would be expected in rhabdomyosarcoma. FP is also discussed in Chap. 8.

9.3.13 Tubulosquamous Polyp

9.3.13.1 General and Clinical Features

Tubulosquamous polyps are benign lesions that are usually diagnosed in postmenopausal or perimenopausal patients.

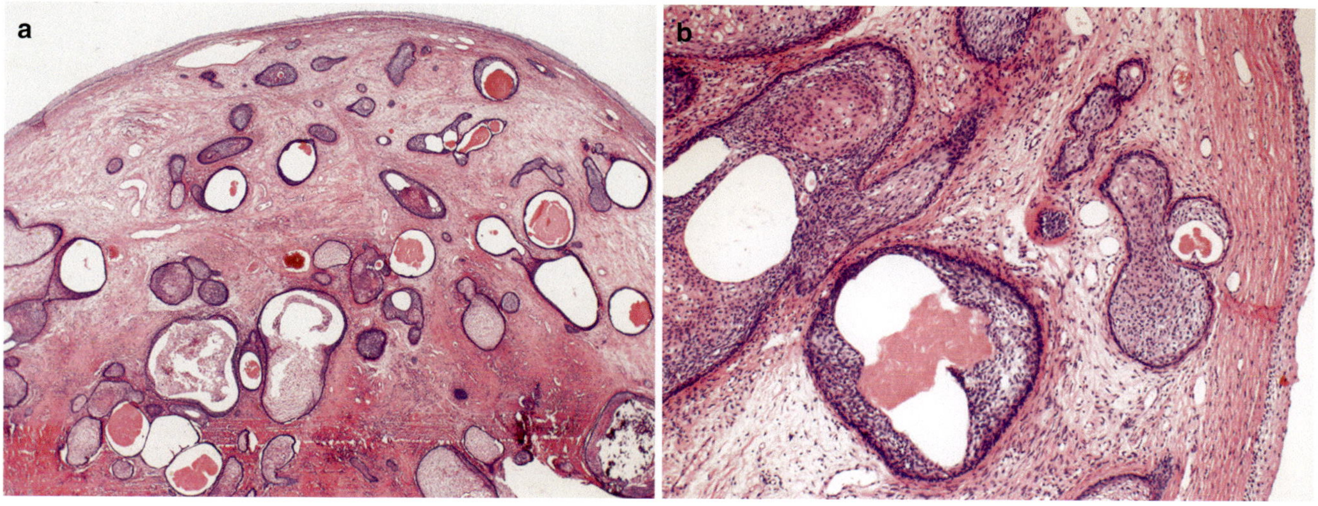

Fig. 9.20 Tubulosquamous polyp. Polypous arrangement of the lesion with apparent epithelial and stromal component (**a**). The epithelial component consists of sharply demarcated nests of cells which are squamous or squamous-transitional in type. Focal tubules can be seen (**b**)

They most commonly occur in the upper vagina and are usually less than 5 cm.

9.3.13.2 Gross and Microscopic Features

Tubulosquamous polyps represent a distinctive entity that is characterized by an admixture of epithelial and stromal components (Fig. 9.20a, b) [141]. The stromal component is in most cases fibrous and rather hypocellular. The epithelial component consists of well-demarcated nests of cells, which are predominantly squamous or squamo-transitional in type, with a minor component of tubules. The tubules are usually small and located at the periphery of squamous nests but may be placed more centrally as well. These tubules are lined by cuboidal cells with scarce clear or eosinophilic cytoplasm [141, 142]. There are also reports of unusual variants of tubulosquamous polyp with a basaloid epithelial component and the presence of sebaceous, mucinous and goblet-cell differentiation [143–145]. Common finding in the glandular component is the immunohistochemical expression of PSA of PrAP [141, 146]. Given this fact, possible histogenetic theories include an origin in [or differentiation towards] ectopic prostatic glands or paraurethral Skene glands [141].

9.3.13.3 Differential Diagnosis

The differential diagnosis for tubulosquamous polyps includes fibroepithelial polyp, vaginal Brenner tumour and mixed tumour of the vagina (spindle cell epithelioma).

Spindle cell epithelioma is also composed of an admixture of epithelial and stromal elements [147]. However, in this entity the stromal component predominates and consists of numerous spindle cells without atypia, which are usually strongly immunoreactive for cytokeratins. In addition, this tumour is usually well circumscribed and occurs in young to middle-aged women, with a predilection for the hymenal region. In contrast, tubulosquamous polyps show a predominance of epithelial cells and the stroma is usually hypocellular. Moreover, the stromal component is cytokeratin negative, and the lesions are usually non-circumscribed and occur in older females, in the upper part of the vagina.

Vaginal Brenner tumour has been rarely reported [148]. Based on the morphology of the reported cases, it is probable that at least some of them could represent tubulosquamous polyp with transitional rather than squamous morphology.

9.3.14 Endocervicosis

By definition, endocervicosis is characterized by the presence of benign glands of endocervical type (probably arising from pelvic or abdominal peritoneum) which are found in ectopic sites, mostly the urinary bladder. Rarely, the cervix, pelvic peritoneum and lymph nodes may also be involved [149, 150]. In the vagina, only two cases have been described, one of them being associated with adenocarcinoma [151, 152].

9.3.15 Endometriosis

Vaginal endometriosis is uncommon and occurs in about 2% of patients with surgically confirmed endometriosis [153]. Based on its location, it can be divided into superficial and deep endometriosis [154]. Superficial endometriosis is associated with direct implantation of endometrial tissue fragments and typically affects the vaginal vault or vaginal stump. Usually, this type of endometriosis is located in areas of prior traumatization, including surgical procedures such as hysterectomy. More common is deep

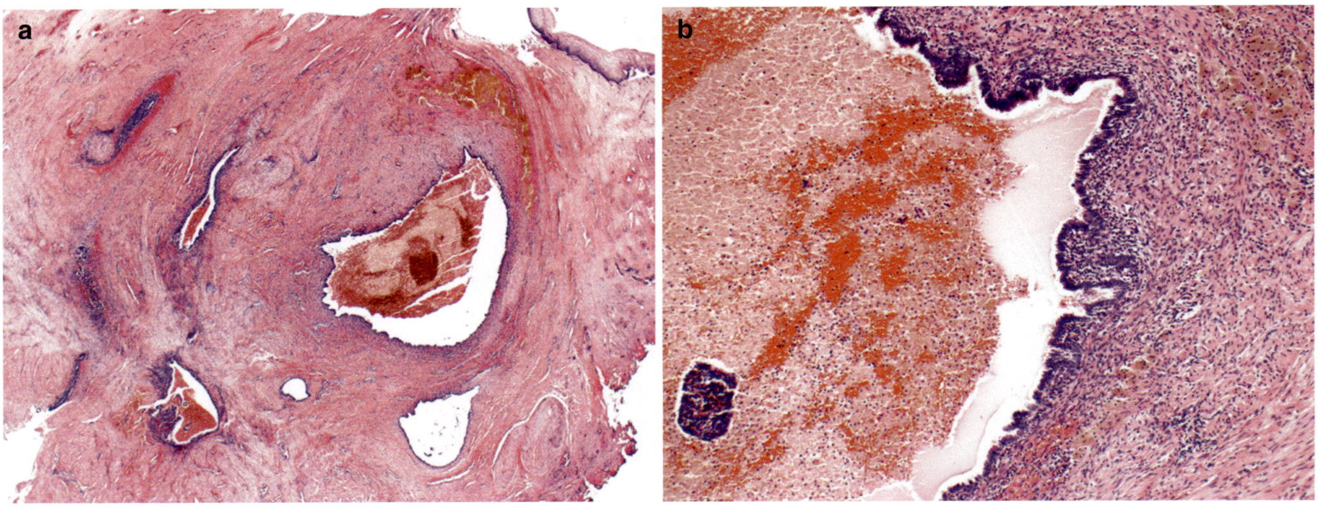

Fig. 9.21 Endometriosis. Presence of endometrial glands and stroma in the vaginal wall (**a**). Inside the dilated endometrial gland, haemolysed blood can be seen. In the surrounding stroma, groups of siderophages with mild inflammatory infiltration are present (**b**)

vaginal endometriosis, which is typically associated with pelvic endometriosis and involves the posterior vaginal fornix. Vaginal endometriosis, as endometriosis in other locations, can give rise to malignant tumours including endometrioid and clear cell carcinoma, adenosarcoma, carcinosarcoma and endometrial stromal sarcoma [155, 156].

Histologically, vaginal endometriosis shows the same features as endometriosis in other locations (Fig. 9.21a, b). Typically there is the presence of both endometrial glands and endometrial stroma, although this is not always the case. Secondary changes such as bleeding and an inflammatory reaction can occur. The diagnosis is usually straightforward; however, in certain cases it may be complicated by secondary changes obscuring the stromal component. In such cases the differential diagnosis of superficial endometriosis and vaginal adenosis can be difficult. The possibility of adenocarcinoma should also be ruled out, especially in cases of deeply infiltrative endometriosis.

9.3.16 Vaginal Adenosis

9.3.16.1 General and Clinical Features

The most common and currently well-known cause of vaginal adenosis is in utero exposure to oral non-steroidal estrogens, such as diethylstilbestrol (DES). The use of these estrogens started in the late 1940s, and before this era, vaginal adenosis was rarely diagnosed [157]. The increased incidence of clear cell adenocarcinoma (CCA) in the offspring of women treated by non-steroidal estrogens during pregnancy led, during the 1970s, to the discovery of the association between these estrogens and both vaginal adenosis and CCA [158].

Vaginal adenosis occurs in 30–45% of women with intrauterine exposure to DES. Experimental studies have shown that the effect of DES is probably related to the influence on urogenital sinus, from which the stratified squamous epithelium (forming the squamous plate in the upper thirds of vagina) arises. Moreover, there is a blockage of the normal segregation of the stroma into the inner and outer layers in the upper genital tract [159, 160]. This knowledge was soon followed by the cessation of non-steroidal estrogen use during pregnancy, and vaginal adenosis related to DES exposure is not a serious issue anymore. Today, vaginal adenosis can occur sporadically in women without any known risk factors, and its incidence has been estimated between 2 and 10% of women. However, adenosis may also be associated with some local therapeutical procedures associated with mucosal injury, such as CO_2 laser vaporization or topical 5-fluorouracil treatment. The etiopathogenetic mechanism of this type of adenosis remains unknown. A possible association between tamoxifen therapy and adenosis has also been described [161].

9.3.16.2 Gross and Microscopic Features

Most cases of adenosis occur in the upper third of the vagina; however, the lesion may occur in the middle and rarely the lower third of the vagina as well. Three main types of adenosis have been described, based on their microscopic features. The most common is endocervical mucinous adenosis, characterized by the presence of endocervical-type mucinous epithelium, which accounts for about 60–75% of cases (Fig. 9.22a, b) [162]. The second type is tuboendometrial adenosis, which is characterized by epithelium with features of endometrial or tubal cells and accounts for about 20% of cases. Rarely, the third type of adenosis may be encountered, consisting of smaller cubic cells usually arranged in small

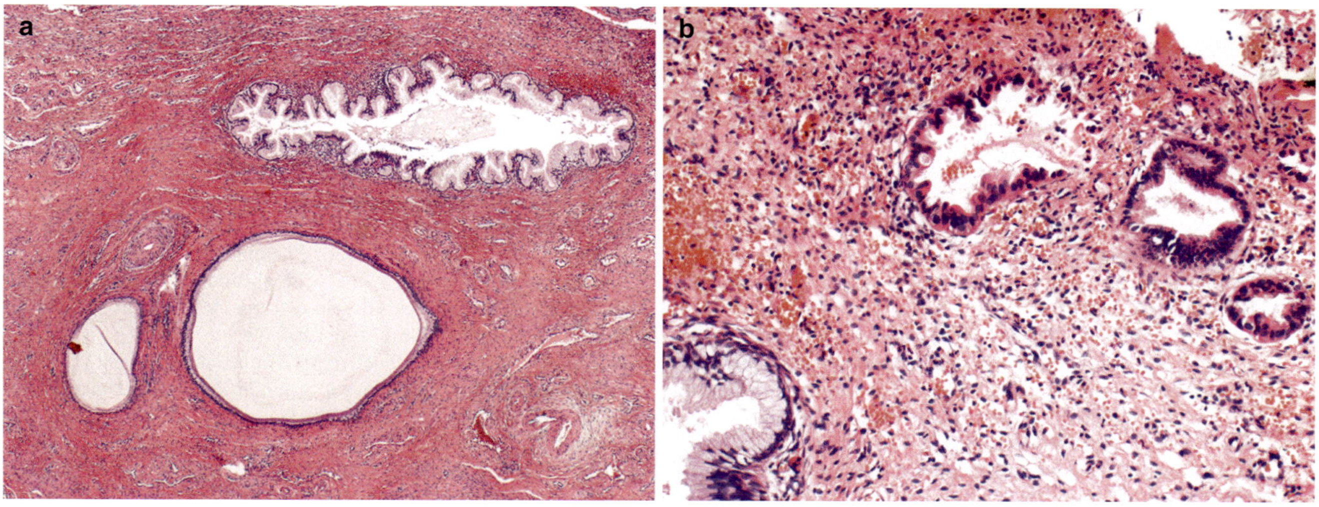

Fig. 9.22 Vaginal adenosis. Mucinous type of adenosis characterized by endocervical-type epithelium with bland nuclear features (**a**). Endometrioid type of adenosis (upper right) consists of smaller glands formed by cells with eosinophilic cytoplasm (**b**)

tubules. Additionally, rare cases of adenosis with intestinal metaplasia have been described [163, 164].

Typically, adenosis affects the superficial vaginal wall, i.e. surface mucosa and/or lamina propria. According to one study, the surface mucosa is involved in about 75% of cases [165]. Adenosis, especially its tuboendometrial variant, may also be located in the lamina propria only. The architecture of adenosis varies from simple glands, which can be cystically dilated, to more complex glandular proliferation. Common change occurring in the areas of adenosis is squamous metaplasia, which can be extensive and can lead to a complete replacement of the antecedent glandular epithelium [166].

9.3.16.3 Atypical Adenosis

Atypical adenosis is characterized by adenosis concurrent with nuclear atypia, including their enlargement, hyperchromasia, irregularity in size and shape, prominent nucleoli and increased mitotic activity. Most cases of atypical adenosis are of the tuboendometrial type [167, 168]. Due to the common association of atypical adenosis with adenocarcinoma, extensive sampling is needed to rule out any presence of invasive growth.

9.3.16.4 Differential Diagnosis

The differential diagnosis of adenosis includes endometriosis, endocervicosis and well-differentiated adenocarcinomas. Endometriosis can be distinguished based on the presence of endometrial stroma, signs of repeated bleeding and, in cases affecting the deeper parts of the vagina, location. Endocervicosis is exceedingly rare and typically affects the deeper parts of the vaginal wall. Well-differentiated adenocarcinoma is usually easily recognized, based on the infiltrative growth pattern and presence of atypia and mitoses.

Acknowledgements This chapter was supported by Ministry of Health, Czech Republic—conceptual development of research organization 64165, General University Hospital in Prague, Czech Republic.

References

1. Weber AM, Walters MD, Schover LR, Mitchinson A. Vaginal anatomy and sexual function. Obstet Gynecol. 1995;86(6):946–9.
2. Levin RJ. Sex and the human female reproductive tract--what really happens during and after coitus. Int J Impot Res. 1998;10(Suppl 1):S14–21.
3. Hodgins MB, Spike RC, Mackie RM, MacLean AB. An immunohistochemical study of androgen, oestrogen and progesterone receptors in the vulva and vagina. Br J Obstet Gynaecol. 1998;105(2):216–22.
4. Miyagawa S, Iguchi T. Epithelial estrogen receptor 1 intrinsically mediates squamous differentiation in the mouse vagina. Proc Natl Acad Sci U S A. 2015;112(42):12986–91.
5. Blakeman PJ, Hilton P, Bulmer JN. Cellular proliferation in the female lower urinary tract with reference to oestrogen status. BJOG. 2001;108(8):813–6.
6. Bachmann GA, Nevadunsky NS. Diagnosis and treatment of atrophic vaginitis. Am Fam Physician. 2000;61(10):3090–6.
7. Simon JA. Identifying and treating sexual dysfunction in postmenopausal women: the role of estrogen. J Womens Health (Larchmt). 2011;20(10):1453–65.
8. Kurman RJ. Blaustein's pathology of the female genital tract. New York: Springer; 2011.
9. Miller EA, Beasley DE, Dunn RR, Archie EA. Lactobacilli dominance and vaginal pH: why is the human vaginal microbiome unique? Front Microbiol. 2016;7:1936.
10. Fettweis JM, Serrano MG, Girerd PH, Jefferson KK, Buck GA. A new era of the vaginal microbiome: advances using next-generation sequencing. Chem Biodivers. 2012;9(5):965–76.
11. Kovachev S. Defence factors of vaginal lactobacilli. Crit Rev Microbiol. 2018;44(1):31–9.
12. Kurman RJ, Hedrick Ellenson L, Ronnett BM. Blaustein's pathology of the female genital tract. 6th ed. New York: Springer; 2011. p. 1246.

13. Bertuccini L, Russo R, Iosi F, Superti F. Effects of Lactobacillus rhamnosus and Lactobacillus acidophilus on bacterial vaginal pathogens. Int J Immunopathol Pharmacol. 2017;30(2):163–7.
14. Nwankwo TO, Aniebue UU, Umeh UA. Syndromic diagnosis in evaluation of women with symptoms of vaginitis. Curr Infect Dis Rep. 2017;19(1):3.
15. Mills BB. Vaginitis: beyond the basics. Obstet Gynecol Clin N Am. 2017;44(2):159–77.
16. Cauci S, Driussi S, De Santo D, Penacchioni P, Iannicelli T, Lanzafame P, et al. Prevalence of bacterial vaginosis and vaginal flora changes in peri- and postmenopausal women. J Clin Microbiol. 2002;40(6):2147–52.
17. Cauci S, Monte R, Driussi S, Lanzafame P, Quadrifoglio F. Impairment of the mucosal immune system: IgA and IgM cleavage detected in vaginal washings of a subgroup of patients with bacterial vaginosis. J Infect Dis. 1998;178(6):1698–706.
18. Gravett MG, Nelson HP, DeRouen T, Critchlow C, Eschenbach DA, Holmes KK. Independent associations of bacterial vaginosis and Chlamydia trachomatis infection with adverse pregnancy outcome. JAMA. 1986;256(14):1899–903.
19. Hillier SL, Nugent RP, Eschenbach DA, Krohn MA, Gibbs RS, Martin DH, et al. Association between bacterial vaginosis and preterm delivery of a low-birth-weight infant. The Vaginal Infections and Prematurity Study Group. N Engl J Med. 1995;333(26):1737–42.
20. Morris M, Nicoll A, Simms I, Wilson J, Catchpole M. Bacterial vaginosis: a public health review. BJOG. 2001;108(5):439–50.
21. Gillet E, Meys JF, Verstraelen H, Verhelst R, De Sutter P, Temmerman M, et al. Association between bacterial vaginosis and cervical intraepithelial neoplasia: systematic review and meta-analysis. PLoS One. 2012;7(10):e45201.
22. Nucci MR, Oliva E. In: Goldblum JR, editor. Gynecologic pathology, vol. 592. 1st ed. Spain: Churchill Livingstone; 2009.
23. Bitew A, Abebaw Y, Bekele D, Mihret A. Prevalence of bacterial vaginosis and associated risk factors among women complaining of genital tract infection. Int J Microbiol. 2017;2017:4919404.
24. Gaydos CA, Beqaj S, Schwebke JR, Lebed J, Smith B, Davis TE, et al. Clinical validation of a test for the diagnosis of vaginitis. Obstet Gynecol. 2017;130(1):181–9.
25. Amsel R, Totten PA, Spiegel CA, Chen KC, Eschenbach D, Holmes KK. Nonspecific vaginitis. Diagnostic criteria and microbial and epidemiologic associations. Am J Med. 1983;74(1):14–22.
26. Nugent RP, Krohn MA, Hillier SL. Reliability of diagnosing bacterial vaginosis is improved by a standardized method of gram stain interpretation. J Clin Microbiol. 1991;29(2):297–301.
27. Sodhani P, Garg S, Bhalla P, Singh MM, Sharma S, Gupta S. Prevalence of bacterial vaginosis in a community setting and role of the pap smear in its detection. Acta Cytol. 2005;49(6): 634–8.
28. Sodhani P, Gupta S, Gupta R, Mehrotra R. Bacterial vaginosis and cervical intraepithelial neoplasia: is there an association or is co-existence incidental? Asian Pac J Cancer Prev. 2017;18(5): 1289–92.
29. Donders GGG, Bellen G, Grinceviciene S, Ruban K, Vieira-Baptista P. Aerobic vaginitis: no longer a stranger. Res Microbiol. 2017;168(9–10):845–58.
30. Donders G, Bellen G, Rezeberga D. Aerobic vaginitis in pregnancy. BJOG. 2011;118(10):1163–70.
31. Rumyantseva TA, Bellen G, Savochkina YA, Guschin AE, Donders GG. Diagnosis of aerobic vaginitis by quantitative real-time PCR. Arch Gynecol Obstet. 2016;294(1):109–14.
32. Geng N, Wu W, Fan A, Han C, Wang C, Wang Y, et al. Analysis of the risk factors for aerobic vaginitis: a case-control study. Gynecol Obstet Investig. 2016;81:148–54.
33. Han C, Wu W, Fan A, Wang Y, Zhang H, Chu Z, et al. Diagnostic and therapeutic advancements for aerobic vaginitis. Arch Gynecol Obstet. 2015;291(2):251–7.
34. Fan A, Yue Y, Geng N, Zhang H, Wang Y, Xue F. Aerobic vaginitis and mixed infections: comparison of clinical and laboratory findings. Arch Gynecol Obstet. 2013;287(2):329–35.
35. Jahic M, Mulavdic M, Nurkic J, Jahic E, Nurkic M. Clinical characteristics of aerobic vaginitis and its association to vaginal candidiasis, trichomonas vaginitis and bacterial vaginosis. Med Arch. 2013;67(6):428–30.
36. Sonnex C. Genital streptococcal infection in non-pregnant women: a case-note review. Int J STD AIDS. 2013;24(6):447–8.
37. Regan JA, Klebanoff MA, Nugent RP, Eschenbach DA, Blackwelder WC, Lou Y, et al. Colonization with group B streptococci in pregnancy and adverse outcome. VIP Study Group. Am J Obstet Gynecol. 1996;174(4):1354–60.
38. Leclair CM, Hart AE, Goetsch MF, Carpentier H, Jensen JT. Group B streptococcus: prevalence in a non-obstetric population. J Low Genit Tract Dis. 2010;14(3):162–6.
39. Savini V, Marrollo R, D'Antonio M, D'Amario C, Fazii P, D'Antonio D. Streptococcus agalactiae vaginitis: nonhemolytic variant on the Liofilchem(R) Chromatic StreptoB. Int J Clin Exp Pathol. 2013;6(8):1693–5.
40. Verkaeren E, Epelboin L, Epelboin S, Boddaert N, Brossier F, Caumes E. Recurrent Streptococcus pyogenes genital infection in a woman: test and treat the partner! Int J Infect Dis. 2014;29:37–9.
41. Verstraelen H, Verhelst R, Vaneechoutte M, Temmerman M. Group A streptococcal vaginitis: an unrecognized cause of vaginal symptoms in adult women. Arch Gynecol Obstet. 2011;284(1):95–8.
42. Meltzer MC, Schwebke JR. Lactational amenorrhea as a risk factor for group a streptococcal vaginitis. Clin Infect Dis. 2008;46(10):e112–5.
43. Chua WC, Mazlan MZ, Ali S, Che Omar S, Wan Hassan WMN, Seevaunnantum SP, et al. Post-partum streptococcal toxic shock syndrome associated with necrotizing fasciitis. IDCases. 2017;9:91–4.
44. Shalaby T, Anandappa S, Pocock NJ, Keough A, Turner A. Lesson of the month 2: toxic shock syndrome. Clin Med (Lond). 2014;14(3):316–8.
45. Schlievert PM, Nemeth KA, Davis CC, Peterson ML, Jones BE. Staphylococcus aureus exotoxins are present in vivo in tampons. Clin Vaccine Immunol. 2010;17(5):722–7.
46. MacPhee RA, Miller WL, Gloor GB, McCormick JK, Hammond JA, Burton JP, et al. Influence of the vaginal microbiota on toxic shock syndrome toxin 1 production by Staphylococcus aureus. Appl Environ Microbiol. 2013;79(6):1835–42.
47. Vostral SL. Rely and toxic shock syndrome: a technological health crisis. Yale J Biol Med. 2011;84(4):447–59.
48. Bhagat N, Karthikeyan A, Kalkur S. Toxic shock syndrome within 24 H of an office hysteroscopy. J Midlife Health. 2017;8(2):92–4.
49. McDermott C, Sheridan M. Staphylococcal toxic shock syndrome caused by tampon use. Case Rep Crit Care. 2015;2015:640373.
50. Ameen F, Moslem M, Al Tami M, Al-Ajlan H, Al-Qahtani N. Identification of Candida species in vaginal flora using conventional and molecular methods. J Mycol Med. 2017;27(3):364–8.
51. Kalaiarasan K, Singh R, Chaturvedula L. Fungal profile of vulvovaginal Candidiasis in a Tertiary Care Hospital. J Clin Diagn Res. 2017;11(3):DC06–DC9.
52. Mtibaa L, Fakhfakh N, Kallel A, Belhadj S, Belhaj Salah N, Bada N, et al. Vulvovaginal candidiasis: etiology, symptomatology and risk factors. J Mycol Med. 2017;27(2):153–8.
53. Nakamura-Vasconcelos SS, Fiorini A, Zanni PD, Bonfim-Mendonca PS, Godoy JR, Almeida-Apolonio AA, et al. Emergence of Candida glabrata in vulvovaginal candidiasis should be attributed to selective pressure or virulence ability? Arch Gynecol Obstet. 2017;296(3):519–26.
54. Mandelblat M, Frenkel M, Abbey D, Ben Ami R, Berman J, Segal E. Phenotypic and genotypic characteristics of Candida albicans isolates from bloodstream and mucosal infections. Mycoses. 2017;60(8):534–45.

55. Matheson A, Mazza D. Recurrent vulvovaginal candidiasis: a review of guideline recommendations. Aust N Z J Obstet Gynaecol. 2017;57(2):139–45.
56. Cauchie M, Desmet S, Lagrou K. Candida and its dual lifestyle as a commensal and a pathogen. Res Microbiol. 2017;168(9–10):802–10.
57. Yano J, Noverr MC, Fidel PL Jr. Vaginal heparan sulfate linked to neutrophil dysfunction in the acute inflammatory response associated with experimental vulvovaginal candidiasis. MBio. 2017;8:2.
58. Asia AJ, Tapre VN. Primary actinomycosis of vulva with inguinal lymphadenopathy. Indian Dermatol Online J. 2016;7(5):402–5.
59. Hagiya H, Ogawa H, Takahashi Y, Kimura K, Hasegawa K, Otsuka F. Actinomyces turicensis bacteremia secondary to pyometra. Intern Med. 2015;54(21):2775–7.
60. Khodavaisy S, Zibafar E, Hashemi SJ, Narenji H, Daie Ghazvini R. Actinomycosis in Iran: short narrative review article. Iran J Public Health. 2014;43(5):556–60.
61. Arora BB, Maheshwari M, Devgan N, Arora DR. Prevalence of trichomoniasis, vaginal candidiasis, genital herpes, chlamydiasis, and actinomycosis among urban and rural women of Haryana, India. J Sex Transm Dis. 2014;2014:963812.
62. Mutter GL, Prat J. Pathology of the female reproductive tract. 3rd ed. Spain: Churchill Livingstone; 2014. p. 904.
63. Yilmaz M, Akbulut S, Samdanci ET, Yilmaz S. Abdominopelvic actinomycosis associated with an intrauterine device and presenting with a rectal mass and hydronephrosis: a troublesome condition for the clinician. Int Surg. 2012;97(3):254–9.
64. Westhoff C. IUDs and colonization or infection with Actinomyces. Contraception. 2007;75(6 Suppl):S48–50.
65. Clement PB, Young RH. Atlas of gynecologic surgical pathology. 3rd ed. Philadelphia, PA: Saunders; 2013. p. 584.
66. Kaya D, Demirezen S, Hascelik G, Gulmez Kivanc D, Beksac MS. Comparison of PCR, culturing and Pap smear microscopy for accurate diagnosis of genital Actinomyces. J Med Microbiol. 2013;62(Pt 5):727–33.
67. Edwards T, Burke P, Smalley H, Hobbs G. Trichomonas vaginalis: clinical relevance, pathogenicity and diagnosis. Crit Rev Microbiol. 2016;42(3):406–17.
68. Fichorova R, Fraga J, Rappelli P, Fiori PL. Trichomonas vaginalis infection in symbiosis with Trichomonasvirus and Mycoplasma. Res Microbiol. 2017;168(9–10):882–91.
69. Fichorova RN. Impact of T. vaginalis infection on innate immune responses and reproductive outcome. J Reprod Immunol. 2009;83(1–2):185–9.
70. Kirkcaldy RD, Augostini P, Asbel LE, Bernstein KT, Kerani RP, Mettenbrink CJ, et al. Trichomonas vaginalis antimicrobial drug resistance in 6 US cities, STD Surveillance Network, 2009–2010. Emerg Infect Dis. 2012;18(6):939–43.
71. Jenniskens ML, Veerbeek JH, Deurloo KL, van Hannen EJ, Thijsen SF. Routine testing of Mycoplasma genitalium and Trichomonas vaginalis. Infect Dis (Lond). 2017;49(6):461–5.
72. Kissinger P. Trichomonas vaginalis: a review of epidemiologic, clinical and treatment issues. BMC Infect Dis. 2015;15:307.
73. Madico G, Quinn TC, Rompalo A, McKee KT Jr, Gaydos CA. Diagnosis of Trichomonas vaginalis infection by PCR using vaginal swab samples. J Clin Microbiol. 1998;36(11):3205–10.
74. Fonseca THS, Oliveira FMS, Alacoque M, Rocha MI, Leite HV, Santos JFG, et al. Immunocytochemistry improving the diagnosis of trichomonas vaginalis infections. Biomed Res Int. 2017;2017:5642535.
75. Van Der Pol B. Sexually transmitted infections in women. Scand J Clin Lab Invest Suppl. 2014;244:68–74. discussion 3
76. Crum CP, Nucci MR, Lee KR. Diagnostic gynecologic and obstetric pathology. 2nd ed. Philadelphia, PA: Elsevier Saunders; 2011. p. 1216.
77. CDC. Sexually transmitted disease surveillance 2014. Atlanta: US Department of Health and Human Services; 2015.
78. Smith L, Angarone MP. Sexually transmitted infections. Urol Clin North Am. 2015;42(4):507–18.
79. Abou M, Dallenbach P. Acute cervicitis and vulvovaginitis may be associated with Cytomegalovirus. BMJ Case Rep. 2013;2013:bcr2013008884.
80. Sobel JD. Gynecologic infections in human immunodeficiency virus-infected women. Clin Infect Dis. 2000;31(5):1225–33.
81. Kemal KS, Foley B, Burger H, Anastos K, Minkoff H, Kitchen C, et al. HIV-1 in genital tract and plasma of women: compartmentalization of viral sequences, coreceptor usage, and glycosylation. Proc Natl Acad Sci U S A. 2003;100(22):12972–7.
82. Herold BC, Keller MJ, Shi Q, Hoover DR, Carpenter CA, Huber A, et al. Plasma and mucosal HIV viral loads are associated with genital tract inflammation in HIV-infected women. J Acquir Immune Defic Syndr. 2013;63(4):485–93.
83. Spear GT, St John E, Zariffard MR. Bacterial vaginosis and human immunodeficiency virus infection. AIDS Res Ther. 2007;4:25.
84. Nardis C, Mosca L, Mastromarino P. Vaginal microbiota and viral sexually transmitted diseases. Ann Ig. 2013;25(5):443–56.
85. Newman L, Rowley J, Vander Hoorn S, Wijesooriya NS, Unemo M, Low N, et al. Global estimates of the prevalence and incidence of four curable sexually transmitted infections in 2012 based on systematic review and global reporting. PLoS One. 2015;10(12):e0143304.
86. Juzlova K, Rob F, Zakoucka H, Kubatova A, Secnikova Z, Krasova M, et al. The first case of lymphogranuloma venereum in a woman in East-Central Europe and its multiple co-infections. Folia Microbiol (Praha). 2018;63(1):93–5.
87. Ceovic R, Gulin SJ. Lymphogranuloma venereum: diagnostic and treatment challenges. Infect Drug Resist. 2015;8:39–47.
88. Gray DJ, Ross AG, Li YS, McManus DP. Diagnosis and management of schistosomiasis. BMJ. 2011;342:d2651.
89. Kjetland EF, Leutscher PD, Ndhlovu PD. A review of female genital schistosomiasis. Trends Parasitol. 2012;28(2):58–65.
90. Kjetland EF, Poggensee G, Helling-Giese G, Richter J, Sjaastad A, Chitsulo L, et al. Female genital schistosomiasis due to Schistosoma haematobium. Clinical and parasitological findings in women in rural Malawi. Acta Trop. 1996;62(4):239–55.
91. Swai B, Poggensee G, Mtweve S, Krantz I. Female genital schistosomiasis as an evidence of a neglected cause for reproductive ill-health: a retrospective histopathological study from Tanzania. BMC Infect Dis. 2006;6:134.
92. Kjetland EF, Kurewa EN, Ndhlovu PD, Midzi N, Gwanzura L, Mason PR, et al. Female genital schistosomiasis--a differential diagnosis to sexually transmitted disease: genital itch and vaginal discharge as indicators of genital Schistosoma haematobium morbidity in a cross-sectional study in endemic rural Zimbabwe. Tropical Med Int Health. 2008;13(12):1509–17.
93. Poggensee G, Feldmeier H. Female genital schistosomiasis: facts and hypotheses. Acta Trop. 2001;79(3):193–210.
94. Helling-Giese G, Sjaastad A, Poggensee G, Kjetland EF, Richter J, Chitsulo L, et al. Female genital schistosomiasis (FGS): relationship between gynecological and histopathological findings. Acta Trop. 1996;62(4):257–67.
95. Midzi N, Ndhlovu PD, Nyanga L, Kjetland EF, Reimert CM, Vennervald BJ, et al. Assessment of eosinophil cationic protein as a possible diagnostic marker for female genital schistosomiasis in women living in a Schistosoma haematobium endemic area. Parasite Immunol. 2003;25(11–12):581–8.
96. Norseth HM, Ndhlovu PD, Kleppa E, Randrianasolo BS, Jourdan PM, Roald B, et al. The colposcopic atlas of schistosomiasis in the lower female genital tract based on studies in Malawi, Zimbabwe, Madagascar and South Africa. PLoS Negl Trop Dis. 2014;8(11):e3229.
97. Dennie J, Grover SR. Distressing perineal and vaginal pain in prepubescent girls: an aetiology. J Paediatr Child Health. 2013;49(2):138–40.

98. Kashyap B, Samantray JC, Kumar S, Jhamb R, Singh AK, Kaur IR. Recurrent paediatric pinworm infection of the vagina as a potential reservoir for Enterobius vermicularis. J Helminthol. 2014;88(3):381–3.
99. Tsai CY, Junod R, Jacot-Guillarmod M, Beniere C, Ziadi S, Bongiovanni M. Vaginal Enterobius vermicularis diagnosed on liquid-based cytology during papanicolaou test cervical cancer screening: a report of two cases and a review of the literature. Diagn Cytopathol. 2018;46(2):179–86.
100. Ngui R, Ravindran S, Ong DB, Chow TK, Low KP, Nureena ZS, et al. Enterobius vermicularis salpingitis seen in the setting of ectopic pregnancy in a Malaysian patient. J Clin Microbiol. 2014;52(9):3468–70.
101. Garden AS. Vulvovaginitis and other common childhood gynaecological conditions. Arch Dis Child Educ Pract Ed. 2011;96(2):73–8.
102. Deshpande AD. Enterobius vermicularis live adult worms in the high vagina. Postgrad Med J. 1992;68(802):690–1.
103. Mehrotra S, Young SL, Wojcik EM. Brown oval structures in vaginal Thin Prep smear: What could they be? Diagn Cytopathol. 2007;35(10):651–2.
104. Raju K, Verappa S, Venkataramappa SM. Enterobius vermicularis infestation masquerading as cervical carcinoma: a cytological diagnosis. J Nat Sci Biol Med. 2015;6(2):476–9.
105. Richens J. Genital manifestations of tropical diseases. Sex Transm Infect. 2004;80(1):12–7.
106. Nopdonrattakoon L. Amoebiasis of the female genital tract: a case report. J Obstet Gynaecol Res. 1996;22(3):235–8.
107. Munguia H, Franco E, Valenzuela P. Diagnosis of genital amebiasis in women by the standard Papanicolaou technique. Am J Obstet Gynecol. 1966;94(2):181–8.
108. Foda AA, El-Malky MM. Prevalence of genital tract infection with Entamoeba gingivalis among copper T 380A intrauterine device users in Egypt. Contraception. 2012;85(1):108–12.
109. Hyun KH, Shin HD, Kim DH. Malakoplakia in a healthy young female patient. Korean J Intern Med. 2013;28(4):475–80.
110. Jimerson SD, Becker JD. Vaginal ulcers associated with tampon usage. Obstet Gynecol. 1980;56(1):97–9.
111. LeRiche T, Black AY, Fleming NA. Toxic shock syndrome of a probable gynecologic source in an adolescent: a case report and review of the literature. J Pediatr Adolesc Gynecol. 2012;25(6):e133–7.
112. Tang YW, Himmelfarb E, Wills M, Stratton CW. Characterization of three Staphylococcus aureus isolates from a 17-year-old female who died of tampon-related toxic shock syndrome. J Clin Microbiol. 2010;48(5):1974–7.
113. Ghoniem GM, Warda HA. The management of genitourinary fistula in the third millennium. Arab J Urol. 2014;12(2):97–105.
114. Morris L, Do V, Chard J, Brand AH. Radiation-induced vaginal stenosis: current perspectives. Int J Womens Health. 2017;9:273–9.
115. Haylen BT, Maher CF, Barber MD, Camargo S, Dandolu V, Digesu A, et al. An International Urogynecological Association (IUGA)/International Continence Society (ICS) joint report on the terminology for female pelvic organ prolapse (POP). Int Urogynecol J. 2016;27(2):165–94.
116. Iglesia CB, Smithling KR. Pelvic organ prolapse. Am Fam Physician. 2017;96(3):179–85.
117. Tjugum J, Jonassen F, Olsson JH. Vaginitis emphysematosa in a renal transplant patient. Acta Obstet Gynecol Scand. 1986;65(4):377–8.
118. Gardner HL, Fernet P. Etiology of vaginitis emphysematosa: report of ten cases and review of literature. Am J Obstet Gynecol. 1964;88:680–94.
119. Reichman O, Sobel J. Desquamative inflammatory vaginitis. Best Pract Res Clin Obstet Gynaecol. 2014;28(7):1042–50.
120. Mitchell L, King M, Brillhart H, Goldstein A. Cervical ectropion may be a cause of desquamative inflammatory vaginitis. Sex Med. 2017;5(3):e212–4.
121. Shaw JL, Diamandis EP. A potential role for tissue kallikrein-related peptidases in human cervico-vaginal physiology. Biol Chem. 2008;389(6):681–8.
122. Chen S, Ge R, Zhu L, Yang S, Wu W, Yang Y, et al. Giant primary vaginal calculus secondary to vesicovaginal fistula with partial vaginal outlet obstruction in a 12-year-old girl. Urology. 2011;78(4):908–10.
123. Malhotra N, Kumar S, Roy KK, Agarwal R, Verma V. Vaginal calculus secondary to vaginal outlet obstruction. J Clin Ultrasound. 2004;32(4):204–6.
124. Rahn DD, Carberry C, Sanses TV, Mamik MM, Ward RM, Meriwether KV, et al. Vaginal estrogen for genitourinary syndrome of menopause: a systematic review. Obstet Gynecol. 2014;124(6):1147–56.
125. Pradhan S, Tobon H. Vaginal cysts: a clinicopathological study of 41 cases. Int J Gynecol Pathol. 1986;5(1):35–46.
126. Steinberg BJ, Mapp T, Mama S, Echols KT. Surgical treatment of persistent vaginal granulation tissue using CO(2) laser vaporization under colposcopic and laparoscopic guidance. JSLS. 2012;16(3):488–91.
127. Proppe KH, Scully RE, Rosai J. Postoperative spindle cell nodules of genitourinary tract resembling sarcomas. A report of eight cases. Am J Surg Pathol. 1984;8(2):101–8.
128. Zhao J, Ping H, Xing N. Postoperative spindle cell nodule of the bladder: a case report and review of the literature. Oncol Lett. 2014;7(5):1507–10.
129. Alderman M, Kunju LP. Inflammatory myofibroblastic tumor of the bladder. Arch Pathol Lab Med. 2014;138(10):1272–7.
130. Harik LR, Merino C, Coindre JM, Amin MB, Pedeutour F, Weiss SW. Pseudosarcomatous myofibroblastic proliferations of the bladder: a clinicopathologic study of 42 cases. Am J Surg Pathol. 2006;30(7):787–94.
131. Song YS, Kang JS, Park MH. Fallopian tube prolapse misdiagnosed as vault granulation tissue: a report of three cases. Pathol Res Pract. 2005;201(12):819–22.
132. Silverberg SG, Frable WJ. Prolapse of fallopian tube into vaginal vault after hysterectomy. Histopathology, cytopathology, and differential diagnosis. Arch Pathol. 1974;97(2):100–3.
133. Wheelock JB, Schneider V, Goplerud DR. Prolapsed fallopian tube masquerading as adenocarcinoma of the vagina in a postmenopausal woman. Gynecol Oncol. 1985;21(3):369–75.
134. Fadare O. Vaginal stromal sclerosis: a distinctive stromal change associated with vaginal atrophy. Int J Gynecol Pathol. 2011;30(3):295–300.
135. Pehlivanov B, Belovegdov V, Ivanov G, Ivancheva H. Primary localised amyloidosis of the vagina. Aust N Z J Obstet Gynaecol. 2008;48(1):120–2.
136. Altinkaya SO, Uzunlar O, Talas BB, Ozat M, Bilge U. Ligneous cervicovaginitis. Taiwan J Obstet Gynecol. 2008;47(3):363–6.
137. Chi AC, Prichard E, Richardson MS, Rasenberger KP, Weathers DR, Neville BW. Pseudomembranous disease (ligneous inflammation) of the female genital tract, peritoneum, gingiva, and paranasal sinuses associated with plasminogen deficiency. Ann Diagn Pathol. 2009;13(2):132–9.
138. Nielsen GP, Young RH. Mesenchymal tumors and tumor-like lesions of the female genital tract: a selective review with emphasis on recently described entities. Int J Gynecol Pathol. 2001;20(2):105–27.
139. Norris HJ, Taylor HB. Polyps of the vagina. A benign lesion resembling sarcoma botryoides. Cancer. 1966;19(2):227–32.
140. Nucci MR, Young RH, Fletcher CD. Cellular pseudosarcomatous fibroepithelial stromal polyps of the lower female genital tract: an underrecognized lesion often misdiagnosed as sarcoma. Am J Surg Pathol. 2000;24(2):231–40.
141. McCluggage WG, Young RH. Tubulo-squamous polyp: a report of ten cases of a distinctive hitherto uncharacterized vaginal polyp. Am J Surg Pathol. 2007;31(7):1013–9.

142. Dundr P, Povysil C, Mara M, Kuzel D. Tubulo-squamous polyp of the vagina. Cesk Patol. 2008;44(2):45–7.
143. Chaturvedi A, Padel A. Tubulo-squamous polyp of the vagina with sebaceous glands: novel features in an uncommon recently described entity. Int J Gynecol Pathol. 2010;29(5):494–6.
144. Tong B, Clarke BA, Ghazarian D. Tubulo-squamous polyp with mucinous and goblet cell differentiation: a unique morphologic variant. Int J Gynecol Pathol. 2011;30(5):518–9.
145. Stewart CJ. Tubulo-squamous vaginal polyp with basaloid epithelial differentiation. Int J Gynecol Pathol. 2009;28(6):563–6.
146. Kazakov DV, Stewart CJ, Kacerovska D, Leake R, Kreuzberg B, Chudacek Z, et al. Prostatic-type tissue in the lower female genital tract: a morphologic spectrum, including vaginal tubulosquamous polyp, adenomyomatous hyperplasia of paraurethral Skene glands (female prostate), and ectopic lesion in the vulva. Am J Surg Pathol. 2010;34(7):950–5.
147. Berdugo J, Gauthier P, Provencher D, Matte C, Piche J, Rahimi K. Spindle cell epithelioma of the vagina: report of two cases, literature review, and new immunohistochemical markers. Int J Surg Pathol. 2015;23(8):677–81.
148. Park S, Cho MS. Vaginal Brenner tumor with literature review: does this tumour originate from Walthard nests? Malays J Pathol. 2017;39(1):89–93.
149. Young RH, Clement PB. Endocervicosis involving the uterine cervix: a report of four cases of a benign process that may be confused with deeply invasive endocervical adenocarcinoma. Int J Gynecol Pathol. 2000;19(4):322–8.
150. Clement PB, Young RH. Endocervicosis of the urinary bladder. A report of six cases of a benign mullerian lesion that may mimic adenocarcinoma. Am J Surg Pathol. 1992;16(6):533–42.
151. Martinka M, Allaire C, Clement PB. Endocervicosis presenting as a painful vaginal mass: a case report. Int J Gynecol Pathol. 1999;18(3):274–6.
152. McCluggage WG, Price JH, Dobbs SP. Primary adenocarcinoma of the vagina arising in endocervicosis. Int J Gynecol Pathol. 2001;20(4):399–402.
153. Stern RC, Dash R, Bentley RC, Snyder MJ, Haney AF, Robboy SJ. Malignancy in endometriosis: frequency and comparison of ovarian and extraovarian types. Int J Gynecol Pathol. 2001;20(2):133–9.
154. Gardner HL. Cervical and vaginal endometriosis. Clin Obstet Gynecol. 1966;9(2):358–72.
155. Liu L, Davidson S, Singh M. Mullerian adenosarcoma of vagina arising in persistent endometriosis: report of a case and review of the literature. Gynecol Oncol. 2003;90(2):486–90.
156. Nomoto K, Hori T, Kiya C, Fukuoka J, Nakashima A, Hidaka T, et al. Endometrioid adenocarcinoma of the vagina with a microglandular pattern arising from endometriosis after hysterectomy. Pathol Int. 2010;60(9):636–41.
157. Guercio F. Adenosis of the vagina and its consequences. Arch Ostet Ginecol. 1959;64:588–600.
158. Scully RE, Robboy SJ, Herbst AL. Vaginal and cervical abnormalities, including clear-cell adenocarcinoma, related to prenatal exposure to stilbestrol. Ann Clin Lab Sci. 1974;4(4):222–33.
159. Robboy SJ, Taguchi O, Cunha GR. Normal development of the human female reproductive tract and alterations resulting from experimental exposure to diethylstilbestrol. Hum Pathol. 1982;13(3):190–8.
160. Forsberg JG. Animal model of human disease: adenosis and clear-cell carcinomas of vagina and cervix. Am J Pathol. 1976;84(3):669–72.
161. Ganesan R, Ferryman SR, Waddell CA. Vaginal adenosis in a patient on Tamoxifen therapy: a case report. Cytopathology. 1999;10(2):127–30. discussion 31
162. Goodman A, Zukerberg LR, Nikrui N, Scully RE. Vaginal adenosis and clear cell carcinoma after 5-fluorouracil treatment for condylomas. Cancer. 1991;68(7):1628–32.
163. Lu W, Zhang X, Lu B. Benign intestinal glandular lesions in the vagina: a possible correlation with implantation. Diagn Pathol. 2016;11(1):52.
164. Merchant WJ, Gale J. Intestinal metaplasia in stilboestrol-induced vaginal adenosis. Histopathology. 1993;23(4):373–6.
165. Antonioli DA, Burke L. Vaginal adenosis. Analysis of 325 biopsy specimens from 100 patients. Am J Clin Pathol. 1975;64(5):625–38.
166. Hart WR, Townsend DE, Aldrich JO, Henderson BE, Roy M, Benton B. Histopathologic spectrum of vaginal adenosis and related changes in stilbestrol-exposed females. Cancer. 1976;37(2):763–75.
167. Robboy SJ, Noller KL, O'Brien P, Kaufman RH, Townsend D, Barnes AB, et al. Increased incidence of cervical and vaginal dysplasia in 3,980 diethylstilbestrol-exposed young women. Experience of the National Collaborative Diethylstilbestrol Adenosis Project. JAMA. 1984;252(21):2979–83.
168. Antonioli DA, Rosen S, Burke L, Donahue V. Glandular dysplasia in diethylstilbestrol-associated vaginal adenosis. A case report and review of the literature. Am J Clin Pathol. 1979;71(6):715–21.

10 Vaginal Neoplasia

Debra S. Heller

Abstract

This chapter covers benign, premalignant, and malignant neoplasms of the vagina. The coverage includes epithelial, mixed epithelial/mesenchymal tumors, lymphoid and myeloid tumors, melanocytic tumors, and a variety of other primary and secondary neoplasms that may involve the vagina. Many of the tumors that arise in the vagina are also seen in other lower genital sites, but the clinical features occasionally differ at this site. Primary carcinoma of the vagina is rare and spread from cervical or vulvar primaries, or metastatic disease must always be considered in the differential diagnosis.

Keywords

Squamous papilloma · Müllerian papilloma
Fibroepithelial polyps · Vaginal adenoma
Vaginal intraepithelial neoplasia · Squamous cell carcinoma · Adenocarcinoma · Adenosquamous carcinoma · Adenoid cystic carcinoma
Adenoid basal carcinoma · Neuroendocrine carcinoma
Mixed tumor · Carcinosarcoma · Adenosarcoma

10.1 Epithelial Tumors of the Vagina

10.1.1 Benign Epithelial Tumors

10.1.1.1 Squamous Papilloma

A variety of polypoid lesions may arise in the vagina (Table 10.1). Squamous papillomas may be single or multiple. When multiple, this version is been called micropapillomatosis labialis (Fig. 10.1a). Micropapillomatosis labialis occurs at the introitus, involving the vestibule. It is considered a normal anatomic variant, unrelated to human papillomavirus, and does not require treatment [1]. It is grossly composed of multiple fingerlike projections of mucosa of normal color, each with a distinct base (Fig. 10.1a), distinguishing it from condyloma accuminatum, which has branching from a common base. Histologically the projections are composed of unremarkable or mildly thickened squamous epithelium devoid of koilocytosis or atypia lining fibrovascular tissue (Fig. 10.1b).

Table 10.1 Polypoid lesions of the vagina

Squamous papilloma
Fibroepithelial polyp
Müllerian papilloma
Vaginal adenoma
Condyloma accuminatum
Brenner tumor
Tubulosquamous vaginal polyp
Sarcoma botryoides
Yolk sac tumor
Adenocarcinoma
Müllerian adenosarcoma
Carcinosarcoma

10.1.1.2 Fibroepithelial Polyps

Fibroepithelial polyps, also known as mesodermal stromal polyps, occur across a wide age range, predominantly reproductive and midlife, but are seen in postmenopausal women as well. While often asymptomatic, the lesions may present with bleeding or local discomfort [2]. Fibroepithelial polyps are single lesions on a stalk, although grossly there may be some branching at the tip. Histologically, the lesions are composed of benign squamous mucosa lining a stroma which is usually of low cellularity (Fig. 10.2); however, there may be hypercellularity, mitotic activity, multinucleation, and atypia of stromal cells [3, 4], which should not be mistaken for malignancy. This finding has led to the term "pseudosarcoma botryoides," which should be avoided in clinical reports. Lack of a cambium layer of condensed stroma under

D. S. Heller (✉)
Department of Pathology, Immunology, and Laboratory Medicine, Rutgers New Jersey Medical School, Newark, NJ, USA
e-mail: hellerds@njms.rutgers.edu

W. Zheng et al. (eds.), *Gynecologic and Obstetric Pathology, Volume 1*, https://doi.org/10.1007/978-981-13-3016-2_10

Fig. 10.1 (**a**) Micropapillomatosis labialis, composed of multiple fingerlike projections with individual bases, arising in the introitus. Copyright Libby Edwards, MD. Used with Permission. (**b**) Squamous papilloma. Fibrovascular core lined by benign squamous epithelium

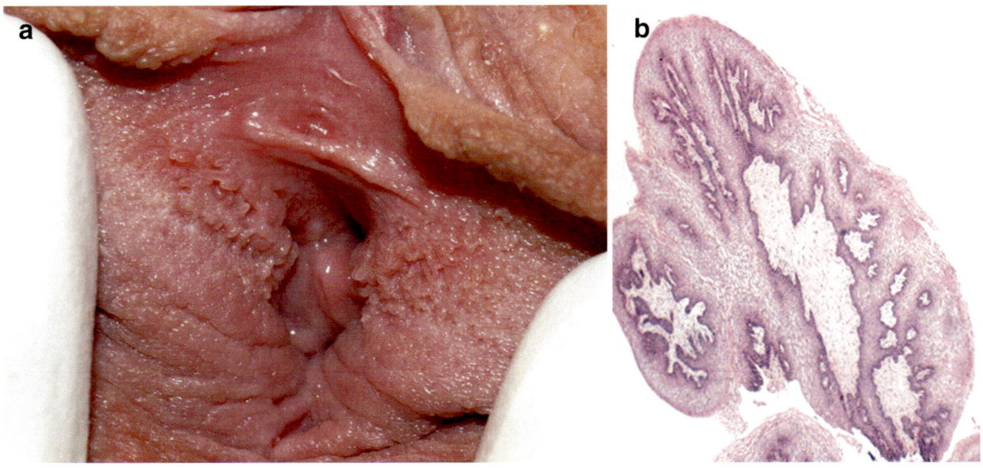

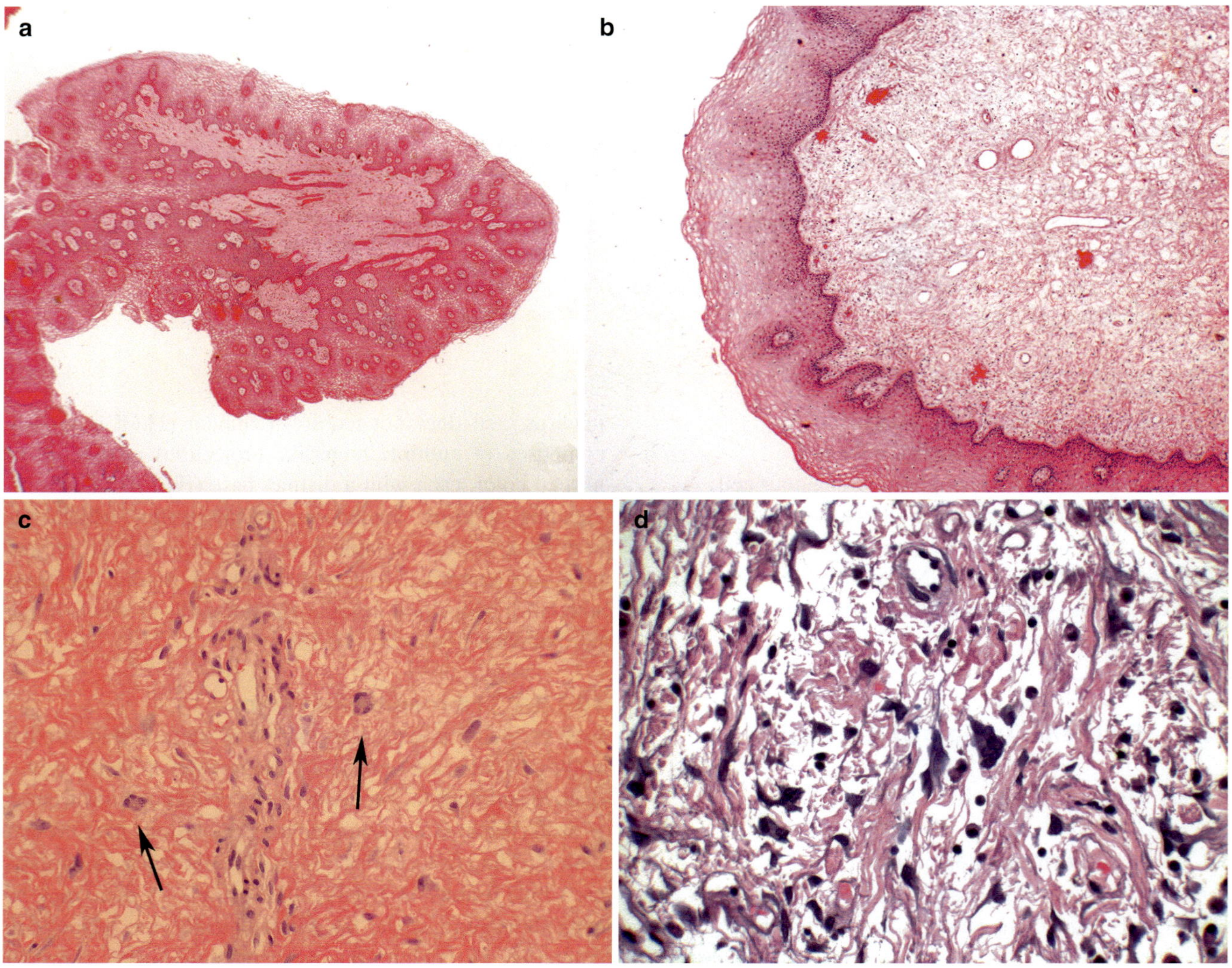

Fig. 10.2 Fibroepithelial polyp squamous lined fibroepithelial polyp on a stalk (**a**). At higher power (**b**), a low cellularity stroma is seen. Occasional rosettes (**c**) (arrows) and atypical stromal cells (**d**) may be seen and should not be mistaken for malignancy

the surface epithelium helps distinguish fibroepithelial polyps from true sarcoma botryoides. The stroma of fibroepithelial polyps is thought to contain myoepithelial cells, as well as estrogen and progesterone receptors [2, 5], and the lesion is frequently associated with pregnancy or hormone therapy [4]. Treatment is simple excision. They can

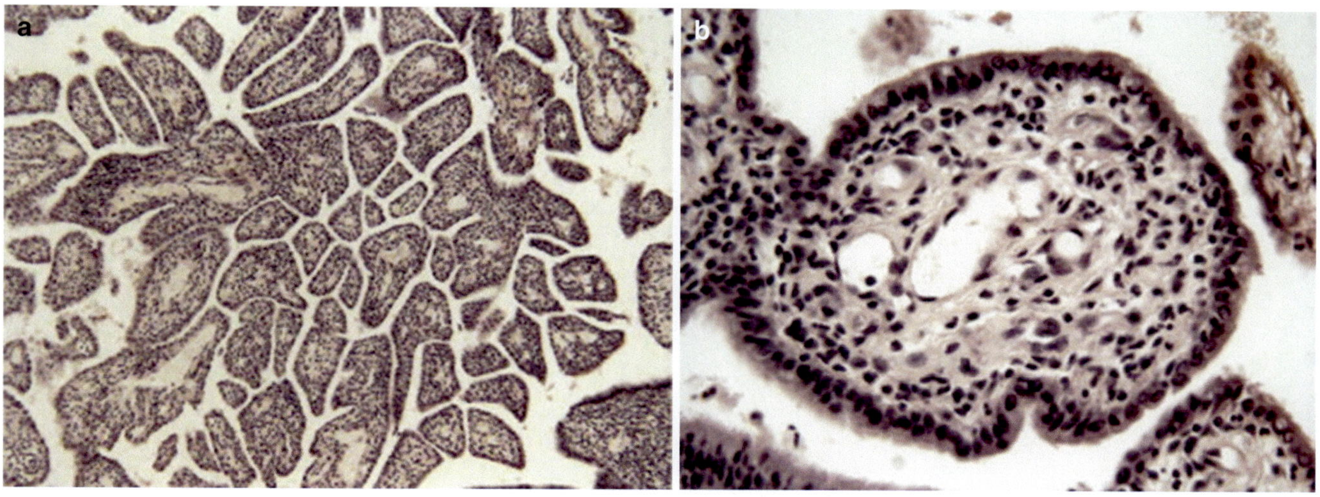

Fig. 10.3 Müllerian papilloma. The lesion is composed of multiple fronds (**a**), lined by a simple cuboidal epithelium (**b**). Reprinted from Journal of Pediatric and Adolescent Gynecology, Carlos A. Reck-Burneo, J Villanueva, FT Velcek. Vaginal Müllerian Papilloma: An Unusual Cause of Vaginal Bleeding in a Toddler. 2009 Oct;22(5):e124–6., with permission from Elsevier (**a**, **b**)

occasionally recur [3]. Fibroepithelial polyps are further discussed in Chaps. 8 and 9.

10.1.1.3 Müllerian Papilloma

Müllerian papillomas are rare benign polypoid neoplasms usually seen in children and adolescents, which may present with vaginal bleeding [6]. They can occur in the cervix as well as the vagina. They are composed of multiple complex branching fronds of fibrovascular tissue lined by a cuboidal to columnar epithelium (Fig. 10.3). Treatment is simple excision. These lesions can rarely recur [7]; however, one case, in a patient with cerebral palsy in a nursing home treated with numerous excisions, showed evolutionary changes over a 40-year period ranging from borderline to frank clear cell carcinoma [8].

10.1.1.4 Vaginal Adenoma

Polypoid lesions resembling colonic adenomatous polyps can occur in the vagina and may be tubular, villous, or tubulovillous. These lesions, common in the colon, are exceptionally rare in the vagina, with only a few case reports. They have similar histology to the intestinal lesions (Fig. 10.4). Reported cases have mostly occurred in the lower vagina of postmenopausal women, although younger patients have also been reported [9, 10], and may present with bleeding. Histologically, they are lined by enteric-type epithelium, which may have arisen from cloacal remnants [10]. The lesions should be considered premalignant, as there has been a report of an enteric-type vaginal adenocarcinoma arising in an adenoma [11], as well as a case with high-grade dysplasia [9], and so these should be excised. The differential diagnosis includes colonic adenocarcinoma, metastatic endocervical or endometrial carcinoma, prolapsed fallopian tube, and endometriosis [9]. Cytokeratin 7 and 20 expression profiles have been variable.

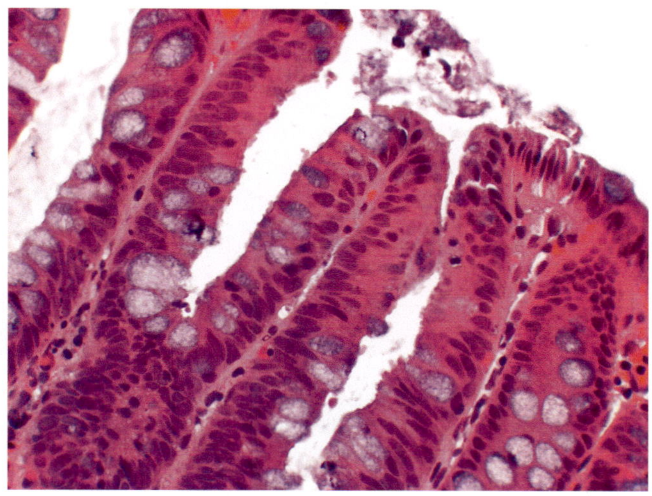

Fig. 10.4 Tubulovillous adenoma. This colonic lesion shows the typical architecture of tubules and villous structures lined by enteric-type tall columnar epithelium with goblet cells

10.1.1.5 Brenner Tumor

Brenner tumors represent about 1–2% of ovarian neoplasms, but only a few case reports describe a vaginal location for this benign neoplasm [12]. Most described cases have been small polypoid lesions found incidentally in elderly women and have been described at all levels of the vagina [12]. Histologically, the appearance is similar to the ovarian counterpart (Fig. 10.5), with nests of epithelium with squamotransitional features, including nuclear grooves, embedded in a fibroconnective tissue stroma. Cystic spaces containing eosinophilic secretions can be seen in the epithelial nests. The origin of vaginal Brenner tumor is unknown, but it has been postulated that they arise from metaplasia of Müllerian epithelium [12]. A benign polypoid lesion in the upper

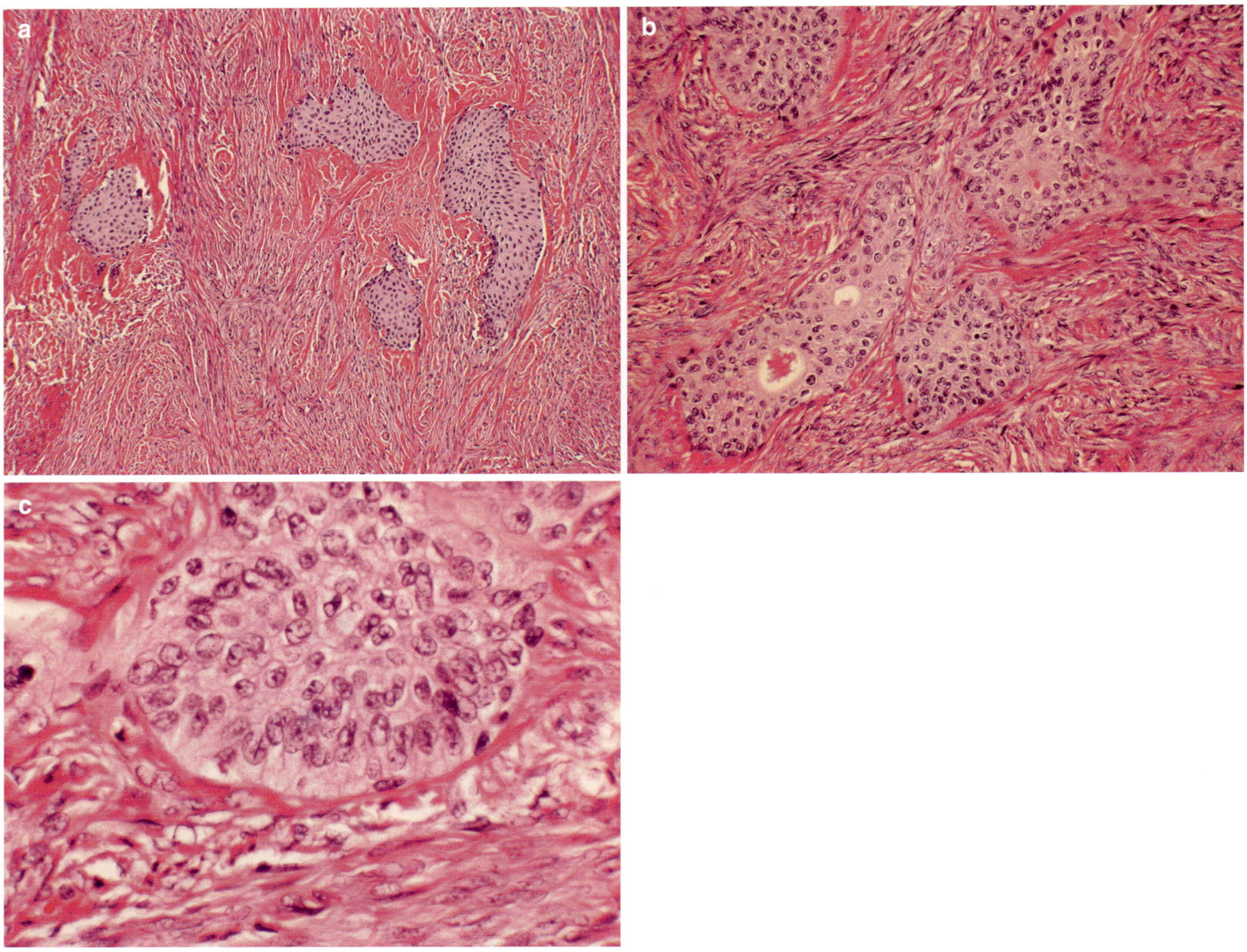

Fig. 10.5 Brenner tumor. The lesion shows nests of epithelial cells in a fibrous stroma (**a**). At higher power, the epithelium resembles squamotransitional epithelium, and the cells show nuclear grooves. Glandular lumens may be seen (**b**, **c**)

vagina of postmenopausal women termed the tubulosquamous vaginal polyp contains nests of cells with overlapping squamous and transitional cell features and may be the same lesion as some of the reported Brenner tumors [13, 14].

10.1.2 Premalignant Vaginal Tumors

10.1.2.1 Vaginal Intraepithelial Neoplasia

Low-Grade Squamous Intraepithelial Lesion (LSIL or Vaginal Intraepithelial Neoplasia [VaIN] 1)

Low-grade squamous intraepithelial lesions are less common in the vagina than the cervix; however, as HPV infection can affect the entire lower genital field, vaginal involvement must be considered in patients with HPV-related disease elsewhere in the lower genital tract. LSIL can be caused by both high-risk and low-risk HPV subtypes. As in other lower genital sites, LSIL is considered low risk for progression and often regresses. Hence, expectant management with follow-up is a reasonable option [15]. LSIL is often not grossly visible, but may be seen on colposcopy, and most often involves the upper vagina [16]. Grossly, the lesions are flat and may be multifocal. Similarly, histology shows that most of the lesions are flat, although condylomatous features are possible both grossly and microscopically. Morphologic changes are as described elsewhere in the lower female genital tract. There is koilocytosis, but maturation of the squamous epithelium is present (Fig. 10.6). In general, the composition of the vagina differs due to a relatively large amount of elastic tissue, when compared to the cervix. This imparts a corrugated architecture, especially when the tissue is removed by biopsy, which may mimic the papillary architecture seen in some dysplastic lesions; therefore, diagnosis of dysplasia requires well-defined nuclear atypia to avoid overcalling this normal finding.

High-Grade Squamous Intraepithelial Lesion (HSIL, VaIN 2/3)

HSIL (VaIN 2/3) of the vagina is considerably less common than HSIL of the cervix. It is seen in midlife and in older women, with a peak age in the 70s, and is frequently associated with lower genital tract neoplasia at other sites [15]. The most commonly associated HPV subtype is HPV 16 [15]. HSIL of the vagina is often discovered during the evaluation of an abnormal cervical cytology, evaluation of cervical HPV disease, or after an abnormal cytology in a woman with a prior hysterectomy related to HPV disease (HSIL or cancer). Usually vaginal HSIL is asymptomatic, although postcoital bleeding or discharge may be reported [15].

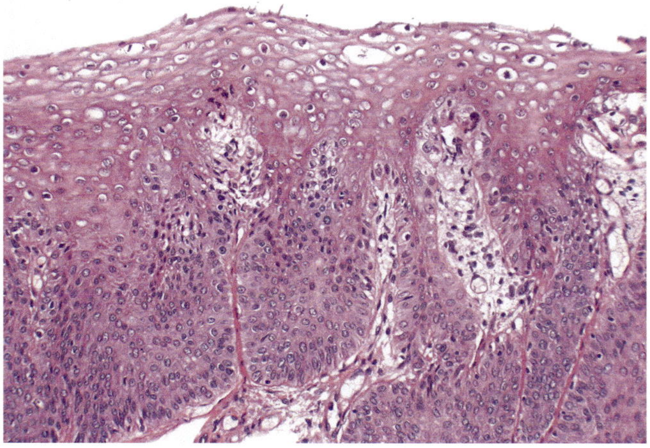

Fig. 10.6 Low-grade squamous intraepithelial lesion. Koilocytosis with epithelial maturation is present

As vaginal HSIL is considered preinvasive, therapy is indicated. Therapy is often individualized, and a variety of pharmacologic agents have been used, although they are not FDA-approved specifically for vaginal lesions, in addition to surgical excision or laser ablation [15]. The disease can be difficult to treat and can recur, particularly in immunosuppressed patients.

Histologically, HSIL of the vagina is similar in appearance to HSIL in other sites, with squamous maturation abnormality extending upward through at least two thirds of epithelium (Fig. 10.7). Some maturation is seen in VaIN 2 and generally none in VaIN 3; however, there is sufficient overlap, and the distinction between VaIN 2 and VaIN 3 is not reliably reproducible. Lesions may be pigmented and may show a predominantly basaloid or warty histology. The LAST project recommends the use of biomarkers for specific diagnostic scenarios, as opposed to routine or reflexive use [17]. P16, when diffusely block positive, is a surrogate marker of high-risk HPV and as such can be useful for distinguishing HSIL from benign mimics such as atrophy (Fig. 10.7e–g). Ki-67 activity above the basal layers is indicative of SIL; however, this does not correlate with grade (Table 10.2). The risk of developing an invasive carcinoma from VaIN is unknown [18].

Squamous neoplasia of the vagina is often associated with other lower genital tract squamous neoplasia, including the vulva, cervix, and anus. Human papillomavirus causes disease in a field effect, and hence, the entire region needs to be evaluated. This is particularly true in immunosuppressed patients, including those with HIV and status post organ transplantation.

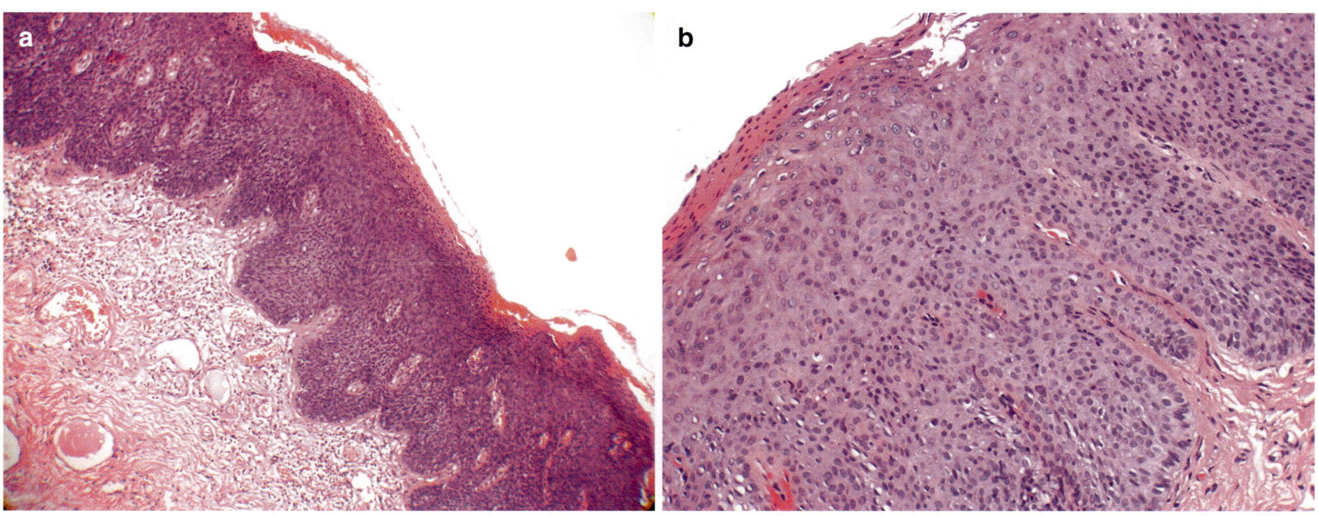

Fig. 10.7 High-grade squamous intraepithelial lesion. At low power (**a**), the epithelium is acanthotic, and parakeratosis is seen. Full thickness maturation abnormality is present (**b**, **c**). The lesions may be pigmented (**d**). There are times where it is difficult on H&E to separate HSIL from atrophy (**e**). This case was determined to be HSIL based on full thickness staining of Ki-67 (**f**) and block positivity for p16 (**g**)

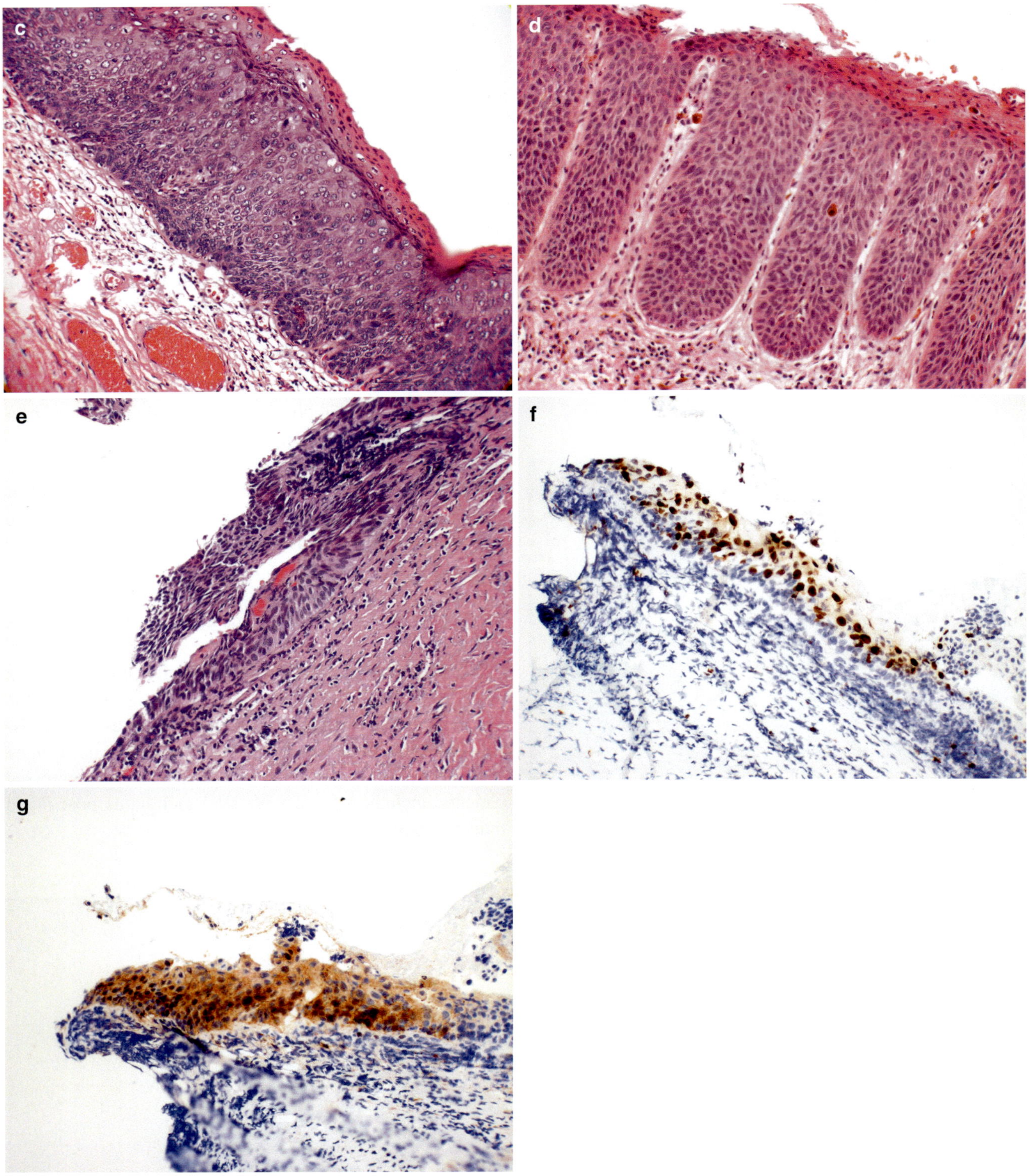

Fig. 10. 7 (continued)

Table 10.2 Immunohistochemistry of SIL (VaIN)

	P16	Ki-67
LSIL	+/–	Above basal layers
HSIL	Usually + diffusely (block positive)	Above basal layers
Atrophy	–	Confined to basal layers

10.1.3 Malignant Epithelial Tumors

10.1.3.1 Squamous Cell Carcinoma

Vaginal carcinoma represents about 2% of gynecologic malignancies for an incidence of about 3000 new cases per year in the USA [18]. Most lesions arise in the upper vagina of elderly women, although younger patients are occasionally affected. The vast majority of cases are squamous, and HPV is the causative agent in about 70–80% of cases [19] (most often HPV16) [20, 21]. Vaginal squamous cell carcinoma is considerably less frequent than cervical squamous cell carcinoma, and many patients with vaginal squamous cell carcinoma have a prior history of cervical disease, although it can be remote. As such, it is not always possible to diagnose a vaginal squamous cell carcinoma as a primary lesion.

While some attempts at defining superficially invasive squamous cell carcinoma of the vagina have been made, the LAST project made no recommendations on a definition for superficial invasion, as there was insufficient data in the group's opinion [17]. Some invasive carcinomas arise from HSIL, but the exact percentages are not known. Patients with invasive carcinoma tend to be about 10 years older than HSIL patients [18]. Interestingly, about half of vaginal carcinoma patients have had a prior hysterectomy [19].

Presenting symptoms of invasive vaginal carcinoma include bleeding, discharge, pain, or discomfort; however, the lesions may be asymptomatic [22]. Biopsy can be difficult, as it is technically challenging to acquire a deep enough biopsy to establish invasion (Fig. 10.8a, b). Histologically, the appearance is similar to squamous cell carcinoma in other lower genital tract locations and may sometimes appear warty or basaloid (Fig. 10.8c, d). Vaginal lesions are difficult to treat surgically, and thus, surgery is used predominantly for early lesions, with radiotherapy for more advanced disease, although treatment is variable [18, 22]. The increased benefit of chemotherapy is unclear, although it has been used with radiotherapy [19]. Stage is the most important prognostic factor [18]. Other poor indicators are size >4 cm, location outside the upper third of the vagina, and older age at presentation. The role of tumor grade is unclear. The presence of high-risk HPV appears to be associated with better clinical outcome [18]. Stage I disease has a 5-year survival rate of about 70% which drops rapidly with more advanced stage disease [22]. Staging is based on the 2009 FIGO system, which is clinical, as well as the AJCC TNM system, which incorporates pathologic findings [23, 24] (Table 10.3). The vagina has a rich lymphatic drainage system, which may be part of the explanation for the relatively poor prognosis. Upper vaginal lesions spread to iliac lymph nodes, and lower two thirds of the vagina lesions spread to inguinal nodes [20]. Distant metastases are uncommon, but the most common sites are the lung, liver, and bone [19].

A variant of squamous cell carcinoma, squamotransitional cell carcinoma, which may be papillary in architecture, and resembling the same neoplasm in the cervix, has been described [25]. It can be distinguished from a metastasis of a bladder primary transitional cell carcinoma by immunohistochemistry. Squamotransitional cell carcinomas of the vagina are typically CK7+/CK20- and stain for p16 reflecting association with high-risk HPV, while transitional cell carcinoma extending from bladder would be CK7+/CK20+, and does not demonstrate evidence of HPV infection [25].

10.1.3.2 Adenocarcinoma

Most vaginal carcinomas are squamous cell carcinomas, but adenocarcinoma represents about 2–10% of vaginal malignancies (Table 10.4) [18, 20]. Because of the rarity of these lesions, large case series are not available for treatment protocols and prognosis. In one series of mixed non-squamous cases, local control was achievable, but distant metastasis remained an issue [26]. In this series, many of the cases were clear cell adenocarcinoma, in spite of the lack of diethylstilbestrol (DES) exposure history [26]. Metastatic disease must be considered, as only about 20% of vaginal adenocarcinomas are primary [27]. Primary adenocarcinomas may be related to in utero exposure to DES or may be unrelated. Clear cell adenocarcinomas have most often arisen previously in association with DES exposure. This is becoming a less significant contributor to cases, as DES is no longer used in pregnancy, having been banned for use in pregnancy in 1971 [28]. Reported DES-associated clear cell adenocarcinomas usually occurred in younger women, in the anterior upper vaginal wall [21]. As many of these reported patients with DES-associated tumors were already under surveillance, their carcinomas were detected early and carried a good prognosis [21]. Late recur-

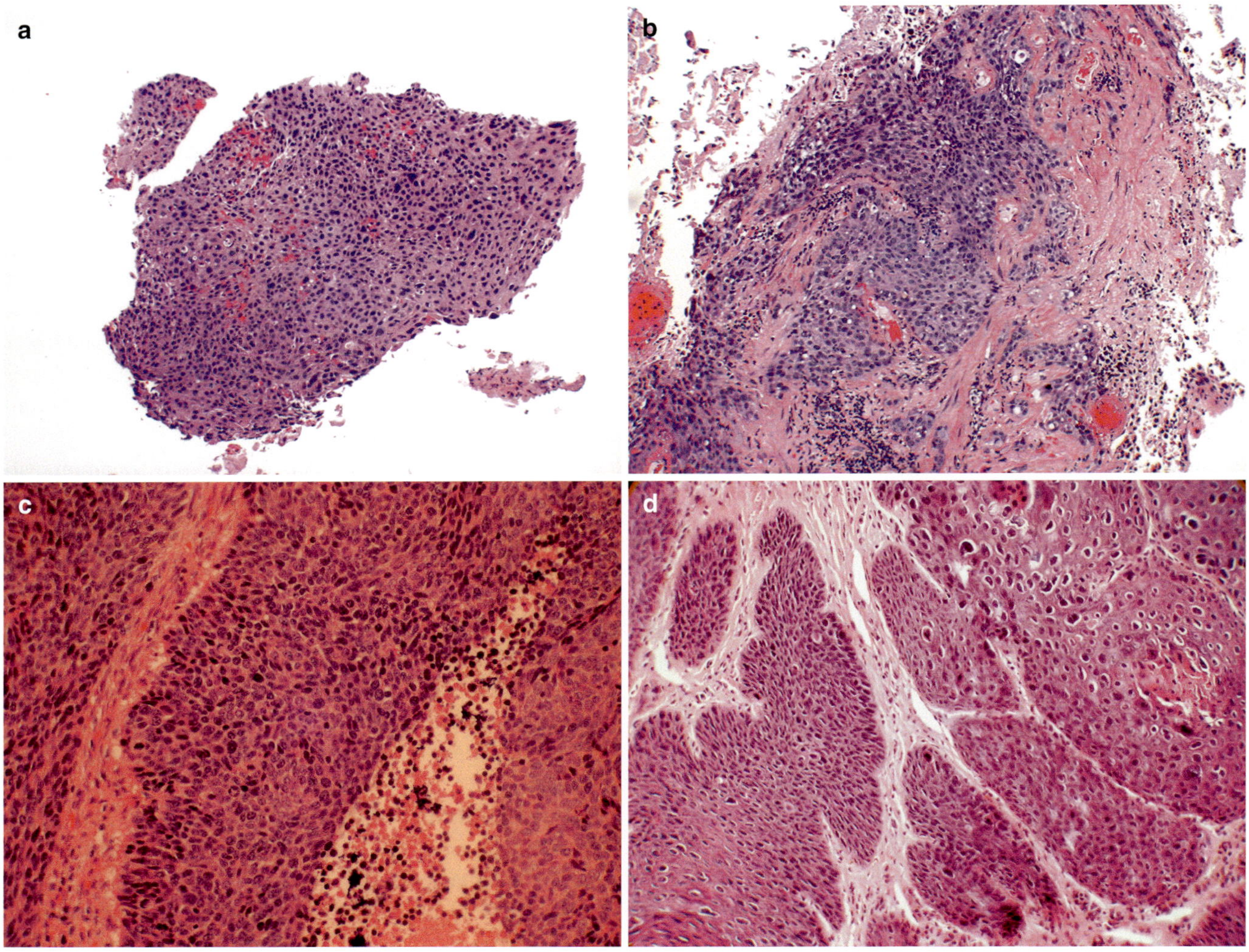

Fig. 10.8 Squamous cell carcinoma of the vagina. Superficial biopsies without underlying stroma may not be diagnostic (**a**), and a deep enough biopsy to show stromal invasion is needed (**b**). Some cases of squamous cell carcinoma may be basaloid (**c**) or warty (**d**)

Table 10.3 FIGO staging of carcinoma of the vagina[a]

FIGO stage	Description
I	The carcinoma is limited to the vaginal wall
II	The carcinoma has involved the subvaginal tissue but has not extended to the pelvic wall
III	The carcinoma has extended to the pelvic wall
IV	The carcinoma has extended beyond the true pelvis or has involved the mucosa of the bladder or rectum; bullous edema as such does not permit a case to be allotted to Stage IV
IVA	Tumor invades the bladder and/or rectal mucosa and/or direct extension beyond the true pelvis
IVB	Spread to distant organs

[a]From: Hacker NF, Eifel PJ, van der Velden J (2015). Cancer of the Vagina. Int J Gynaecol Obstet.131 Suppl 2:S84–7. doi: https://doi.org/10.1016/j.ijgo.2015.06.003

Table 10.4 Adenocarcinoma of the vagina

Primary
DES-associated
Clear cell adenocarcinoma
DES-unassociated
Clear cell adenocarcinoma
Mucinous adenocarcinoma
Intestinal type
Endocervical type
Endometrioid adenocarcinoma
Mesonephric adenocarcinoma
Serous adenocarcinoma
Metastatic

rences dictated prolonged follow-up [21]. Clear cell adenocarcinomas can arise in the absence of DES. Histologically, they appear similar to clear cell adenocarcinomas in other genital

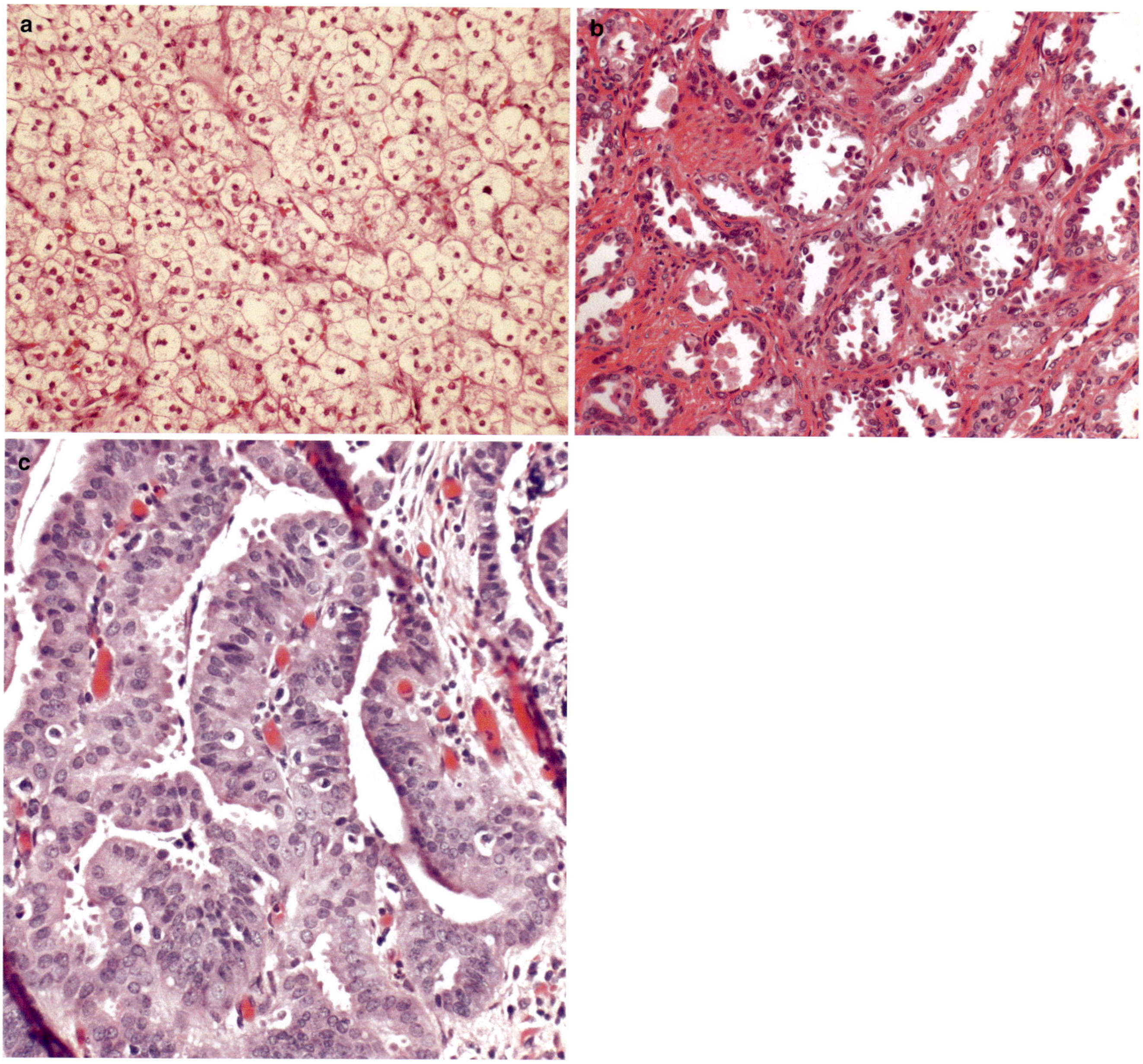

Fig. 10.9 Adenocarcinoma of the vagina. Clear cell adenocarcinoma may appear as sheets of cells with clear cytoplasm (**a**) or have a tubulopapillary architecture (**b**). Other types of adenocarcinoma include endometrioid (**c**), as well as endocervical and intestinal types (not shown)

sites and may have a clear cell or tubulopapillary appearance (Fig. 10.9). Adenocarcinoma can also rarely arise from endometriosis [20].

Adenocarcinomas not associated with DES have been reported in late reproductive and postmenopausal patients but can also occur in younger patients [11, 29]. Mucinous adenocarcinomas may be of endocervical or intestinal type. Primary vaginal adenocarcinoma of intestinal type is a rare tumor that must be distinguished from metastatic disease, particularly from the gastrointestinal tract [11]. This can be challenging, as the primary vaginal colonic-type lesions stain for CK20 and CEA, as well as CDX2 [30], but are negative for CK7, similar to a colonic neoplasms [11]. Theories of the origin of these lesions include gastrointestinal metaplasia, heterotopia, adenosis, mesonephric or cloacal remnants, or evolution from metaplastic endometriosis [11]. Endocervical-type adenocarcinoma has been theorized to arise from adenosis or endocervicosis [31]. Adenocarcinoma arising in the vagina may also be of the endometrioid type (Fig. 10.9c), as well as of serous, mucinous, or mesonephric types [26, 31–33]. The morphologic and immunophenotypic features of the various histotypes of primary vaginal adenocarcinomas are as described for these histotypes at other locations of the gynecologic tract.

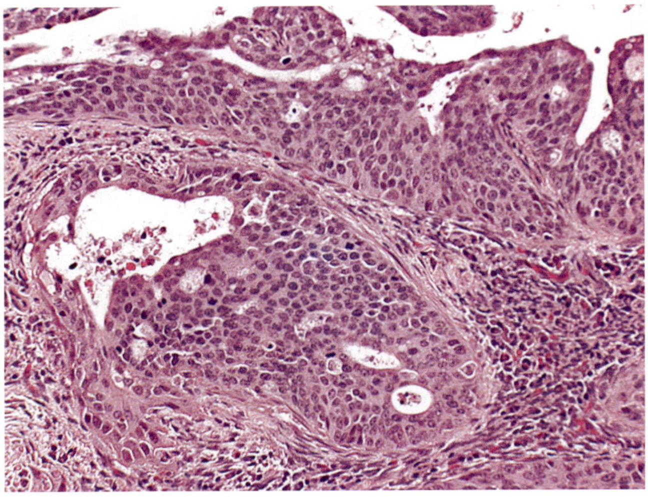

Fig. 10.10 Adenosquamous carcinoma, showing both squamous and glandular features

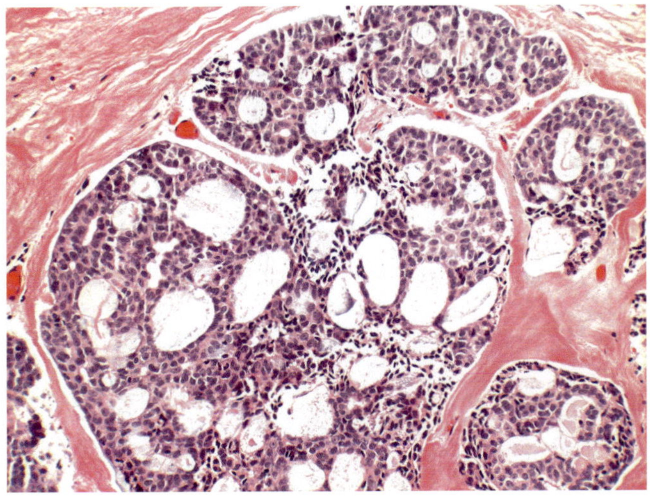

Fig. 10.11 Adenoid cystic carcinoma. The lesion is composed of "cookie cutter" round spaces in the epithelium, filled with basement membrane material

10.1.3.3 Adenosquamous Carcinoma

Adenosquamous carcinoma, containing both glandular and squamous differentiation (Fig. 10.10), has been reported as isolated cases [34, 35]. In one series, it represented about 4% of all primary vaginal cancers [35]. Lesions are most likely to arise on the anterior vagina [36]. The tumor has been described as locally aggressive with metastatic potential, as lung metastases have been described [35, 36]. Theories of origin have included adenosis, endometriosis, or growth from minor vestibular glands, misplaced Bartholin's glands, or glands of cloacogenic origin [36]. Glassy cell carcinoma, the most poorly differentiated aggressive form of adenosquamous carcinoma, which is usually seen in the cervix, has rarely been reported to arise primarily in the vagina [37].

10.1.3.4 Adenoid Cystic Carcinoma

Adenoid cystic carcinomas are classically described as tumors of the salivary glands, but rare cases have arisen in Bartholin's glands [38] and the vagina [39]. The tumors are composed of bland epithelial nests with cribriform architecture, embedded in an eosinophilic stroma composed of basement membrane material (Fig. 10.11). A tumor in the differential diagnosis of adenoid cystic carcinoma is polymorphous low-grade adenocarcinoma, another salivary gland neoplasm which has been reported to arise in the vulva and vagina [40]. It can be distinguished from adenoid cystic by its mixed pattern of cribriform (resembling adenoid cystic), papillary, and cystic growth [40]. Both lesions arise too infrequently in the vagina to establish prognosis; however, in the salivary glands, adenoid cystic carcinomas can metastasize, while polymorphous low-grade adenocarcinoma can recur locally [40].

10.1.3.5 Adenoid Basal Carcinoma

Adenoid basal carcinoma is a rare cervical lesion, with only sporadic case reports in the vagina [39, 41]. Nave's case [41] arose in the posterior upper third of the vagina in a 46-year-old woman who presented with abnormal bleeding. The lesions are composed of subepithelial nests of basaloid cells with no stromal reaction. The center of the nests may show glandular or squamous differentiation [36, 41](Fig. 10.12). A benign lesion in the differential diagnosis is a tubulosquamous vaginal polyp, which may contain abundant basaloid nests [14, 42]. However, tubulosquamous vaginal polyps can be differentiated from adenoid basal carcinoma by areas of frank squamous differentiation, as well as the presence of a tubular component. Basaloid nests, when present, are less likely to show prominent palisading in tubulosquamous vaginal polyps [42].

10.1.3.6 Neuroendocrine Carcinoma

Neuroendocrine carcinoma is more common in the cervix but can rarely arise in the vagina. The lesions may be of either small cell or large cell type.

Extrapulmonary small cell carcinoma is unusual. It can arise in the cervix, endometrium, ovary, vulva, and vagina [43]. Small cell neuroendocrine carcinoma of the vagina was first described by Scully et al. [44]. At the time of Bing's series, there were 25 described cases of small cell neuroendocrine carcinoma primary in the vagina [45]. Small cell neuroendocrine carcinoma is similar to the lung primary, with sheets of small cells with minimal cytoplasm, granular "salt and pepper" chromatin, and inconspicuous nucleoli [45]. There is often abundant necrosis and mitotic activity and a feature known as "crush artifact" (Fig. 10.13a, b).

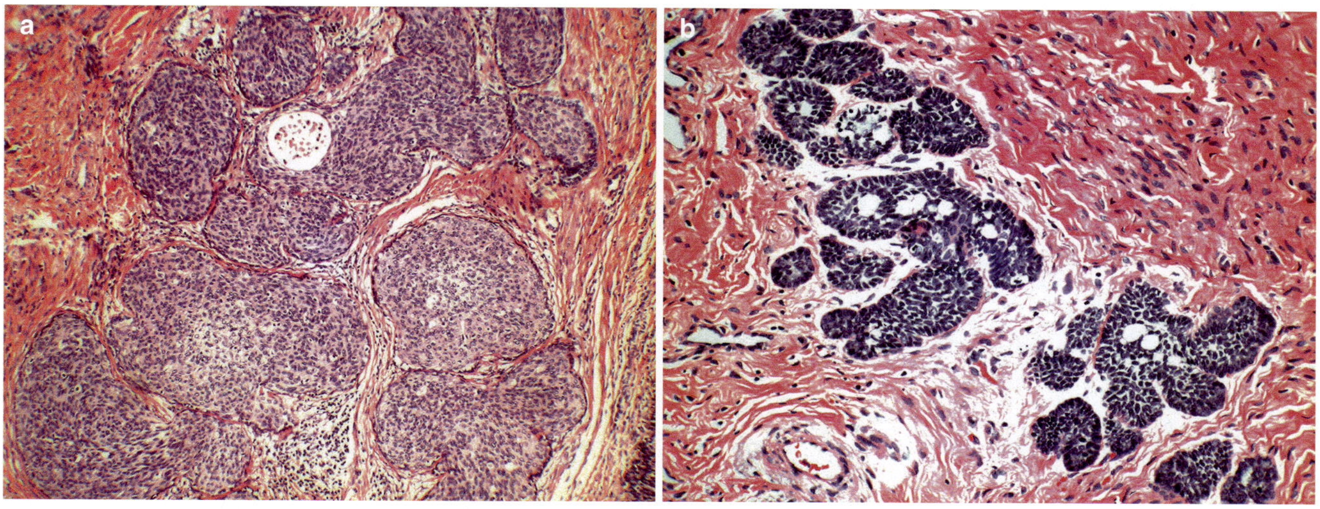

Fig. 10.12 Adenoid basal carcinoma. The lesion is composed of well-circumscribed nests of basaloid cells without a stromal reaction (**a**). Cystic spaces are often seen (**b**)

The tumors stain with neuroendocrine markers such as chromogranin and synaptophysin. Small cell carcinoma is a very aggressive tumor, typically presenting at an advanced stage with symptoms of bleeding, pain, and dysuria. A few cases have been associated with Cushing's syndrome due to ectopic ACTH production [46]. The lesions are often ulcerated and variable in size [36, 45]. Because of the rarity of the lesion, standardized therapy has not been established; however, they are typically treated with similar chemotherapeutic regimens as pulmonary tumors [47]. The origin of these tumors is not known; however, the lesion has been described with coexisting atypical adenosis of the vagina [48]. Coleman's case was described as having a Merkel cell carcinoma phenotype, based on positive CK20 staining, which was not investigated in many of the reported cases [49]. Merkel cell carcinoma is a neuroendocrine carcinoma of the skin.

Large cell neuroendocrine carcinoma (LNEC) is exceptionally rare, with only one case having been previously described [50]. The patient presented at an advanced stage, and histologically, the tumor was composed of sheets or organoid arrangements of poorly differentiated malignant cells with more cytoplasm that the small cell tumor. There was no nuclear molding, and nucleoli were prominent [50] (Fig. 10.13c–e). Neuroendocrine markers are expected to be positive as they are in the small cell variant.

10.1.3.7 Undifferentiated Carcinoma

Carcinomas lacking specific differentiation can occur in the vagina [39]. Undifferentiated carcinomas are composed of sheets of primitive undifferentiated cells with no evidence of specific phenotype by histology or immunohistochemistry.

10.2 Mixed Epithelial and Mesenchymal Tumors

10.2.1 Mixed Tumor

Mixed tumors of the vagina are rare benign lesions seen predominantly in premenopausal women and tend to occur in the lower vagina near the hymenal ring [14]. These lesions differ in appearance from the salivary gland tumors of the same name, which are thought to be of myoepithelial origin. Their origin in the vagina is unclear [51]. Vaginal mixed tumors are well circumscribed but not encapsulated [21]. The lesion is composed of both epithelial and stromal elements, with a mix of squamous, glandular, and spindle cells, which, although mesenchymal in appearance, stain with cytokeratin [14] (Fig. 10.14). In a series of cases, it was shown that these lesions have coexpression for epithelial and mesenchymal markers, without a specific immunoprofile, and therefore, diagnosis should rely on histology [51]. The authors felt the tumor may arise from pluripotential cells. Treatment is excision, although rarely these can recur [21].

10.2.2 Vaginal Adenosarcoma

Extrauterine adenosarcomas, including those arising in the vagina, are very rare lesions. Reported cases have occurred in midlife or postmenopausal women, with an association with prior hysterectomy [52]. Vaginal adenosarcoma has been proposed to arise from endometriosis [53, 54] or, alternatively, from pluripotential cells [53]. The tumors, like the uterine counterpart, are mixed epithelial-stromal tumors

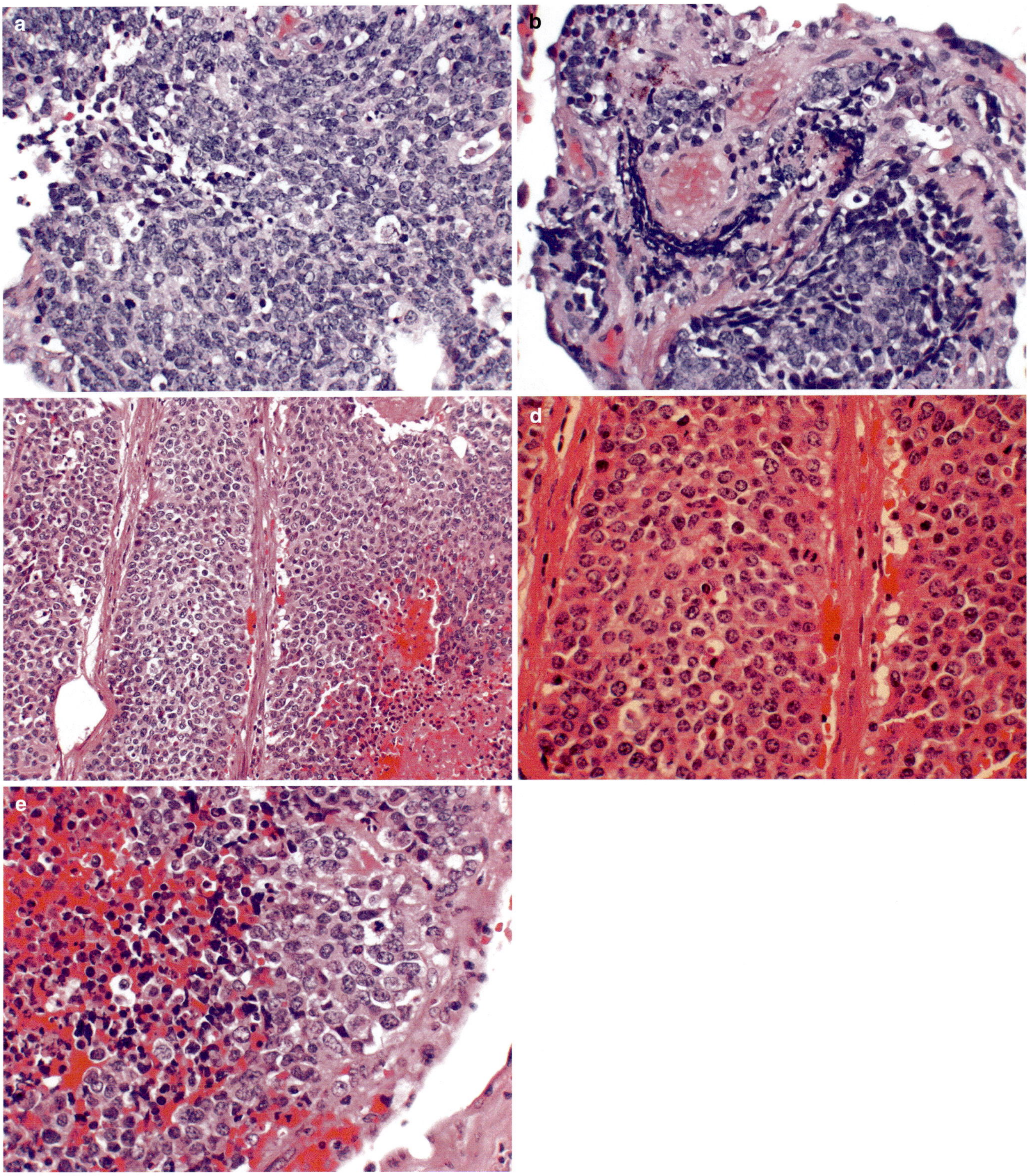

Fig. 10.13 Neuroendocrine carcinoma. The features of neuroendocrine carcinoma are demonstrated in these lung neoplasms. Small cell neuroendocrine carcinoma showing diffuse sheets of small cells with minimal cytoplasm and dispersed chromatin (**a**). Small cell carcinomas often show "crush artifact" (**b**). Large cell neuroendocrine carcinomas contain more cytoplasm than small cell neuroendocrine tumors (**c**–**e**) and may be arranged in organoid clusters (**c**, **d**) with areas of necrosis (**e**)

composed of benign glands in a malignant stroma. The lesions are often bulky and polypoid and may have a "phyllodes" (leaflike) architecture of epithelium lining sarcomatous projections. Histologically, the tumors are composed of benign-appearing endometrial-type glands and surface epithelium in a malignant spindle cell stroma, which has a

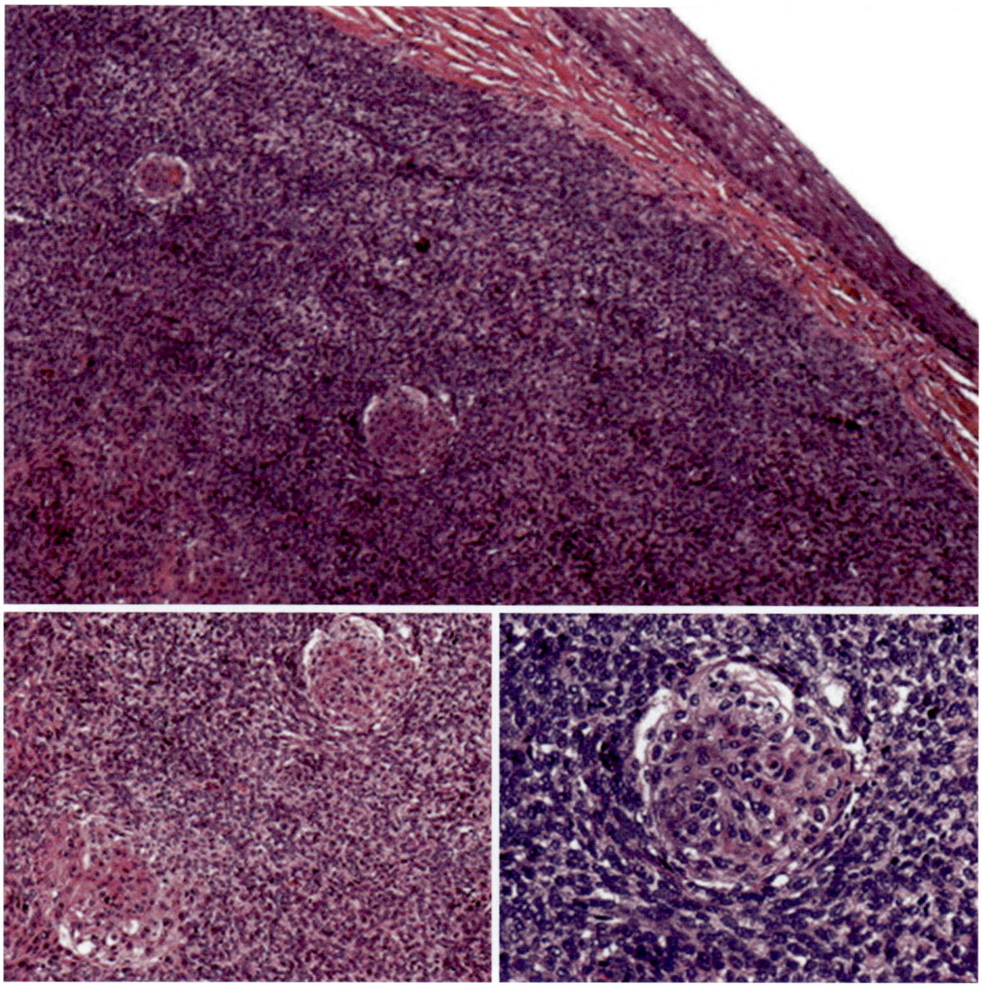

Fig. 10.14 Mixed tumor of the vagina. The lesion is composed of squamoid nests surrounded by spindle cells. The lesion is seen arising under the epithelium. Reprinted from Pathology Research and Practice 208(7) Mahe E, Bishara M, El Demellawy D, DeNardi F, Alowami S. The vaginal spindle cell epithelioma: A case report, review of the literature and discussion of potential histogenesis. p. 424–32, 2012 with permission from Elsevier

tendency to cuff around the glands under the surface in a "cambium" layer (Fig. 10.15). Heterologous elements such as rhabdomyosarcoma, chondrosarcoma, or liposarcoma can be present [55]. Although malignant, adenosarcomas usually are indolent; however, if sarcomatous overgrowth occurs, the tumor is aggressive with a poor prognosis [53].

10.2.3 Carcinosarcoma

Carcinosarcomas of the female genital tract usually arise from the endometrium of postmenopausal women. Primary vaginal carcinosarcomas are rare with only a few reports in the literature. They generally occur as a polypoid mass in postmenopausal women [56, 57]. The tumor is composed of malignant, high-grade epithelial and stromal elements, like its uterine counterpart; however, the epithelial component in vaginal tumors is more likely to be squamous as opposed to the more likely endometrioid epithelial component in the uterus (Fig. 10.16a) [56]. A previously described case was described as a polypoid lesion that was positive for HPV 31/33/51 by in situ hybridization in both the epithelial and mesenchymal components, favoring a metaplastic carcinoma for origin of the tumor [56]. Primary vaginal lesions appear to be aggressive [56, 57]. A diagnosis of carcinosarcoma should be made on the histologic presence of unequivocal, high-grade epithelial and mesenchymal components. This may be difficult in select cases, and immunohistochemistry may help; however, a diagnosis should never be made on immunohistochemical grounds alone. Sarcomatoid carcinoma is one of the most difficult entities to rule out in the differential diagnosis; however, sarcomatoid carcinoma (Fig. 10.16b) typically does not display vimentin expression as would be seen in the mesenchymal portion of carcinosarcoma [56].

10.2.4 Mixed Tumor Resembling Synovial Sarcoma

Synovial sarcoma is a soft tissue tumor that has overlapping epithelial and mesenchymal immunohistochemical markers. It may be monophasic with spindle cells, or biphasic, with a glandular or papillary epithelial component. Some cases may

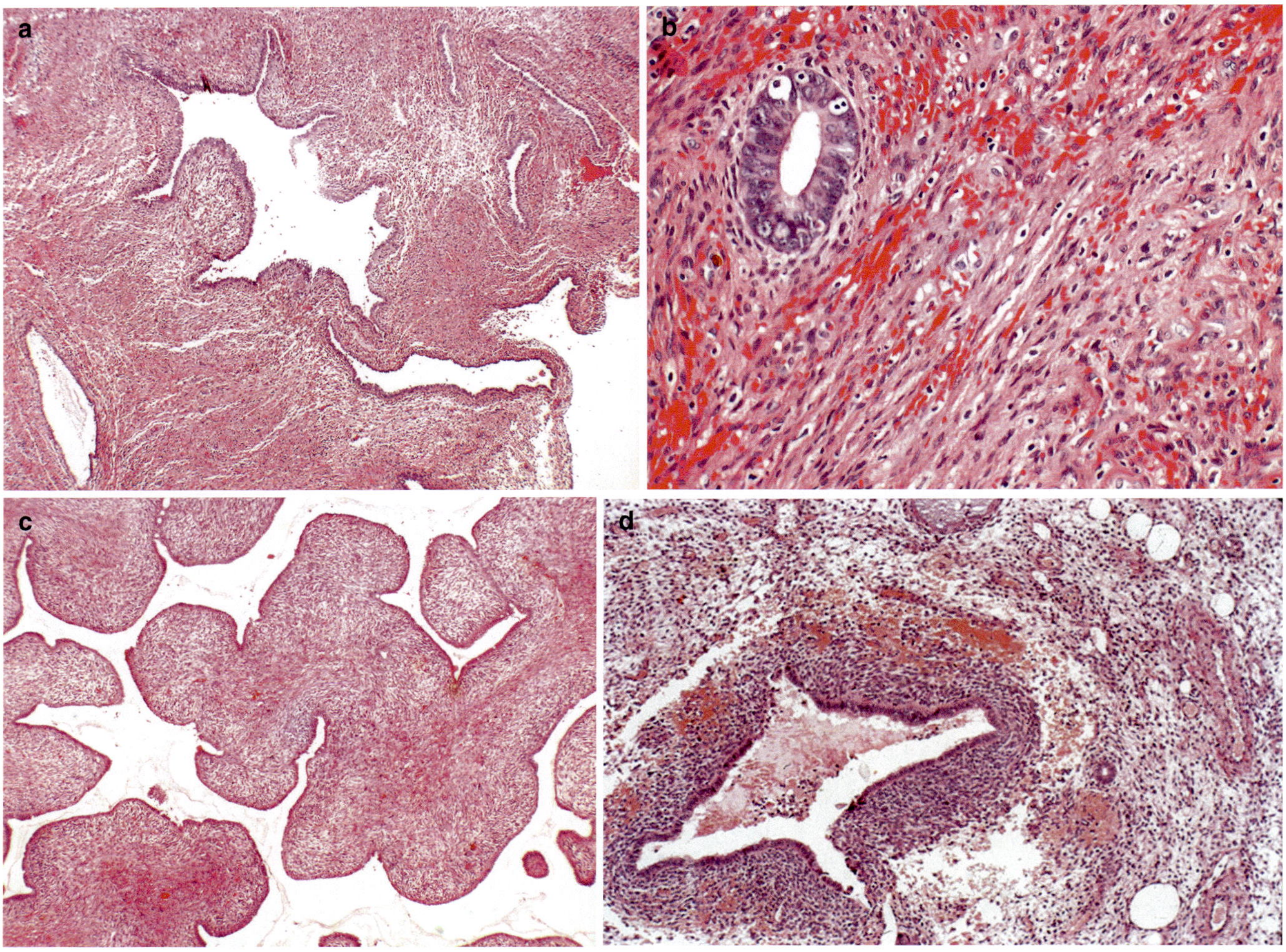

Fig. 10.15 Adenosarcoma. The lesions are composed of benign glands in a malignant stroma (**a**, **b**) and may have a leaflike (phyllodes) architecture (**c**). The malignant stromal cells may cuff under the glands in a "cambium" layer (**d**); (Part label **d** with permission from Heller DS, Handbook of Endometrial Pathology. London: JP Medical, 2012)

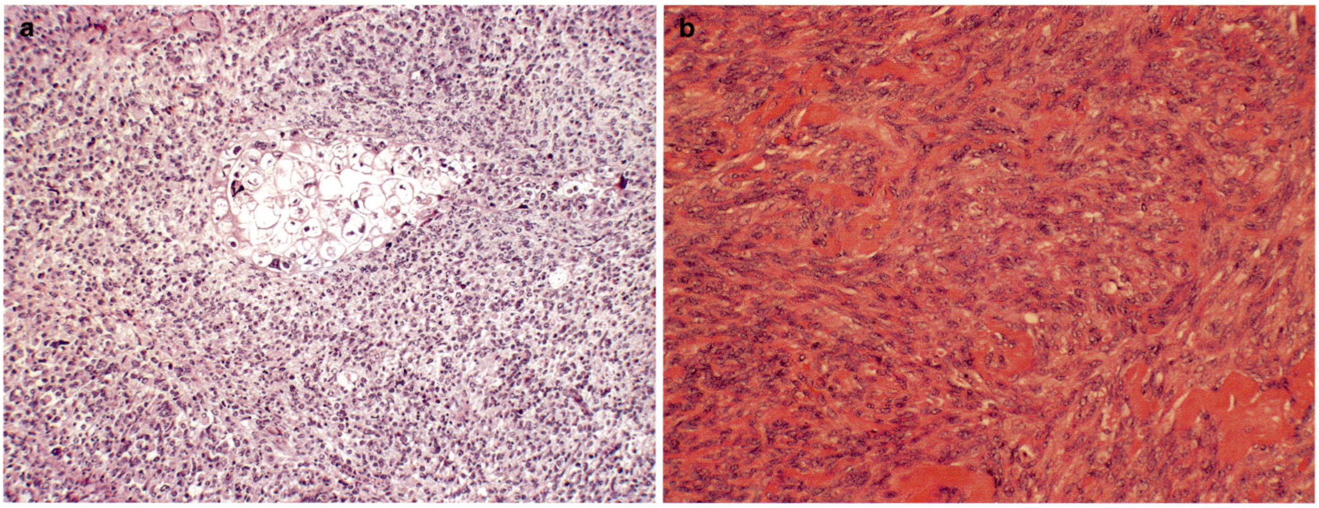

Fig. 10.16 Carcinosarcoma. Vaginal carcinosarcomas are more likely to have squamous epithelial elements rather than the endometrioid elements seen in the uterine counterpart (Part label **a**, With permission from Heller DS, Handbook of Endometrial Pathology. London: JP Medical, 2012). This needs to be distinguished from sarcomatoid carcinoma (**b**) which stains for keratins but not vimentin

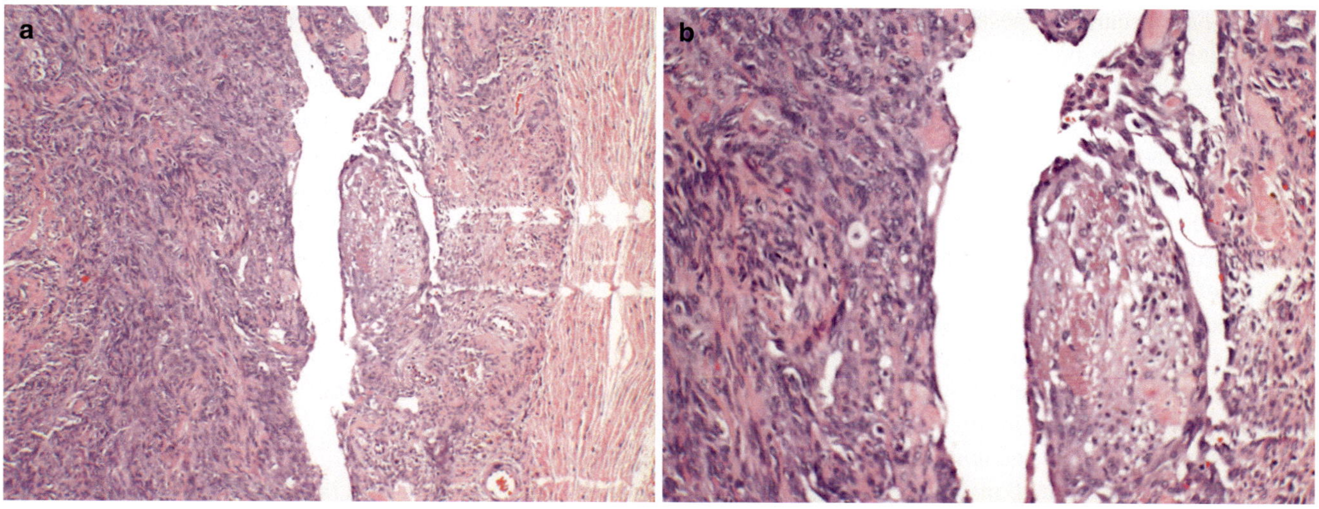

Fig. 10.17 Synovial sarcoma – this soft tissue lesion is spindle cell predominant, with only a minor epithelial component (**a**, **b**)

contain poorly differentiated sheets of pleomorphic tumor cells. In 1976, Okagaki et al. described a tumor arising in the upper vagina of a 24-year-old woman with a mixed pattern of tubular epithelial elements and spindle cell elements resembling fibrosarcoma, which they felt resembled synovial sarcoma [58]. They considered the tumor likely malignant, but did not provide follow-up. Since then, rare case reports of vaginal synovial sarcomas have appeared, with some of them having confirmatory molecular testing showing the characteristic X;18 translocation, as well as the overlapping immunoprofile of vimentin, cytokeratin, and epithelial membrane antigen [59]. Malignant behavior has been demonstrated, as proven in one case, where the patient developed lung metastases 11 months after initial surgery [60]. Additionally, another reported patient suffered multiple local recurrences and eventually died of disease 8 years after diagnosis [59]. The differential diagnosis of this lesion includes carcinosarcoma. Synovial sarcoma arising in the vagina has been described in younger women than carcinosarcoma, with one patient in her 20s and two in their 40s [58–60]. Additionally, the epithelial and mesenchymal components of carcinosarcoma are usually of higher grade than synovial sarcoma [59], which is often predominantly composed of a bland spindle cell proliferation (Fig. 10.17). This distinction, however, may be difficult, as both neoplasms tend to show sharp demarcation of epithelial and mesenchymal elements, overlapping immunoprofiles, and both may have heterologous elements [59]. Mixed tumor of the vagina is also in the differential diagnosis but usually has both squamous and glandular epithelial elements, with a spindle cell component that is usually bland with no mitotic activity. Mixed tumors are more likely to be diffusely positive for cytokeratin, while the spindle cell component of synovial sarcoma is usually focally positive for cytokeratin [59]. Monophasic spindle cell synovial sarcoma raises a wide differential of spindle cell lesions that can occur in the vagina, which can be distinguished by immunohistochemistry and molecular genetic studies.

10.3 Other Rare Tumors

10.3.1 Melanocytic Lesions

10.3.1.1 Melanocytic Nevus

The vagina does not usually contain melanocytes; however, rare benign pigmentation of the vagina has been reported [61]. Although theoretically possible, no well-documented melanocytic nevus has been reported in the literature [36]. Melanocytic nevi are composed of nests of melanocytes, which may be intradermal, junctional, or compound, based on the location of the cells.

10.3.1.2 Blue Nevus

Blue nevi are so termed because grossly they display a blue hue. This gross feature is because of the clusters of spindle-shaped dendritic melanocytes that comprise these lesions that are located deep in the dermis [36] with no junctional activity. Vaginal blue nevi have been occasionally reported [62]. These benign lesions may be biopsied over concern of melanoma (Fig. 10.18).

10.3.1.3 Malignant Melanoma

Vaginal melanoma represents about 3% of malignant vaginal tumors [28]. This aggressive neoplasm is usually diagnosed late, with poor outcome, presenting symptoms including bleeding, mass, or discharge [22]. In one reported case, the patient developed a paraneoplastic syndrome comprised of paraneoplastic cerebellar degeneration with opsoclonus myoclonus [63]. The lesions tend to arise in the lower vagina, and most have occurred in postmenopausal women [22]. As in other areas of the body, mucosal melanomas tend to be more aggressive than their cutaneous counterparts; hence, vaginal melanoma typically behaves more aggressively than the more common vulvar melanoma [22]. Compared with an overall 50–60% 5-year survival in vulvar melanoma, vaginal melanoma has an overall 15% 5-year survival, with frequent local recurrences and distant metastasis (lung and liver) [63]. Because of the rarity of the lesion, treatment has been individualized. Radical surgery has not been shown to improve outcomes [64]; however, surgical excision as primary treatment seems to be the best option when possible, with radiotherapy sometimes used in nonresectable disease [65]. Adjunctive chemotherapy and immunotherapy are also used. In evaluation of a vaginal melanoma excised specimen, tumor size and Breslow thickness should be provided, as they are with the vulvar tumor. Tumor thickness has been described as an indicator of disease-free interval but not survival in one meta-analysis, with size less than 3 cm a significant survival factor [66]. Fortunately, most vaginal melanomas are pigmented [64]. Histologically, vaginal melanoma is similar to other locations, with either an epithelioid, spindle cell, or mixed histology (Fig. 10.19). Prominent nucleoli are often seen in epithelioid lesions, as well as scattered mitotic figures and a loss of cellular maturation in the submucosal connective tissue. Tumors are immunoreactive for melanocytic markers such as S100, HMB 45, SOX10, tyrosinase, miTF, and Melan-A.

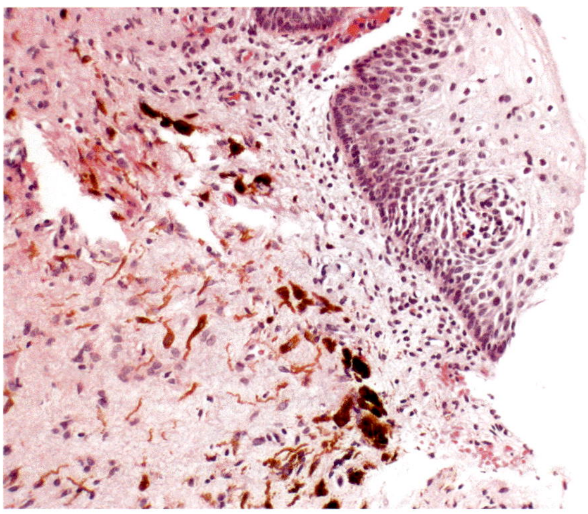

Fig. 10.18 Blue nevus. Dendritic melanocytes are seen in the submucosa

10.3.2 Germ Cell Tumors

10.3.2.1 Dermoid Cyst

Vaginal dermoid cysts are rare, although they have been known since biblical times [67]. The term is used as it is in cutaneous dermoids, rather than as it is for ovarian "dermoids" which are composed of all three germ cell layers. In skin and vaginal dermoids, ectodermal cells are entrapped during embryogenesis [68]. The differential diagnosis includes vaginal cysts, paravaginal cysts including embryologic remnants (Gartner's duct and Müllerian cysts), and epidermal inclusion cysts [69], the last two of which are similar on ultrasound [70]. As several of the reported cases of dermoid cyst of the vagina occurred in women with prior episiotomy, it is possible that dermal appendages became entrapped and that dermoid cysts are actually a type of epidermal inclusion cyst [70].

10.3.2.2 Yolk Sac Tumor or Endodermal Sinus Tumor

Extragonadal yolk sac tumor (endodermal sinus tumor) most commonly arises in the vagina [21], but it is an uncommon lesion with less than 100 cases reported [71]. The clinical differential diagnosis includes the more common rhabdomyosarcoma, which can be distinguished on histopathology. Yolk sac tumor is usually seen in girls under 3 years of age,

Fig. 10.19 Melanoma. Sheets of cells with prominent nucleoli (**a**, **b**) and melanin pigment (**b**) are seen

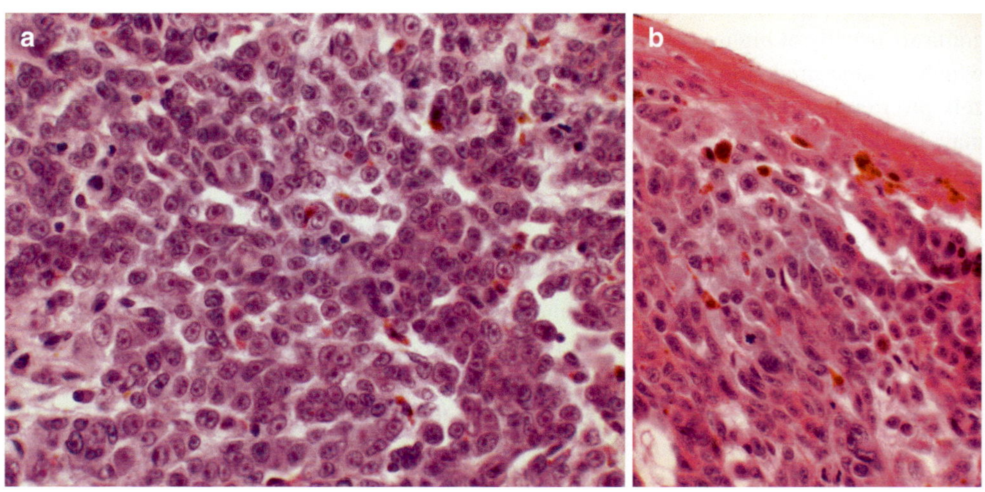

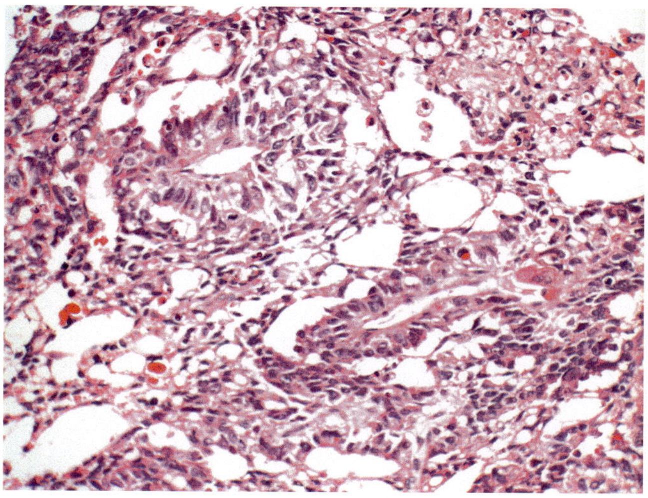

Fig. 10.20 Yolk sac tumor. The lesion is comprised of a reticular pattern. Two Schiller-Duval bodies are seen. Eosinophilic globules positive for AFP (not shown) are often present

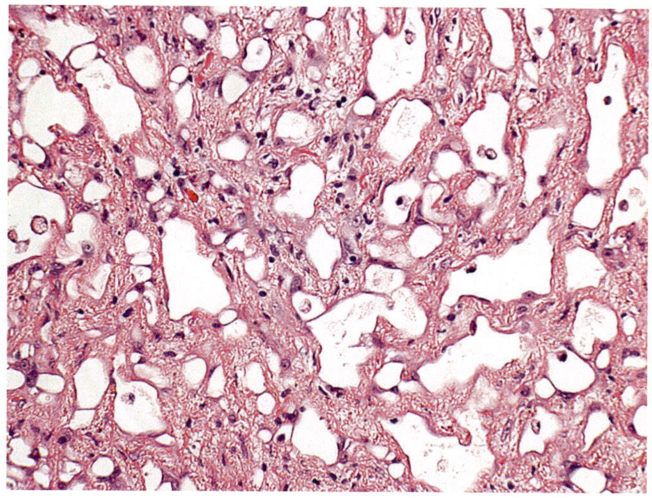

Fig. 10.21 Adenomatoid tumor, comprised of tubules lined by flattened mesothelial cells

presenting as a polypoid lesion [21, 72]. With improved chemotherapy, survival is much improved, and there has been a move away from radical surgery and toward either conservative surgery with chemotherapy or sometimes chemotherapy alone [71, 72]. Histologically, the tumor is similar to the ovarian counterpart, with a reticular pattern containing Schiller-Duval bodies and PAS- and AFP-positive globules (Fig. 10.20).

10.3.3 Other Tumors

10.3.3.1 Adenomatoid Tumor

Adenomatoid tumors are benign neoplasms occasionally seen as incidental findings in the uterus or fallopian tubes. Rarely, they can arise in the vagina (Fig. 10.21). They are of mesothelial origin and hence stain for mesothelial markers such as calretinin, D2-40, and WT-1 [73]. The lesions are composed of tubules lined by a flattened epithelium.

10.3.3.2 Neuroectodermal Tumors

Neuroectodermal tumors (peripheral neuroectodermal tumor (PNET), Ewing's sarcoma) are most often lesions of the bone and soft tissue, but rare cases have been reported in the vagina [74, 75]. These lesions fall under the category of small round blue cell tumors, requiring immunohistochemistry and molecular studies to establish the diagnosis. Membranous CD99 and Fli-1 immunostaining are expected, but may not be specific. Epithelial and neuroendocrine markers may be positive. A characteristic t11;22 (q24;q12) translocation is seen in most of these lesions [74, 75] and serves to confirm the diagnosis. In one series of seven cases [74], patient age ranged from 28 to 47 years. Lesions presented as masses of variable size, with vaginal bleeding in some cases.

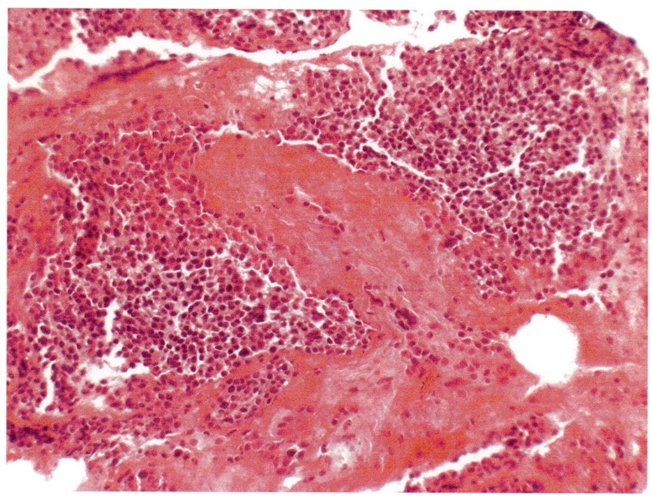

Fig. 10.22 Ewing's sarcoma. This lesion of the bone shows the characteristic sheets of small blue cells with minimal cytoplasm

All patients were alive 3–48 months after diagnosis. Histologically the tumors are composed of lobulated sheets of small blue cells with coarse chromatin and small nucleoli [75] (Fig. 10.22).

10.3.3.3 Lymphoma and Leukemia

Primary vaginal lymphoma is exceptionally rare, although it is not an unusual site in disseminated disease [76]. Presenting symptoms of primary vaginal lymphoma have included pain, bleeding, discharge, and a mass lesion, although they may be asymptomatic. Most cases are composed of diffuse large B cell lymphoma, which may present as multiple subepithelial nodules [76]. Histologically the lesions are similar to lymphomas elsewhere in the body (Fig. 10.23a), and adjunctive studies including cytogenetics, FISH, flow cytometry, and

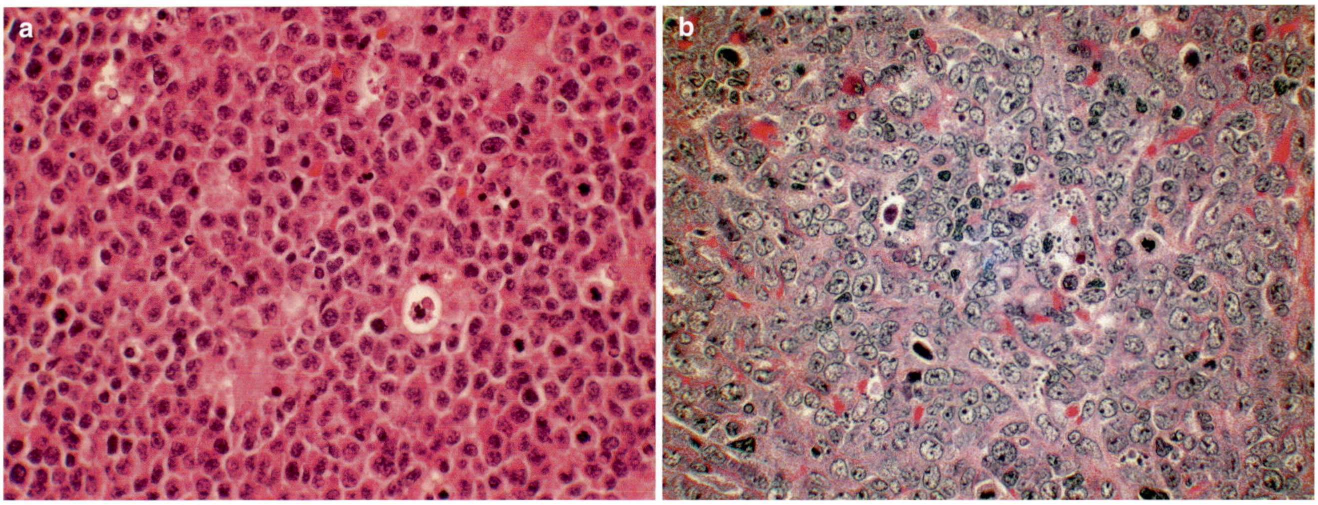

Fig. 10.23 Hematologic neoplasms. The vagina is a rare site for lymphoma (**a**) and myeloid sarcoma (**b**), both falling under the small round blue cell tumor category, requiring adjunct studies to elucidate the lineage

immunohistochemistry are useful adjuncts in the workup of such a lesion. Therapy is nonsurgical and utilizes chemotherapy [76]. Distinguishing lymphoma from other small blue cell lesions that can occur in the vagina, such as small cell neuroendocrine carcinoma, is critical as treatment modalities differ drastically between most of the tumors in this differential diagnosis.

Myeloid (granulocytic) sarcomas are solid masses composed of myeloid precursor cells and may be associated with a myeloproliferative disorder or rarely predate a leukemia [77]. Its occurrence in the vagina is exceptionally rare, with one case presenting with vaginal bleeding [77]. Historically, these tumors were termed "chloroma" referring to the green color that can be seen grossly due to myeloperoxidase. The lesions usually arise as submucosal nodules. The tumor is composed of sheets of mononuclear cells (Fig. 10.23b) and falls into the small round blue cell category. It has been suggested that therapy be individualized in these rare cases [77]. Overall prognosis is poor [78].

10.3.3.4 Secondary Tumors

80–90% of vaginal malignancies are secondary to metastatic disease, with primaries arising from the vulva, cervix, bladder, or rectum [20]. Metastatic disease may be from both genital tract and extragenital primaries [79]. Metastatic diseases from endometrial and ovarian primaries are not infrequent. According to one study, the most common primary site of metastatic carcinoma is the cervix, followed by the endometrium, colon, ovary, vulva, and urinary tract [27]; however, another series [79] found that the most common primary sites were the colon and rectum (Fig. 10.24). It is important to have the patient's prior history and to employ adjunctive immunohistochemistry in these cases to avoid errors in diagnosis and therapy.

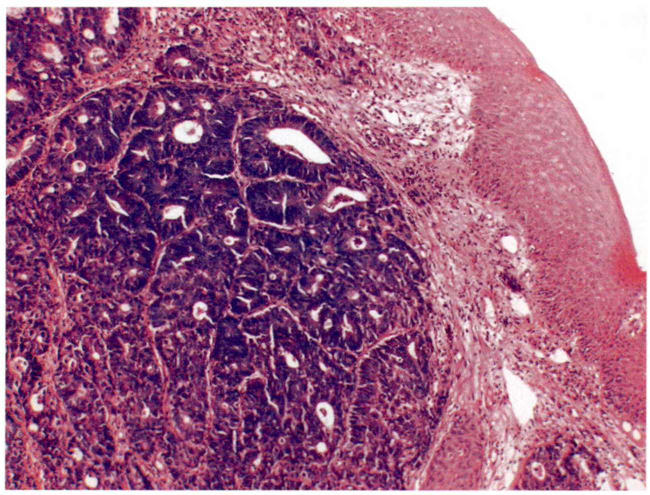

Fig. 10.24 Colonic adenocarcinoma metastatic to vaginal submucosa

References

1. Diaz Gonzales JM, Martinez Luna E, Pena Romero A, Molina Hernandez A, Dominguez Cherit J. Vestibular papillomatosis as a normal vulvar anatomical condition. Dermatol Online J. 2013;19(10):20032.
2. Rollason TP, Byrne P, Williams A. Immunohistochemical and electron microscopic findings in benign fibroepithelial vaginal polyps. Am J Clin Pathol. 1990;43(3):224–9.
3. Nucci MR, Young RH, Fletcher CDM. Cellular pseudosarcomatous fibroepithelial stromal polyps of the lower female genital tract: an under recognized lesion often misdiagnosed as sarcoma. Am J Surg Pathol. 2000;24:231–40.
4. Heller A, Ukazu A, Wang Q. Pseudosarcomatous vaginal polyp: a benign mimic of malignancy. Int J Surg Pathol. 2017;2:54–5.
5. Hartmann CA, Sperling M, Stein H. So-called fibroepithelial polyps of the vagina exhibiting an unusual but uniform antigen profile characterized by expression of desmin and steroid hormone recep-

tors but no muscle specific actin or macrophage markers. Am J Clin Pathol. 1990;93:604–8.
6. Reck-Burneo CA, Villanueva J, Velcek FT. Vaginal Müllerian papilloma: an unusual cause of vaginal bleeding in a toddler. J Pediatr Adolesc Gynecol. 2009;22:e124–6.
7. Luttges JE, Lubke M. Recurrent benign Mullerian papilloma of the vagina. Arch Gynecol Obstet. 1994;225:157–60.
8. Abu J, Nunns D, Ireland D, Brown L. Malignant progression through borderline changes in recurrent Mullerian papilloma of the vagina. Histopathology. 2003;42:510–7.
9. Pena-Fernandez M, Abdulkader-Nallib I, Novo-Dominguez A, et al. Vaginal tubulovillous adenoma: a clinicopathologic and molecular study with review of the literature. Int J Gynecol Pathol. 2012;32:131–6.
10. Lee SE, Park NH, Park IA, Kang SB, Lee HP. Tubulovillous adenoma of the vagina. Gynecol Oncol. 2005;96:556–8.
11. Mudhar HS, Smith JH, Tidy J. Primary vaginal adenocarcinoma of intestinal type arising from an adenoma: case report and review of the literature. Int J Gynecol Pathol. 2001;20:204–9.
12. Shaco-Levy R, Benharroch D. Vaginal Brenner tumor. Int J Gynecol Pathol. 2013;32:238–41.
13. Stewart CJR. Tubulosquamous vaginal polyp with basaloid epithelial features. Int J Gynecol Pathol. 2009;28:563–6.
14. McCluggage WG, Young RH. Tubulo-squamous polyp: a report of ten cases of a distinctive hitherto uncharacterized vaginal polyp. Am J Surg Pathol. 2007;31:1013–9.
15. Nelson EL, Stockdale CK. Vulvar and vaginal HPV disease. Obstet Gynecol Clin N Am. 2013;40:359–76.
16. Srodon M, Stoler MH, Baber GB, Kurman RJ. The distribution of low and high-risk HPV types in vulvar and vaginal intraepithelial neoplasia (VIN and VAIN). Am J Surg Pathol. 2006;30:1513–8.
17. Darragh TM, Colgan TJ, Cox JT, et al. The lower anogenital squamous terminology standardization project for HPV-associated lesions: background and consensus recommendations from the College of American Pathologists, and the American Society for Colposcopy and Cervical Pathology. J Low Genit Tract Dis. 2012;16:205–42.
18. Gadducci A, Fabrini MG, Lanfredini N, Sergiampietri C. Squamous cell carcinoma of the vagina: natural history, treatment modalities, and prognostic factors. Crit Rev Oncol Hematol. 2015;93:211–24.
19. Hiniker SM, Roux A, Murphy JD, et al. Primary squamous cell carcinoma of the vagina: prognostic factors, treatment patterns, and outcomes. Gynecol Oncol. 2013;131:380–5.
20. Elsayes KM, Narra VR, Dillman JR, et al. Vaginal masses: magnetic resonance imaging features with pathologic correlation. Acta Radiol. 2007;48(8):921–33.
21. Robboy SJ, Welch WR. Selected topics in the pathology of the vagina. Hum Pathol. 1991;22:868–76.
22. Benedet JL. Vaginal malignancy. Curr Opin Obstet Gynecol. 1991;3:73–7.
23. Rajaram S, Maheshwari A, Srivastava A. Staging for vaginal cancer. Best Pract Res Clin Obstet Gynaecol. 2015;29:822–32.
24. http://www.cap.org/ShowProperty?nodePath=/UCMCon/Contribution%20Folders/WebContent/pdf/cp-vagina-16protocol-3200.pdf
25. Patrelli TS, Silini EM, Berretta R, et al. Squamotransitional cell carcinoma of the vagina: diagnosis and clinical management. Pathol Oncol. 2011;17:149–53.
26. Nomura H, Matoda M, Okamoto S, et al. Clinical characteristics of non-squamous cell carcinoma of the vagina. Int J Gynecol Cancer. 2015;25:320–4.
27. Nomoto K, Hori T, Kiya C, et al. Endometrioid adenocarcinoma of the vagina with a microglandular pattern arising from endometriosis after hysterectomy. Pathol Int. 2010;60:636–41.
28. Wilkinson EJ. Pathology of the vagina. Curr Opin Obstet Gynecol. 1991;3:553–60.
29. Tjalma WA, Colpaert CG. Primary vaginal adenocarcinoma of intestinal type arising from a tubulovillous adenoma. Int J Gynecol Cancer. 2006;16:1461–5.
30. Ditto A, Martinelli F, Carcangiu M, et al. Incidental diagnosis of primary vaginal adenocarcinoma of intestinal type: a case report and review of the literature. Int J Gynecol Pathol. 2007;26:490–3.
31. Tatsumi K, Schlappe B, Everett EN, Gibson PC, Mount SL. Primary vaginal mucinous adenocarcinoma of intestinal type, associated with intestinal metaplasia of Skene ducts in a diethylstilbestrol-exposed woman. Am J Clin Pathol. 2015;144:790–5.
32. Riva C, Fabbri A, Facco C, Tibiletti MG, Guglielmin P, Capella C. Primary serous papillary adenocarcinoma of the vagina: a case report. Int J Gynecol Pathol. 1997;16:286–90.
33. Heller DS, Merrell M, Sama J, Anderson J, Cracchiolo B. Periurethral vaginal adenocarcinoma of the intestinal type: report of two cases and review of the literature. Gynecol Oncol. 2000;77(3):478–81.
34. Nomura H, Matoda M, Okamoto S, et al. Clinical characteristics of non-squamous cell carcinoma of the vagina. Int J Gynecol Cancer. 2015;25:320–4.
35. Sulak P, Barnhill D, Heller P, et al. Nonsquamous cancer of the vagina. Gynecol Oncol. 1988;29:309–20.
36. Kurman RJ, Carcangiu ML, Herrington CS, Young RH. WHO classification of tumors of the female reproductive organs. Geneva: WHO Press; 2014. p. 217.
37. Nasu K, Hamasaki C, Takai N, Narahara H. Glassy cell carcinoma arising in the vagina. Acta Obstet Gynecol. 2008;87:982–4.
38. Sahincioğlu O, Berker B, Güngör M, Kankaya D, Sertçelik A. Adenoid cystic carcinoma of the Bartholin's gland: a rare tumor unmarked by persistent vulvar pain in a postmenopausal woman. Arch Gynecol Obstet. 2008;278:473–6.
39. Kurman RJ, Norris HJ, Wilkinson E. Atlas of tumor pathology-tumors of the cervix, vagina, and vulva. 3rd ed. Washington, DC: American Registry of Pathology; 1992. p. 157–8.
40. Young S, Leon M, Talerman A, Teresi M, Emmadi R. Polymorphous low-grade adenocarcinoma of the vulva and vagina: a tumor resembling adenoid cystic carcinoma. Int J Surg Pathol. 2003;11:43–9.
41. Naves AE, Monti JA, Chichoni E. Basal cell-like carcinoma in the upper third of the vagina. Am J Obstet Gynecol. 1980;137:136–7.
42. Stewart CJ. Tubulo-squamous vaginal polyp with basaloid epithelial differentiation. Int J Gynecol Pathol. 2009;28:563–6.
43. Bhalodia JN, Kapapura DV, Parekh MN. Primary small cell neuroendocrine carcinoma of the vagina: a rare case report. Path Res Int. 2011;2011:306921.
44. Scully RE, Aguirre P, DeLellis RA. Argyrophilia, serotonin, and peptide hormones in the female genital tract and its tumors. Int J Gynecol Pathol. 1984;3:51–70.
45. Bing Z, Levine L, Lucci JA, Hatch SS, Eltorky MA. Primary small cell neuroendocrine carcinoma of the vagina: a clinicopathologic study. Arch Pathol Lab Med. 2004;128:857–62.
46. Colleran KM, Burge MR, Crooks LA, et al. Small cell carcinoma of the vagina causing Cushing's syndrome by ectopic production and secretion of ACTH: a case report. Gynecol Oncol. 1997;65:526–9.
47. Tamura R, Yokoyama Y, Kobayashi A, et al. A case of small cell carcinoma of the vagina. Rare Tumors. 2013;5:e58.
48. Khurana A, Gupta G, Gupta M, Kaur M. Primary neuroendocrine carcinoma of the vagina coexistent with atypical vaginal adenosis: a rare entity. J Cancer Res Ther. 2013;9:328–30.
49. Coleman NM, Smith-Zagone MJ, Tanyi J, et al. Primary neuroendocrine carcinoma of the vagina with Merkel cell carcinoma phenotype. Am J Surg Pathol. 2006;30:405–10.
50. Jin B, Pickens A, Shah MB, Turrisi A, Saleh H. Primary large cell neuroendocrine carcinoma of the vagina: cytomorphometry of previously unreported case. Diagn Cytopathol. 2010;38:925–8.
51. Oliva E, Gonzalez L, Dionigi A, Young RH. Mixed tumors of the vagina: an immunohistochemical study of 13 cases with emphasis

on the cell of origin and potential aid in differential diagnosis. Mod Pathol. 2004;17:1243–50.
52. Liu L, Davidson S, Singh M. Müllerian adenosarcoma of vagina arising in persistent endometriosis: report of a case and review of the literature. Gynecol Oncol. 2003;90:486–90.
53. Toyoshima M, Akahira J, Moriya T, Hayakawa S, Yaegashi N. Primary vaginal adenosarcoma with sarcomatous overgrowth. Gynecol Oncol. 2004;95:759–61.
54. Han X, Leng J, Guo L, Xiang Y, Lang J. Vaginal adenosarcoma arising from refractory endometriosis: a case report. Aust N Z J Obstet Gynaecol. 2010;50:574–6.
55. McCluggage WG. Mullerian adenosarcoma of the female genital tract. Adv Anat Pathol. 2010;17:122–9.
56. Sebenkik M, Yan Z, Khalbuss WE, Mittal K. Malignant mixed mullerian tumor of the vagina: case report and review of the literature, immunohistochemical study, and evaluation for human papilloma virus. Hum Pathol. 2007;38:1282–8.
57. Ahuja A, Safaya R, Prakash G, Kumar L, Shukla NK. Primary mixed mullerian tumor of the vagina-a case report with review of the literature. Pathol Res Pract. 2011;207:253–5.
58. Okagaki T, Ishida T, Hilgers RD. A malignant tumor of the vagina resembling synovial sarcoma. Cancer. 1976;37:2306–20.
59. Sumathi VP, Fisher C, Williams A, et al. Synovial sarcoma of the vulva and vagina: a clinicopathologic and molecular genetic study of 4 cases. Int J Gynecol Pathol. 2010;30:84–91.
60. Pelosi G, Luzzatto F, Landoni F, et al. Poorly differentiated synovial sarcoma of the vagina: first reported case with immunohistochemical, molecular, and ultrastructural data. Histopathology. 2007;50:808–10.
61. Toncini C, Innocenti S. Two pigmented lesions of the female genital system-blue nevus of the uterine endocervix and melanin pigmentation of the vagina. Eur J Gynaecol Oncol. 1984;5:76–84.
62. Fitzhugh VA, Houck K, Heller DS. Vaginal blue nevus: report of a case and review of the literature. J Low Genit Tract Dis. 2011;15:325–7.
63. Hauspy J, Nevin A, Harly I, et al. Paraneoplastic syndrome in vaginal melanoma: a case report and review of the literature. Int J Gynecol Cancer. 2007;17:1159–63.
64. Stefanovic A, Jeremic J, Jeremic K, Likic I, Mitrovic M, Stojnic J. Primary melanoma of the vagina: a case report and review of the literature. Eur J Gynaecol Oncol. 2015;36:755–7.
65. Miner TJ, Delgado R, Zeisler J, et al. Primary vaginal melanoma: a critical analysis of therapy. Ann Surg Oncol. 2004;11:34–9.
66. Reid GC, Schmidt RW, Roberts JA, Hopkins MP, Barrett RJ, Morley GW. Primary melanoma of the vagina: a clinicopathologic analysis. Obstet Gynecol. 1989;74:190–9.
67. Steinfeld AD, McDuff HC. An ancient report of a dermoid cyst of the vagina. Surg Gynecol Obstet. 1980;150:95–6.
68. Heller DS. Vaginal cysts-a pathology review. J Lower Gen Tract D. 2012;16:140–4.
69. Hirose R, Imai A, Kondo H, Itoh K, Tamaya T. A dermoid cyst of the paravaginal space. Acta Gynecol Obstet. 1991;249:39–41.
70. Siu S-S, Tam W-H, To K-F, Yuen P-M. Is vaginal dermoid cyst a rare occurrence or a misnomer? A case report and review of the literature. Ultrasound Obstet Gynecol. 2003;21:404–6.
71. Rajagopal R, Ariffin H, Krishnan S, Abdullah WA, Lin HP. Pediatric vaginal yolk sac tumor: reappraisal of treatment strategy in a rare tumor in a unique location. J Pediatr Hematol Oncol. 2015;37:391–5.
72. Bhatt MD, Braga LH, Stein N, Terry J, Portwine C. Vaginal yolk sac tumor in an infant: a case report and literature review of the last 30 years. J Pediatr Hematol Oncol. 2015;37:e336–40.
73. Sangoi AR, McKenney JK, Schwartz EJ, Rouse RV, Longacre TA. Adenomatoid tumors of the female and male genital tracts: a clinicopathological and immunohistochemical study of 44 cases. Mod Pathol. 2009;22:1228–35.
74. Bancalari E, de Alava E, Tardio JC. Primary vaginal Ewing sarcoma: case report and review of the literature. Int J Surg Pathol. 2012;20:305–10.
75. McCluggage WG, Sumathi VP, Nucci MR, et al. Ewing family of tumours involving the vulva and vagina: a report of a series of four cases. J Clin Pathol. 2007;60:674–80.
76. Guastafierro S, Tedeschi A, Criscuolo C, et al. Primary extranodal non-Hodgkin's lymphoma: a case report and a review of the literature. Acta Haematol. 2011;128:33–8.
77. Modi G, Madabhavi I, Panchal H, et al. Primary vaginal myeloid sarcoma: a rare case report and review of the literature. Case Rep Obstet Gynecol. 2015;2015:957490. https://doi.org/10.1155/2015/957490. Epub 2015 Jan 18
78. Skeete DH, Cesar-Rittenberg P, Jong R, Murray SK, Colgan TJ. Myeloid sarcoma of the vagina: a report of 2 cases. J Low Genit Tract Dis. 2010;14:136–41.
79. Mazur MT, Hsueh S, Gersell DJ. Metastases to the female genital tract. Analysis of 325 cases. Cancer. 1984;53:1978–84.

Cervical Carcinogenesis, Early Detection and Prevention

11

Sharon J. Song, Diane Bruyere, Kyle Devins, Alizee Lebeau, M. Carolina Reyes, and Michael Herfs

Abstract

Cervical carcinoma is a major cause of morbidity and mortality in the United States and throughout the world. Associated to the infection with one or several high-risk human papillomavirus (HPV) genotypes, the incidence of cervical cancer increases progressively from age 30 and peaks between 45 and 50. Due to the implementation of screening programs, the number of diagnosed invasive cervical neoplasms has significantly decreased in the last decades in developed countries. The present chapter summarizes the current knowledge on HPV-related carcinogenesis, discusses the histology, diagnosis and outcome of HPV-positive cervical (pre)neoplastic lesions and, finally, reviews the different methods of cervical cancer screening/prevention.

Keywords

Human papillomavirus · Cervical cancer · Molecular mechanisms · Diagnosis · Screening · Prevention

11.1 Risk Factors of Cervical Cancer Development

11.1.1 HPV Infections

Cervical carcinoma is a major cause of morbidity and mortality in the United States and throughout the world. In the USA, cervical cancer ranks below uterine and ovarian cancers as the third most common gynecologic malignancy and the third highest cause of gynecologic cancer-related mortality [1–3]. Approximately 13,000 new US cases are diagnosed each year, with 4000 annual cancer-related deaths [1, 2]. However, cervical cancer is much more common in underdeveloped areas. In Africa and Central America, for example, it remains the leading cause of cancer-related death in women. Access to screening programs is the major reason for this disparity. Developed nations have experienced a 75% decrease in incidence and mortality from cervical cancer over the past 50 years due to the implementation of screening programs [4]. Racial and ethnic factors also appear to influence both incidence and mortality, with the highest rates occurring among black and Hispanic populations [1, 2] (see table). Cervical cancer has a bimodal age distribution, with most cases occurring in the fifth decade of life. However, older women remain at risk [5].

11.1.1.1 Risk Factors

The major risk factor for cervical cancer is infection with high-risk strains of human papillomavirus (HPV). In the cervix, high-risk HPV (hr-HPV) are associated with nearly all cases of cervical carcinoma, particularly squamous cell carcinoma (SCC) and conventional endocervical adenocarcinomas, the most common histologic subtypes. Studies using rigorous detection methods have identified hr-HPV in 99.7% of squamous cell carcinomas and >80% of cervical adenocarcinomas [6, 7].

HPV infection is spread primarily through sexual intercourse. As a result, most risk factors for cervical carcinoma are related to sexual exposure [8]. Women with multiple sexual partners, early age of first sexual intercourse, early age of first pregnancy, and coinfection with other sexually transmitted infections are at higher risk of HPV infection and subsequent carcinoma. As previously mentioned, access to screening programs is a major risk determinate. Women of poor socioeconomic status are therefore at increased risk [4].

Although infection with hr-HPV is a requisite step in most cases of cervical carcinogenesis, it does not appear to

M. Carolina Reyes and Michael Herfs are co-last authors.

S. J. Song · K. Devins · M. Carolina Reyes (✉)
Department of Pathology, Hospital of the University of Pennsylvania, Philadelphia, PA, USA
e-mail: Carolina.Reyes@uphs.upenn.edu

D. Bruyere · A. Lebeau · M. Herfs (✉)
Laboratory of Experimental Pathology, GIGA-Cancer, University of Liege, Liege, Belgium
e-mail: M.Herfs@uliege.be

W. Zheng et al. (eds.), *Gynecologic and Obstetric Pathology, Volume 1*, https://doi.org/10.1007/978-981-13-3016-2_11

be independently sufficient to cause invasive carcinoma [8]. This is evidenced by the high rate of clearance following initial HPV infection, suggesting other factors such as host immune response may play a role. The increased incidence of cervical carcinoma in HIV-infected individuals and women with other forms of immunosuppression further supports this concept [9, 10]. In addition, numerous studies have identified HLA antigen groups which positively or negatively affect the risk of cervical cancer development [10].

Obesity, tobacco and estrogen exposure have also been identified as independent risk factors for HPV-mediated cervical cancer [11, 12]. Women who smoke tobacco are twice as likely to develop cervical carcinoma than nonsmokers. Women with increased parity or long-term exposure to oral contraceptives may be at increased risk due to the effects of estrogens on the cervical transformation zone in conjunction with HPV infection. Women with a family history of cervical cancer are also at increased risk, suggesting genetic factors beyond those explained by HLA type [13].

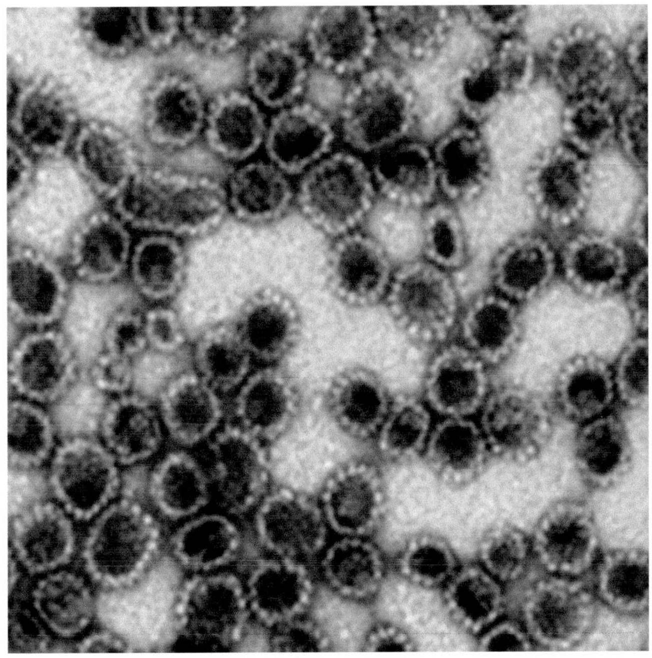

Fig. 11.1 Electron micrograph depicting HPV viral capsids (virus-like particles). Source: Courtesy of Prof. Antoine Touze, University of Tours, France

11.2 Non-HPV Risk Factors-Mediated Carcinogenesis

While the vast majority of cervical carcinomas are related to infection with hr-HPV, occasional HPV-negative cases occur. These carcinomas are typically adenocarcinomas of unusual histologic subtype, including clear cell, minimal deviation (adenoma malignum), gastric-type, and mesonephric [14]. These subtypes are rare, and their pathogenesis is poorly understood. They tend to occur in women of younger age and appear unrelated to HPV.

A subset of cases of clear cell adenocarcinoma is associated with exposure to diethylstilbestrol (DES) in utero [15]. DES is an estrogenic agent given to some pregnant women in the 1940s to 1970s. Women who were exposed to DES in utero have a 40× increased risk of vaginal and cervical clear cell carcinoma; however, the overall risk in exposed women remains low (approximately 1.6 per 1000) [16]. Minimal deviation adenocarcinoma is often associated with Peutz–Jeghers syndrome [17]. Exceptionally rare cases of HPV-negative squamous cell carcinoma of the cervix have been reported. In these cases, disease pathogenesis and risk factors remain unknown [18].

11.3 Human Papillomavirus

11.3.1 Structure and Classification of HPV

Belonging to the papovaviridae family, HPVs are non-enveloped and icosahedral viruses of approximately 55 nm in diameter. All HPV genotypes contain a circular double-stranded DNA (~8 Kb). This viral genome is divided into three parts [19]:

- A noncoding regulatory region [Long Control Region (LCR)] of about 1000 base pairs containing the origin of replication (Ori), the early promoter (p97), and encapsulation sequences.
- An "early" region coding for six early proteins (E1, E2, E4, E5, E6, E7). These proteins are involved in viral replication (E1, E2), amplification (E4), and cell immortalization/transformation (E5, E6, E7).
- A "late" region coding for two late proteins. Together, the major (L1) and minor (L2) structural proteins form 72 pentameric capsomeres constituting the viral capsid (Fig. 11.1).

To date, more than 220 different HPV genotypes have been identified on the basis of genomic differences [20]. The World Health Organization (WHO) divides HPVs according to their carcinogenic potential. Twelve viral strains (HPV16, 18, 31, 33, 35, 39, 45, 51, 52, 56, 58, 59) are designated as "high-risk." These oncogenic HPV are the causative agents of most (if not all) cervical cancers and precursors. In contrast, other genotypes (mainly HPV6 and 11) are only involved in the development of condylomas and benign genital warts.

Based on their L1 sequence similarity, virologists usually separate HPV genotypes into five groups: α-, β-, γ-, μ-, and ν-papillomaviruses [21]. To be part of the same genus, two viruses must display a genetic similarity of at least 60%. Within each of these five groups, HPVs that differ by more than 10% are considered as separated genotypes. The HPV community recently qualified sequences differing by less than 10% as variants (designated by A, B, C, D) [22]. These small variations in the HPV DNA sequences are thought to have occurred during human evolution and are presumed to have an impact in cancer development. Indeed, variants of the same HPV strain could have different oncogenic potentials as recently highlighted with both HPV16 and 18 (further information in *Epidemiology of HPV infection*).

11.3.2 Life Cycle of HPV

In the preceding decades, basal keratinocytes were considered as the only HPV-target cells. These latter cells were vulnerable to HPV infection following microtraumas or abrasions into the squamous epithelium lining the external part of the uterine cervix and the transformation zone [23]. This paradigm was recently undermined by accumulating evidence supporting the critical role of discrete populations of "junctional" cells in the pathogenesis of both cervical and anal (pre)cancers. Exhibiting intriguing phenotypic/transcriptomic similarities with the large majority (~90%) of cervical cancers and high-grade (pre)neoplastic lesions, these immature cuboidal cells located within the squamocolumnar (SC) junction were shown to be actively involved in cervical carcinogenesis [24] (Fig. 11.2). Following HPV infection, these cytokeratin7 (krt7)-positive

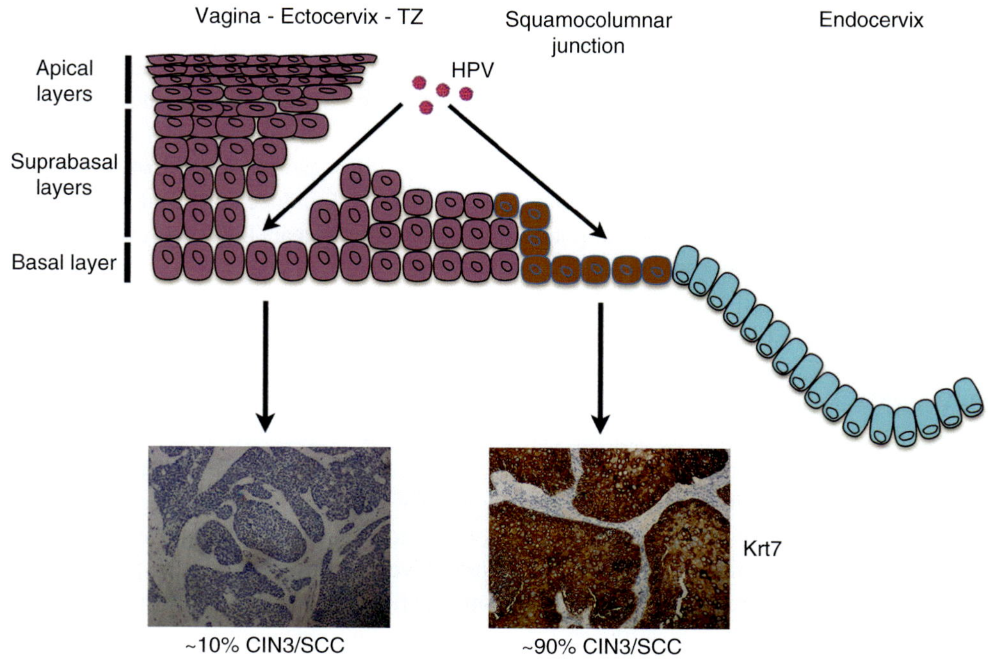

Fig. 11.2 HPV target cells in the uterine cervix. Following microtraumas into the squamous epithelium lining the ectocervix and the transformation zone, basal keratinocytes are vulnerable to HPV infection and related carcinogenesis. Based on phenotypic/transcriptomic analysis, this model of HPV infection is responsible for ~10% of all CIN3 and cancers. In contrast, ~90% CIN3 and invasive neoplasms are caused by the direct infection of a discrete population of cells located within or close to the squamocolumnar junction. *TZ* transformation zone, *Krt7* keratin 7 (adapted from Herfs and Crum, Nat Rev Clin Oncol 2015)

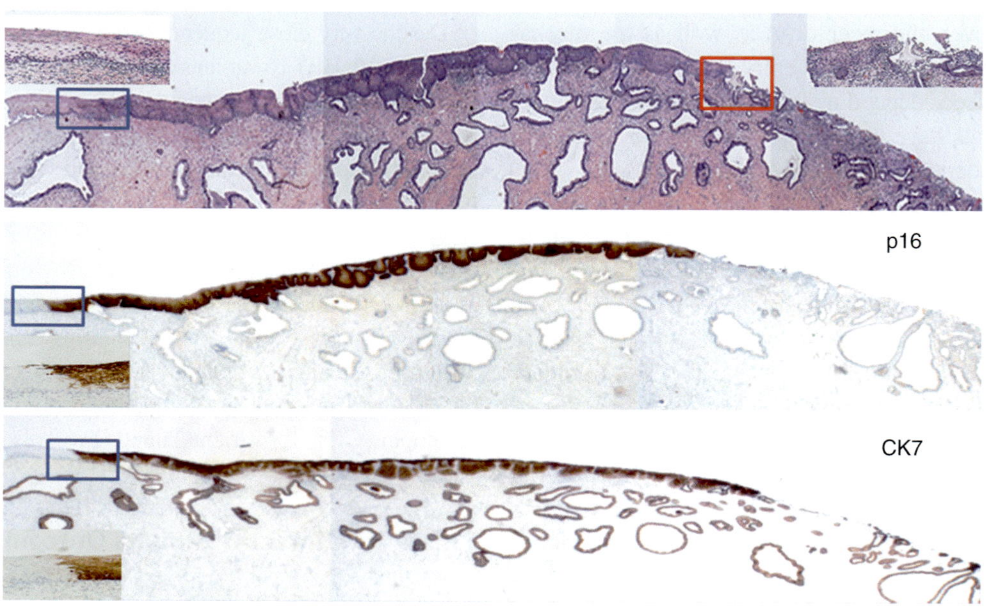

Fig. 11.3 Representative example of high-grade CIN developing at the squamocolumnar junction (SCJ), 4×. The upper left corner shows previous or old SCJ as shown in blue squared area, which is magnified in the left top corner, while the current SCJ is illustrated in upper right red squared area and magnified in the right top. Transformation zone is defined by the area between previous and current SCJ, which contains a high-grade intraepithelial lesion (HSIL) or precancerous lesion. This HSIL is highlighted by intense p16 stain (mid-panel) and Krt 7 overexpression (low panel). Such commonly clinically encountered findings support that the Krt7-positive cuboidal cells located within or in close proximity to the SCJ are the most vulnerable cells for HPV infection. (Figure contributed by Dr. W Zheng)

cells give rise to infected reserve cells. The proliferation of these progeny cells results in the development of (pre)cancerous lesions associated with a higher risk of progression [25] (Fig. 11.3). This model was named "top-down differentiation" due to the apical location of progenitor cells [26]. Explaining the high susceptibility of the uterine cervix for (pre)cancer development (cervical SCC is up to 25-fold more prevalent than vaginal/vulvar neoplasms [27]), the essential role of "junctional" cells in HPV-induced carcinogenesis was further highlighted by recent studies evaluating the expression profile of several biomarkers specifically expressed (or overexpressed) by these latter cells [i.e., Krt7 or cystic fibrosis transmembrane conductance regulator (CFTR)] in large series of cervical intraepithelial lesions [25, 28]. Intriguingly, HPV-positive adenocarcinomas also display a strong positivity for these biomarkers and were shown to mainly develop within the SC junction microenvironment [24, 29]. Although the differentiation potential of SC junction cells is still unknown, these results argue for the multipotent potential of these latter cells. Finally, one main question remains unsolved: what are the reasons for the high vulnerability of "junctional" cells to HPV infection and related carcinogenesis? Although a few explanations were recently proposed (i.e., the stabilization of HPV mRNA by some overexpressed keratin filaments such as Krt7 or the alteration of antiviral peptide expression), the subject still deserves further investigations [30].

Whatever the cell initially infected, the entry of HPV into host cells is initiated by the binding of the viral capsid to the basement membrane, rich in heparan sulfate proteoglycans. Cell surface cyclophilin B then mediates a conformational change in the viral capsid, resulting in the exposure of the minor capsid protein (L2). A highly conserved L2 site is finally cleaved by a convertase (furin) before cell internalization [31]. However, the receptor(s) as well as the mechanisms responsible for the HPV entry are still a matter of debate [32]. Indeed, depending on the experimental model used, two theories have been proposed: clathrin-dependent versus caveolin-dependent endocytosis.

After internalization, both the separation of L1 capsomers and a subviral complex of L2/viral DNA occur in late endosomes. The viral genome is then trafficked to the Golgi network before entering in the nucleus of the host cell where viral genome transcription starts [31]. Access to a cell able to undergo epithelial differentiation is mandatory for a productive viral cycle. The first viral mRNAs detected in the infected cells encode for both E1 and E2 proteins. The main role of these proteins is to initiate viral replication, bringing the viral load to around 100 copies per cell [20]. At this step, the infection is considered as nonproductive given that no new virion is produced yet. In infected basal cells, the viral and the host DNA are replicated at the same time and distributed equally between daughter cells. Within the upper cell layers of the squamous epithelium, a pattern of viral gene expression is executed to amplify viral genome and to express late viral proteins (caused by a switch towards late promoter activation). The last step of the viral cycle is the icosahedral particle formation. L1 and L2 proteins spontaneously assemble to form the capsid containing one copy of the viral genome. Given that HPV is a non-lytic virus, it takes advantage of the epithelium upper layer's peeling to be released into the extracellular environment and, eventually, to reinfect other epithelial cells [20].

11.3.3 Epidemiology of HPV Infection

HPV is the most common sexually transmitted infectious agent in industrialized countries and spreads by direct contact between infected sexual partners. The number of new HPV infections is estimated to reach 30 million per year worldwide. Most infections (>90%) are asymptomatic or induce epithelial lesions that regress spontaneously within 2 years [33]. However, a persistent (5–10 years) high-risk HPV infection may progress to invasive cancer. Each year, ~630,000 HPV-related neoplasms are diagnosed worldwide, including 520,000 cervical squamous cell carcinoma (SCC) [27]. Very rare before the age of 25, the incidence of cervical cancer increases progressively from age 30 and peaks between 45 and 50. Besides cervical carcinogenesis, oncogenic HPV genotypes (most notably HPV16) are also involved in a significant percentage of cancers occurring in the vulva (~40%), vagina (~80%), anal canal (~90%), penis (~50%), and oropharynx (~40%) [27]. It is important to note that a large disparity in terms of cancer risk is observed between countries. Indeed, as previously mentioned, ~85% of cervical cancers occur in developing countries due to a lack of prevention and insufficient screening measures.

Despite very close sequences (see *Structure and classification of HPV*), HPV16 variants could be associated with different cancer risks. Indeed, recent epidemiological studies highlighted that European variants (A) tend to be less carcinogenic than their non-European counterparts (B and C for African, D for Asian-American). The persistence of non-European HPV16 variants is approximately twice as long and associated with a two- to fourfold increased risk of CIN3 outcome [34, 35]. Moreover, for unclear reasons, D variants seem to be more commonly found in glandular neoplasms (adenocarcinomas) whereas A variants are mainly detected in SCC [36]. Regarding HPV18, evidences are less compelling but an increased risk of developing CIN3 for variants A and D was also reported [35].

11.3.4 HPV Infection and Its Outcome

Histologically, HPV-related preneoplastic lesions are divided into three groups. When atypical cells are only detected in the bottom third of the infected epithelium, a Cervical

Intraepithelial Neoplasia I (CIN I, also called mild dysplasia) is diagnosed. CIN II (moderate dysplasia) or III (severe dysplasia) are considered when atypical cells are observed in two-third or the entire epithelium, respectively. Besides this CIN classification, the Bethesda system is increasingly favored. With this latter, abnormal results include LSIL (Low-Grade Squamous Intraepithelial Lesions which correspond to CIN I) and HSIL (High-Grade Squamous Intraepithelial Lesions which contain both CIN II and CIN III) [37] (further information in *Terminology*).

About 75% of sexually active women will be infected by HPV during their lifetime but, as mentioned above, the large majority eliminates the virus within 2 years post infection. Based on large epidemiological studies, only ~10% of LSIL progress to HSIL and only one-third of these untreated high-grade lesions progress to invasive cancer [33].

11.4 Carcinogenesis After HPV Infection

11.4.1 Direct Tumorigenic Effects of HPV

The mechanism by which a high-risk HPV infection induces malignant transformation is complex but has been progressively elucidated during the last two decades [38]. E6 and E7 are the two major HPV oncoproteins (the role of E5 is more controversial). Globally, E6 interferes with cell survival pathways and E7 promotes cell proliferation, leading to cell immortalization.

The main E6 target protein is p53. Actually, this interaction is not direct and requires an E3 ubiquitin ligase called E6AP. Interestingly, the affinity of this latter protein with p53 is modified upon its binding with HPV E6. The related increased ubiquitination of p53 leads to its degradation and impedes the apoptosis of infected cells [39]. E6 is also known to interact with other pro-apoptotic proteins such as Bak, FADD, and procaspase 8 [40–42] as well as with other proteins implicated in protein degradation by the proteasome (UBR5/EDD, HERC2, S5a proteasome subunit) [43, 44]. Moreover, E6 derived from carcinogenic HPV genotypes activates hTERT (telomerase reverse transcriptase), therefore maintaining telomerase length at the end of the chromosome and contributing to cell immortalization [38].

The most described function for E7 is its capacity to directly interact with the pocket family proteins such as p107, p130, and pRb. The direct interaction between E7 and pRb induces both the ubiquitination and degradation of this latter protein by the proteasome [45]. No longer repressed by pRb, the transcription factor E2F can then induce the expression of Cyclin A and E as well as $p16^{ink4a}$. This creates a feedback loop, trying to restore the inhibitory function of pRb. Indeed, $p16^{ink4a}$ inhibits the phosphorylation of CDK4/6 and cyclin D complex and an imbalance towards activation of pRb arises. In the case of HPV infection and constant degradation of pRb, this loop is inefficient and leads to an overexpression of $p16^{ink4a}$ which is well known to be used as a standardized indirect method for oncogenic HPV detection [46] (see below). Besides the pocket family proteins, approximately 150 other host proteins (i.e., p21, p27, NuMa, …) were also reported to interact with the E7 oncoprotein [38, 47, 48].

Although collected results are unclear and/or still controversial, E5 from high-risk HPV genotypes could have a weak oncogenic potential and, in combination with E6 and E7 activities, might contribute to cell transformation. For example, E5 reduces endosomal acidification by inhibiting the vacuolar ATPase proton pump, which would promote EGFR activation and cell proliferation [49]. E5 was also shown to affect the KGFR (keratinocyte growth factor receptor)-mediated epithelial growth and deregulate cell autophagy [50]. Altogether, E5 would lead to the hyperproliferation of basal cells and to a decreased proliferation of the suprabasal layers of the squamous epithelium.

During early stages of HPV-related carcinogenesis, E6 and E7 oncoproteins are downregulated by E2, ensuring a balance between cell death and cell immortality. In contrast, in late stages (CIN III and cancer), an overexpression of viral oncoproteins occurs frequently. This phenomenon is explained by the integration of viral DNA into the host genome. During this process, the circular viral DNA becomes linear and the break is usually located in the E2 open reading frame (ORF) [51], preventing the transcription of this latter gene. Upon integration, the infected cells also stop producing viral particles. However, it is important to note that ~20% of cervical cancers still carry an episomal form of HPV, suggesting that viral integration is not necessary for cancer development.

11.4.2 Indirect Tumorigenic Effects of HPV

In addition to their direct carcinogenic effects, HPV E6 and E7 oncoproteins indirectly modify the immune microenvironment by various mechanisms.

11.4.2.1 Decreased Expression of Key Innate Immune Sensors

Viral DNA molecules are sensed by several families of pathogen recognition receptors. Among these latter, the Toll-like receptor (TLR) family (especially TLR9) was shown to initiate the secretion of proinflammatory cytokines as well as type I interferon (IFN) upon recognition of HPV genome. Interestingly, recent studies demonstrated that E7 oncoprotein inhibits TLR9 at the mRNA level through the formation of a transcriptional repressor complex [52]. The subsequent downregulation of TLR9 participates undoubtedly to the immune escape of HPV.

11.4.2.2 Alteration of the IFN Signaling Pathway

By interacting with several host proteins, E6 and E7 collectively interfere with the response to IFN. Indeed, E6 was shown to target IRF3 and Tyk2, inducing their degradation. As for E7, a strong interaction with IRF1 and p48 was reported. Altogether, HPV-infected cells become progressively resistant to IFN-induced growth arrest [53].

11.4.2.3 Alteration of Antigen-Presenting Cell Trafficking and Maturation

In squamous epithelia, the adhesion between keratinocytes and antigen-presenting cells (mostly Langerhans cells) is largely mediated by the E-cadherin protein expressed by both immune and epithelial cells. By promoting the hypermethylation of *CDH1* promoter, E7 reduces E-cadherin expression at the keratinocyte surface [54]. The subsequent downregulation of this protein was shown to impair not only the adhesion but also the maturation of Langerhans cells. Indeed, a tolerogenic phenotype was demonstrated following E-cadherin disruption [55]. Interestingly, through the inhibition of several chemokines involved in cellular chemotaxis (i.e., CCL20), E6 also indirectly reduces the density of antigen-presenting cells in the HPV-infected microenvironment [56].

11.4.2.4 Alteration of NF-κB Signaling Pathway

Although the molecular mechanism is still unclear (impaired acetylation and/or nuclear translocation of p65) [57], both E6 and E7 oncoproteins were shown to alter this signaling pathway involved in the expression of numerous proinflammatory cytokines (i.e., IL1β, IL-6, IL-8, and TNF-α). The subsequent reduced secretion of inflammatory mediators contributes to the creation of an immunosuppressive microenvironment promoting both the persistence and progression of HPV-related lesions.

11.5 Cell Morphological Changes After HPV Infection

11.5.1 Gross Pathology

Colposcopy, performed with a binocular instrument, is the gold standard for evaluating abnormal cervical cytology. Normal cervical squamous epithelium is smooth and pale pink, while columnar epithelium appears red due to its thinness and the proximity of blood vessels to the surface. As cervical lesions are often not grossly visible, unless they are papillary or exophytic as in condyloma acuminatum, 3–5% acetic acid is applied to the cervix to visualize precursor lesions. The acetic acid solution acts as a mucolytic agent, causing coagulation of nuclear chromatin and preventing transmission of light through the epithelium. In neoplastic lesions where the level of nuclear protein is high, this process manifests as an acetowhite lesion. Low-grade intraepithelial lesions appear bright white or translucent, with vague, feathery, or irregular geographic borders. High-grade intraepithelial lesions, in contrast, demonstrate a longer-lasting, duller hue of white and are characterized by sharply demarcated margins. The vascular pattern within the acetowhite area is important to note, as higher-grade lesions tend to produce an increase in local growth factors. Abnormal surface vasculature may demonstrate a stippled and dot-like appearance, referred to as punctation, and cobbled mosaicism, which represents interconnecting blood vessels surrounding the rete pegs of the epithelium. Punctation and mosaicism look fine in low-grade lesions and coarser with increasing severity of dysplasia.

11.5.2 Low-Grade Squamous Intraepithelial Lesion

LSIL is the morphologic manifestation of HPV infection in terminally differentiated squamous cells, the majority of which (up to 85%) are due to high-risk HPV types [58, 59]. Most will spontaneously regress (60 to >90%) if left untreated and approximately 10% will progress to HSIL within 2 years [60–62]. The hallmark features include changes to the lower third of the squamous epithelium and koilocytosis of the superficial or intermediate cells where the highest viral loads are found. On scanning power, the mucosa can appear thickened with proliferation of basal-like squamous cells extending up to a third of the epithelial thickness (Fig. 11.4). Nuclear atypia is minimal to mild and mitotic figures, if present, are confined to the lower part of the epithelium. The cells mature as they reach the surface, but superficial and intermediate cells show at least threefold nuclear enlargement with relatively low nuclear-to-

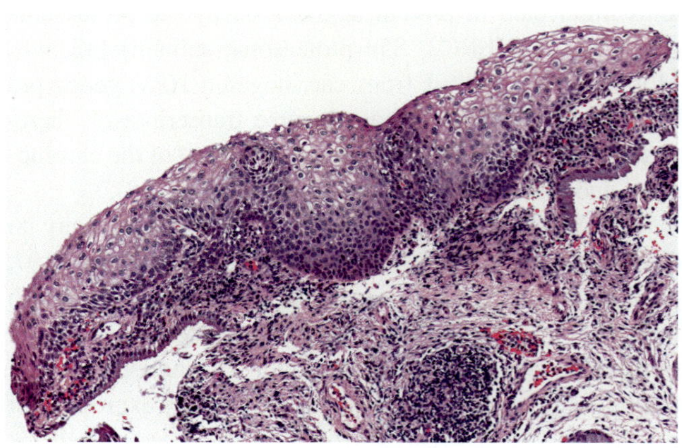

Fig. 11.4 CIN1, 10×. Low-grade squamous intraepithelial lesion (CIN1). At low power surface koilocytes and mild proliferation of basaloid cells within the lower third of the epithelium are seen

cytoplasmic ratios, raisinoid nuclear membranes, and dark chromatin. The nonspecific features of perinuclear halos and bi- or multinucleation are commonly seen. The halo typically displays sharply defined, irregularly shaped outlines while surrounding an off-centered nucleus. Nucleoli are rare and a more prevalent finding in reactive atypia. Collectively, these cytologic features represent HPV cytopathic effect and are referred to as koilocytosis. Other findings include hyperkeratosis or parakeratosis. Comparison with adjacent normal epithelium at low magnification accentuates the architectural and cytologic abnormalities associated with LSIL.

Condyloma acuminatum, a benign morphologic variant of LSIL associated with low-risk HPV types, usually HPV 6 or 11, manifests as multiple wart-like growths most commonly in external genital sites like the vagina and vulva. The lesion is composed of papillary fronds containing arborizing fibrovascular cores (papillomatosis), lined by hyperplastic squamous epithelium (acanthosis) showing hyperkeratosis, parakeratosis, and classic koilocytic atypia as described above (Fig. 11.5a, b). The parabasal layer is increased and cells may show mild cytologic atypia.

Reactive changes that can be seen in the squamous epithelium associated with infections, inflammation or repair, can mimic LSIL. These changes include cytoplasmic glycogenation, mild nuclear enlargement, the presence of nucleoli, and an altered chromatin pattern ranging from vesicular to hyperchromatic. Glycogenation can mimic koilocytosis, but in the reactive setting the perinuclear halo is round, less distinct, and uniformly centered around the nucleus (Fig. 11.6).

11.5.3 High-Grade Squamous Intraepithelial Lesion

HSIL is the result of HPV viral DNA integration into the host DNA and subsequent overexpression of E6 and E7 oncoproteins in proliferating cells. These lesions are precursors to invasive squamous cell carcinoma with a progression risk of 31% over a 30-year period [63]. The morphology is characterized by clonal expansion of immature, atypical cells from the basal layer into the middle third of the epithelium in CIN2 (Fig. 11.7) and the superficial third in CIN3 (Fig. 11.8). Variable maturation or koilocytic atypia may be present at the surface. On low power, the cells appear crowded, disorderly, and oftentimes syncytial with indistinct intercellular borders. Nuclei are enlarged and hyperchromatic and show increased nuclear-to-cytoplasmic ratios, irregular nuclear membranes, finely to coarsely granular chromatin, and inconspicuous nucleoli. Cases with the overall morphology of LSIL but with the additional features of marked cytologic atypia in the lower epithelium, including nuclear enlargement of at least 5 times the size of an intermediate cell nucleus or multinucleation, or atypical mitoses at any level represent DNA instability and aneuploidy and are upgraded to HSIL [64, 65].

11.5.4 P16 Immunohistochemistry

In difficult cases, immunohistochemistry may aid in the diagnosis of cervical dysplasias. According to findings from the LAST project, sufficient evidence is only available for use of p16 as a marker of oncogenic HPV infection [66]. P16 is a cyclin-dependent kinase (CDK) 4 inhibitor which binds to cyclin D-CDK4/6 complexes to control the cell cycle, at the G1-S interphase [67]. Normally, when p16 binds to CDK, the phosphorylation of pRb is inhibited, preventing cell cycle activation. However, when high-risk HPV integrates in the cell, viral oncoprotein E7 binds to pRb, rendering it inactive, and resulting in p16 overexpression. This manifests as diffuse cytoplasmic and/or nuclear p16 staining of the affected epithelium (Fig. 11.9).

Strong and diffuse block-positive p16 staining supports a diagnosis of CIN2 or CIN3 whereas negative, cytoplasmic

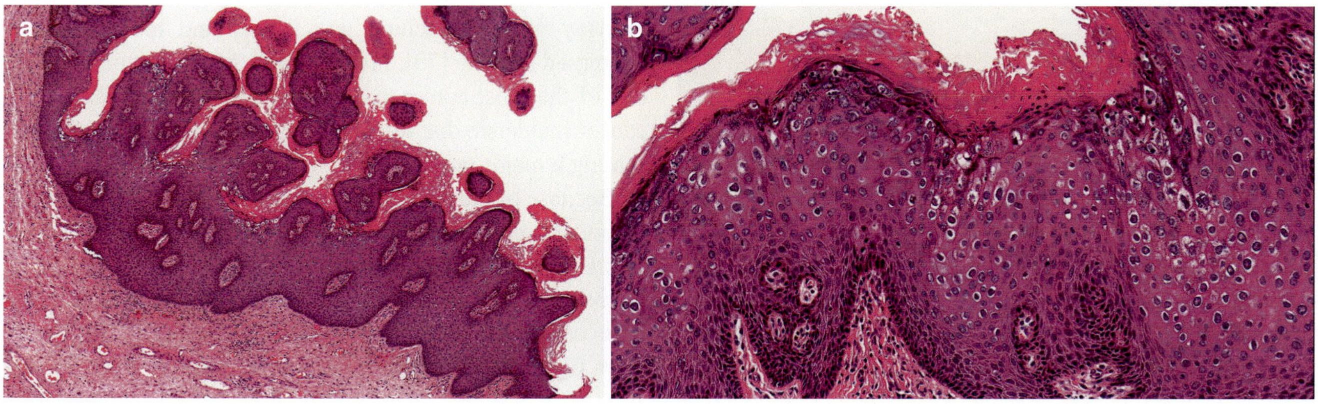

Fig. 11.5 (**a**) VIN1, 5×. Condyloma acuminatum. Acanthotic epithelium with hyperkeratotic, papillomatous, and koilocytic changes. (**b**) VIN1, 20×. Condyloma acuminatum. Note the koilocytic atypia

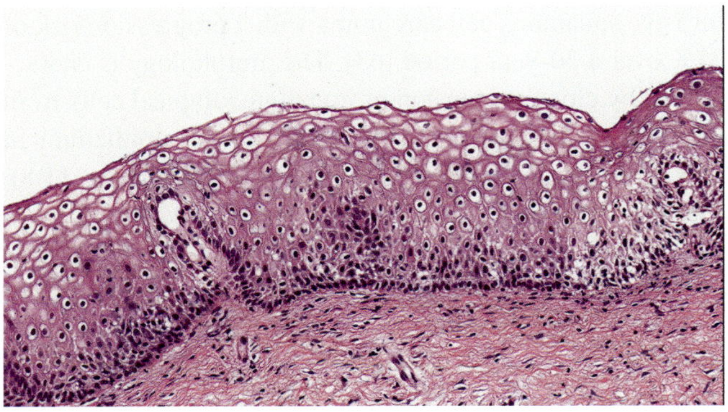

Fig. 11.6 Reactive changes, 20×. Reactive changes. Glycogenated superficial and intermediate cells mimicking koilocytes

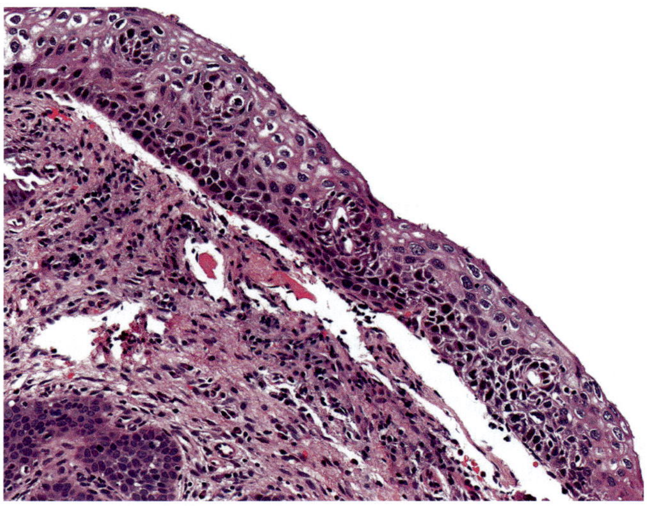

Fig. 11.7 CIN2, 20×. High-grade squamous intraepithelial lesion (CIN2). Atypical hyperchromatic basaloid cells extend into the mid epithelium

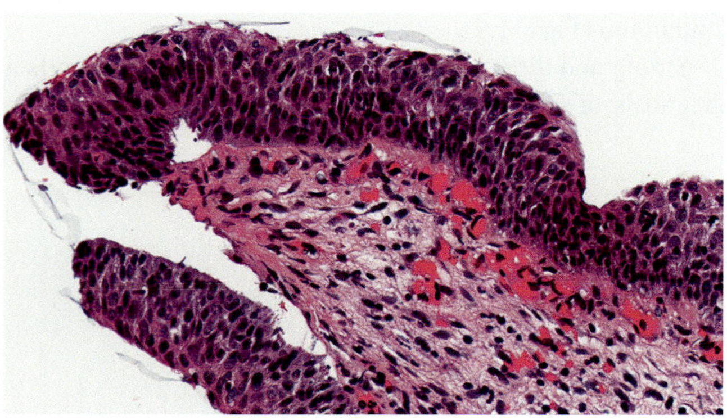

Fig. 11.8 CIN3, 40×. High-grade squamous intraepithelial lesion (CIN3). Crowded, atypical cells with high N:C ratios, pleomorphic and hyperchromatic nuclei and loss of polarity involving full thickness of epithelium

only, or focal and patchy, non-block staining is interpreted as negative. Metaplastic and reparative processes and atrophic epithelium do not stain for p16. However, caution is advised

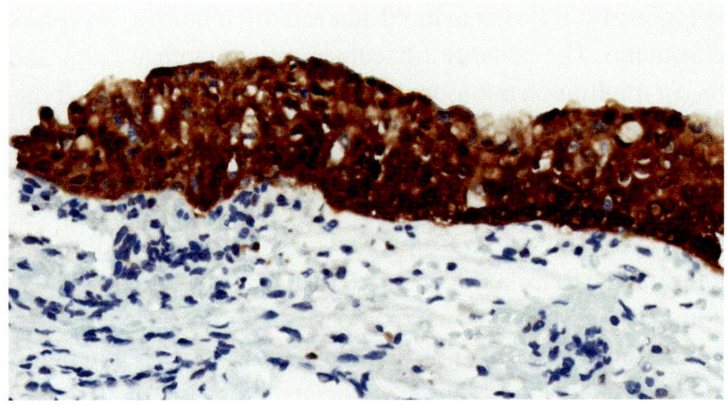

Fig. 11.9 P16/CIN3, 40×. This high-grade squamous intraepithelial lesion shows strong and diffuse block-positive p16 staining

as block-positive staining can also be observed in 39% of LSIL cases, and ultimately histomorphology should dictate the grade of the lesion in these cases [68, 69]. Additionally, the LAST project recommends against using p16 routinely in cases where the diagnosis is unequivocally negative, CIN1 or CIN3, in order to avoid overusing and misinterpreting cases on the basis of the p16.

11.6 Cervical Cancer Screening

11.6.1 Screening with Cytology

The Papanicolaou (Pap) cytology test is inexpensive, easily administered, and well tolerated by patients, making it an ideal screening test. Since its introduction in the mid-twentieth century to screen for cervical cancer and its precursor lesions, the number of squamous cervical cancers has markedly decreased, particularly in areas where effective screening and intervention programs are available to women [70–72]. This correlation is illustrated well in a study of screening practices in Nordic countries. In Iceland where screening was highest, death rates fell by 84% in contrast to Norway where screening was lowest and mortality only decreased by 11% [73]. In the United States, what used to be one of the most common causes of cancer now ranks 21 in cancer incidence due to the efforts of screening [74], representing a major public health milestone.

Because of the difficulties in implementing a primary and secondary prevention program in areas lacking advanced infrastructure, cervical cancer is still the fourth leading cause of cancer deaths worldwide [75] and the second most common cancer in underdeveloped countries [76]. Mortality rates range from less than 2 per 100,000 to over 20 per 100,000 worldwide [76]. Adherence to screening guidelines is essential for cervical cancer prevention. Among women with invasive cervical cancer, over 50% have received inadequate screening, including 41.5% who have never been screened [77].

The major professional societies—U.S. Preventive Services Task Force (USPSTF), American Congress of Obstetricians and Gynecologists (ACOG), and a consortium of the American Cancer Society, the American Society for Colposcopy and Cervical Pathology, and the American Society for Clinical Pathology (ACS/ASCCP/ASCP)—have issued cervical cancer screening guidelines for average-risk women. Withstanding minor differences, there is general agreement that screening should begin at the age of 21 regardless of sexual activity or HPV vaccination status. Modalities include cytology alone every 3 years, or, for women between the ages of 30 and 65 who prefer a longer screening interval, by the cytology and HPV co-test (with Hr-HPV DNA) every 5 years. Beyond the age of 65, women with three consecutive negative Pap results or two consecutive negative co-test results in the prior 10 years may discontinue screening. Women who have undergone a total hysterectomy but who do not have a history of high-grade cervical dysplasia may also discontinue screening. Higher-risk women with cervical cancer, immunosuppression, HIV, or exposure to diethylstilbestrol in utero may benefit from more frequent screening.

11.7 Sampling Methods

There are two methods for obtaining cervical cytology specimens. For both, a plastic or wooden spatula is rotated 360° to collect cells from the transformation zone and adjacent ectocervical squamous mucosa and a brush is used to sample the endocervical canal. The more traditional technique of creating a conventional smear then requires the clinician to transfer the collected cells directly onto a slide, followed by spray fixation of the smear. Limitations of this method include failure to transfer all of the cells onto the slide, inadequate specimen fixation, air-drying artifact, poor visibility due to obscuring elements, and technical variability in the quality of the smear.

Liquid-based cytology preparations like ThinPrep and Surepath were developed as an alternative to address some of these problems and provide a better platform for computer-based automated screening devices. While more expensive, this newer technology was quickly embraced by the medical community, currently accounting for more than 90% of the Pap tests performed in the United States. In this technique, the cells are rinsed in a liquid preservative following collection and subsequently processed in a lab for slide preparation. This method ensures that the majority of cells captured at the time of collection are transferred into the liquid media, fixed immediately, and homogeneously distributed throughout the specimen. The remaining portion of the sample can be used for ancillary testing such as reflex human papillomavirus DNA or chlamydia and gonorrhea testing. Other advantages of liquid-based cytology include the ability to prepare duplicate slides or a cell block, remove obscuring material such as blood, inflammation, and debris, and create a thinner cell preparation that is easier for cytopathologists and technologists to read than smears. Despite these benefits, there are no significant differences in accuracy between a conventional smear and liquid-based cytology for detecting cervical intraepithelial neoplasia, and both are considered acceptable for use in screening [78–80].

11.8 Pap Test Accuracy

Despite its impact on reducing cancer incidence and mortality, the performance characteristics of the Pap test are limited. The sensitivity of cytology is low (48–61%) and specificity ranges from 82 to 97% [81–83]. False-negative smears account for a proportion of cervical cancer cases, attributable to sampling error or failure to detect abnormal cells [77]. False-positive results can be seen in the setting of reparative changes and exfoliating high-grade squamous intraepithelial lesions, particularly when keratinized or occurring in an atrophic or necrotic background [84, 85].

The interobserver reproducibility of Pap test interpretations is also only moderate. In the Bethesda Interobserver Reproducibility Study, a web-based format was used to see how pathologists and cytotechnologists assessed a range of images compared to panel review of these images [86]. Exact agreement with the panel was achieved only 55.3% of the time, which improved to 84.1% when distinguishing negative from nonnegative results. Agreement was lowest for the diagnostic categories of atypical squamous cells of undetermined significance (ASC-US, 39.9%) and atypical squamous cells, cannot exclude high-grade squamous intraepithelial lesion (ASC-H, 22.4%), and highest for low-grade squamous intraepithelial lesion (LSIL, 54.1%) and negative for intraepithelial lesion or malignancy (NILM, 67.9%). In this study, morphology was a more important predictor of agreement than participants' training, experience level, or practice settings. Another study echoed these findings with a quality control group only agreeing with 43% of ASC-US and 47% of HSIL clinical center interpretations [87].

11.8.1 Screening by Detecting HPV

Persistent HPV infection of the cervix with carcinogenic HPV types is required for the development of invasive cervical cancer [6]. As previously mentioned, 12 HPV genotypes are considered oncogenic, and these hrHPV types are associated with the majority of all cervical cancers [88, 89]. While these infections are common, the majority of women clear the infection with no development of clinical lesions. A small group of women may develop persistent hrHPV infections and these are the women at risk for development of invasive cervical cancer and precursor lesions. The recognition of the relationship between persistent infection of the uterine cervix with hrHPV types and cancer development has resulted in the development of various HPV DNA or HPV RNA detection systems for screening [90]. Numerous societies and organizations recommend reflex hrHPV DNA testing in women with equivocal cytology (i.e., atypical squamous cells of undetermined significance or AS-CUS) and as an adjunct to cytology when screening women 30 years and older (cotesting) [78]. A negative hrHPV test in patients with abnormal cytology correlates with the absence of cervical dysplasia [91]. However, detection of hrHPV positivity alone with a negative cytology may lead clinicians to aggressive and perhaps unnecessary treatments [92]. This is the reason why the 2011 guidelines do not recommend HPV testing alone for women 30–65 in most clinical settings [93, 94].

Detection of hrHPV DNA could be considered useful in three clinical settings: as a primary screening test (by itself or in combination with a Pap smear) to detect CIN2/3 lesions; as a triage test to detect minor cytologic abnormalities in Pap smears (equivocal or low-grade abnormalities) needing referral for diagnosis and treatment; and potentially as a follow-up test for women treated for CIN2/CIN3 lesions [95].

Although sensitivity of hrHPV DNA testing is higher when compared with cytology [95, 96], a high specificity should also be achieved with hrHPV testing to avoid unnecessary colposcopies. Although there are some benefits for hrHPV DNA testing in patients with equivocal/low-grade smears and in the surveillance of women after treatment of CIN [96], there are issues regarding how to use hrHPV DNA testing as a primary screening test. Primary screening with Hybrid Capture 2 (HC2) is more sensitive than cytology but suffers from lower specificity. Several approaches to deal with the lower specificity of hrHPV DNA testing have been considered: HPV typing for HPV16 and 18/45 and mRNA coding for the viral E6 and/or E7 proteins.

Even though hrHPV DNA testing suffers from a low specificity when compared with cytology, the Food and Drug Administration (FDA) approved the modified labeling of a hrHPV assay (cobas HPV Test) as a primary hrHPV screening modality for women 25 years and older in April 2014 [62]. The test reports 12 oncogenic HPV genotypes including genotypes 16 and 18. This new approval was based on long-term findings from the ATHENA trial, a clinical trial that included more than 47, 000 women [97]. The trial showed that the cobas HPV Test performed better than the Pap test at identifying women at risk for developing cervical dysplasia. However, the pap test still remains the first screening method to detect cervical dysplasia and HPV testing has not been incorporated in the regular screening guidelines.

11.9 Cervical Cancer Prevention

Cervical cancer and its precursors can be prevented in two ways: with screening tools such as cytology and/or hrHPV DNA testing and with HPV vaccines. Development of various HPV vaccines to prevent HPV infection came as a result of the causal relationship between HPV infection and cervical dysplasia/cancer development. Currently, there are three HPV vaccines: a bivalent vaccine that protects against HPV16 and HPV18; a quadrivalent vaccine that protects against HPV16, HPV18, and non-oncogenic HPV types 6 and 11; and a 9-valent vaccine that protects against those in the quadrivalent vaccine and five additional oncogenic HPV types (HPV31, 33, 45, 52, and 58) [98]. Only the 9-valent vaccine (Gardasil 9) is available in the United States. Currently, the World Health Organization (WHO) recommends two doses of HPV vaccine for children 9–14 years of age. Only 37% of countries worldwide have introduced the HPV vaccine, leaving many yet to take this important step in prevention [98].

References

1. National Cancer Institute. Surveillance, Epidemiology, and End Results (SEER) Program SEER*Stat Database: Incidence – SEER 9 Regs Research Data. 2017. http://www.seer.cancer.gov. Accessed 11 Oct 2017.
2. National Cancer Institute. Surveillance, Epidemiology, and End Results (SEER) Program Stat Database: Mortality – All COD, Aggregated With State, Total U.S. (1969–2014). http://www.seer.cancer.gov.
3. Centers for Disease Control and Prevention NCI. U.S. Cancer Statistics Working Group. United States Cancer Statistics: 1999–2014 Incidence and Mortality Web-based Report. http://www.cdc.gov/uscs. Accessed 11 Oct 2017.
4. Torre LA, Bray F, Siegel RL, et al. Global cancer statistics, 2012. CA Cancer J Clin. 2015;65:87–108.
5. Adegoke O, Kulasingam S, Virnig B. Cervical cancer trends in the United States: a 35-year population-based analysis. J Womens Health (Larchmt). 2012;21:1031–7.
6. Walboomers JM, Jacobs MV, Manos MM, et al. Human papillomavirus is a necessary cause of invasive cervical cancer worldwide. J Pathol. 1999;189:12–9.
7. Zielinski GD, Snijders PJ, Rozendaal L, et al. The presence of high-risk HPV combined with specific p53 and p16INK4a expression patterns points to high-risk HPV as the main causative agent for adenocarcinoma in situ and adenocarcinoma of the cervix. J Pathol. 2003;201:535–43.
8. Snijders PJ, Steenbergen RD, Heideman DA, et al. HPV-mediated cervical carcinogenesis: concepts and clinical implications. J Pathol. 2006;208:152–64.
9. Hosono S, Kawase T, Matsuo K, et al. HLA-A alleles and the risk of cervical squamous cell carcinoma in Japanese women. J Epidemiol. 2010;20:295–301.
10. Hubert P, Herman L, Roncarati P, et al. Altered alpha-defensin 5 expression in cervical squamocolumnar junction: implication in the formation of a viral/tumour-permissive microenvironment. J Pathol. 2014;234:464–77.

11. Ramachandran B. Functional association of oestrogen receptors with HPV infection in cervical carcinogenesis. Endocr Relat Cancer. 2017;24:R99–R108.
12. Fonseca-Moutinho JA. Smoking and cervical cancer. ISRN Obstet Gynecol. 2011;2011:847684.
13. Zoodsma M, Sijmons RH, de Vries EG, et al. Familial cervical cancer: case reports, review and clinical implications. Hered Cancer Clin Pract. 2004;2:99–105.
14. Park KJ, Kiyokawa T, Soslow RA, et al. Unusual endocervical adenocarcinomas: an immunohistochemical analysis with molecular detection of human papillomavirus. Am J Surg Pathol. 2011;35:633–46.
15. Hoover RN, Hyer M, Pfeiffer RM, et al. Adverse health outcomes in women exposed in utero to diethylstilbestrol. N Engl J Med. 2011;365:1304–14.
16. Troisi R, Hatch EE, Titus-Ernstoff L, et al. Cancer risk in women prenatally exposed to diethylstilbestrol. Int J Cancer. 2007;121:356–60.
17. McGowan L, Young RH, Scully RE. Peutz-Jeghers syndrome with "adenoma malignum" of the cervix. A report of two cases. Gynecol Oncol. 1980;10:125–33.
18. Casey S, Harley I, Jamison J, et al. A rare case of HPV-negative cervical squamous cell carcinoma. Int J Gynecol Pathol. 2015;34:208–12.
19. Johansson C, Schwartz S. Regulation of human papillomavirus gene expression by splicing and polyadenylation. Nat Rev Microbiol. 2013;11:239–51.
20. Doorbar J, Quint W, Banks L, et al. The biology and life-cycle of human papillomaviruses. Vaccine. 2012;30(Suppl 5):F55–70.
21. Egawa N, Egawa K, Griffin H, et al. Human papillomaviruses; epithelial tropisms, and the development of neoplasia. Viruses. 2015;7:3863–90.
22. Chen Z, Schiffman M, Herrero R, et al. Evolution and taxonomic classification of human papillomavirus 16 (HPV16)-related variant genomes: HPV31, HPV33, HPV35, HPV52, HPV58 and HPV67. PLoS One. 2011;6:e20183.
23. Woodman CB, Collins SI, Young LS. The natural history of cervical HPV infection: unresolved issues. Nat Rev Cancer. 2007;7:11–22.
24. Herfs M, Yamamoto Y, Laury A, et al. A discrete population of squamocolumnar junction cells implicated in the pathogenesis of cervical cancer. Proc Natl Acad Sci U S A. 2012;109:10516–21.
25. Mills AM, Paquette C, Terzic T, et al. CK7 immunohistochemistry as a predictor of CIN1 progression: a retrospective study of patients from the quadrivalent HPV vaccine trials. Am J Surg Pathol. 2017;41:143–52.
26. Herfs M, Vargas SO, Yamamoto Y, et al. A novel blueprint for 'top down' differentiation defines the cervical squamocolumnar junction during development, reproductive life, and neoplasia. J Pathol. 2013;229:460–8.
27. de Martel C, Plummer M, Vignat J, et al. Worldwide burden of cancer attributable to HPV by site, country and HPV type. Int J Cancer. 2017;141:664–70.
28. Paquette C, Mills AM, Stoler MH. Predictive value of cytokeratin 7 immunohistochemistry in cervical low-grade squamous intraepithelial lesion as a marker for risk of progression to a high-grade lesion. Am J Surg Pathol. 2016;40:236–43.
29. Lee KR, Flynn CE. Early invasive adenocarcinoma of the cervix. Cancer. 2000;89:1048–55.
30. Herfs M, Soong TR, Delvenne P, et al. Deciphering the multifactorial susceptibility of mucosal junction cells to HPV infection and related carcinogenesis. Viruses. 2017;9:E85.
31. Day PM, Schelhaas M. Concepts of papillomavirus entry into host cells. Curr Opin Virol. 2014;4:24–31.
32. Horvath CA, Boulet GA, Renoux VM, et al. Mechanisms of cell entry by human papillomaviruses: an overview. Virol J. 2010;7:11.
33. Holowaty P, Miller AB, Rohan T, et al. Natural history of dysplasia of the uterine cervix. J Natl Cancer Inst. 1999;91:252–8.
34. Schiffman M, Rodriguez AC, Chen Z, et al. A population-based prospective study of carcinogenic human papillomavirus variant lineages, viral persistence, and cervical neoplasia. Cancer Res. 2010;70:3159–69.
35. Xi LF, Koutsky LA, Hildesheim A, et al. Risk for high-grade cervical intraepithelial neoplasia associated with variants of human papillomavirus types 16 and 18. Cancer Epidemiol Biomarkers Prev. 2007;16:4–10.
36. Mirabello L, Yeager M, Cullen M, et al. HPV16 sublineage associations with histology-specific cancer risk using HPV whole-genome sequences in 3200 women. J Natl Cancer Inst. 2016;108:djw100.
37. Solomon D, Davey D, Kurman R, et al. The 2001 Bethesda system: terminology for reporting results of cervical cytology. JAMA. 2002;287:2114–9.
38. Moody CA, Laimins LA. Human papillomavirus oncoproteins: pathways to transformation. Nat Rev Cancer. 2010;10:550–60.
39. Martinez-Zapien D, Ruiz FX, Poirson J, et al. Structure of the E6/E6AP/p53 complex required for HPV-mediated degradation of p53. Nature. 2016;529:541–5.
40. Thomas M, Banks L. Human papillomavirus (HPV) E6 interactions with Bak are conserved amongst E6 proteins from high and low risk HPV types. J Gen Virol. 1999;80(Pt 6):1513–7.
41. Filippova M, Parkhurst L, Duerksen-Hughes PJ. The human papillomavirus 16 E6 protein binds to Fas-associated death domain and protects cells from Fas-triggered apoptosis. J Biol Chem. 2004;279:25729–44.
42. Filippova M, Johnson MM, Bautista M, et al. The large and small isoforms of human papillomavirus type 16 E6 bind to and differentially affect procaspase 8 stability and activity. J Virol. 2007;81:4116–29.
43. Tomaic V, Pim D, Thomas M, et al. Regulation of the human papillomavirus type 18 E6/E6AP ubiquitin ligase complex by the HECT domain-containing protein EDD. J Virol. 2011;85:3120–7.
44. Tomaic V, Ganti K, Pim D, et al. Interaction of HPV E6 oncoproteins with specific proteasomal subunits. Virology. 2013;446:389–96.
45. Munger K, Werness BA, Dyson N, et al. Complex formation of human papillomavirus E7 proteins with the retinoblastoma tumor suppressor gene product. EMBO J. 1989;8:4099–105.
46. Sano T, Oyama T, Kashiwabara K, et al. Expression status of p16 protein is associated with human papillomavirus oncogenic potential in cervical and genital lesions. Am J Pathol. 1998;153:1741–8.
47. Nguyen CL, Munger K. Human papillomavirus E7 protein deregulates mitosis via an association with nuclear mitotic apparatus protein 1. J Virol. 2009;83:1700–7.
48. Groves IJ, Coleman N. Pathogenesis of human papillomavirus-associated mucosal disease. J Pathol. 2015;235:527–38.
49. Schapiro F, Sparkowski J, Adduci A, et al. Golgi alkalinization by the papillomavirus E5 oncoprotein. J Cell Biol. 2000;148:305–15.
50. Belleudi F, Leone L, Purpura V, et al. HPV16 E5 affects the KGFR/FGFR2b-mediated epithelial growth through alteration of the receptor expression, signaling and endocytic traffic. Oncogene. 2011;30:4963–76.
51. Pett M, Coleman N. Integration of high-risk human papillomavirus: a key event in cervical carcinogenesis? J Pathol. 2007;212:356–67.
52. Hasan UA, Zannetti C, Parroche P, et al. The human papillomavirus type 16 E7 oncoprotein induces a transcriptional repressor complex on the toll-like receptor 9 promoter. J Exp Med. 2013;210:1369–87.
53. Beglin M, Melar-New M, Laimins L. Human papillomaviruses and the interferon response. J Interferon Cytokine Res. 2009;29:629–35.
54. Laurson J, Khan S, Chung R, et al. Epigenetic repression of E-cadherin by human papillomavirus 16 E7 protein. Carcinogenesis. 2010;31:918–26.

55. Jiang A, Bloom O, Ono S, et al. Disruption of E-cadherin-mediated adhesion induces a functionally distinct pathway of dendritic cell maturation. Immunity. 2007;27:610–24.
56. Caberg JH, Hubert P, Herman L, et al. Increased migration of Langerhans cells in response to HPV16 E6 and E7 oncogene silencing: role of CCL20. Cancer Immunol Immunother. 2009;58:39–47.
57. Vandermark ER, Deluca KA, Gardner CR, et al. Human papillomavirus type 16 E6 and E 7 proteins alter NF-kB in cultured cervical epithelial cells and inhibition of NF-kB promotes cell growth and immortalization. Virology. 2012;425:53–60.
58. Arbyn M, Benoy I, Simoens C, et al. Prevaccination distribution of human papillomavirus types in women attending at cervical cancer screening in Belgium. Cancer Epidemiol Biomarkers Prev. 2009;18:321–30.
59. Arbyn M, Martin-Hirsch P, Buntinx F, et al. Triage of women with equivocal or low-grade cervical cytology results: a meta-analysis of the HPV test positivity rate. J Cell Mol Med. 2009;13:648–59.
60. Schlecht NF, Platt RW, Duarte-Franco E, et al. Human papillomavirus infection and time to progression and regression of cervical intraepithelial neoplasia. J Natl Cancer Inst. 2003;95:1336–43.
61. Ostor AG. Natural history of cervical intraepithelial neoplasia: a critical review. Int J Gynecol Pathol. 1993;12:186–92.
62. Wright TC Jr, Massad LS, Dunton CJ, et al. 2006 consensus guidelines for the management of women with cervical intraepithelial neoplasia or adenocarcinoma in situ. J Low Genit Tract Dis. 2007;11:223–39.
63. McCredie MR, Sharples KJ, Paul C, et al. Natural history of cervical neoplasia and risk of invasive cancer in women with cervical intraepithelial neoplasia 3: a retrospective cohort study. Lancet Oncol. 2008;9:425–34.
64. Aoyama C, Peters J, Senadheera S, et al. Uterine cervical dysplasia and cancer: identification of c-myc status by quantitative polymerase chain reaction. Diagn Mol Pathol. 1998;7:324–30.
65. Park K, Ellenson LH, Pirog EC. Low-grade squamous intraepithelial lesions of the cervix with marked cytological atypia-clinical follow-up and human papillomavirus genotyping. Int J Gynecol Pathol. 2007;26:457–62.
66. Darragh TM, Colgan TJ, Cox JT, et al. The lower anogenital squamous terminology standardization project for HPV-associated lesions: background and consensus recommendations from the College of American Pathologists and the American Society for Colposcopy and Cervical Pathology. Arch Pathol Lab Med. 2012;136:1266–97.
67. Klaes R, Friedrich T, Spitkovsky D, et al. Overexpression of p16(INK4A) as a specific marker for dysplastic and neoplastic epithelial cells of the cervix uteri. Int J Cancer. 2001;92:276–84.
68. Keating JT, Cviko A, Riethdorf S, et al. Ki-67, cyclin E, and p16INK4 are complimentary surrogate biomarkers for human papilloma virus-related cervical neoplasia. Am J Surg Pathol. 2001;25:884–91.
69. Galgano MT, Castle PE, Atkins KA, et al. Using biomarkers as objective standards in the diagnosis of cervical biopsies. Am J Surg Pathol. 2010;34:1077–87.
70. Peto J, Gilham C, Fletcher O, et al. The cervical cancer epidemic that screening has prevented in the UK. Lancet. 2004;364:249–56.
71. Gustafsson L, Ponten J, Zack M, et al. International incidence rates of invasive cervical cancer after introduction of cytological screening. Cancer Causes Control. 1997;8:755–63.
72. Kulasingam SL, Havrilesky L, Ghebre R, et al. Screening for cervical cancer: a decision analysis for the US preventive services task force. Rockville, MD: Agency for Healthcare Research and Quality (US); 2011.
73. Laara E, Day NE, Hakama M. Trends in mortality from cervical cancer in the Nordic countries: association with organised screening programmes. Lancet. 1987;1:1247–9.
74. Siegel RL, Miller KD, Jemal A. Cancer statistics, 2017. CA Cancer J Clin. 2017;67:7–30.
75. Serrano B, Brotons M, Bosch FX, et al. Epidemiology and burden of HPV-related disease. Best Pract Res Clin Obstet Gynaecol. 2018;47:14–26.
76. Ferlay J, Soerjomataram I, Dikshit R, et al. Cancer incidence and mortality worldwide: sources, methods and major patterns in GLOBOCAN 2012. Int J Cancer. 2015;136:E359–86.
77. Spence AR, Goggin P, Franco EL. Process of care failures in invasive cervical cancer: systematic review and meta-analysis. Prev Med. 2007;45:93–106.
78. Moyer VA, Force USPST. Screening for cervical cancer: U.S. Preventive Services Task Force recommendation statement. Ann Intern Med. 2012;156:880–91. W312
79. Arbyn M, Bergeron C, Klinkhamer P, et al. Liquid compared with conventional cervical cytology: a systematic review and meta-analysis. Obstet Gynecol. 2008;111:167–77.
80. Siebers AG, Klinkhamer PJ, Grefte JM, et al. Comparison of liquid-based cytology with conventional cytology for detection of cervical cancer precursors: a randomized controlled trial. JAMA. 2009;302:1757–64.
81. Mayrand MH, Duarte-Franco E, Rodrigues I, et al. Human papillomavirus DNA versus Papanicolaou screening tests for cervical cancer. N Engl J Med. 2007;357:1579–88.
82. Kulasingam SL, Hughes JP, Kiviat NB, et al. Evaluation of human papillomavirus testing in primary screening for cervical abnormalities: comparison of sensitivity, specificity, and frequency of referral. JAMA. 2002;288:1749–57.
83. Wright TC, Stoler MH, Behrens CM, et al. Primary cervical cancer screening with human papillomavirus: end of study results from the ATHENA study using HPV as the first-line screening test. Gynecol Oncol. 2015;136:189–97.
84. Mount S, Harmon M, Eltabbakh G, et al. False positive diagnosis in conventional and liquid-based cervical specimens. Acta Cytol. 2004;48:363–71.
85. Levine PH, Elgert PA, Mittal K. False-positive squamous cell carcinoma in cervical smears: cytologic-histologic correlation in 19 cases. Diagn Cytopathol. 2003;28:23–7.
86. Sherman ME, Dasgupta A, Schiffman M, et al. The Bethesda Interobserver Reproducibility Study (BIRST): a web-based assessment of the Bethesda 2001 system for classifying cervical cytology. Cancer. 2007;111:15–25.
87. Stoler MH, Schiffman M, Atypical Squamous Cells of Undetermined Significance-Low-grade Squamous Intraepithelial Lesion Triage Study G. Interobserver reproducibility of cervical cytologic and histologic interpretations: realistic estimates from the ASCUS-LSIL Triage Study. JAMA. 2001;285:1500–5.
88. Munoz N, Bosch FX, de Sanjose S, et al. Epidemiologic classification of human papillomavirus types associated with cervical cancer. N Engl J Med. 2003;348:518–27.
89. Wheeler CM, Hunt WC, Schiffman M, et al. Human papillomavirus genotypes and the cumulative 2-year risk of cervical precancer. J Infect Dis. 2006;194:1291–9.
90. Bosch FX, Lorincz A, Munoz N, et al. The causal relation between human papillomavirus and cervical cancer. J Clin Pathol. 2002;55:244–65.

91. Sherman ME, Lorincz AT, Scott DR, et al. Baseline cytology, human papillomavirus testing, and risk for cervical neoplasia: a 10-year cohort analysis. J Natl Cancer Inst. 2003;95:46–52.
92. Rao A, Sandri MT, Sideri M, et al. Comparison of hybrid capture 2 high-risk HPV results in the low positive range with cobas(R) HPV test results from the ATHENA study. J Clin Virol. 2013;58:161–7.
93. Huh WK, Ault KA, Chelmow D, et al. Use of primary high-risk human papillomavirus testing for cervical cancer screening: interim clinical guidance. Gynecol Oncol. 2015;136:178–82.
94. Saslow D, Solomon D, Lawson HW, et al. American Cancer Society, American Society for Colposcopy and Cervical Pathology, and American Society for Clinical Pathology screening guidelines for the prevention and early detection of cervical cancer. Am J Clin Pathol. 2012;137:516–42.
95. Arbyn M, Sasieni P, Meijer CJ, et al. Chapter 9: clinical applications of HPV testing: a summary of meta-analyses. Vaccine. 2006;24(Suppl 3):S3/78–89.
96. Cuzick J, Clavel C, Petry KU, et al. Overview of the European and North American studies on HPV testing in primary cervical cancer screening. Int J Cancer. 2006;119:1095–101.
97. Stoler MH, Wright TC Jr, Sharma A, et al. High-risk human papillomavirus testing in women with ASC-US cytology: results from the ATHENA HPV study. Am J Clin Pathol. 2011;135:468–75.
98. Senkomago V, Duran D, Loharikar A, et al. CDC activities for improving implementation of human papillomavirus vaccination, cervical cancer screening, and surveillance worldwide. Emerg Infect Dis. 2017;23:S101–7.

Cervical Squamous Neoplasia

12

Eric C. Huang and Deyin Xing

Abstract

Cervical squamous neoplasia is the most common lesion of the cervix and is caused by human papillomavirus infection at the squamocolumnar junction. In this chapter, we describe the histologic features of low- and high-grade squamous intraepithelial lesions, superficially invasive (microinvasive) and invasive squamous cell carcinomas. Diagnostic mimics and differential diagnosis are discussed for each section followed by management algorithms. Immunohistochemical markers useful for cervical squamous neoplasia are also described. The goal of the chapter is to provide readers with a concise reference and better understanding of these lesions when encountered in a routine pathology practice.

Keywords

Cervical squamous neoplasia · squamous intraepithelial lesion · squamous cell carcinoma · human papillomavirus

12.1 Cervical Precancerous Lesions—Squamous Intraepithelial Lesion (SIL)

12.1.1 The Concept and the Nomenclature/Vulnerable Anatomic Location

Cervical squamous intraepithelial neoplasia is defined as squamous alterations caused by human papillomavirus (HPV) infection at the cervical transformation zone or squamocolumnar junction (discussed in Chap. 11 for more details). In 1887, Williams first described intraepithelial precancer of the cervix [1]. Broders later described lesions that look like cancer, but have not penetrated the basement membrane as "carcinoma in situ" (CIS) [2]. This early description led to hysterectomy as treatment of choice for women with CIS. By the early 1950s, pathologists began to realize that there are lesions that behave in a less aggressive fashion and do not fulfill the criteria of CIS. Reagan et al. then introduced the term "dysplasia" and graded them as mild, moderate, and severe [3]. Richart proposed the term "cervical intraepithelial neoplasia" (CIN) and suggested that cervical carcinogenesis was a continuum from mild dysplasia to cervical cancer [4, 5]. This concept was accepted by the International Society of Gynecological Pathologists in 1980s and the term CIS was retired; however, due to the concept of CIN as a continuum to cancer, treatment for all of these lesions became common practice.

It became increasingly understood that the biology of cervical dysplasia is caused by HPV infection [6]. Furthermore, it became apparent that the grading of cervical dysplasia suffered from low reproducibility, and that a 2-tiered system would be more reproducible among pathologists and be more biologically relevant for management [7, 8]. A 2-tiered system (low- vs. high-grade squamous intraepithelial lesion) was adopted by the Bethesda system for cervical cytology in 1988 [9]. In the 1990s, histologic CIN1 (low-grade squamous intraepithelial lesion/LSIL) was managed with observation while CIN2–3 (high-grade squamous intraepithelial lesion/HSIL) was excised with a loop electrosurgical excision procedure (LEEP); this further reinforced the 2-tiered system. Time has proven the 2-tiered system to be more biologically relevant and histologically more reproducible, and to that end the Lower Anogenital Squamous Terminology (LAST) Project proposed the standardization of the histologic diagnosis of all cervical dysplasia into a 2-tiered system (except in young women where a 3-tier system is clinically relevant for appropriate management) [10]. Of note, the term "young women" has no age threshold and generally refers to patients who desire fertility, and as a result, conservative management of their disease [11].

E. C. Huang (✉)
Department of Pathology, University of Washington School of Medicine, Seattle, WA, USA
e-mail: ecchuang@uw.edu

D. Xing
Department of Pathology, The Johns Hopkins University School of Medicine, Baltimore, MD, USA
e-mail: dxing2@jhmi.edu

W. Zheng et al. (eds.), *Gynecologic and Obstetric Pathology, Volume 1*, https://doi.org/10.1007/978-981-13-3016-2_12

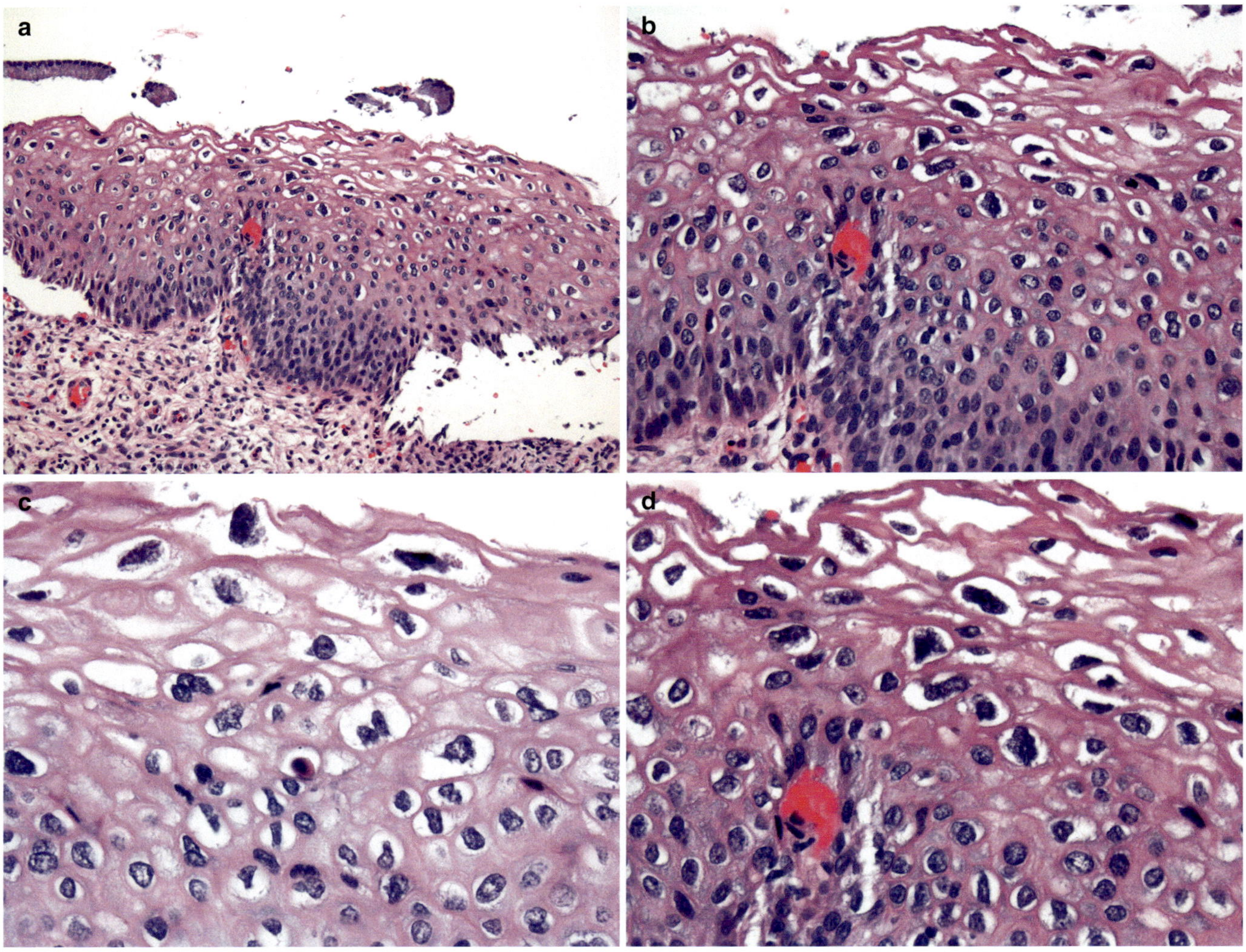

Fig. 12.1 Low-grade squamous intraepithelial lesion. (**a**, **b**) The superficial squamous epithelium shows nuclear atypia and koilocytosis. The basal layer demonstrates subtle disorganization of the normal "picket-fence" architecture. (**c**) Binucleation and multinucleation are common findings in LSILs. (**d**) The nuclei are hyperchromatic and irregular, and are commonly said to have the appearance of raisins

12.1.2 Pathological Diagnosis and Grading

12.1.2.1 Low-Grade Squamous Intraepithelial Lesion (LSIL/CIN1)

The main diagnostic criterion of LSIL is the identification of koilocytes, which are defined by their atypical nuclei and perinuclear halos. The features of atypical nuclei in this setting include nuclear enlargement, variations in size (at least 3 times larger than normal size of an intermediate squamous cell nuclei), variable nuclear hyperchromasia, coarse chromatin, and irregular nuclear contours (raisinoid appearance) (Fig. 12.1). Generally a low nuclear-to-cytoplasmic ratio is seen. Binucleation or multinucleation is another feature that can be observed in LSIL (Fig. 12.1). Basal and parabasal cells proliferate and stratify upward to involve more than three cell layers, but less than half of the epithelial thickness. Mitoses may be seen within the lower one-third of the epithelium. Atypical mitoses are uncommon. Many of these features may be seen in reactive lesions and more severe dysplasia; therefore, it is important to remember that no single feature is specific, and it is important to consider a combination of various features when rendering a diagnosis of LSIL.

Two different patterns of LSILs can exist. The most common is flat LSIL (or flat condyloma). It has features of LSIL while lacking an exophytic, or papillary, growth pattern (Fig. 12.2). Changes in this pattern of LSIL are most pronounced in the upper third of the epithelium, while the lower two-thirds exhibit mild to minimal changes. Flat condylomata are often associated with high-risk HPV infection; hence, it is not uncommon to see diffuse p16 in this lesion. Alternatively, LSIL may have an exophytic or wart-like pattern; these are classic examples of condyloma acuminatum (Fig. 12.3), which are strongly associated with HPV types 6 and 11. In these cases the p16 stain will usually demonstrate patchy cytoplasmic staining that is weak

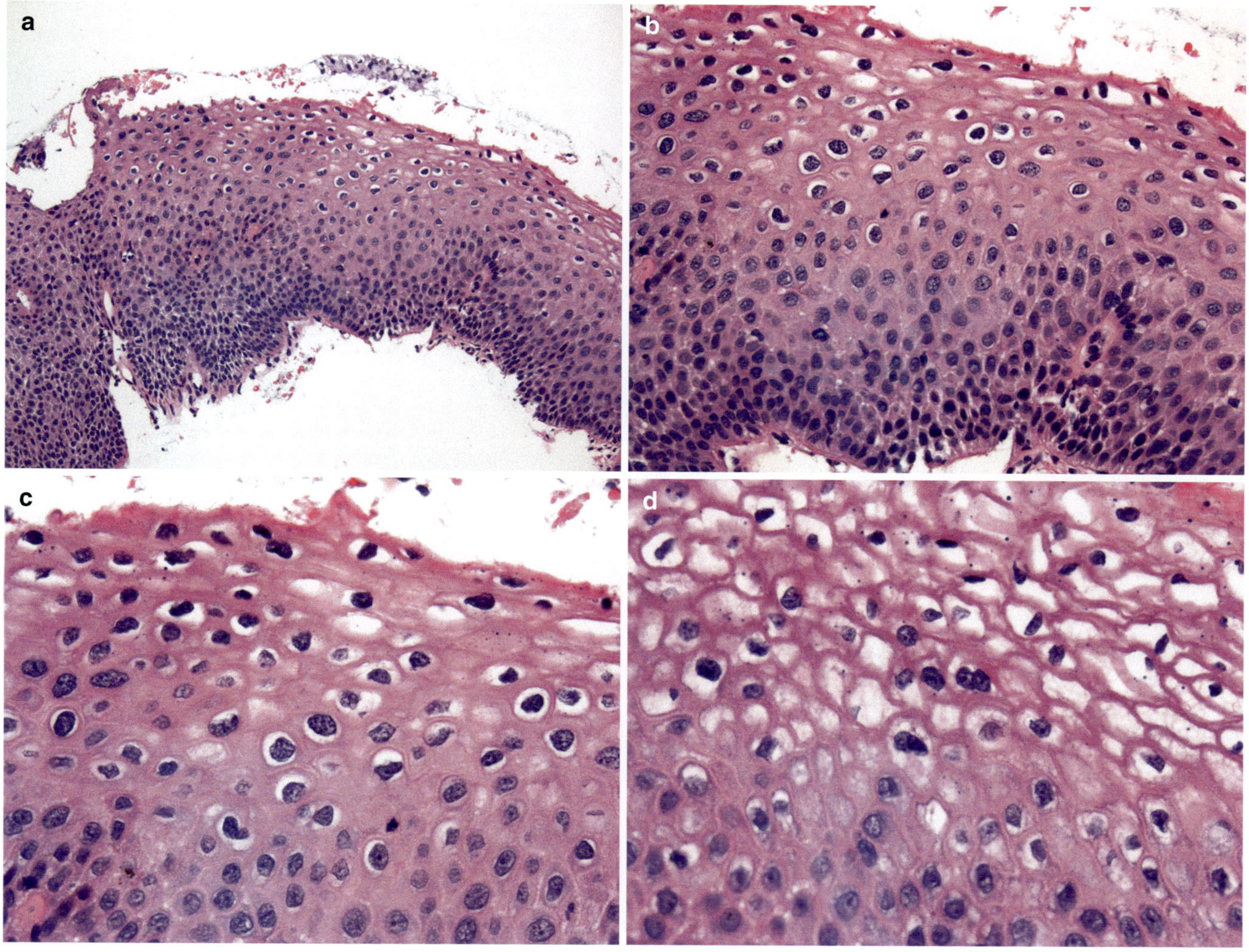

Fig. 12.2 Flat low-grade squamous intraepithelial lesion/condyloma. (**a–d**) Similar features are seen when compared to Fig. 12.1. Note the hyperchromatic nuclei, coarse chromatin, irregular nuclear contours, and perinuclear halos, all features of LSIL

or may be completely negative. Condyloma acuminatum exhibits a verrucous growth pattern, often with prominent papillomatosis (Fig. 12.3a), koilocytic atypia (Fig. 12.3b), acanthosis, hyperkeratosis (Fig. 12.3c), and parakeratosis (Fig. 12.3d).

When interpreting cervical biopsies, it is important to identify alterations in the lower third of the epithelium when considering a diagnosis of LSIL. In the setting of LSIL, the basal layer will often demonstrate a subtle loss of its picket-fence arrangement and some alterations in nuclear size and shape (Figs. 12.1 and 12.2). Most koilocytosis is present in the upper two-thirds of the epithelium.

12.1.2.2 High-Grade Squamous Intraepithelial Lesion (HSIL/CIN2–3)

High-grade lesions have a high nuclear-to-cytoplasmic ratio, hyperchromatic nuclei, and irregular nuclear contours, yet are often more monomorphic than their low-grade counterparts (Fig. 12.4a, b). There is a lack of maturation, with increased nuclear density and atypia, in both the upper and lower epithelial layers. Importantly, overlapping nuclei are commonly seen and abnormal mitotic figures can be present. The basal layer will display marked nuclear crowding and overlap, as well as loss of maturation extending into the upper half of the epithelium (Fig. 12.4c). This can be an important feature to help differentiating HSILs from LSILs (Fig. 12.4d).

The most disagreement in classifying SILs is associated with the diagnosis of CIN2. It has low reproducibility, especially among relatively inexperienced pathologists [12, 13]. In some cases, it is difficult to precisely separate CIN1 from CIN2, especially among pathologists, as interpretative thresholds vary among pathologists and practice groups. In certain challenging cases, some pathologists may opt to use diagnostic terminology such as "SIL of indeterminate grade (CIN1-CIN2)"; however, this is discouraged as it may lead to a management conundrum. A special comment or communication with the treating

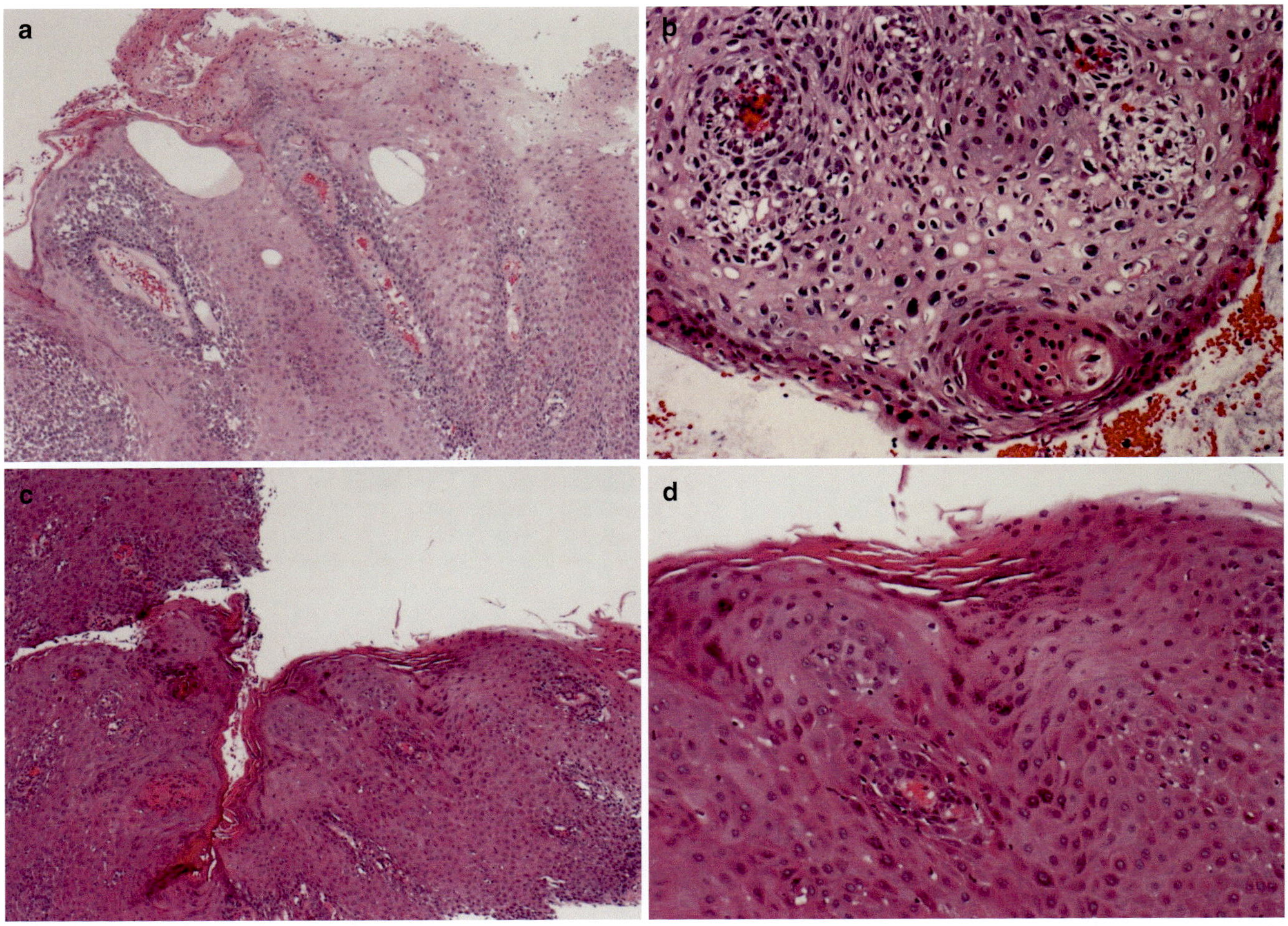

Fig. 12.3 Condyloma acuminatum. (**a**) An exophytic, or verrucous, growth pattern is the first sign of condyloma at low power. (**b**) On higher power, nuclear atypia with prominent koilocytosis are typically present. (**c**) Hyperkeratosis and (**d**) parakeratosis can be easily appreciated

clinician is recommended to help guide the most appropriate follow-up for these patients.

While the distinction of CIN2 and CIN3 may not be critical, as they are both considered high-grade lesions, the identification of CIN2 should be undertaken as some young patients with that diagnosis may be conservatively managed [11]. In principle, these two lesions are distinguished based on the degree of dysmaturation, or atypia, within the epithelium. In CIN2, the nuclear atypia is present in the lower two-thirds of the epithelium (Fig. 12.4e). Some degree of maturation or koilocytic atypia can be seen in the upper one-third. In CIN3, there is minimal to no maturation as the immature cells occupy the full thickness of the epithelium (Fig. 12.4a, b); mitoses can be seen at all levels. Although a defining feature of CIN1, there are no koilocytes present in CIN3 lesions. Figure 12.5 illustrates examples of normal, low-grade and high-grade squamous intraepithelial lesions.

Eosinophilic dysplasia of the cervix is a variant of CIN2 that contains both metaplastic features and a moderate degree of atypia [14]. This lesion is defined by (1) absence of normal maturation; (2) an increased amount of eosinophilic cytoplasm and distinct cell borders when compared with a conventional HSIL; (3) a mildly to moderately increased nuclear-to-cytoplasmic ratio; and (4) focal dysplastic nuclei with enlargement and hyperchromasia, irregular nuclear membranes, and appreciable nucleoli (Fig. 12.6). These lesions are subtle and can easily be mistaken as reactive squamous metaplasia.

12.1.3 Common Diagnostic Problems and Differential Diagnosis

Reactive atypia due to inflammation or a variety of infections are commonly misinterpreted as LSILs. In reactive epithelium, the cells can show nuclear enlargement (usually <3 times of the intermediate size squamous nuclei) and variation in nuclear size is minimal to absent (monotonous changes among neighboring cells) (Fig. 12.7). Perinuclear halos can be identified (particularly in *Candida* infections); however, no associated atypical nuclei should be present, and the demarcation of the cytoplasmic halo is not as sharp and distinct as the halo seen in HPV infection. The chroma-

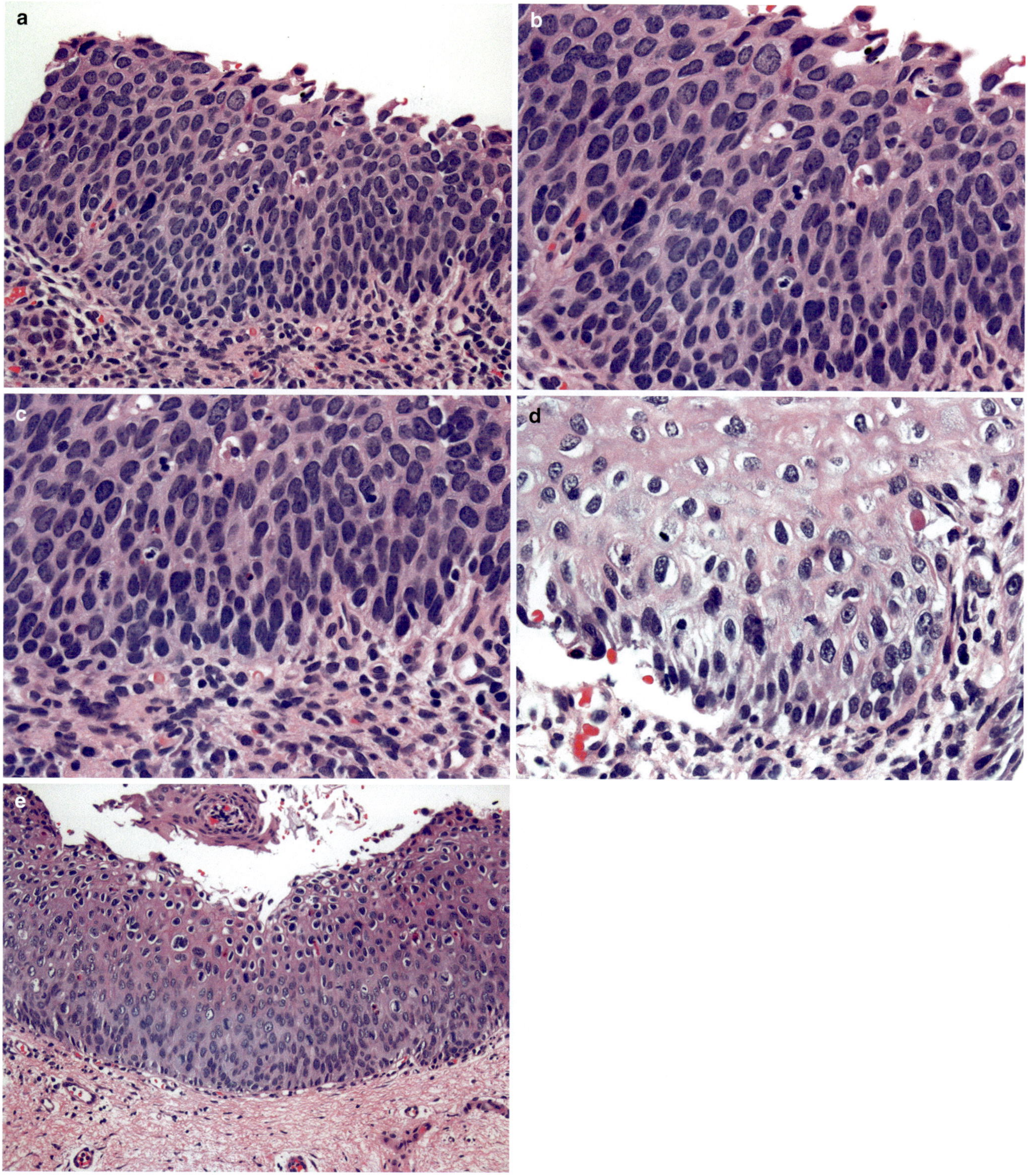

Fig. 12.4 High-grade squamous intraepithelial lesion. (**a**, **b**) The squamous epithelium shows full-thickness atypia with nuclear crowding and overlap. (**c**) The basal layer extends upward, throughout the entire thickness of the epithelium in this example. (**d**) Compared to HSIL, the basal layer of LSIL has subtle disorganization. (**e**) CIN2 with atypia involving the lower two-thirds of the epithelium. Note the disorganization of the basal layer when compared to LSIL

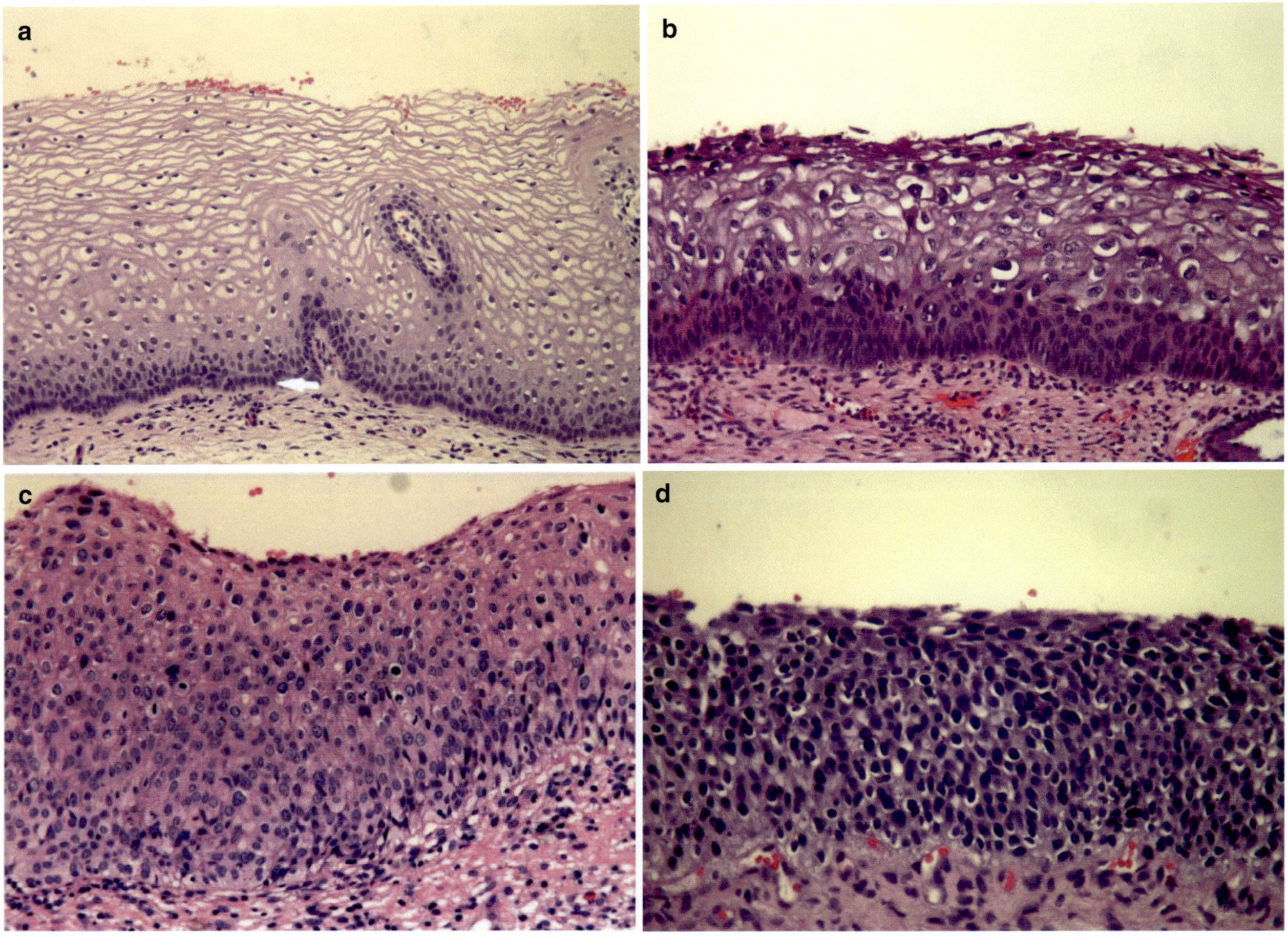

Fig. 12.5 The full spectrum of squamous epithelial lesions. (**a**) Normal. (**b**) LSIL/CIN1. (**c**) HSIL/CIN2. (**d**) HSIL/CIN3

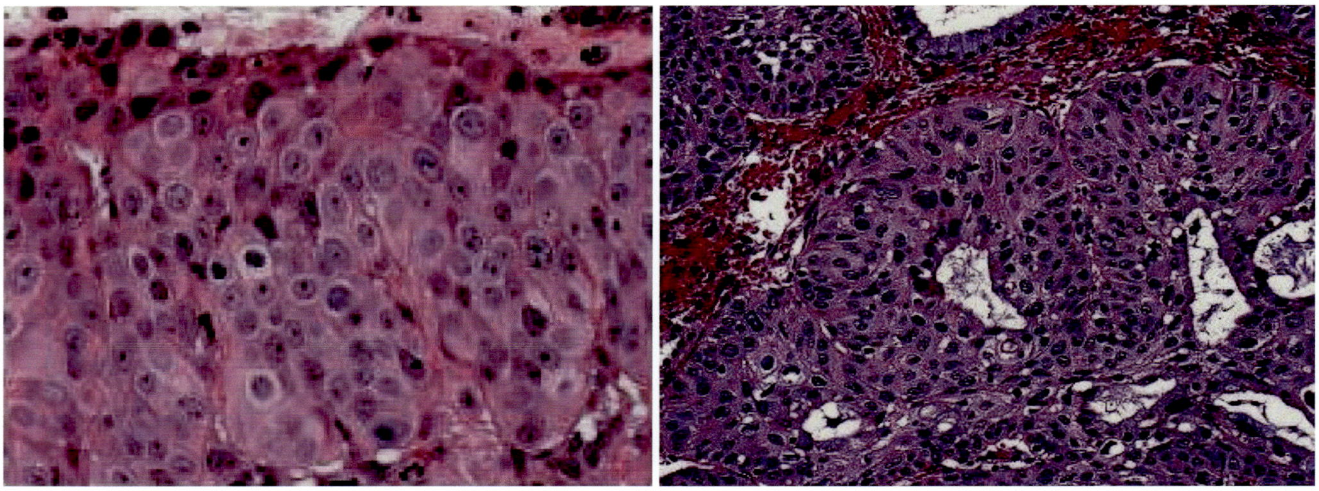

Fig. 12.6 Eosinophilic dysplasias have a metaplastic appearance with abundant eosinophilic cytoplasm. This is a rare variant of CIN2 and can often be confused with metaplastic changes

tin is more open and vesicular (as opposed to hyperchromatic and coarse) and multiple small nucleoli may be present in reactive epithelial changes.

LSILs can sometimes be difficult to differentiate from CIN2, especially in flat lesions. CIN2 is the therapeutic threshold for excision, but also the least reproducible diag-

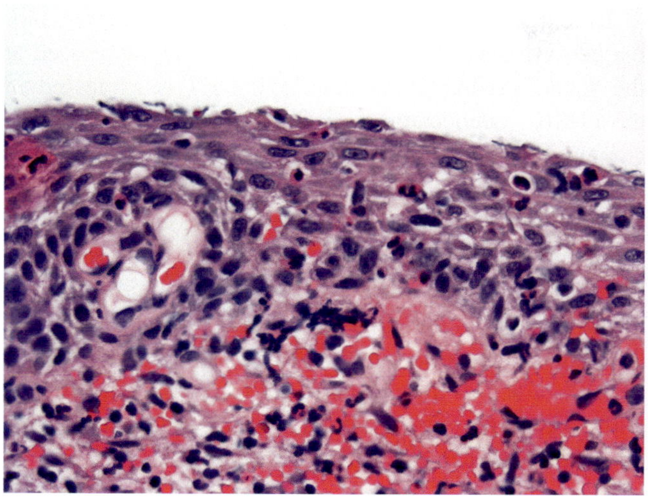

Fig. 12.7 Reactive changes consist of enlarged nuclei and slight nuclear irregularities. Note the presence of neutrophils and the uniformity of the changes among the cells. Prominent nuclei should alert the pathologists that the irregularities are reactive rather than lesional

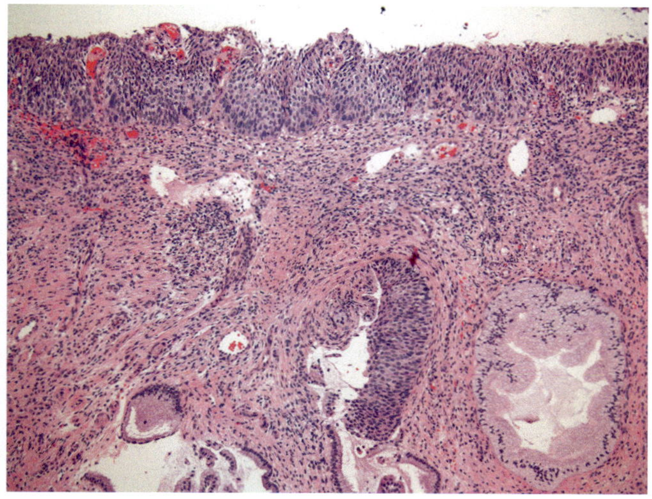

Fig. 12.8 High-grade squamous intraepithelial lesion with gland (crypt) involvement. HSIL can track into endocervical glands deep within the stroma; however, adjacent endocervical epithelium, the presence of smooth contours, and lack of desmoplastic response confirm the absence of invasion

nostic grade in cervical biopsies; therefore, its existence is not without controversy [15]. Young women with CIN2 can be followed conservatively with observation; therefore, it is important for pathologists to render this diagnosis accurately when necessary. As discussed earlier, CIN2 is characterized by squamous atypia in the lower two-thirds of the epithelium. Occasionally, koilocytic atypia maybe present in the superficial layer, which makes the distinction from LSIL difficult. Helpful features include the presence of mitoses within the upper half of the epithelium, nuclear crowding within the lower half of the epithelium, and the loss of the "picket-fence" configuration of a normal basal layer.

Dysplasia, especially high-grade dysplasia, extending into the crypts is frequently encountered in cervical lesions (Fig. 12.8). It can occasionally cause a diagnostic conundrum and be overdiagnosed as superficially invasive squamous cell carcinoma. The presence of rounded outer contours and a smooth basement membrane, as well as a lack of desmoplastic stromal changes, typically excludes invasion. This issue is discussed in more detail later in this chapter.

Another diagnostic challenge is differentiating atrophy and transitional metaplasia from HSIL. Similar to HSIL, atrophy contains squamous cells with hyperchromatic nuclei and a high nuclear-to-cytoplasmic ratio due to the relative loss of cytoplasm (Fig. 12.9). In transitional metaplasia, the cells stratify with some nuclear crowding, resembling urothelium. Both scenarios can be misclassified as HSIL; however, in these lesions, the cells are monotonous with very little anisonucleosis, and essentially no mitotic activity. In difficult cases p16 is a helpful marker as HSILs are positive while the mimics are negative.

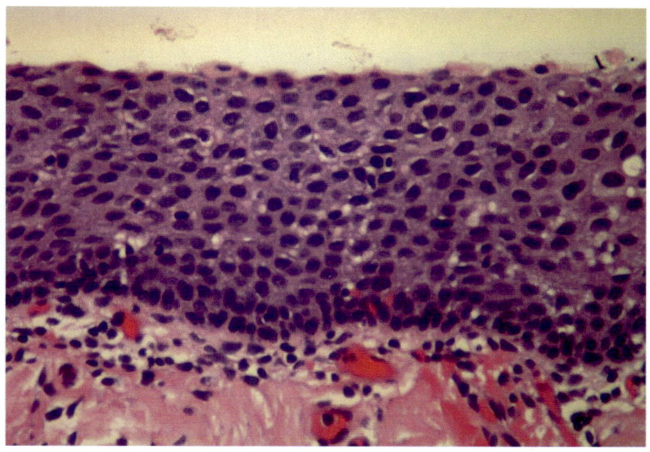

Fig. 12.9 Atrophy. The cells in atrophic epithelium have increased nuclear-to-cytoplasmic ratio, making them appear crowded and hyperchromatic. There is lack of nuclear membrane irregularities and the cell size is more or less uniform

12.1.4 Immunohistochemical Markers Useful for the Diagnosis and Possible Prognosis

p16ink4 (p16), a surrogate marker for HPV infection, is a cyclin-dependent kinase inhibitor that is overexpressed in the presence of high-risk HPVs (hrHPV) [16]. p16 is considered positive when it demonstrates strong and diffuse nuclear and cytoplasmic staining involving at least the lower one-third of the epithelium (Fig. 12.10) [10]. Focal, or patchy, staining is considered nonspecific and can be present in LSILs associated with low-risk HPV infection. p16 is most useful in differentiating HSILs from metaplastic changes, atrophy, and reactive atypia as previously discussed (Fig. 12.10a, b). When differentiating LSILs from HSILs, p16 should be used with caution. LAST recommends that histologically suspected CIN2 lesions be confirmed with a positive p16 [10]. This is a helpful recommendation to prevent overinterpretation of LSILs as CIN2 since most HSILs should be p16 positive. That being said, the use of p16 as an adjudicate marker between LSIL and CIN2 should be interpreted with caution as 20–70% of LSILs show strong p16 positivity [16, 17]. As a result, p16 does not distinguish LSIL from HSIL; however, p16 has a high negative predictive value, as p16 negative lesions are unlikely to be HSILs. Classic histologic CIN1 and CIN3 lesions should not be stained with p16.

Recent attention has shifted to another emerging biomarker, cytokeratin 7 (CK7), which is highly expressed at the squamocolumnar junction [17]. CK7 is expressed in most HSILs, adenocarcinoma in situ, and squamous cell carcinomas [17]. HPV-related lesions located within the mature metaplastic or ectocervical epithelium are CK7 negative. Interestingly, lesions that are CK7 negative correlate with a lower histological grade and, presumably, a lower risk of progression to malignancy [18]. Furthermore, LSILs that are negative for CK7 are less likely to have a subsequent HSIL diagnosis in follow-up samples [15, 19]. As a result, CK7 has been identified as a potential triage tool for LSIL patients, with CK7 negativity conferring a better prognosis (Fig. 12.11). When assessing CK7 staining, strong expres-

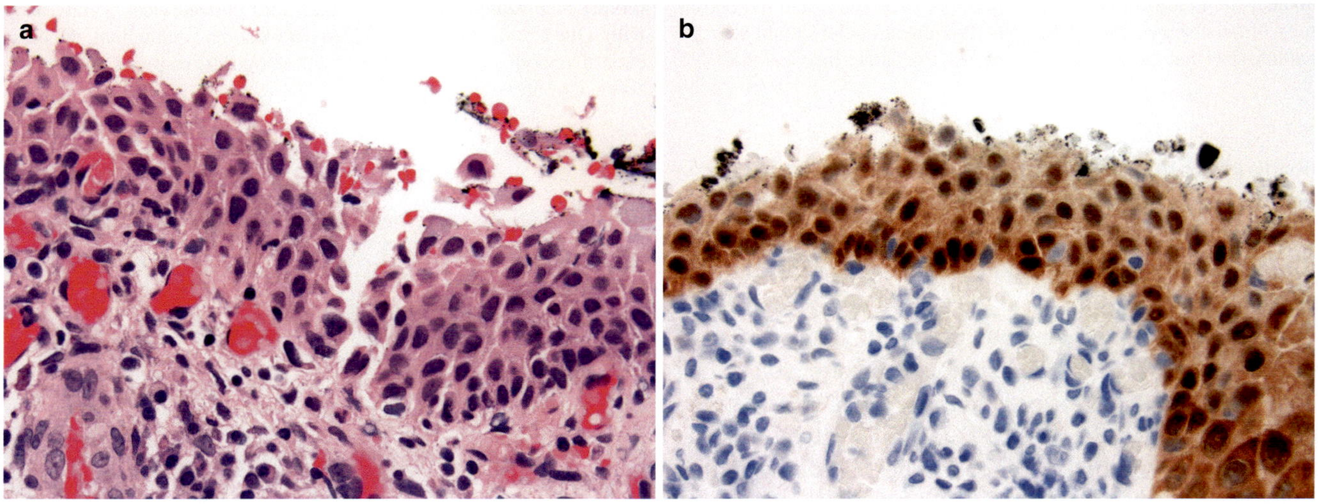

Fig. 12.10 High-grade squamous intraepithelial lesion. (**a**) This example demonstrates squamous epithelium with nuclear atypia and eosinophilic metaplastic changes. (**b**) A p16 stain is diffusely positive, supporting an HSIL diagnosis

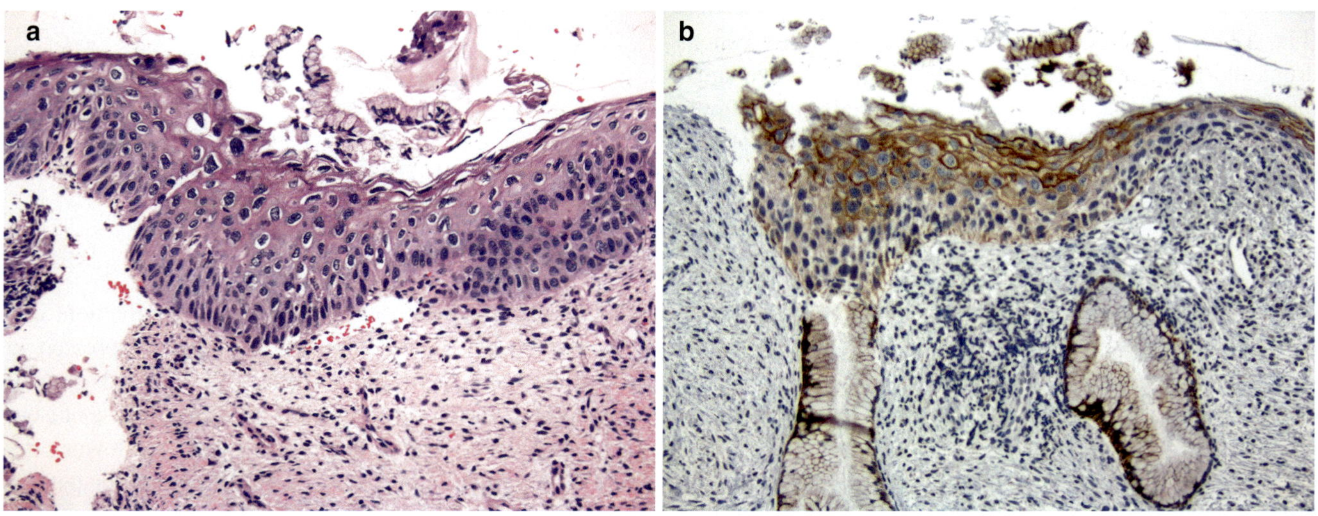

Fig. 12.11 Low-grade squamous intraepithelial lesion. (**a**) The squamous epithelium demonstrates the classic features of nuclear enlargement, raisinoid nuclei, and koilocytosis. (**b**) CK7 is positive in this lesion and the patient developed HSIL upon follow-up

sion of CK7 in multiple contiguous cells in at least the superficial epithelial layers is considered positive.

Additional immunohistochemical markers are discussed in greater detail in later sections.

12.1.5 Clinical Impact of the Pathology Report

It is important for pathologists to clearly delineate LSIL from HSIL as management significantly differs between the two groups. The American Society of Colposcopy and Cervical Pathology (ASCCP) is the leading organization in cervical management recommendations and its guidelines are discussed in the following section [11].

12.1.6 Outcome of Lesions, General Principles, and Management Options for Patients

12.1.6.1 LSIL/CIN1

Since approximately 90% of patients with LSIL will spontaneously regress and clear the HPV infection in 2 years, it is important not to overtreat these patients [20]. Patients with biopsy-proven LSIL can be followed at 1 year intervals with repeat co-testing (Papanicolaou test and HPV testing). If LSIL persists for more than 2 years, the clinician may choose to continue following the patient or excise the lesion for definitive treatment, particularly when hrHPV is positive.

In patients with LSIL on biopsy, with previous cytologic HSILs or atypical squamous cells, cannot exclude HSILs (ASC-H), recommendations include either following these patients conservatively with co-testing at 12 and 24 months, or treating these patients aggressively with immediate excision for women who have completed child bearing or if the patient is at a significant risk of being lost to follow-up. It is also acceptable to rereview the Papanicolaou smear if available. If upon rereview, the cytologic interpretation is changed to LSIL or less, then patients can be followed with repeat co-testing in 1 year.

12.1.6.2 HSIL/CIN2–3

CIN2 remains the diagnostic threshold for treatment; therefore, excision is recommended in women with HSIL/CIN2; however, as LEEP is associated with obstetric complications and a greater risk of premature delivery due to cervical incompetence, ASCCP has recommended different management options for these patients.

CIN2

In patients with CIN2, up to two-thirds of lesions will regress spontaneously [20, 21]. Further complicating the issue CIN2 is a poorly reproducible diagnostic entity. In the ASCCP management guidelines, CIN2 patients can be managed conservatively with colposcopic examination every 6 months for 2 years, or the lesion can be excised if immediate treatment is desired. In women who still desire fertility, a conservative approach is reasonable as excision can lead to pregnancy complications.

CIN3

CIN3 is less likely to regress and has high risk of developing into invasive squamous cell carcinoma; therefore, these patients should not be observed, but treated immediately with LEEP.

Margin Status After Excision

If HSIL is present at a tissue margin on a LEEP or conization specimen, or within the endocervical curettage (ECC), the preferred follow-up method is with cytology and ECC at 4–6 months. If the patient or the clinician is uncomfortable with the positive margins, repeat excision is acceptable. Hysterectomy is an option if a repeat excision is not feasible, and repeat excision or hysterectomy is acceptable for recurrent or persistent HSIL.

12.1.6.3 Management Options for Patients in Pregnancy

As most LSILs will regress, follow-up without treatment is recommended for pregnant patients with LSIL. In pregnant patients with HSIL, in the absence of invasive disease, additional colposcopy and Papanicolaou testing is acceptable at 12 weeks or greater intervals. Deferring reevaluation until at least 6 weeks postpartum is also an option. During reevaluation, if the colposcopic appearance worsens or if the Papanicolaou test is suggestive of invasive disease, a repeat biopsy is recommended. Excision is only recommended if invasion is suspected. It is important to remember that an ECC should not be performed on a pregnant patient.

12.2 Superficially Invasive (Microinvasive) Squamous Cell Carcinoma

12.2.1 The Concept and the Nomenclature

A unified concept for prognostically favorable early invasive squamous cell carcinoma is not widely accepted, illustrated by the fact that the definition of this entity has changed over time according to the International Federation of Obstetrics and Gynecology (FIGO) cancer staging system. In a 1937 FIGO staging system all cancer confined within the uterine cervix was considered stage I. By the year 1964, Stage I lesions were divided into Stage IA (early stromal invasion) and Stage IB (invasive tumor confined within the cervix other than IA). In 1973, Stage IA disease was further defined as early invasive carcinoma that could only be diagnosed microscopically. In 1985, this early lesion was subclassified as Stage IA1 and Stage IA2: the former referred to those small tumor foci breaking through the basement membrane with a depth of stromal invasion no more than 3 mm; the latter with the depth of invasion less than or equal to 5 mm and the horizontal extent no more than 7 mm. This classification was revised in 1994 as the following: Stage IA1 was defined a depth of invasion ≤3 mm and a horizontal extent ≤7 mm; Stage IA2 with a depth of invasion >3 mm but ≤5 mm, along with a horizontal extent ≤7 mm [22]. It has been emphasized that the presence of lymphovascular space invasion has no effect on staging. Despite detailed descriptions of histopathologic features of early invasive squamous cell carcinoma in the FIGO staging system, a formal concept/nomenclature has not been provided. Historically, different terms have been used to describe this constellation of entities, including microinvasive carcinoma, early invasive carcinoma, early invasive preclinical carcinoma, very small carcinoma, and covert invasive carcinoma, among others.

The concept of microinvasive carcinoma of the uterine cervix was first introduced in 1947 by Mestwerdt, in 1953, who further described it as a lesion with a stromal invasion ≤5 mm measured from the basement membrane. In 1974, The Society of Gynecological Oncologists (SGO) in the United States adopted the concept of microinvasive carcinoma and proposed a more restricted definition similar to that of FIGO Stage IA1 disease, i.e., a histologic lesion with ≤3 mm stromal invasion but no lymphovascular space invasion [23]. Unlike FIGO classification, the horizontal extent of the lesion was not defined in the SGO system. The depth of stromal invasion remains the most important factor for staging and prognosis in these classification systems; while there are obvious differences regarding whether the horizontal extent and lymphovascular space invasion are included during staging, the depth of stromal invasion is strictly defined in both FIGO and SGO classification system (Table 12.1).

Table 12.1 Diagnostic criteria and nomenclature of early stage of invasive squamous cell carcinoma of the cervix

	FIGO Stage	SGO *nomenclature*
Depth of invasion ≤3 mm	IA1	Microinvasive carcinoma
Depth of invasion >3 but ≤5 mm	IA2	Stage IB (not microinvasive carcinoma)
Horizontal extent ≤7 mm	IA1 or IA2	N/A
Horizontal extent >7 mm	IB	N/A
Lymphovascular space invasion	No effect	Not microinvasive carcinoma
Pattern of invasion	N/A	If confluent growth, not microinvasive carcinoma

In the third edition of the World Health Organization (WHO) classification of tumors of female genital organs, the term "microinvasive squamous cell carcinoma" is a synonym for "early invasive squamous cell carcinoma" for which the definition is "a squamous cell carcinoma with early stromal invasion, the extent of which has not been precisely defined, and a low risk of local lymph node metastasis." This entity has not been listed as a separate category in the fourth edition of WHO classification of tumors [24]. In 2012, the LAST Project [10] made recommendations for the utilization of the term "superficially invasive squamous cell carcinoma of the cervix" that is defined as an invasive squamous carcinoma that: (1) is not a grossly visible lesion; (2) has an invasive depth of ≤3 mm from the basement membrane of the point of origin; (3) demonstrates horizontal spread of ≤7 mm in maximal extent; and (4) is completely excised. In our opinion, this terminology best reflects the nature of the disease, from the histopathologic features to the clinical outcome.

12.2.2 General Morphologic Features

Not surprisingly, nearly all superficially invasive squamous cell carcinoma arises in a background of extensive HSIL, and, in most instances, is associated with endocervical gland involvement. The involved glands are sometimes deeply situated with central luminal necrosis. While HSILs usually display a smooth epithelial-stromal border, superficial stromal invasion is characterized by the presence of a focally disrupted and ragged basement membrane. Within the invasive foci, the cells usually display a well-differentiated morphology with abundant, eosinophilic cytoplasm, prominent nucleoli, and, occasionally, keratin pearl formation, in comparison to the adjacent HSIL, a phenomenon called "reversed" or "paradoxical maturation." In addition to features of cytologic atypia, loss of polarity, and paradoxical maturation, another important morphologic feature indicating invasion is the presence of a stromal reaction composed of desmoplasia, edema, and inflammatory infiltrates.

Superficially invasive squamous cell carcinoma usually displays three invasive patterns: budding growth, "spray bud" growth, and tongue-like growth. Among them, budding growth is thought to be the earliest recognizable form of invasion and is characterized by a tiny bud of invasive cells arising from a background of HSIL/CIN3. This bud penetrates through the basement membrane and pushes into the underlying stroma (Fig. 12.12a). While budding invasion usually manifests with a single focus, this type of invasion can also be multifocal. Whether single or multiple, the farthest distance from the basement membrane to the tip of bud is usually less than 1 mm; therefore, patients with this type of invasion generally have a very favorable prognosis. As the

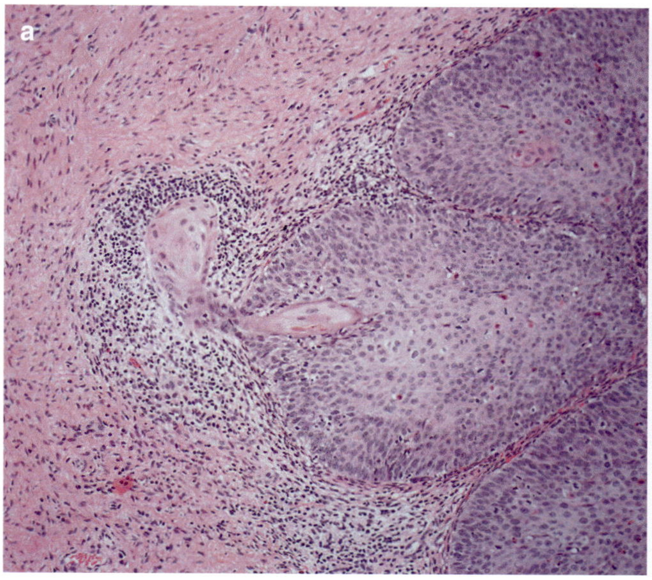

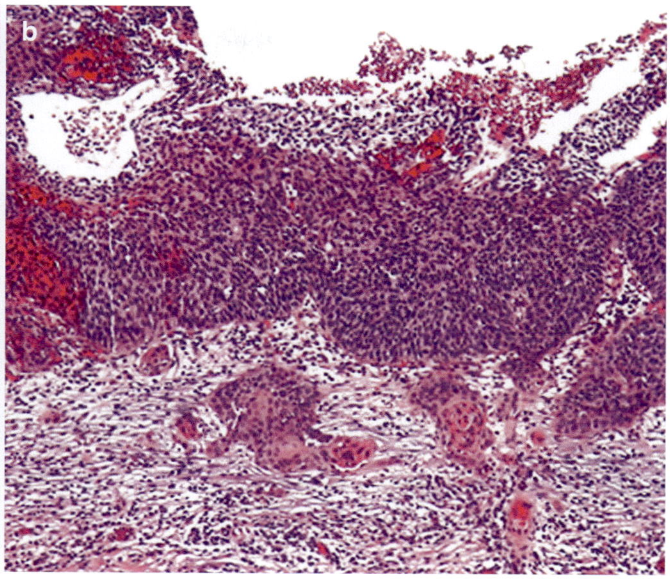

Fig. 12.12 Superficially invasive squamous cell carcinoma. (**a**) Budding growth, characterized by a tiny bud of invasive cells penetrating through the basement membrane, arising from a background of HSIL/CIN3. (**b**) Spray bud growth, characterized by deeper invasion with several nests of tumor separated from the basement membrane and extending into the stroma

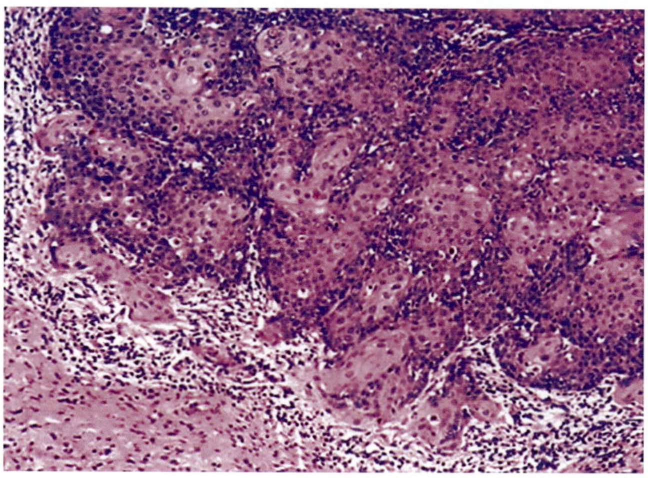

Fig. 12.13 Superficially invasive squamous cell carcinoma, tongue/confluent growth pattern invasion. The lesion merges into a tongue-like growth pattern

depth of invasion increases, the nests of tumor cells separate from the basement membrane, extending into the stroma, forming a "spray bud" pattern of invasion that is usually 1–2 mm in depth, but may rarely exceed 3 mm (Fig. 12.12b). Once invasive foci become larger, longer, and wider, the lesion may gradually merge into a tongue-like growth pattern, also referred to in the literature as "confluent growth" (Fig. 12.13). This pattern has been defined as a solid nest with a size more than 1 mm, or anastomosing tongues of epithelium with pushing border. It has been recommended that, from the pathologic point of view, when the confluent growth pattern of invasion is present, the lesion needs to be well sampled in order to identify other possible features that may affect the stage and prognosis. Typically, this consists of ordering deeper levels; however, submission of all of the cervical tissue should be undertaken if not already accomplished.

12.2.3 Measurement of Superficially Invasive Squamous Cell Carcinoma

The diagnosis of superficially invasive squamous cell carcinoma is primarily based on the depth and width of the invasive focus. Although the specific depth and width of this entity varies in the different systems, it is very important to provide an accurate measurement that is reflected in the pathology report.

12.2.3.1 Measurement of Depth of Invasion

1. If the origin of the invasive foci arises from HSIL, the depth of invasion is measured from the point of the origin in the basement membrane, vertically downward to the deepest point of the invasive focus (Fig. 12.14).
2. If the invasive foci arises from endocervical glands involved by HSIL, the depth of invasion is measured to the deepest point from the nearest overlying basement membrane of the involved gland.
3. If the invasive foci are present in the area surrounding endocervical glands involved by HSIL, but not continuous with either surface HSIL or the involved glands, the depth is measured from the deepest lesion to the basement membrane of the involved gland.

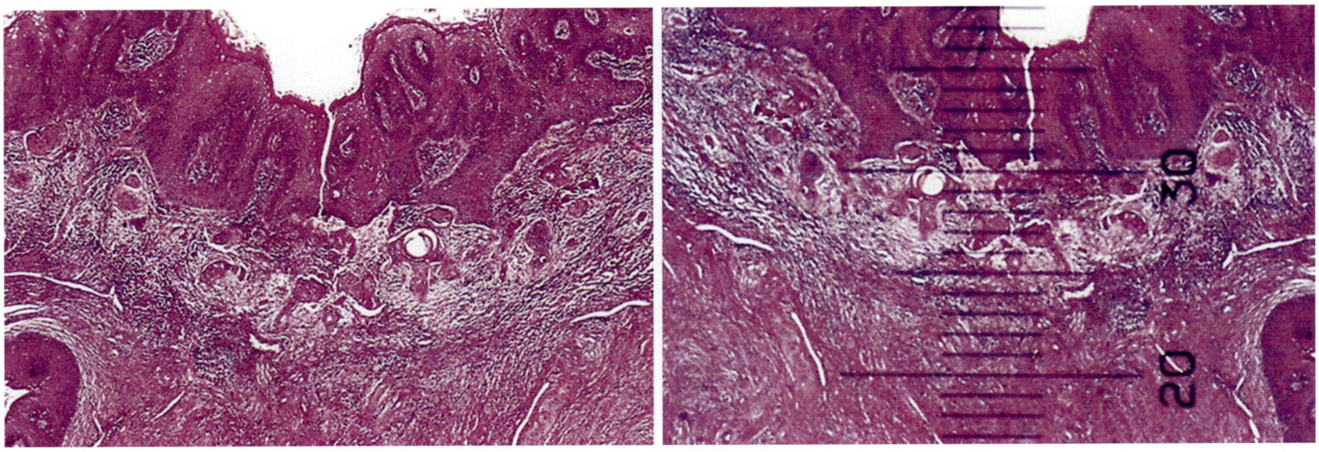

Fig. 12.14 Measurement of the depth of invasion of superficially invasive squamous cell carcinoma. This tumor displays multiple invasive foci, and the depth of invasion is measured from the point origin within the basement membrane, vertically downward to the farthest point of the invasive focus; in this case the depth of invasion is nearly 5 mm

Fig. 12.15 Measurement of horizontal extent. This figure contains two low-power fields (2×). The measurement was performed from one edge (left, dotted) to another (right, dotted) that covers the entire area including the normal interstitial stroma

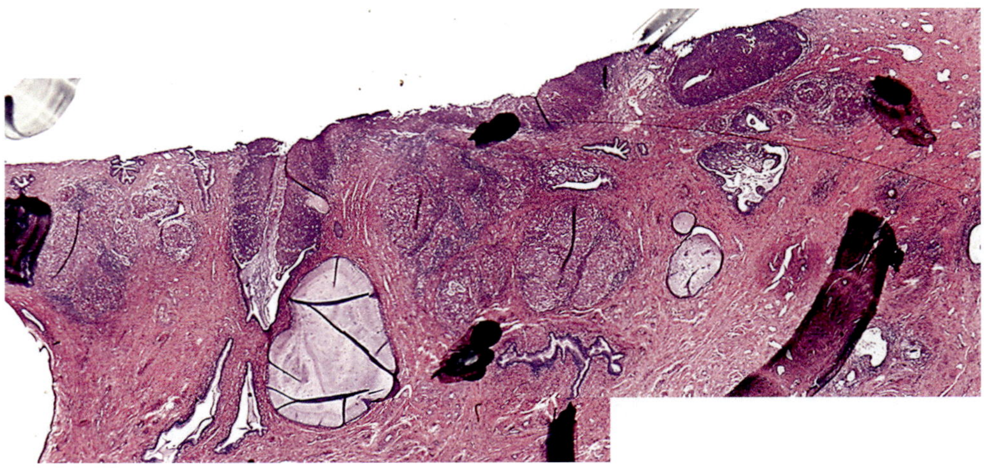

4. If the origin of invasion is not seen (no overlying HSIL or an ulcerated/eroded surface), depth of invasion is measured from the basement membrane of the most adjacent normal squamous epithelium or from the surface of the area of ulceration.
5. If multiple invasive foci are present simultaneously, the measurement should be performed from the point of the deepest invasive focus.

It is important to emphasize that a cervical biopsy is a rather limited specimen. The size/depth/extent of the invasive component in this specimen cannot be guaranteed to represent the entire invasive lesion. Accordingly, if one desires to use this diagnostic category, we recommend that a diagnosis of superficially invasive squamous cell carcinoma should only be rendered on a LEEP, cold knife cone resection, or hysterectomy specimen. Additionally, precise measurements should be included in the pathology report either within the diagnostic line or in synoptic templates.

12.2.3.2 Measurement of Horizontal Extent

While horizontal measurement of a single lesion is relatively straightforward (from one side to the other), measurement of multifocal lesions can be performed in three different ways:

1. Budding pattern invasion: If the invasive foci arise from overlying HSIL, then the horizontal extent is a sum of width of individual invasive foci, excluding the normal stroma between the lesions.
2. If both budding and spray bud pattern invasion are present simultaneously, the measurement should be performed from one edge to another that cover the entire area (one or more low-power fields) including the normal interstitial stroma (Fig. 12.15).
3. If the invasive foci are present in multiple sections, the measurement needs to be performed in each section, and meanwhile the distance between each section should also be measured; however, a well-accepted criteria for this scenario are not available.

12.2.3.3 Measurement of Volume

Some studies have demonstrated that the volume of invasive lesions, rather than the depth and/or width, can more accurately predict the clinical outcome. Carcinoma rarely undergoes metastasis if the volume is less than 500 mm^3 [25]; however, in reality, measurement of volume is not widely used in daily practice due to its complexity. Recently developed tissue clearing technology allowing for 3-dimensional measurement may facilitate clinical application of this method.

12.2.4 Lymphovascular Space Invasion (LVSI)

The prognostic value of LVSI in superficially invasive squamous cell carcinoma is less evident in comparison to the depth of invasion and lymph node metastases. It has been reported that the presence of LVSI may indicate a retained lesion in the subsequent hysterectomy specimen [26]. While the presence/absence of LVSI has no effect on the FIGO staging system, a diagnosis of superficially invasive carcinoma can only be rendered without LVSI by SGO criteria [10]. In fact, many studies indicate that the presence of LVSI is an adverse prognostic factor for superficially invasive squamous cell carcinoma and should be addressed if present [26–28]. In general, LVSI is readily recognizable (Fig. 12.16). The diagnosis of LVSI is defined as the presence of the tightly clustered tumor cell nests in a well-bordered lymphovascular space, lacking a surrounding stromal reaction. Immunohistochemical staining for CD34, CD31, Factor VIII, and D2–40 (more specific for lymphatic endothelia) can be used to aid in the recognition of LVSI when morphologically ambiguous.

In the daily practice, it is worth noting that the determination of LVSI should mainly rely on the H&E section with immunohistochemical staining as only an ancillary method [29, 30]. In fact, it has been shown that immunostains do not appear to be superior to routine H&E sections for the assessment of LVSI [30]. This is due to several factors: different antibodies with different sensitivities for recognizing endothelial or lymphatic endothelium; frequent high-background, nonspecific staining; and depletion of tiny invasive foci in the deeper levels when immunostains are performed. Some reports have proposed evaluation of the amount of LVSI. While the value of quantitative assessment of LVSI remains controversial, these reports demonstrate a positive relationship between the amount of LVSI and recurrence/lymph node metastasis. Under their proposed schema, utilization of terms such as "focal LVSI" and "extensive LVSI" has been proposed where 1–2 foci of LVSI is considered focal and ≥3 foci would be considered extensive [31, 32]. It is reasonable to state that no definitive LVSI is identified when the confidence level of true LVSI is low.

12.2.5 Differential Diagnosis

12.2.5.1 Artifacts

Tissue retraction artifacts

Artifactual retraction of stroma around aggregates of tumor cells, mostly due to tissue processing, may simulate LVSI, leading to a misdiagnosis (Fig. 12.17).

Tumor epithelial displacement

Epithelial displacement is mostly seen in stromal tissues in association with prior biopsy or anesthesia injection site changes including hemorrhage, fibrosis, and hemosiderin-laden macrophages. Likewise, displaced epithelium may

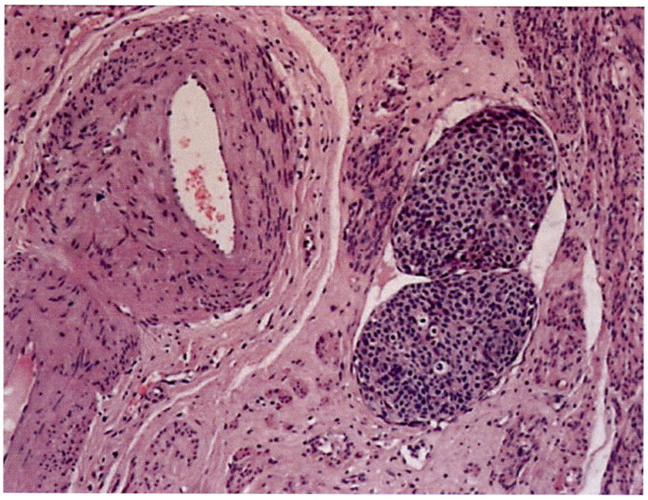

Fig. 12.16 Lymphovascular space invasion by carcinoma. A tumor thrombus fills a vascular space lined by endothelial cells

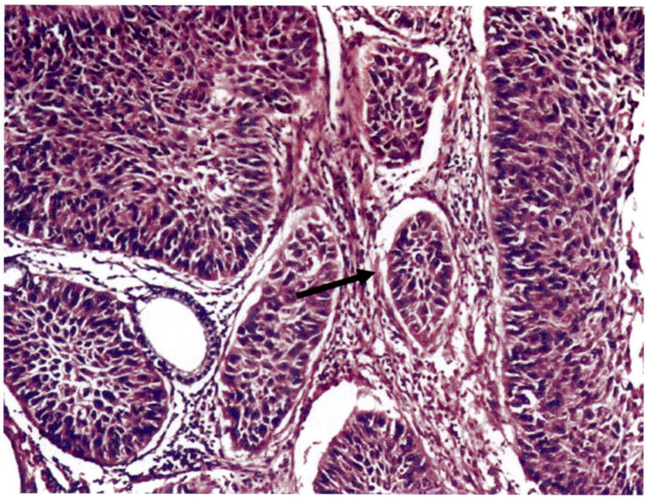

Fig. 12.17 Pseudo lymphovascular space invasion caused by tissue processing. Note that the cells within the space appear intact and that extensive cleft formation is present in other spaces as well

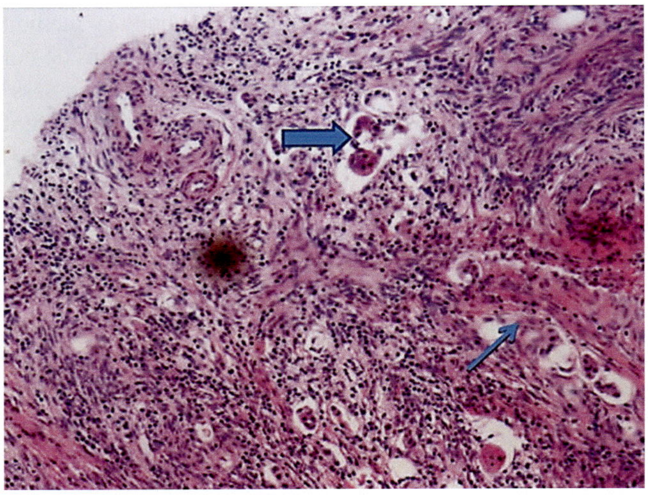

Fig. 12.18 Residual/retained epithelial elements and a foreign body giant cell reaction in the cervical stroma following conization

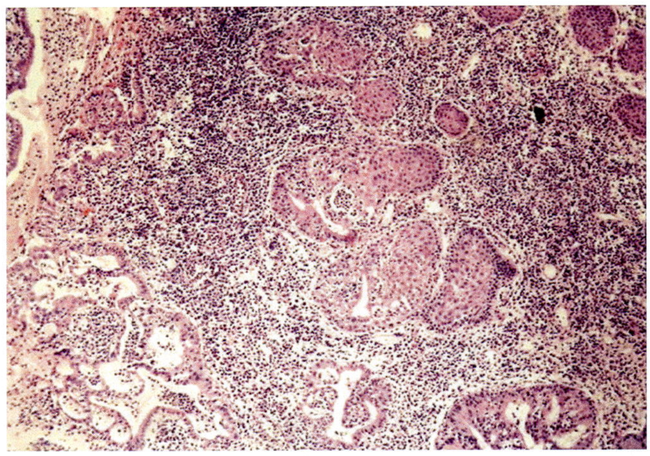

Fig. 12.19 Extensive squamous metaplasia within endocervical glands. The extensive inflammatory cell infiltrate causes the basement membrane to display an irregular contour, mimicking superficial invasion. Cytologic atypia, a desmoplastic reaction, and an overlying squamous intraepithelial lesion are absent

also be located within lymphovascular spaces, leading to misinterpretation as LVSI. This can be even more problematic when the displaced epithelia happen to be malignant cells or cells with reactive/reparative atypia. In general, as a result of injection, the blood vessels in this area are usually dilated, the epithelial cells have different contours, and the surface damage caused by the injection may be evident. If immunohistochemistry is used to confirm the endothelium of blood vessels or lymphatic vessels, the focus of the interest may disappear in the deeper levels. Accordingly, the discrimination of epithelial displacement into lymphovascular spaces from true LVSI may mainly rely on the H&E slides, in combination with the patient's history. Care should be taken when dealing with a specimen in a patient with a prior biopsy or LEEP/cold knife cone, as some displacement of the epithelium into the stroma may occur after these operations (Fig. 12.18). The main clue is a lack of fibrosis and desmoplasia around the displaced tissue.

12.2.5.2 Inflammatory Changes

Chronic inflammation can lead to reactive squamous hyperplasia, squamous metaplasia, and inflammatory cell infiltration in the mucosa and underlying stroma. As a result, the basement membrane may display an irregular contour, mimicking superficial invasion (Fig. 12.19). Features arguing against true invasion include the absence of cytologic atypia and the lack of a desmoplastic reaction. Care should be exercised when evaluating for invasion in heavily inflamed specimen, and if there is any doubt to the presence of true invasion, then a descriptive diagnosis is appropriate.

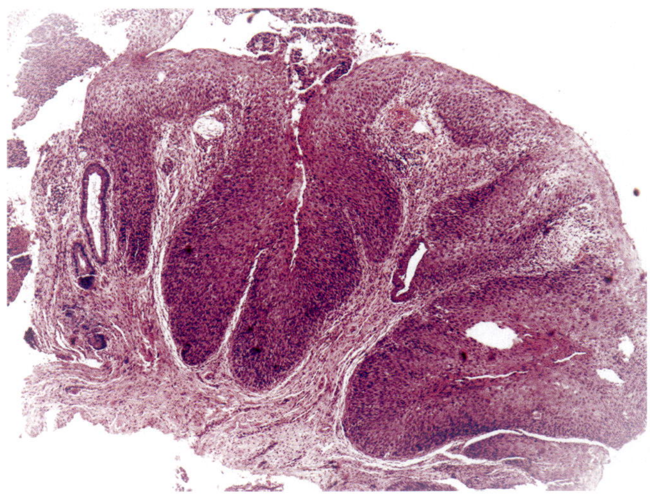

Fig. 12.20 HSIL/CIN3 involving endocervical glands. This morphology can be very deceptive, and confused with superficial/early invasive carcinoma, especially when the lesion becomes solid, completely replaces the glandular epithelium, and is tangentially sectioned

12.2.5.3 HSIL/CIN3 Involving Endocervical Glands

Colonization of glands by high-grade dysplasia can be very deceptive and cause confusion with superficial/early invasive carcinoma, especially when HSIL completely replaces the glandular epithelium with tangential sections. In fact, a misdiagnosis is more likely when it is difficult to appreciate the relationship between the involved glands and the HSIL/CIN3 in the surface squamous epithelium, and when the lesions become solid (Fig. 12.20). Endocervical gland involvement by HSIL usually displays a clear-cut contour with a smooth border, and will lack a desmoplastic stromal reaction, paradoxical maturation, and an irregular margin or scalloping of the epithelial nest. On the other hand, a subset of invasive squamous cell carcinoma (ISCC), classified as "CIN3-like growth pattern ISCC," presents diagnostic difficulty and may be misinterpreted as a noninvasive lesion leading to inappropriate management [33, 34]. This entity will be further discussed in the next section.

12.2.5.4 Placental Site Nodule (PSN)

Placental site nodules (PSN or plaques) are benign, well-circumscribed nodules or plaques characterized by nodular aggregates of chorionic-type intermediate trophoblast that are embedded in a hyalinized stroma (Fig. 12.21). PSNs are usually incidental findings in endometrial or endocervical curettings, cervical biopsies, and occasionally in fallopian tubes (probably a consequence of prior ectopic pregnancy). The presence of a PSN in the uterine cervix and its association with HSIL might prompt an erroneous diagnosis of cervical ISCC. The combination of morphology, clinical data, and immunohistochemical studies are mandatory for a correct diagnosis.

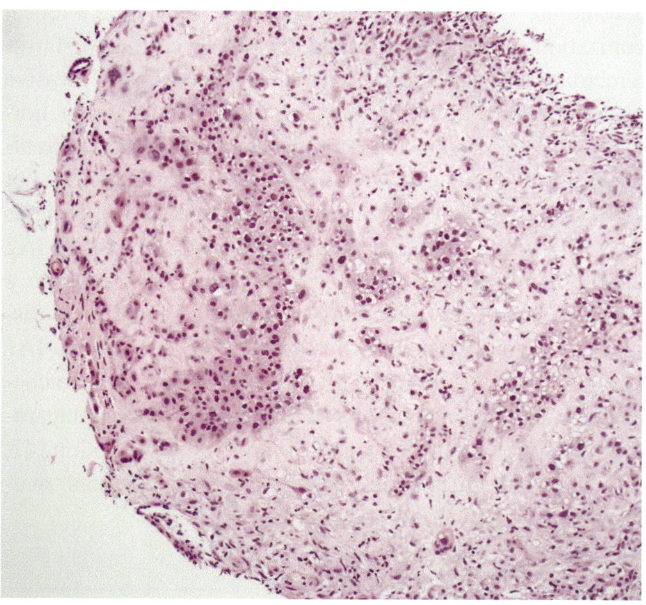

Fig. 12.21 Placental site nodule. A benign, well-circumscribed lesion, placental site nodules are characterized by nested aggregates of chorionic-type intermediate trophoblast embedded in a hyalinized stroma

12.2.6 Prognosis

The prognosis of superficially invasive squamous cell carcinoma of the cervix (FIGO grade IA1) is excellent, with a 5-year survival rate of nearly 99%. Factors affecting prognosis are as follows.

12.2.6.1 Depth of Invasion and Horizontal Extent

The depth of invasion is thought to be the most important prognostic factor for superficially invasive squamous cell carcinoma. While there is almost no risk of lymph node metastasis, LVSI is reported to occur in 4.4% of cases if the depth of stromal invasion is <1 mm. When the depth of invasion ranges from 2 to 3 mm, LVSI incidence increases to 16.4% despite a relatively low rate of lymph node metastasis (from 1 to 5.3%). Not surprisingly, LVSI is reported to occur in 19.7% of invasive carcinoma when the depth of invasion reaches 3–5 mm [35].

There is a growing body of evidence that the horizontal extent of invasive carcinoma may be as important as the depth of invasion. In one report, when controlling for depth of invasion, the lymph node metastasis rate was 3.4% if the width of the horizontal extent was <7 mm; however, the rate increased to 9.1% when the width was >7 mm [36].

12.2.6.2 Tumor Volume

The concept of tumor volume in superficially invasive carcinoma was introduced to by Burghardt and Holzer in 1977 [25]. Based on a large case series, they concluded that microinvasive carcinoma with a tumor volume of less than 500 mm^3 is generally not associated with metastasis, and thus may be treated with conservative excision. Interestingly, they also concluded that the depth of invasion alone is of little value for the assessment of the biologic potency of the tumor. The topic of volumetric evaluation of these tumors has been relatively unstudied and the value of these criteria remains debatable; however, in recent years, the concept of tumor volume has gained more attention. Some authors postulate that it represents a reliable parameter for the prediction of clinical outcome. Measurement of tumor volume by serially sectioning LEEP/cone specimens is very time-consuming and not practical, and thus unlikely to become a routine laboratory method; however, progress with a rapid and easy-to-implement dibenzyl ether-based technique to clear thick sections of surgically resected specimens, allowing 3-dimensional visualization of the lesion, and thus tumor volume, may change the field in the future [37].

12.2.6.3 Lymphovascular Space Invasion (LVSI)

The clinical significance of LVSI in superficially invasive carcinoma is not clear. A study by Ostor et al. [36] failed to observe a relationship between LVSI and lymph node metastases. Yet, Raspagliesi et al. [28] found that the presence of LVSI was significantly related with recurrence. In a review article [27], it has been reported that 0.8% of patients had lymph node metastasis when the depth of invasion was ≤3 mm and LVSI was present. Conversely, the lymph node metastasis rate increased 10 times (8.3%) in patients with a similar depth of invasion but no LVSI. These results indicate that LVSI is of importance in predicting nodal disease and prognosis. Simply put, the lymph node metastasis and recurrence rates in patients with LVSI is higher than in patients without LVSI. Accordingly, microinvasive carcinoma is defined as being devoid of LVSI by the SGO.

On the other hand, some studies have found that the prognostic significance of LVSI is associated with the size of the tumor. For example, small tumors, even with LVSI, have a lower risk of metastasis than large ones [35]. Without consideration of the depth of invasion and tumor volume, patients with LVSI do not appear to have an increased lymph node metastasis and recurrence rate. Accordingly, the presence/absence of LVSI has no direct impact on FIGO staging.

12.2.6.4 Surgical Margins

It has been suggested that one of the most important parameters for the subsequent management of superficially invasive squamous cell carcinoma is evaluation of the surgical margins. A study by Roman et al. [38] demonstrated that residual invasive carcinoma in a repeat conization or hysterectomy specimen was present in 22% of women with an involved surgical margin versus 3% in those with a negative margin. When the status of both the surgical margin and post-conization ECC were considered, residual invasion was present in 4% of patients if both were negative, 13% if one was positive, and 33% if both were positive. The authors concluded that if either the margin or the post-conization ECC contains HSIL or carcinoma, the risk of residual carcinoma is high and repeat conization or hysterectomy are warranted.

12.2.6.5 Tumor Differentiation

As a general rule, poorly differentiated tumors have a poor prognosis; however, the correlation between the degree of tumor differentiation and the prognosis of superficially invasive squamous cell carcinoma remains elusive.

12.2.7 Immunohistochemical Markers

In recent years, a number of immunohistochemical markers, such as p16, Ki-67 (MIB-1), ProExC, pRb, hTERC as well as different methods for HPV detection have been applied to diagnose SIL. It should be noted that these markers are of very little help in distinguishing HSIL/CIN3 from superficially invasive squamous cell carcinoma. It has been postulated that epithelial-mesenchymal transition (EMT) may be a mechanism of invasion in HSIL and expression of EMT-associated proteins could be useful in the differential diagnosis between in situ and invasive carcinoma. In fact, Koay et al. [39] demonstrated that most invasive tumor cells expressed Cyclin D1 and showed a reduction in E-cadherin and beta-catenin staining. In another study, they found that fascin was overexpressed in most SILs, suggesting that it may be a marker of increased invasive potential in HSIL [40], but that its expression does not distinguish LSIL from HSIL or dysplasia from invasive squamous cell carcinoma.

12.2.8 Treatment

As mentioned previously, invasive squamous cell carcinoma with ≤3 mm of stromal invasion without LVSI is rarely metastatic or recurrent; therefore, in the current guidelines for the treatment of the superficially invasive squamous cell carcinoma, LEEP/conization is acceptable management for the patients who desire fertility if: (1) the depth of invasion ≤3 mm from the basement membrane, (2) no LVSI is present, and the (3) surgical margin is uninvolved by HSIL or carcinoma. When the surgical margins are involved a repeat conization should be performed, otherwise, simple total hysterectomy is adequate treatment for superficially invasive squamous cell carcinoma. Because these lesions are not hormonally dependent, oophorectomy is not required for treatment in premenopausal women, despite a low risk (3.5%) of the lesion to be potentially metastatic. Accordingly, patients with FIGO stage IA1 carcinoma with LVSI, or a stage IA2 lesion, as suggested by most authorities, may undergo a modified radical hysterectomy with pelvic lymph node dissection. If young patients who have a 1A2 lesion, or a IA1 tumor with LVSI, desire to preserve fertility, radical trachelectomy and parametrectomy with extraperitoneal or laparoscopic pelvic lymphadenectomy is an alternative option [41, 42]. Once lymph node metastasis is present, additional treatment such as pelvic radiation is required.

12.3 Invasive Squamous Cell Carcinoma (ISCC)

Cervical cancer is among one of the most common cancers in women. Cervical cancer incidence and mortality rates are highest in sub-Saharan Africa, Southeast Asia, Latin America, and Central and Eastern Europe. The incidence is also endemically influenced by a high prevalence of HIV infection, which has been found to promote progression of cancerous lesions. In the United States, the incidence of cervical carcinoma has declined by about one-third over the past several decades, mostly due to the success of screening with the Papanicolaou test. Despite the decrease in overall incidence rates, it has been estimated that there will be approximately 13,240 new cases diagnosed and roughly 4170 deaths due to cervical cancer in 2018 [43]. In women aged from 21 to 39 in the United States, cervical cancer is the second leading cause of mortality. We expect that increasing vaccination rates will decrease the overall incidence of cervical cancer in the future.

12.3.1 Clinicopathologic Features of Invasive Squamous Cell Carcinoma

12.3.1.1 General Features

Accounting for approximately 70–75% of all cervical cancers (up to 90% in developing countries), nearly all ISCCs are caused by one of carcinogenic types of hrHPV, with HPV16 and HPV18 most prevalent. This carcinoma can occur in a wide age range but the majority of patients diagnosed are 40 to 55 years old; for women younger than age 40 years, 78% of the cervical cancer cases are diagnosed in women aged 30–39, 21% are diagnosed in women 20–29 years of age, and 1% diagnosed in women younger than age 20 years [44]. Evolution of ISCC from its precursor lesion, LSIL and HSIL, occurs in a stepwise fashion. Patients with ISCC are usually 20 years older than patients with HSIL and 8 years older than patients with superficially ISCC. At the time of diagnosis, about 50% have stage I carcinoma, of which, about 15% are stage IA1 (superficially ISCC) that is usually asymptomatic. Abnormal vaginal bleeding and discharge can occur when the tumor grows to form a mass. With extra-cervical extension (lateral growth into the parametrium, anterior tumor growth involving bladder, posterior tumor growth involving rectum), symptoms may include anuria, uremia, urinary frequency, bladder pain, hematuria, tenesmus, rectovaginal fistula, vesicovaginal fistula, and lymphedema of the lower extremities. Pelvic sidewall involvement can cause sciatic pain.

12.3.1.2 Macroscopic Findings

In its early stage, ISCC can present as mucosal roughness, a papillary or polypoid excrescence, or as a focally indurated, ulcerated, or granular area. Endophytic carcinomas can be grossly normal or present with surface ulceration. These tumors usually develop in the endocervical canal with frequent infiltration into the cervical stroma, producing an enlarged, hard, barrel-shaped cervix. Alternatively, the majority of ISCCs display an exophytic growth pattern with a red, friable, and polypoid appearance (Fig. 12.22). Advanced stage tumors extend to the pelvic wall and/or the lower third of the vagina, and may cause hydronephrosis or nonfunctioning kidneys. In addition, with further growth, the tumor may invade the mucosa of the bladder or rectum (Fig. 12.23), or extend beyond the true pelvis, with or without regional lymph node metastasis and distant metastasis.

12.3.1.3 Microscopic Findings

ISCC of the uterine cervix can display variable patterns of growth, cell type, and degree of differentiation, and further classification of the following variants is based on those features; however, the stage and grade, rather than histologic subtype, impacts therapy and clinical outcomes.

Keratinizing Squamous Cell Carcinoma

By definition, keratinizing squamous cell carcinomas contain keratin pearls, a keratinized structure composed of well-differentiated squamous cells arranged in concentric nests

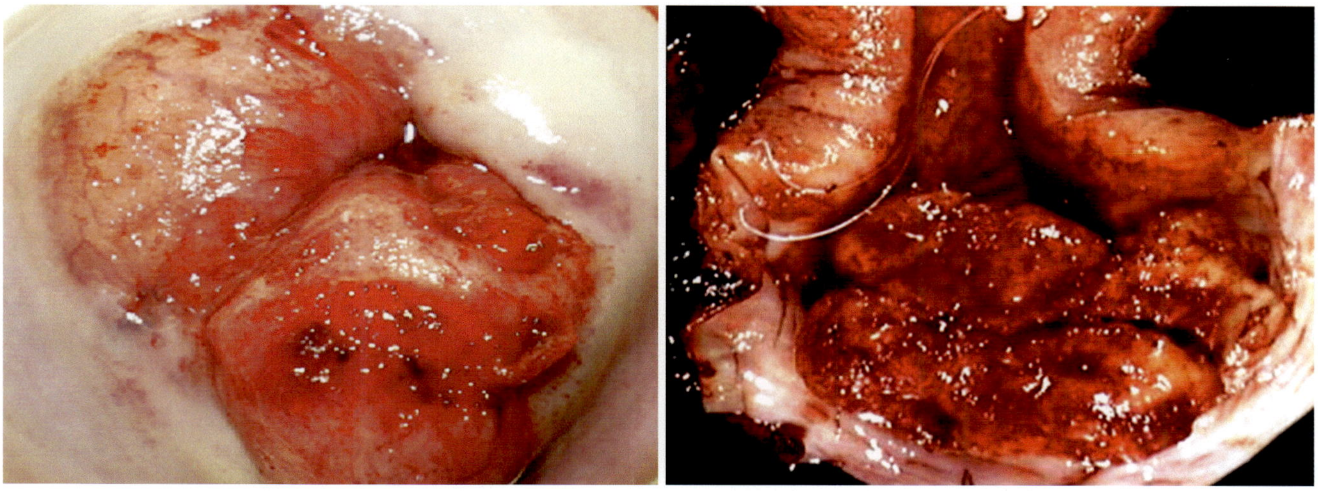

Fig. 12.22 Gross appearance of invasive squamous cell carcinoma with an exophytic growth pattern and a red, friable, polypoid appearance

that have undergone keratinization with abundant *keratohyalin granules and dense cytoplasmic keratin* (Fig. 12.24). The tumor cells usually contain abundant eosinophilic cytoplasm, notable intracellular bridges, and occasional mitosis. The nuclei are often pleomorphic, enlarged and hyperchromatic with coarse chromatin. It has been emphasized that grading these tumors cannot solely rely on the presence of keratin pearls; in other words, keratinizing squamous cell carcinoma should be graded based on nuclear grade rather than on the cytoplasmic differentiation or the presence of keratin pearls. One point that should be emphasized is that the incidence of keratinizing squamous cell carcinoma of the cervix is very low compared to the corresponding cancer in the vulva, although it remains listed as a histologic type.

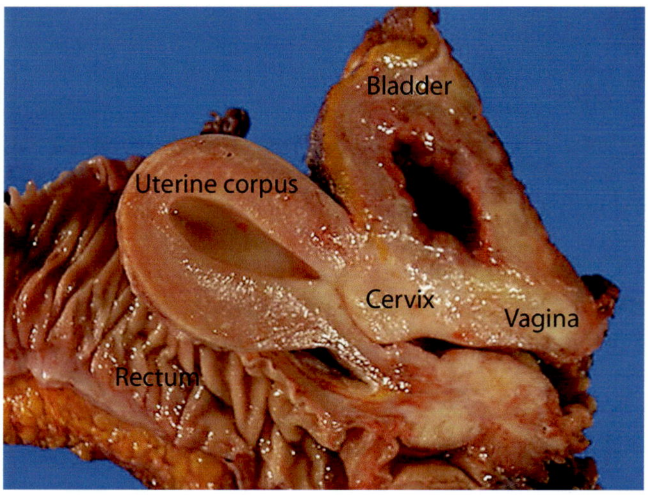

Fig. 12.23 Diffusely invasive squamous cell carcinoma infiltrating into the bladder, vagina, and rectosigmoid colon

Differential diagnosis. The differential diagnosis for this type of tumor is limited. This tumor is relatively easy to classify as it is defined by the presence of keratin pearls, the characteristic feature of keratinizing ISCC.

Nonkeratinizing Squamous Cell Carcinoma

Nonkeratinizing squamous cell carcinoma, by far the most common subtype of ISCC of the cervix, is characterized by neoplastic squamous cells arranged in sheets or nests that may undergo individual cell keratinization but without keratin pearl formation (Fig. 12.25). The tumor may take on a heterogeneous morphology. In some areas, the polygonal tumor cells display distinct cell borders, variable cytologic atypia, enlarged nuclei with coarse chromatin, and intercellular bridges. In high-grade, poorly differentiated regions, the tumor is composed of smaller cells with indistinct cell borders, a very high nuclear-to-cytoplasmic ratio, less prominent nucleoli, and readily recognizable mitosis.

Differential diagnosis. The morphologic features of this tumor may overlap with basaloid squamous cell carcinoma (discussed in the next section) and, occasionally, small cell neuroendocrine carcinoma. The latter is composed of monotonous small cells with enlarged ovoid hyperchromatic nuclei, nuclear molding, finely stippled chromatin, inconspicuous nucleoli, and scanty cytoplasm. Abundant mitotic figures, apoptotic bodies, extensive necrosis, and crush artifact are characteristic features seen in neuroendocrine carcinoma. The tumor cells are usually positive for synaptophysin, chromogranin, and INSM1. Ancillary studies such as immunohistochemical stains might be necessary for definitive classification in difficult cases.

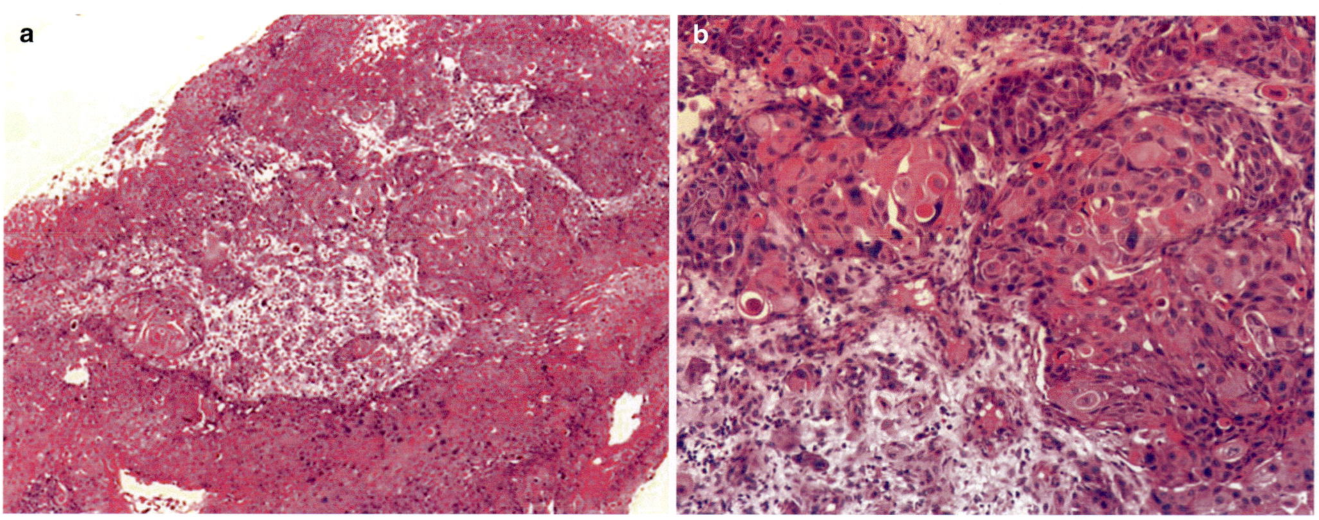

Fig. 12.24 Keratinizing squamous cell carcinoma. (**a**) Well-differentiated squamous cells are arranged in concentric nests and demonstrate keratinization with abundant *keratohyalin granules and dense, eosinophilic cytoplasm*. On higher power (**b**), the tumor cells contain abundant eosinophilic cytoplasm, enlarged, hyperchromatic nuclei with coarse chromatin, and notable intracellular bridges

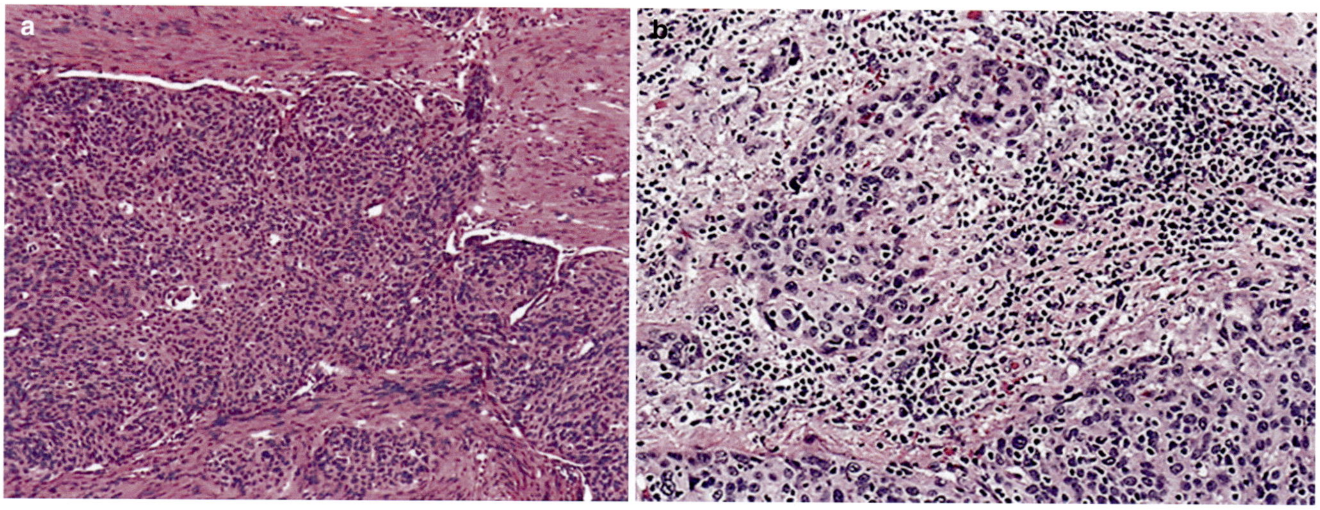

Fig. 12.25 Nonkeratinizing squamous cell carcinoma. (**a**) Within the high-grade, poorly differentiated regions, the tumor is composed of smaller cells with indistinct cell borders, a high nuclear-to-cytoplasmic ratio and less prominent nucleoli. (**b**) Comparatively, this relatively low-grade area demonstrates cells with polygonal distinct cell borders, variable cytologic atypia, enlarged nuclei with coarse chromatin, and intercellular bridges

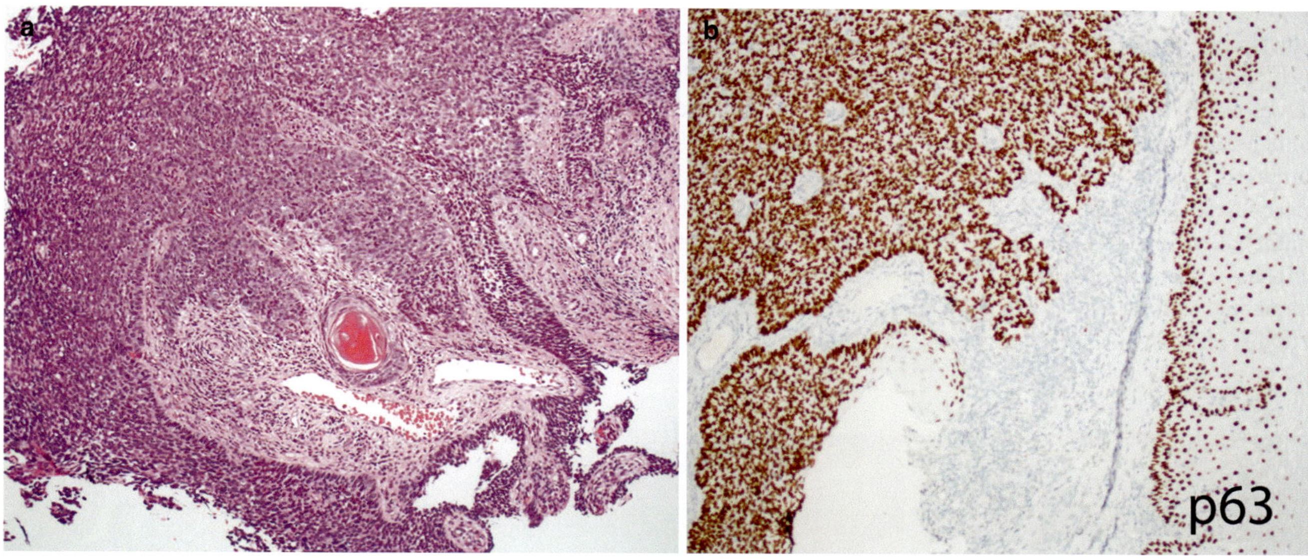

Fig. 12.26 Basaloid squamous cell carcinoma. (**a**) This tumor consists of clusters and nests of basaloid squamous cells with oval/round nuclei and scant cytoplasm. (**b**) The tumor expresses p63

Basaloid Squamous Cell Carcinoma

Basaloid squamous cell carcinoma, an under-recognized high-grade tumor, poses diagnostic challenges. This tumor consists of clusters and nests of basal type squamous cells with a high nuclear-to-cytoplasmic ratio, which closely resembles the cells of HSIL/CIN3 (Fig. 12.26). Occasionally, some keratinization can be encountered in individual cells but no keratin pearls are seen. Not uncommonly, brisk mitotic activity and tumor necrosis are present, suggesting aggressive behavior. It has been postulated that basaloid squamous cell carcinoma, similar to adenoid basal carcinoma/epithelioma and adenoid cystic carcinoma of the uterine cervix, arises from "reserve cells" that have features of progenitor cells which have the ability to give rise to a variety of tumors [45].

Differential diagnosis. Basaloid ISCC, adenoid cystic carcinoma, and adenoid basal carcinoma/epithelioma sometimes coexist; however, because basaloid squamous cell carcinoma and adenoid cystic carcinomas are associated with a distinctly unfavorable prognosis, they should be distinguished from adenoid basal carcinoma/epithelioma. Basaloid ISCC lacks the organized growth pattern of adenoid basal carcinoma/epithelioma which usually displays lobular clusters of basaloid nests with bland cytology; rather, basaloid

ISCC is composed of mitotically active, hyperchromatic tumor cells, forming solid islands with peripheral palisading. Adenoid cystic carcinoma can display cribriform, nested, solid, trabecular, and corded patterns of growth. Basement membrane material is usually seen within acini or in a trabecular pattern separating the tumor cells. Overlapping features can also be encountered between basaloid ISCC and small cell neuroendocrine carcinoma (see above section). The distinction may be difficult on a small biopsy, and most times ancillary studies are necessary.

Verrucous Carcinoma

Verrucous carcinoma is a rare variant of squamous cell carcinoma that most commonly involves the vulva in elderly women, but can also occur in the cervix. It remains controversial whether verrucous carcinoma is etiologically related to HPV infection. While some literature has shown that low- and high-risk HPV types were identified in verrucous carcinoma, overt evidence of HPV cytopathic effect (koilocytosis) was not usually found [46]. Furthermore, given the prevalence of HPV infection, it is unclear if the detected HPV is causal or incidental. This entity presents as a well-differentiated, slow-growing, locally invasive squamous cell carcinoma that has a hyperkeratotic and undulating surface and invades into the underlying stroma with a well-circumscribed pushing margin (Fig. 12.27). Often, there is a conspicuous inflammatory and desmoplastic reaction at the epithelial stromal junction, indicating invasion. The tumor cells have abundant cytoplasm but lack significant cytologic atypia and mitotic activity. Patients with verrucous carcinomas usually have a good prognosis. The tumor has a tendency to recur locally after excision but does not metastasize.

Differential diagnosis. The differential diagnosis includes condyloma acuminatum and more common types of squamous cell carcinoma. The former usually displays koilocytosis and fibrovascular cores but lacks broad papillae. The latter commonly shows cytologic atypia and infiltrative growth pattern, both of which should be absent in a verrucous carcinoma.

Warty or Condylomatous Carcinoma

This lesion is a variant of squamous cell carcinoma with morphology and architecture similar to that of a condyloma or Bowenoid lesion of the vulva. Microscopically the tumor cells may display koilocytic atypia, characteristic of HPV infection.

Differential diagnosis. The differential diagnosis includes condyloma acuminatum and verrucous carcinoma. Warty carcinoma is set apart by its infiltrative growth pattern at the deep margin, and greater degree of atypia (especially when compared to verrucous carcinoma).

Papillary Squamous Carcinoma and Squamotransitional Cell Carcinoma

In the 2003 and 2014 WHO classification of tumors of female reproductive organs, cervical papillary squamous cell carcinoma and squamotransitional cell carcinoma were classified separately. Both are variant forms of squamous cell carcinoma that have morphological overlap, and sometimes are difficult to distinguish from each other. Because they demonstrate a spectrum of histologic appearance, these

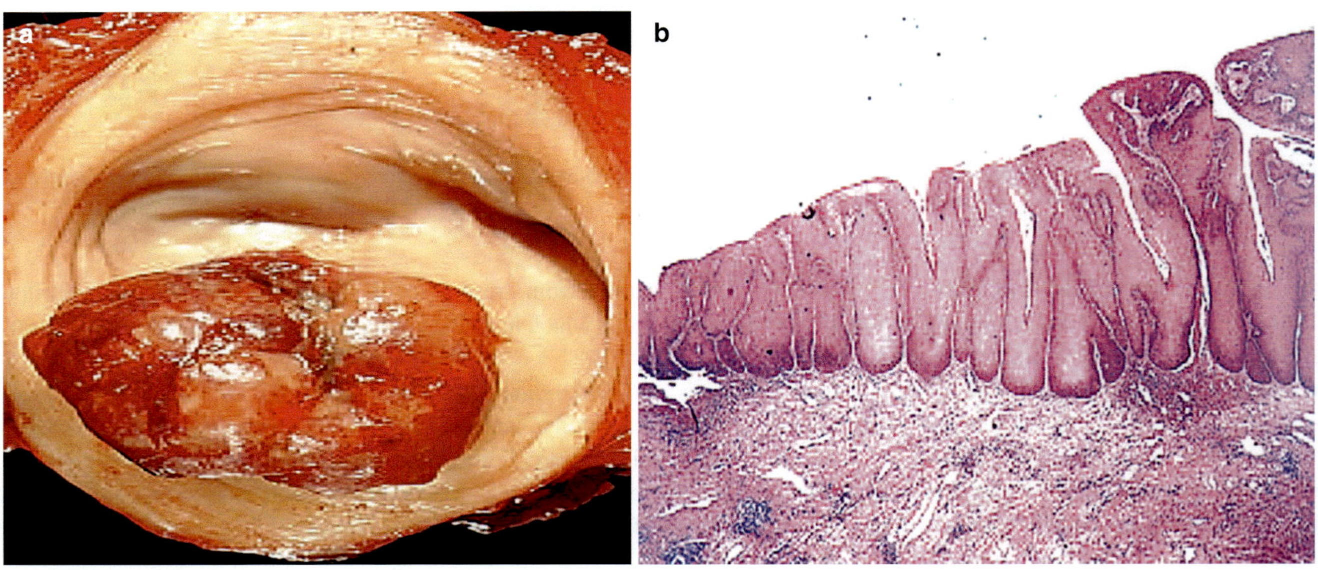

Fig. 12.27 Verrucous carcinoma. (**a**) Grossly this tumor consists of cauliflower-like lesions with papillary surfaces. (**b**) Histologically, the tumor is well differentiated and has a hyperkeratotic and undulating surface that invades into the underlying stroma with a well-circumscribed pushing margin. Note the lack of atypia throughout the lesion

tumors have been referred to, by some authorities, as papillary squamotransitional carcinoma which can be subdivided into three groups: predominately squamous, predominantly transitional, and mixed squamous and transitional.

Microscopically, papillary squamous cell carcinoma is composed of broad or thin papillae with fibrous stroma covered by epithelium resembling HSIL/CIN3 (Fig. 12.28). Mitosis is easily recognized. To diagnose a papillary squamous cell carcinoma the specimen needs to be thoroughly assessed for stromal invasion. In general, typical features of ISCC can be seen at the base of this tumor. Accordingly, papillary squamous cell carcinoma can be misdiagnosed as an in situ lesion on a superficial biopsy that may not reveal clear-cut invasion. Unlike warty carcinoma, this tumor lacks typical features of HPV infection.

Squamotransitional carcinoma has been described analogous to its counterparts in the urinary bladder. The lesion resembles transitional cell epithelium and is composed of oval cells with their long axis oriented perpendicular to the surface with minimal flattening as they extend upward into the epithelium. This tumor differs from transitional cell carcinoma by its occasional squamous differentiation and immunostaining profile (CK7 positive and CK20 negative).

Differential diagnosis. A major differential diagnostic consideration is papillary immature metaplasia (immature condyloma) that typically forms thin, papillary projections with an architecture similar to that of papillary squamous cell carcinoma. The key difference is that the lesional cells have a metaplastic phenotype with minimal koilocytosis and lack significant cytologic atypia or readily recognizable mitosis. These lesions occur in the transformation zone and are associated with HPV 6 or 11, thus lacking a "block positive pattern" of p16 expression with immunohistochemical stains.

Lymphoepithelioma-Like Carcinoma

This tumor is thought to be a distinct subtype of squamous cell carcinoma that displays morphology similar to that of the nasopharyngeal tumor of the same name. The tumor consists of large, atypical, discohesive cells simulating lymphoma, in a background of a stromal inflammatory infiltrate composed of lymphocytes, plasma cells, and eosinophils. The tumor cells appear to be poorly differentiated with indistinct borders and moderate amounts of slightly eosinophilic cytoplasm with uniform vesicular nuclei and prominent nucleoli (Fig. 12.29). Despite having a high-grade morphology, these tumors appear to have a better prognosis than typical squamous cell carcinoma [47, 48]. Whether the Epstein-Barr virus (EBV) plays a role in the genesis of lymphoepithelioma-like carcinoma remains elusive. While EBV has been detected in these tumors in Asian women [47, 49], a similar result was not reported in women in Western countries. Rather, these tumors are likely HPV-related as are nearly all cervical squamous cell carcinomas.

Differential diagnosis. This lesion can be mistaken for a severe inflammatory process, a true lymphoproliferative disorder, or glassy cell carcinoma. Benign inflammatory processes contain mixed populations of lymphocytes and other inflammatory cells but lack epithelial cells, which can be proven with cytokeratin staining. Unlike lymphomas that are immunoreactive for lymphocytic markers and contain a monoclonal population of neoplastic lymphocytic cells, lymphoepithelioma-like carcinoma consists of large epithelial cells that are immunoreactive for high molecular-weight keratins. Glassy cell carcinomas are characterized by distinct cell borders, ground glass cytoplasm, and prominent nucleoli. While glassy cell carcinoma may be inflamed, the degree

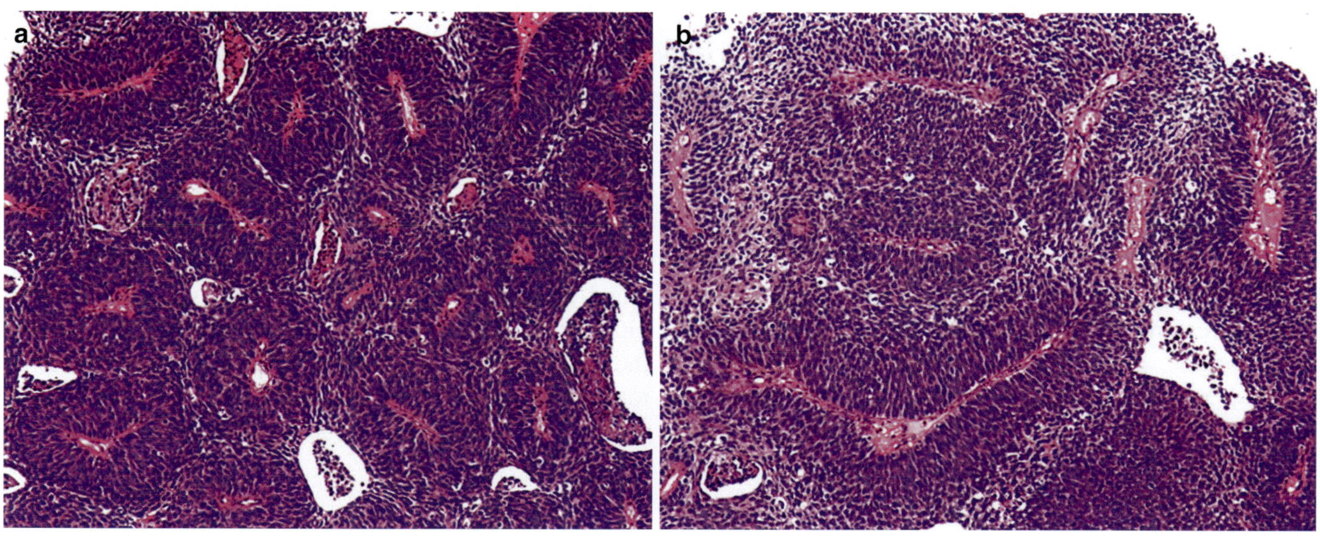

Fig. 12.28 Papillary squamous cell carcinoma. (**a**, **b**) The tumor is composed of broad or thin papillae with fibrous stroma covered by epithelium that lacks maturation, resembling HSIL/CIN3

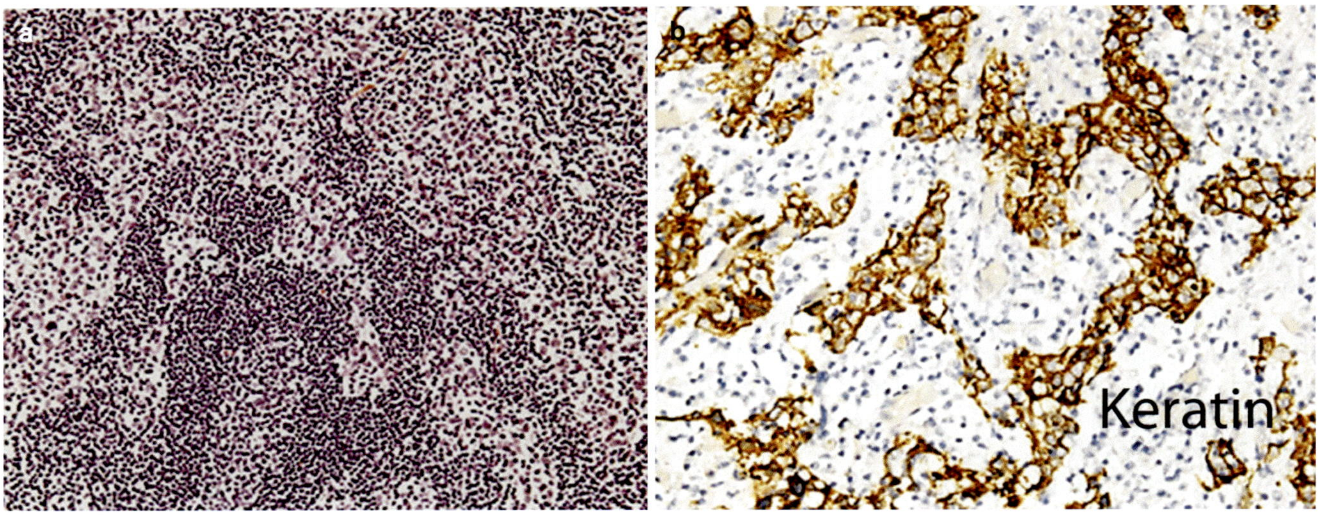

Fig. 12.29 Lymphoepithelioma-like carcinoma. (**a**) The tumor contains abundant lymphocytes. (**b**) The large, atypical, discohesive tumor cells are immunoreactive for cytokeratin

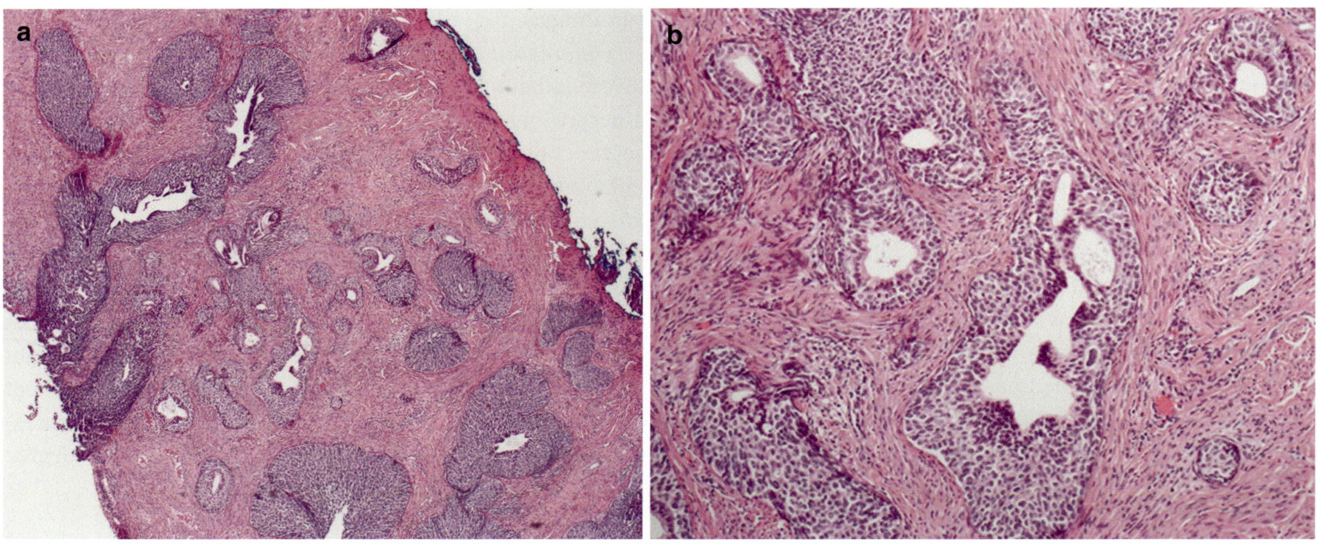

Fig. 12.30 CIN3-like squamous cell carcinoma. (**a**, **b**) The tumor usually invades deeply into the stroma and demonstrates a growth pattern that mimics endocervical gland involvement by HSIL/CIN 3

of inflammation typically falls far short of that seen in lymphoproliferative disorders and lymphoepithelial carcinoma.

CIN3-Like Squamous Cell Carcinoma

This entity may represent an architectural variant of squamous cell carcinoma of the cervix rather than a histopathologic subtype. Regardless, it seems that this lesion has received relatively limited attention in the literature. Histologically, the tumor is characterized by well-circumscribed cellular aggregates that invade deeply into the stroma, often associated with a mild stromal and inflammatory reaction (Fig. 12.30). It has been speculated that CIN3-like growth represents an example of collective cellular invasion or migration, a process in which malignant cells invade as relatively large cohesive aggregates [50].

Differential diagnosis. The invasive tumor deceptively demonstrates a growth pattern that mimics endocervical gland involvement by HSIL/CIN3, thus posing diagnostic pitfall, particularly in small biopsy specimens [33, 34]. By thorough examination of the specimen (LEEP or hysterectomy), many cases show a variable component of conventional ISCC that may be helpful in establishing the diagnosis.

Spindle Cell (Sarcomatoid) Squamous Cell Carcinoma

Spindle cell, or sarcomatoid, squamous cell carcinoma is distinctly rare. Despite sharing a similar etiology to usual type of ISCC, this tumor usually has a poorer prognosis, and behaves in an aggressive fashion, with early recurrence following treatment and a short disease-free survival [51]. Most patients present at an advanced stage at the time of hysterectomy. Due to its rarity, there are no well-established guidelines for treatment; most cases are managed similar to common types of ISCC. Histologically, the tumor is composed of fascicles of spindle-shaped neoplastic squamous cells with readily recognized mitoses and moderate to severe cytologic atypia (Fig. 12.31). The sarcomatoid tumor cells are immunoreactive for CK5/6, p40, p63 and p16 (diffuse) but negative for mesenchymal markers. Conventional morphologic features of ISCC are usually present.

Differential diagnosis. Associated with sarcoma-like stroma, spindle cell ISCC may mimic a sarcoma, as such, the differential diagnosis for this lesion includes malignant mixed mullerian tumor (MMMT, carcinosarcoma) and mesenchymal spindle cell tumors, including leiomyosarcoma, fibrosarcoma, spindle cell malignant melanoma (extremely rare in the cervix), and transitional cell carcinoma with spindle cell features. The neoplastic cells of spindle cell carcinoma are immunoreactive for keratin and p16, and high-risk HPV can be commonly detected, which can set this tumor apart from the previously mentioned entities.

12.3.2 Prognostic Factors

Stage is considered the most important prognostic factor for cervical ISCC. As noted in the following sections, studies have shown a 5-year survival rate for Stage II patients of 70%, while survival in Stage III patients drops to only 30–35%. Other prognostic factors include age, tumor size, depth of invasion, and LVSI.

12.3.2.1 Age

Some evidence has suggested that age is a poor prognostic factor. In a population-based study of 10,022 cases, Meanwell

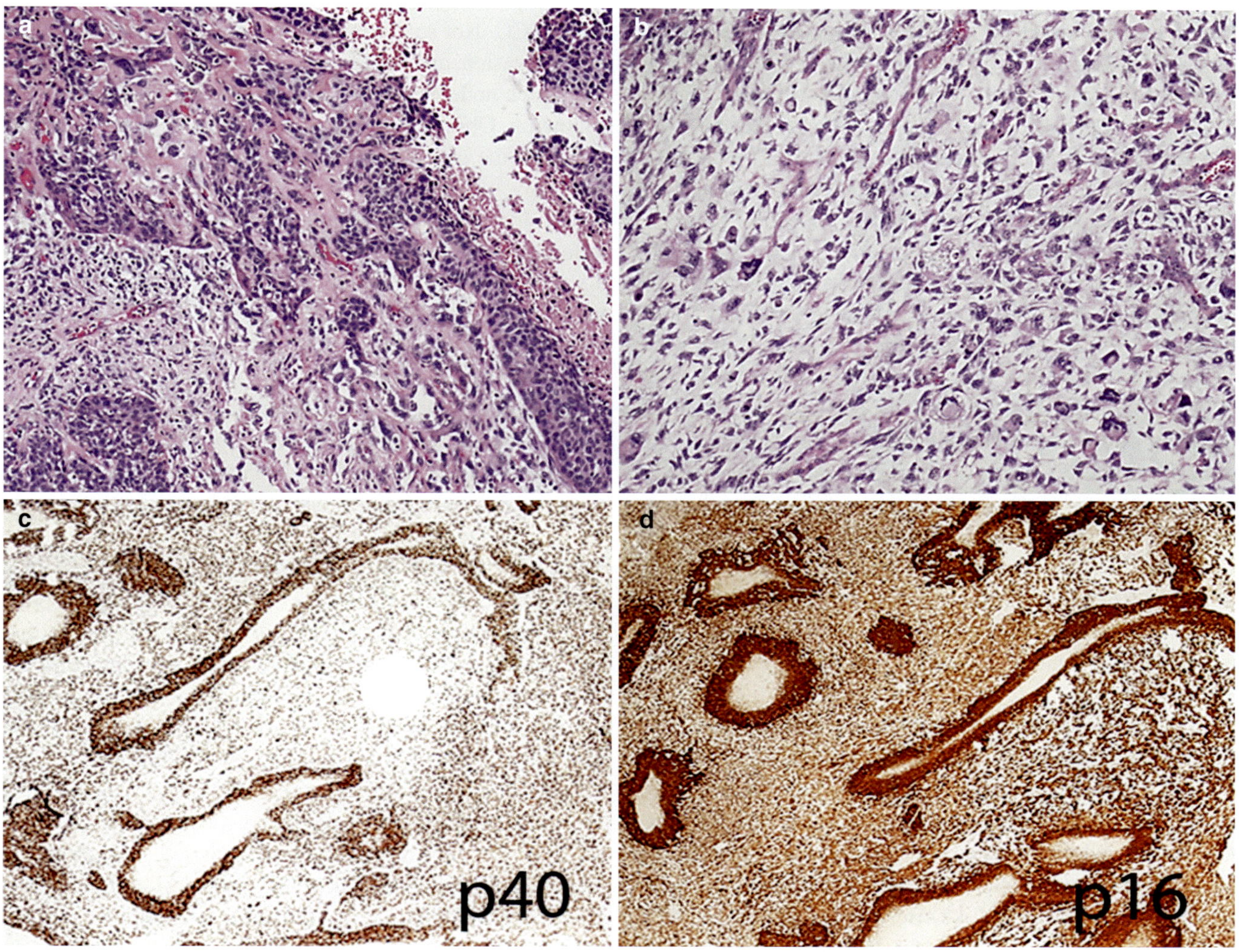

Fig. 12.31 (**a**, **b**) Spindle cell/sarcomatoid squamous cell carcinoma is composed of spindle-shaped neoplastic squamous cells with readily recognized mitoses and moderate to severe cytologic atypia. The sarcomatoid tumor cells are immunoreactive for (**c**) p40 and (**d**) p16

et al. [52] reported that the 5-year survival rate was 69% for patients under 40 and 45% for those 40 or older. After adjusting for confounding factors, young age remained a significant positive factor. Kokawa et al. [53] systemically analyzed the clinical stage, histologic type, treatment, and prognosis of a total of 4975 cases in a Japanese cohort, including 441 patients less than 35 years old. They found that the prognosis of cervical ISCC tends to be better in young women than in older patients, illustrated by 5-year survival rates that were nearly two times higher for patients under 35 when compared with that of patients older than 35.

12.3.2.2 Histopathologic Type and Grade

While verrucous carcinoma, as an exception, may be associated with a very favorable prognosis, other histological subtypes or grades of ISCC of the cervix do not appear to be strong independent predictive variables. In fact, recent studies have shown that there is no significant difference in the survival rate between different histopathologic types of ISCC of the cervix, barring a few types that are not associated with HPV infection and have a worse prognosis. Due to the lack of standardized criteria, and heterogeneity of the tumors, the data on the correlation between histopathologic type and prognosis in the current literature varies significantly. To standardize the diagnostic criteria, Stendahl [54] has proposed a detailed grading system for ISCC of the uterine cervix. This system was based upon evaluation of tumor differentiation, structure/architecture, nuclear polymorphism, frequency of mitotic figures, mode of invasion, stage of invasion, vascular invasion, and the degree of lymphoplasmacytic infiltration. These features were graded on a 1 to 3 point scale (with 1 being papillary architecture and solid growth, large cells, few enlarged nuclei, single mitosis, well defined borders, superficial invasion, no LVSI, and a marked lymphoplasmacytic response while a score of 3 indicated marked cellular dissociation, small cells, numerous irregular or anaplastic nuclei, numerous mitoses, diffuse growth, massive invasion, presence of LVSI, and no lymphoplasmacytic response). Scoring totals 8 to 24 points, with cases scoring 24 being associated with a worse outcome. This scoring method appears to correlate with clinical outcome; however, it is not practical due to its complexity.

12.3.2.3 Tumor Volume and Depth of Invasion

As discussed previously, many studies have shown that tumor size is a relatively important prognostic factor. A recent study by Lee et al. [55] demonstrated that mid-radiation tumor volume was an independent and strong prognostic parameter for patients with cervical ISCC and was associated with longer progression-free survival. Likewise, a large series (1178 cases) by Perez et al. [56] found that the 10-year treatment failure rate in Stage IB patients was 6% for tumors less than 3 cm, 15% for tumors 3–5 cm, and 30% for tumors more than 5 cm. In terms of tumor volume, tissue sections are routinely cut at 4–5 μm, resulting in a two-dimensional (2D) histologic assessment. Currently, three-dimensional microscopic tissue reconstruction is mostly carried out by serial sectioning, and thus is laborious and sensitive to tissue deformation. As it currently stands, the process is complicated and not practical. Recent progress with a rapid tissue clearing technique in combination with confocal laser scanning microscopy (CLSM) allows measurement of tumor volume in its actual 3-dimensional context [37].

The depth of invasion, the most readily available parameter in surgical specimens, is usually positively correlated with tumor volume, and thus indirectly reflects the volume of tumor. It has been documented that the most important prognostic factors in women with stage IB and IIA ISCC are tumor size, depth of invasion, parametrial involvement, and lymph node metastasis. If the lymph nodes are negative, the depth of invasion is the most important independent prognostic factor.

12.3.2.4 Lymphovascular Space Invasion (LVSI)

The lymphatic system is the main metastatic pathway of cervical ISCC. Not surprisingly, LVSI is a sign of surrounding tissue invasion, and thus confers a poor prognosis even without lymph node metastasis. In a recent study with long-term follow-up, Obrzut et al. [57] demonstrated that the presence of LVSI, the only prognostic factor by univariate analysis, adversely affected the 10-year overall survival. In a Gynecologic Oncology Group (GOG) study, Zaino et al. [58] found that LVSI was marginally associated with a decreased 5-year progression-free interval (70% in tumors with LVSI vs. 83% without LVSI). While LVSI appears to be somewhat less important than tumor size and depth of invasion, this parameter has been proven to have correlation with the depth of invasion and lymph node metastasis (see next section). It has been documented that presence of LVSI is associated with a three- to fourfold increase in risk of pelvic lymph node metastases in patients with early disease [59].

12.3.2.5 Lymph Node Metastasis

Lymph node metastasis is a very powerful indicator of poor prognosis. In a population-based Surveillance, Epidemiology, and End Results Program (SEER) study, Macdonald et al. [60] analyzed 4559 patients and found that the 5-year rates of cause specific survival and overall survival were 94% and 91%, 76% and 69%, 62% and 58%, and 41% and 35%, for patients with 0, 1 to 2, 3 to 9 and ≥10 positive lymph nodes. The study demonstrated that lymph node metastasis in carcinoma of the cervix predicts a prognosis that is inversely related to the number of involved nodes. Moreover, tumor grade, size, and FIGO stage were associated with increasing risk for lymph node metastases. Likewise, in an early GOG study of 732 stage IB patients, Delgado et al. [61] found that the 3-year disease-free interval was 85.6% for patients with negative pelvic nodes, and 74.4% for patients with positive pelvic nodes. Unlike the Macdonald's study, the latter failed to conclude a relationship between the number of involved nodes and the prognosis. In order to assess micrometastases in lymph nodes, especially sentinel nodes, some studies have applied molecular and/or immunohistochemical methods to detect HPV virus or keratin proteins [62, 63]; however, the prognostic and therapeutic value of micrometastases and isolated tumor cells is debatable.

12.3.2.6 Margin Status

The relationship between margin status and prognosis in hysterectomy specimen is still controversial. Some studies suggest that a positive margin is related to local recurrence [64–66]. Carballo et al. [67] reported that tumor coming to within <3 mm of a negative surgical margin is a significant adverse prognostic factor for patients with Stage IB and IIA disease. Of note, a negative margin in a conization specimen does not guarantee the absence of residual tumor in the subsequent hysterectomy specimen.

12.3.3 Treatment

In general, radical hysterectomy is still the first choice for treatment of cervical cancer. The 5-year disease-free survival rate in young patients with a small (<2 cm) stage IA or IB1 tumors was nearly 100% when radical hysterectomy and pelvic lymphadenectomy are performed. Radical trachelectomy combined with laparoscopic pelvic lymphadenectomy is also acceptable for the treatment of such patients. For patients with tumors larger than 4 cm and/or LVSI, radical hysterectomy plus postoperative adjuvant radiotherapy and/or chemotherapy can reduce the risk of recurrence. In fact, a reported clinical trial incorporating radiotherapy and concurrent platinum-based chemotherapy for stage II and stage III cancers has shown significant improvements in survival compared to radiation alone [68]. Moreover, for patients with early-stage cervical cancer and risk factors for recurrence, the addition of platinum-based chemotherapy to radiotherapy may offer clinical benefit. In contrast, a recent study has shown that a combination of external radiotherapy, intracavitary radiation and platinum-based chemotherapy versus surgery produce similar results for stage IB cancer [69]. Finally, it is widely accepted that advanced tumors are usually treated with aggressive surgery and chemoradiation [70].

12.3.4 Biomarkers and Molecular Genetics of Cervical Squamous Cell Carcinoma

Over decades, pathologists and molecular biologists have been focusing on identification of biological markers that are able to potentially predict the progression of precancerous SIL to carcinoma. Currently there is no such a marker that is superior to morphology, but progress has been made to facilitate the diagnosis of potentially progressive lesions.

12.3.4.1 Ki-67

Ki-67 is a nuclear protein that is associated with cellular proliferation. Unlike metaphase-specific markers, this protein is present during all active phases of the cell cycle (G_1, S, G_2, and M), but is absent in resting (G_0) cells. As such, it has been postulated that the expression levels in women with CIN2 might predict their prognosis. A study by Miyamoto et al. [71] showed that positive Ki-67 staining in more than 50% of cells was significantly more common among women with progression than among those with regression. Similarly, Portari et al. [72] found that p16, Ki-67, p21, and p53 positivity increased in vertical distribution within the epithelium with increasing SIL severity, with the strongest correlations being observed for p16 and Ki-67. To quantitatively assess Ki-67 in the prediction of disease progression, Kruse et al. [73] proposed the concept of MIDTHIRD (Ki-67-positive cells located in the middle third layer of the epithelium) and SI90 (the 90th percentile of the stratification index). The combination of these parameters was best for predicting progression. In daily practice, due to the computational complexity and obvious interobserver variability, application of this index is not practical.

12.3.4.2 p16

p16 is a cell cycle-dependent kinase inhibitor that plays an important role in cell cycle regulation by decelerating cell cycle progression from the G1 checkpoint to the S phase. Physiologically, p16 binds to CDK4/6, inhibiting its kinase activity and preventing pRb phosphorylation. High-risk HPV E7 oncoproteins target pRb, disrupting growth-suppressive pRB-E2F complexes by releasing E2F and inducing p16 overexpression through a pRb/p16 feedback-loop mechanism. Accordingly, p16 is a surrogate marker for hrHPV infection.

Per the LAST consensus guidelines [10], p16 immunohistochemistry is recommended to adjudicate those SILs for which a diagnosis of HSIL/CIN2 is being considered—that is, those that are considered morphologically borderline between LSIL/CIN1 and precancer (HSIL/CIN2–3). As discussed earlier, p16 should be used with caution in this situation as a significant proportion (20–70%) of adjudicated LSIL/CIN1 demonstrates diffuse p16 expression. Therefore, a subset of hrHPV-related SILs are allowed to be p16-positive yet maintain classification as LSIL/CIN1. Of note, positive p16 expression should be contiguous ("block positive") in at least the lower one-third to one-half of the lesion epithelium, and does need not be full thickness (Fig. 12.32a, b). Negative or patchy p16 expression in this setting supports interpretation as LSIL/CIN1, but may be seen in reactive lesions and metaplasia as well (Fig. 12.32c, d).

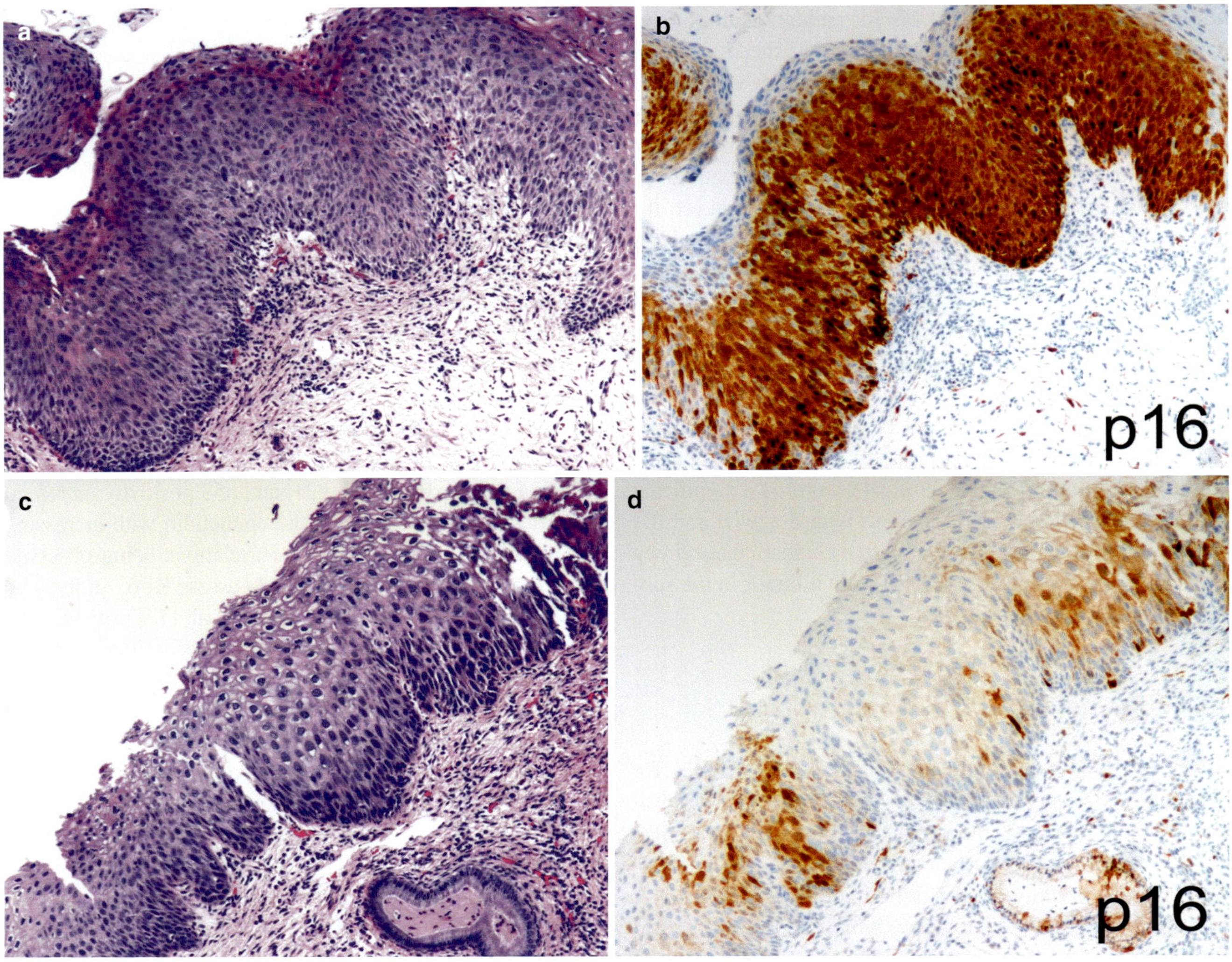

Fig. 12.32 (**a**, **b**) p16 expression secondary to High-risk HPV should be contiguous ("block positive" pattern) in at least the lower one-third to one-half of the lesional epithelium. (**c**, **d**) Negative or patchy p16 expression in this example supports a diagnosis of a low-grade lesion or normal/reactive changes

It has been recommended to perform both p16 and Ki-67 to address the differential diagnosis of HSIL versus immature metaplasia. This approach allows for resolution of most cases of "atypical immature metaplasia" into positive (HSIL) and negative (immature metaplasia). Most cases stain in a concordant fashion with these markers (i.e., p16 diffuse/strong positive and Ki-67 notably increased to more than 30% of labeling index in HSIL; p16 negative/focal weak and Ki-67 low/confined to basal/parabasal layers or less than 30% labeling index in immature metaplasia), such that one or the other stain can suffice for establishing a diagnosis; however, occasional cases can demonstrate discordant results. For these cases, use of only one marker could lead to underdiagnosis of the lesion; therefore, having both results provides more data to guide interpretation of the combined morphologic and immunohistochemical findings. Interestingly, p16 immunostaining can display a completely negative pattern in rare hrHPV-related lesions, likely due to gene promoter methylation or gene deletion.

While some data may suggest that p16-positive LSIL/CIN1 might be a higher risk category than p16-negative LSIL/CIN1, studies of cases with adjudicated LSIL/CIN1 have determined that p16 immunohistochemistry does not stratify risk of future/concurrent HSIL/CIN2–3 among patients with LSIL/CIN1 [15, 74]. Therefore, in the case of an unequivocal case of LSIL/CIN1 based on morphology, p16 should not be ordered.

12.3.4.3 ProEx C

ProEx C is an antibody cocktail labeling topoisomerase IIα (Top2α) and minichromosome maintenance protein-2 (MCM2). Both proteins are overexpressed in the nucleus during aberrant S-phase induction of neoplastic cells, which leads to cell proliferation. Top2α opens the double strands of DNA during replication; MCM2 is a component of the pre-replication complex that facilitates the early G1 phase of cell division.

HPV viral oncoproteins E6 and E7 bind and disrupt cell cycle regulatory proteins p53 and pRB, leading to secondary imbalances in the levels of numerous cell cycle proteins including overexpression of Top2α and MCM2. ProEx C is an immunohistochemical marker that contains monoclonal antibodies against these two proteins and functions as a surrogate marker of HPV infection [75]; however, some studies have shown that p16 is superior to ProExC in identifying HSIL. Therefore, it is rarely used in pathology daily practice, although ProExc is still being used in recognition of HPV-related anal lesions [76].

12.3.4.4 hTERC

It has been reported that HSIL and ISCC of the cervix are frequently associated with the amplification of chromosome 3q, which harbors the hTERC (human telomerase RNA component, 3q26.3) gene. In one study, He et al. [77] found that the frequency of genomic amplification of hTERC increased with the severity of the disease, illustrated by significant differences between LSIL, HSIL, and squamous cell carcinoma. As such, some pathologists have proposed that assessment of hTERC amplification within cervical lesions by fluorescence in situ hybridization (FISH) analysis may be clinically applied to differentiate between LSILs and HSILs. From a prognostic point, Alameda et al. [78] demonstrated statistically significant differences of *hTERC* copies between cases with persistence or progression of LSIL/CIN1, and cases with regression. Accordingly, it has been proposed that determination of 3q26 gains (hTERC copy number) in LSIL could be useful to predict the persistence and/or progression of these lesions [78, 79].

12.3.4.5 Cytokeratin (CK)

Cytokeratins are cytoskeleton proteins (molecular weight 44-66KDa) in the cytoplasm of epithelial cells, that allow for resistance of mechanical stress. Endocervical glandular epithelium usually expresses CK 7, 8, 18, 19 and variable amount of CK 4. Interestingly, squamous epithelium expresses keratins in relation to the level of its maturation. In the immature form, CK 5, 8, 17, and 18 are expressed, while CK 4, 13, and 14 appear in more mature forms [80]. It has been well demonstrated that the squamocolumnar junction (SCJ) is the most common location where HPV infection causes cancers and precancerous lesions [17]. The cervical SCJ cells are the putative residual embryonic stem cells near the cervical transformation zone [17]. Interestingly, LSILs not expressing SCJ biomarkers, such as CK7, are unlikely to be followed by the development of HSIL [15, 81]. A follow-up study to evaluate CK7 expression on adjudicated CIN1 tissue from women in the placebo arm of the HPV vaccine trials found that full-thickness CK7 staining showed the highest correlation with progression to HSIL, confirming the data by Huang et al. [15] that CK7 staining may risk stratify LSIL/CIN1 [82]. However, it is important to remember that CK7 is most useful when it is completely negative as this pattern correlates strongly with a lower risk of progression to HSIL [15]. Recently, Lee et al. [83] reported positive CK7 expression in 100% of CIN3 cases and in 20/30 (66%) SCCs; within their study, patchy staining of CK7 and episomal HPV DNA overlapped in the upper layers of CIN3 lesions and in the central portion of invasive nests in SCC, suggesting that CK7 may be more related with viral episomal replication. Furthermore since CK19 expression may correlate with p16 staining and HPV DNA integration, they proposed that coordinated CK7/CK19 staining may be used as a marker for identifying the physical presence of hrHPV and E7 oncoprotein in cervical ISCC (Figs. 12.33 and 12.34).

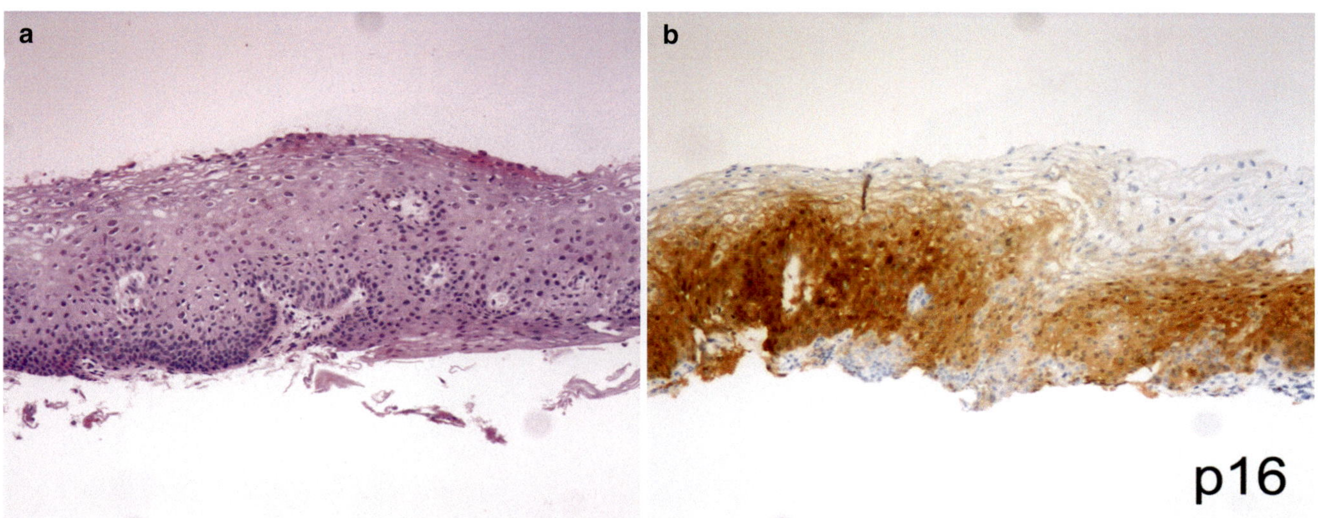

Fig. 12.33 LSIL/CIN 1. (**a**) Squamous epithelium with koilocytic atypia. (**b**) Patchy p16 staining, confined to the middle and lower layer of the epithelium. (**c**) Weak and focal CK7 expression in the superficial layer of the squamous epithelium. (**d**) Patchy CK19 expression in the basal layer of the epithelium

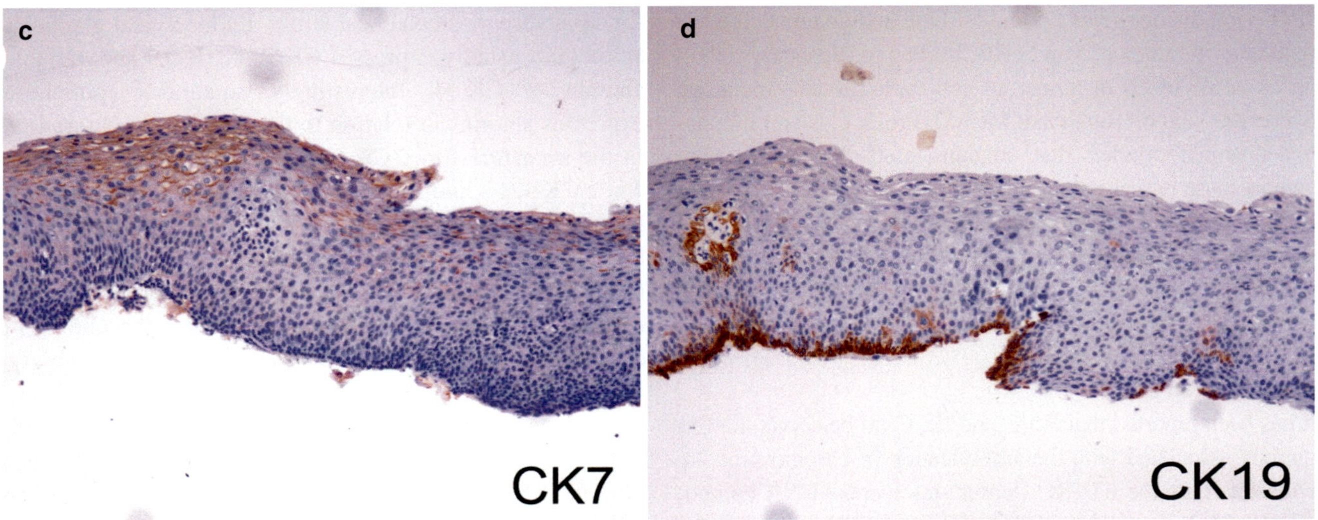

Fig. 12.33 (continued)

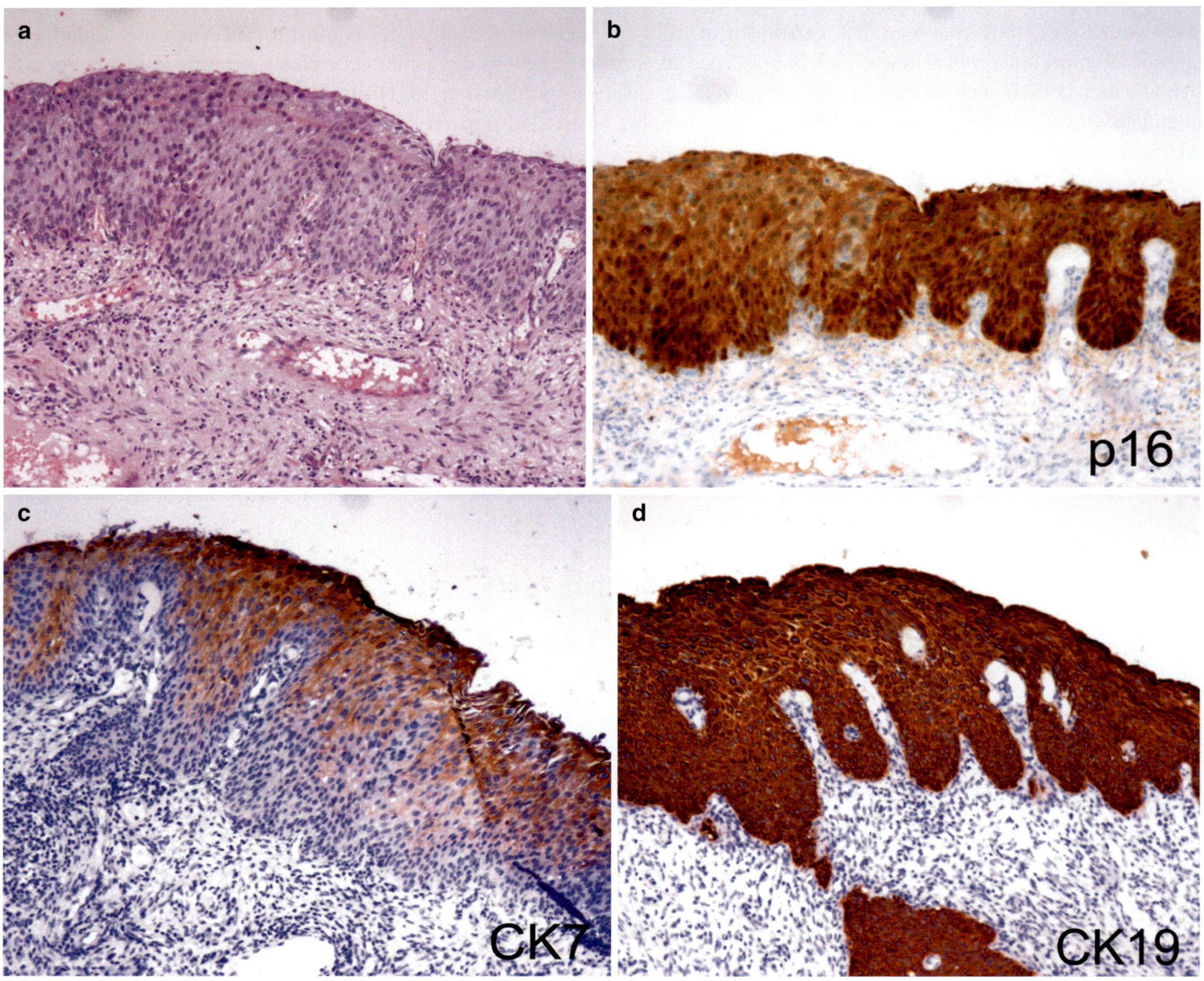

Fig. 12.34 HSIL/CIN 2-3. (**a**) This HSIL demonstrates nuclear crowding and overlap with loss of maturation extending into the upper half of the epithelium. (**b**) Strong and diffuse p16 immunoreactivity. (**c**) CK7 expression in the middle and upper layers of the epithelium. (**d**) Strong and diffuse CK19 expression similar to that of p16

12.3.4.6 IMP3

IMP3 (insulin-like growth factor II mRNA binding protein 3), an oncofetal protein, has been shown to correlate with aggressive behavior in certain cancers, thus serving as a biomarker. In a large case series (1249 patients with no cervical lesion; 710 patients with CIN2–3), Lu et al. [84] found invasive cancer was present only in patients with IMP3-positive CIN2–3, whereas no invasive cancer was detected in follow-up resections in patients with IMP3-negative CIN2–3. As such, IMP3 can be used at the time of initial diagnosis to triage a group of patients with an increased chance of developing invasive cancer. Further studies are needed to confirm the findings.

12.3.4.7 HPV

Almost all SILs and ISCCs of the uterine cervix are HPV related; therefore, the detection of HPV plays a critical role in the screening and early diagnosis of these lesions. Currently, there are nearly 200 molecular tests that are commercially available on the global market for the detection of HPV. While the principles for detection of HPV viral infection vary among methods, all are based on molecular mechanisms that can be placed in the following categories [85]:

1. Non-amplified hybridization assays (direct probe), such as Southern blot, dot blot hybridization (DB), and in situ hybridization (ISH of both DNA and RNA). Southern blot requires large amounts of DNA, is laborious and not reproducible; DNA ISH has only moderate sensitivity and low specificity for HPV, although recent development of RNAscope has shown better results.
2. Signal amplified hybridization assays, such as hybrid capture assays (digene HC2) and the Cervista HPV test. The former is based on signal amplification using RNA probes to target the entire hrHPV genome of 18 types of HPV (13 high risk and 5 low risk).
3. Target amplification assays, such as polymerase chain reaction (PCR) and in situ PCR. In comparison to other methods, PCR-based detection is both highly sensitive and specific. Another advantage of this method is that very small amounts of DNA are sufficient. As this is a very sensitive test, care for cross-contamination needs to be kept in mind. Cobas 4800 is a target amplification HPV test that uses multiplex real-time PCR and nucleic acid hybridization with four different fluorescent reporter probes that concurrently detect the L1 gene of HPV16 and HPV18 individually, as well as 12 other HPVs as a pooled result.

It is well accepted that overexpression of HPV E6 and E7 oncoproteins is a marker for increased risk of cervical cancer, as such, detection of E6 and E7 oncogene expression could serve as a predictor of cervical cancer risk [86, 87]. The Aptima HPV assay is a target amplification nucleic acid probe test for the in vitro qualitative detection of E6/E7 viral messenger RNA (mRNA) from 14 hrHPVs [88]. The PreTect HPV-Proofer test is another E6/E7 mRNA-based assay that detects E6/E7 mRNA from five high-risk HPVs. Recently, next generation ISH-based RNAscope has been developed based on Advanced Cell Diagnostics (ACD) unique, patented probe design that enables simultaneous signal amplification and background noise suppression. In a study using RNAscope technology, 126 cervical biopsies originally diagnosed as LSIL/CIN1 were compared to HPV RNA ISH results to assess whether this assay can attain the existing "gold standard" of morphologic consensus diagnosis [89]. It was found that integrating RNA ISH into morphologic review led to reclassification of 10% of cases, resulting in improvement of the accuracy of LSIL/CIN1 diagnosis in morphologically ambiguous cases.

12.3.5 Molecular Genetics of Invasive Squamous Cell Carcinoma

12.3.5.1 HPV-induced genetic alterations

Nobel laureate winner Dr. Harald Zur Hausen and his group identified HPV16 in cervical cancer in 1983 [90] and HPV18 in 1984 [91]. These two culprits are responsible for approximately 75% of human cervical cancers. To this date, approximately 200 different HPVs have been identified, and new types are regularly being added to this list. More than 40 HPV types can easily be spread through direct sexual contact as HPVs are epitheliotropic viruses in which the infection is transmitted to the basal cells of skin and mucous membranes through minor abrasions or epithelial trauma. HPV-mediated transformation represents a consequence of viral replication, integration of viral genomes into the host cell, and oncoprotein-induced genomic instability.

The hrHPV E1 and E2 proteins play important roles in viral genome replication. Early viral transcription is repressed by high levels of E2 protein. E2 also interacts with the viral DNA helicase E1 to form a complex that is necessary for efficient origin recognition and viral genome replication. The E4 protein probably plays a role in virion release by disrupting the intermediate filaments of the host cells. L1 and L2 are capsid proteins involved in virion packaging. The two primary oncogenic proteins of hrHPV are E6 and E7. It has been demonstrated that overexpression of these proteins promotes cellular proliferation and confers malignant transformation of the host cells by inactivation of p53 (inactivated by E6) and pRb (inactivated by E7). Briefly, E6 and E6-associated protein ubiquitinate p53 via their ubiquitin ligase activity, leading to proteasomal degradation. E7 protein competes for pRb binding, thus releasing transcription factor E2F to activate its targets, pushing the cell cycle transition from G1 to S phase. p16 is a tumor suppressor protein that inhibits cyclin-dependent kinases-4 and -6 (CDK-4 and CDK-6), thus regulating the G1 checkpoint. The CDKs phosphorylate pRb, leading to a conformational change and release of E2F from the pRb. Thus, inactivation of pRb function through HPV E7 protein may cause p16 expression through feedback regulatory mechanisms.

12.3.5.2 Molecular genetics in the host cells

While hrHPV infection is the most important carcinogenic factor in cervical cancer, not all individuals infected with HPVs will develop cancer. Oncogenesis is closely related to the individual's immune status, hormone levels, environmental factors such as smoking, and molecular genetic characteristics.

Genetic studies have demonstrated that somatic mutations in PIK3CA, ERBB2, PTEN, TP53, STK11, MAPK1, and KRAS, as well as several gain-of and loss-of-function and copy-number alterations, play a role in the development of cervical cancer. A recent study employed whole-exome sequencing, transcriptome sequencing, and whole-genome sequencing to investigate the genetic alterations at the genome level [92]. This study revealed novel somatic mutations including recurrent E322K substitutions in the MAPK1 gene, inactivating mutations in the HLA-B gene, and mutations in EP300, FBXW7, NFE2L2, TP53, and ERBB2. In another study, the authors identified *SHKBP1, ERBB3, CASP8, HLA-A*, and *TGFBR2* as novel mutated genes in cervical cancer [93]. Importantly, they also discovered amplifications in immune targets PD-L1 and PD-L2, implicating significant therapeutic value with checkpoint inhibitors. The presence of genetic and epigenetic alterations that are amenable to targeted therapy in cervical cancers offers the potential for individualized management strategies for treatment of this aggressive tumor.

References

1. Williams J. Harveian lectures on cancer of the uterus. Br Med J. 1887;1(1359):100–1.
2. Broders AC. Carcinoma in situ contrasted with benign penetrating epithelium. J Am Med Assoc. 1932;99:1670–4.
3. Reagan JW, Seidemann IL, Saracusa Y. The cellular morphology of carcinoma in situ and dysplasia or atypical hyperplasia of the uterine cervix. Cancer. 1953;6(2):224–34.
4. Richart RM, Barron BA. A follow-up study of patients with cervical dysplasia. Am J Obstet Gynecol. 1969;105(3):386–93.
5. Richart RM. Influence of diagnostic and therapeutic procedures on the distribution of cervical intraepithelial neoplasia. Cancer. 1966;19(11):1635–8.
6. Crum CP, et al. Human papillomavirus type 16 and early cervical neoplasia. N Engl J Med. 1984;310(14):880–3.
7. Ismail SM, et al. Reporting cervical intra-epithelial neoplasia (CIN): intra- and interpathologist variation and factors associated with disagreement. Histopathology. 1990;16(4):371–6.
8. Robertson AJ, et al. Observer variability in histopathological reporting of cervical biopsy specimens. J Clin Pathol. 1989;42(3):231–8.
9. The 1988 Bethesda system for reporting cervical/vaginal cytological diagnoses. National Cancer Institute workshop. JAMA. 1989;262(7):931–4.
10. Darragh TM, et al. The lower Anogenital squamous terminology standardization project for HPV-associated lesions: background and consensus recommendations from the College of American Pathologists and the American Society for Colposcopy and Cervical Pathology. J Low Genit Tract Dis. 2012;16(3):205–42.
11. Massad LS, et al. 2012 updated consensus guidelines for the management of abnormal cervical cancer screening tests and cancer precursors. J Low Genit Tract Dis. 2013;17(5 Suppl 1):S1–S27.
12. Stoler MH, Schiffman M, Atypical Squamous G. Cells of undetermined significance-low-grade squamous intraepithelial lesion triage study, *Interobserver reproducibility of cervical cytologic and histologic interpretations: realistic estimates from the ASCUS-LSIL Triage Study*. JAMA. 2001;285(11):1500–5.
13. Galgano MT, et al. Can HPV-16 genotyping provide a benchmark for cervical biopsy specimen interpretation? Am J Clin Pathol. 2008;130(1):65–70.
14. Ma L, et al. Eosinophilic dysplasia of the cervix: a newly recognized variant of cervical squamous intraepithelial neoplasia. Am J Surg Pathol. 2004;28(11):1474–84.
15. Huang EC, et al. p16ink4 and cytokeratin 7 immunostaining in predicting HSIL outcome for low-grade squamous intraepithelial lesions: a case series, literature review and commentary. Mod Pathol. 2016;29(12):1501–10.
16. Sano T, et al. Expression status of p16 protein is associated with human papillomavirus oncogenic potential in cervical and genital lesions. Am J Pathol. 1998;153(6):1741–8.
17. Herfs M, et al. A discrete population of squamocolumnar junction cells implicated in the pathogenesis of cervical cancer. Proc Natl Acad Sci U S A. 2012;109(26):10516–21.
18. Yang EJ, et al. Microanatomy of the cervical and anorectal squamocolumnar junctions: a proposed model for anatomical differences in HPV-related cancer risk. Mod Pathol. 2015;28(7):994–1000.
19. Herfs M, et al. Cervical squamocolumnar junction-specific markers define distinct, clinically relevant subsets of low-grade squamous intraepithelial lesions. Am J Surg Pathol. 2013;37(9):1311–8.
20. Moscicki AB, et al. Regression of low-grade squamous intraepithelial lesions in young women. Lancet. 2004;364(9446):1678.
21. Moscicki AB, et al. Rate of and risks for regression of cervical intraepithelial neoplasia 2 in adolescents and young women. Obstet Gynecol. 2010;116(6):1373–80.
22. Creasman WT. New gynecologic cancer staging. Gynecol Oncol. 1995;58(2):157–8.
23. Berchuck A. Society of gynecologic oncologists. J Cancer Res Clin Oncol. 1994;120(9):562–3.
24. Kurman RJ, et al. WHO classification of tumors of female reproductive organs. Lyon: IARC; 2014.
25. Burghardt E, Holzer E. Diagnosis and treatment of microinvasive carcinoma of the cervix uteri. Obstet Gynecol. 1977;49(6):641–53.
26. Bai H, et al. Accuracy of conization procedure for predicting pathological parameters of radical hysterectomy in stage Ia2-Ib1 (</=2 cm) cervical cancer. Sci Rep. 2016;6:25992.
27. Benedet JL, Anderson GH. Stage IA carcinoma of the cervix revisited. Obstet Gynecol. 1996;87(6):1052–9.
28. Raspagliesi F, et al. Prognostic factors in microinvasive cervical squamous cell cancer: long-term results. Int J Gynecol Cancer. 2005;15(1):88–93.
29. Ostör AG. Studies on 200 cases of early squamous cell carcinoma of the cervix. Int J Gynecol Pathol. 1993;12(3):193.
30. Lim CS, et al. Clinical value of immunohistochemically detected lymphovascular space invasion in early stage cervical carcinoma. Ann Surg Oncol. 2008;15(9):2581–8.

31. Chernofsky MR, et al. Influence of quantity of lymph vascular space invasion on time to recurrence in women with early-stage squamous cancer of the cervix. Gynecol Oncol. 2006;100(2):288–93.
32. Urabe A, et al. Grading system of lymphatic invasion according to D2-40 immunostaining is useful for the prediction of nodal metastasis in squamous cell carcinoma of the uterine cervix. Histopathology. 2006;49(5):493–7.
33. Al-Nafussi AI, Monaghan H. Squamous carcinoma of the uterine cervix with CIN 3-like growth pattern: an under-diagnosed lesion. Int J Gynecol Cancer. 2000;10(2):95–9.
34. Stewart CJ, Crook ML. Cervical intraepithelial neoplasia (CIN) 3-like squamous cell carcinoma of the cervix: a review of 14 cases with comparison of E-cadherin and cyclin D1 expression in the CIN 3-like and infiltrative tumour elements. Histopathology. 2017;70(3):367–74.
35. Raspagliesi F, et al. Microinvasive squamous cell cervical carcinoma. Crit Rev Oncol Hematol. 2003;48(3):251–61.
36. Östör AG, Rome RM. Micro-invasive squamous cell carcinoma of the cervix: a clinico-pathologic study of 200 cases with long-term follow-up. Int J Gynecol Cancer. 1994;4(4):257.
37. Noe M, et al. Immunolabeling of cleared human pancreata provides insights into three-dimensional pancreatic anatomy and pathology. Am J Pathol. 2018;188(7):1530–5.
38. Roman LD, et al. Risk of residual invasive disease in women with microinvasive squamous cancer in a conization specimen. Obstet Gynecol. 1997;90(5):759–64.
39. Koay MH, Crook M, Stewart CJ. Cyclin D1, E-cadherin and beta-catenin expression in FIGO stage IA cervical squamous carcinoma: diagnostic value and evidence for epithelial-mesenchymal transition. Histopathology. 2012;61(6):1125–33.
40. Koay MH, Crook M, Stewart CJ. Fascin expression in cervical normal squamous epithelium, cervical intraepithelial neoplasia, and superficially invasive (stage IA1) squamous carcinoma of the cervix. Pathology. 2014;46(5):433–8.
41. Mota F. Microinvasive squamous carcinoma of the cervix: treatment modalities. Acta Obstet Gynecol Scand. 2003;82(6):505.
42. Diaz JP, et al. Oncologic outcome of fertility-sparing radical trachelectomy versus radical hysterectomy for stage IB1 cervical carcinoma. Gynecol Oncol. 2008;111(2):255–60.
43. Siegel RL, Miller KD, Jemal A. Cancer statistics, 2018. CA Cancer J Clin. 2018;68(1):7–30.
44. Benard VB, et al. Cervical carcinoma rates among young females in the United States. Obstet Gynecol. 2012;120(5):1117–23.
45. Grayson W, Taylor LF, Cooper K. Adenoid cystic and adenoid basal carcinoma of the uterine cervix: comparative morphologic, mucin, and immunohistochemical profile of two rare neoplasms of putative 'reserve cell' origin. Am J Surg Pathol. 1999;23(4):448–58.
46. Kurman RJ, et al. WHO classification of tumours of female reproductive organs. Lyon: IARC; 2014.
47. Tseng CJ, et al. Lymphoepithelioma-like carcinoma of the uterine cervix: association with Epstein-Barr virus and human papillomavirus. Cancer. 1997;80(1):91–7.
48. Weinberg E, et al. Uterine cervical lymphoepithelial-like carcinoma. Absence of Epstein-Barr virus genomes. Am J Clin Pathol. 1993;99(2):195–9.
49. Martinez-Leandro EP, et al. Lymphoepithelial-like carcinoma of the uterine cervix. Study of a case with in situ hybridization of the Epstein-Barr virus genome and the human papillomavirus genome. Acta Obstet Gynecol Scand. 1994;73(7):589–92.
50. Friedl P, et al. Classifying collective cancer cell invasion. Nat Cell Biol. 2012;14(8):777–83.
51. Brown J, et al. Sarcomatoid carcinoma of the cervix. Gynecol Oncol. 2003;90(1):23–8.
52. Meanwell CA, et al. Young age as a prognostic factor in cervical cancer: analysis of population based data from 10,022 cases. Br Med J (Clin Res Ed). 1988;296(6619):386–91.
53. Kokawa K, et al. The incidence, treatment and prognosis of cervical carcinoma in young women: a retrospective analysis of 4,975 cases in Japan. Eur J Gynaecol Oncol. 2010;31(1):37.
54. Stendahl U, Willen H, Willen R. Classification and grading of invasive squamous cell carcinoma of the uterine cervix. Acta Radiol Oncol Radiat Phys Biol. 1979;18(6):481–96.
55. Lee JH, et al. Tumour size, volume, and marker expression during radiation therapy can predict survival of cervical cancer patients: a multi-institutional retrospective analysis of KROG 16-01. Gynecol Oncol. 2017;147(3):577–84.
56. Perez CA, et al. Effect of tumor size on the prognosis of carcinoma of the uterine cervix treated with irradiation alone. Cancer. 1992;69(11):2796–806.
57. Obrzut B, et al. Prognostic parameters for patients with cervical Cancer FIGO stages IA2-IIB: a long-term follow-up. Oncology. 2017;93(2):106–14.
58. Zaino RJ, et al. Histopathologic predictors of the behavior of surgically treated stage IB squamous cell carcinoma of the cervix. A Gynecologic Oncology Group Study. Cancer. 1992;69(7):1750–8.
59. Delgado G, et al. A prospective surgical pathological study of stage I squamous carcinoma of the cervix: a gynecologic oncology group study. Gynecol Oncol. 1989;35(3):314–20.
60. Macdonald OK, et al. Prognostic significance of histology and positive lymph node involvement following radical hysterectomy in carcinoma of the cervix. Am J Clin Oncol. 2009;32(4):411–6.
61. Delgado G, et al. Prospective surgical-pathological study of disease-free interval in patients with stage IB squamous cell carcinoma of the cervix: a gynecologic oncology group study. Gynecol Oncol. 1990;38(3):352–7.
62. Yamashita T, et al. Management of pelvic lymph nodes by sentinel node navigation surgery in the treatment of invasive cervical cancer. Int J Gynecol Cancer. 2009;19(6):1113–8.
63. Lindell G, et al. Presence of human papillomavirus (HPV) in vulvar squamous cell carcinoma (VSCC) and sentinel node. Gynecol Oncol. 2010;117(2):312–6.
64. Papakonstantinou K, et al. Management of stage Ia1 squamous cervical cancer and the importance of excision margins: a retrospective study of long-term outcome after 25 years of follow-up. Am J Obstet Gynecol. 2014;211(6):625.e1–6.
65. Kwon J, et al. The prognostic impact of the number of metastatic lymph nodes and a new prognostic scoring system for recurrence in early-stage cervical Cancer with high risk factors: a multicenter cohort study (KROG 15-04). Cancer Res Treat. 2018;50(3):964–74.
66. Hartman CA, et al. Analysis of conservative surgical treatment and prognosis of microinvasive squamous cell carcinoma of the cervix stage IA1: results of follow-up to 20 years. Int J Gynecol Cancer. 2017;27(2):357–63.
67. Carballo N, et al. Indications for adjuvant radiotherapy treatment after surgery and novel modalities for treatment. Gynecol Oncol. 2008;110(2):41–4.
68. Monk BJ, Tewari KS, Koh WJ. Multimodality therapy for locally advanced cervical carcinoma: state of the art and future directions. J Clin Oncol. 2007;25(20):2952–65.
69. Matsuo K, et al. Effectiveness of adjuvant systemic chemotherapy for intermediate-risk stage IB cervical cancer. Oncotarget. 2017;8(63):106866–75.
70. Rose PG, et al. Long-term follow-up of a randomized trial comparing concurrent single agent cisplatin, cisplatin-based combination chemotherapy, or hydroxyurea during pelvic irradiation for locally advanced cervical cancer: a gynecologic oncology group study. J Clin Oncol. 2007;25(19):2804–10.
71. Miyamoto S, et al. The association between p16 and Ki-67 immunohistostaining and the progression of cervical intraepithelial neoplasia grade 2. Int J Gynaecol Obstet. 2016;134(1):45–8.

72. Portari EA, et al. Immunohistochemical expression of cyclin D1, p16Ink4a, p21WAF1, and Ki-67 correlates with the severity of cervical neoplasia. Int J Gynecol Pathol. 2013;32(5):501–8.
73. Kruse AJ, et al. Ki67 predicts progression in early CIN: validation of a multivariate progression-risk model. Cell Oncol. 2004;26(1–2):13–20.
74. Sagasta A, et al. p16 staining has limited value in predicting the outcome of histological low-grade squamous intraepithelial lesions of the cervix. Mod Pathol. 2015;29(1):51.
75. Guo M, et al. Efficacy of p16 and ProExC immunostaining in the detection of high-grade cervical intraepithelial neoplasia and cervical carcinoma. Am J Clin Pathol. 2011;135(2):212–20.
76. Bala R, et al. p16 is superior to ProEx C in identifying high-grade squamous intraepithelial lesions (HSIL) of the anal canal. Am J Surg Pathol. 2013;37(5):659–68.
77. He C, et al. Genomic amplification of hTERC in paraffin-embedded tissues of cervical intraepithelial neoplasia and invasive cancer. Int J Gynecol Pathol. 2012;31(3):280–5.
78. Alameda F, et al. 3q26 (hTERC) gain studied by fluorescence in situ hybridization as a persistence-progression indicator in low-grade squamous intraepithelial lesion cases. Hum Pathol. 2009;40(10):1474–8.
79. Caraway NP, et al. Gain of the 3q26 region in cervicovaginal liquid-based pap preparations is associated with squamous intraepithelial lesions and squamous cell carcinoma. Gynecol Oncol. 2008;110(1):37–42.
80. Smedts F, et al. Keratin expression in cervical cancer. Am J Pathol. 1992;141(2):497–511.
81. Paquette C, Mills AM, Stoler MH. Predictive value of cytokeratin 7 immunohistochemistry in cervical low-grade squamous intraepithelial lesion as a marker for risk of progression to a high-grade lesion. Am J Surg Pathol. 2016;40(2):236–43.
82. Mills AM, et al. CK7 immunohistochemistry as a predictor of CIN1 progression: a retrospective study of patients from the Quadrivalent HPV vaccine trials. Am J Surg Pathol. 2017;41(2):143–52.
83. Lee H, Lee H, Cho YK. Cytokeratin7 and cytokeratin19 expression in high grade cervical intraepithelial neoplasm and squamous cell carcinoma and their possible association in cervical carcinogenesis. Diagn Pathol. 2017;12(1):40.
84. Lu D, et al. IMP3, a new biomarker to predict progression of cervical intraepithelial neoplasia into invasive cancer. Am J Surg Pathol. 2012;35(11):1638–45.
85. Zaravinos A, et al. Molecular detection methods of human papillomavirus (HPV). Int J Biol Markers. 2009;24(4):215–22.
86. Broccolo F, et al. Comparison of oncogenic HPV type-specific viral DNA load and E6/E7 mRNA detection in cervical samples: results from a multicenter study. J Med Virol. 2013;85(3):472–82.
87. Duvlis S, et al. HPV E6/E7 mRNA versus HPV DNA biomarker in cervical cancer screening of a group of Macedonian women. J Med Virol. 2015;87(9):1578–86.
88. Ratnam S, et al. Aptima HPV E6/E7 mRNA test is as sensitive as hybrid capture 2 assay but more specific at detecting cervical precancer and cancer. J Clin Microbiol. 2011;49(2):557–64.
89. Mills AM, et al. HPV E6/E7 mRNA in situ hybridization in the diagnosis of cervical low-grade squamous intraepithelial lesions (LSIL). Am J Surg Pathol. 2018;42:192.
90. Durst M, et al. A papillomavirus DNA from a cervical carcinoma and its prevalence in cancer biopsy samples from different geographic regions. Proc Natl Acad Sci U S A. 1983;80(12):3812–5.
91. Boshart M, et al. A new type of papillomavirus DNA, its presence in genital cancer biopsies and in cell lines derived from cervical cancer. EMBO J. 1984;3(5):1151–7.
92. Ojesina AI, et al. Landscape of genomic alterations in cervical carcinomas. Nature. 2014;506(7488):371–5.
93. Cancer Genome Atlas Research N, et al. Integrated genomic and molecular characterization of cervical cancer. Nature. 2017;543(7645):378–84.

13 Glandular Neoplasia of the Uterine Cervix and Its Related Lesions

Carlos Parra-Herran

Abstract

This chapter describes the pathology of glandular neoplasia of the uterine cervix. The spectrum of endocervical glandular malignancy is wide and sometimes diagnostically challenging. While most cervical adenocarcinomas are secondary to Human Papillomavirus infection, some tumors are unrelated to it; these lesions are now recognized for their aggressive clinical behavior and still obscure pathogenesis. The description of each adenocarcinoma type in this chapter follows an etiology (HPV-related versus unrelated) and traditional morphology-based approach. Important diagnostic situations such as diagnosis of stromal invasion, pattern-based assessment, and staging are also discussed. The chapter also presents the pathology of mixed lesions with a glandular component and benign glandular proliferations that need to be distinguished from preinvasive and invasive endocervical malignancy.

Keywords

Adenocarcinoma · Cervix · Endocervical · HPV · Early invasive adenocarcinoma · Pattern-based classification · International Endocervical Adenocarcinoma Classification and Criteria · Adenocarcinoma in situ · Lobular endocervical glandular hyperplasia · Usual-type adenocarcinoma · Signet-ring cell · Intestinal · Stratified mucin producing carcinoma · Adenoma malignum · Minimal deviation adenocarcinoma · Gastric type adenocarcinoma · Endometrioid carcinoma · Clear cell carcinoma · Mesonephric carcinoma · Serous carcinoma · Mixed adenocarcinoma · Adenosquamous carcinoma · Glassy cell carcinoma · Metastatic adenocarcinoma · Endocervical polyp · Nabothian cyst · Tunnel cluster · Diffuse laminar endocervical hyperplasia · Endometriosis · Endocervicosis · Tubo-endometrioid metaplasia · Microglandular hyperplasia · Arias-Stella reaction · Mesonephric hyperplasia

C. Parra-Herran (✉)
Department of Laboratory Medicine and Pathobiology, University of Toronto, Toronto, ON, Canada

Sunnybrook Health Sciences Centre, Toronto, ON, Canada
e-mail: carlos.parraherran@sunnybrook.ca

13.1 Introduction

13.1.1 The Normal Endocervix

Our current understanding of the development, anatomy, and histology of the normal endocervix is based on the initial models by *C. F. Fluhmann*, who described the endocervical mucosa as a complex system of mucosal infoldings [1, 2]. Unlike other mucosal linings such as the endometrium, the basic structural unit of the endocervix is not a vertical tube but a series of mucosal infoldings coursing in various directions (Fig. 13.1). Folding occurs due to epithelial proliferation driven by hormonal stimulation, and leads to the formation of clefts and grooves [1, 2]. The haphazard distribution and orientation of the endocervical mucosal clefts and grooves is reflected in the heterogeneous architecture seen in routine bidimensional tissue preparations of the cervix. This complexity contributes to our difficulty in distinguishing between abnormal proliferations confined to the epithelial compartment (in situ) and those invading cervical stroma, as discussed further in this chapter.

13.1.2 Endocervical Adenocarcinoma: Epidemiologic and Classification Trends

Compared to invasive squamous cell carcinoma, screening strategies have been less effective at detecting endocervical glandular malignancies around the globe. Indeed, the relative incidence of adenocarcinoma has increased from ~5% to ~20% between the 1960s and the 2000s [3, 4]. Cumulative incidence rates have increased internationally, particularly in women 30 years of age and older [5]. In the United States,

W. Zheng et al. (eds.), *Gynecologic and Obstetric Pathology, Volume 1*, https://doi.org/10.1007/978-981-13-3016-2_13

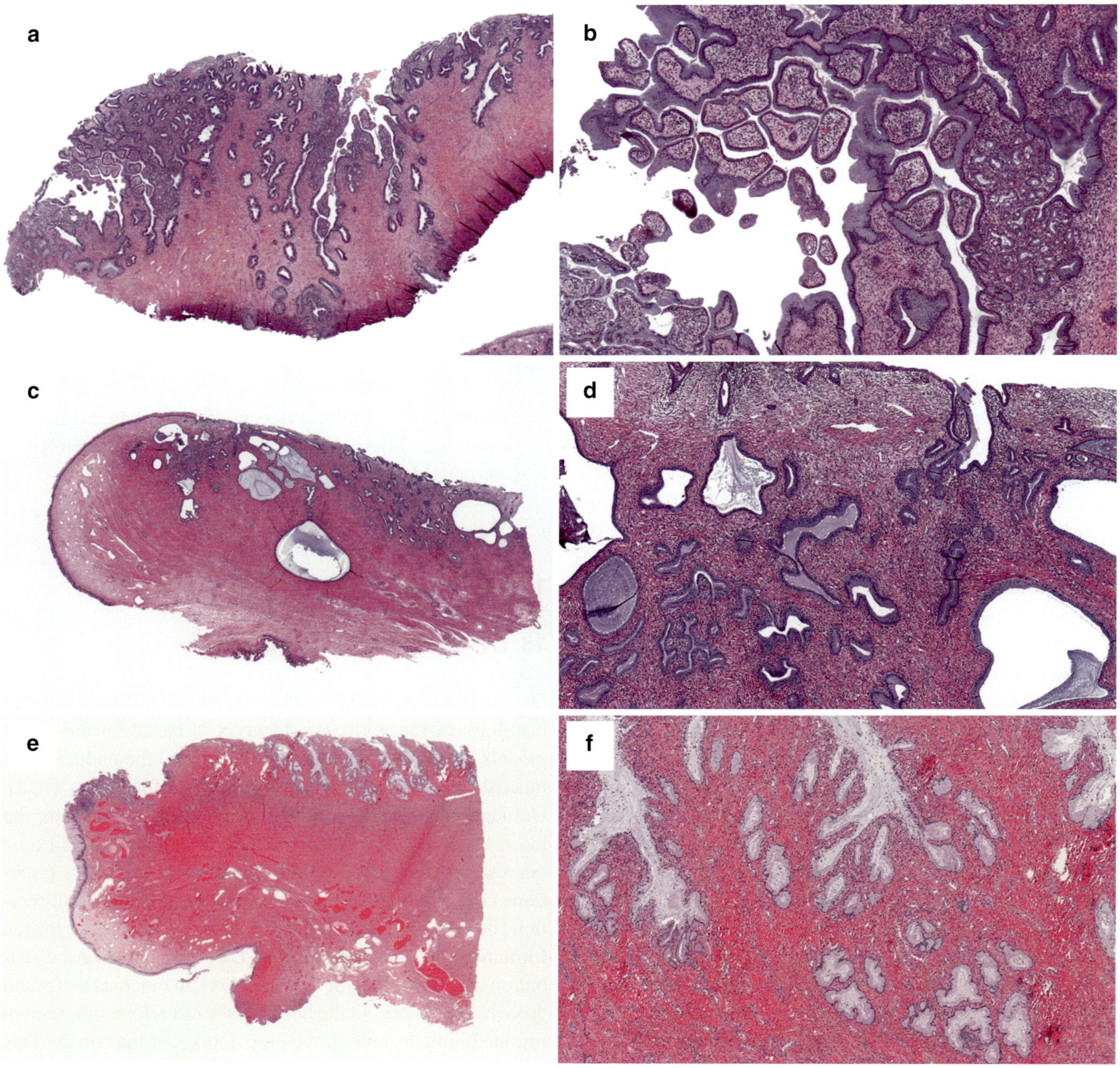

Fig. 13.1 Normal endocervix. The Endocervical mucosa is comprised of numerous surface infoldings, which gradually leads to the formation of clefts and grooves (seen as "glandular" structures in routine preparations) (**a**). The distribution of these structures is rather haphazard (**b**). Communication with the canal can eventually become obliterated, leading to the formation of cystically dilated glands (**c**, **d**). A more lobulated pattern can also be seen, with a centrally dilated cleft and peripheral grooves organized in a uniform "lobular" distribution (**e**, **f**)

incidence rates of endocervical adenocarcinoma have shown an increment of 32.2%, from 1.09/100,000 women in 1975 to 1.44/100,000 women in 2007 [6]. Similar increases have been documented in more recent literature from Denmark and the Netherlands, despite well-established screening programs [7, 8]. These surge in incidence can be attributed to differences in the diagnostic performance of the Pap test for glandular (versus squamous) lesions or may be caused by increased detection in some populations. However, the growing case numbers suggest that screening methods may not be adequate to detect adenocarcinoma in situ (AIS), as supported by the significant number of women with negative or low-risk Pap results before the glandular neoplasm is identified [9]. From an epidemiologic perspective, endocervical neoplasia is associated with higher socioeconomic and educational levels than squamous neoplasia. In addition, risk factors for squamous malignancy such as early and frequent sexual activity and smoking are less frequently associated with glandular lesions [10].

Virtually all squamous cell carcinomas and high-grade squamous intraepithelial lesions of the uterine cervix are related to high-risk Human Papilloma Virus (HPV) infections [11]. While the same was previously presumed for endocervical glandular neoplasms [12], recent evidence reveals a more heterogeneous landscape:

- The majority (85–90%) of adenocarcinoma in situ and invasive adenocarcinoma cases are indeed related to high-risk HPV, mainly HPV18 and HPV16, the rest being positive for HPV45 and other more rare HPV subtypes [13–15]. Coexistence of HPV-related glandular and squamous neoplasia is a common occurrence [16].
- A minor proportion of endocervical adenocarcinomas (10–15%) is negative for HPV [13, 17, 18]. Most of these cases belong to certain adenocarcinoma subtypes, including gastric, clear cell, and mesonephric categories. This subset of HPV-negative carcinomas has distinct morphology and clinical behavior compared to HPV-related lesions.

This chapter presents the relevant pathologic and clinical features of the diverse forms of endocervical glandular neoplasia. While the terminology employed mirrors the current World Health Organization (WHO) classification, cervical glandular proliferations covered here are categorized based on: (a) their pathogenesis (HPV-dependent versus independent) and (b) recent biology-based criteria and classification proposals. The chapter also covers the most common benign endocervical proliferations as they pertain to the differential diagnosis of preinvasive and invasive glandular malignancy.

13.2 Preinvasive Glandular Neoplasia

13.2.1 Nomenclature

In the last two decades, the terminology used for the categorization of endocervical adenocarcinoma precursors has shifted towards simplification. Formerly proposed terms such as cervical intraepithelial glandular neoplasia (CIGN), glandular atypia, and glandular hyperplasia have been largely abandoned given the lack of data proving an association with AIS and with invasive adenocarcinoma [19]. Unlike squamous lesions, there is currently no evidence that the cervical in situ glandular neoplasia spectrum includes a definable low-grade category.

The term "*Endocervical Glandular Dysplasia*" (EGD), proposed for noninvasive lesions with features bordering on but not diagnostic of AIS [20], suffers from significant interobserver variation especially in its distinction from benign cervix [21]. Moreover, its biologic and clinical significance has not been firmly established. Its occurrence in patients with concurrent AIS or invasive adenocarcinoma is rare; in this scenario, most EGD harbor an HPV infection, implying that they are subtle forms of AIS [22]. In contrast, isolated EGD is usually negative for HPV and p16, contradicting its alleged role as a precursor [22, 23]. Currently available ancillary tools such as p16 and Ki67 immunohistochemistry and HPV testing have improved the stratification of lesions with equivocal features into benign or AIS categories, further obviating the need for an intermediate category like EGD [24]. Given the lack of evidence-based support for alternative / supplementary terminology, the 2014 WHO of Tumours of Female Reproductive Organs eliminated EGD and other categories and recommends the use of AIS as the only established precursor of invasive endocervical glandular malignancy [11].

13.2.2 Adenocarcinoma In Situ, Conventional (HPV-Related) Type

Initially described in 1953 [25], AIS of the cervix is now regarded as a precursor of invasive endocervical adenocarcinoma. This precursor role has been attributed based on the following evidence: (1) women with AIS have a mean age of 35 years at presentation, 10–20 years younger than those with invasive adenocarcinoma; (2) AIS is frequently found adjacent to invasive adenocarcinoma [26]; (3) the spectrum of HPV types in AIS and invasive adenocarcinoma is similar; and (4) invasive endocervical adenocarcinoma has been documented in patients with previous AIS either missed in biopsy or curettage, or diagnosed and left untreated [26, 27].

Clinical Features

AIS is not symptomatic and its diagnosis is made in the context of cytologic screening abnormalities. AIS does not produce a macroscopic abnormality in most cases as the presence of a lesion on colposcopy and/or pathologic gross examination is usually related to a coexistent squamous lesion, an exophytic papillary component (either squamous or glandular) or invasive carcinoma.

Pathologic Features

AIS is defined by the following histologic features [11, 27, 28] (Fig. 13.2):

(a) Columnar epithelium with pseudostratified, enlarged, elongated, hyperchromatic nuclei and variable loss of intracytoplasmic mucin.
(b) Easily identifiable apical mitotic figures and apoptotic bodies (at least one in each gland).
(c) Preservation of the normal glandular architecture, since the neoplastic proliferation is, by definition, restricted to the preexisting endocervical epithelial compartment; architectural complexity is allowed (papillary, micro-

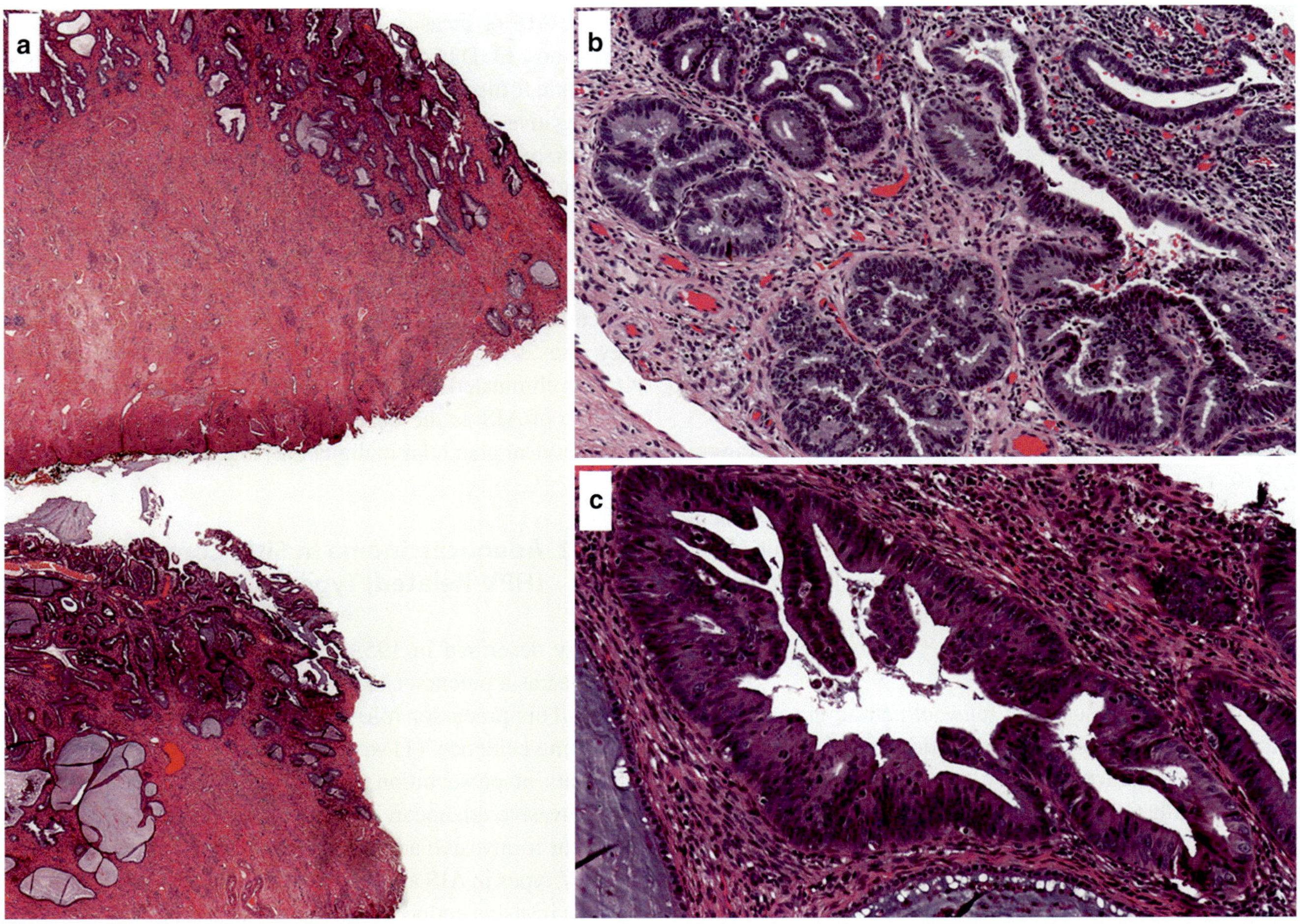

Fig. 13.2 Adenocarcinoma in situ, HPV-related (AIS). The neoplastic glandular proliferation in (**a**) (lower half) has the same density and architecture of the normal endocervix (upper half), in keeping with an in situ process. AIS is characterized by columnar cells with hyperchromatic nuclei, conspicuous apical mitoses and apoptosis, and mucin depletion (**b**, **c**)

papillary, or cribriform growth) as long as it is either confined to the surface or intraglandular (similar size and shape of other AIS glands and normal endocervix).

The lesion is usually centered in the squamous–columnar junction; it can, however, occur in the proximal endocervical canal, as far as 3 cm from the junction in one series [16]. Multifocality is seen in two-thirds of AIS cases.

Similar to its invasive counterparts, the most frequent histologic types of AIS are usual (intracytoplasmic mucin in <50% of the cells) and mucinous endocervical (intracytoplasmic mucin in >50% of cells). Since its original characterization, several other variants of AIS have been described including endometrioid (smaller, rounder nuclei with little to no mucin production), intestinal (goblet cell differentiation, Paneth cells), and tubal. All these variants are related to HPV infection and constitute part of the morphologic spectrum of AIS, commonly seen within the same lesion / patient in varying proportions [29–31].

A less frequent but challenging type of AIS is seen in the form of simple frond-like projections confined to the surface of the cervix. This growth pattern is termed exophytic or villoglandular, and can be seen in usual, mucinous or endometrioid AIS. The exophytic component is comprised of papillary structures lined by abnormal AIS-type epithelium.

Ancillary Studie

P16/*CDKN2A* is a tumor suppressor protein/gene that inhibits cyclin-dependent kinase 4A (*CDK4A*). p16 protein expression with cell cycle progression is mediated by the transcriptional activator E2F and promotes production of the retinoblastoma protein (Rb), which binds to E2F, thus stopping cell cycle progression. In the presence of transcriptionally active HPV, the viral oncoprotein E7 binds competitively to Rb, inactivating it. Rb inactivation causes an increase in free E2F leading to activation of cell cycle progression pathways; this also disrupts the negative feedback loop for p16, which consequently accumulates within the cell. Thus, overexpression of p16 by immunohistochemistry has become an excellent surrogate marker of high-risk HPV infection. Indeed, p16 is identified at high levels in most AIS lesions [23, 32–34]. P16 overexpression is strictly defined as strong, cytoplasmic *and* nuclear staining in the majority of abnormal cells, which results in a "block" pattern of positivity.

The majority of AIS cells exhibit increased expression of proliferation markers. Ki67 is elevated with a labeling index usually greater than 30%. ProEx C labels nuclear proteins (mini-chromosome maintenance protein 2, MCM2 and topoisomerase II-alpha, TOP2A) that are overexpressed during the aberrant S-phase induction of HPV infected and neoplastic cells; this marker is consistently positive in AIS [34, 35]. Loss of estrogen and progesterone receptor expression is also a common event in AIS, thus ER/PR negativity by immunohistochemistry is helpful in excluding benign mimics and endometrial endometrioid neoplasia which are ER/PR positive [36].

High-risk HPV can be detected in conventional AIS by in situ hybridization or sequencing methods [18, 37]. The most common types are HPV16, HPV18, HPV45, and HPV35 [15, 17, 38]. HPV testing is increasingly available, and should be considered if the differential includes AIS versus benign proliferations or HPV-independent neoplasia.

Differential Diagnosis

The most critical differential diagnoses of AIS are invasive adenocarcinoma, HPV-negative endocervical neoplasia, and certain benign cervical lesions. The latter two scenarios will be discussed here; the distinction between in situ and invasive carcinoma will be explored in the next section.

Rare and under-recognized (until recently), HPV-independent AIS is an important form of cervical glandular neoplasia, given its association with aggressive types of invasive adenocarcinoma, most importantly gastric-type adenocarcinoma [39, 40]. Mucin depletion, or presence of endocervical-type mucin, is more in keeping with conventional-type AIS. In addition, nuclei in HPV-related AIS tends to be elongated and hyperchromatic, compared to the more round nuclei with vesicular chromatin of gastric-type AIS. HPV testing is helpful in this distinction.

A range of benign cervical proliferations can mimic AIS, both architecturally and cytologically. In all these, p16 staining is normal (negative or patchy), which constitutes a valuable tool in the differential exercise. The most relevant entities are listed here, with useful features in their distinction from AIS in parenthesis: (a) tubo-endometrioid metaplasia (absence or paucity of mitoses; lack of hyperchromasia; nuclear expression of estrogen receptor and Bcl-2), (b) endometriosis (overall absence of mucinous differentiation; absence of nuclear atypia and hyperchromasia; presence of endometrial-type stroma and hemosiderin deposition; expression of hormone receptors), (c) immature squamous metaplasia (stratification and orderly, albeit incomplete, squamous differentiation; absence of nuclear atypia; expression of squamous cell markers), and (d) mesonephric remnants (flat to cuboidal cells, less frequently columnar; round, bland nuclei with absence of mitoses; eosinophilic luminal secretions).

Management and Prognosis

In the past, hysterectomy was recommended as the standard treatment for AIS; it is still recommended in patients with other comorbidities benefiting from removal of the uterus (e.g., menorrhagia), those without the need to preserve fertility and those with factors complicating follow-up (e.g., cervical stenosis). Given its safety and superior fertility-related outcomes, conservative management with conization and loop electrosurgical excisional procedure (LEEP) has been increasingly performed. However, the possibility of incomplete excision and recurrence in these treatment modalities warrants close surveillance with cytology and colposcopy [41]. The type of procedure and the margin status are the most important predictive factors of residual disease and recurrence. LEEP is more frequently associated with residual disease (51%) compared to conization (30%) [42]. The prevalence of residual AIS after cold knife conization or LEEP is 16% for excisions with negative margins versus 49% for those with positive margins [42]. Similarly, the prevalence of invasive carcinoma after cold knife conization / LEEP for AIS is 0.1–0.6% for excisions with negative margins versus 5–6% for those with positive margins [42, 43]. AIS recurrence in patients on surveillance after conization is 3% when margins are negative and 17–19% when margins are positive [42, 43].

13.2.2.1 Stratified Mucin-Producing Intraepithelial Lesion (HPV-Related AIS, Stratified Variant)

The stratified variant of AIS was initially described by *Park et al.* as stratified mucin producing intraepithelial lesion (SMILE) [44]. As the name implies, SMILE is characterized by its stratified appearance. From low-power magnification, the stratified epithelial architecture is reminiscent of a squamous intraepithelial lesion. However, examination under high-power magnification reveals intracytoplasmic mucin throughout the entire epithelial thickness (Fig. 13.3). SMILE frequently coexists with HSIL and/or conventional AIS. When present, an invasive carcinoma component has glandular, adenosquamous or stratified mucin-producing appearance [44].

Like conventional AIS, SMILE is characterized by p16 overexpression and high Ki67 proliferation index; conversely p63 is negative in columnar cells, and only positive in the basal layer (likely residual reserve cells) [44, 45]. HPV is consistently detected, mostly types 16 and 18. The ultrastructure of SMILE has revealed presence of microvilli, vacuolar structures, and mitochondria in the absence of tonofilaments, supporting the hypothesis that this lesion belongs to the spectrum of endocervical glandular neoplasia [45].

The differential diagnosis of SMILE includes a high-grade squamous intraepithelial lesion (HSIL) undermining normal endocervix, in which the mucinous cells are dispersed and displaced towards the lumen. This contrasts with the diffuse and full-thickness distribution of mucin-producing

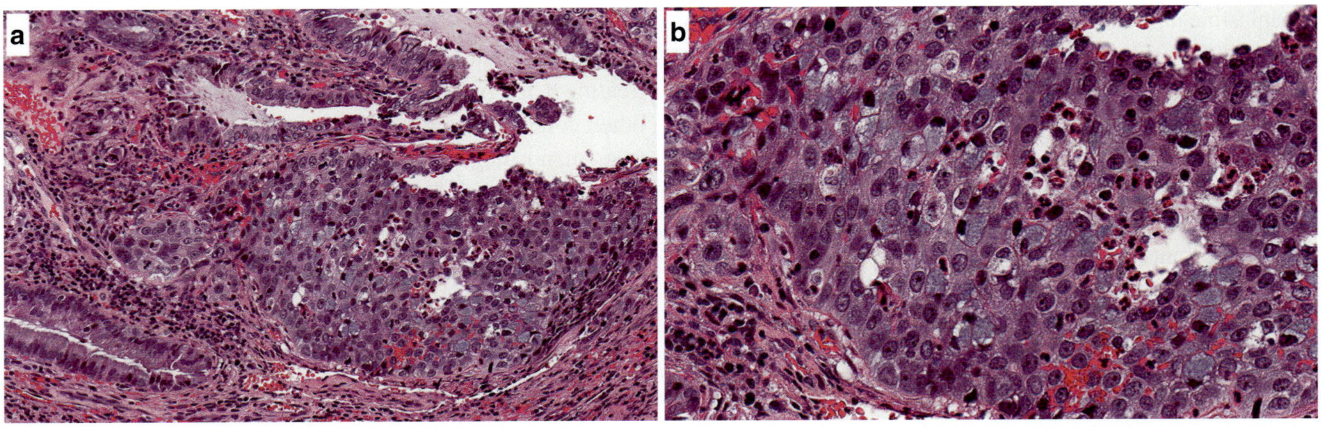

Fig. 13.3 Stratified mucin-producing intraepithelial lesion. This in situ proliferation is stratified, resembling a squamous intraepithelial lesion (A). However, intracytoplasmic mucin can be observed throughout the lesion on high-power view

cells in SMILE. The nuclei of the endocervical mucinous cells surrounded by HSIL have a bland appearance. In contrast, dysplastic nuclear morphology of the mucin-producing population should raise the possibility of SMILE. Conventional AIS can harbor areas of intraglandular complexity that may appear stratified, and both stratified and conventional morphologies can coexist. Finally, immature squamous metaplasia should also be considered; the retained polarization and lack of nuclear dysplasia indicate a benign diagnosis. P16 and Ki67 stains can be performed in equivocal instances.

13.2.3 Adenocarcinoma In Situ, Gastric Type and Lobular Endocervical Glandular Hyperplasia

Compared to HPV-related adenocarcinoma, the pathogenesis of cervical malignancies not related to high-risk HPV infection is less characterized. Nonetheless, the spectrum of gastric differentiation in the endocervix is well recognized; within it, certain lesions are now understood as likely precursors of gastric-type endocervical neoplasia.

Benign gastric (pyloric) metaplasia has been described in the endocervix in two forms:

- Simple gastric metaplasia: Simple gastric-type mucinous epithelium lining otherwise unremarkable endocervical glands [46].
- Tunnel clusters type A [47].

An architecturally more complex gastric-type proliferation, lobular endocervical glandular hyperplasia (LEGH, namely complex gastric metaplasia), was initially described by *Nucci et al.* [48]. Although by itself a benign process, LEGH is included in this section because of its association with gastric-type adenocarcinomas including adenoma malignum: LEGH has been identified in up to 20% of gastric type adenocarcinomas and 50% minimal deviation adenocarcinomas [49–51]. Moreover, gains of chromosome 3q and a loss of 1p (which are common in minimal deviation adenocarcinoma) have been detected in a subset of LEGH (21%) [52]. This evidence suggests that LEGH is a nonobligatory precursor of endocervical gastric-type malignancy.

LEGH is usually an incidental finding; however, it may present as a mass or cyst detected on imaging or examination. Histologically, LEGH is a well-demarcated lesion with lobular/acinar architecture. It is composed of a central gland, sometimes with cystic dilation, surrounded by smaller glands and cysts arranged in a floret-like pattern (Fig. 13.4). Central and peripheral glands are lined by low columnar cells with pale eosinophilic cytoplasm [48, 49]. Cells are mucinous with a similar appearance than the normal endocervix. Nonetheless, the mucin profile, characterized by pale or eosinophilic staining, is different from the slightly basophilic (blue-purple) appearance of the normal mucinous endocervical cell.

Atypical LEGH is a related lesion, also strongly associated with minimal deviation adenocarcinoma (seen in ~30% of cases). Atypical LEGH is characterized by an elevated Ki67 index and abnormal p53 immunohistochemical expression [53]. Furthermore, it shares similar molecular alterations with minimal deviation adenocarcinoma (MDA), in particular 3q gain and 1p loss [51]. From this perspective, atypical LEGH may be considered an immediate precursor of MDA (e.g., pre-cancerous). Atypical LEGH is architecturally consistent with LEGH, but with four or more of the following features:

- Nuclear enlargement.
- Irregular nuclear contours.
- Distinct nucleoli and coarse chromatin.
- Loss of polarity.
- Mitotic figures (occasional).

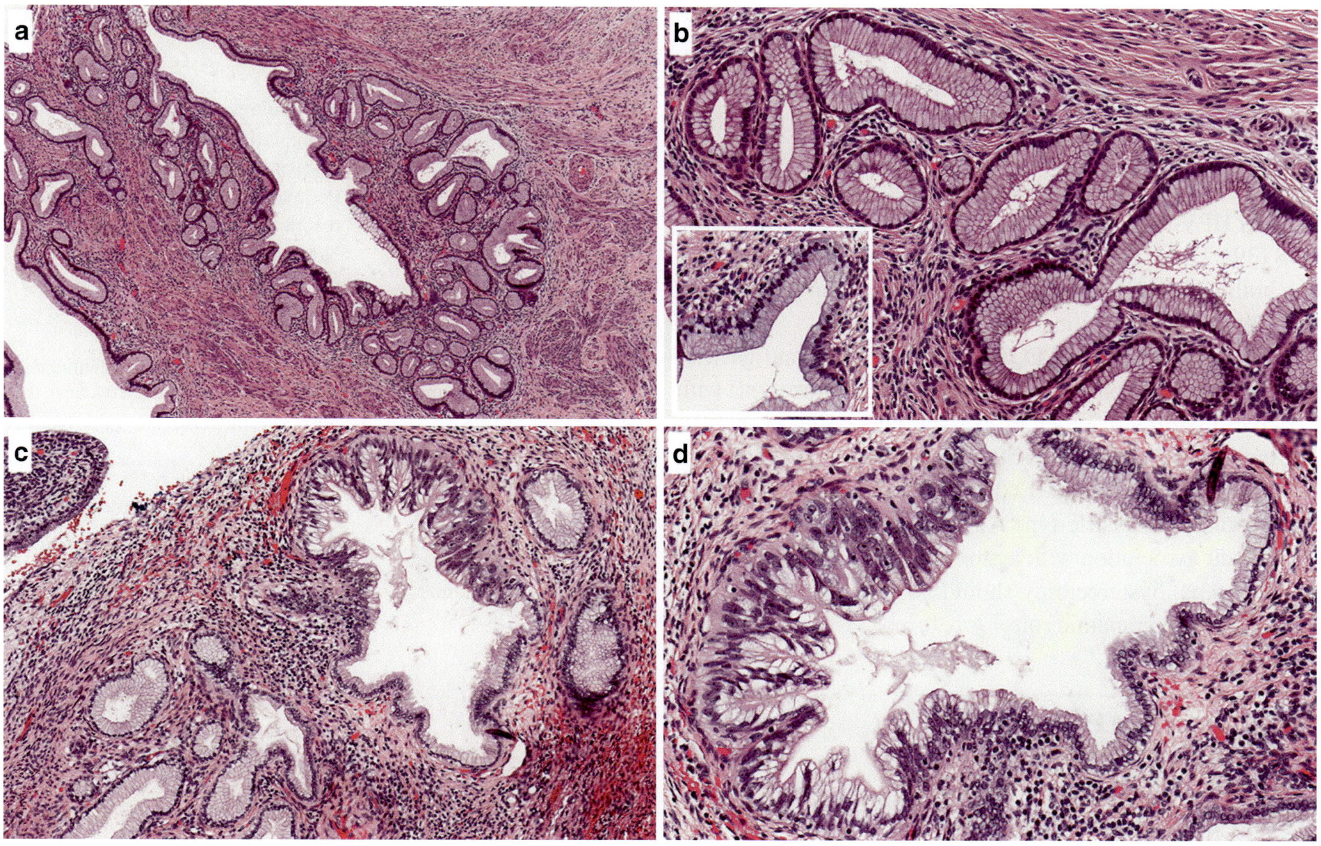

Fig. 13.4 Lobular endocervical glandular hyperplasia (LEGH). A central dilated cleft is surrounded by small, round to tubular glands in a floret pattern (**a**). Lining epithelium is mucinous columnar and highly resembles the normal endocervix (**b**); however, cytoplasm is less basophilic and cell borders are more accentuated (compare to normal endocervix from the same patient, insert). Atypical LEGH; this example is characterized by severe nuclear atypia partially involving a dilated duct in an area of otherwise typical LEGH (**c**, **d**)

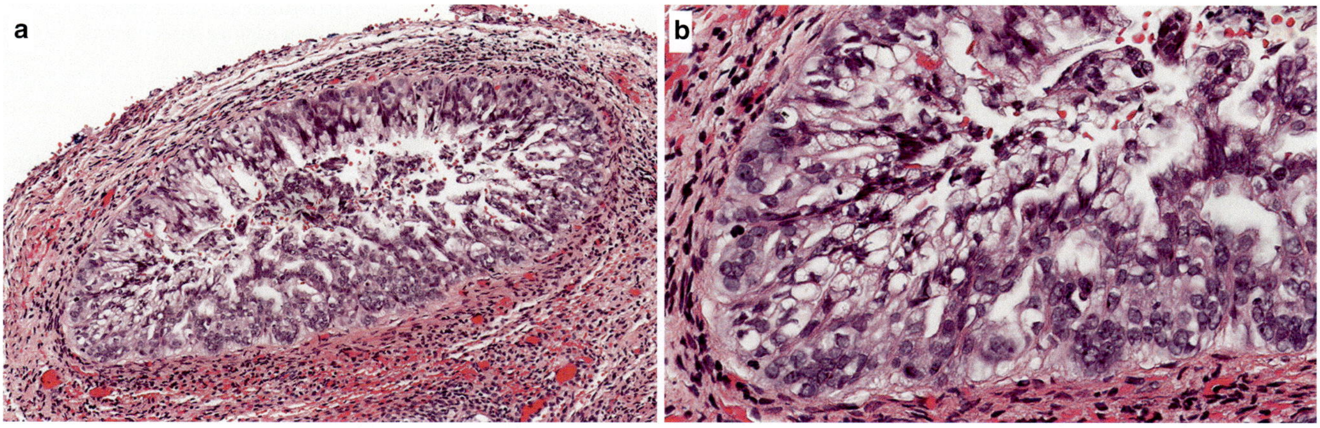

Fig. 13.5 Adenocarcinoma in situ, gastric type. Intraglandular proliferation with micropapillary architecture (**a**), comprised of cells with round, enlarged nuclei and abundant clear cytoplasm (different from the elongated, hyperchromatic nuclei and mucin-depleted cytoplasm of HPV-related AIS) (**b**). This lesion was negative for p16 and HPV testing

- Apoptotic bodies or luminal nuclear debris.
- Intraluminal papillary projections.

Gastric-type adenocarcinoma in situ is also comprised of atypical cells as outlined above, but without the classic lobular architecture of atypical LEGH [46]. The neoplastic cells display evident pleomorphism and cytological features of gastric differentiation; namely abundant, vacuolated, clear to eosinophilic and/or mucinous cytoplasm and distinct cell borders (Fig. 13.5).

The differential diagnosis of atypical LEGH and gastric-type AIS includes: (a) invasive gastric-type adenocarcinoma, in which destructive stromal invasion is evident (marked desmoplasia, solid growth, architectural complexity); (b) HPV-related AIS, which is typically mucin-depleted and contains elongated hyperchromatic nuclei; mitotic activity is conspicuous in HPV-related AIS, and less prominent in gastric-type AIS [39]; HPV-related AIS can be confirmed by demonstrating both p16 IHC overexpression *and* detection of high-risk HPV by molecular testing.

The management of LEGH, atypical LEGH and gastric-type AIS found in biopsy involves excision (conization) with negative margins in order to exclude concomitant invasive malignancy. LEGH can be safely monitored. In reproductive age women, follow-up after conservative excision of atypical LEGH and even gastric-type AIS may be prudent. However, given their association with aggressive types of invasive adenocarcinoma, hysterectomy should be considered as it may have a better therapeutic role.

13.3 Invasive Endocervical Adenocarcinoma

13.3.1 General Considerations

13.3.1.1 Diagnosis of Invasion by Endocervical Adenocarcinoma

Stromal invasion by endocervical adenocarcinoma acquires a variety of histologic patterns, some easily identified as invasive and some with significant overlap with the architecture of the normal cervix, and therefore difficult to assess. HPV-negative invasive endocervical adenocarcinoma tends to be widely infiltrative, and diagnosis of invasion in these lesions is usually straightforward. HPV-positive adenocarcinoma is more heterogeneous, and not infrequently displays more subtle patterns of glandular proliferation referred to by some authors as "AIS-like." Table 13.1 summarizes the morphologic spectrum of stromal invasion by endocervical glandular neoplasia [27, 54].

Common circumstances in which distinction between AIS and invasive adenocarcinoma is particularly challenging (and useful hints on how to approach them) include (Fig. 13.6):

Table 13.1 Morphologic spectrum of stromal invasion by endocervical adenocarcinoma

Pattern of invasion	Type	Morphologic spectrum
Destructive	Infiltrative growth	Glands with irregular and angulated contours
		Periglandular stromal desmoplastic reaction
		Non-gland forming elements (individual cells; cell clusters, buds or nests)
	Complex/ confluent architecture	Anastomosed, fused or interconnected glandular elements (scant to no stroma in between)
		Seen as cribriform, labyrinth-like or solid patterns
		Endophytic papillary/ micropapillary (within cervical wall)
AIS-like	Increased glandular density	Gland crowding that exceeds the density of the adjacent normal cervix (or in its absence, the expected glandular density in a normal cervix)
		Tight clustering of small glands, sometimes with small and focal gland fusion
	Deep glandular proliferation	Gland extension into deep cervical stroma
		Haphazard distribution (lack of lobulation)
		Close proximity to thick-walled vessels
	Exophytic complex growth	Exophytic papillary or villoglandular growth with epithelial complexity (cribriforming, anastomosing within papillae spaces and/or stroma)

- Extensive AIS with lobulated proliferation, increased glandular density and/or areas of complexity are suggestive but not diagnostic of invasion. In these situations, neoplastic glands are superficially located or organized in well-formed lobules, mirroring to an extent the normal cervix architecture. These types of neoplastic growth appear to be relatively indolent with nil risk of nodal metastases (see pattern-based classification section). However, ovarian spread has been documented in these otherwise "borderline" or "in situ like" tumors, indicating that they can potentially behave in a malignant fashion, and therefore are best categorized as invasive carcinoma [55].
- Presence of distorting elements such as inflammation, mucosal erosion / ulceration, previous biopsy site reaction and edema, when prominent, can obscure the presence of invasive elements. Conversely, they can also distort the contours of AIS glands making assessment of invasion difficult. When possible, evaluation should be made in areas away from these changes (which are usually superficial).
- Papillary/villoglandular growth. As mentioned previously, endocervical adenocarcinoma can grow predominantly or exclusively in the surface and acquire an exophytic appearance. When simple (small, non-branching or confluent papillae, stroma devoid of complex glands), such proliferations are most in keeping with AIS. More complex

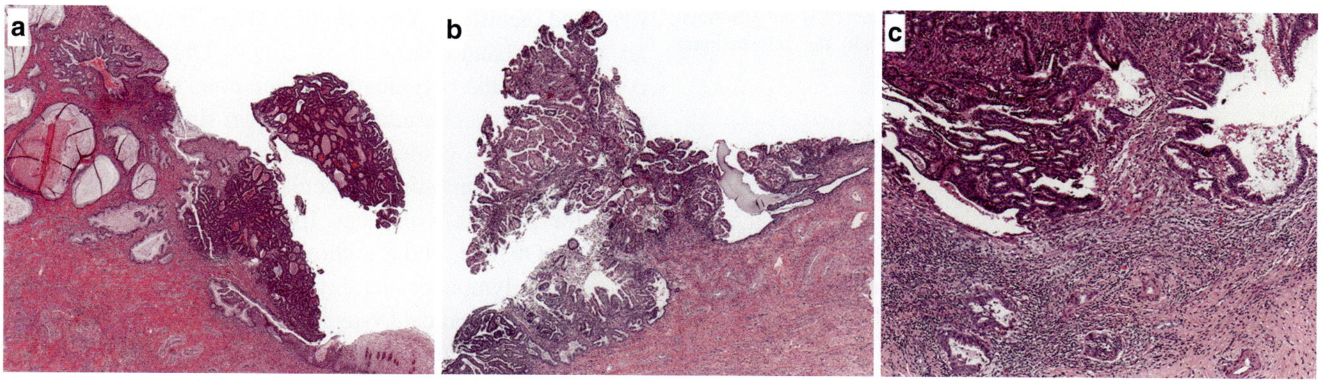

Fig. 13.6 Assessment of stromal invasion by endocervical adenocarcinoma can be challenging when proliferation is well differentiated (purely glandular). Diagnosis of invasion is warranted when the glandular density obviously exceeds that of the adjacent normal cervix (**a**) and when papillary growth is not only in the surface but also involves stroma within papillae or in the cervix per se) (**b**). It is recommended that horizontal extent and depth measurements encompass the entire lesion in these instances. Chronic inflammation can be unrelated to the tumor, and does not necessarily constitute a sign of invasion (**c**). If possible, assessment of invasion should be made in areas devoid of obscuring inflammation; however, densely inflamed areas should be carefully examined for the presence of unequivocal invasive foci (single cells, clusters, LVI, etc.)

degrees of epithelial proliferation encountered include branching and confluent papillae/micropapillae as well as cribriform or confluent glandular elements within the papillary stroma; most pathologists will accept such complexity as a form of invasive adenocarcinoma. Categorization of papillary lesions as in situ or invasive is difficult, particularly in biopsy material. A final diagnosis of AIS should only be made after assessing the underlying stroma and excluding endophytic papillary growth or any other sign of unequivocal stromal invasion [54].

The above situations illustrate the challenge of diagnosing invasion by endocervical adenocarcinoma, which has been stated as difficult or impossible to determine in about 20% of cases [56]. This is likely explained by the architectural overlap between the normal cervix, AIS, and certain forms of nondestructive neoplasia traditionally deemed as invasive, which cannot be reliably distinguished by pathologists [57]. In this exercise, consensus review with colleagues may help reach a defensible diagnosis. If uncertainty persists, a less definitive diagnosis indicating concern for early stromal invasion in the setting of florid AIS may be the best approach.

When diagnosing invasion by endocervical adenocarcinoma, the terms "microinvasive" and "superficially invasive" should be avoided; the former is no longer recommended in cervical neoplasia, while the latter is reserved for squamous tumors and is not suitable for endocervical adenocarcinoma. The main reasons for this include the difficulty of estimating the invasive component in cases with "AIS-like" invasion and in the diagnostic situations outlined above. When the in situ and invasive components cannot be reliably separated, the dimensions of the entire lesion should be provided. This includes the thickness measured from the surface, which replaces the depth parameter, and the horizontal dimensions (measured from the slides and / or estimated from the number of blocks involved). Other estimations of size such as percentage of the cervical circumference involved or the quadrant extension are helpful (but frequently imprecise) additions to the standard tumor size measurements.

13.3.1.2 Staging

Staging definitions as per the latest recommendations from the American Joint Committee on Cancer (AJCC) and the International Collaboration on Cancer Reporting (ICCR). are listed in Table 13.2. Of note, the International Federation of Obstetrics and Gyneaocology (FIGO) recently changed the staging system for cervical cancer; a critical change is that in stage I lesions the horizontal extent criterion was abolished and stage was redefined as Ia1 (depth of invasion <3 mm), Ia2 (depth 3-5 mm), Ib1 (depth > 5 mm or grossly visible lesions <2 cm in size), Ib2 (size 2-4 cm) and Ib3 (size >4 cm). Both staging systems equally apply to squamous, glandular, mixed, and miscellaneous cervical malignancies. Special mention will be given to stage T1a/IA adenocarcinoma, since it is, by definition, based on assessment of microscopic size.

Early (Minimally) Invasive Adenocarcinoma (Stage T1A/IA)

Stage IA lesions are less than 5 mm in depth and 7 mm in horizontal spread. These have a negligible risk of nodal spread compared to tumors of stage IB or larger. Studies addressing the biological behavior of early stage adenocarcinoma have different definitions for what constitutes early invasion. Perhaps the most comprehensive analysis of the literature was performed by *Östör* [56], who studied 436 lesions with an invasive depth of <5 mm. Of these, 126 were

Table 13.2 Staging of carcinoma of the uterine cervix as per American Joint Committee on Cancer (IAJCC), 8th ed and the International Collaboration on Cancer Reporting (ICCR)

TNM	Definition
TX	Primary tumor cannot be assessed
T0	No evidence of primary tumor
Tis	Carcinoma in situ (preinvasive carcinoma)
T1	Tumor confined to the cervix (extension to corpus should be disregarded)
T1a	Invasive carcinoma diagnosed only by microscopy. Stromal invasion with a maximal depth of 5.0 mm measured from the base of the epithelium and a horizontal spread of 7.0 mm or less[a]
T1a1	Measured stromal invasion 3.0 mm or less in depth and 7.0 mm or less in horizontal spread
T1a2	Measured stromal invasion more than 3.0 mm and not more than 5.0 mm in depth, with a horizontal spread of 7.0 mm or less
T1b	Clinically visible lesion confined to the cervix or microscopic disease greater than T1a/IA2
T1b1	Clinically visible lesion 4.0 cm or less in greatest dimension
T1b2	Clinically visible lesion more than 4.0 cm in greatest dimension
T2	Tumor invades beyond uterus but not to pelvic wall or lower third of vagina
T2a	Tumor without parametrial invasion
T2a1	Clinically visible lesion 4.0 cm or less in greatest dimension
T2a2	Clinically visible lesion more than 4.0 cm in greatest dimension
T2b	Tum or with parametrial invasion
T3	Tumor extends to pelvic wall, involves lower one-third of vagina, causes hydronephrosis or nonfunctioning kidney
T3a	Tumor involves lower one-third of vagina
T3b	Tumor extends to pelvic wall, causes hydronephrosis or nonfunctioning kidney
T4	Tumor invades mucosa of the bladder or rectum, or extends beyond true pelvis
NX	Regional lymph nodes cannot be assessed
N0	No regional lymph node metastases
N1	Regional lymph node metastases
MX	Distant metastases cannot be assessed
M0	No distant metastases
M1	Distant metastases (includes inguinal lymph nodes and intraperitoneal disease except metastases to pelvic serosa). It excludes metastases to vagina, pelvic serosa and adnexa

[a]All macroscopically visible lesions, even with superficial invasion, are T1b/IB
[b]Vascular space involvement, venous or lymphatic, does not affect classification
[c]Bullous edema is not sufficient to classify a tumor as T4
[d]Invasion of bladder or rectal mucosa should be biopsy proven

treated by radical hysterectomy, and none had parametrial involvement. Moreover, 155 patients underwent bilateral oophorectomy and none had ovarian metastases. Of the 219 cases in this cohort with pelvic lymph node dissection, five (2%) had metastasis. Overall, there were 15 recurrences and six tumor-related deaths in the cohort. Only 21 cases had conization as the only treatment, and none suffered a recurrence. More recent studies have shown similar results, providing further evidence to recommend conservative management, consisting of conization with negative margins, for patients with stage IA invasive adenocarcinoma [58–60]. Of note, some authors recommend consideration for pelvic lymphadenectomy and conventional surgery (trachelectomy, radical hysterectomy) for patients with stage IA2 tumors *and* lymphovascular space invasion [60, 61].

13.3.1.3 Management

Primary surgery is the treatment of choice for patients with endocervical adenocarcinoma confined to the uterus; in this subset, surgery is superior to primary radiation [62]. Adjuvant systemic treatment is reserved for patients with upstage after pathologic examination of the resected specimen (parametrial involvement, lymph node metastases); in these patients, combination of chemotherapy and radiation is superior to radiation alone [63]. High-risk factors in the excised tumor such as high grade, deep cervical stromal infiltration, uterine corpus involvement, and extensive lymphovascular space invasion should also prompt consideration for systemic adjuvant treatment. Patients with disease beyond the uterus on clinical and radiologic examination undergo primary radiation and chemotherapy [64]. The latter includes Platinum derivatives (Cisplatin, Carboplatin) usually combined with Paclitaxel or other agents.

13.3.1.4 Genetic Profile

Infection by oncogenic HPV is the main causative event in most endocervical adenocarcinomas. Infection occurs in the squamous–columnar junction which harbors a recently characterized reserve cell precursor [65]. As outlined previously for AIS, active HPV infection leads to p16 overexpression. Other than the integration of HPV DNA into the host cell genome, prevalent genetic alterations in endocervical adenocarcinoma include mutations in *PIK3CA*, *KRAS*, and *PTEN*, all members of the *PI3K/Akt/mTOR* signaling cascade [66–69]. Remarkably, these mutations have predictive and prognostic value as they are amenable to targeted therapies [70] and are associated with tumors with destructive invasion [71]. Moreover, *KRAS* mutations are associated with advanced stage and tumor recurrence [71, 72]. Little is known of the molecular landscape of HPV-unrelated endocervical adenocarcinoma types.

13.3.1.5 Pattern-Based Classification

Risk stratification of early (FIGO stage I) invasive endocervical adenocarcinoma is currently based on measurement of tumor width and depth of invasion, as outlined above [73]. A novel classification system based on the pattern, rather than

Table 13.3 Pattern-based classification of HPV-related endocervical adenocarcinoma

Pattern A	Well-demarcated glands with rounded contours, frequently forming groups.
	No destructive stromal invasion.
	No single cells or cell detachment.
	No Lymphovascular invasion.
	Complex intraglandular growth acceptable (i.e., cribriform, papillae).
	Lack of solid growth (i.e., architecture well-moderately differentiated).
	Depth of tumor or relationship to large cervical vessels not relevant.
Pattern B	*Localized* (limited, early) *destructive stromal invasion* arising from pattern A glands (well-demarcated glands).
	Individual or small groups of tumor cells, separated from the rounded gland, often in a focally desmoplastic or inflamed stroma.
	Foci may be single, multiple or linear at base of tumor.
	Lymphovascular invasion +/−.
	Lack of solid growth (i.e., architecturally well-moderately differentiated).
Pattern C	*Diffuse destructive invasion*, characterized by:
	Diffusely infiltrative glands with associated extensive desmoplastic response.
	Glands often angulated or with canalicular pattern, with interspersed open glands.
	Confluent growth filling a 4× field (5 mm): glands, papillae (stroma only within papillae), or mucin lakes.
	Solid, poorly differentiated component (architecturally high grade); nuclear grade is disregarded.
	Lymphovascular invasion +/−.

the size of the invasive component, has been proposed as an alternative for risk stratification that obviates the well-known challenges of size measurement and invasion assessment [74–76]. The classification applies only to HPV-related endocervical adenocarcinoma (see *Nomenclature* section below). It divides invasive tumors into three groups according to the histologic pattern of stromal invasion (Table 13.3, Fig. 13.7).

Initial studies demonstrated that tumors with a nondestructive pattern of invasion (pattern A) were not associated with lymph node metastases, whereas tumors with focally (B) and diffusely (C) destructive patterns had 4% and 23% rates of nodal involvement, respectively [74, 75]. Tumor recurrence was seen in 0%, 1.2 and 22.1% of patients with patterns A, B, and C, respectively, and death of disease was exclusively seen in patients with pattern C tumors (8.8%) [74]. Other studies have found similar findings [77–79]. Pattern of stromal invasion also correlates with tumor size (horizontal spread and depth of invasion): in one study, 90% of pattern A tumors were stage IA, whereas 76% of pattern B and 80% of pattern C tumors were stage IB [78]. Differences in clinical presentation and outcome may have a genetic correlation: mutations in *KRAS*, *PIK3CA*, and other oncogenes commonly altered in endocervical adenocarcinoma are significantly more frequent in destructively invasive (B and C) tumors [71].

Application of the pattern-based classification requires evaluation of the entire tumor. However, pattern evaluation in cone and LEEP specimens has utility, since it is predictive of the final pattern in hysterectomy. Pattern evaluation in biopsy material, however, is less optimal with significant rates of upgrade (from A to C) on excision [78].

The overall interobserver reproducibility of the pattern-based classification is good [79, 80]. The highest level of concordance lies in the distinction between destructive (patterns B and C) and nondestructive patterns (pattern A, adenocarcinoma in situ) [79, 81]. Contrarily, the reproducibility of in situ versus invasive adenocarcinoma (particularly pattern A) diagnosis is poor [79]. Certain circumstances make pattern assessment difficult: tumors with an exophytic papillary component, tumors with brisk inflammation obscuring glandular contours, and tumors with a cellular periglandular stroma suggestive but not definitive for desmoplasia.

13.3.1.6 Nomenclature

The current WHO classification of tumors of the female reproductive system categorizes endocervical adenocarcinoma based on architectural and cytological morphologic features [11]. Histologic subtypes of endocervical adenocarcinoma (usual, mucinous, villoglandular, endometrioid) have been treated over the decades as distinct variants based on their peculiar histologic features. However, their biological and clinical significance has been questioned as multivariate analyses have shown no significant impact of major histologic types of HPV-related adenocarcinoma on patient survival [82].

Our growing knowledge of the etiology and clinical behavior of this disease now serves as a tool to refine classification. From an etiologic point of view, the majority (85–90%) of adenocarcinomas of the cervix are caused by high-risk HPV infection and originate from conventional AIS as their precursor. These tumors are detected at early stages with screening cytology and HPV-testing initiatives [9, 83]. The remaining (10–15%) comprise a heterogeneous group of lesions with a more aggressive clinical behavior, obscure pathogenesis, and need of better early detection tools.

The International Endocervical Adenocarcinoma Classification and Criteria (IECC) has been recently introduced as a more biologically and clinically congruent system to stratify invasive endocervical glandular malignancy, compared to the morphology-based WHO classification [84]. This system divides adenocarcinomas into HPV-related and HPV-unrelated. Subdivision of HPV-unrelated tumors into pertinent subtypes (gastric, clear cell, mesonephric) is important because of their distinct clinico-pathologic features. HPV-related adenocarcinoma subtypes, on the other hand, are similar from a demo-

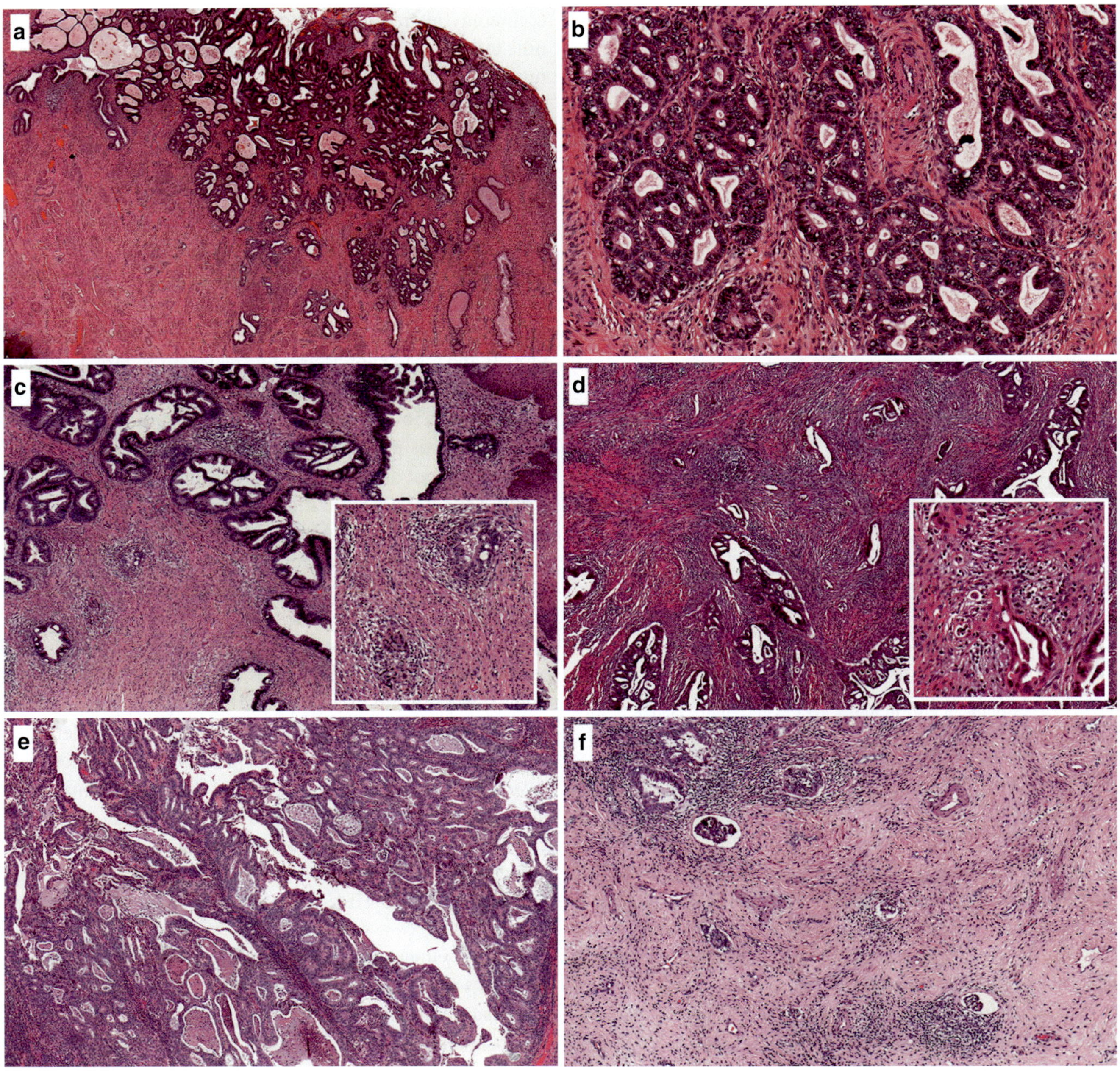

Fig. 13.7 Pattern-based classification. Pattern A (nondestructive) adenocarcinoma is well differentiated and diagnosed purely on the basis of glandular density and distribution (**a**, **b**). Focal destructive invasion, categorized as pattern B, arises from nondestructive glands (**c**); it is seen under high-power magnification as irregular glands and epithelial clusters (insert in C). Diffuse destructive invasion defines pattern C tumors; it can be seen as stromal desmoplasia (**d**), angulated and fragmented glands (insert in D), confluent solid, cribriform of papillary growth (**e**) and lymphovascular space invasion (**f**)

graphic and immunophenotypic perspective. A third group corresponds to rare tumors with unclear relationship to HPV infection (serous carcinoma), as well as unclassifiable and mixed lesions. Each subtype has an expected expression profile of immunohistochemical markers (mainly p16, progesterone receptor, vimentin and p53, see Table 13.4) [84].

It has been recently shown that compared to the WHO system, the IECC approach has superior interobserver agreement among gynecologic pathologists [85]. Importantly, agreement is substantial when distinguishing HPV-related from HPV-unrelated tumors, and in the diagnosis of important HPV-unrelated categories, which carry a more aggressive behavior (gastric). Conversely, the diagnosis of HPV-positive morphologic variants shows inferior reproducibility [85, 86]. Classification by pathologists as per the IECC also showed high correlation with HPV molecular

Table 13.4 Immunohistochemical profile of major types of endocervical adenocarcinoma

	HPV	p16	ER/PR	p53	Vimentin	mCEA
HPV-related	Positive	Overexpressed	Negative	Wild type	Negative	Positive
Gastric-type	Negative	Negative/patchy[a]	Negative	Abnormal[b]	Negative	Positive
Clear cell	Negative	Negative/patchy[a]	Negative	Wild type	Negative	Negative
Mesonephric	Negative	Negative/patchy[a]	Negative	Wild type	Negative	Positive
Endometrioid	Negative	Negative/patchy[a]	Positive	Wild type	Positive	Positive
Serous	Negative	Overexpressed	Pos/Neg	Abnormal	Pos/Neg	Positive

[a]p16 overexpression, independent from HPV infection, can be seen in these categories, particularly in poorly differentiated tumors
[b]Abnormal p53 staining (overexpression or complete absence) is seen in approximately 50% of gastric type tumors

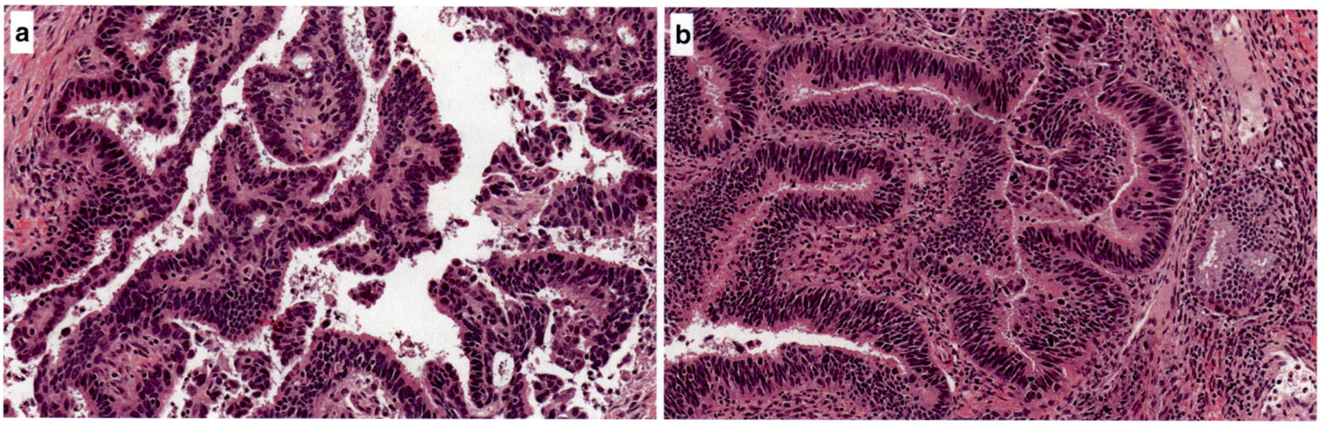

Fig. 13.8 Endocervical adenocarcinoma, usual type. Cytologically, this tumor type displays mucin depletion, nuclear hyperchromasia, and elongation similar to conventional AIS (**a**, **b**)

results. This suggests that the IECC is a more biologically congruent and clinically valuable system in the pathologic approach to endocervical adenocarcinoma.

The following paragraphs describe the pathology of invasive endocervical adenocarcinoma classified as per the IECC scheme (HPV-related and unrelated) and elaborates on the traditional WHO categories when appropriate. Miscellaneous lesions, including those with mixed or unusual patterns of glandular differentiation, are also covered here.

13.3.2 HPV-Related Endocervical Adenocarcinoma

By IECC definition, HPV-related adenocarcinoma contains *apical mitotic figures* and *apoptotic bodies*, easily identifiable at scanning magnification [84]. Well- to moderately differentiated forms of this adenocarcinoma type are characterized by columnar epithelium forming glandular structures of varying sizes and shapes; the luminal borders tend to be smooth. Solid nests, solid conglomerates, and individual cells are seen in poorly differentiated tumors. Morphologic variants are defined by the amount of intracytoplasmic mucin (usual versus mucinous) or by the architecture (villoglandular).

13.3.2.1 Usual Adenocarcinoma

Clinical Features

This subtype is, by far, the most common histologic type of adenocarcinoma of the cervix, accounting for 74–80% of cases [84, 87]. In fact, our cumulative knowledge of HPV-related adenocarcinoma is largely representative of usual-type lesions, by virtue of their frequency. While some patients present with symptoms (abnormal bleeding or pain), nowadays most cases are detected by screening cervicovaginal cytology.

Pathologic Features

Usual-type endocervical adenocarcinoma is comprised of columnar glandular epithelium with pseudostratified, elongated, and hyperchromatic nuclei and cytoplasmic mucin "depletion" (appreciable mucinous cytoplasm in 0–50% of cells only, Fig. 13.8).

Differential Diagnosis

Since usual-type adenocarcinoma has mucin depletion and consequently a pseudo-endometrioid phenotype, the most important differential diagnosis is with endometrioid carcinoma, either of cervical or endometrial origin. True endometrioid neoplastic proliferations display round, low-grade nuclei and generally lack the hyperchromasia and conspicuous mitotic activity seen in HPV-related endocervical lesions. In addition, the presence of "confirmatory endometrioid" features is in keeping with an endometrioid carcinoma (low-grade glands, squamous differentiation, and adjacent endometriosis) [84, 88]. The value of immunohistochemistry in distinguishing between endometrial and HPV-related usual endocervical adenocarcinoma is discussed later (see "Metastatic adenocarcinoma to the cervix").

13.3.2.2 Mucinous Adenocarcinoma

Counterintuitive to the mucinous nature of the normal endocervix, predominantly or purely mucinous tumors represent only a minority of all cervical adenocarcinomas [87]. They are divided based on the appearance of the intracytoplasmic mucin. It is now recognized that gastric mucinous carcinoma is a biologically separate entity; thus, it will be discussed later.

Mucinous Adenocarcinoma, Not Otherwise Specified

The mucinous variant, not otherwise specified, displays intracytoplasmic mucin in ≥50% of neoplastic cells, usually with a minor component of usual-type (mucin depleted) adenocarcinoma (Fig. 13.9). Mucin is of *endocervical type* (acid-type mucin with pale blue color in H&E preparations and dark purple staining in Alcian blue-PAS stain, akin to the normal endocervix).

Intestinal Type

Pathologic Features

A minority of HPV-related glandular malignancies of the uterine cervix display intestinal differentiation in the form of goblet cells, Paneth cells, and other entero-endocrine cells [89, 90] (Fig. 13.10). These tumors are relatively infrequent, described mostly in case reports and small series. While the biologic behavior of this subtype does not seem to differ from other HPV-related types, one study found that intestinal-type adenocarcinoma in situ was more likely to be associated with early invasive adenocarcinoma than usual-type adenocarcinoma in situ (31% vs. 17%) [30]. By immunohistochemistry, intestinal-type adenocarcinoma is positive for CK7 and negative/patchy for CK20. CDX2 is frequently positive, in keeping with an enteric phenotype [30].

Differential Diagnosis

When diffuse, intestinal differentiation and HPV-related adenocarcinoma may be confused with clear cell or gastric-type adenocarcinoma. It is important to note that gastric-type adenocarcinoma can contain goblet or neuroendocrine cells; thus, attention to the distinct cytologic features of this neoplasm is key (see description later). In addition, gastric-type tumors produce neutral-type mucin, which stains red in PAS-Alcian blue preparations; conversely, acid-type mucins characteristic of intestinal-type epithelium stain dark blue [47]. Another important consideration is secondary (metastatic) involvement of the cervix by an intestinal carcinoma. Primary endocervical tumors will show diffuse and strong p16 staining and are positive for high-risk HPV detection; in addition, patchy CK20 may help exclude colorectal metastases. CDX2 has been negative in intestinal-type endocervical adenocarcinoma in some series [91]; however, it's been shown to be frequently positive in others, limiting its diagnostic value [30, 92].

Signet-Ring Cell Type

Pathologic Features

This variant is exceedingly rare with less than 20 cases reported according to recent English literature reviews [93]. It is characterized by the presence of loose (non-cohesive) round cells with a mucinous vacuole that displaces the

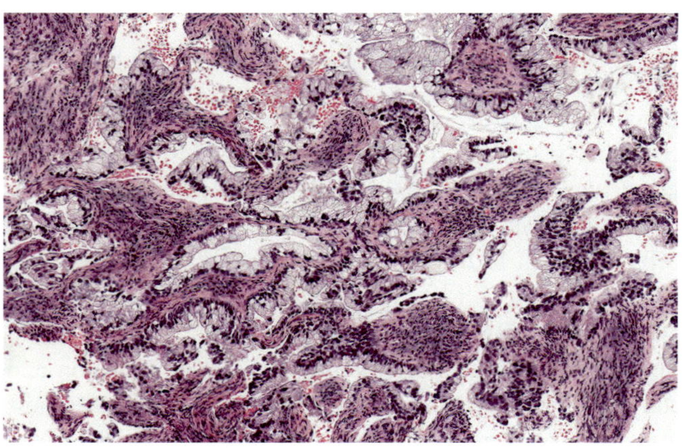

Fig. 13.9 Endocervical adenocarcinoma, mucinous endocervical type. This subtype is diagnosed when more than 50% of tumor cells contain endocervical-type mucin

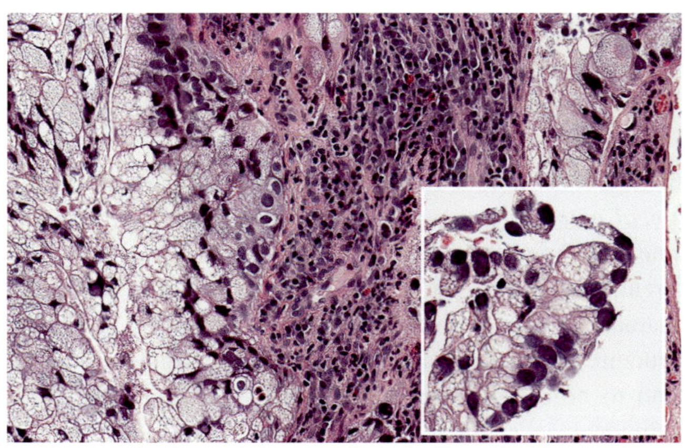

Fig. 13.10 Endocervical adenocarcinoma, mucinous intestinal type. This type is characterized by signs of intestinal differentiation including goblet cells (insert). This lesion was positive for p16 overexpression and high-risk HPV

nucleus to the side (imparting the classic appearance of a signet ring). These cells can grow in confluent sheets or be scattered throughout the stroma, which may appear normal if careful observation at high magnification is not performed. In adjacent areas usual or mucinous NOS morphology can be found. Interestingly, almost all cases subjected to HPV testing in the literature have revealed HPV type 18 DNA [93].

Differential Diagnosis

When encountering a cervical adenocarcinoma with signet-ring cell differentiation, a metastatic carcinoma from gastrointestinal or breast origin should be considered. Actually, this scenario may be even more frequent than a primary endocervical signet-ring cell carcinoma. It is important to know that not all metastatic cases have a previous or concurrent history of gastric or mammary cancer, and the cervical lesion may be the presenting sign / symptom [94, 95]. Features suggestive of metastases include extensive cervical involvement with prominent lymphatic vascular invasion and absence of an intraepithelial precursor (AIS or HSIL). Conversely, detection of HPV DNA can confirm a primary cervical origin. Immunohistochemistry has a value in excluding a breast primary; signet-ring mammary carcinomas are almost always of lobular type, and will express hormone receptors and GATA3. Unfortunately, the immunophenotype of cervical and gastrointestinal signet-ring cell carcinomas overlaps, since both are positive for CK7 and show variable expression of CK20, CDX2, and mucins [96]. In HPV-negative and equivocal cases, the pathologist should raise the possibility of metastases and prompt clinical and radiologic investigations to exclude it.

Prognosis and Management

Prognosis is very poor in patients with advanced stage at presentation. Early stage tumors, on the other hand, tend to be associated with good prognosis after surgical +/− adjuvant systemic treatment [97, 98].

Stratified Mucin-Producing Carcinoma

Pathologic Features

Recently, an invasive carcinoma with morphology reminiscent of SMILE has been described under the name "invasive stratified mucin-producing carcinoma" (ISMC) [99]. Most of these carcinomas are associated with adjacent SMILE. The invasive lesion is comprised of stratified, immature nuclei with variable intracytoplasmic mucin, usually with solid and/or nested tumor architecture (Fig. 13.11). Most of these lesions are architecturally moderately or poorly differentiated; however, cytologic features tend to be low grade (nuclei similar to other HPV-related variants, intracytoplasmic mucin), which is a helpful diagnostic clue. Like SMILE, electron microscopy studies of ISMC showed ultrastructural evidence of glandular differentiation with microvilli, vacuolar structures, and mitochondria, supporting the hypothesis that these lesions represent stratified variants of endocervical glandular malignancy [45].

Differential Diagnosis

The differential diagnosis of ISMC includes adenosquamous carcinoma, since both lesions display a stratified neoplastic population. Adenosquamous carcinoma is comprised of distinct glandular and squamous populations. The presence of a definitive squamous cell component (keratinization, intercellular junctions) will favor this entity. Absence of squamous differentiation, diffuse scattered presence of mucin-producing cells, and adjacent SMILE are features more consistent with ISMC.

13.3.2.3 Villoglandular Carcinoma

Pathologic Features

This adenocarcinoma type is characterized by its prominent exophytic papillary growth. Villoglandular adenocarcinoma

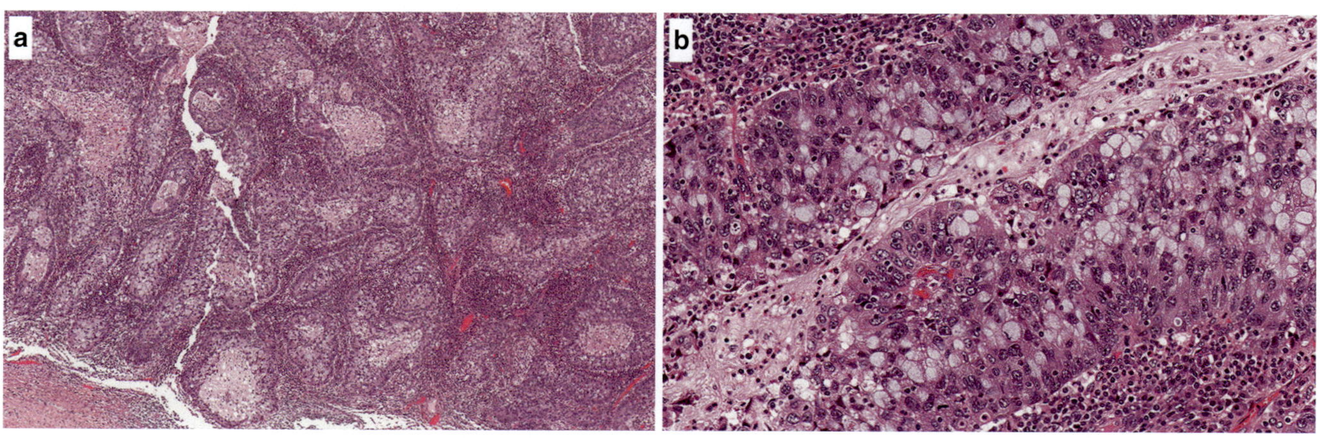

Fig. 13.11 Invasive stratified mucin-producing carcinoma. Gland formation is retained in this invasive tumor; however, lining epithelium is stratified (**a**) and comprised of mucin-producing atypical cells (**b**)

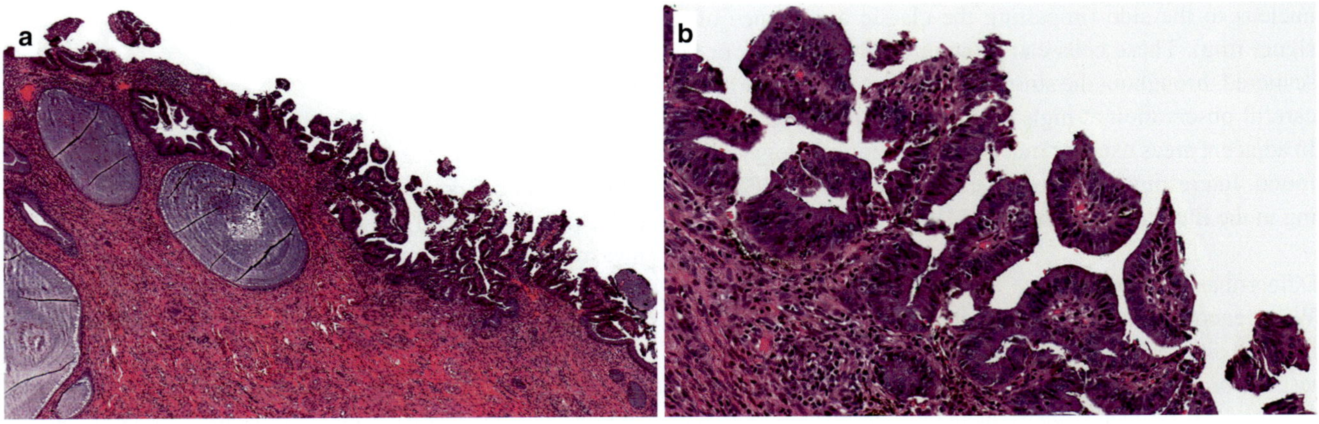

Fig. 13.12 Endocervical adenocarcinoma, villoglandular type. The lesion is usually superficial and exophytic (**a**); papillary-like projections are lined by columnar epithelium akin to usual-type adenocarcinoma (**b**)

is described as predominantly superficial and composed of papillae of varying thickness and length, containing central fibrous cores with numerous inflammatory cells [100, 101] (Fig. 13.12). Papillae are lined by columnar pseudostratified epithelial cells similar to adenocarcinoma of the usual- or mucinous-types. The deep aspect of the tumor consists of branching tubular glands, well demarcated from the adjacent cervical stroma.

Differential Diagnosis

Similar to other types of HPV-related adenocarcinoma, the differential diagnosis includes endometrial endometrioid carcinoma involving the cervix, since some endometrial endometrioid carcinomas display villoglandular growth. The presence of HPV-related features (apical mitoses, apoptosis, and hyperchromatic elongated nuclei) should suggest an endocervical process. Immunohistochemistry can be helpful to differentiate cervical primary from endometrial metastasis (see "metastatic carcinoma to cervix"). Other primary cervical lesions can display prominent exophytic papillary growth, importantly serous and clear cell carcinoma. Unlike high-grade forms of adenocarcinoma, nuclear atypia in villoglandular carcinoma is at most moderate and the nuclear-to-cytoplasmic ratio is low. An abnormal p53 stain argues against villoglandular carcinoma, and suggests a serous neoplasm (less likely clear cell). Napsin-A expression should raise concern for clear cell carcinoma.

Prognosis and Management

The prognosis of villoglandular adenocarcinoma was traditionally considered excellent, and conservative management with simple excision was advocated [100, 101]. More recently, however, tumor recurrence and death from disease have been documented in a significant proportion of cases [102–104], and survival analyses have shown similar trends between villoglandular and other subtypes [82, 105]. In a relatively large recent cohort, the overall and disease-free 5-year survival was 82% and 75%, respectively [106]. Importantly, several pathologic features are associated with poor prognosis, including involvement of the deep cervical stroma, lymphovascular space invasion, lymph node metastases, and advanced stage at presentation [102, 107]. Consequently, conservative surgical treatment should only be considered after cone / LEEP evaluation demonstrates negative margins and tumor restricted to the surface / superficial stroma [106, 108]. Standard treatment, akin to other adenocarcinoma types, is the norm for patients with clinical or pathologic adverse factors.

13.3.3 HPV-Unrelated Endocervical Adenocarcinoma

13.3.3.1 Gastric Mucinous Adenocarcinoma (Including Minimal Deviation Adenocarcinoma)

Awareness of the existence of HPV-unrelated neoplasms has markedly increased over the last decade, greatly due to the advances in our understanding of gastric-type differentiation in the endocervix. Indeed, according to recent classifications, gastric type adenocarcinoma is the most frequent type of HPV-independent endocervical adenocarcinoma.

Clinical Features

The median age of patients with gastric type adenocarcinoma is 49 years (range 37–84) [109]. Presenting symptoms include bleeding, watery vaginal discharge, and cytologic abnormalities (atypical cells with yellowish-orange intracytoplasmic mucin) [46]. A latex agglutination test using HIK1083 (a marker of pyloric gland mucin) is available as a screening tool for patients with watery discharge; initial studies on this tool demonstrated high sensitivity and specificity for gastric-type proliferations (LEGH, atypical LEGH and MDA) [110].

Pathologic Features

Macroscopically, the lesion can be polypoid or ulcerated; in typical cases the cervical wall is indurated and expanded in a circumferential fashion (so-called "barrel" shaped cervix) [111].

Gastric differentiation in the cervix is defined as conversion towards a gastric, "pyloric" type mucinous phenotype. Gastric mucins are neutral, whereas endocervical mucins are acidic. Neutral mucins stain pale red in Alcian blue/PAS special stain, whereas acid mucins stain dark purple/blue [47]. On H&E preparations, gastric-type epithelium is characterized by cells with *clear or pale eosinophilic cytoplasm* and *distinct cell borders* [109]. The reproducibility of the diagnosis of gastric-type adenocarcinoma as defined is substantial [112]. On the other hand, interobserver agreement of the distinction between minimal deviation adenocarcinoma and benign endocervical proliferations is poor, likely due to its deceptively bland morphology [113].

Gastric-type adenocarcinoma is classified into two groups: MDA (also known as Adenoma Malignum) and gastric adenocarcinoma not otherwise specified (GA-NOS). MDA is characterized by (Fig. 13.13):

- *Low-grade morphology:* minimal to absent cytologic atypia, abundant apical mucin, well-defined glands with a claw-like pattern.
- Deep haphazard gland distribution with minimal to no desmoplastic reaction.

This low-grade morphology must be present in 90% or more of the tumor. If less, the tumor is classified as GA-NOS [114, 115] (Fig. 13.14). GA-NOS tumors are usually moderately to poorly differentiated with destructive and florid stromal invasion. Lymphovascular space invasion is frequent (48% of cases).

Ancillary Studies

By immunohistochemistry, tumor cells are frequently positive for markers of gastric epithelial differentiation MUC6 and HIK1083, although expression can be focal [109, 116]. Other frequently positive markers include PAX8, carbonic anhydrase IX, CA19-9, CK7, CK20 (focal), and CDX2 (focal) [117]. PAX2 expression is lost in most cases [117, 118]. Unlike HPV-related tumors, GAS and MDA usually lack p16 overexpression (stain is either negative or patchy); however, high-grade GAS and occasional MDA cases can demonstrate p16 overexpression, unrelated to HPV [84, 119]. In such instance, HPV detection studies should be considered. p53 expression is abnormal in approximately 45% of gastric-type tumors, whereas most (~100%) HPV-related carcinomas show normal (wild type) expression [120]. Loss of PAX2 expression has been documented in MDA but not in benign lesions [118]. Estrogen and progesterone receptors are typically negative.

Gastric mucinous adenocarcinoma has been found to be negative for HPV infection in numerous studies [114, 121, 122]. Besides this, the molecular mechanisms underlying the pathogenesis of gastric-type adenocarcinoma are still largely unknown. MDA has been described in patients with Peutz-Jeghers syndrome, which is related to alterations in the *LKB1/STK11* gene [111]. Interestingly, *LKB1/STK11* mutations have also been identified in sporadic MDA [123].

Differential Diagnosis

The differential diagnosis of gastric mucinous endocervical adenocarcinoma is wide. MDA can be mistaken as benign endocervical tissue, even in resection specimens. A haphazard arrangement of the glands, extension into deep stroma, and circumferential cervical involvement are all abnormal features that should raise suspicion for a malignant process. While subtle, the clear to eosinophilic mucinous profile of MDA and GAS glands can be appreciated by an attentive eye and contrasted with the mucin of the normal endocervix.

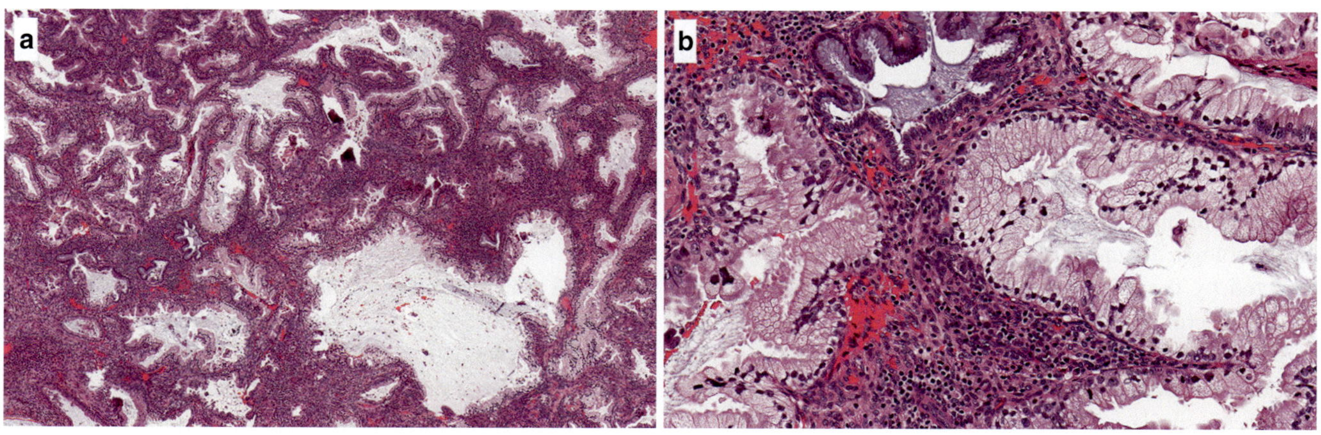

Fig. 13.13 Gastric-type endocervical adenocarcinoma, minimal deviation type. Well-formed glands haphazardly distributed throughout the cervical wall (**a**); neoplastic glands display "gastric" features including abundant pale vacuolated cytoplasm and distinct cell borders (**b**); epithelium is extremely bland (compare to normal cervical gland on top center)

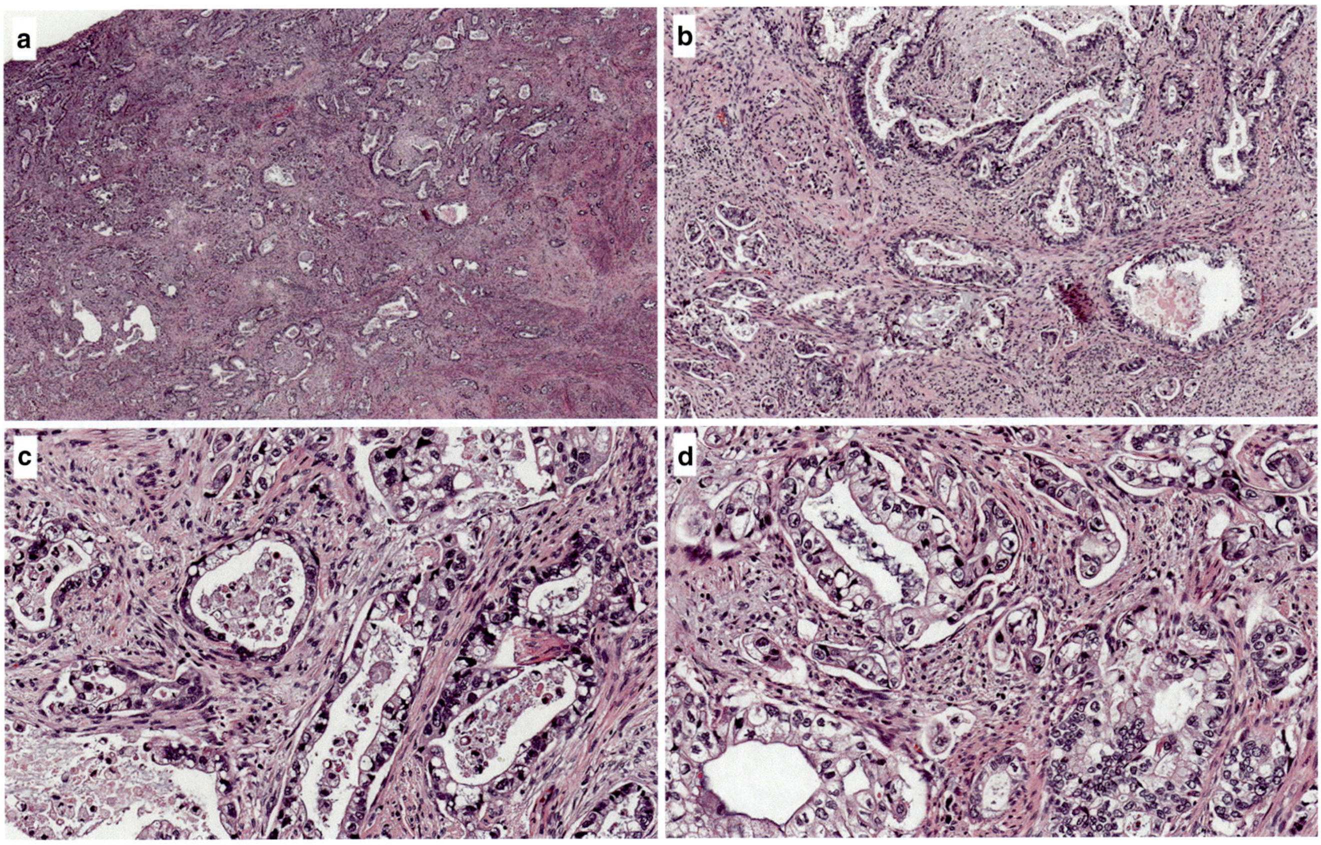

Fig. 13.14 Gastric-type endocervical adenocarcinoma, not otherwise specified. These tumors tend to be widely infiltrative (**a**) and less differentiated, at least focally (**b**, lower left). Gland forming epithelium displays marked nuclear pleomorphism and abundant vacuolated mucinous cytoplasm (**c** and **d**)

Unlike LEGH, MDA lacks a lobulated architecture and often extends beyond the superficial stroma.

Tumors in the GAS spectrum can be easily recognized as malignant; however, distinction from a HPV-related lesion can be difficult. In fact, adenocarcinomas with mixed morphology have been described; these cases display areas with usual-type morphology (mucin-depleted cells with apical mitoses and apoptosis) admixed with areas of gastric-type morphology (abundant, pale to eosinophilic cytoplasm) [124]. These cases demonstrate either a gastric (most commonly) or a usual phenotype by ancillary studies (HIK1083, p53, p16, and HPV molecular studies) indicating that they are tumors with variant morphology instead of truly "mixed" lesions. This highlights the importance of ancillary testing in the pathologic diagnosis of endocervical adenocarcinoma, as depicted by the IECC. Another important, although infrequent, differential is a metastatic gastric carcinoma to the cervix. These lesions usually have signet-ring cells, which are not typical of GAS. However, morphologic and immunophenotypic similarity exists, and exclusion of a gastrointestinal tract primary should be recommended to the treating physician if one cannot be convinced that a gastric-type malignancy is primary cervical or metastatic in origin.

Prognosis and Management

Gastric-type endocervical mucinous adenocarcinoma is a biologically aggressive neoplasm. Compared to usual-type adenocarcinoma, it has significantly higher rates of ovarian, pelvic, and abdominal metastases as well as regional and distal lymph node involvement [114]. Up to 60% of cases present at stage II or higher. 5-year disease-free survival is 30%, and overall survival is 42% (compared to 77 and 91% for usual-type tumors, respectively) [109, 114]. Importantly, this tumor has a poor prognosis regardless of the degree of differentiation. In fact, similarly to poorly differentiated tumors, extremely well differentiated forms (MDA) have high rates of extra-uterine spread with up to 50% mortality rate [114].

13.3.3.2 Endometrioid Adenocarcinoma

In this textbook, this tumor type is defined following the IECC recommendations which differ from the WHO classification. The latter defines endometrioid carcinoma as "morphologically similar to endometrioid adenocarcinomas of the uterine corpus" and divides it etiologically into HPV-related and endometriosis-related (HPV-negative) categories [11]. Unfortunately, this WHO definition, as with prior literature,

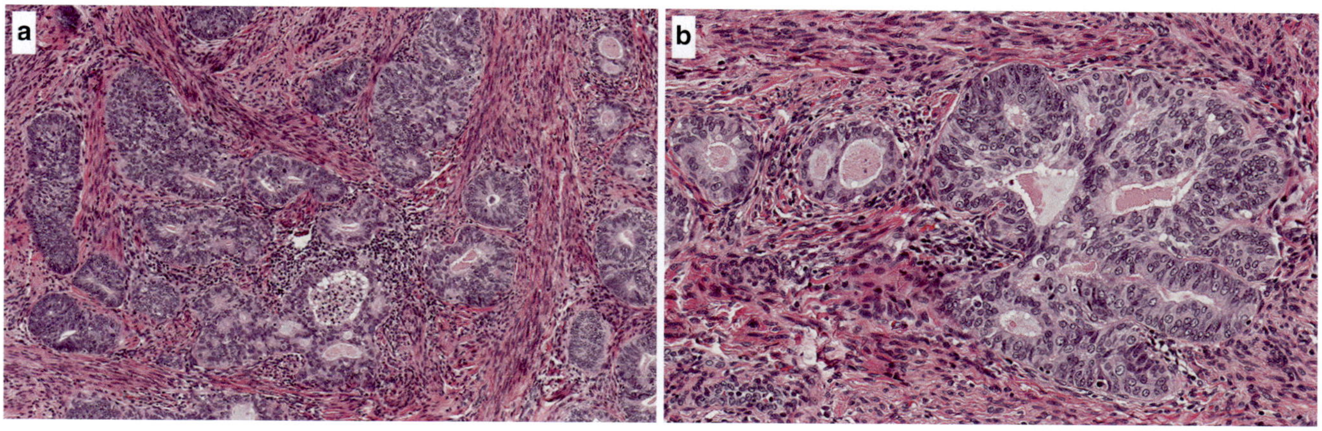

Fig. 13.15 Endometrioid endocervical adenocarcinoma. The morphology is identical to that seen in endometrial endometrioid carcinoma (see Fig. 13.19a,b). Cells are columnar and mucin-depleted, but lack the hyperchromasia, elongation, and mitotic activity of HPV-related adenocarcinoma (**a**, **b**)

is vague, greatly overlapping with the description of usual-type and endometrioid-type carcinomas. Not surprisingly, the diagnosis of endometrioid endocervical adenocarcinoma is one that often causes confusion among pathologists and treating clinicians. The IECC approach is preferred because it separates true "endometrioid" morphology from the spectrum of HPV-related cervical glandular neoplasia.

Pathologic Features

The term endometrioid carcinoma, as per IECC, is reserved for tumors with low-grade endometrioid glands *and* confirmatory endometrioid features (squamous metaplasia, endometriosis, Fig. 13.15). Under this definition, endometrioid carcinoma is rare, representing ~1% of cervical adenocarcinomas [84]. It is suggested to originate from endometriosis or other type of endometrioid-type precursor in the cervix, and is unrelated to HPV infection [125].

A similar entity is the so-called "minimal deviation endometrioid adenocarcinoma" [126, 127]. This term refers to neoplasms with bland glandular endometrioid cytomorphology and deceptively well-differentiated architecture; usually located in the upper endocervix/lower uterine segment [128, 129].

Differential Diagnosis

The chief differential diagnosis is a primary endometrial endometrioid carcinoma with a "minimal deviation" pattern of spreading into cervical stroma [130, 131]. The immunophenotype of these lesions mirrors that of an endometrial endometrioid carcinoma (ER positive, vimentin positive, CEA negative) [128]. Given the considerable histologic and immunophenotypic overlap, determination of origin (endocervical or endometrial) in this context can be quite difficult in biopsy material, thus deferral to assessment on hysterectomy is recommended. One last consideration is the occurrence of synchronous primary endometrial and endocervical endometrioid carcinomas, which has been suggested in a few patients based on DNA clonality and loss of heterozygosity [132].

13.3.3.3 Clear Cell Adenocarcinoma

Clinical Features

Clear cell carcinoma of the uterine cervix accounts for 4% of all cervical adenocarcinomas [133]. An association with in utero exposure to diethylstilbestrol (DES) has been described; in patients with such exposure, incidence peaks at young age (median age 26 years) and again later in life (median age 71 years) [134, 135]. Use of DES during pregnancy has been long discontinued. Nowadays, only a minority of clear cell carcinomas are related to DES exposure (6% in one study) [136]. Median age of patients with clear cell carcinoma is 53 years. Most patients present with vaginal bleeding. Cervicovaginal cytology is abnormal only in a small proportion of cases (18%), limiting its screening value for this entity [136].

Pathologic Features

Histologically, clear cell carcinoma is arranged in tubulocystic, papillary and solid patterns, similar to its ovarian and endometrial counterparts [137]. Papillae usually have hyalinized fibrovascular cores. The cytomorphology of clear cell carcinoma is distinctive: tumor cells are cuboidal, have clear (translucent) cytoplasm and enlarged nuclei that protrude towards the luminal aspect, giving a "hobnail" appearance (Fig. 13.16). Cells with clear cytoplasm can be only focal or absent (their presence is not required for this diagnosis). "Non-clear" cells have a vaguely eosinophilic and granular cytoplasm.

Ancillary Studies

Unlike usual-type adenocarcinoma, cervical clear cell carcinoma is unrelated to HPV infection [138]. Microsatellite instability and somatic mutations of microsatellite repeats

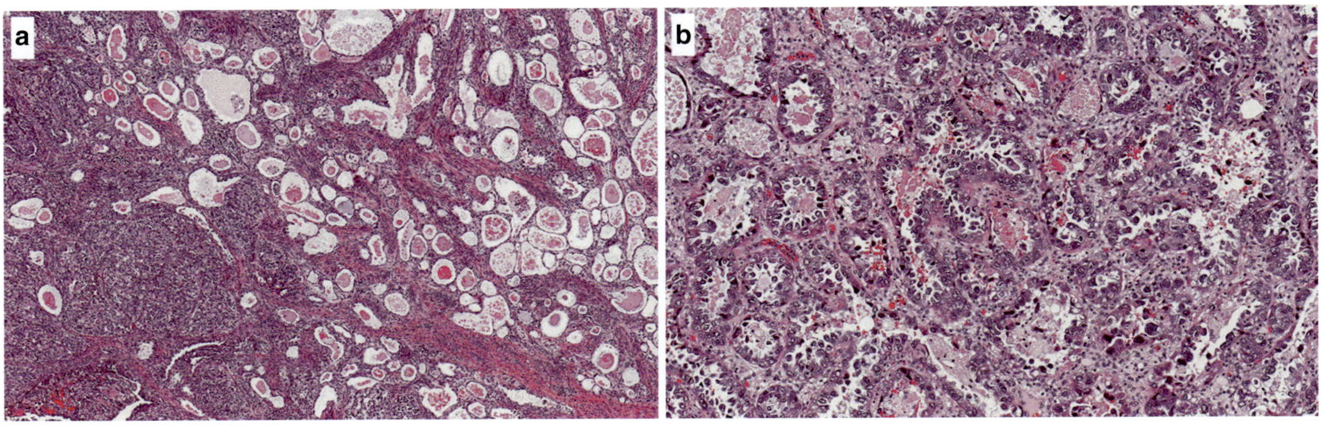

Fig. 13.16 Clear cell endocervical adenocarcinoma. The lesion usually has varying architecture with tubulocystic (**a**, right) and solid (**a**, left) patterns. Tumor cells have scant cytoplasm and highly atypical nuclei protruding towards the lumen (hobnail pattern) (**b**). Notice the absence of clear cytoplasm in this area of the tumor (clear cytoplasm is not a requirement for this diagnosis)

has been documented in clear cell carcinoma, predominantly in cases associated with DES exposure [139]. EGFR and HER2 overexpression has been observed in 75% and 25% of cases, respectively, as well as activation of *AKT* and *mTOR* in 58% and 50% of cases, respectively [138].

While unrelated to HPV infection, p16 is frequently strongly and diffusely positive in clear cell carcinoma [120]. Also, like most other types of endocervical adenocarcinoma, estrogen and progesterone receptors are negative in this tumor. On the other hand, monoclonal carcinoembryonic antigen (CEA) appears to be consistently negative in clear cell carcinoma, and may be of value in distinguishing clear cell from other subtypes [120]. Napsin-A is frequently positive in endocervical clear cell carcinoma [140]; however, Arias-Stella reaction can also express this marker [141].

Differential Diagnosis

The differential diagnosis includes not only other types of cervical glandular malignancy but also benign lesions, most importantly microglandular hyperplasia and Arias-Stella reaction. Microglandular hyperplasia can have a complex architectural appearance with back-to-back glands mimicking a tubulocystic clear cell carcinoma. However, cells in microglandular hyperplasia contain mucinous cytoplasm and lack nuclear atypia. Arias-Stella reaction is an important differential. Although it is usually seen in the context of pregnancy or high-dose progestin exposure, such history may not be apparent in all cases. Arias-Stella reaction is characterized by cells with abundant cytoplasm and markedly enlarged nuclei. However, unlike clear cell carcinoma, the nuclear-to-cytoplasmic ratio remains low (since cytoplasm is abundant) and there is no mitotic activity. Rare malignant lesions in the differential, particularly in the pediatric population, include yolk sac tumor (reticular pattern, Schiller-Duval bodies, α-fetoprotein expression) and alveolar soft part sarcoma (PAS-positive intracytoplasmic crystals).

Prognosis and Management

The majority of patients with cervical clear cell carcinoma are diagnosed at early stage (FIGO stage I or II) and have an overall good prognosis. Pelvic lymph node involvement is seen in 25% of patients and is associated with lymphovascular space invasion. Chemotherapy and radiation has been reported to be useful in advanced-stage tumors or with high-risk factors (lymphatic vascular invasion, parametrial involvement, tumor size >4 cm, >2/3 cervical stromal invasion, positive margins) [133, 136].

13.3.3.4 Mesonephric Adenocarcinoma

Clinical Features

Mesonephric carcinoma of the cervix represents less than 1% of all cervical carcinomas [142]. The morphologic and immunohistochemical similarities with mesonephric remnants support a mesonephric derivation [143, 144]. Patient age at presentation ranges from 24 to 72 years (median age 43–52 years) [144–146]. Most patients present with abnormal bleeding, abnormal Pap smear, or with a mass detected on examination.

Pathologic Features

Macroscopically, the tumor presents in the lateral aspect of the cervix or with circumferential cervical involvement. Microscopically, mesonephric carcinoma characteristically shows a spectrum of architectural patterns including tubuloglandular, ductal, retiform, solid, spindle cell, and sex cord-like (Fig. 13.17). Better differentiated areas have small, round, glandular, and tubular structures containing eosinophilic luminal secretions, resembling benign mesonephric structures. A retiform pattern is characterized by slit-like spaces outlined by branching papillae. Solid and spindle cell components are usually present in variable proportions. When present, the spindle cell component usually has malig-

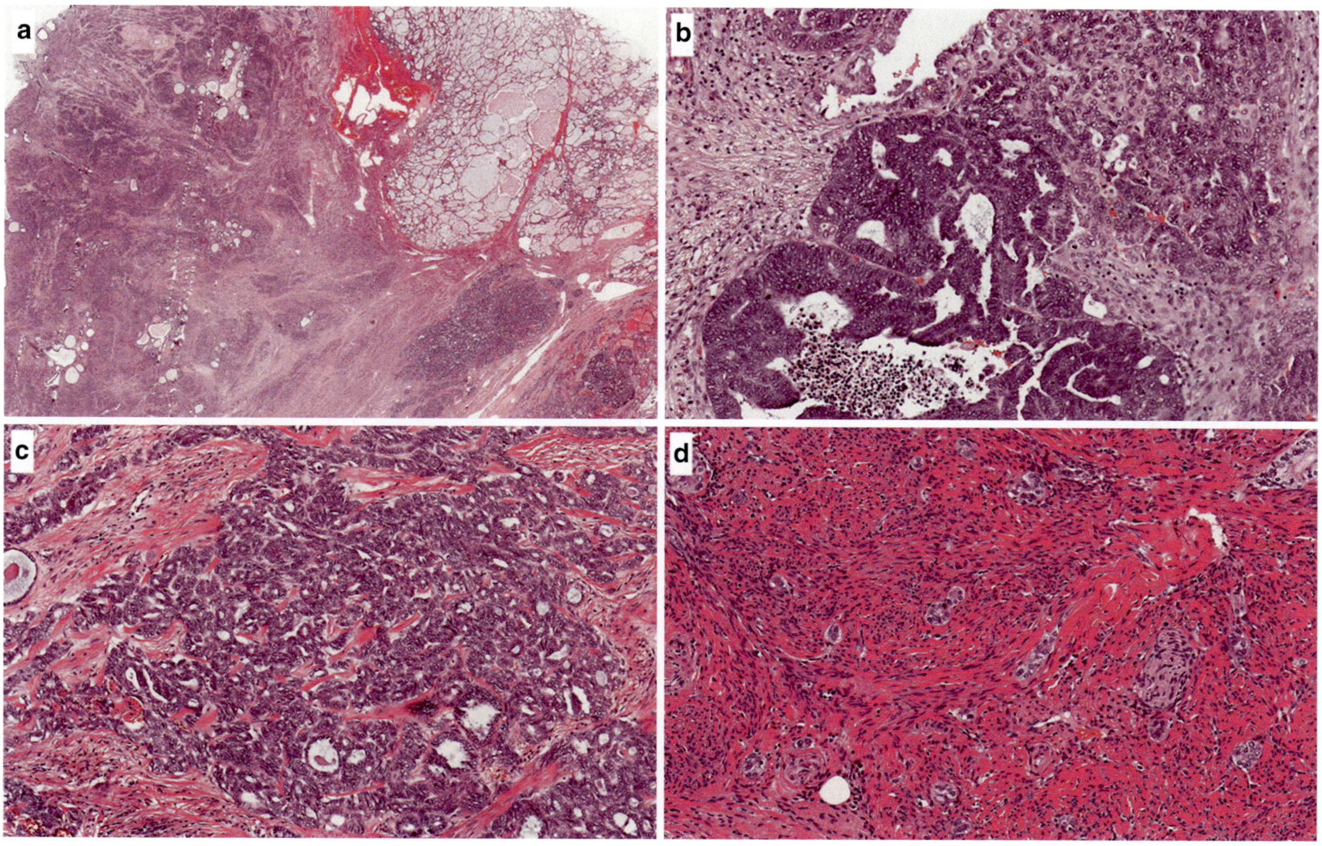

Fig. 13.17 Mesonephric adenocarcinoma. This tumor was located in the deep cervical and uterine wall. Carcinoma typically has a range of architectural patterns including tubulo-glandular (**a**), ductal (**b**), and retiform (**c**). Deceptively bland infiltration, mimicking mesonephric hyperplasia, can be observed (**d**)

nant features resembling an endometrial stromal sarcoma. In these cases, the term "malignant mixed mesonephric tumor" has been used [145, 146].

Ancillary Studies

By immunohistochemistry, mesonephric carcinoma cells are positive for keratins, calretinin, vimentin, CD10 (apical staining), and GATA3; conversely, they lack estrogen and progesterone receptor expression [144, 147]. Of importance, this tumor is also positive for PAX8 and can express p16, although focally in most cases [148]. At the molecular level, mesonephric carcinoma is characterized by recurrent *KRAS* mutations, detected in 81% of cases [142]. HPV has not been detected in this tumor [148].

Differential Diagnosis

The differential diagnosis mainly includes Müllerian (endocervical or endometrial) adenocarcinoma and mesonephric remnants. A deep cervical or uterine wall location and a variety of architectural patterns will be more in keeping with a mesonephric neoplasm. Conversely, definitive mucinous, tubal, or endometrioid morphology indicates a Müllerian tumor. In challenging cases, immunohistochemistry can help; the most useful markers, as described above, are GATA3, CD10, calretinin, p16, and ER/PR.

Prognosis and Management

The biologic behavior of mesonephric carcinoma appears to be better than Müllerian cervical adenocarcinomas when adjusted for stage. Nonetheless, recurrences have been reported in early stage cases and adverse outcome is usually seen in cases with advanced stage [144]. Malignant mixed mesonephric tumors tend to present at advanced stage suggesting a more aggressive course [146].

13.3.4 Other Adenocarcinoma Types

13.3.4.1 Serous Carcinoma

Primary cervical serous carcinoma is rare; in fact, some authors believe that its occurrence is debatable and that cases reported actually represent either lower uterine segment endometrial tumors or cervical metastases of endometrial, tubal, ovarian or peritoneal origin [149, 150]. This derives from the observation that, by using strict current morphologic and immunohistochemical criteria, such diagnosis is hardly ever encountered nowadays [84]. As a counterargument, misdiagnosis may explain some but not all cases of endocervical serous carcinoma reported in the literature [151–153]. For instance, 3 out of 10 endocervical serous carcinomas studied by *Nofech-Mozes et al.* underwent hysterectomy or pelvic exenteration, and no endometrial or tubo-ovarian malignancy was identified; these tumors were included following strict criteria (high-grade, pleomorphic nuclei and focal papillary tufting in at least 50% of its mass) [154]. Therefore, endocervical serous carcinoma as an entity remains in the current IECC and WHO classification systems.

Clinical Features

In its initial descriptions, the age at presentation of cervical serous carcinoma was wide, with a peak in young patients (<40 years old) followed by a second peak after 65 years of age [152]. Most patients present with abnormal vaginal bleeding and abnormal cytologic findings.

Pathologic Features

Microscopically, serous carcinoma of the cervix displays the characteristic papillary and micropapillary tufting seen in other sites. Severe nuclear atypia is a requirement for this diagnosis; it is usually evident at low-power magnification as pleomorphic cells with loss of polarity, high nuclear-to-cytoplasmic ratio, and prominent eosinophilic nucleoli (Fig. 13.18). Mitotic activity is usually high, >10 mitoses per 10 HPFs [152]. Psammoma bodies are observed in a minority of cases.

Ancillary Studies

Mutation of the *TP53* gene is an early carcinogenic event in serous carcinoma of the female genital tract, and abnormal expression of p53 has been reported in endocervical serous carcinoma [154, 155]. WT1 expression has been observed in only a few patients; in fact, when encountered, this finding should raise suspicion for a tubo-ovarian primary. Only 6 out of 17 (35%) cases in the pooled literature were positive for high-risk HPV DNA [155–158].

Differential Diagnosis

Given its rarity, the diagnosis of endocervical serous carcinoma is one of exclusion. Clear cell and gastric type endocervical adenocarcinomas usually display marked nuclear pleomorphism. The architecture of clear cell carcinoma is usually distinct, characterized by the presence of tubulocystic areas or simple papillae with hyalinized cores. Gastric type adenocarcinoma has a more columnar glandular architecture and cells contain abundant, vacuolated mucinous cytoplasm. Ancillary studies have limited value: abnormal p53 expression and p16 overexpression can be seen in serous, gastric, and clear cell types. Other markers such as Napsin-A (for clear cell) and HIK1083 (for gastric type) can be considered. HPV-related endocervical adenocarcinoma of the usual (endocervical) type can also mimic serous carcinoma, especially if having solid or papillary architecture; these lesions tend to have a lower nuclear-to-cytoplasmic ratio and lesser degrees of atypia. Importantly, p53 will help in this differential as staining is normal in usual-type endocervical adenocarcinoma. Lastly, in the presence of an unequivocal serous carcinoma based on morphology and immunophenotype, endocervical origin should only be entertained after an endo-

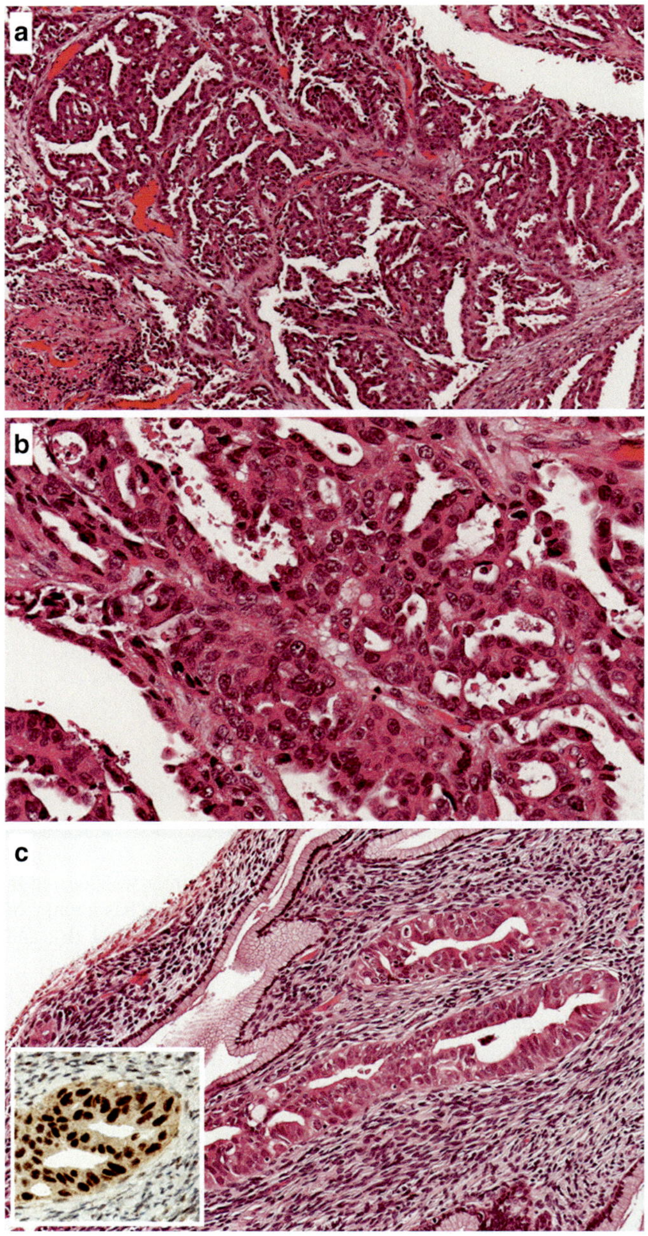

Fig. 13.18 Serous endocervical carcinoma. Tumor in this case was confined to the cervix; endometrium, ovaries and tubes were unremarkable. It is possible, however, the the tumor originated in the lower uterine segment. Tumor shows complex micropapillary growth with slit-like spaces (**a**); tumor cells have high-grade features including prominent nucleoli and high nuclear-to-cytoplasmic ratio (**b**). An intraglandular component with similar morphology and p53 overexpression was also identified (**c**, insert). This lesion was negative for p16 and HPV molecular studies

metrial or upper genital serous carcinoma has been thoroughly excluded.

Prognosis and management

Prognosis largely depends on tumor stage with tumors showing extra-uterine spread at presentation (FIGO stage II or greater) having dismal 5-year survival [153, 159]. Radical surgery followed by radiation and/or chemotherapy is the standard of treatment. Upfront chemoradiation, usually recommended in patients with advanced disease, can have a significant response [160, 161].

13.3.4.2 Metastatic Adenocarcinoma to the Cervix

Secondary involvement of the uterine cervix by carcinoma is, in most instances, caused by an endometrial malignancy. Metastases from other genital organs and from extra-genital sites are, in comparison, quite uncommon [162]. The relatively small size of the cervix and its limited vasculature relative to the volume of stroma are possible explanations for the rarity of this scenario [163, 164]. Not surprisingly, misdiagnosis of a metastatic cervical lesion as primary endocervical adenocarcinoma occurs commonly (up to 42% of cases) [162].

Endometrial Adenocarcinoma

Involvement of cervical stroma by endometrial carcinoma is an important diagnosis, since it influences staging and subsequent patient management. Well-differentiated endometrioid carcinoma can mimic an HPV-related usual-type endocervical carcinoma; both are mucin-depleted and display glands with tall columnar to cuboidal cells (Fig. 13.19). Features that should raise the possibility of an endometrial primary are: round nuclei with less conspicuous pseudostratification and relative hypochromasia, squamous differentiation that appears bland morphologically, secretory differentiation and foamy histiocytes within the periglandular stroma. The presence of a precursor lesion is also a helpful clue in determining origin (AIS versus endometrioid intraepithelial neoplasia, especially in biopsy material). Microglandular hyperplasia can be cribriform, mimicking endometrioid carcinoma involving the cervix. Nonetheless, microglandular hyperplasia has a characteristic stratification pattern (with a layer of basal reserve cells underneath a layer of columnar mucinous to clear cells) and bland nuclear morphology. As discussed previously, a primary cervical endometrioid carcinoma is a rare but documented event, and should be considered if definitive endometrioid features are present in a background of cervical endometriosis.

Immunohistochemistry for ER, p16, vimentin, and mCEA is widely used to assist in the distinction between endometrioid endometrial carcinoma and HPV-related endocervical adenocarcinoma (either usual or mucinous type). The expected profile of HPV-related endocervical adenocarcinoma is p16 overexpressed (diffuse and strong, nuclear and cytoplasmic), ER negative, vimentin negative, and mCEA positive (membranous); the opposite profile is expected in endometrioid tumors: p16 negative or patchy, ER positive (any nuclear staining, typically diffuse—50% or more), vimentin positive (membranous), and mCEA negative [36, 165–167]. Nonetheless, as many as 50% of endocervical and 30% of endometrial carcinomas deviate from the expected profile at least in one marker [168]. It is important to note that high-grade endometrial carcinomas can have p16 over-

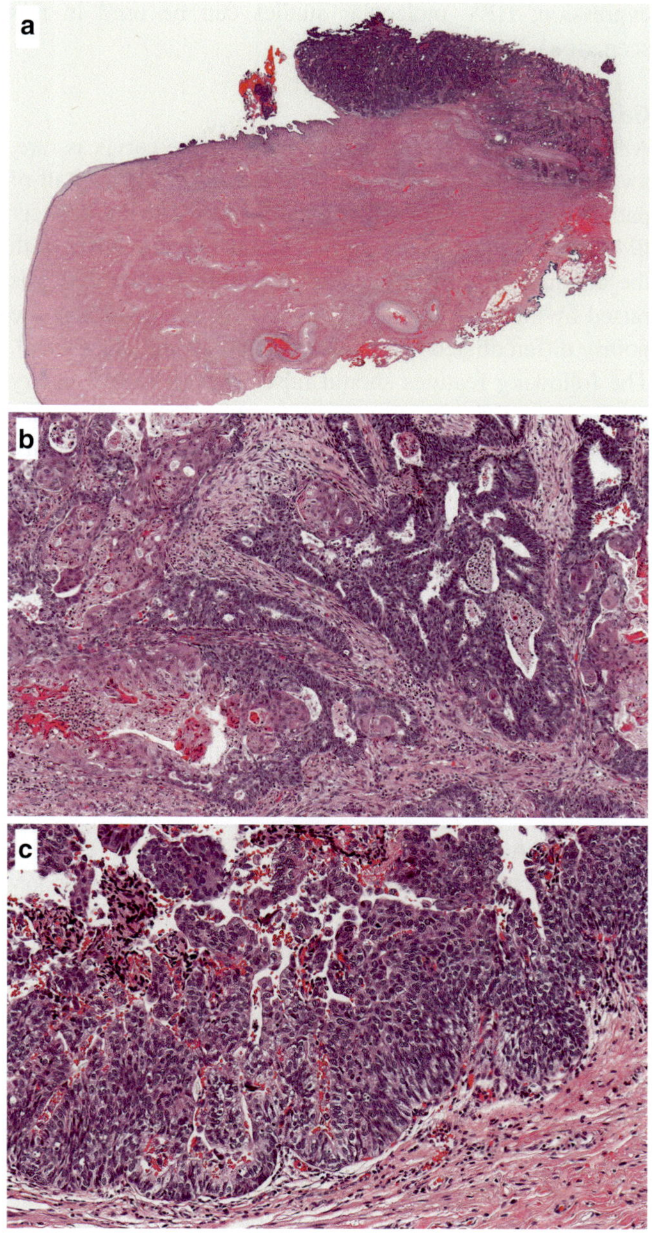

Fig. 13.19 Metastatic adenocarcinoma to the cervix. The most common carcinoma secondarily involving the cervix is endometrial, usually by direct extension from the corpus (**a**); classic endometrioid morphology is observed, including squamous differentiation (**b**). Urothelial carcinoma can spread to the cervix in a pagetoid fashion mimicking a primary cervical malignancy (**c**)

expression; HPV molecular studies can be used in this scenario.

Gastric Adenocarcinoma

Although gastric carcinoma metastatic to the cervix is rare, awareness of its occurrence is important since almost half of patients present without previous history of gastric cancer [94, 95] and the primary is discovered synchronously with the cervical lesion or after the possibility of metastases is raised by the pathologist [163]. Most metastatic tumors are poorly differentiated and have a signet-ring cell component. The following features should raise concern for secondary origin: poor differentiation, extensive lymphovascular space invasion, multifocality, and extension to other pelvic organs. When a tumor with signet-ring morphology is encountered, the possibility of a primary cervical signet-ring cell mucinous carcinoma should be considered and investigated with p16 staining and HPV molecular testing. Primary endocervical gastric-type adenocarcinoma can also mimic metastases, both histologically and immunophenotypically; sometimes, distinction cannot be made with certainty, and correlation with clinical and radiologic findings is required. Prognosis of patients with metastatic gastric carcinoma to the cervix is poor with rapid (<1 year) progression and death of disease.

Colorectal Adenocarcinoma

Patients are usually postmenopausal and present with abnormal bleeding; the cervical lesion can be the presenting sign [163, 169]. The clinical course is aggressive, with a median survival of 11 months (range 1–60) [169, 170]. As a diagnostic pitfall, the tumor frequently displays features mimicking a cervical or endometrial endometrioid carcinoma in surgical material. The tumor appearance ranges from well to poorly differentiated (some with signet-ring cell component); cells form pseudo-endometrioid glands with striking atypia and luminal necrosis. Wide infiltration into the cervical wall, prominent lymphatic vascular invasion and signet-ring morphology should raise concern for metastases. Markers of colorectal origin can be of value, particularly CK20 and SATB2 which are negative or patchy in primary cervical while diffusely positive in colorectal tumors. In addition, p16 and HPV testing can provide further evidence of cervical origin.

Urothelial Carcinoma

Spread of urothelial carcinoma to female reproductive organs is a very rare event [171–173]. The malignant process usually arises in the urinary bladder, and reaches the cervix in a pagetoid fashion either by direct intraepithelial spread or seeding; indeed, most lesions involving the cervix are in situ or only superficially invasive [171, 174]. Cervical involvement tends to manifest with bleeding or cytologic abnormalities, months to years after the diagnosis of urothelial carcinoma. However, cervical manifestations can be the presenting sign of malignancy. The prognosis is dictated by the stage and histologic grade of the primary urothelial malignancy [171].

The microscopic appearance is that of an intraepithelial proliferation with stratified transitional cytomorphology and papillary or flat architecture. Metastatic urothelial carcinoma to the cervix can closely resemble a primary cervical neoplasm, either in situ (AIS, squamous intraepithelial lesion) or invasive. This potential pitfall is particularly important in urothelial carcinomas with squamous or glandular differentiation [175, 176] (Fig. 13.19). By immunohistochemistry, urothelial carcinoma co-expresses CK7 and CK20 [177], which helps in its distinction from primary cervical lesions (CK20 negative). P16 may be of value, although it can also be overexpressed in high-grade urothelial carcinoma, and HPV testing should be considered since high-grade urothelial lesions are unrelated to HPV infection [178]. GATA3 is usually diffusely positive in urothelial lesions, and only focally positive in cervical squamous malignancies [179]. Nonetheless, it is important to note that urothelial carcinomas with squamous and / or glandular differentiation have lower rates of GATA3 expression [180, 181]. S-100 appears to have superior sensitivity in this group of urothelial carcinomas with variant morphology [181].

13.4 Mixed and Miscellaneous Cervical Neoplasms

13.4.1 Adenosquamous Carcinoma

13.4.1.1 Clinical Features

This type of mixed carcinoma represents ~4% of all cervical malignancies [182]. Age at presentation is similar to patients with squamous cell carcinoma, with a median of 46 years [182]. Most patients present with bleeding and/or cytologic abnormalities, and an exophytic or ulcerated lesion macroscopically.

13.4.1.2 Pathologic Features

By definition, adenosquamous carcinoma has areas of both *squamous* and *glandular* differentiation; the former tends to be poorly differentiated, but can be recognized by the presence of intercellular tight junctions and keratinization; the latter is seen as recognizable glands with lumen formation (Fig. 13.20). A clear cell variant has been described; the clear cell change involves the squamous component and is secondary to glycogenization [183].

13.4.1.3 Ancillary Studies

Adenosquamous carcinoma is related to high-risk HPV infection; HPV18 is the most common type identified, followed by HPV16 [184]. It is believed that adenosquamous cell carcinoma may represent a variant of cervical adenocar-

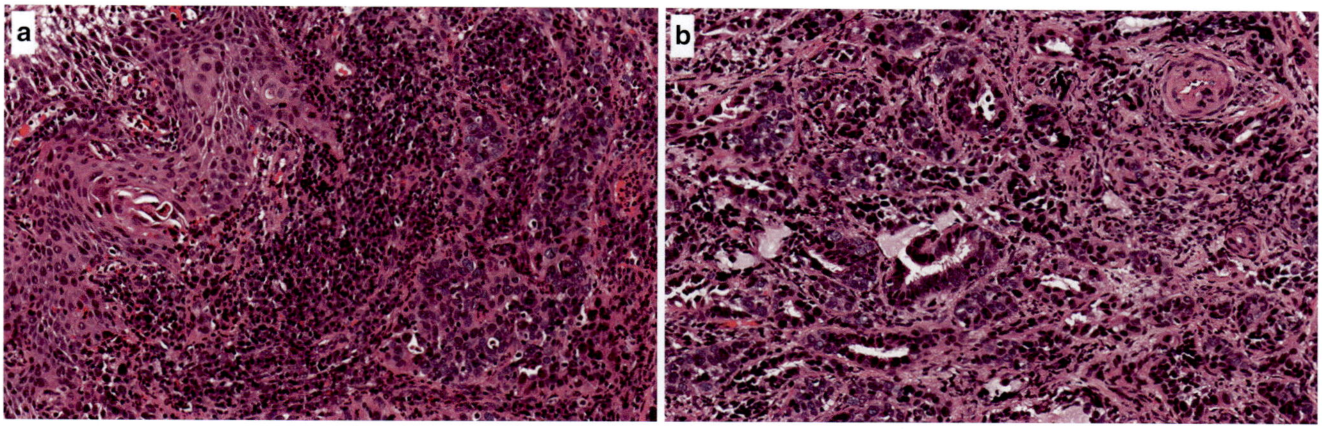

Fig. 13.20 Adenosquamous carcinoma. Unequivocal squamous (**a**) and glandular (**b**) differentiation is required for this diagnosis, the former tends to be poorly differentiated

cinoma. Interestingly, HPV and DNA clonality are identical in both squamous and glandular elements, suggesting biphasic differentiation of an HPV-infected common epithelial precursor [185]. This also correlates with the diffuse and strong p16 expression seen in both tumor components. Expression of squamous (p63, p40, CK5) and glandular (mucins) markers may vary, particularly in poorly differentiated lesions; moreover, they can highlight benign elements admixed with the tumor (areas of entrapped benign glands or squamous metaplasia) and caution in their interpretation is advised. Compared to squamous cell carcinoma, adenosquamous carcinoma shows absent to low ARID1A expression more frequently [186]. Expression of EGFR and PDGFRA is common; however, it does not correlate with *EGFR* and *PDGFRA* activating mutations [187].

13.4.1.4 Differential Diagnosis

The differential diagnosis of adenosquamous carcinoma includes: endometrioid adenocarcinoma with squamous differentiation (glandular component is low grade, squamous component lacks cytologic atypia and retains organization), invasive stratified mucin-producing carcinoma (absence of squamous differentiation), poorly differentiated squamous cell carcinoma (absence of glandular differentiation), adenoid basal carcinoma (basaloid component, squamous and glandular differentiation restricted to the center of the basaloid clusters, lack of desmoplasia or single-cell infiltration), and clear cell carcinoma (cytoplasmic clearing in glandular cells, absence of malignant squamous elements).

Prognosis and Management

Treatment usually involves chemoradiation. Patient outcome, in terms of overall and disease-free survival, is significantly worse in cases of adenosquamous carcinoma compared to squamous cell carcinoma regardless of stage [188–190]. When matched to those with pure endocervical adenocarcinoma, patients with advanced-stage disease adenosquamous carcinoma also have a worse prognosis [191, 192]. Early stage adenosquamous carcinoma, treated with radical surgery, is comparable to adenocarcinoma in terms of outcome [193].

13.4.1.5 13.4.1.1.Glassy Cell Carcinoma

Clinical Features

Glassy cell carcinoma, representing 0.2–9.3% of cervical cancers, is considered by some as a poorly differentiated variant of adenosquamous carcinoma [194]. It is seen in patients on average 10 years younger than those with cervical cancer [195].

Pathologic Features

Microscopically, tumor cells have sharp borders that stain with periodic acid-Schiff (PAS), large round nuclei with visible nucleoli, and eosinophilic cytoplasm with a "ground glass" appearance (hence the glassy cell denomination) (Fig. 13.21). There is no apparent squamous or glandular differentiation [196]. A brisk inflammatory eosinophilic infiltrate is characteristic. This morphology is usually diffuse; nonetheless, the presence of minor "glassy cell" features in otherwise conventional adenosquamous carcinomas and in poorly differentiated non-keratinizing carcinomas has been noted [197].

Ancillary Studies

By immunohistochemistry, glassy cell carcinoma expresses both squamous and glandular markers [198]. Estrogen and progesterone receptors are negative [199]. HPV types 18 and 16 have been demonstrated in both glassy cell carcinomas and adenosquamous carcinomas with focal glassy cell morphology [198, 200].

Differential Diagnosis

Glassy cell carcinoma is in essence a morphologic diagnosis. It can be distinguished from conventional squamous cell car-

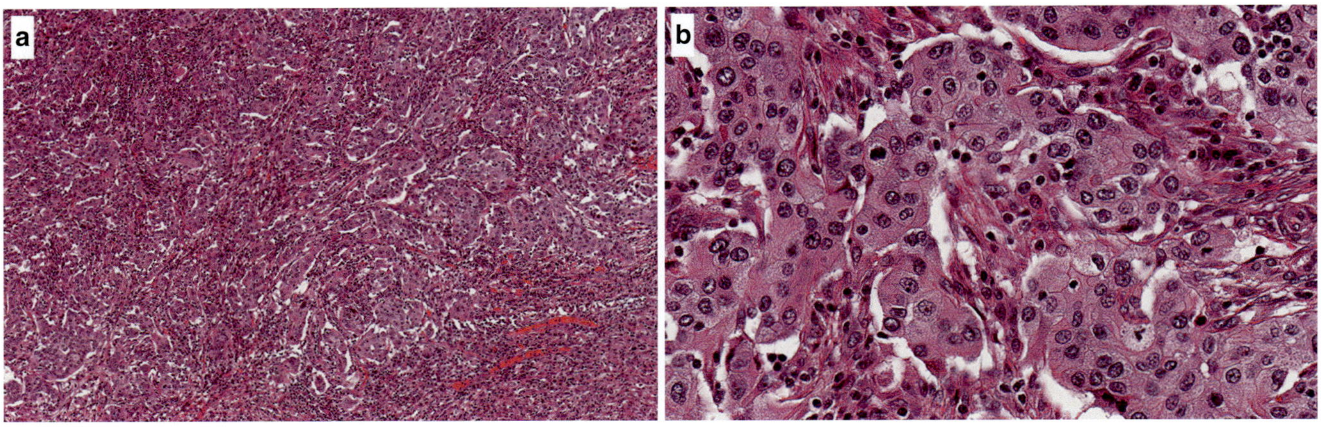

Fig. 13.21 Glassy cell carcinoma. This poorly differentiated tumor has a solid appearance (**a**) and contains pleomorphic cells with abundant polygonal "ground glass" cytoplasm (**b**)

cinoma and poorly differentiated adenocarcinoma by following strict morphologic criteria. An important differential is with epithelioid trophoblastic tumor, since both neoplasms have solid growth and contain cells with eosinophilic cytoplasm and round nuclei. The presence of a syncytial arrangement, abundant necrosis, lack of distinct cell borders, and strong GATA3 and cyclin E expression are features more in keeping with epithelioid trophoblastic tumor.

Prognosis and Management

Glassy cell carcinoma often has an aggressive clinical course with rapid progression and extrapelvic metastases [201]. Overall, 5-year survival is lower for glassy cell carcinoma compared to other cervical cancers (55% vs. 75%, respectively); survival is also poorer when adjusted for stage [194]. Systemic treatment is usually indicated.

13.4.1.6 Mucoepidermoid Carcinoma

This neoplasm is morphologically identical to its counterpart in the salivary glands and is defined by the presence of three cell types (epidermoid, intermediate, and mucin producing) [202]. These cells appear in varying proportions, organized in nests or solid sheets, rudimentary duct-like structures and cysts. Epidermoid cells display eosinophilic cytoplasm but lack keratinization and overt intercellular junctions, unlike adenosquamous carcinoma. Furthermore, mucinous cells are intermixed with other cell types with no definitive gland formation. Intermediate cells are usually the most prominent population; they have basaloid appearance and aggregate in clusters [202].

The main differential diagnosis is with conventional adenosquamous carcinoma. The diagnosis of cervical mucoepidermoid carcinoma should be contemplated only in cases with the classic microscopic appearance. Overt squamous or glandular differentiation and absence of an intermediate cell population are more in keeping with adenosquamous carcinoma. Since the morphologic appearance of mucoepidermoid carcinoma can be bland, it can be confused with a benign proliferation (squamous metaplasia, microglandular hyperplasia); mass forming or infiltrative growth, and haphazard organization of the diverse cell types should raise concern for malignancy rather than a benign process.

Although mucoepidermoid carcinoma falls into the spectrum of adenosquamous differentiation, there is evidence that it is a distinct biologic entity since it harbors recurrent abnormalities in the *CRTC1* and *MAML2* genes (fusion or rearrangements) similar to salivary gland mucoepidermoid carcinomas [202].

13.4.2 Adenoid Basal Cell Carcinoma (Epithelioma)

13.4.2.1 Clinical Features

This rare tumor, representing less than 1% of cervical cancers, is composed of nests of bland basaloid cells with variable glandular and squamous differentiation. Like tumors with adenoid cystic differentiation, adenoid basal lesions can be divided into two groups: pure adenoid basal tumors and mixed tumors, the latter having a second component, such as squamous cell carcinoma, adenoid cystic carcinoma small cell carcinoma or, rarely, carcinosarcoma [203, 204].

Adenoid basal carcinomas usually occur in postmenopausal women (median age 66 years, range 19–91) [203]. They are frequently associated with a high-grade squamous intraepithelial lesion (HSIL); in fact, most cases are discovered incidentally on LEEP or cone after a biopsy diagnosis of HSIL [205].

13.4.2.2 Pathologic Features

Histologically, adenoid basal carcinoma is composed of small round nests of basaloid cells with peripheral palisading. Although growth and distribution are haphazard, there is no stromal desmoplastic reaction. Towards the central/lumi-

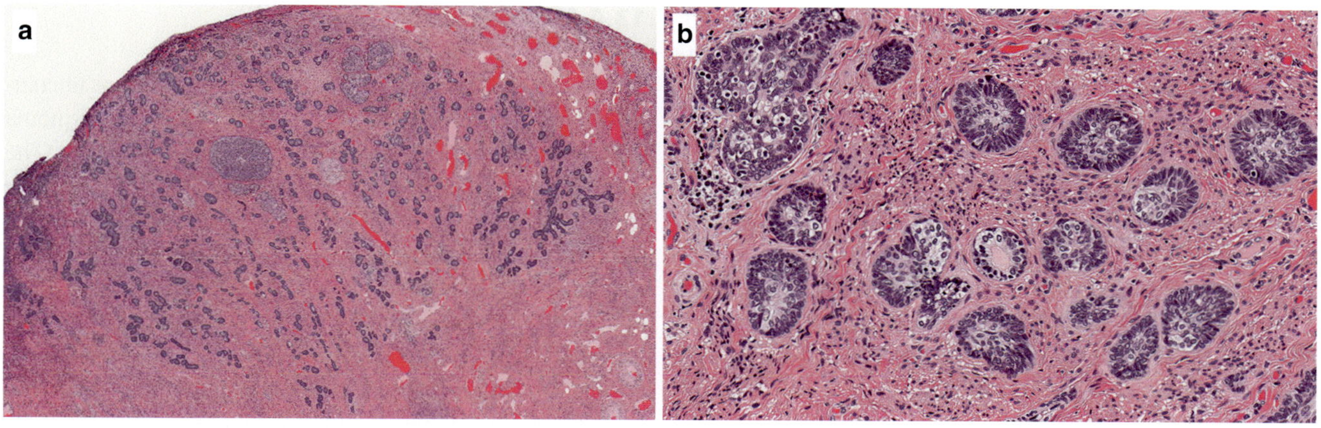

Fig. 13.22 Adenoid basal carcinoma. This basaloid proliferation is haphazardly distributed throughout the cervical stroma; however, there is no desmoplasia (**a**). Nests have smooth outer contours; they may have central squamous or glandular differentiation, however the periphery retains a basaloid appearance (**b**)

nal portion of the nests, squamous and glandular differentiation can be appreciated (Fig. 13.22). The tumor lacks lymphovascular and perineural invasion [206]. High-risk HPV is detected in the vast majority of lesions [203, 205].

13.4.2.3 Differential Diagnosis

The differential diagnosis includes adenoid cystic carcinoma, squamous cell carcinoma, and adenosquamous carcinoma, although it is important to bear in mind that these lesions can coexist. These malignancies tend to present clinically as a mass. In addition, identification of the distinct nested architecture and basaloid pattern with palisading in adenoid basal carcinoma suffices in most instances. Immunohistochemistry for CAM5.2 highlights the basaloid cell population in the periphery of the nests, and can be of value in distinguishing squamous cell carcinoma from adenoid basal carcinoma with extensive squamous metaplasia [207].

Adenoid basal hyperplasia, an allegedly related lesion, has been described as a superficial proliferation extending less than 1 mm from the superficial epithelial basement membrane at the level of the squamous–columnar junction [208]. Unlike adenoid basal carcinoma, HPV testing is negative in adenoid basal hyperplasia.

13.4.2.4 Prognosis and Management

Pure adenoid basal carcinoma has a benign behavior with no metastases, lymph node involvement, recurrences, or deaths reported to date [203]. Hence, the term "epithelioma" is favored by many authors over the term "carcinoma." Mixed lesions also have an excellent prognosis, likely because most are diagnosed and treated at an early stage. Nonetheless, the presence of a second malignant component may have an adverse prognostic impact. Thus, after a biopsy diagnosis of adenoid basal carcinoma, surgical excision with negative margins and evaluation of the entire tumor is warranted in order to exclude a second component.

Table 13.5 Classification of adenoid cystic carcinomas of the female lower genital tract

Taken from Xing et al. [205]	Pure adenoid cystic carcinoma	Mixed carcinoma with adenoid cystic differentiation
Patient age	Median 48 years, range 27–74	Median 76 years, range 50–86
Adenoid cystic component	100%	Usually <25%
High-risk HPV	Not detected	Detected (usually HPV16)
P16 immunohistochemistry	Non-diffuse	Diffuse and strong
Perineural invasion	~50%	Absent

13.4.3 Adenoid Cystic Carcinoma

13.4.3.1 Clinical Features

Tumors of the lower genital tract with adenoid cystic differentiation can be divided in two groups: pure adenoid cystic carcinomas and adenoid cystic carcinomas mixed with a second component, usually squamous cell carcinoma or adenoid basal carcinoma [209]. The main differences between these types are depicted in Table 13.5. Mixed tumors occur in older patients and are usually related to high-risk HPV infection; in these, the adenoid cystic component is usually minor and less than 50% of the tumor volume.

13.4.3.2 Pathologic Features

Adenoid cystic carcinoma of the uterine cervix displays the same morphologic features as its counterparts in the salivary gland, upper respiratory tract, breast, and vulva. The tumor is composed of basaloid cells arranged in cribriform, tubular, and solid growth patterns [210]. Tumors with cribriform architecture have cystic areas containing mucinous or eosinophilic secretions, alternating with pseudo-cystic areas containing basement membrane-like material, positive for collagen type IV and PAS stain [210] (Fig. 13.23). Tumors with solid growth also have basement membrane-like material around tumor nests and cords [211].

13.4.3.3 Ancillary Studies

By immunohistochemistry, adenoid cystic carcinoma is negative for hormone receptors. In addition, MYB expression has been documented. This finding may be related to translocation of the *MYB* and/or *NFIB* transcription factors, which has been documented in adenoid cystic carcinomas of the salivary gland, breast and vulva [212].

13.4.3.4 Differential Diagnosis

The differential diagnosis of adenoid cystic carcinoma includes adenoid basal carcinoma and squamous cell carcinoma. Importantly, all these lesions can coexist. However, distinction between pure adenoid basal and adenoid cystic carcinoma is important, since the former has an indolent prognosis. Both have a basaloid phenotype including expression of basal and myoepithelial markers like S100 [210]. Nonetheless, the histopathology of adenoid cystic carcinoma is usually distinct, and the diagnosis can be ascertained on morphologic grounds in most cases. CD117 (C-KIT) may be of value; its expression is consistently negative in adenoid basal tumors, and appears to be at least focally positive in cervical adenoid cystic carcinoma [213, 214].

13.4.3.5 Prognosis and Management

After a biopsy diagnosis of adenoid cystic carcinoma, the possibility of a second component should be considered. Therefore, excisional sampling with LEEP or cone may be advisable. Initial series of adenoid cystic carcinoma report an aggressive behavior with recurrence or metastases in nearly half of cases at time of follow-up [215]. It remains unclear if prognosis differs between pure and mixed tumors.

13.4.4 Mixed Carcinoma

Truly "mixed" carcinomas of the uterine cervix are uncommon. The usual scenario is of an HPV-related adenocarcinoma with areas of neuroendocrine differentiation (Fig. 13.24). The latter is more commonly of the small cell type. The lesion tends to be large and efface the cervix at the time of presentation. The neuroendocrine component usually comprises the majority of the tumor volume. The prognosis is poor.

Primary carcinosarcoma of the cervix is exceedingly unusual. These lesions occur in a wide age range. They are related to HPV-infection, and frequently are associated with an in situ squamous component [204]. As in the uterine corpus, diagnosis of carcinosarcoma requires the presence of two distinct components: carcinomatous and sarcomatous. The former can be squamous cell, adenoid basal, adenoid cystic, undifferentiated carcinoma, or combinations thereof [204]; the latter is usually homologous. Stage is the most important prognostic factor. Treatment involves primary surgery followed by radiation and chemotherapy [216].

Other rare carcinoma combinations have been reported in the literature, including mesonephric plus neuroendocrine carcinoma [217], villoglandular adenocarcinoma plus transitional cell carcinoma [218, 219], and signet-ring cell adenocarcinoma plus glassy cell carcinoma [220].

13.5 Benign Endocervical Glandular Lesions

The following lesions are covered in this chapter as they usually pertain to the differential diagnosis of preinvasive and invasive endocervical glandular malignancy. Some of these proliferations are reactive in nature (tubo-endometrioid metaplasia); others likely represent embryologic remnants

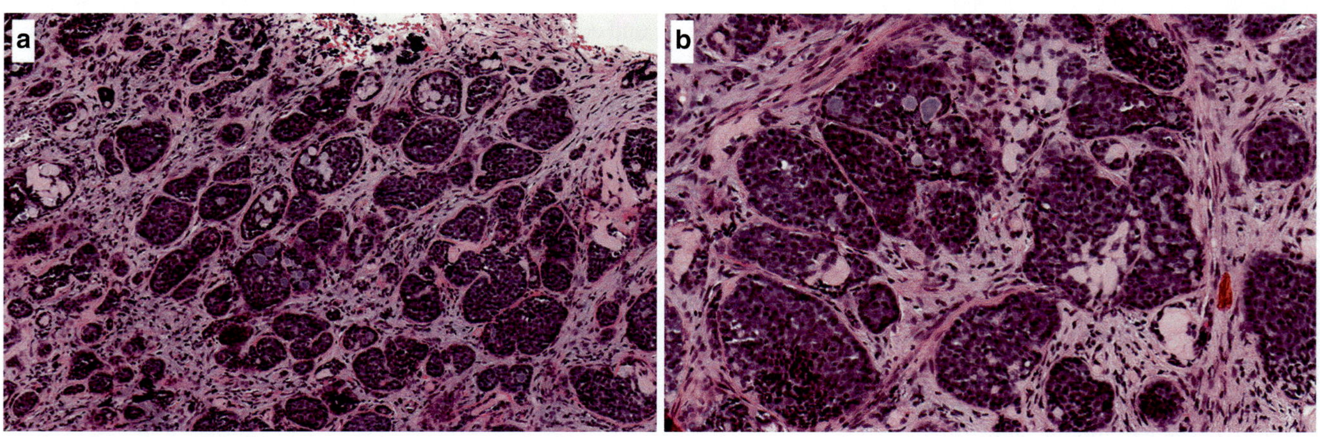

Fig. 13.23 Adenoid cystic carcinoma. Basaloid population with solid and cribriform architecture (**a**). Notice the presence of pseudo-lumens filled with basement membrane material (**b**)

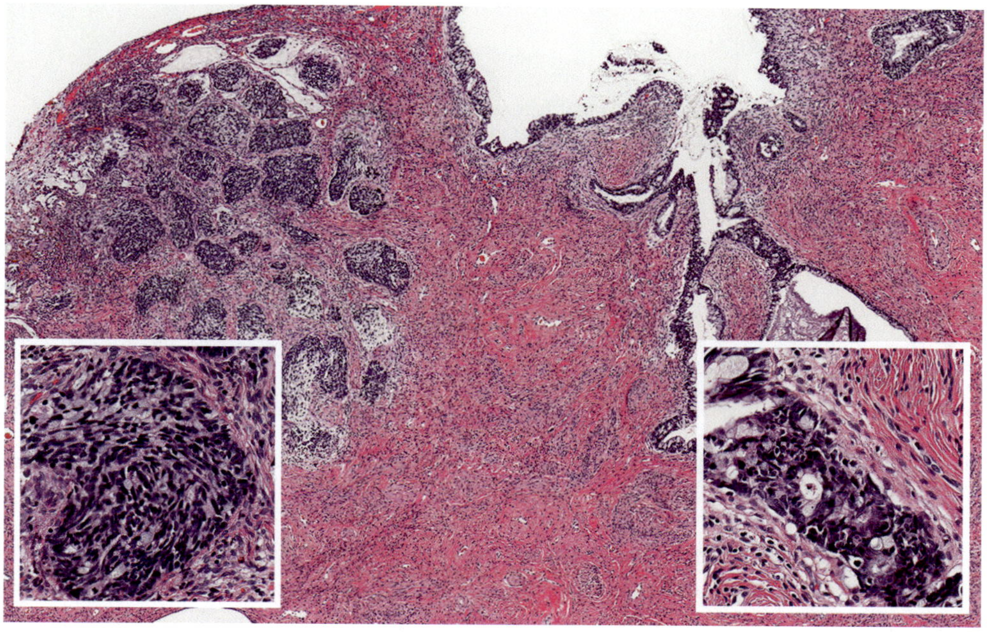

Fig. 13.24 Mixed carcinoma with a glandular (right insert) and neuroendocrine component (left insert); the latter was strongly positive for synaptophysin and chromogranin. The tumor was positive for high-risk HPV

(mesonephric remnants, prostatic tissue) or variations of the normal endocervix (tunnel clusters, nabothian cysts). Some can be secondary to the hormonal background (Arias-Stella reaction). Most are composed of Müllerian epithelium; however, other types of epithelial derivation (mesonephric, epidermal) can be observed.

13.5.1 Endocervical Polyp

13.5.1.1 Clinical Features

Polyps of the uterine cervix are very common, characteristically in adult women. Most cases present with a single polyp, usually are small (1 cm or less), variably located along the endocervical canal.

13.5.1.2 Pathologic Features

Microscopically, the endocervical polyp is defined by an exophytic mucosal lesion containing benign endocervical-type glands and a central / basal fibrovascular core (Fig. 13.25). Variable degrees of inflammation are present in the superficial stroma. Likewise, the overlying epithelium commonly displays reactive changes including squamous metaplasia, tubal metaplasia, or microglandular hyperplasia. Mucosal erosion and granulation tissue is usually a sign of mechanical irritation. Stromal cartilaginous and osseous metaplasia has been described [221]. Epidermoid cysts with keratinization and adnexal structures within an endocervical polyp have also been reported [222, 223].

13.5.1.3 Differential Diagnosis

The main differential of endocervical polyp is from Müllerian adenosarcoma. The glandular component of adenosarcoma usually has a distinct appearance with cystically dilated "rigid" (smooth, concave luminal contours) glands, as well as glands with narrowed lumens due to broad-base protrusions of the stroma, causing a characteristic "leaf-like" pattern. The glands in endocervical polyps show variation in size and shape: their outer contour tends to be festooning and variably convoluted instead of rigid, and glands also tend to retain their lumens. If present, stromal projections do not fully conform to the shape of the space and only fill it partially. The stromal component of the endocervical polyp is non-atypical and lacks the periglandular condensation seen in adenosarcoma; mitoses, if present, are occasional (one per 10 HPFs). Importantly, worrisome indicators for adenosarcoma (rigid glands, leaf-like architecture, periglandular condensation, stromal atypia, 2 or more mitoses/10 HPFs) can be seen *focally* in endocervical polyps. These lesions have been termed "polyps with unusual features", in view of their indolent behavior [224]. If any of these characteristics is present *diffusely* within the tumor, the diagnosis of adenosarcoma must be considered.

Endocervical polyp can also overlap morphologically with other benign conditions, such as endometrial polyp and polypoid endometriosis. In fact, some polyps arise in the upper endocervix/lower uterine segment mucosa, and have mixed endocervical and endometrial features. The term "Müllerian" polyp can be used in this instance. Lastly, the infoldings of the normal endocervical mucosa can appear polypoid in routine preparations from excised material (cone, hysterectomy). The diagnosis of endocervical polyp should be reserved for lesions with truly exophytic architecture and prominent fibro-vasculature stroma within its core.

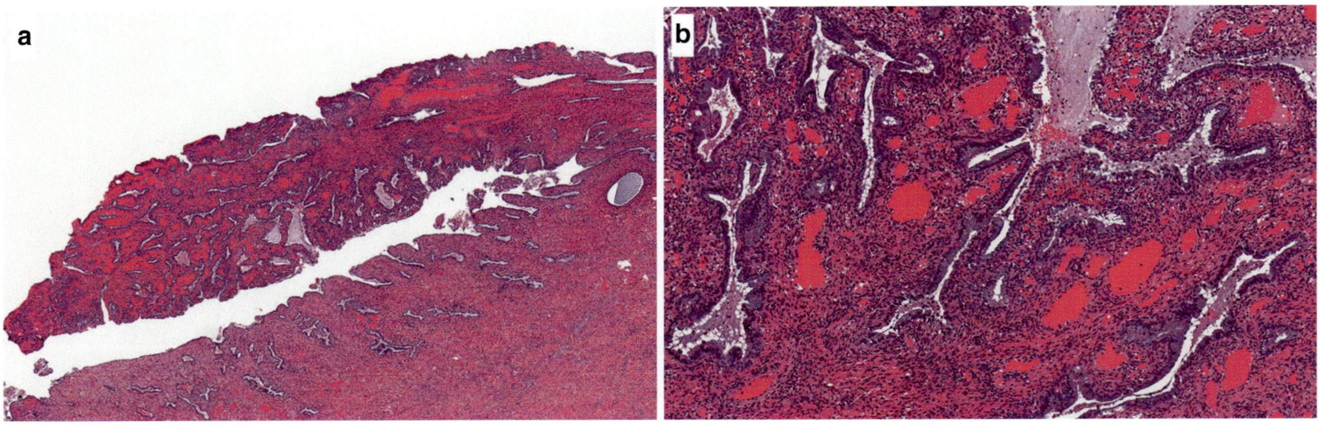

Fig. 13.25 Endocervical polyp. Exophytic proliferation of benign endocervical glands and stroma (**a**), harboring normal mucinous endocervical epithelium and dilated vessels (**b**)

13.5.1.4 Prognosis and Management

Endocervical polyps are indolent lesions; when encountered, simple excisional sampling is sufficient. While benign by definition, endocervical polyps can rarely harbor an intraepithelial lesion or malignancy [225, 226]. Premenopausal women appear to be at higher risk of developing epithelial lesions in a polyp compared to postmenopausal women [227, 228]. It is unclear whether intraepithelial lesions or carcinomas confined to an endocervical polyp carry the same prognosis as early stage cervical carcinoma involving the normal (non-polypoid) cervix. Likewise, sometimes a preexisting endocervical polyp is involved by endometrial carcinoma, which for now should be best interpreted as cervical involvement for staging purposes, even if the rest of the cervix is uninvolved. Whether this situation is clinically different from other forms of cervical involvement is yet to be determined.

13.5.2 Müllerian Papilloma

This very rare lesion typically arises in the posterior vagina or cervix of girls under 10 years of age [229]. Given its exophytic appearance and age distribution, there is commonly clinical concern for botryoid rhabdomyosarcoma. However, the arborizing glandular epithelial morphology of müllerian papilloma makes the distinction straightforward. The lesion is unifocal and small (<2 cm). It is composed of finely branched papillare lined by simple epithelium, typically columnar although a squamous component can be seen [230]. There is no cytologic atypia, stratification, or mitoses. The lesion is benign and local excision is the treatment of choice [231]. Occasional recurrences have been reported [232].

13.5.3 Nabothian Cysts

13.5.3.1 Clinical Features

Nabothian cysts are more prevalent in multiparous women. They are presumably secondary to obstruction of the communication of a cervical crypt with the surface and subsequent cystic enlargement, likely during / after pregnancy. While most are superficial, less than 10 mm in size and asymptomatic, some may acquire significant sizes and involve the deep aspect of the cervical wall. These large cysts may cause a variety of symptoms, ranging from bleeding and discomfort to prolapse, labor passage obstruction, and hematometra [233–235].

13.5.3.2 Pathologic Features

Nabothian cysts are visible grossly as unilocular lesions with thick mucinous to gelatinous material and a smooth lining. Histologically, the cyst is round with concave luminal contours and is lined by a simple layer of columnar to flattened bland mucinous epithelium, cytologically identical to the background normal glands (Fig. 13.26). The surrounding stroma is indistinct from the remaining cervical wall.

13.5.3.3 Differential Diagnosis

Nabothian cysts must be distinguished from minimal deviation adenocarcinoma, particularly when symptomatic, causing cervical enlargement or involving the deep cervix [236, 237]. Minimal deviation adenocarcinoma usually presents as multiple cystic lesions, distorting the cervix but otherwise benign-appearing, both clinically and on pathologic examination. Indicators of minimal deviation adenocarcinoma include: haphazard distribution of cystically dilated glands, usually with accompanying non-cystic glands; different mucin profile compared to the normal cervix, with a paler to vaguely eosinophilic appearance and red staining in PAS-Alcian blue preparations (normal endocervical mucin stains dark blue), nuclear enlargement and atypia, usually very focal and loss of PAX2 expression [118].

13.5.4 Tunnel Clusters

13.5.4.1 Clinical Features

Tunnel clusters are rounded, densely packed aggregates of glands in the endocervical wall. They are vastly more com-

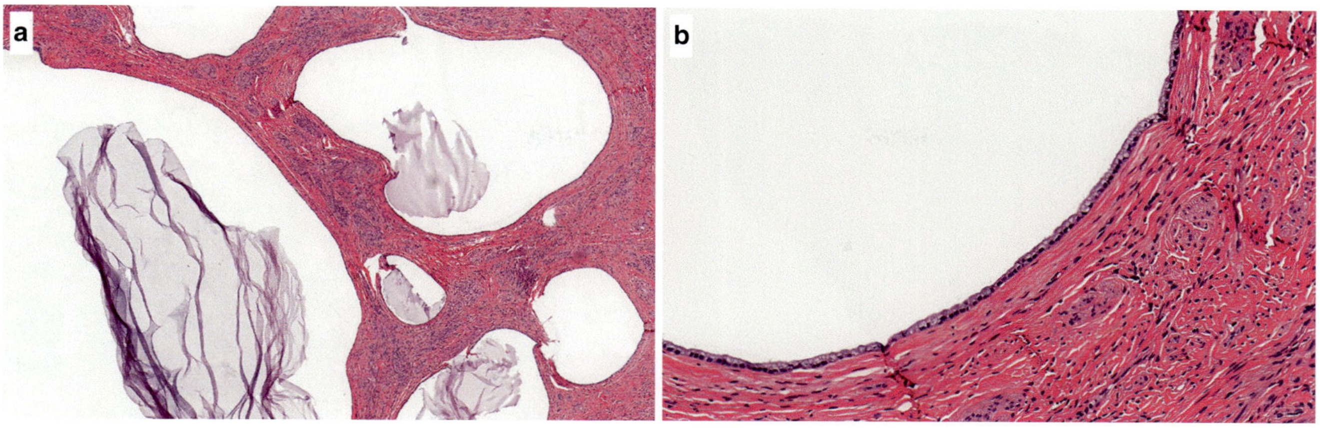

Fig. 13.26 Nabothian cysts. Cystically dilated endocervix, sometimes producing a grossly visible lesion (**a**); cysts are lined by flattened but otherwise unremarkable endocervical epithelium (**b**)

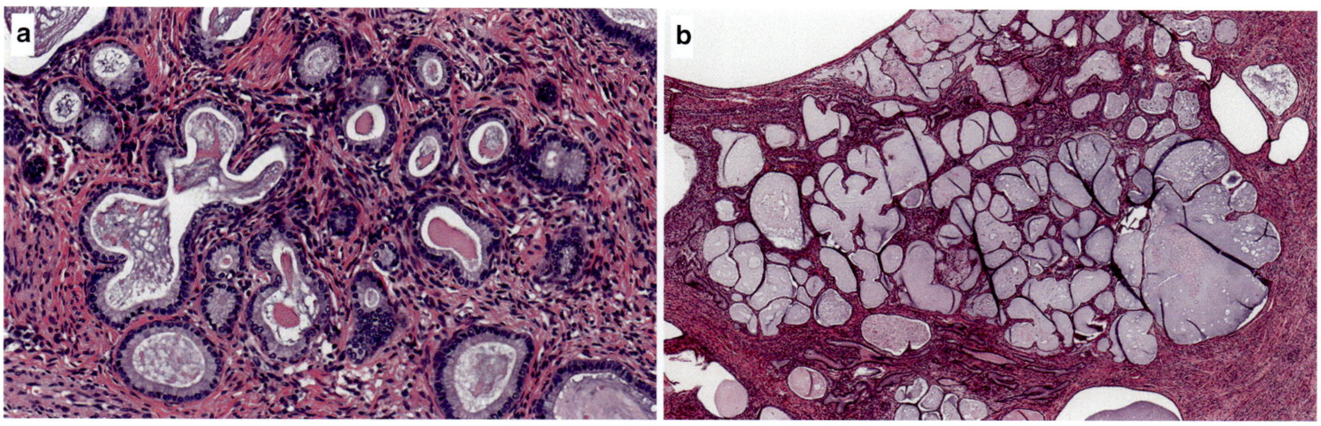

Fig. 13.27 Tunnel clusters. Type-A tunnel clusters appear as well-contoured tight glandular conglomerates (**a**). Type-B tunnel clusters have the same crowded density and smooth contour appearance, but glands have cystic dilation (**b**)

mon in multiparous women. They can present with mucoid discharge, but are usually asymptomatic and only incidentally noted on excision material.

13.5.4.2 Pathologic Features

Tunnel clusters are divided into type-A (non-cystic) and type-B (cystic) [238]. The former are comprised of small glands arranged around a central cleft in a lobulated pattern, all with undulated contours and lined by simple low cuboidal mucinous epithelium [239]. A subset of type-A tunnel clusters has been shown to express gastric (neutral) mucins, and thus thought to belong to the spectrum of endocervical gastric metaplasia [47]. Type-B tunnel clusters tend to be multifocal and, given their larger size, may cause distortion of the mucosa [240]. They are composed of round and dilated glandular structures, also arranged in a tightly packed lobular arrangement which distinguishes them from the normal endocervix (Fig. 13.27).

13.5.4.3 Differential Diagnosis

Similar to nabothian cysts, the differential of tunnel clusters includes endocervical adenocarcinoma, importantly of the gastric (minimal deviation) type. A superficial location, organized lobular architecture and lack of nuclear atypia and proliferation are indicative of tunnel clusters.

13.5.5 Diffuse Laminar Endocervical Hyperplasia

This highly uncommon type of endocervical glandular proliferation is seen as densely packed glands and clefts, concentrated in the superficial mucosal aspect in a band-like fashion and sharply separated from the underlying stroma [241, 242]. Lining epithelium has an endocervical mucinous profile (Fig. 13.28). Due to striking glandular crowding and variable mucosal thickening, diffuse laminar endocervical hyperplasia can be mistaken for malignancy, either endocervical (minimal deviation adenocarcinoma) or endometrial endometrioid. This pitfall applies in particular to biopsy material [243]. Attention to the normal endocervical mucinous profile will aid in identifying this benign process. In excision material, the diagnosis of diffuse laminar endocervical hyperplasia is easier to ascertain based on the superficial location of the glands, its sharp demarcation from the underlying stroma and the absence of significant atypia.

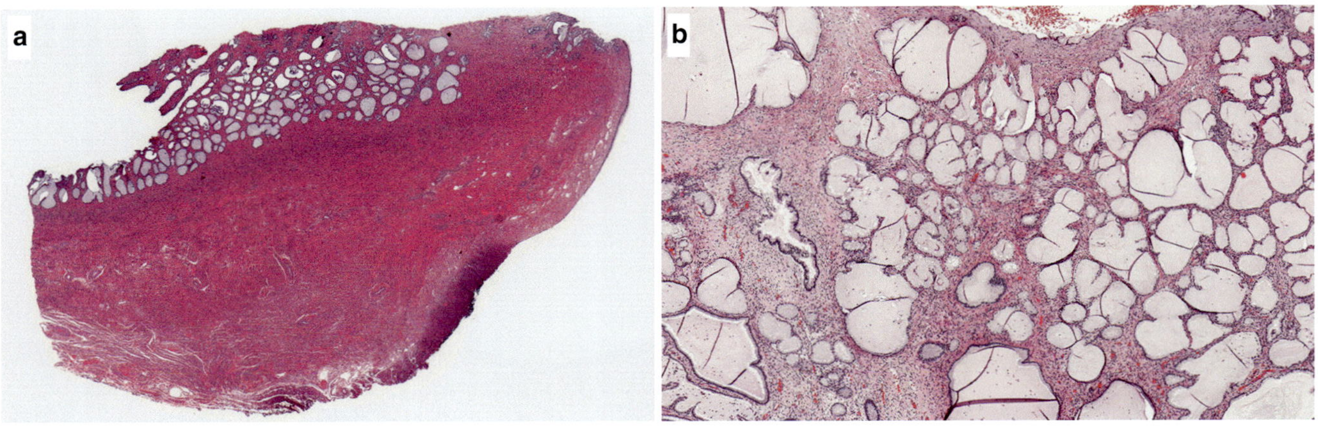

Fig. 13.28 Diffuse laminar endocervical hyperplasia. Increase in glandular density uniformly and diffusely involving the mucosa (**a**), comprised of densely packed glands of varying sizes and shapes (**b**)

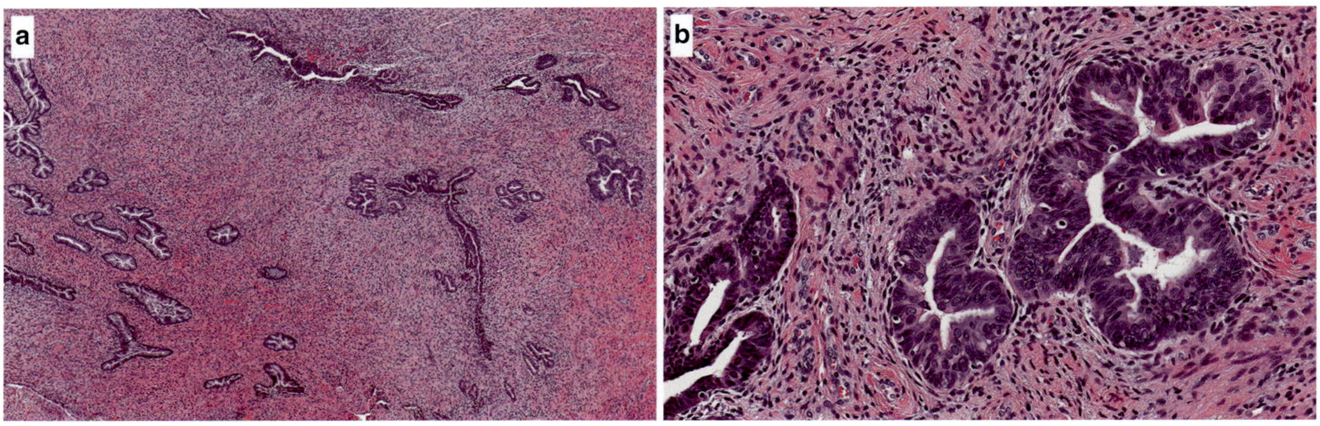

Fig. 13.29 Tubo-endometrioid metaplasia. Glandular proliferation associated with reactive ("pseudo-desmoplastic") stroma in a patient with previous cervical conization (**a**). The proliferation is composed of glands with tubal and endometrioid differentiation and bland morphology (**b**)

13.5.6 Tubo-Endometrioid Metaplasia

13.5.6.1 Clinical Features

Tubo-endometrioid metaplasia (TEM) can pose diagnostic difficulty, since it has some morphologic overlap with endocervical adenocarcinoma of the usual type. TEM is a frequent finding, incidental in most cases: it is seen in 21% cone biopsies and 62% of hysterectomy specimens [244]. An association with previous cone procedure has been reported [245].

13.5.6.2 Pathologic Features

TEM is characterized by columnar glandular epithelium with elongated, cigar-shaped nuclei and uniform cytoplasm with scant to absent cytoplasmic mucin (Fig. 13.29). These features recapitulate the appearance of inactive or proliferative phase endometrium. Tubal differentiation is evident in the form of ciliated cells interspersed with non-ciliated and peg cells. Mitotic activity can be observed, but is usually scant. Involved glands have similar size and distribution to the normal endocervix, usually confined to the superficial layer; however, deep cervical involvement has been reported [246]. The stroma around the glands can be hypercellular, edematous, or myxoid, mimicking desmoplastic reaction [246].

13.5.6.3 Differential Diagnosis

TEM can mimic endocervical adenocarcinoma in situ of the usual (endocervical) type, either in situ or invasive. Both entities depict "mucin-depleted" cells, variable proliferation, and may display reactive stroma. Unlike TEM, endocervical adenocarcinoma has enlarged hyperchromatic nuclei with irregular chromatin distribution, prominent pseudostratification and loss of polarity. Moreover, apical mitoses are usually brisk in adenocarcinoma, and occasional in TEM. In difficult cases, immunohistochemistry is useful. Usual-type endocervical adenocarcinoma is typically positive for p16 overexpression and negative for estrogen receptor and vimentin; BCL-2 is either negative of patchy. The opposite profile is characteristic of TEM (negative or patchy p16, estrogen receptor and vimentin positive, diffuse BCL-2 expression) [118, 247–249].

13.5.7 Endometriosis

13.5.7.1 Clinical Features

Endometriosis, although a very common affliction, rarely occurs in the cervix, representing only 0.2% of all endometriosis cases in a recent single-institution series [250]. History of previous vaginal pregnancy and/or curettage is seen in most, but not all patients [250, 251]. While many cases are only identified incidentally on pathologic examination, about half present with symptoms (bleeding, pain). Some patients present with atypical glandular cells in screening cytology [252]. Given its rarity, this diagnosis is usually unsuspected clinically.

13.5.7.2 Pathologic Features

The histologic appearance of endometriosis is similar to other sites, harboring endometrial-type glands, stroma, and frequent evidence of hemorrhage (hemosiderin-laden macrophages, Fig. 13.30). Tubal differentiation may also be seen. The lesion is usually located in the mucosal surface [253], but can be present anywhere in the cervical stroma or the paracervical soft tissue.

13.5.7.3 Differential Diagnosis

While there is morphologic overlap between tubo-endometrioid metaplasia and endometriosis, the former lacks the dense endometrial-type stroma of the latter. More importantly, endometriosis can mimic endocervical adenocarcinoma, especially if the endometrial glands display proliferative characteristics (mitoses, elongated and pseudostratified nuclei) and when it infiltrates deeply into the wall [253]. Attention to the presence of endometrial-type stroma and hemosiderin-laden macrophages is very important. Negative / patchy p16 and positive hormone receptors by immunohistochemistry are also in keeping with endometriosis.

13.5.7.4 Prognosis and Management

Instances of microscopic endometrioid and clear cell adenocarcinoma arising in cervical endometriosis have been reported [125, 254]; nonetheless, this appears to be an exceedingly rare phenomenon, as previously discussed (see "endometrioid carcinoma"). Simple excision appears to be sufficient for superficial lesions, with nil recurrence rates reported [250]. On occasion, endometriosis is extensive (deep infiltrating endometriosis) requiring radical excision (trachelectomy, hysterectomy) and close surveillance [255, 256].

13.5.8 Endocervicosis

13.5.8.1 Clinical Features

This rare phenomenon is more frequent in the bladder [257]; however, it can also occur in other pelvic tissues including the anterior outer cervical wall and paracervical soft tissue [258, 259]. It is thought to be a form of Müllerianosis. A role for Cesarean section has been implied in its pathogenesis, which suggests mechanical displacement of endocervical cells and implantation into the outer cervical wall [260].

13.5.8.2 Pathologic Features

The lesion can be grossly visible, measuring up to 3 cm. Endocervicosis is a benign mucinous glandular proliferation, haphazardly oriented within the connective tissue but not infiltrative. Stromal reaction can be seen if there is mucin extravasation [258]. Glandular elements are lined by bland and non-proliferative endocervical-type mucinous epithelium (Fig. 13.31). Expression of estrogen and progesterone receptors has been reported [260].

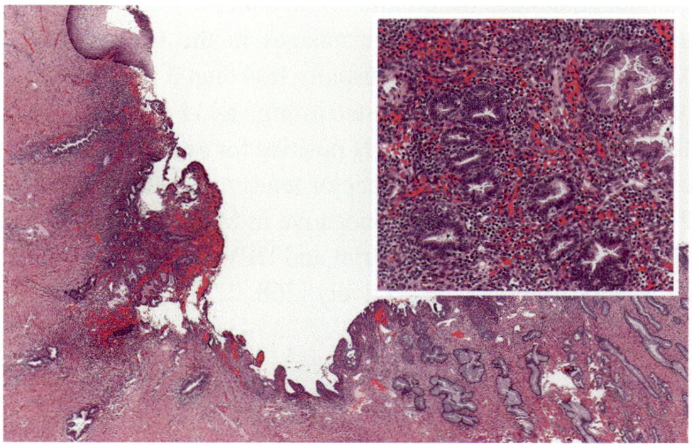

Fig. 13.30 Endometriosis. This lesion is seated in the squamous-columnar junction and depicts endometrial-type glands and stroma (insert)

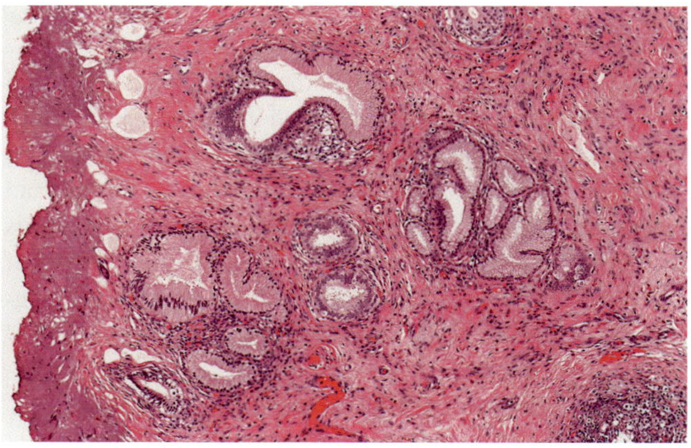

Fig. 13.31 Endocervicosis. This benign proliferation, resembling endocervical epithelium, was identified in the bladder wall

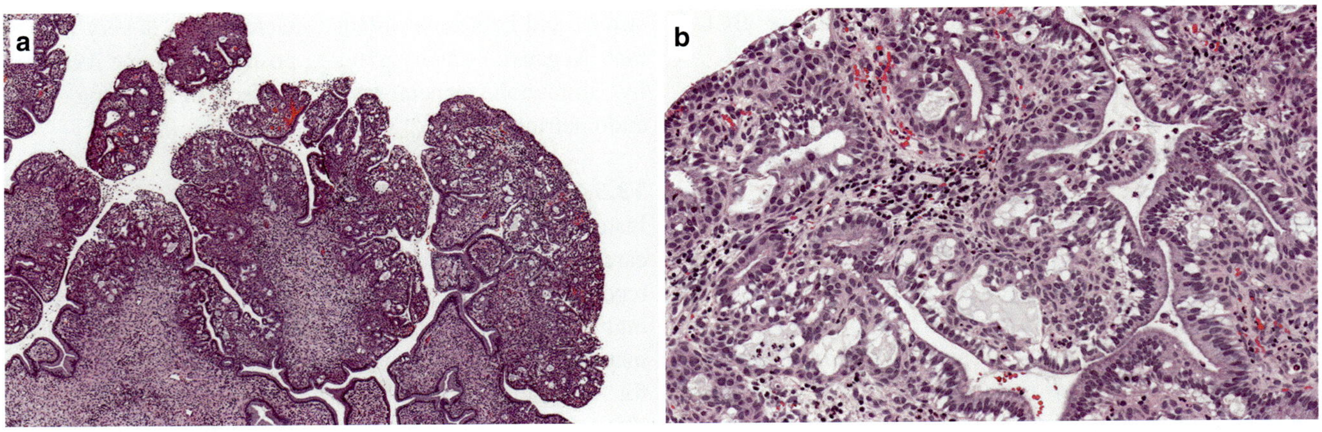

Fig. 13.32 Microglandular hyperplasia (MGH). This change is seen as an area of epithelial crowding, usually in the mucosal surface (**a**). The intraglandular cribriforming and glandular confluence may raise concern for malignancy, particularly endometrioid carcinoma; the presence of a basal (reserve) cell layer is typical of MGH and excludes an endometrial endometrioid neoplasm (**b**)

13.5.8.3 Differential Diagnosis

When encountered, the diagnosis of endocervicosis requires exclusion of adenocarcinoma, especially the minimal deviation type. Endocervicosis is typically confined to the outer cervical wall and paracervical soft tissue, and the stroma between it and the endocervical mucosa is spared. In contrast, a malignant process would feature transmural involvement. The mucin profile of endocervicosis is identical to the native endocervix, which, with a trained eye, can be distinguished from the gastric-type mucinous appearance of minimal deviation adenocarcinoma. Lastly, hormone receptor immunohistochemistry can also be of aid.

13.5.8.4 Prognosis and Management

Endocervicosis is a benign condition with no recurrences reported following surgical excision. Cases of malignant transformation into mucinous adenocarcinoma have been described in extra-cervical locations [261, 262].

13.5.9 Microglandular Hyperplasia

13.5.9.1 Clinical Features

Initial descriptions of this phenomenon attributed it to oral contraceptive use and other hormonal imbalances [263, 264]. However, a subsequent study by *Greeley et al.* showed no association between microglandular hyperplasia (MGH) and exogenous hormonal therapy or pregnancy [265]. Indeed, this lesion is commonly encountered in patients with no history of oral contraceptive use. Inflammation is usually present, suggesting that MGH can be reparative or metaplastic in nature.

13.5.9.2 Pathologic Features

MGH usually does not have a macroscopic correlate; however, it is sometimes identified as areas of erosion or polypoid friable tissue. Microscopically, it is defined as a superficial benign proliferation of endocervical glands with significant crowding and confluent appearance, which imparts a characteristic microacinar and cribriform architecture. The population is bland, composed of uniform columnar or cuboidal glandular cells with vacuolization, usually admixed with a prominent reserve cell layer and immature metaplastic squamous epithelium towards the epithelial base (Fig. 13.32).

13.5.9.3 Differential Diagnosis

The chief differential diagnosis of MGH is adenocarcinoma of endocervical and endometrial origin. The bland cytomorphology of MGH contrasts with the variable but consistent nuclear atypia is seen in most endocervical adenocarcinoma types. Given its striking mixture of complex architecture with bland cytology, MGH can resemble endometrial carcinoma. This is an important differential, especially when endometrial carcinoma displays mucinous differentiation or a microglandular growth pattern, which has been described [266, 267]. Features in keeping with MGH include: uniform subnuclear vacuolization, reserve cell hyperplasia and squamous metaplasia of *basal location* (versus the *superficial / luminal* squamous differentiation in endometrial carcinoma) and absence of foamy macrophages in the stroma [268]. Mitotic activity in MGH is usually less than 3 per 10 HPFs, but it has been recently reported as high as 11 mitoses per 10 HPFs [269]. MGH is diffusely positive for estrogen receptor; conversely, progesterone receptor tends to be negative [268, 270]. Vimentin and p16 are negative in MGH, which aids in its distinction from endometrial and HPV-related endocervical adenocarcinoma, respectively [268, 271].

13.5.10 Arias-Stella Reaction

13.5.10.1 Clinical Features

Arias-Stella reaction is a characteristic change of the endocervical and endometrial glandular epithelium secondary to high circulating progesterone levels. Thus, it is typically seen during/

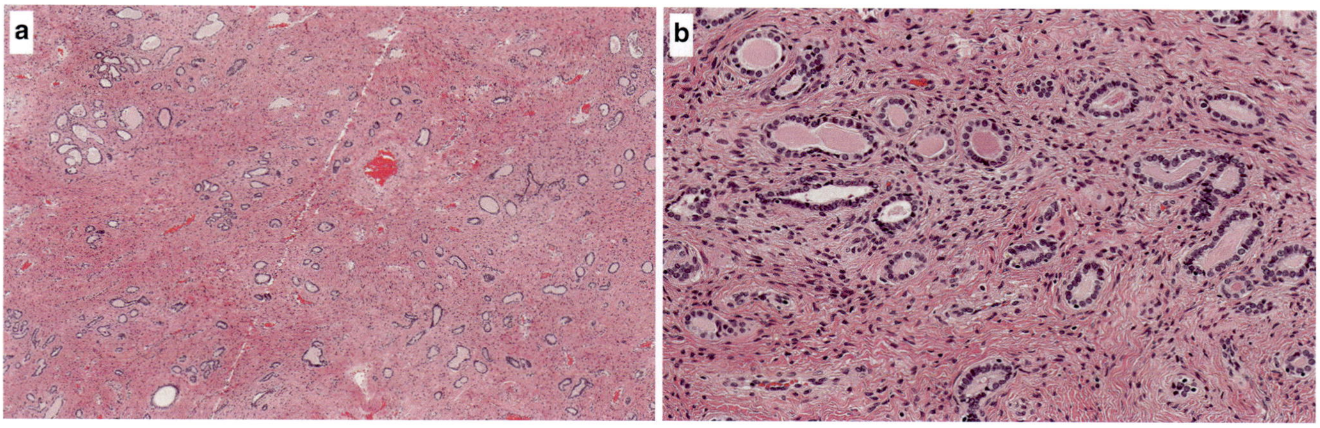

Fig. 13.33 Mesonephric hyperplasia. This lesion can be superficial or deep; glands are haphazardly distributed and display variation of size and shape (**a**). They are lined by flat to cuboidal epithelium without tubal or mucinous differentiation; lumens typically contain eosinophilic material (**b**)

shortly after pregnancy and in patients on exogenous progestin treatment or contraceptive use [272]. Arias-Stella reaction is commonly incidental, but can present as a polyp or a "lesion" detected on gynecologic exam [272]. It usually affects the upper endocervical canal, and it can be multifocal [273].

13.5.10.2 Pathologic Features

On histologic examination, Arias-Stella reaction is characterized by tortuous, "hypersecretory" glands with festooning or ruffled luminal borders, sometimes quite florid with papillary or cribriform patterns. Epithelial cells are large and tall with abundant clear (secretory) cytoplasm and markedly enlarged nuclei. The latter are usually hyperchromatic and irregular in shape, and can protrude towards the lumen ("hobnail" appearance). Mitotic activity is absent to scant.

13.5.10.3 Differential Diagnosis

The striking nuclear features of Arias-Stella commonly raise concern for clear cell carcinoma. This type of malignancy typically has high-grade pleomorphic cells with high nuclear-to-cytoplasmic ratio; conversely, the nuclear-to-cytoplasmic ratio in Arias-Stella reaction remains low (since cytoplasm is abundant) and there is no mitotic activity. P53 can be of aid, since it can be abnormal in clear cell carcinoma [274]. Napsin-A is frequently present in Arias-Stella reaction, limiting the role of this marker in the above differential [141]. Likewise, glands displaying Arias-Stella reaction may have low to absent expression of hormone receptors, limiting their value in separating it from endocervical adenocarcinoma [274, 275].

13.5.11 Mesonephric Remnants and Mesonephric Hyperplasia

13.5.11.1 Clinical Features

Remnants of the mesonephric duct are commonly seen in resection specimens, particularly in the cervical stroma and in the adnexal (paratubal) region. In the cervix, they are most commonly seen in cone and LEEP excisions [143].

13.5.11.2 Pathologic Features

Mesonephric duct remnants appear as groups of round glands and tubules, lined by simple flat to low cuboidal epithelium. The glandular lumen is usually filled with a dense eosinophilic PAS positive, diastase resistant material [143]. Mucinous or ciliated cells are not identified (Fig. 13.33). Hyperplasia of mesonephric ducts is characterized by a glandular population similar to mesonephric remnants, but larger, more irregular and haphazardly distributed [143]. It has been described in a number of architectural patterns, most frequently lobular but also ductal and diffuse. While most cases of mesonephric hyperplasia are incidental, some can be grossly identified as areas of induration or nodularity. They can be as large as 2.5 cm and extend to the deep cervical stroma.

13.5.11.3 Differential Diagnosis

The main differential diagnosis of mesonephric hyperplasia includes mesonephric carcinoma and endocervical adenocarcinoma. Unlike mesonephric hyperplasia, carcinoma produces mass-related symptoms. While the contour of mesonephric hyperplasia can be irregular, a frankly infiltrative border should raise concern for malignancy. Mesonephric carcinoma typically displays marked cytologic atypia, solid and confluent growth, mitotic activity and lymphatic vascular invasion. Endocervical adenocarcinoma typically displays mucinous differentiation at least focally, and lacks the eosinophilic secretions characteristic of mesonephric glands.

Mesonephric hyperplasia can overlap morphologically with tunnel clusters and lobular endocervical glandular hyperplasia. The presence of intra and extracellular mucin in these two entities should be indicative of the correct diagnosis. The distinction between mesonephric remnants and hyperplasia is not only subjective but also inconsequential, since both entities are benign.

13.5.11.4 Prognosis and Management

Mesonephric hyperplasia is regarded as a benign lesion, with no documented progression to malignancy following initial diagnosis [276]. Nonetheless, mesonephric hyperplasia has been found in the vicinity of most mesonephric carcinomas suggesting a potential role as a precursor lesion [144].

References

1. Fluhmann CF. The cervix uteri and its diseases. 1st ed. Philadelphia, PA: W. B. Saunders Company; 1961.
2. Fluhmann CF. The nature and development of the so-called glands of the cervix uteri. Am J Obstet Gynecol. 1957;74:753–66; discussion 766–768
3. Wang SS, Sherman ME, Hildesheim A, et al. Cervical adenocarcinoma and squamous cell carcinoma incidence trends among white women and black women in the United States for 1976–2000. Cancer. 2004;100:1035–44. https://doi.org/10.1002/cncr.20064.
4. Smith HO, Tiffany MF, Qualls CR, Key CR. The rising incidence of adenocarcinoma relative to squamous cell carcinoma of the uterine cervix in the United States--a 24-year population-based study. Gynecol Oncol. 2000;78:97–105. https://doi.org/10.1006/gyno.2000.5826.
5. Vizcaino AP, Moreno V, Bosch FX, et al. International trends in the incidence of cervical cancer: I. Adenocarcinoma and adenosquamous cell carcinomas. Int J Cancer. 1998;75:536–45.
6. Adegoke O, Kulasingam S, Virnig B. Cervical cancer trends in the United States: a 35-year population-based analysis. J Women's Health. 2012;21:1031–7. https://doi.org/10.1089/jwh.2011.3385.
7. Baldur-Felskov B, Munk C, Nielsen TSS, et al. Trends in the incidence of cervical cancer and severe precancerous lesions in Denmark, 1997–2012. Cancer Causes Control. 2015;26:1105–16. https://doi.org/10.1007/s10552-015-0603-7.
8. van der Horst J, Siebers AG, Bulten J, et al. Increasing incidence of invasive and in situ cervical adenocarcinoma in the Netherlands during 2004–2013. Cancer Med. 2017;6:416–23. https://doi.org/10.1002/cam4.971.
9. Moukarzel LA, Angarita AM, VandenBussche C, et al. Preinvasive and invasive cervical adenocarcinoma: preceding low-risk or negative pap result increases time to diagnosis. J Low Genit Tract Dis. 2017;21:91–6. https://doi.org/10.1097/LGT.0000000000000286.
10. Korhonen MO. Epidemiological differences between adenocarcinoma and squamous cell carcinoma of the uterine cervix. Gynecol Oncol. 1980;10:312–7.
11. Kurman R, Carcangiu M, Herrington C, Young R. World Health Organization classification of tumours of female reproductive organs. 4th ed. Geneva: WHO Press; 2014.
12. Zielinski GD, Snijders PJF, Rozendaal L, et al. The presence of high-risk HPV combined with specific p53 and p16INK4a expression patterns points to high-risk HPV as the main causative agent for adenocarcinoma in situ and adenocarcinoma of the cervix. J Pathol. 2003;201:535–43. https://doi.org/10.1002/path.1480.
13. Andersson S, Rylander E, Larsson B, et al. The role of human papillomavirus in cervical adenocarcinoma carcinogenesis. Eur J Cancer. 2001;37:246–50.
14. Monsonego J, Cox JT, Behrens C, et al. Prevalence of high-risk human papilloma virus genotypes and associated risk of cervical precancerous lesions in a large U.S. screening population: data from the ATHENA trial. Gynecol Oncol. 2015;137:47–54. https://doi.org/10.1016/j.ygyno.2015.01.551.
15. Clifford G, Franceschi S. Members of the human papillomavirus type 18 family (alpha-7 species) share a common association with adenocarcinoma of the cervix. Int J Cancer. 2008;122:1684–5. https://doi.org/10.1002/ijc.23282.
16. Bertrand M, Lickrish GM, Colgan TJ. The anatomic distribution of cervical adenocarcinoma in situ: implications for treatment. Am J Obstet Gynecol. 1987;157:21–5.
17. Holl K, Nowakowski AM, Powell N, et al. Human papillomavirus prevalence and type-distribution in cervical glandular neoplasias: results from a European multinational epidemiological study. Int J Cancer. 2015;137:2858–68. https://doi.org/10.1002/ijc.29651.
18. Sheng Z, Minato H, Sasagawa T, et al. Detection of high-risk human papillomavirus subtypes in cervical glandular neoplasia by in situ hybridization. Int J Clin Exp Pathol. 2013;6:2168–77.
19. Lee KR. Symposium part 4: should pathologists diagnose endocervical preneoplastic lesions "less than" adenocarcinoma in situ?: counterpoint. Int J Gynecol Pathol. 2003;22:22–4.
20. Gloor E, Hurlimann J. Cervical intraepithelial glandular neoplasia (adenocarcinoma in situ and glandular dysplasia). A correlative study of 23 cases with histologic grading, histochemical analysis of mucins, and immunohistochemical determination of the affinity for four lectins. Cancer. 1986;58:1272–80.
21. Ioffe OB, Sagae S, Moritani S, et al. Symposium part 3: should pathologists diagnose endocervical preneoplastic lesions "less than" adenocarcinoma in situ?: point. Int J Gynecol Pathol. 2003;22:18–21.
22. Lee KR, Sun D, Crum CP. Endocervical intraepithelial glandular atypia (dysplasia): a histopathologic, human papillomavirus, and MIB-1 analysis of 25 cases. Hum Pathol. 2000;31:656–64. https://doi.org/10.1053/hupa.2000.7644.
23. Lu X, Shiozawa T, Nakayama K, et al. Abnormal expression of sex steroid receptors and cell cycle-related molecules in adenocarcinoma in situ of the uterine cervix. Int J Gynecol Pathol. 1999;18:109–14.
24. Murphy N, Heffron CCBB, King B, et al. p16INK4A positivity in benign, premalignant and malignant cervical glandular lesions: a potential diagnostic problem. Virchows Arch. 2004;445:610–5. https://doi.org/10.1007/s00428-004-1111-4.
25. Friedell GH, McKay DG. Adenocarcinoma in situ of the endocervix. Cancer. 1953;6:887–97.
26. Boon ME, Baak JP, Kurver PJ, et al. Adenocarcinoma in situ of the cervix: an underdiagnosed lesion. Cancer. 1981;48:768–73.
27. Zaino RJ. Symposium part I: adenocarcinoma in situ, glandular dysplasia, and early invasive adenocarcinoma of the uterine cervix. Int J Gynecol Pathol. 2002;21:314–26.
28. Moritani S, Ioffe OB, Sagae S, et al. Mitotic activity and apoptosis in endocervical glandular lesions. Int J Gynecol Pathol. 2002;21:125–33.
29. Jaworski RC. Endocervical glandular dysplasia, adenocarcinoma in situ, and early invasive (microinvasive) adenocarcinoma of the uterine cervix. Semin Diagn Pathol. 1990;7:190–204.
30. McCluggage WG, Shah R, Connolly LE, McBride HA. Intestinal-type cervical adenocarcinoma in situ and adenocarcinoma exhibit a partial enteric immunophenotype with consistent expression of CDX2. Int J Gynecol Pathol. 2008;27:92–100. https://doi.org/10.1097/pgp.0b013e31815698e7.
31. Schlesinger C, Silverberg SG. Endocervical adenocarcinoma in situ of tubal type and its relation to atypical tubal metaplasia. Int J Gynecol Pathol. 1999;18:1–4.
32. Negri G, Egarter-Vigl E, Kasal A, et al. p16INK4a is a useful marker for the diagnosis of adenocarcinoma of the cervix uteri and its precursors: an immunohistochemical study with immunocytochemical correlations. Am J Surg Pathol. 2003;27:187–93.
33. Schorge JO, Lea JS, Elias KJ, et al. P16 as a molecular biomarker of cervical adenocarcinoma. Am J Obstet Gynecol. 2004;190:668–73. https://doi.org/10.1016/j.ajog.2003.09.038.
34. Negri G, Bellisano G, Carico E, et al. Usefulness of p16ink4a, ProEX C, and Ki-67 for the diagnosis of glandu-

lar dysplasia and adenocarcinoma of the cervix uteri. Int J Gynecol Pathol. 2011;30:407–13. https://doi.org/10.1097/PGP.0b013e31820a79b0.
35. Aximu D, Azad A, Ni R, et al. A pilot evaluation of a novel immunohistochemical assay for topoisomerase II-alpha and minichromosome maintenance protein 2 expression (ProEx C) in cervical adenocarcinoma in situ, adenocarcinoma, and benign glandular mimics. Int J Gynecol Pathol. 2009;28:114–9. https://doi.org/10.1097/PGP.0b013e3181895573.
36. McCluggage WG, Sumathi VP, McBride HA, Patterson A. A panel of immunohistochemical stains, including carcinoembryonic antigen, vimentin, and estrogen receptor, aids the distinction between primary endometrial and endocervical adenocarcinomas. Int J Gynecol Pathol. 2002;21:11–5.
37. Gradíssimo A, Burk RD. Molecular tests potentially improving HPV screening and genotyping for cervical cancer prevention. Expert Rev Mol Diagn. 2017;17:379–91. https://doi.org/10.1080/14737159.2017.1293525.
38. Quint KD, de Koning MNC, van Doorn L-J, et al. HPV genotyping and HPV16 variant analysis in glandular and squamous neoplastic lesions of the uterine cervix. Gynecol Oncol. 2010;117:297–301. https://doi.org/10.1016/j.ygyno.2010.02.003.
39. Talia KL, Stewart CJR, Howitt BE, et al. HPV-negative gastric type adenocarcinoma in situ of the cervix: a spectrum of rare lesions exhibiting gastric and intestinal differentiation. Am J Surg Pathol. 2017;41:1023–33. https://doi.org/10.1097/PAS.0000000000000855.
40. Hasumi K, Ehrmann RL. Clear cell carcinoma of the uterine endocervix with an in situ component. Cancer. 1978;42:2435–8.
41. Kim J-H, Park J-Y, Kim D-Y, et al. The role of loop electrosurgical excisional procedure in the management of adenocarcinoma in situ of the uterine cervix. Eur J Obstet Gynecol Reprod Biol. 2009;145:100–3. https://doi.org/10.1016/j.ejogrb.2009.04.011.
42. Baalbergen A, Helmerhorst TJM. Adenocarcinoma in situ of the uterine cervix-a systematic review. Int J Gynecol Cancer. 2014;24:1543–8. https://doi.org/10.1097/IGC.0000000000000260.
43. Salani R, Puri I, Bristow RE. Adenocarcinoma in situ of the uterine cervix: a metaanalysis of 1278 patients evaluating the predictive value of conization margin status. Am J Obstet Gynecol. 2009;200:182.e1–5. https://doi.org/10.1016/j.ajog.2008.09.012.
44. Park JJ, Sun D, Quade BJ, et al. Stratified mucin-producing intraepithelial lesions of the cervix: adenosquamous or columnar cell neoplasia? Am J Surg Pathol. 2000;24:1414–9.
45. Onishi J, Sato Y, Sawaguchi A, et al. Stratified mucin-producing intraepithelial lesion with invasive carcinoma: 12 cases with immunohistochemical and ultrastructural findings. Hum Pathol. 2016;55:174–81. https://doi.org/10.1016/j.humpath.2016.05.007.
46. Mikami Y, McCluggage WG. Endocervical glandular lesions exhibiting gastric differentiation: an emerging spectrum of benign, premalignant, and malignant lesions. Adv Anat Pathol. 2013;20:227–37. https://doi.org/10.1097/PAP.0b013e31829c2d66.
47. Kondo T, Hashi A, Murata S-I, et al. Gastric mucin is expressed in a subset of endocervical tunnel clusters: type A tunnel clusters of gastric phenotype. Histopathology. 2007;50:843–50. https://doi.org/10.1111/j.1365-2559.2007.02705.x.
48. Nucci MR, Clement PB, Young RH. Lobular endocervical glandular hyperplasia, not otherwise specified: a clinicopathologic analysis of thirteen cases of a distinctive pseudoneoplastic lesion and comparison with fourteen cases of adenoma malignum. Am J Surg Pathol. 1999;23:886–91.
49. Mikami Y, Hata S, Melamed J, et al. Lobular endocervical glandular hyperplasia is a metaplastic process with a pyloric gland phenotype. Histopathology. 2001;39:364–72.
50. Ohta Y, Suzuki T, Hamatani S, et al. Lobular endocervical glandular hyperplasia might become a precursor of adenocarcinoma with pyloric gland features. Pathol Res Pract. 2008;204:683–7. https://doi.org/10.1016/j.prp.2008.02.009.
51. Mikami Y, Kiyokawa T, Hata S, et al. Gastrointestinal immunophenotype in adenocarcinomas of the uterine cervix and related glandular lesions: a possible link between lobular endocervical glandular hyperplasia/pyloric gland metaplasia and "adenoma malignum.". Mod Pathol. 2004;17:962–72. https://doi.org/10.1038/modpathol.3800148.
52. Kawauchi S, Kusuda T, Liu X-P, et al. Is lobular endocervical glandular hyperplasia a cancerous precursor of minimal deviation adenocarcinoma?: a comparative molecular-genetic and immunohistochemical study. Am J Surg Pathol. 2008;32:1807–15. https://doi.org/10.1097/PAS.0b013e3181883722.
53. Mikami Y, Kojima A, Kiyokawa T, Manabe T. Ki67 labelling index and p53 status indicate neoplastic nature of atypical lobular endocervical glandular hyperplasia (ALEGH). Histopathology. 2009;55:362–4. https://doi.org/10.1111/j.1365-2559.2009.03346.x.
54. Ronnett BM. Endocervical adenocarcinoma: selected diagnostic challenges. Mod Pathol. 2016;29(Suppl 1):S12–28. https://doi.org/10.1038/modpathol.2015.131.
55. Ronnett BM, Yemelyanova AV, Vang R, et al. Endocervical adenocarcinomas with ovarian metastases: analysis of 29 cases with emphasis on minimally invasive cervical tumors and the ability of the metastases to simulate primary ovarian neoplasms. Am J Surg Pathol. 2008;32:1835–53. https://doi.org/10.1097/PAS.0b013e3181758831.
56. Ostör AG. Early invasive adenocarcinoma of the uterine cervix. Int J Gynecol Pathol. 2000;19:29–38.
57. Douglas G, Howitt BE, Schoolmeester JK, et al. Architectural overlap between benign endocervix and pattern-A endocervical adenocarcinoma: Are all pattern-A tumors invasive? Pathol Res Pract. 2017;213(7):799–803. https://doi.org/10.1016/j.prp.2017.03.008.
58. Buchanan T, Pierce JY, Graybill W, et al. Why do we continue to overtreat stage Ia carcinoma of the cervix? Am J Obstet Gynecol. 2017;217:413–7. https://doi.org/10.1016/j.ajog.2017.05.020.
59. Reynolds EA, Tierney K, Keeney GL, et al. Analysis of outcomes of microinvasive adenocarcinoma of the uterine cervix by treatment type. Obstet Gynecol. 2010;116:1150–7. https://doi.org/10.1097/AOG.0b013e3181f74062.
60. Baalbergen A, Smedts F, Helmerhorst TJM. Conservative therapy in microinvasive adenocarcinoma of the uterine cervix is justified: an analysis of 59 cases and a review of the literature. Int J Gynecol Cancer. 2011;21:1640–5. https://doi.org/10.1097/IGC.0b013e3182262059.
61. Bisseling KCHM, Bekkers RLM, Rome RM, Quinn MA. Treatment of microinvasive adenocarcinoma of the uterine cervix: a retrospective study and review of the literature. Gynecol Oncol. 2007;107:424–30. https://doi.org/10.1016/j.ygyno.2007.07.062.
62. Baalbergen A, Veenstra Y, Stalpers L. Primary surgery versus primary radiotherapy with or without chemotherapy for early adenocarcinoma of the uterine cervix. Cochrane Database Syst Rev. 2013;1:CD006248. https://doi.org/10.1002/14651858.CD006248.pub3.
63. Peters WA, Liu PY, Barrett RJ, et al. Concurrent chemotherapy and pelvic radiation therapy compared with pelvic radiation therapy alone as adjuvant therapy after radical surgery in high-risk early-stage cancer of the cervix. J Clin Oncol. 2000;18:1606–13. https://doi.org/10.1200/JCO.2000.18.8.1606.
64. Osman M. The role of neoadjuvant chemotherapy in the management of locally advanced cervix cancer: a systematic review. Oncol Rev. 2014;8:250. https://doi.org/10.4081/oncol.2014.250.

65. Herfs M, Yamamoto Y, Laury A, et al. A discrete population of squamocolumnar junction cells implicated in the pathogenesis of cervical cancer. Proc Natl Acad Sci U S A. 2012;109:10516–21. https://doi.org/10.1073/pnas.1202684109.
66. Ojesina AI, Lichtenstein L, Freeman SS, et al. Landscape of genomic alterations in cervical carcinomas. Nature. 2014;506:371–5. https://doi.org/10.1038/nature12881.
67. Wright AA, Howitt BE, Myers AP, et al. Oncogenic mutations in cervical cancer: genomic differences between adenocarcinomas and squamous cell carcinomas of the cervix. Cancer. 2013;119:3776–83. https://doi.org/10.1002/cncr.28288.
68. Lou H, Villagran G, Boland JF, et al. Genome analysis of latin American cervical cancer: frequent activation of the PIK3CA pathway. Clin Cancer Res. 2015;21:5360–70. https://doi.org/10.1158/1078-0432.CCR-14-1837.
69. Tornesello ML, Annunziata C, Buonaguro L, et al. TP53 and PIK3CA gene mutations in adenocarcinoma, squamous cell carcinoma and high-grade intraepithelial neoplasia of the cervix. J Transl Med. 2014;12:255. https://doi.org/10.1186/s12967-014-0255-5.
70. Chappell WH, Steelman LS, Long JM, et al. Ras/Raf/MEK/ERK and PI3K/PTEN/Akt/mTOR inhibitors: rationale and importance to inhibiting these pathways in human health. Oncotarget. 2011;2:135–64. https://doi.org/10.18632/oncotarget.240.
71. Hodgson A, Amemiya Y, Seth A, et al. Genomic abnormalities in invasive endocervical adenocarcinoma correlate with pattern of invasion: biologic and clinical implications. Mod Pathol. 2017;30:1633–41. https://doi.org/10.1038/modpathol.2017.80.
72. Xiang L, Li J, Jiang W, et al. Comprehensive analysis of targetable oncogenic mutations in chinese cervical cancers. Oncotarget. 2015;6:4968–75. https://doi.org/10.18632/oncotarget.3212.
73. Pecorelli S, Zigliani L, Odicino F. Revised FIGO staging for carcinoma of the cervix. Int J Gynaecol Obstet. 2009;105:107–8. https://doi.org/10.1016/j.ijgo.2009.02.009.
74. Diaz De Vivar A, Roma AA, Park KJ, et al. Invasive endocervical adenocarcinoma: proposal for a new pattern-based classification system with significant clinical implications: a multi-institutional study. Int J Gynecol Pathol. 2013;32:592–601. https://doi.org/10.1097/PGP.0b013e31829952c6.
75. Roma AA, Diaz De Vivar A, Park KJ, et al. Invasive endocervical adenocarcinoma: a new pattern-based classification system with important clinical significance. Am J Surg Pathol. 2015;39:667–72. https://doi.org/10.1097/PAS.0000000000000402.
76. Roma AA, Mistretta T-A, Diaz De Vivar A, et al. New pattern-based personalized risk stratification system for endocervical adenocarcinoma with important clinical implications and surgical outcome. Gynecol Oncol. 2016;141:36–42. https://doi.org/10.1016/j.ygyno.2016.02.028.
77. Jeffus SK, Quick CM, Stolnicu S, et al. Tumor growth pattern can predict nodal metastasis: a study of 130 cases of endocervical adenocarcinoma. Mod Pathol. 2015;28:292A.
78. Djordjevic B, Parra-Herran C. Application of a pattern-based classification system for invasive endocervical adenocarcinoma in cervical biopsy, cone and loop electrosurgical excision (LEEP) material: pattern on cone and LEEP is predictive of pattern in the overall tumor. Int J Gynecol Pathol. 2016;35:456–66. https://doi.org/10.1097/PGP.0000000000000264.
79. Parra-Herran C, Taljaard M, Djordjevic B, et al. Pattern-based classification of invasive endocervical adenocarcinoma, depth of invasion measurement and distinction from adenocarcinoma in situ: interobserver variation among gynecologic pathologists. Mod Pathol. 2016;29:879–92. https://doi.org/10.1038/modpathol.2016.86.
80. Rutgers JKL, Roma AA, Park KJ, et al. Pattern classification of endocervical adenocarcinoma: reproducibility and review of criteria. Mod Pathol. 2016;29:1083–94. https://doi.org/10.1038/modpathol.2016.94.
81. Paquette C, Jeffus SK, Quick CM, et al. Interobserver variability in the application of a proposed histologic subclassification of endocervical adenocarcinoma. Am J Surg Pathol. 2014;39(1):93–100. https://doi.org/10.1097/PAS.0000000000000316.
82. Alfsen GC, Kristensen GB, Skovlund E, et al. Histologic subtype has minor importance for overall survival in patients with adenocarcinoma of the uterine cervix: a population-based study of prognostic factors in 505 patients with nonsquamous cell carcinomas of the cervix. Cancer. 2001;92:2471–83.
83. Castanon A, Landy R, Sasieni PD. Is cervical screening preventing adenocarcinoma and adenosquamous carcinoma of the cervix? Int J Cancer. 2016;139:1040–5. https://doi.org/10.1002/ijc.30152.
84. Stolnicu S, Barsan I, Hoang L, et al. International endocervical adenocarcinoma criteria and classification (IECC): a new pathogenetic classification for invasive adenocarcinomas of the endocervix. Am J Surg Pathol. 2018;42(2):214–26. https://doi.org/10.1097/PAS.0000000000000986.
85. Hodgson A, Park KJ, Djordjevic B, et al. International classification of endocervical adenocarcinoma: validation and interobserver reproducibility. Mod Pathol. 2018:31.
86. Alfsen GC, Reed W, Abeler VM. Reproducibility of classification in non-squamous cell carcinomas of the uterine cervix. Gynecol Oncol. 2003;90:282–9.
87. Young RH, Clement PB. Endocervical adenocarcinoma and its variants: their morphology and differential diagnosis. Histopathology. 2002;41:185–207.
88. Lim D, Murali R, Murray MP, et al. Morphological and immunohistochemical reevaluation of tumors initially diagnosed as ovarian endometrioid carcinoma with emphasis on high-grade tumors. Am J Surg Pathol. 2016;40:302–12. https://doi.org/10.1097/PAS.0000000000000550.
89. Lee KR, Trainer TD. Adenocarcinoma of the uterine cervix of small intestinal type containing numerous paneth cells. Arch Pathol Lab Med. 1990;114:731–3.
90. Shintaku M, Kushima R, Abiko K. Colloid carcinoma of the intestinal type in the uterine cervix: mucin immunohistochemistry. Pathol Int. 2010;60:119–24. https://doi.org/10.1111/j.1440-1827.2009.02485.x.
91. Raspollini MR, Baroni G, Taddei A, Taddei GL. Primary cervical adenocarcinoma with intestinal differentiation and colonic carcinoma metastatic to cervix: an investigation using Cdx-2 and a limited immunohistochemical panel. Arch Pathol Lab Med. 2003;127:1586–90. https://doi.org/10.1043/1543-2165(2003)127<1586:PCAWID>2.0.CO;2.
92. Howitt BE, Herfs M, Brister K, et al. Intestinal-type endocervical adenocarcinoma in situ: an immunophenotypically distinct subset of AIS affecting older women. Am J Surg Pathol. 2013;37:625–33. https://doi.org/10.1097/PAS.0b013e318285be00.
93. Sal V, Kahramanoglu I, Turan H, et al. Primary signet ring cell carcinoma of the cervix: a case report and review of the literature. Int J Surg Case Rep. 2016;21:1–5. https://doi.org/10.1016/j.ijscr.2016.02.007.
94. Imachi M, Tsukamoto N, Amagase H, et al. Metastatic adenocarcinoma to the uterine cervix from gastric cancer. A clinicopathologic analysis of 16 cases. Cancer. 1993;71:3472–7.
95. Suárez-Peñaranda JM, Abdulkader I, Barón-Duarte FJ, et al. Signet-ring cell carcinoma presenting in the uterine cervix: report of a primary and 2 metastatic cases. Int J Gynecol Pathol. 2007;26:254–8. https://doi.org/10.1097/01.pgp.0000236949.49161.31.
96. Washimi K, Yokose T, Noguchi A, et al. Diagnosis of primary pure signet-ring cell carcinoma of the cervix. Pathol Int. 2015;65:393–5. https://doi.org/10.1111/pin.12275.
97. Giordano G, Pizzi S, Berretta R, D'Adda T. A new case of primary signet-ring cell carcinoma of the cervix with prominent endometrial and myometrial involvement: Immunohistochemical and molecular studies and review of the literature. World J Surg Oncol. 2012;10:7. https://doi.org/10.1186/1477-7819-10-7.

98. Cracchiolo B, Kuhn T, Heller D. Primary signet ring cell adenocarcinoma of the uterine cervix—A rare neoplasm that raises the question of metastasis to the cervix. Gynecol Oncol Rep. 2016;16:9–10. https://doi.org/10.1016/j.gore.2016.01.004.
99. Lastra RR, Park KJ, Schoolmeester JK. Invasive stratified mucin-producing carcinoma and stratified mucin-producing intraepithelial lesion (SMILE): 15 cases presenting a spectrum of cervical neoplasia with description of a distinctive variant of invasive adenocarcinoma. Am J Surg Pathol. 2016;40:262–9. https://doi.org/10.1097/PAS.0000000000000543.
100. Young RH, Scully RE. Villoglandular papillary adenocarcinoma of the uterine cervix. A clinicopathologic analysis of 13 cases. Cancer. 1989;63:1773–9.
101. Jones MW, Silverberg SG, Kurman RJ. Well-differentiated villoglandular adenocarcinoma of the uterine cervix: a clinicopathological study of 24 cases. Int J Gynecol Pathol. 1993;12:1–7.
102. Kim H-J, Sung J-H, Lee E, et al. Prognostic factors influencing decisions about surgical treatment of villoglandular adenocarcinoma of the uterine cervix. Int J Gynecol Cancer. 2014;24:1299–305. https://doi.org/10.1097/IGC.0000000000000197.
103. Macdonald RD, Kirwan J, Hayat K, et al. Villoglandular adenocarcinoma of the cervix: clarity is needed on the histological definition for this difficult diagnosis. Gynecol Oncol. 2006;100:192–4. https://doi.org/10.1016/j.ygyno.2005.07.133.
104. Bouman A, Oosterhuis GJ, Naudin ten Cate L, van Doorn GA. Villoglandular papillary adenocarcinoma of the cervix. Beware of a wolf in sheep's clothing. Eur J Obstet Gynecol Reprod Biol. 1999;87:183–9.
105. Heatley MK. Villoglandular adenocarcinoma of the uterine cervix-a systematic review of the literature. Histopathology. 2007;51:268–9. https://doi.org/10.1111/j.1365-2559.2007.02759.x.
106. Lataifeh IM, Al-Hussaini M, Uzan C, et al. Villoglandular papillary adenocarcinoma of the cervix: a series of 28 cases including two with lymph node metastasis. Int J Gynecol Cancer. 2013;23:900–5. https://doi.org/10.1097/IGC.0b013e31828efcaa.
107. Khunamornpong S, Maleemonkol S, Siriaunkgul S, Pantusart A. Well-differentiated villoglandular adenocarcinoma of the uterine cervix: a report of 15 cases including two with lymph node metastasis. J Med Assoc Thail. 2001;84:882–8.
108. Stanley-Christian H, Heim BK, Hines JF, et al. Villoglandular adenocarcinoma of the cervix: a report of three cases and review of the literature. Gynecol Oncol. 1997;66:327–30. https://doi.org/10.1006/gyno.1997.4747.
109. Kojima A, Mikami Y, Sudo T, et al. Gastric morphology and immunophenotype predict poor outcome in mucinous adenocarcinoma of the uterine cervix. Am J Surg Pathol. 2007;31:664–72. https://doi.org/10.1097/01.pas.0000213434.91868.b0.
110. Omori M, Hashi A, Ishii Y, et al. Clinical impact of preoperative screening for gastric mucin secretion in cervical discharge by HIK1083-labeled latex agglutination test. Am J Clin Pathol. 2008;130:585–94. https://doi.org/10.1309/L8XME5JVEJ74C3F1.
111. Kwon SY, Choe MS, Lee HW, et al. Minimal deviation adenocarcinoma of the cervix and tumorlets of sex-cord stromal tumor with annular tubules of the ovary in Peutz-Jeghers syndrome. J Gynecol Oncol. 2013;24:92–5. https://doi.org/10.3802/jgo.2013.24.1.92.
112. Kawakami F, Mikami Y, Kojima A, et al. Diagnostic reproducibility in gastric-type mucinous adenocarcinoma of the uterine cervix: validation of novel diagnostic criteria. Histopathology. 2010;56:551–3. https://doi.org/10.1111/j.1365-2559.2010.03500.x.
113. Tsuda H, Mikami Y, Kaku T, et al. Interobserver variation in the diagnosis of adenoma malignum (minimal deviation adenocarcinoma) of the uterine cervix. Pathol Int. 2003;53:440–9.
114. Karamurzin YS, Kiyokawa T, Parkash V, et al. Gastric-type endocervical adenocarcinoma: an aggressive tumor with unusual metastatic patterns and poor prognosis. Am J Surg Pathol. 2015;39:1449–57. https://doi.org/10.1097/PAS.0000000000000532.
115. Tsuda H, Mikami Y, Kaku T, et al. Reproducible and clinically meaningful differential diagnosis is possible between lobular endocervical glandular hyperplasia and "adenoma malignum" based on common histopathological criteria. Pathol Int. 2005;55:412–8. https://doi.org/10.1111/j.1440-1827.2005.01846.x.
116. Pirog EC. Diagnosis of HPV-negative, gastric-type adenocarcinoma of the endocervix. Methods Mol Biol. 2015;1249:213–9. https://doi.org/10.1007/978-1-4939-2013-6_16.
117. Carleton C, Hoang L, Sah S, et al. A detailed immunohistochemical analysis of a large series of cervical and vaginal gastric-type adenocarcinomas. Am J Surg Pathol. 2016;40:636–44. https://doi.org/10.1097/PAS.0000000000000578.
118. Rabban JT, McAlhany S, Lerwill MF, et al. PAX2 distinguishes benign mesonephric and mullerian glandular lesions of the cervix from endocervical adenocarcinoma, including minimal deviation adenocarcinoma. Am J Surg Pathol. 2010;34:137–46. https://doi.org/10.1097/PAS.0b013e3181c89c98.
119. Peng W-X, Kure S, Ishino K, et al. P16-positive continuous minimal deviation adenocarcinoma and gastric type adenocarcinoma in a patient with Peutz-Jeghers syndrome. Int J Clin Exp Pathol. 2015;8:5877–82.
120. Park KJ, Kiyokawa T, Soslow RA, et al. Unusual endocervical adenocarcinomas: an immunohistochemical analysis with molecular detection of human papillomavirus. Am J Surg Pathol. 2011;35:633–46. https://doi.org/10.1097/PAS.0b013e31821534b9.
121. Houghton O, Jamison J, Wilson R, et al. p16 Immunoreactivity in unusual types of cervical adenocarcinoma does not reflect human papillomavirus infection. Histopathology. 2010;57:342–50. https://doi.org/10.1111/j.1365-2559.2010.03632.x.
122. Kusanagi Y, Kojima A, Mikami Y, et al. Absence of high-risk human papillomavirus (HPV) detection in endocervical adenocarcinoma with gastric morphology and phenotype. Am J Pathol. 2010;177:2169–75. https://doi.org/10.2353/ajpath.2010.100323.
123. Kuragaki C, Enomoto T, Ueno Y, et al. Mutations in the *STK11* gene characterize minimal deviation adenocarcinoma of the uterine cervix. Lab Investig. 2003;83:35. https://doi.org/10.1097/01.LAB.0000049821.16698.D0.
124. Wada T, Ohishi Y, Kaku T, et al. Endocervical adenocarcinoma with morphologic features of both usual and gastric types: clinicopathologic and immunohistochemical analyses and high-risk HPV detection by in situ hybridization. Am J Surg Pathol. 2017;41:696–705. https://doi.org/10.1097/PAS.0000000000000833.
125. Park HM, Lee SS, Eom DW, et al. Endometrioid adenocarcinoma arising from endometriosis of the uterine cervix: a case report. J Korean Med Sci. 2009;24:767–71. https://doi.org/10.3346/jkms.2009.24.4.767.
126. Rahilly MA, Williams AR, al-Nafussi A. Minimal deviation endometrioid adenocarcinoma of cervix: a clinicopathological and immunohistochemical study of two cases. Histopathology. 1992;20:351–4.
127. Young RH, Scully RE. Minimal-deviation endometrioid adenocarcinoma of the uterine cervix. A report of five cases of a distinctive neoplasm that may be misinterpreted as benign. Am J Surg Pathol. 1993;17:660–5.
128. Landry D, Mai KT, Senterman MK, et al. Endometrioid adenocarcinoma of the uterus with a minimal deviation invasive pattern. Histopathology. 2003;42:77–82.
129. Nanbu K, Konishi I, Yamamoto S, et al. Minimal deviation adenocarcinoma of endometrioid type may arise in the isthmus: clinicopathological and immunohistochemical study of two cases. Gynecol Oncol. 1995;58:136–41.
130. Tambouret R, Clement PB, Young RH. Endometrial endometrioid adenocarcinoma with a deceptive pattern of spread to the uterine cervix: a manifestation of stage IIB endometrial carcinoma liable to be misinterpreted as an independent carcinoma or a benign lesion. Am J Surg Pathol. 2003;27:1080–8.

131. Mai KT, Perkins DG, Yazdi HM, Thomas J. Endometrioid carcinoma of the endometrium with an invasive component of minimal deviation carcinoma. Hum Pathol. 2002;33:856–8.
132. Jiang L, Malpica A, Deavers MT, et al. Endometrial endometrioid adenocarcinoma of the uterine corpus involving the cervix: some cases probably represent independent primaries. Int J Gynecol Pathol. 2010;29:146–56. https://doi.org/10.1097/PGP.0b013e3181b8e951.
133. Hasegawa K, Nagao S, Yasuda M, et al. Gynecologic Cancer InterGroup (GCIG) consensus review for clear cell carcinoma of the uterine corpus and cervix. Int J Gynecol Cancer. 2014;24:S90–5. https://doi.org/10.1097/IGC.0000000000000297.
134. Hanselaar A, van Loosbroek M, Schuurbiers O, et al. Clear cell adenocarcinoma of the vagina and cervix. An update of the central Netherlands registry showing twin age incidence peaks. Cancer. 1997;79:2229–36.
135. Smith EK, White MC, Weir HK, et al. Higher incidence of clear cell adenocarcinoma of the cervix and vagina among women born between 1947 and 1971 in the United States. Cancer Causes Control. 2012;23:207–11. https://doi.org/10.1007/s10552-011-9855-z.
136. Thomas MB, Wright JD, Leiser AL, et al. Clear cell carcinoma of the cervix: a multi-institutional review in the post-DES era. Gynecol Oncol. 2008;109:335–9. https://doi.org/10.1016/j.ygyno.2008.02.007.
137. Reich O, Tamussino K, Lahousen M, et al. Clear cell carcinoma of the uterine cervix: pathology and prognosis in surgically treated stage IB-IIB disease in women not exposed in utero to diethylstilbestrol. Gynecol Oncol. 2000;76:331–5. https://doi.org/10.1006/gyno.1999.5700.
138. Ueno S, Sudo T, Oka N, et al. Absence of human papillomavirus infection and activation of PI3K-AKT pathway in cervical clear cell carcinoma. Int J Gynecol Cancer. 2013;23:1084–91. https://doi.org/10.1097/IGC.0b013e3182981bdc.
139. Boyd J, Takahashi H, Waggoner SE, et al. Molecular genetic analysis of clear cell adenocarcinomas of the vagina and cervix associated and unassociated with diethylstilbestrol exposure in utero. Cancer. 1996;77:507–13. https://doi.org/10.1002/(SICI)1097-0142(19960201)77:3<507::AID-CNCR12>3.0.CO;2-8.
140. Ju B, Wang J, Yang B, et al. Morphologic and immunohistochemical study of clear cell carcinoma of the uterine endometrium and cervix in comparison to ovarian clear cell carcinoma. Int J Gynecol Pathol. 2018;37(4):388–96. https://doi.org/10.1097/PGP.0000000000000430.
141. Fadare O. Expression of Napsin A is common in Arias-Stella reaction. Hum Pathol. 2016;54:202. https://doi.org/10.1016/j.humpath.2016.02.028.
142. Mirkovic J, Sholl LM, Garcia E, et al. Targeted genomic profiling reveals recurrent KRAS mutations and gain of chromosome 1q in mesonephric carcinomas of the female genital tract. Mod Pathol. 2015;28:1504–14. https://doi.org/10.1038/modpathol.2015.103.
143. Ferry JA, Scully RE. Mesonephric remnants, hyperplasia, and neoplasia in the uterine cervix. A study of 49 cases. Am J Surg Pathol. 1990;14:1100–11.
144. Silver SA, Devouassoux-Shisheboran M, Mezzetti TP, Tavassoli FA. Mesonephric adenocarcinomas of the uterine cervix: a study of 11 cases with immunohistochemical findings. Am J Surg Pathol. 2001;25:379–87.
145. Clement PB, Young RH, Keh P, et al. Malignant mesonephric neoplasms of the uterine cervix. A report of eight cases, including four with a malignant spindle cell component. Am J Surg Pathol. 1995;19:1158–71.
146. Bagué S, Rodríguez IM, Prat J. Malignant mesonephric tumors of the female genital tract: a clinicopathologic study of 9 cases. Am J Surg Pathol. 2004;28:601–7.
147. Howitt BE, Emori MM, Drapkin R, et al. GATA3 is a sensitive and specific marker of benign and malignant mesonephric lesions in the lower female genital tract. Am J Surg Pathol. 2015;39:1411–9. https://doi.org/10.1097/PAS.0000000000000471.
148. Kenny SL, McBride HA, Jamison J, McCluggage WG. Mesonephric adenocarcinomas of the uterine cervix and corpus: HPV-negative neoplasms that are commonly PAX8, CA125, and HMGA2 positive and that may be immunoreactive with TTF1 and hepatocyte nuclear factor 1-β. Am J Surg Pathol. 2012;36:799–807. https://doi.org/10.1097/PAS.0b013e31824a72c6.
149. McCluggage WG, Hurrell DP, Kennedy K. Metastatic carcinomas in the cervix mimicking primary cervical adenocarcinoma and adenocarcinoma in situ: report of a series of cases. Am J Surg Pathol. 2010;34:735–41. https://doi.org/10.1097/PAS.0b013e3181d6b8fd.
150. Kos Z, Broaddus RR, Djordjevic B. Fallopian tube high-grade serous carcinoma with intramucosal spread and presenting as a malignancy on pap smear. Int J Gynecol Pathol. 2014;33:443–8. https://doi.org/10.1097/PGP.0b013e31829c728b.
151. Gilks CB, Clement PB. Papillary serous adenocarcinoma of the uterine cervix: a report of three cases. Mod Pathol. 1992;5:426–31.
152. Zhou C, Gilks CB, Hayes M, Clement PB. Papillary serous carcinoma of the uterine cervix: a clinicopathologic study of 17 cases. Am J Surg Pathol. 1998;22:113–20.
153. Togami S, Kasamatsu T, Sasajima Y, et al. Serous adenocarcinoma of the uterine cervix: a clinicopathological study of 12 cases and a review of the literature. Gynecol Obstet Investig. 2012;73:26–31. https://doi.org/10.1159/000329319.
154. Nofech-Mozes S, Rasty G, Ismiil N, et al. Immunohistochemical characterization of endocervical papillary serous carcinoma. Int J Gynecol Cancer. 2006;16(Suppl 1):286–92. https://doi.org/10.1111/j.1525-1438.2006.00514.x.
155. Togami S, Sasajima Y, Kasamatsu T, et al. Immunophenotype and human papillomavirus status of serous adenocarcinoma of the uterine cervix. Pathol Oncol Res. 2015;21:487–94. https://doi.org/10.1007/s12253-014-9854-y.
156. Nofech-Mozes S, Khalifa MM, Ismiil N, et al. Detection of HPV-DNA by a PCR-based method in formalin-fixed, paraffin-embedded tissue from rare endocervical carcinoma types. Appl Immunohistochem Mol Morphol. 2010;18:80–5. https://doi.org/10.1097/PAI.0b013e3181ae7240.
157. Pirog EC, Kleter B, Olgac S, et al. Prevalence of human papillomavirus DNA in different histological subtypes of cervical adenocarcinoma. Am J Pathol. 2000;157:1055–62. https://doi.org/10.1016/S0002-9440(10)64619-6.
158. Watrowski R, Striepecke E, Jäger C, et al. Papillary-serous adenocarcinoma of the uterine cervix during tamoxifen therapy after bilateral breast cancer. Anticancer Res. 2012;32:5075–8.
159. Costa MJ, McIlnay KR, Trelford J. Cervical carcinoma with glandular differentiation: histological evaluation predicts disease recurrence in clinical stage I or II patients. Hum Pathol. 1995;26:829–37.
160. Ueda M, Koshiyama M, Yamaguchi A, et al. Advanced papillary serous carcinoma of the uterine cervix: a case with a remarkable response to paclitaxel and carboplatin combination chemotherapy. Rare Tumors. 2012;4:e1. https://doi.org/10.4081/rt.2012.e1.
161. Khan M, Gilman AD, Nizami S, et al. Papillary serous carcinoma of the uterine cervix with lung metastasis. Case Rep Oncol Med. 2014;2014:683103. https://doi.org/10.1155/2014/683103.
162. Mazur MT, Hsueh S, Gersell DJ. Metastases to the female genital tract. Analysis of 325 cases. Cancer. 1984;53:1978–84.
163. Pérez-Montiel D, Serrano-Olvera A, Salazar LC, et al. Adenocarcinoma metastatic to the uterine cervix: a case series. J Obstet Gynaecol Res. 2012;38:541–9. https://doi.org/10.1111/j.1447-0756.2011.01747.x.
164. Esposito JM, Zarou DM, Zarou GS. Extragenital adenocarcinoma metastatic to the cervix uteri: a diagnostic problem. Am J Obstet Gynecol. 1965;92:792–5.

165. Castrillon DH, Lee KR, Nucci MR. Distinction between endometrial and endocervical adenocarcinoma: an immunohistochemical study. Int J Gynecol Pathol. 2002;21:4–10.
166. Staebler A, Sherman ME, Zaino RJ, Ronnett BM. Hormone receptor immunohistochemistry and human papillomavirus in situ hybridization are useful for distinguishing endocervical and endometrial adenocarcinomas. Am J Surg Pathol. 2002;26:998–1006.
167. Kamoi S, AlJuboury MI, Akin M-R, Silverberg SG. Immunohistochemical staining in the distinction between primary endometrial and endocervical adenocarcinomas: another viewpoint. Int J Gynecol Pathol. 2002;21:217–23.
168. Han C-P, Lee M-Y, Kok L-F, et al. Adding the p16(INK4a) marker to the traditional 3-marker (ER/Vim/CEA) panel engenders no supplemental benefit in distinguishing between primary endocervical and endometrial adenocarcinomas in a tissue microarray study. Int J Gynecol Pathol. 2009;28:489–96. https://doi.org/10.1097/PGP.0b013e31819e8ab4.
169. Nakagami K, Takahashi T, Sugitani K, et al. Uterine cervix metastasis from rectal carcinoma: a case report and a review of the literature. Jpn J Clin Oncol. 1999;29:640–2.
170. Kapoor R, Khosla D, Gupta R, et al. Uterine cervix metastasis from primary colorectal carcinoma: a report of two cases with review of literature. J Gastrointest Cancer. 2013;44:231–3. https://doi.org/10.1007/s12029-012-9437-7.
171. Reyes MC, Park KJ, Lin O, et al. Urothelial carcinoma involving the gynecologic tract: a morphologic and immunohistochemical study of 6 cases. Am J Surg Pathol. 2012;36:1058–65. https://doi.org/10.1097/PAS.0b013e318251eade.
172. Salem H, El-Mazny A. A clinicopathologic study of gynecologic organ involvement at radical cystectomy for bladder cancer. Int J Gynaecol Obstet. 2011;115:188–90. https://doi.org/10.1016/j.ijgo.2011.05.026.
173. Varkarakis IM, Pinggera G, Antoniou N, et al. Pathological review of internal genitalia after anterior exenteration for bladder cancer in women. Evaluating risk factors for female organ involvement. Int Urol Nephrol. 2007;39:1015–21. https://doi.org/10.1007/s11255-006-9158-6.
174. Herawi M, Leppert JT, Thomas GV, et al. Implants of noninvasive papillary urothelial carcinoma in peritoneum and ileocolonic neobladder: support for "seed and soil" hypothesis of bladder recurrence. Urology. 2006;67:746–50. https://doi.org/10.1016/j.urology.2005.10.023.
175. Behzatoğlu K. Malignant glandular lesions and glandular differentiation in invasive/noninvasive urothelial carcinoma of the urinary bladder. Ann Diagn Pathol. 2011;15:422–6. https://doi.org/10.1016/j.anndiagpath.2011.06.003.
176. Lee YJ, Moon KC, Jeong CW, et al. Impact of squamous and glandular differentiation on oncologic outcomes in upper and lower tract urothelial carcinoma. PLoS One. 2014;9:e107027. https://doi.org/10.1371/journal.pone.0107027.
177. Hodges KB, Lopez-Beltran A, Emerson RE, et al. Clinical utility of immunohistochemistry in the diagnoses of urinary bladder neoplasia. Appl Immunohistochem Mol Morphol. 2010;18:401–10. https://doi.org/10.1097/PAI.0b013e3181e04816.
178. Piaton E, Casalegno J-S, Advenier A-S, et al. p16(INK4a) overexpression is not linked to oncogenic human papillomaviruses in patients with high-grade urothelial cancer cells. Cancer Cytopathol. 2014;122:760–9. https://doi.org/10.1002/cncy.21462.
179. Chang A, Amin A, Gabrielson E, et al. Utility of GATA3 immunohistochemistry in differentiating urothelial carcinoma from prostate adenocarcinoma and squamous cell carcinomas of the uterine cervix, anus, and lung. Am J Surg Pathol. 2012;36:1472–6. https://doi.org/10.1097/PAS.0b013e318260cde7.
180. Verduin L, Mentrikoski MJ, Heitz CT, Wick MR. The utility of GATA3 in the diagnosis of urothelial carcinomas with variant morphologic patterns. Appl Immunohistochem Mol Morphol. 2016;24:509–13. https://doi.org/10.1097/PAI.0000000000000221.
181. Paner GP, Annaiah C, Gulmann C, et al. Immunohistochemical evaluation of novel and traditional markers associated with urothelial differentiation in a spectrum of variants of urothelial carcinoma of the urinary bladder. Hum Pathol. 2014;45:1473–82. https://doi.org/10.1016/j.humpath.2014.02.024.
182. Amălinei C, Balan R, Stolnicu S, et al. Adenosquamous cervical carcinoma morphological characteristics. Rev Med Chir Soc Med Nat Iasi. 2005;109:343–6.
183. Garg MM, Arora VK. Clear cell adenosquamous carcinoma of the cervix: a case report with discussion of the differential diagnosis. Int J Gynecol Pathol. 2012;31:294–6. https://doi.org/10.1097/PGP.0b013e31823b6f37.
184. Yoshida T, Sano T, Oyama T, et al. Prevalence, viral load, and physical status of HPV 16 and 18 in cervical adenosquamous carcinoma. Virchows Arch. 2009;455:253–9. https://doi.org/10.1007/s00428-009-0823-x.
185. Ueda Y, Miyatake T, Okazawa M, et al. Clonality and HPV infection analysis of concurrent glandular and squamous lesions and adenosquamous carcinomas of the uterine cervix. Am J Clin Pathol. 2008;130:389–400. https://doi.org/10.1309/ERR93AF840YYNDRQ.
186. Solakoglu Kahraman D, Diniz G, Sayhan S, et al. Differences in the ARID-1 alpha expressions in squamous and adenosquamous carcinomas of uterine cervix. Acta Pathol Microbiol Immunol Scand. 2015;123:847–50. https://doi.org/10.1111/apm.12435.
187. Longatto-Filho A, Pinheiro C, Martinho O, et al. Molecular characterization of EGFR, PDGFRA and VEGFR2 in cervical adenosquamous carcinoma. BMC Cancer. 2009;9:212. https://doi.org/10.1186/1471-2407-9-212.
188. Rose PG, Java JJ, Whitney CW, et al. Locally advanced adenocarcinoma and adenosquamous carcinomas of the cervix compared to squamous cell carcinomas of the cervix in gynecologic oncology group trials of cisplatin-based chemoradiation. Gynecol Oncol. 2014;135:208–12. https://doi.org/10.1016/j.ygyno.2014.08.018.
189. Zhou J, Wu S-G, Sun J-Y, et al. Comparison of clinical outcomes of squamous cell carcinoma, adenocarcinoma, and adenosquamous carcinoma of the uterine cervix after definitive radiotherapy: a population-based analysis. J Cancer Res Clin Oncol. 2017;143:115–22. https://doi.org/10.1007/s00432-016-2246-9.
190. Yokoi E, Mabuchi S, Takahashi R, et al. Impact of histological subtype on survival in patients with locally advanced cervical cancer that were treated with definitive radiotherapy: adenocarcinoma/adenosquamous carcinoma versus squamous cell carcinoma. J Gynecol Oncol. 2017;28:e19. https://doi.org/10.3802/jgo.2017.28.e19.
191. Lee J-Y, Lee C, Hahn S, et al. Prognosis of adenosquamous carcinoma compared with adenocarcinoma in uterine cervical cancer: a systematic review and meta-analysis of observational studies. Int J Gynecol Cancer. 2014;24:289–94. https://doi.org/10.1097/IGC.0000000000000063.
192. Farley JH, Hickey KW, Carlson JW, et al. Adenosquamous histology predicts a poor outcome for patients with advanced-stage, but not early-stage, cervical carcinoma. Cancer. 2003;97:2196–202. https://doi.org/10.1002/cncr.11371.
193. Baek M-H, Park J-Y, Kim D, et al. Comparison of adenocarcinoma and adenosquamous carcinoma in patients with early-stage cervical cancer after radical surgery. Gynecol Oncol. 2014;135:462–7. https://doi.org/10.1016/j.ygyno.2014.10.004.
194. Guitarte C, Alagkiozidis I, Mize B, et al. Glassy cell carcinoma of the cervix: a systematic review and meta-analysis. Gynecol Oncol. 2014;133:186–91. https://doi.org/10.1016/j.ygyno.2014.01.048.
195. Zolciak-Siwinska A, Jonska-Gmyrek J. Glassy cell carcinoma of the cervix: a literature review. Eur J Obstet Gynecol Reprod Biol. 2014;179:232–5. https://doi.org/10.1016/j.ejogrb.2014.03.035.

196. Ulbright TM, Gersell DJ. Glassy cell carcinoma of the uterine cervix. A light and electron microscopic study of five cases. Cancer. 1983;51:2255–63.
197. Costa MJ, Kenny MB, Hewan-Lowe K, Judd R. Glassy cell features in adenosquamous carcinoma of the uterine cervix. Histologic, ultrastructural, immunohistochemical, and clinical findings. Am J Clin Pathol. 1991;96:520–8.
198. Kato N, Katayama Y, Kaimori M, Motoyama T. Glassy cell carcinoma of the uterine cervix: histochemical, immunohistochemical, and molecular genetic observations. Int J Gynecol Pathol. 2002;21:134–40.
199. Atlas I, Gajewski W, Falkenberry S, et al. Absence of estrogen and progesterone receptors in glassy cell carcinoma of the cervix. Obstet Gynecol. 1998;91:136–8.
200. Kenny MB, Unger ER, Chenggis ML, Costa MJ. In situ hybridization for human papillomavirus DNA in uterine adenosquamous carcinoma with glassy cell features ("glassy cell carcinoma"). Am J Clin Pathol. 1992;98:180–7.
201. Littman P, Clement PB, Henriksen B, et al. Glassy cell carcinoma of the cervix. Cancer. 1976;37:2238–46.
202. Lennerz JKM, Perry A, Mills JC, et al. Mucoepidermoid carcinoma of the cervix: another tumor with the t(11;19)-associated CRTC1-MAML2 gene fusion. Am J Surg Pathol. 2009;33:835–43. https://doi.org/10.1097/PAS.0b013e318190cf5b.
203. Russell MJ, Fadare O. Adenoid basal lesions of the uterine cervix: evolving terminology and clinicopathological concepts. Diagn Pathol. 2006;1:18. https://doi.org/10.1186/1746-1596-1-18.
204. Grayson W, Taylor LF, Cooper K. Carcinosarcoma of the uterine cervix: a report of eight cases with immunohistochemical analysis and evaluation of human papillomavirus status. Am J Surg Pathol. 2001;25:338–47.
205. Parwani AV, Smith Sehdev AE, Kurman RJ, Ronnett BM. Cervical adenoid basal tumors comprised of adenoid basal epithelioma associated with various types of invasive carcinoma: clinicopathologic features, human papillomavirus DNA detection, and P16 expression. Hum Pathol. 2005;36:82–90. https://doi.org/10.1016/j.humpath.2004.08.015.
206. Brainard JA, Hart WR. Adenoid basal epitheliomas of the uterine cervix: a reevaluation of distinctive cervical basaloid lesions currently classified as adenoid basal carcinoma and adenoid basal hyperplasia. Am J Surg Pathol. 1998;22:965–75.
207. Hart WR. Symposium part II: special types of adenocarcinoma of the uterine cervix. Int J Gynecol Pathol. 2002;21:327–46.
208. Kerdraon O, Cornélius A, Farine M-O, et al. Adenoid basal hyperplasia of the uterine cervix: a lesion of reserve cell type, distinct from adenoid basal carcinoma. Hum Pathol. 2012;43:2255–65. https://doi.org/10.1016/j.humpath.2012.03.023.
209. Xing D, Schoolmeester JK, Ren Z, et al. Lower female genital tract tumors with adenoid cystic differentiation: P16 expression and high-risk HPV detection. Am J Surg Pathol. 2016;40:529–36. https://doi.org/10.1097/PAS.0000000000000565.
210. Grayson W, Taylor LF, Cooper K. Adenoid cystic and adenoid basal carcinoma of the uterine cervix: comparative morphologic, mucin, and immunohistochemical profile of two rare neoplasms of putative "reserve cell" origin. Am J Surg Pathol. 1999;23:448–58.
211. Albores-Saavedra J, Manivel C, Mora A, et al. The solid variant of adenoid cystic carcinoma of the cervix. Int J Gynecol Pathol. 1992;11:2–10.
212. Xing D, Bakhsh S, Melnyk N, et al. Frequent NFIB-associated gene rearrangement in adenoid cystic carcinoma of the vulva. Int J Gynecol Pathol. 2017;36(3):289–93. https://doi.org/10.1097/PGP.0000000000000324.
213. Chen T-D, Chuang H-C, Lee L. Adenoid basal carcinoma of the uterine cervix: clinicopathologic features of 12 cases with reference to CD117 expression. Int J Gynecol Pathol. 2012;31:25–32. https://doi.org/10.1097/PGP.0b013e31822103a1.
214. Shi X, Wu S, Huo Z, et al. Co-existing of adenoid cystic carcinoma and invasive squamous cell carcinoma of the uterine cervix: a report of 3 cases with immunohistochemical study and evaluation of human papillomavirus status. Diagn Pathol. 2015;10:145. https://doi.org/10.1186/s13000-015-0376-z.
215. Ferry JA, Scully RE. "Adenoid cystic" carcinoma and adenoid basal carcinoma of the uterine cervix. A study of 28 cases. Am J Surg Pathol. 1988;12:134–44.
216. Kimyon Comert G, Turkmen O, Karalok A, et al. Therapy modalities, prognostic factors, and outcome of the primary cervical carcinosarcoma: meta-analysis of extremely rare tumor of cervix. Int J Gynecol Cancer. 2017;27:1957–69. https://doi.org/10.1097/IGC.0000000000001086.
217. Cavalcanti MS, Schultheis AM, Ho C, et al. Mixed mesonephric adenocarcinoma and high-grade neuroendocrine carcinoma of the uterine cervix: case description of a previously unreported entity with insights into its molecular pathogenesis. Int J Gynecol Pathol. 2017;36:76–89. https://doi.org/10.1097/PGP.0000000000000306.
218. Robinson CE, Sarode VR, Albores-Saavedra J. Mixed papillary transitional cell carcinoma and adenocarcinoma of the uterine cervix: a clinicopathologic study of three cases. Int J Gynecol Pathol. 2003;22:220–5. https://doi.org/10.1097/01.PGP.0000070853.25718.7E.
219. Murata S, Miyata K, Takaishi K, et al. Mixed papillary adenocarcinoma and transitional cell carcinoma of the uterine cervix. Pathol Int. 2004;54:63–6.
220. Moritani S, Ichihara S, Kushima R, et al. Combined signet ring cell and glassy cell carcinoma of the uterine cervix arising in a young Japanese woman: a case report with immunohistochemical and histochemical analyses. Pathol Int. 2004;54:787–92. https://doi.org/10.1111/j.1440-1827.2004.01756.x.
221. Terada T. Large endocervical polyp with cartilaginous and osseous metaplasia: a hitherto unreported entity. Int J Gynecol Pathol. 2009;28:98–100. https://doi.org/10.1097/PGP.0b013e31817eb796.
222. Angra S, McCluggage WG. Endocervical polyp with florid "epidermal metaplasia": report of a previously undescribed phenomenon. Int J Gynecol Pathol. 2016;35:478–81. https://doi.org/10.1097/PGP.0000000000000288.
223. Tran TAN. Endocervical polyp with florid "epidermal metaplasia": report of a previously undescribed phenomenon from a dermatopathologic view: is it an epidermal inclusion cyst or a dermoid cyst. Int J Gynecol Pathol. 2017;36:528–9. https://doi.org/10.1097/PGP.0000000000000363.
224. Howitt BE, Quade BJ, Nucci MR. Uterine polyps with features overlapping with those of Müllerian adenosarcoma: a clinicopathologic analysis of 29 cases emphasizing their likely benign nature. Am J Surg Pathol. 2015;39:116–26. https://doi.org/10.1097/PAS.0000000000000303.
225. Berzolla CE, Schnatz PF, O'Sullivan DM, et al. Dysplasia and malignancy in endocervical polyps. J Women's Health. 2007;16:1317–21. https://doi.org/10.1089/jwh.2007.0408.
226. Chin N, Platt AB, Nuovo GJ. Squamous intraepithelial lesions arising in benign endocervical polyps: a report of 9 cases with correlation to the Pap smears, HPV analysis, and immunoprofile. Int J Gynecol Pathol. 2008;27:582–90. https://doi.org/10.1097/PGP.0b013e31817e0928.
227. Long ME, Dwarica DS, Kastner TM, et al. Comparison of dysplastic and benign endocervical polyps. J Low Genit Tract Dis. 2013;17:142–6. https://doi.org/10.1097/LGT.0b013e318260e32f.
228. Schnatz PF, Ricci S, O'Sullivan DM. Cervical polyps in postmenopausal women: is there a difference in risk? Menopause. 2009;16:524–8. https://doi.org/10.1097/gme.0b013e3181927286.
229. Lane BR, Ross JH, Hart WR, Kay R. Müllerian papilloma of the cervix in a child with multiple renal cysts. Urology. 2005;65:388. https://doi.org/10.1016/j.urology.2004.08.023.

230. Kumar A, Kumar A. Benign müllerian papilloma of the cervix. J Minim Invasive Gynecol. 2012;19:541–2. https://doi.org/10.1016/j.jmig.2011.11.004.
231. Schmedding A, Zense M, Fuchs J, Glüer S. Benign papilloma of the cervix in childhood: immunohistochemical findings and review of the literature. Eur J Pediatr. 1997;156:320–2.
232. Smith YR, Quint EH, Hinton EL. Recurrent benign müllerian papilloma of the cervix. J Pediatr Adolesc Gynecol. 1998;11: 29–31.
233. Nigam A, Choudhary D, Raghunandan C. Large nabothian cyst: a rare cause of nulliparous prolapse. Case Rep Obstet Gynecol. 2012;2012:192526. https://doi.org/10.1155/2012/192526.
234. Vural F, Sanverdi I, Coskun ADE, et al. Large nabothian cyst obstructing labour passage. J Clin Diagn Res. 2015;9(10):QD06–7. https://doi.org/10.7860/JCDR/2015/15191.6630.
235. Torky HA. Huge nabothian cyst causing hematometra (case report). Eur J Obstet Gynecol Reprod Biol. 2016;207:238–40. https://doi.org/10.1016/j.ejogrb.2016.10.042.
236. Clement PB, Young RH. Deep nabothian cysts of the uterine cervix. A possible source of confusion with minimal-deviation adenocarcinoma (adenoma malignum). Int J Gynecol Pathol. 1989;8:340–8.
237. Sui M, Pei Y, Li D, et al. Misdiagnosis analysis of cervical minimal deviation adenocarcinoma: a report of three rare cases and literature review. Ann Clin Lab Sci. 2016;46:680–90.
238. Fluhmann CF. Focal hyperplasis (tunnel clusters) of the cervix uteri. Obstet Gynecol. 1961;17:206–14.
239. Jones MA, Young RH. Endocervical type A (noncystic) tunnel clusters with cytologic atypia. A report of 14 cases. Am J Surg Pathol. 1996;20:1312–8.
240. Segal GH, Hart WR. Cystic endocervical tunnel clusters. A clinicopathologic study of 29 cases of so-called adenomatous hyperplasia. Am J Surg Pathol. 1990;14:895–903.
241. Jones MA, Young RH, Scully RE. Diffuse laminar endocervical glandular hyperplasia. A benign lesion often confused with adenoma malignum (minimal deviation adenocarcinoma). Am J Surg Pathol. 1991;15:1123–9.
242. Maruyama R, Nagaoka S, Terao K, et al. Diffuse laminar endocervical glandular hyperplasia. Pathol Int. 1995;45:283–6.
243. Dainty LA, Krivak TC, Webb JC, et al. Diffuse laminar endocervical glandular hyperplasia: a case report. Int J Gynecol Cancer. 2009;19:1091–3. https://doi.org/10.1111/IGC.0b013e3181a839d3.
244. Jonasson JG, Wang HH, Antonioli DA, Ducatman BS. Tubal metaplasia of the uterine cervix: a prevalence study in patients with gynecologic pathologic findings. Int J Gynecol Pathol. 1992;11:89–95.
245. Ismail SM. Cone biopsy causes cervical endometriosis and tubo-endometrioid metaplasia. Histopathology. 1991;18:107–14.
246. Oliva E, Clement PB, Young RH. Tubal and tubo-endometrioid metaplasia of the uterine cervix. Unemphasized features that may cause problems in differential diagnosis: a report of 25 cases. Am J Clin Pathol. 1995;103:618–23.
247. Cameron RI, Maxwell P, Jenkins D, McCluggage WG. Immunohistochemical staining with MIB1, bcl2 and p16 assists in the distinction of cervical glandular intraepithelial neoplasia from tubo-endometrial metaplasia, endometriosis and microglandular hyperplasia. Histopathology. 2002;41:313–21.
248. El-Ghobashy AA, Shaaban AM, Innes J, et al. Differential expression of cyclin-dependent kinase inhibitors and apoptosis-related proteins in endocervical lesions. Eur J Cancer. 2007;43:2011–8. https://doi.org/10.1016/j.ejca.2007.06.019.
249. Stewart CJR, Little L. Diagnostic value and implications of vimentin expression in normal, reactive and neoplastic endocervical epithelium. Pathology (Phila). 2010;42:217–23. https://doi.org/10.3109/00313021003631353.
250. Wang S, Li XC, Lang JH. Cervical endometriosis: clinical character and management experience in a 27-year span. Am J Obstet Gynecol. 2011;205:452.e1–5. https://doi.org/10.1016/j.ajog.2011.06.070.
251. Wolfe SA, Mackles A, Greene HJ. Endometriosis of the cervix. Classification and analysis of 17 cases. Am J Obstet Gynecol. 1961;81:111–23.
252. Szyfelbein WM, Baker PM, Bell DA. Superficial endometriosis of the cervix: a source of abnormal glandular cells on cervicovaginal smears. Diagn Cytopathol. 2004;30:88–91. https://doi.org/10.1002/dc.10418.
253. Baker PM, Clement PB, Bell DA, Young RH. Superficial endometriosis of the uterine cervix: a report of 20 cases of a process that may be confused with endocervical glandular dysplasia or adenocarcinoma in situ. Int J Gynecol Pathol. 1999;18:198–205.
254. Hiromura T, Tanaka YO, Nishioka T, et al. Clear cell adenocarcinoma of the uterine cervix arising from a background of cervical endometriosis. Br J Radiol. 2009;82:e20–2. https://doi.org/10.1259/bjr/75304693.
255. Rodolakis A, Akrivos N, Haidopoulos D, et al. Abdominal radical trachelectomy for treatment of deep infiltrating endometriosis of the cervix. J Obstet Gynaecol Res. 2012;38:729–32. https://doi.org/10.1111/j.1447-0756.2011.01768.x.
256. Richard F, Canlorbe G, Bazot M, Daraï E. Management of pregnancy in woman with suspected malignant deep infiltrating endometriosis fistulised to the uterine cervix. BMJ Case Rep. 2014;2014 https://doi.org/10.1136/bcr-2014-204978.
257. Humphrey PA. Endometriosis, endocervicosis and müllerianosis of the bladder. J Urol. 2014;192:1523–4. https://doi.org/10.1016/j.juro.2014.08.012.
258. Young RH, Clement PB. Endocervicosis involving the uterine cervix: a report of four cases of a benign process that may be confused with deeply invasive endocervical adenocarcinoma. Int J Gynecol Pathol. 2000;19:322–8.
259. Lee SH, Park J-W, Oh SR, Rha SH. Diagnostic dilemma in cervical endocervicosis. Obstet Gynecol Sci. 2017;60:396–400. https://doi.org/10.5468/ogs.2017.60.4.396.
260. Mobarki M, Karpathiou G, Forest F, et al. Endocervicosis of the uterine cervix. Int J Gynecol Pathol. 2016;35:475–7. https://doi.org/10.1097/PGP.0000000000000277.
261. Kruse A-J, Slangen B, Dunselman GA, et al. Neoplastic transformation of endocervicosis into an extraovarian mucinous cystadenocarcinoma. Hum Pathol. 2011;42:743–8. https://doi.org/10.1016/j.humpath.2010.08.017.
262. Nakaguro M, Tsuzuki T, Shimada S, et al. Adenocarcinoma arising in urinary bladder endocervicosis. Pathol Int. 2016;66:108–13. https://doi.org/10.1111/pin.12375.
263. Gondos B. Histologic changes associated with oral contraceptive usage. Ann Clin Lab Sci. 1976;6:291–9.
264. Wilkinson E, Dufour DR. Pathogenesis of microglandular hyperplasia of the cervix uteri. Obstet Gynecol. 1976;47:189–95.
265. Greeley C, Schroeder S, Silverberg SG. Microglandular hyperplasia of the cervix: a true "pill" lesion? Int J Gynecol Pathol. 1995;14:50–4.
266. Zaloudek C, Hayashi GM, Ryan IP, et al. Microglandular adenocarcinoma of the endometrium: a form of mucinous adenocarcinoma that may be confused with microglandular hyperplasia of the cervix. Int J Gynecol Pathol. 1997;16:52–9.
267. Zamecnik M, Skalova A, Opatrny V. Microglandular adenocarcinoma of the uterus mimicking microglandular cervical hyperplasia. Ann Diagn Pathol. 2003;7:180–6.
268. Qiu W, Mittal K. Comparison of morphologic and immunohistochemical features of cervical microglandular hyperplasia with low-grade mucinous adenocarcinoma of the endometrium. Int J Gynecol Pathol. 2003;22:261–5. https://doi.org/10.1097/01.PGP.0000071043.12278.8D.

269. Abi-Raad R, Alomari A, Hui P, Buza N. Mitotically active microglandular hyperplasia of the cervix: a case series with implications for the differential diagnosis. Int J Gynecol Pathol. 2014;33:524–30. https://doi.org/10.1097/PGP.0000000000000086.
270. Zamecnik M. Hormone receptors in microglandular hyperplasia of the uterine cervix. Int J Gynecol Pathol. 2002;21:424–5.
271. Stewart CJR, Crook ML. PAX2 and cyclin D1 expression in the distinction between cervical microglandular hyperplasia and endometrial microglandular-like carcinoma: a comparison with p16, vimentin, and Ki67. Int J Gynecol Pathol. 2015;34:90–100. https://doi.org/10.1097/PGP.0000000000000107.
272. Nucci MR, Young RH. Arias-Stella reaction of the endocervix: a report of 18 cases with emphasis on its varied histology and differential diagnosis. Am J Surg Pathol. 2004;28:608–12.
273. Schneider V. Arias-Stella reaction of the endocervix: frequency and location. Acta Cytol. 1981;25:224–8.
274. Vang R, Barner R, Wheeler DT, Strauss BL. Immunohistochemical staining for Ki-67 and p53 helps distinguish endometrial Arias-Stella reaction from high-grade carcinoma, including clear cell carcinoma. Int J Gynecol Pathol. 2004;23:223–33.
275. Arias-Stella J. The Arias-Stella reaction: facts and fancies four decades after. Adv Anat Pathol. 2002;9:12–23.
276. Seidman JD, Tavassoli FA. Mesonephric hyperplasia of the uterine cervix: a clinicopathologic study of 51 cases. Int J Gynecol Pathol. 1995;14:293–9.

14 Cervical Neuroendocrine Tumours, Mixed Epithelial/Mesenchymal and Mesenchymal Tumours and Other Miscellaneous Lesions

Anthony T. Williams and Raji Ganesan

Abstract

Cervical cancers are the third most common cancers of the female genital tract. Most of these neoplasms are human papillomavirus (HPV)-related squamous cell carcinomas and adenocarcinomas, but in addition a wide range of uncommon and rare tumours may occur. These may present particular diagnostic challenges resulting from their rarity and the differential diagnoses which may arise at this site.

Neuroendocrine carcinomas (NEC) are not uncommonly encountered in routine practice. They are aetiologically related to HPV and may be associated with squamous and adenocarcinoma or their precursors. Diagnosis of NEC is important as it has a poorer outcome and is treated aggressively with non-surgical modalities. Mixed tumours include the common cervical polyps and the rarer adenosarcomas. The latter has a potential for recurrence and sarcomatous overgrowth. Of the cervical sarcomas, embryonal rhabdomyosarcoma is the commonest at this site and has distinctive appearance and clinical profile.

In general, accurate diagnosis of these entities is important in determining optimal patient management since some tumours may be associated with tumour syndromes and extracervical disease.

Keywords

Neuroendocrine carcinoma · Sarcoma · Mixed tumour Adenosarcoma · Rhabdomyosarcoma · Immunohisto chemistry · Classification

A. T. Williams · R. Ganesan (✉)
Birmingham Women's Hospital, Birmingham, UK
e-mail: anthony.williams@bsuh.nhs.uk; r.ganesan@nhs.net

14.1 Neuroendocrine Tumours

Neuroendocrine cancers of the cervix (NEC) account for less than 5% of all cervical carcinomas [1]. The diagnosis is based on accurate histopathological recognition of neuroendocrine features. The nomenclature of these tumours has changed several times over the years. The present (2014) WHO classification of cervical carcinomas [2] is similar to that used for gastro-entero-pancreatic neuroendocrine carcinomas (Table 14.1). Low-grade neuroendocrine tumours are extremely rare in the cervix and are primarily defined by the same architectural and cytological features used in diagnosis of these neoplasms at other sites. High-grade neuroendocrine carcinomas are more commonly encountered. Up to 25% of neuroendocrine carcinomas are associated with intraepithelial or invasive squamous cell carcinomas or adenocarcinomas [3].

14.1.1 Low-Grade Neuroendocrine Tumours

These are very rare tumours in the cervix [4]. Most reported cases have been in 1970s and 1980s and diagnostic parameters have altered with the widespread use of immunohistochemistry and recognition of high-grade neuroendocrine carcinomas [5]. The diagnosis is made using the same parameters as for carcinoids and atypical carcinoids of the gut. Care should be taken to sample widely to ensure no

Table 14.1 Classification of neuroendocrine carcinomas of the cervix (based on present WHO classification)

Type	Morphology
Low-grade neuroendocrine tumour	Carcinoid
	Atypical carcinoid
High-grade neuroendocrine carcinoma	Small cell neuroendocrine carcinoma
	Large cell neuroendocrine carcinoma

W. Zheng et al. (eds.), *Gynecologic and Obstetric Pathology, Volume 1*, https://doi.org/10.1007/978-981-13-3016-2_14

high-grade features such as mitotic activity, apoptosis or necrosis are overlooked. There is no prescribed treatment for these rare tumours.

14.1.2 High-Grade Neuroendocrine Carcinoma (Small Cell Type, SCNEC)

14.1.2.1 Clinical Features

These are the most common type of neuroendocrine tumour in the cervix. SCNEC mostly occurs in young women. They usually present with irregular vaginal bleeding and may or may not have a cervical mass. They are rarely detected by cervical screening and often present at an advanced stage.

14.1.2.2 Gross Findings

These carcinomas are usually visible at the time of diagnosis. They present as friable cervical masses that tend to ulcerate easily.

14.1.2.3 Microscopic Findings

Fairly monotonous cells that show round to oval nuclei, nuclear hyperchromasia, high nucleocytoplasmic ratio and scant cytoplasm characterize SCNEC. The chromatin pattern appears stippled. Nuclear moulding is seen (Fig. 14.1). There may be streaming artefact, which is a basophilic streak of nuclear material that has been sheared due to crushing of the neoplastic tissue. The carcinomas, typically, show brisk mitotic and apoptotic activity and often exhibit areas of necrosis (Fig. 14.2). Lymphovascular and perineural invasion are often present [6].

14.1.2.4 Immunohistochemical Features

Immunohistochemical staining for neuroendocrine markers aids the diagnosis of SCNEC. The commonly used markers are chromogranin (granular, cytoplasmic), synaptophysin (cytoplasmic), CD56 (membranous with weaker cytoplasmic expression) (Fig. 14.3), and PGP 9.5 (cytoplasmic). In most cases, the staining is diffuse. Chromogranin staining may be focal and appreciated only on high-power examination as punctate, cytoplasmic staining. CD56 and synaptophysin are more sensitive but CD56 lacks contextual specificity, as it can be positive in squamous and adenocarcinomas. Broad-spectrum cytokeratins such as AE1/AE3 (cytoplasmic) are usually positive. Dot-like para-nuclear cytoplasmic staining (Fig. 14.4) may be seen with antibodies to low molecular weight cytokeratins such as CAM 5.2

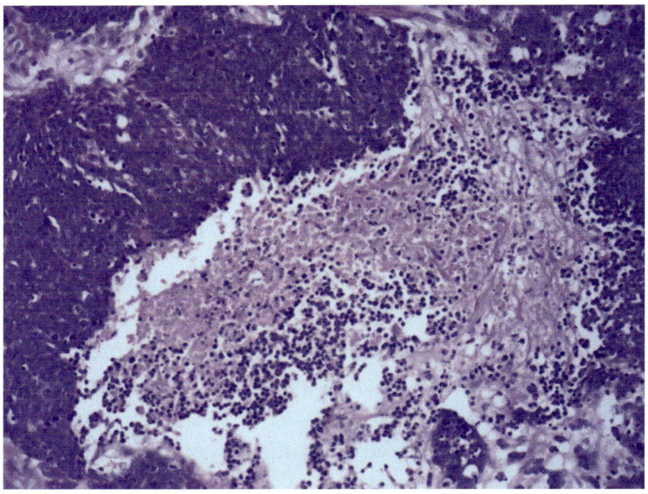

Fig. 14.2 SCNEC showing areas of necrosis

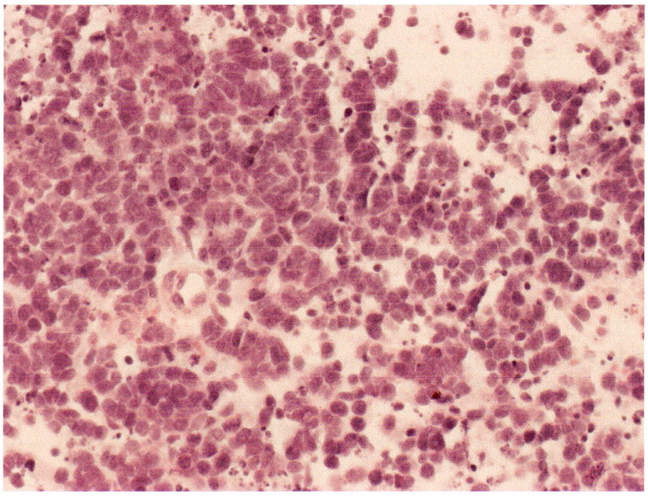

Fig. 14.1 SCNEC showing small ovoid cells with nuclear hyperchromasia, nuclear moulding, apoptosis and mitotic figures

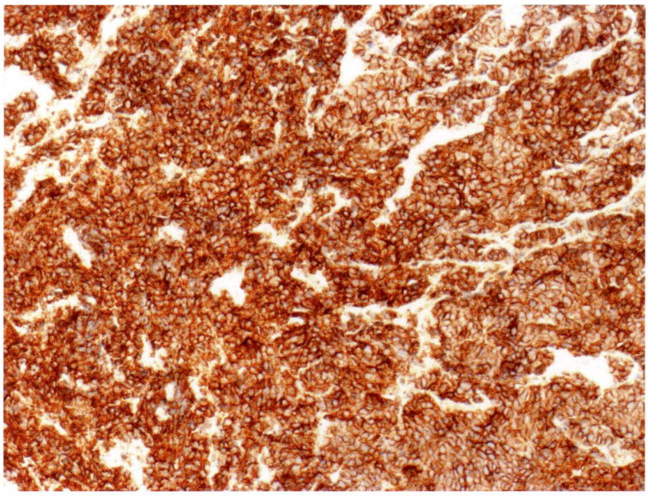

Fig. 14.3 CD56 staining of SCNEC showing strong, diffuse, membranous positivity

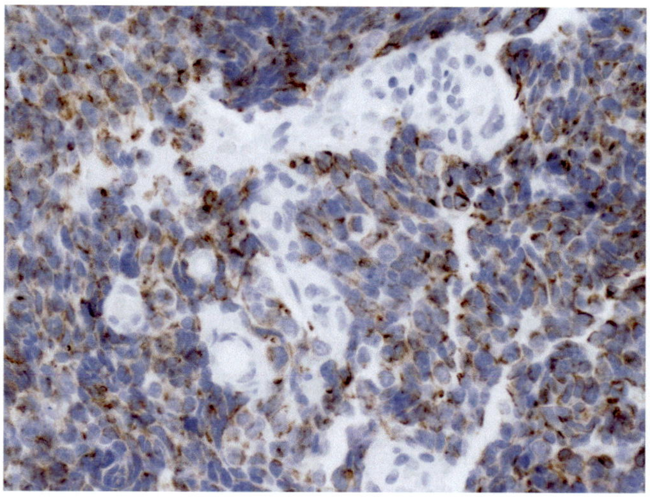

Fig. 14.4 Typical dot-like, paranuclear staining of SCNEC with CAM 5.2

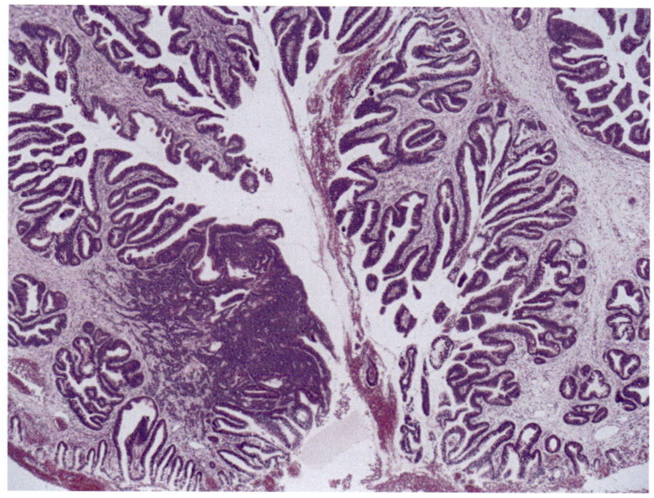

Fig. 14.5 SCNEC associated with high-grade CGIN/AIS (adenocarcinoma in situ)

(cytoplasmic). Unlike neuroendocrine carcinomas from other sites, there are no established criteria of Ki67 labelling index and mitotic count in neuroendocrine neoplasms of the cervix [7].

Once the diagnosis of SCNEC is made on a cervical biopsy, it is appropriate to confirm a cervical origin. Use of TTF-1 (nuclear) to exclude a lung primary is not reliable as non-pulmonary SCNECs can be positive with the marker. SCNECs are generally CK7 positive (cytoplasmic); however, they can also be CK20 (cytoplasmic) positive making differential cytokeratin staining unhelpful [8]. PAX8 (nuclear) expression, which is usually used to confirm an origin from the female genital tract, can also be positive in pancreatic neuroendocrine tumours and is, therefore, of limited use in this scenario [9]. SCNEC, like other types of cervical cancer, is associated with high-risk HPV infection, most often with HPV type 18. Overexpression of p16 (cytoplasmic and nuclear) is regarded as a surrogate marker for the presence of high-risk HPV and demonstrated by block staining with p16. This can be useful in confirming a cervical origin [10] as SCNEC of the lung are not aetiologically associated with HPV [11].

SCNEC can coexist with squamous and adenocarcinomas of the cervix and their precursors (Fig. 14.5). In this context, the morphology and immunohistochemistry of the SCNEC remains the same as pure SCNECs; whilst the expression of neuroendocrine markers in the epithelial component is restricted to chromogranin staining of few cells in the neoplastic glands. In the presence of the two distinct components, it is recommended that the diagnostic bottom line states adenocarcinoma or squamous cell carcinoma admixed with neuroendocrine carcinoma [2].

14.1.2.5 Molecular Features

Comprehensive molecular characterization of SCNEC is not available. Due to the rarity of the tumour, the integrated genomic and molecular characterization of cervical cancers does not have a separate subset of neuroendocrine neoplasms. To date, loss of heterozygosity (LOH) at specific gene or chromosomal regions in SCNEC using polymorphic microsatellite markers has been investigated in small studies. The commonest finding was LOH in any region of the short arm of chromosome 3 (3p) [12]. Small studies have shown that the neuroendocrine carcinomas show similar genetic alterations to the squamous and/or glandular component, implying common origin for both [13].

14.1.2.6 Differential Diagnoses

A diagnosis of SCNEC can be made on morphology alone when typical features of hyperchromasia, scant cytoplasm, nuclear moulding, mitosis and apoptosis are present. Marker expression may be focal and difficult to interpret in small biopsies. The main differential diagnoses are other neoplasms composed of small cells including non-keratinizing small cell squamous cell carcinoma, undifferentiated carcinoma, lymphoma, melanoma and rhabdomyosarcoma.

It is perhaps most important to differentiate SCNEC from small cell squamous carcinomas as the latter has a significantly better prognosis [14]. Squamous cell carcinomas can be composed of small cells and, especially when non-keratinizing, can be difficult to differentiate from SCNEC. Cells constituting squamous cell carcinomas are cohesive and intercellular bridges can be seen. Even when the cytoplasm is scanty it tends to surround the nucleus unlike SCNEC where the cytoplasm is eccentrically located.

Squamous cell carcinomas lack the nuclear moulding and apoptosis seen in SCNEC. On immunohistochemistry, squamous cell carcinomas are consistently negative for neuroendocrine markers (CD56, chromogranin, synaptophysin, PGP9.5). Many squamous cell carcinomas will stain for p63 (nuclear). NECs can co-exist with other epithelial malignancies including adenocarcinomas and squamous cell carcinoma. When there are two distinct morphological and immunohistochemical components, it is recommended that the diagnostic bottom line states adenocarcinoma or squamous cell carcinoma admixed with neuroendocrine carcinoma [2] rather than adenocarcinoma or squamous cell carcinoma with neuroendocrine differentiation. The former terminology allows the clinician to manage the patient as a high-grade NEC.

Undifferentiated carcinomas show, at least focal, staining with AE1/AE3 and EMA and lack staining for neuroendocrine markers.

Lymphomas are morphologically more dyshesive than SCNEC. Their nuclei tend to be rounded and do not show the moulding seen with SCNEC. Staining for CD45 (membranous) will be positive with lymphomas.

Melanomas can be composed of small cells. Primary mucosal melanomas of the cervix are rare tumours. They tend to have a junctional component that may not be visible on small biopsies. When amelanotic they pose a difficult differential from SCNEC, as both tumours can be mitotically and apoptotically prodigious. Melanomas are positive for S100 (nuclear), Melan A (membranous) and SOX10 (nuclear).

14.1.2.7 Prognosis and Management

Neuroendocrine tumours of the gynaecologic tract are rare and pose a significant clinical challenge. Management is guided by accurate pathological diagnosis. For early-stage cervical neuroendocrine carcinoma patients, tumour recurrence is significantly associated with the presence of lymph node metastases, depth of invasion, and the presence of lymphovascular space invasion.

Consensus guidelines published by the Society of Gynecologic Oncology (SGO) recommend multimodality treatment for early stage tumours [15]. In the past, 5-year survival rates of 14% to 29% were typical, but more recently 5-year survival of 45% has been reported and this may be likely to the result of aggressive multimodal therapy [16]. Targeted therapies that are being studied include angiogenesis inhibitors, mTOR inhibitors, VEGF inhibitors and tyrosine kinase inhibitors. Irrespective of the stage, the outcome is poorer for neuroendocrine carcinomas compared to squamous cell carcinomas. In pooled studies, the hazard ratio for death in early stages has been noted as 2.96 and in late stages as 1.70 for neuroendocrine carcinoma in comparison with squamous cell carcinoma [17].

14.1.3 High-Grade Neuroendocrine Carcinoma of the Large Cell Type (LCNEC)

14.1.3.1 Clinical Features

LCNEC are rarer than SCNEC, with less than 100 cases reported in literature. They present with clinical symptoms and signs similar to those of SCNEC.

14.1.3.2 Microscopic Findings

LCNEC typically display an organoid pattern, with cells organized in solid, nesting and trabecular patterns. Nuclear moulding is not seen. The neoplastic cells are large polygonal to round cells with eosinophilic cytoplasm (Fig. 14.6). Geographic tumour necrosis is seen in some tumours (Fig. 14.7). Mitotic activity is brisk and numerous mitotic figures are seen. Vascular invasion is common (Fig. 14.8).

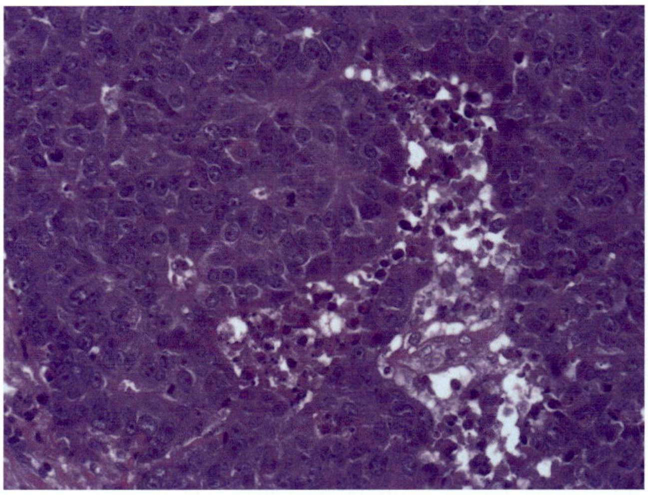

Fig. 14.6 High-power view of LCNEC showing round and polygonal cells with abundant eosinophilic cytoplasm. Mitotic activity, apoptosis and necrosis are also seen

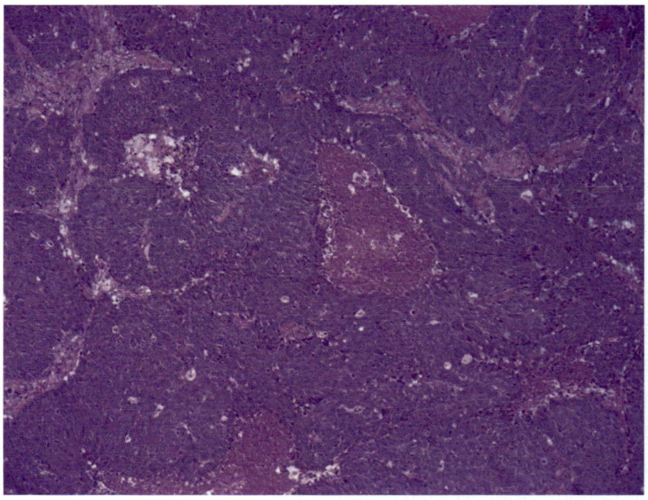

Fig. 14.7 Low-power view of LCNEC showing solid pattern of growth and necrosis

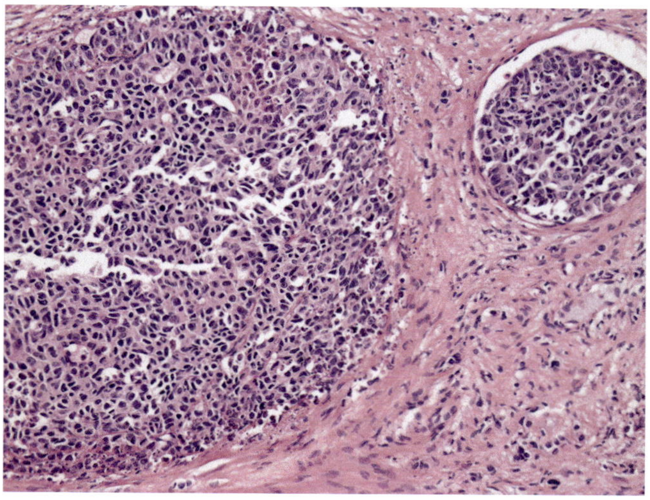

Fig. 14.8 Vascular invasion in LCNEC

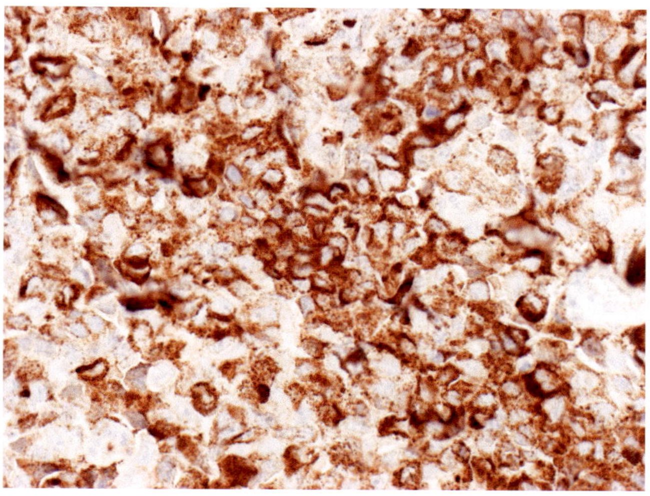

Fig. 14.9 Chromogranin shows granular, cytoplasmic staining in LCNEC

14.1.3.3 Immunohistochemical Features

Immunohistochemical expression of neuroendocrine markers, such as chromogranin (Fig. 14.9), is a requirement for this diagnosis [2]. These carcinomas are also aetiologically associated with high-risk HPV infection [11]. This can be confirmed by block positive staining with p16 (Fig. 14.10). The key features of neuroendocrine carcinomas are summarized in Table 14.2.

14.1.3.4 Differential Diagnoses

The presence of high-grade nuclear atypia in large cells with eosinophilic cytoplasm, brisk mitosis and necrosis should raise the suspicion of LCNEC. The main differential diagnosis is poorly differentiated squamous or adenocarcinomas. Expression of neuroendocrine markers, even focally, should prompt a diagnosis of LCNEC. Presence of glandular or squamous areas indicates a co-existent squamous or adenocarcinomas and does not detract from the diagnosis of LCNEC.

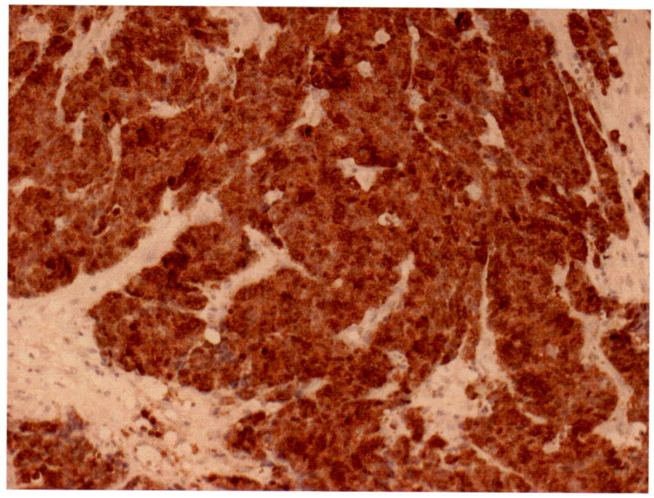

Fig. 14.10 P16 shows nuclear and cytoplasmic staining in LCNEC

Table 14.2 Summary of key features of SCNEC and LCNEC

Features	SCNEC	LCNEC
Clinical presentation	Abnormal vaginal bleeding Cervical mass	Abnormal vaginal bleeding Cervical mass
Morphology	Small cells Scanty cytoplasm Solid and trabecular patterns common Nuclear moulding Basophilic streaks Brisk mitotic activity Necrosis Can be associated with squamous carcinoma and adenocarcinoma	Large cells Abundant eosinophilic cytoplasm Solid and trabecular patterns common Nuclear moulding Brisk mitotic activity Necrosis Can be associated with squamous carcinoma and adenocarcinoma
IHC	Not mandatory for diagnosis *Positive:* Chromogranin Synaptophysin CD56 PGP 9.5 P16 TTF1 Cytokeratins CAM5.2—paranuclear dot-like *Negative* p63	Mandatory for diagnosis *Positive:* Chromogranin Synaptophysin CD56 PGP 9.5 P16 TTF1 Cytokeratins *Generally negative* p63
Differential diagnosis	Other small, round, blue cell tumours—lymphoma, melanoma, rhabdomyosarcoma, small cell squamous carcinoma	Poorly differentiated squamous carcinoma and adenocarcinoma

14.1.3.5 Prognosis and Management

Management and prognosis of these tumours is similar to that of SCNEC, not least because clinical guidelines and trials do not separate these rare neoplasms from SCNEC.

14.2 Mixed Epithelial—Mesenchymal Tumours

14.2.1 Endocervical Polyp

14.2.1.1 Clinical Features

Endocervical polyps are common lesions that occur mostly in peri- and postmenopausal women. Most polyps are not symptomatic [18]; however, some patients present with intermenstrual, post-coital or postmenopausal bleeding.

14.2.1.2 Microscopic Findings

Endocervical polyps are fibroepithelial lesions whose surfaces are covered by endocervical mucinous epithelium that commonly shows squamous metaplasia or microglandular hyperplasia. Surface ulceration, papillation and inflammation are commonly seen (Fig. 14.11 inset). The core often contains dilated cystic glands. The stroma can show foci of decidualization during pregnancy or with exogenous progesterone use. Scattered "atypical" stromal cells are usually present in variable numbers.

14.2.1.3 Differential Diagnoses

The main differential diagnoses are cervical adenomyomas and cervical adenosarcomas. The former are distinguished by the presence of smooth muscle in their stroma. Cervical adenosarcomas (discussed later) show increased cellularity of stroma immediately underlying the epithelium—a feature that is not seen in cervical polyps. Endocervical polyps may recur and in such cases careful examination is required to rule out an adenosarcoma.

14.2.2 Other Polypoid Lesions

Mullerian papillomas are benign polypoid lesions that occur in the cervix and vagina of children—the average age of presentation being 5 years. They present with vaginal bleeding and are no more than 2 cm in greatest dimension [19]. They are composed of fine, branching, fibrous papillae lined by non-atypical, cuboidal or hobnail epithelium. The mucinous epithelium that is seen in endocervical polyps is not a feature of this entity (Fig. 14.12 inset).

Giant cervical polyps are distinguished by their size—greater than 4 cm. They are rare and have a benign outcome after removal [20]. Rarely, metastatic malignancies may present as endocervical polyps [21].

Endocervical polyps are managed by removal, often in an outpatient setting. Although the vast majority are benign, histopathological examination is required to rule out the possibility of a more sinister lesion [22].

14.2.3 Endocervical Adenomyoma

14.2.3.1 Clinical Features

These are uncommon tumours that present as polypoid lesions. They may present with abnormal vaginal bleeding but are often asymptomatic. In reported cases, the age range is between 21 and 55 years of age [23].

14.2.3.2 Microscopic Findings

Endocervical adenomyomas are relatively well-circumscribed lesions that blend, at the periphery, with the surrounding cervical stroma. The lesional glands are widely

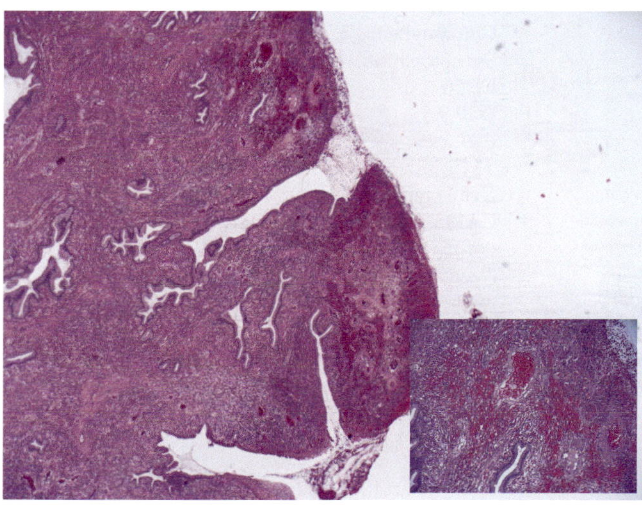

Fig. 14.11 Low-power view of a benign endocervical polyp showing inflammation and ulceration. The stromal cells in the area of ulceration show reactive atypia (inset)

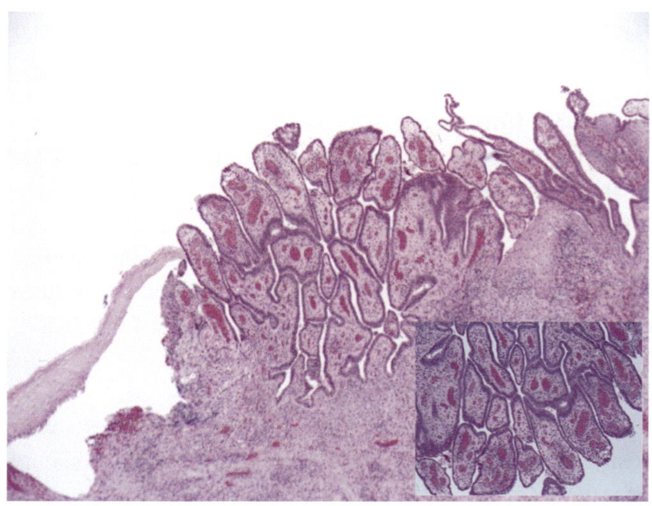

Fig. 14.12 Low-power view of a Mullerian papilloma with blunt papillae lined by non-atypical cuboidal cells. The cuboidal cells do not contain mucin (inset)

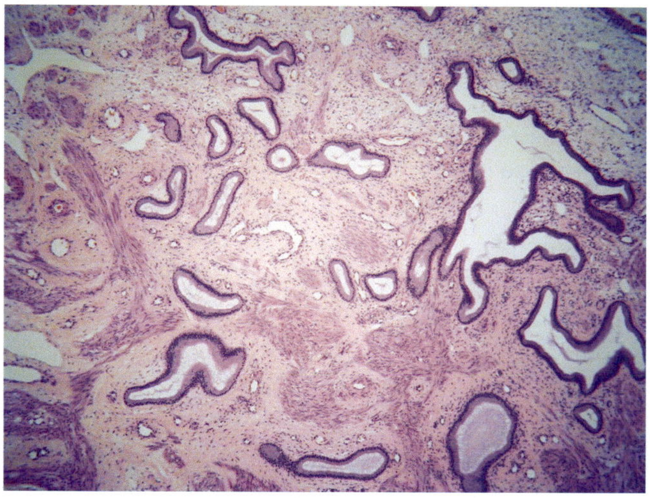

Fig. 14.13 A cervical adenomyoma showing glands widely separated by stroma that contains smooth muscle. (Courtesy Professor WG McCluggage, Belfast, UK)

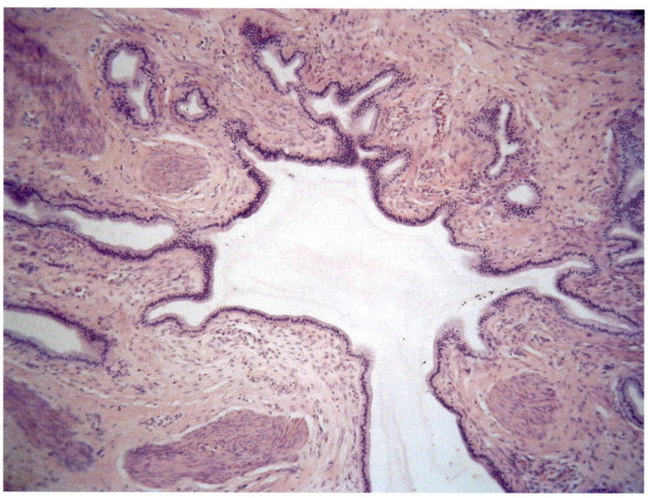

Fig. 14.14 The glands have a lobular architecture with a centrally dilated gland. (Courtesy Professor WG McCluggage, Belfast, UK)

spaced and separated by smooth muscle (Fig. 14.13). The latter may show foci with bizarre nuclei. The glands often have a lobular architecture with a centrally dilated gland surrounded by smaller glands (Fig. 14.14).

14.2.3.3 Differential Diagnoses

The most important differential diagnosis is adenoma malignum or minimal deviation adenocarcinoma. Both adenomyomas and minimal deviation adenocarcinoma are characterized by the presence of bland mucinous glands in smooth muscle. In the carcinoma, this is a manifestation of deep invasion of the cervical stroma [24]. In differentiation between these entities it is helpful to note that adenomyomas commonly present as polyps whilst adenoma malignum is a deeply invasive mural lesion. Features favouring the diagnosis of an adenomyoma are the lobularity of glandular architecture, absence of nuclear atypia, desmoplastic response lymphovascular or perineural invasion, although these features may be absent, or not focally seen in minimal deviation adenocarcinoma. Use of PAX2 (nuclear) staining may be helpful. PAX2 stains benign Mullerian epithelial proliferations but staining is lost in minimum deviation adenocarcinomas [25].

Some benign endocervical polyps may contain small amounts of smooth muscle in their stroma. The smooth muscle component in these situations is wispy and is not organized enough to consider a diagnosis of adenomyoma.

14.2.3.4 Prognosis and Management

Initial management of adenomyomas is by polypectomy. Recurrences are not uncommon and hysterectomy may be done. Examination of the hysterectomy specimens generally show that residual polyp, if any, is confined to the cervix.

14.2.4 Atypical Polypoid Adenomyoma

14.2.4.1 Clinical Features

These tumours are rare in the cervix and occur more commonly in the corpus. They present as polyps.

14.2.4.2 Microscopic Features

These are polypoid tumours in which the glands are lined by endometrioid-type epithelium exhibiting extensive squamous metaplasia and foci of luminal necrosis. The glands are often closely packed and the stromal component is often more cellular and shows a low degree of mitotic activity.

14.2.4.3 Differential Diagnosis

Adenomyomas of usual type are considered in the differential, as they contain endometrioid-type glands and smooth muscle. In atypical polypoid adenomyomas, the glands are closely packed with very scanty intervening stroma.

The other diagnostic consideration is adenosarcoma. On low-power examination, adenosarcomas show a club-like/leaf-like (phyllodes-like) growth pattern. The stroma, especially subepithelially, shows some atypia and mitotic activity and they lack a significant smooth muscle stromal component.

14.2.4.4 Prognosis and Management

Most cases are treated by polypectomy. Very few case reports are found in the literature [26] and therefore their behaviour, assumed to be benign, cannot be robustly evidenced.

14.2.5 Adenosarcoma

14.2.5.1 Clinical Features

These are biphasic tumours that occur most often in the uterine corpus and less commonly in the cervix. With cervical tumours, the patients present in the reproductive age. Presenting symptoms include vaginal bleeding, polyp detected on routine examination and abdominal pain. A history of recurrent polyps may be obtained in some cases [27].

14.2.5.2 Microscopic Features

Cervical adenosarcomas are polypoid lesions. They have a characteristic appearance on low-power examination with glands of varying shapes and variably conspicuous leaf-like, intraglandular projections secondary to stromal excess (Fig. 14.15). The lining epithelium is often mucinous, endocervical in type, but any form of Mullerian differentiation can be seen. On higher magnification, the stromal cells show mild atypia and mitotic activity and these features are most appreciable in the immediately subepithelial stroma—the so-celled cambium layer. According to the World Health Organisation definition, mitotic activity of 2 or more per 10 high-power fields, in the stroma, is required for a diagnosis of adenosarcoma. In practice the diagnosis is less dependent on the mitotic count and most pathologists will make the diagnosis when the characteristic architecture and cambium layer is present [27]. Cervical adenosarcomas may contain heterologous elements such as cartilage and rhabdomyoblasts. Sarcomatous overgrowth (Fig. 14.16) is defined as the presence of pure sarcoma, often high-grade, in at least 25% of the lesion [28].

14.2.5.3 Differential Diagnosis

Benign endocervical polyps and cervical adenomyomas—both of which lack the characteristic architecture of adenosarcomas. The category of adenofibromas is not included in the mixed epithelial and mesenchymal tumours of the cervix as the so-called adenofibromas can behave as low-grade malignancies [29].

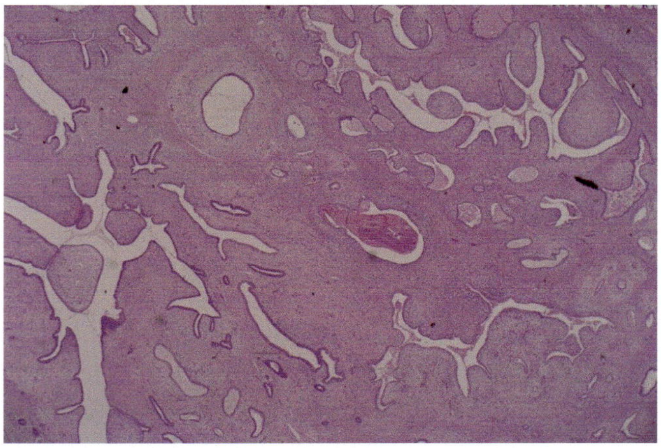

Fig. 14.15 Low-power view of an adenosarcoma showing the stromal excess resulting in a leaf-like pattern of the glands. Periglandular stromal condensation is seen

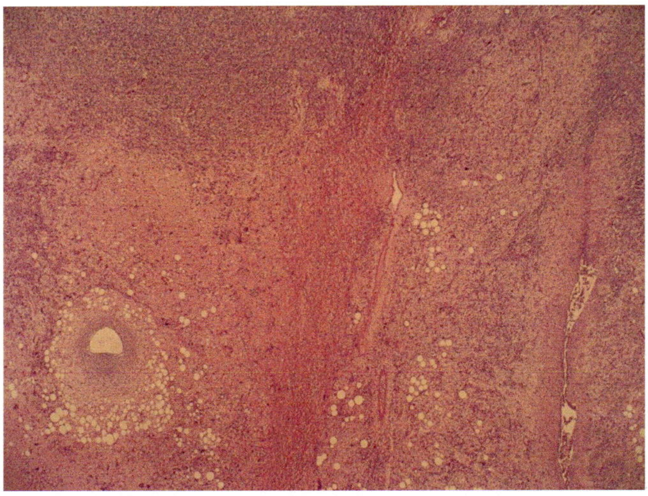

Fig. 14.16 Sarcomatous overgrowth in adenosarcoma. The latter is recognizable by the small benign gland with periglandular stromal condensation. Heterologous fat component is present

Carcinosarcomas are the main differential diagnosis in cases that show the presence of heterologous elements like rhabdomyoblasts or sarcomatous overgrowth. In adenosarcomas, only the mesenchymal component is malignant, whilst in carcinosarcomas both the epithelial and mesenchymal elements show high-grade malignant changes.

Rhabdomyosarcomas are rare tumours. When they entrapped benign glands, they can be mistaken for an adenosarcoma. They typically show high-grade atypia and will not show the subepithelial stromal condensation that is typically seen in adenosarcomas.

14.2.5.4 Prognosis and Management

Adenosarcomas are treated primarily by surgery in the form of hysterectomy. A decision for radiotherapy or chemotherapy is based on the extent of the primary tumour. Adverse prognostic features include sarcomatous overgrowth and recurrence after primary treatment [30].

14.2.6 Carcinosarcoma

14.2.6.1 Clinical Features

Carcinosarcomas of the uterine cervix are extremely rare. Cervical carcinosarcoma may originate in the endocervical/Mullerian epithelium or in mesonephric duct remnants [31, 32]. The patients are generally postmenopausal and present with a polypoid mass and bleeding.

14.2.6.2 Macroscopic Findings

Grossly, the polyps appear fleshy and often necrotic.

14.2.6.3 Microscopic Findings

The carcinomatous component is usually one that resembles a primary cervical carcinoma such as a squamous cell carcinoma or adenoid basal carcinoma [33]. If the carcinosarcoma is of mesonephric derivation, then the epithelium is usually GATA3 positive and negative for PAX8, oestrogen receptors and p16 [34]. The sarcomatous component is usually homologous.

14.2.6.4 Differential Diagnosis

Distinction from adenosarcoma has already been described. It is important to rule out an origin from the endometrium. Imaging may helpful in the distinction.

14.2.6.5 Prognosis and Management

Radical surgery is the mainstay of treatment. Cervical carcinosarcomas are often confined to the cervix, unlike their corpus counterparts which often present with spread beyond the uterus. This may account for the relatively better prognosis of cervical carcinosarcomas.

Table 14.3 provides a summary of the key features of mixed tumours of the cervix.

Table 14.3 Summary of key features of mixed tumours of the cervix

	Morphology	Clinical behaviour
Endocervical polyp	Polyps Covered by glandular and squamous epithelium Microglandular hyperplasia common	Benign
Mulleria papilloma	Polyps occurring in children Fine, branching, fibrous papillae Cuboidal epithelium	Benign
Endocervical adenomyoma	Circumscribed lesions Glands separated by smooth muscle	Benign, may recur
Atypical polypoid adenomyoma	Endometrioid-type epithelium exhibiting extensive squamous metaplasia Stroma usually muscular	Benign, may recur Need to ensure they are not endometrial in origin
Adenosarcoma	Glands with leaf like, intraglandular projections Periglandular stromal condensation May contain heterologous elements Stromal overgrowth—poor prognosis	Low-grade malignancy
Carcinosarcoma	Both epithelial and stromal elements are malignant	Malignant

Summary of key features of sarcomas of the cervix

	Morphology	IHC	Molecular features
Rhabdomyosarcoma	Polypoid Cellular, mitotically active cambium layer underlining normal epithelium	Myogenin and MyoD1 positive	Up to 20% have germline mutations of DICER 1
ESS	Vasopermeative tumour Low-grade ESS similar to endometrial stroma High-grade ESS shows atypia and mitotic activity	Low-grade ESS—CD10 positive High-grade ESS—Cyclin D1 positive	Low-grade ESS—JAZF1-SUZ12 fusion High-grade ESS—YWHAE-NUTM2 gene fusion
ASPS	Large tumour cells with organoid pattern separated by delicate septa	TFE3 positive	ASPSCR1—TFE3 gene fusion
Leiomyosarcoma	Spindle or epithelioid cells with atypia, mitotic activity and tumour cell necrosis	SMA, Desmin, h-caldesmon positive	
MPNST	Fascicular pattern with atypia and mitosis	S100 positive CD34 positive in fibroblastic variant	
PNET	Sheets of small, round, blue cells with scanty cytoplasm and evenly dispersed chromatin. Brisk mitotic activity	CD99, FLI1 positive	Chromosomal translocation t(11;22)(q24;q12)
PEComa	epithelioid and spindled cells arranged in nests with intervening, delicate vascular network	HMB45, Melan A MiTF, SMA positive	Inactivation of TSC1 or TSC2 genes
Angiosarcoma	Vasoformative malignant tumour	CD31, CD34 and FVIII RA positive	
Liposarcoma	Lipoblasts with atypia and mitosis	S100 positive	
Proximal-type epithelioid sarcoma	Multinodular pattern Large, severely atypical epithelioid cells	Keratin, vimentin, BRG1, FLI1 positive INI 1 negative	SMARCB1 deletions

14.3 Sarcomas

Sarcomas presenting in the uterine cervix are rare, representing less than 1% of all malignancies [35] and available data concerning their behaviour is limited to that from case reports and small case series. A wide range of tumour histotypes are described, including tumours more commonly seen in the uterine corpus and those which normally present at other anatomical sites [36–38]. Whilst the morphologic spectrum of these tumours may be broadly the same as in extra-cervical lesions, they may not be initially considered in the differential diagnosis of cervical samples. Precise classification is of increasing importance as specific tumours may be associated with particular targetable mutations to allow the delivery of precision adjuvant treatment.

14.3.1 Rhabdomyosarcoma/Embryonal Rhabdomyosarcoma

Rhabdomyosarcoma is the most frequent sarcoma to arise within the cervix. The tumour arises in a generally younger group of women (from late teens to early 20s, although is described across a wide age range) [39, 40]. An association with ovarian Sertoli-Leydig cell tumours, pleuropulmonary blastoma and thyroid goitre is recognized, as a result of an underlying germline mutation of DICER1. Up to 20% of women with cervical embryonal rhabdomyosarcoma have other DICER1 associated tumours [40].

Tumours usually present with vaginal bleeding and/or a polypoid mass, which may occasionally be removed by polypectomy. The mass is covered by benign Mullerian glandular epithelium and similarly benign glands may be found buried within the stroma. Occasionally, squamous differentiation of the epithelium may also be present. The tumour stroma may be hypocellular and oedematous, but hypercellular foci are usually evident and increased around the glandular epithelium with the formation of a cambium layer (Fig. 14.17). Mitoses and apoptosis are usually identifiable in these more cellular areas. The stromal cells have small, hyperchromatic nuclei, scant cytoplasm (Fig. 14.18) and fine cytoplasmic processes: some cells with more extensive eosinophilic cytoplasm and cytoplasmic cross-striations may be present but these are not always evident and are not essential for diagnosis.

Islands of hyaline or cellular benign cartilage may be present. Some areas may show features resembling alveolar rhabdomyosarcoma. Areas with red blood cell extravasation, frank haemorrhage or necrosis may be seen. Expression of myogenin (nuclear) and myoD1 (nuclear) may be demonstrable in a proportion of nuclei. Smooth muscle actin (cytoplasmic) and h-caldesmon (cytoplasmic) are usually negative [41, 42].

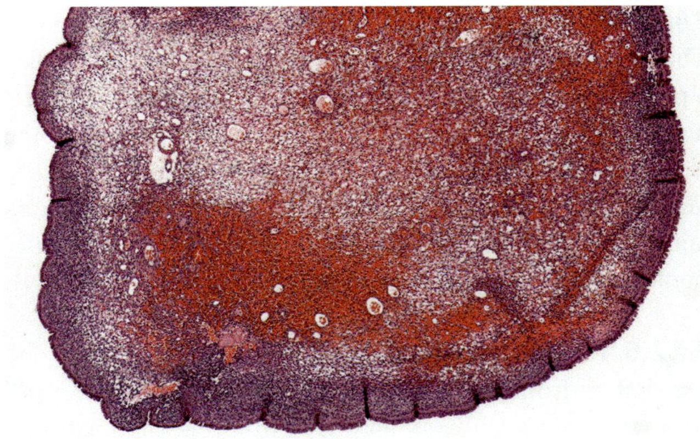

Fig. 14.17 Embryonal rhabdomyosarcoma showing subepithelial hypercellularity—the so-called cambium layer.

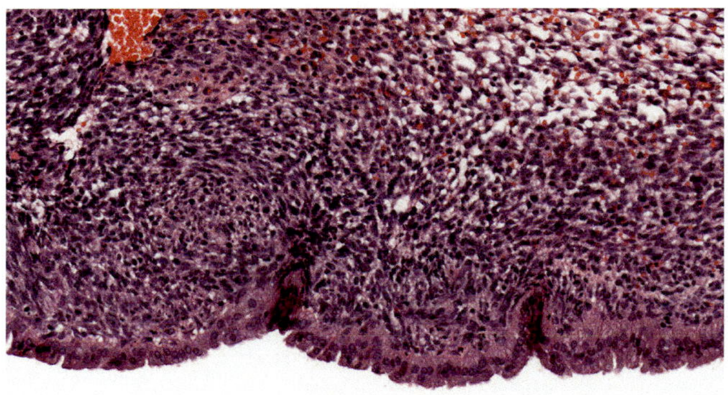

Fig. 14.18 High-power view of cambium layer shows hyperchromatic, small, oval cells with nuclear atypia and mitotic activity

The differential diagnosis includes an endocervical polyp (when paucicellular) and adenosarcoma. Features favouring embryonal rhabdomyosarcoma include the absence of phylloides-like architecture, relative paucity of glands, and high-grade (primitive) appearance of periglandular sarcoma.

14.3.2 Endometrial Stromal Sarcoma

The endometrial stromal sarcomas (ESS) are a diverse group of mesenchymal tumours, which are infrequently reported in the cervix, despite the cervix being a relatively common site of endometriosis, from which these tumours may arise [43].

ESS may be low or high grade. Low-grade ESS are more common, show characteristic morphology and usually present relatively little diagnostic challenge. Tumour cells in low-grade ESS usually show strong, diffuse expression of CD10 (membranous and cytoplasmic), and will often demonstrate expression of smooth muscle actin and, less often, desmin. Diagnostic difficulty may arise when endometrioid-type glands are present within the tumour as this may create morphologic overlap with endometriosis and has been noted to lead to delayed diagnosis in cervical biopsies [44]. Conversely, pauciglandular endometriosis (stromal endometriosis or "stromatosis") may mimic a neoplastic mesenchymal proliferation. The absence of a mass lesion, superficial location and presence of stromal breakdown may aid recognition.

High-grade endometrial stromal sarcoma has more recently been distinguished as a distinct clinico-pathological entity, with a characteristic YWHAE-NUTM2 gene fusion. Presentation as a cervical mass has been described, in a 26-year-old woman, in association with vaginal bleeding [45].

14.3.3 Alveolar Soft Part Sarcoma

Alveolar soft part sarcoma (ASPS) is a rare neoplasm, with distinctive morphology but of uncertain histogenesis, most commonly found in the deep soft tissue of the thigh or buttock in adults or in the head and neck region in infants and children. Small number of cases have been described in the female reproductive tract, including the cervix [46–48]. The natural history of disease typically involves localized disease at the time of presentation, but late recurrence with metastatic disease may occur.

The tumour cells are large, uniform and epithelioid with clearly defined cell borders, copious eosinophilic granular cytoplasm and central bland nuclei with prominent nucleoli. Tumour cells are characteristically arranged with organoid architecture into solid nests, separated by delicate septa containing sinusoidal vascular channels. Loss of cohesion or necrosis of the cells in the centre of the nests frequently (although not always) results in a pseudo-alveolar appearance (Fig. 14.19). Tumour cells often contain

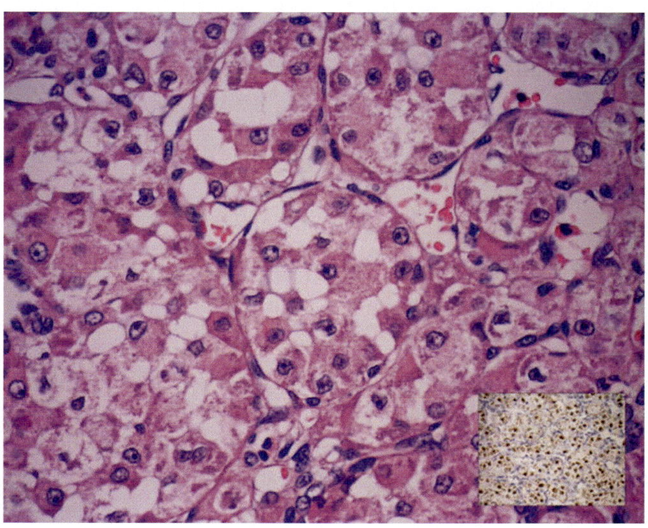

Fig. 14.19 ASPS with uniform and epithelioid cells, clearly defined cell borders, copious eosinophilic granular cytoplasm arranged with organoid architecture into solid nests, separated by delicate septa. The cells are positive for TFE-3 (inset)

rhomboid- or rod-shaped intracytoplasmic inclusions, or coarse intracytoplasmic granules, highlighted by staining for diastase-PAS.

Tumour cells show strong nuclear staining with an antibody to the c-terminal portion of TFE3 (nuclear) which is retained in the fusion protein, where most normal cells show only weak or no nuclear reactivity [49]. As a note of caution, TFE staining may also be seen in granular cell tumours that show morphologic overlap with ASPS (and are described in the cervix). Focal staining with immunohistochemistry for desmin (cytoplasmic) and HMB45 (cytoplasmic) is also described.

There is a characteristic gene fusion between ASPSCR1 and TFE3, detection of which by FISH or RT-PCR is confirmatory in diagnostically challenging cases [50]. It is worth noting that this finding may also be present in a subset of renal cell carcinomas. The fusion oncoprotein is a transactivator of the MET (Mesenchymal Epithelial Transition) promoter, suggesting MET inhibitors as potential therapeutic agents in metastatic disease, which is largely resistant to radiotherapy or chemotherapy.

At this site, the main morphologic differential diagnoses are clear cell carcinoma, undifferentiated carcinoma and PEComa, including both conventional and TFE rearranged subtypes, which may show morphologic overlap. A diagnostic immunohistochemistry panel which includes HMB45, MelanA and desmin will aid distinction of these diagnoses [49].

14.3.4 Leiomyosarcoma

Leiomyosarcomas including epithelioid [51–53] and myxoid [54] variants may occasionally occur as primary cervical neoplasms [55] most likely arising from the scattered smooth muscle cells present in the normal cervical stroma. These present as masses which may project into the endocervical canal or vaginal lumen. A case report documents occurrence in the cervical stump following subtotal hysterectomy [56]. The macroscopic appearances resemble those seen in the uterine corpus, with white/grey and fleshy cut surfaces or a gelatinous appearance in myxoid variants. The masses may appear circumscribed or show infiltration into the surrounding stroma. It has been inferred that criteria for malignancy are similar to those seen in the uterine corpus [57].

14.3.5 Malignant Peripheral Nerve Sheath Tumour

A small number of cases of malignant peripheral nerve sheath tumour of the cervix have been described in case reports and one small case series [58, 59]. The tumours form polypoid or mass lesions and show fascicular architecture with alternating hyper and hypocellular areas, composed of spindle cells among which mitotic figures can be identified. Up to 50% show S100 (nuclear) expression on immunohistochemistry.

A variant endocervical fibroblastic malignant peripheral nerve sheath tumour has been reported in a small series of three cases [60]. These tumours presented as polypoid or mass forming lesions and showed fibroblastic, endoneurial-like differentiation. Morphologic features included compact fascicles of spindled cells in herringbone, fascicular and vaguely storiform patterns. Both diffuse S100 and CD34 (membranous) expression were demonstrated, suggesting possible origin from CD34-expressing endocervical fibrocytes.

14.3.6 Ewings Sarcoma/Peripheral Primitive Neuroectodermal Tumour

Ewings Sarcoma (Peripheral primitive neuroectodermal tumour, PNET) has been rarely described arising in the cervix, in sporadic case reports and small series [61–65].

As at other sites the tumours are composed of well demarcated, lobulated sheets of uniform small cells with round hyperchromatic nuclei containing evenly dispersed chromatin. Cytoplasm is scant and mitotic figures are frequent. Occasional rosettes may be seen. The differential diagnosis includes rhabdomyosarcoma; lymphoma; undifferentiated, small cell squamous and neuroendocrine carcinomas; malignant melanoma and endometrial stromal sarcoma. There is diffuse membranous expression of CD99 with FLI1 (nuclear) and cytokeratin expression occasionally demonstrated. The chromosomal translocation t(11;22)(q24;q12) or the EWS/FLI fusion product may be demonstrable.

14.3.7 Perivascular Epithelioid Cell Tumour

A few case reports describe perivascular epithelioid cell tumour (PEComa) arising in the cervix [66] including with TFE3 gene re-arrangement [67]. The tumours presented with abnormal vaginal bleeding or a mass and in one case was identified on cervical cytology [68]. The tumours are circumscribed with occasional tongue-like protrusions into adjacent stroma and are composed of epithelioid and spindled cells with a delicate vascular network. Tumour cells express HMB45, Melan A (cytoplasmic) and MiTF (nuclear) with frequent positivity for smooth muscle actin. Most tumours demonstrate inactivation of TSC1 or TSC2 genes with activation of the mTOR pathway providing a potential focus of targetable therapy [69].

14.3.8 Angiosarcoma

Angiosarcoma is rarely described arising in the cervix, forming a flat or raised violaceous plaque with an ulcerated haemorrhagic surface [70]. The tumours are composed of infiltrative, anastomosing vascular channels with solid poorly differentiated areas, haemorrhage and necrosis. Tumour cells are flat or cuboidal with atypical nuclei and inconspicuous cytoplasm; the epithelioid variant shows epithelioid endothelial cells with copious eosinophilic cytoplasm and large nuclei with prominent nucleoli. Expression of CD31 (membranous), CD34 and Factor VIII related antigen (FVIII RA—cytoplasmic) may be demonstrated on immunohistochemistry.

14.3.9 Liposarcoma

Cervical liposarcoma is exceedingly rare [35] albeit that adipocytes may be considered a normal constituent of the cervical stroma [71]. A recent report describes a cervical pleomorphic liposarcoma in association with small cell carcinoma of the ovary of hypercalcaemic type in a woman with Li Fraumeni syndrome [72].

14.3.10 Proximal-Type Epithelioid Sarcoma

The proximal variant of epithelioid sarcoma is described to occur at a number of sites in the deep pelvic tissues and vulva, and has occasionally been described as arising in the cervix [73, 74]. The tumour shows a multinodular pattern of growth and is composed of large, epithelioid cells with severe cytological atypia, vesicular nuclei and prominent nucleoli. Rhabdoid features may be observed, or predominate such that the main differential diagnosis is extra-renal rhabdoid tumour. Necrosis may be present but is not generally associated with the granuloma-like pattern seen in the conventional, distal form of epithelioid sarcoma.

14.3.11 Undifferentiated Endocervical Sarcoma

A group of high-grade tumours, termed undifferentiated endocervical sarcoma (encompassing lesions also termed endocervical stromal sarcoma), has been previously described. The diagnosis can be established after excluding other specific diagnoses. In addition to lacking morphologically recognizable patterns of differentiation, these showed expression only of vimentin. Patient outcomes have been described as variable, probably reflecting likely histogenetic variability of lesions within this group [35] some reports of which preceded the availability of ancillary immunochemical and molecular genetic markers.

In conclusion, the uterine cervix maybe the site of a number of unusual neoplastic proliferations. Knowledge of their occurrence at this site and their distinctive features aids diagnosis of these tumours.

References

1. Crowder S, Tuller E. Small cell carcinoma of the female genital tract. Semin Oncol. 2007;34:57–63.
2. Kurman RJ, Carcangiu ML, Herrington CS, Young RH. WHO classification of tumours of the female reproductive organs. 4th ed. Lyon: IARC; 2014.
3. Horn LC, Hentschel B, Bilek K, et al. Mixed small cell carcinomas of the uterine cervix: prognostic impact of focal neuroendocrine differentiation but not of Ki-67 labeling index. Ann Diagn Pathol. 2006;10:140–3.
4. Modlin IM, Shapiro MD, Kidd M. An analysis of rare carcinoid tumors: clarifying these clinical conundrums. World J Surg. 2005;29:92–101.
5. Papatsimpas G, Samaras I, Theodosiou P, Papacharalampous K, Maragkouli E, Papadopoulos NV, Tsapakidis K, Litos I, Sogka E, Kostopoulou E, Koukoulis GK. A case of cervical carcinoid and review of the literature. Case Rep Oncol. 2017;10(2):737–42.
6. Rekhi B, Patil B, Deodhar KK, et al. Spectrum of neuroendocrine carcinomas of the uterine cervix, including histopathologic features, terminology, immunohistochemical profile, and clinical outcomes in a series of 50 cases from a single institution in India. Ann Diagn Pathol. 2013;17:1–9.
7. Kim JY, Hong SM, Ro JY. Recent updates on grading and classification of neuroendocrine tumors. Ann Diagn Pathol. 2017;29:11–6.
8. McCluggage WG, Kennedy K, Busam KJ. An immunohistochemical study of cervical neuroendocrine carcinomas: Neoplasms that are commonly TTF1 positive and which may express CK20 and P63. Am J Surg Pathol. 2010;34:525–32.
9. Liau JY, Tsai JH, Jeng YM, et al. The diagnostic utility of PAX8 for neuroendocrine tumors: An immunohistochemical reappraisal. Appl Immunohistochem Mol Morphol. 2016;24:57–63.
10. Atienza-Amores M, Guerini-Rocco E, Soslow RA, et al. Small cell carcinoma of the gynecologic tract: a multifaceted spectrum of lesions. Gynecol Oncol. 2014;134:410–8.
11. Hartley CP, Steinmetz HB, Memoli VA, Tafe LJ. Small cell neuroendocrine carcinomas of the lung do not harbor high-risk human papillomavirus. Hum Pathol. 2015;46:577–82.
12. Wistuba II, Thomas B, Behrens C, Onuki N, et al. Molecular abnormalities associated with endocrine tumors of the uterine cervix. Gynecol Oncol. 1999;72:3–9.
13. Emerson RE, Michael H, Wang M. Cervical carcinomas with neuroendocrine differentiation: A report of 28 cases with immunohistochemical analysis and molecular genetic evidence of common clonal origin with coexisting squamous and adenocarcinomas. Int J Gynecol Pathol. 2016;35:372–84.
14. Ganesan R, Hirschowitz L, Dawson P, et al. Neuroendocrine carcinoma of the cervix: Review of a series of cases and correlation with outcome. Int J Surg Pathol. 2016;24:490–6.
15. Gardner GJ, Reidy-Lagunes D, Gehrig PA. Neuroendocrine tumors of the gynecologic tract: A Society of Gynecologic Oncology (SGO) clinical document. Gynecol Oncol. 2011;122:190–8.
16. Margolis B, Tergas AI, Chen L, et al. Natural history and outcome of neuroendocrine carcinoma of the cervix. Gynecol Oncol. 2016;141:247–54.
17. Intaraphet S, Kasatpibal N, Siriaunkgul S, et al. Prognostic factors for small cell neuroendocrine carcinoma of the uterine cervix: an institutional experience. Int J Gynecol Cancer. 2014;24:272–9.
18. Tirlapur SA, Adeyemo A, O'Gorman N, et al. Clinico-pathological study of cervical polyps. Arch Gynecol Obstet. 2010;282:535–8.
19. McQuillan SK, Grover SR, Pyman J, et al. Literature review of benign Müllerian papilloma contrasted with vaginal rhabdomyosarcoma. J Pediatr Adolesc Gynecol. 2016;29:333–7.
20. Bucella D, Frédéric B, Noël JC. Giant cervical polyp: a case report and review of a rare entity. Arch Gynecol Obstet. 2008;278:295–8.
21. Godfrey GJ, Moore G, Alatassi H. Presentation of renal cell carcinoma as cervical polyp metastasis. J Low Genit Tract Dis. 2010;14:387–9.
22. Levy RA, Kumarapeli AR, Spencer HJ, Quick CM. Cervical polyps: is histologic evaluation necessary? Pathol Res Pract. 2016;212:800–3.
23. Gilks CB, Young RH, Clement PB, et al. Adenomyomas of the uterine cervix of of endocervical type: a report of ten cases of a benign cervical tumor that may be confused with adenoma malignum. Mod Pathol. 1996;9:220–4.
24. Casey S, McCluggage WG. Adenomyomas of the uterine cervix: report of a cohort including endocervical and novel variants. Histopathology. 2015;66:420–9.
25. Rabban JT, McAlhany S, Lerwill MF, Grenert JP, Zaloudek CJ. PAX2 distinguishes benign mesonephric and mullerian glandular lesions of the cervix from endocervical adenocarcinoma, including minimal deviation adenocarcinoma. Am J Surg Pathol. 2010;34:137–46.
26. Bachurska S, Yamakov K, Belovezdov V, et al. Case of atypical polypoid adenomyoma of the uterine cervix. Akush Ginekol (Sofiia). 2013;52:67–70.
27. McCluggage WG. Mullerian adenosarcoma of the female genital tract. Adv Anat Pathol. 2010;17:122–9.
28. Comunoğlu N, Comunoğlu C, Başsüllü N, et al. Müllerian adenosarcoma with sarcomatous overgrowth of the cervix: unusual large polypoid mass. Ups J Med Sci. 2007;112:67–72.
29. Gallardo A, Prat J. Mullerian adenosarcoma: a clinicopathologic and immunohistochemical study of 55 cases challenging the existence of adenofibroma. Am J Surg Pathol. 2009;33:278–88.
30. Verschraegen CF, Vasuratna A, Edwards C, et al. Clinicopathologic analysis of mullerian adenosarcoma: the M.D. Anderson Cancer Center experience. Oncol Rep. 1998;5:939–44.
31. Kim M, Lee C, Choi H, et al. Carcinosarcoma of the uterine cervix arising from Müllerian ducts. Obstet Gynecol Sci. 2015;58:251–5.
32. Meguro S, Yasuda M, Shimizu M, et al. Mesonephric adenocarcinoma with a sarcomatous component, a notable subtype of cervical carcinosarcoma: a case report and review of the literature. Diagn Pathol. 2013;8:74.
33. Grayson W, Taylor LF, Cooper K. Carcinosarcoma of the uterine cervix: a report of eight cases with immunohistochemical analysis and evaluation of human papillomavirus status. Am J Surg Pathol. 2001;25:338–47.
34. Roma AA. Mesonephric carcinosarcoma involving uterine cervix and vagina: report of 2 cases with immunohistochemical positivity for PAX2, PAX8, and GATA-3. Int J Gynecol Pathol. 2014;33:624–9.
35. Fadare O. Uncommon sarcomas of the uterine cervix: a review of selected entities. Diagn Pathol. 2006;1:30.
36. Clement PB. Miscellaneous primary tumors and metastatic tumours of the uterine cervix. Semi Diagn Pathol. 1990;7:228–48.
37. Bansal S, Lewin SN, Burke WM, et al. Sarcoma of the cervix: natural history and outcomes. Gynecol Oncol. 2010;118:134–8.
38. Khosla D, Gupta R, Srinivasan R, et al. Sarcomas of Uterine cervix. Int J Gynecol Cancer. 2012;22:1026–30.
39. Daya D, Scully RE. Sarcoma botyroides of the uterine cervix in young women: a clinicopathological analysis of 13 cases. Gynecol Oncol. 1998;29:290–304.

40. Dehner LP, Jarzebowski JA, Hill DA. Embryonal rhabdomyosarcoma of the uterine cervix: a report of 14 cases and a discussion of its unusual clinicopathological associations. Mod Pathol. 2012;25:602–14.
41. Krissemen ML, Wang WL, Sullinger J, et al. Rhabdomyosarcoma of the cervix in adult women and younger patients. Gynecol Oncol. 2012;126:351–639.
42. Li FL, Gupta M, McCluggage WG, et al. Embryonal rhabdomyosarcoma (botyroid type) of the uterine corpus and cervix in adult women. Am J Surg Pathol. 2013;37:344–55.
43. Boardman CH, Webb MJ, Jefferies JA. Low-grade endometrial stromal sarcoma of the ectocervix after therapy for breast cancer. Gynecol Oncol. 2006;79:120–3.
44. McCluggage WG, Ganesan R, Herrington CS. Endometrial stromal sarcomas with extensive endometrioid glandular differentiation: report of a series with emphasis on the potential for misdiagnosis and discussion of the differential diagnosis. Histopathology. 2009;54:365–73.
45. Cernelc J, Volchek M. YWHAE-FAM22 high grade endometrial stromal sarcoma presenting as a cervical mass. Pathology. 2017;49(s1):S68.
46. Nielsen GP, Oliva E, Young RH, et al. Alveolar soft part sarcoma of the female genital tract: a report of nine cases and review of the literature. Int J Gynecol Pathol. 1995;14:283–92.
47. Feng M, Jian W, He Y, et al. Primary alveolar soft part sarcoma of the uterine cervix. A case report and literature review. Int J Clin Exp Pathol. 2014;7:8223–6.
48. Schoolmeester JK, Carlson J, Keeney GL, et al. Alveolar soft part sarcoma of the female genital tract. Am J Surg Pathol. 2017;41:622–32.
49. Roma AA, Yang B, Senior MR, et al. TFE3 immunoreactivity in alveolar soft part sarcoma of the uterine cervix: a case report. Int J Gynecol Pathol. 2005;24:131–5.
50. Jabbour MN, Seoud M, Al-Ahamadie H, et al. ASPL-TFE3 translocation in vulvovaginal alveolar soft part sarcoma. Int J Gynecol Pathol. 2014;33:263–7.
51. Colombat M, Sevestre H, Gontier MF. Epithelioid leiomyosarcoma of the uterine cervix. Report of a case. Ann Pathol. 2001;21:48–50.
52. Gotoh T, Kikuchi Y, Takano M, et al. Epithelioid leiomyosarcoma of the uterine cervix. Gynecol Oncol. 2001;82:400–5.
53. Fujiwaki R, Yoshida M, Iida K, et al. Epithelioid leiomyosarcoma of the uterine cervix. Acta Obstet Gynecol Scand. 1998;77:246–8.
54. Fraga M, Prieto O, Garcia-Caballero T, et al. Myxoid leiomyosarcoma of the uterine cervix. Histopathology. 1994;25:381–4.
55. Abdul-Karim FW, Bazi TM, Sorensen K. Sarcoma of the uterine cervix: clinicopathologic findings in three cases. Gynecol Oncol. 1987;26:103–11.
56. Zhiqiang L, Bin S, Min F, et al. Leiomyosarcoma of cervical stump following subtotal hysterectomy: a case report and review of literature. Eur J Gynecol Oncol. 2016;37:148–51.
57. Bell SW, Kempson RL, Hendrickson MR. Problematic uterine smooth muscle neoplasms. A clinicopathological study of 213 cases. Am J Surg Pathol. 1994;18:535–58.
58. Bernstein HB, Broman JH, Apicelli A, et al. Primary malignant schwannoma of the uterine cervix: a case report and literature review. Gynecol Oncol. 1999;74:288–92.
59. Keel SB, Clement PB, Prat J, et al. Malignant schwannoma of the uterine cervix: A study of three cases. Int J Gynecol Pathol. 1998;17:223–30.
60. Mills AM, Karamchandani JR, Vogel H, et al. Endocervical fibroblastic malignant peripheral nerve sheath tumour (neurofibrosarcoma): report of a novel entity possibly related to endocervical CD34 fibrocytes. Am J Surg Pathol. 2011;35:404–12.
61. Horn LC, Fischer U, Bilek K. Primitive neuroectodermal tumor of the cervix uteri. A case report. Gen Diagn Pathol. 1997;142:227–30.
62. Pauwels P, Ambros P, Hattinger C, et al. Peripheral primitive neuroectodermal tumour of the cervix. Virchows Arch. 2000;436:68–73.
63. Malpica A, Moran CA. Primitive neuroectodermal tumor of the cervix: A clinicopathologic and immunohistochemical study of two cases. Ann Diagn Pathol. 2002;6:281–7.
64. Snijders-Keilholz A, Ewing P, Seynaeve C, Burger CW. Primitive neuroectodermal tumor of the cervix uteri: a case report-changing concepts in therapy. Gynecol Oncol. 2005;98:516–9.
65. Chiang S, Snuderi M, Kojiro-Sanada S, et al. Primitive neuroectodermal tumours of the female genital tract. Am J Surg Pathol. 2017;41(6):761–72.
66. Kudela E, Biringer K, Kasajova P, et al. Perivascular epithelioid tumours of the uterine cervix. Pathol Res Pract. 2016;212:667–71.
67. Liu F, Zhang R, Wang Z-Y, et al. Malignant perivascular epithelioid cell tumor (PEComa) of cervix with *TFE3* gene rearrangement: a case report. Int J Clin Exp Pathol. 2014;7:6409–14.
68. Tajima S, Koda K. Perivascular epithelioid cell tumour of the uterine cervix identified on a conventional cervical smear. Diagn Cytopathol. 2015;43:1011–6.
69. Thway K, Fisher C. PEComa: morphology and genetics of a complex tumour family. Ann Diagn Pathol. 2015;19:359–68.
70. Ohayi SA, Ezugwu EC, Aderibigbe AS, et al. Angiosarcoma of the cervix: a case and literature review. Niger J Med. 2013;22:362–4.
71. Doldan A, Otis CN, Pantanowitz L. Adipose tissue: a normal constituent of the uterine cervical stroma. Int J Gynecol Pathol. 2009;28:396–400.
72. Tandon B, Hagemann IS, Maluf HM, et al. Association of Li Fraumeni syndrome with small cell carcinoma of the ovary, hypercalcemic type and concurrent pleomorphic liposarcoma of the cervix. Int J Gynecol Pathol. 2017;36:593–9.
73. Suarez-Zamora A, Barrera-Herrera LE, Rodriguez-Urrego PA. Proximal-type epithelioid sarcoma: report of an unusual case in the uterine cervix. Int J Surg Path. 2017;25:468–7471.
74. Jeney H, Heller DS, Hameed M, et al. Epithelioid sarcoma of the uterine cervix. Gynecol Oncol. 2003;89:536–9.

Cyclic Endometrium and Exogenous Hormone Effect

15

Geok Chin Tan and T. Yee Khong

Abstract

The endometrium is a complex tissue that is constantly influenced by ovarian steroid hormones such as oestrogen and progesterone during the reproductive period. It undergoes regular cyclical changes in each menstrual cycle with the exception of early menarche and perimenopausal period when ovulation can be irregular. This chapter provides detail histomorphologic descriptions of the three phases of menstrual cycle, namely proliferative, secretory and menstrual, as well as a discussion on dating of endometrium. These changes are observed in the functional layer, sparing the basal layer of the endometrium. This is followed by a discussion about the different techniques in obtaining an endometrial sample, adequacy of tissue, and artefacts that may be encountered. The determination of sample adequacy can be challenging as calling minimal tissue adequate may result in false negative and on the contrary casual calling of inadequate sample may lead to an unnecessary repeat procedure. In menstrual cycle disorders, depending on whether there is continuous oestrogen stimulation or oestrogen deficiency, the endometrium demonstrates prolonged proliferative activity or atrophic changes, respectively. Anovulatory cycle is normally perceived as continuous proliferative activity even in secretory phase. However, one should interpret this with caution as the duration of proliferative phase differs in women. The effects of endometrium associated with the use of hormone in contraception, hormone replacement in postmenopausal women and receptor-modulation in cancer therapy are also described in this chapter.

Keywords

Endometrium · Histology · Menstrual cycle · Endometrial sampling method · Hormone

15.1 Anatomy and Histology

The endometrium is a complex tissue composed of surface epithelium, glands, stromal and inflammatory cells and blood vessels. It forms the mucosal lining of the uterine cavity between the interstitial segments of the fallopian tubes in the uterine cornua on either side of the fundus and the isthmical portion above the cervix.

During premenarche, the endometrial cavity is lined by cuboidal epithelium with clefts burrowing into spindly stroma (Fig. 15.1). With the onset of puberty, the influence of oestrogen leads to endometrial proliferation and commencement of the cyclical changes. In the early phase of menarche, ovulation is irregular and anovulatory bleeding is frequent. When regular ovulatory cycles are established, the

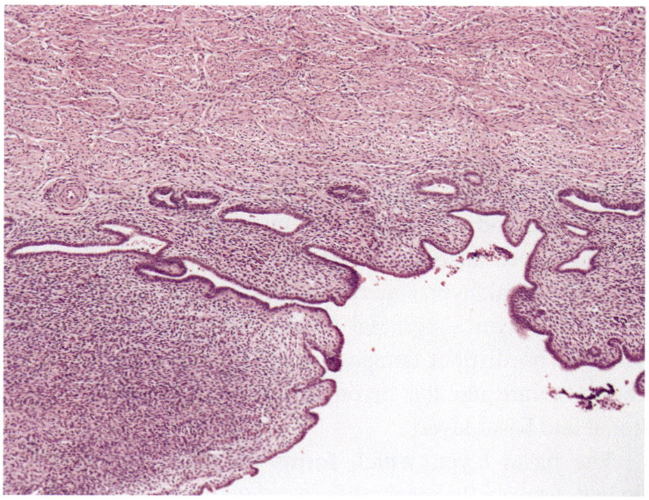

Fig. 15.1 Endometrium in a 3-year-old showing simple glands burrowing into spindly stroma

G. C. Tan
Universiti Kebangsaan Malaysia Hospital,
Kuala Lumpur, Malaysia

T. Yee Khong (✉)
SA Pathology, Women's and Children's Hospital,
North Adelaide, Australia

University of Adelaide, Adelaide, Australia
e-mail: yee.khong@adelaide.edu.au

W. Zheng et al. (eds.), *Gynecologic and Obstetric Pathology, Volume 1*, https://doi.org/10.1007/978-981-13-3016-2_15

endometrium undergoes regular cyclical changes with continuous loops of morphologic changes in response to the recurrent hormonal changes and, except during lactation and pregnancy, true menstruation is experienced. The endometrium will revert to forming a mucous membrane for the myometrium in the postmenopausal period.

The endometrial response to cyclical hormonal changes is crucial to implantation and development of the fertilized ovum. The menstrual cycle encompasses the first day of bleeding until just before the next menstrual period; each cycle lasts for about 28 days. However the length of each cycle can vary from one woman to another and between cycles in the same woman. The menstrual cycle is divided into three phases: follicular (proliferative), ovulatory (interval) and luteal (secretory). In follicular phase, the ovarian follicles are stimulated under the influence of follicle-stimulating hormone (FSH) with a rise in plasma oestrogen. The latter leads to an inhibitory feedback for production of FSH and a positive feedback for the production of luteinizing hormone (LH). A rapid upsurge of the plasma gonadotropins, LH and FSH, results in follicular rupture and ovulation occurs just prior to ovulation. Eventually, the ruptured follicle is converted to a corpus luteum, and starts to produce progesterone, which causes a rapid rise of previously very low plasma progesterone. After ovulation, there is a rapid decline in the plasma LH and FSH levels while the plasma progesterone levels remain high for about 10 days. Oestrogen levels decline for a few days after ovulation but there is a mid-luteal phase rise. If conception does not occur, the corpus luteum regresses and both plasma oestrogen and progesterone levels decline rapidly during the last week of the cycle. Plasma FSH and LH levels rise again before menstruation commences in preparation for the next cycle.

Depending upon the anatomical location of endometrium in uterus, the morphology differs. At the transition between endometrium and endocervical mucosa in the isthmus, the endometrial glands are poorly developed and unresponsive. In biopsy specimens, the clue to this setting is the further it is from the body of the uterus, the stroma tends to become progressively more fibrous and less cellular (Fig. 15.2). Isthmic glands are lined by ciliated epithelial cells. In the fundus and body, the endometrium is generally fairly uniform in appearance and is conventionally divided into two parts: the basal layer, superficial to the myometrium, and the functional layer superficial to the basal layer (Fig. 15.3). There is no distinct demarcation either between the basal endometrium and the myometrium or between the functional and basal layers.

The basal layer, which forms the regenerative layer, does not normally respond to hormonal stimulation. Here, the glands demonstrate no secretory activity and there is absent to minimal mitotic activity. The gland-to-stroma ratio is low, and thus the stroma is relatively more prominent in comparison with the functional layer (Fig. 15.4). The stromal cells mostly have spindled nuclei with scanty cytoplasm.

On the other hand, the more superficial functional layer is responsive to the hormonal changes of the ovulatory cycle. In the reproductive years, it becomes mitotically active in the proliferative phase and is shed during the menstrual period (Fig. 15.5). This layer is further subdivided into the stratum compactum and the stratum spongiosum. This subdivision becomes more obvious during the late secretory phase when the stroma in the spongiosum layer is more oedematous.

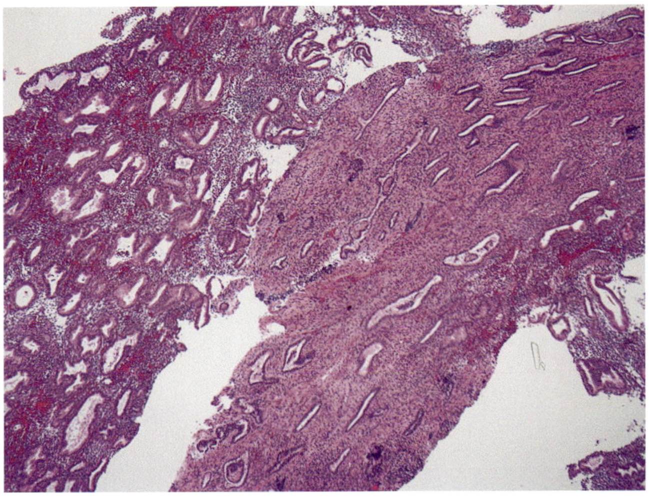

Fig. 15.2 Endometrium in the lower segment (right) showing fibrous stroma and more widely spaced glands in contrast to the body of the endometrium (left) showing secretory-phase endometrium with normal stroma and complement of glands

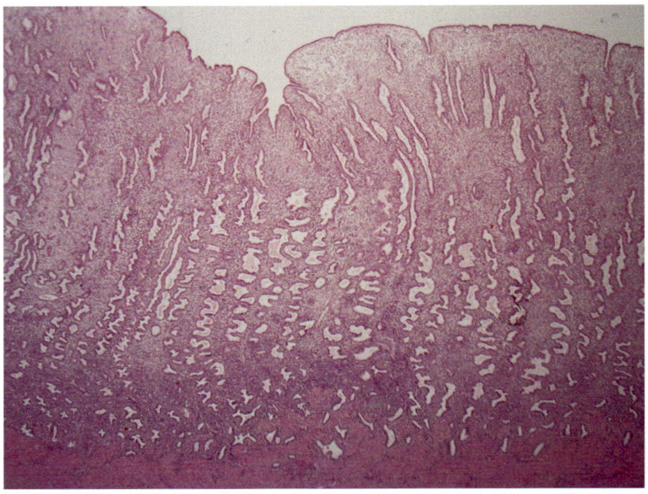

Fig. 15.3 Endometrium in the body of the uterus showing superficial functional zone and deeper basal layer with slightly denser stroma. Note the absence of a clear demarcation between the two layers and between the basal layer and underlying myometrium

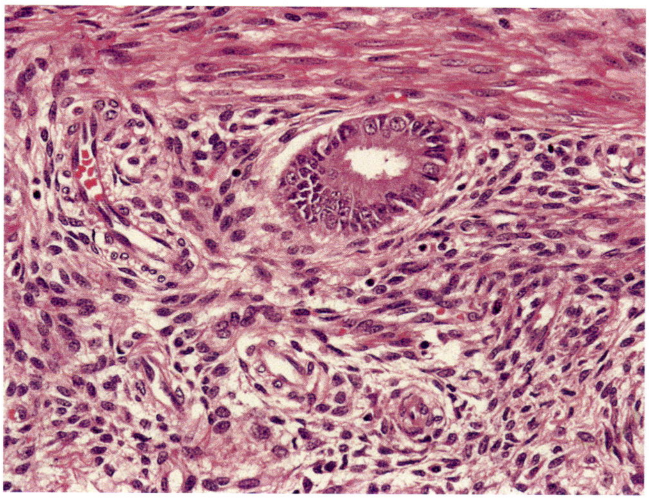

Fig. 15.4 The basal layer in the proliferative phase: the stroma is dense and the stromal cells mostly have spindled nuclei with scanty cytoplasm; the glands demonstrate no secretory activity and there is absent to minimal mitotic activity

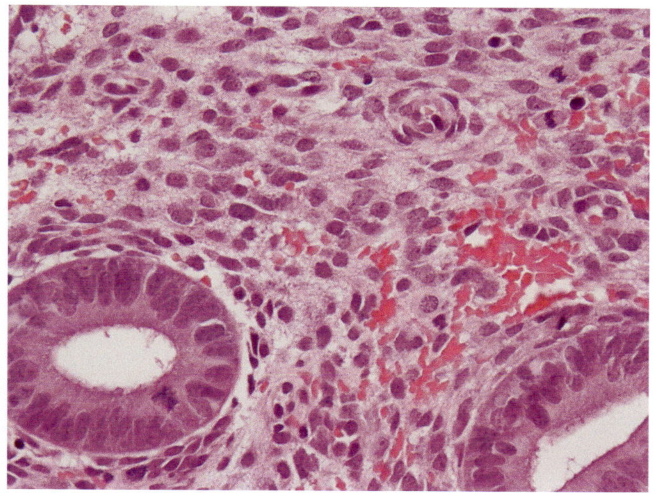

Fig. 15.6 Early proliferative phase: stromal cells with oval nuclei and inconspicuous cytoplasm; mitotic activity is readily seen within stromal cells (upper right) and in the glandular epithelium

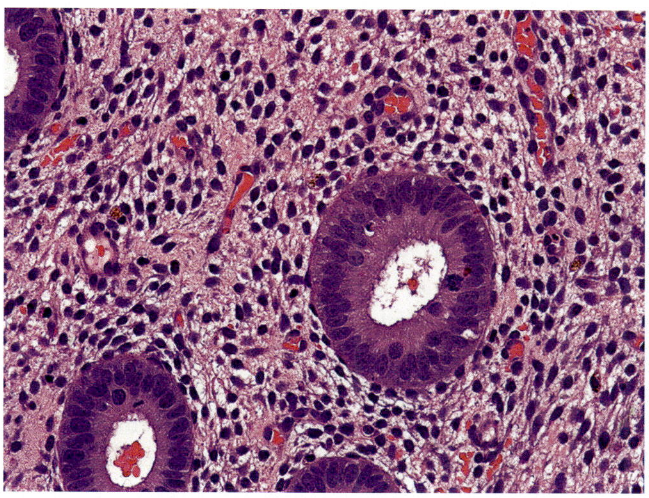

Fig. 15.5 The functional layer in the proliferative phase: the stroma is looser and the stromal cells are less spindly than in the basal layer; the glands demonstrate mitotic activity

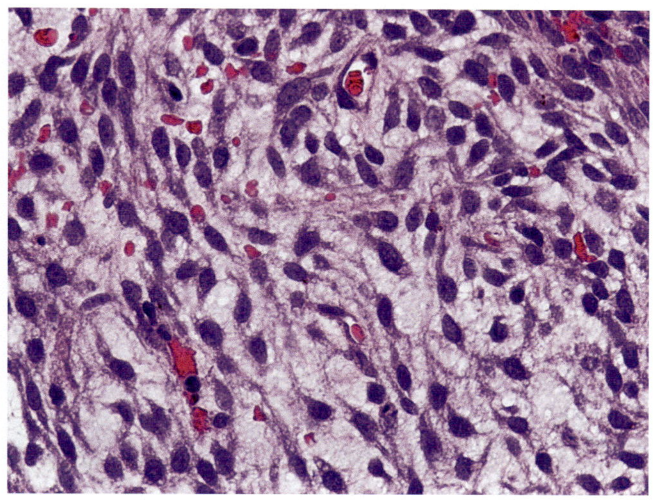

Fig. 15.7 Early secretory phase: stromal cells are spindle-shaped with slightly larger and vesicular nuclei

15.1.1 Endometrial Glands

The glandular epithelium is in continuity with the surface epithelium but the latter is less involved by the cyclical hormonal influence. The morphology of the glandular epithelium changes with the phase of the menstrual cycle, which will be discussed in the later section.

15.1.2 Stroma

The stromal cells demonstrate considerable morphologic changes throughout the endometrial cycle, in particular during the last seven or so days of the normal cycle. During the proliferative phase, they have the appearance of fibroblasts with oval hyperchromatic nuclei and inconspicuous cytoplasm (Fig. 15.6), while in the late proliferative phase and early secretory phase, they display slightly larger nuclei and the cytoplasm becomes more noticeable due to the accumulation of organelles. In the late secretory phase, the nuclei continue to become larger and also vesicular, and the cytoplasm is more abundant with increasing accumulation of glycogen (Fig. 15.7). This pre-decidualization of the stromal cells forms around the spiral arteries and arterioles cuffing those vessels, as a fore-runner of the Streeter's columns of spiral arteries cuffed by decidua in pregnancy (Fig. 15.8). Stromal oedema becomes prominent and delineates the middle of the endometrium into the spongy layer.

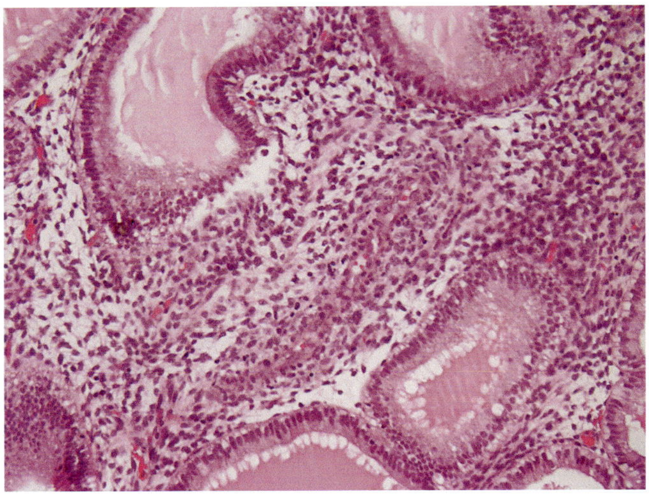

Fig. 15.8 Decidualization of the stromal cells around spiral arteries

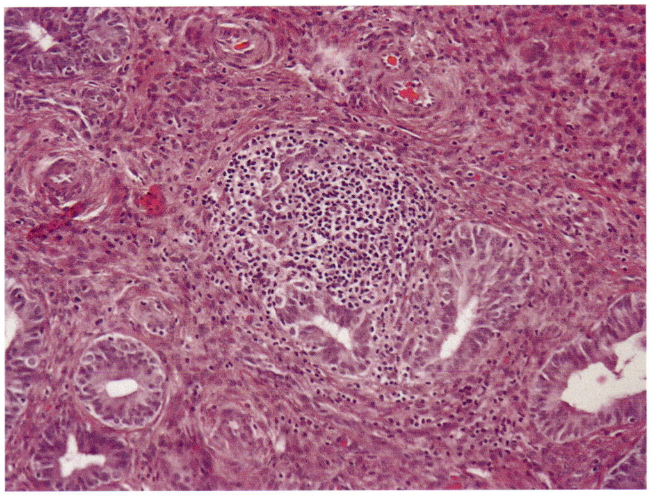

Fig. 15.9 Stroma lymphoid aggregate in proliferative phase endometrium

Pre-decidualization continues into the upper layer of the endometrium to form a more or less compact zone of swollen stromal cells, the compact layer. The stromal cells in the basal and parabasal layers are less responsive to progesterone and remain largely unchanged from those seen in the proliferative phase.

By tradition, the terms used for progestogen-induced stromal changes are influenced by the situation in which it is taking place. By and large, changes seen in stromal cells during pregnancy are called decidualization and decidua. Predecidua is used to describe the stromal change seen during the secretory phase of the menstrual cycle while pseudodecidua refers to those induced by exogenous progesterone therapy. The stromal changes induced by endogenous progesterone during the secretory phase or pregnancy are more extensive and uniform but largely similar to those induced by synthetic progesterone therapy.

15.1.3 Inflammatory Cells

Leucocytes comprise about 10–25% of all endometrial cells. They are most abundant compared to other parts of the female genital tract, and thought to have originated from circulating blood, in situ proliferation of immune cells or recruitment of haemopoietic precursor cells that differentiated within the endometrium [1–3]. The number and distribution of leucocytes vary during the menstrual cycle. Natural killer cells (CD56+ NK cells) constitute the majority of endometrial leucocytes, and this is followed by macrophages that consist of about 30% of the leucocyte population. Majority of the T lymphocytes are CD8+, and they are found in the basal endometrium in lymphoid aggregates, and throughout the endometrial stroma and epithelium (Fig. 15.9). Other less significant inflammatory cells seen in the endometrium are CD83+ dendritic cells, CD16+ natural killer cells and mast cells. In the menstrual phase, neutrophils may be seen. Plasma cells and eosinophils are not common residents in the endometrium but the identification of single or very rare plasma cells is not diagnostic of chronic endometritis. In fetuses, neonates and children, the majority of endometrial inflammatory cells are macrophages and monocytes; CD56+ natural killer cells are only present postnatally and in relatively small numbers [4].

The uterine NK cells are also known as endometrial granulocytes, large granulated lymphocytes or K cells (Körnchenzellen), and are small rounded cells with indented nuclei and eosinophilic intracytoplasmic granules of varying size. The intracytoplasmic granules of these cells may lead the unwary to mistake them for polymorphonuclear leucocytes. During early pregnancy, there is a marked increase in the number of these cells such that they comprise as much as 70–80% of all endometrial leucocytes. It has been suggested that they play a role in implantation and placentation either by acting as cytotoxic effector cells or by secretion of various cytokines [3].

15.1.4 Blood Supply

The uterine artery is the main blood supply to the uterus and arises from the internal iliac artery. It reaches the uterus at the level of the upper cervix where the ascending branch runs lateral to the uterus, and anastomoses with the branches of the ovarian artery at the lateral upper part of the uterus below the isthmic part of the fallopian tube. The uterine artery gives a descending branch that anastomoses with the vaginal artery. These paired uterine arteries that run lateral to the uterus, with anastomotic contributions from the ovarian arteries, predominantly supply the uterus. Branches from this utero-ovarian anastomosis penetrate the serosa and form a circular arcuate system in the outer myometrium. Arteries from the arcuate arterial system radiate into the inner myometrium. These radial arteries terminate, just proximal to the junction of the endometrium and myometrium, as the basal arteries and the spiral arteries. The basal or straight arteries ramify in the innermost layers of the myometrium and terminate in the basal endometrium, which they supply. The spiral or coiled arteries that are destined to become the uteroplacental arteries during pregnancy traverse the endometrium in their course towards the uterine lumen. The spiral arteries give off anastomosing branches to the glands and stroma of the functional layer and they terminate in a complex anastomotic network in the superficial layer of the endometrium (Fig. 15.10). The venous drainage from the endometrium, in general, follows the arterial supply. The human endometrium also contains lymphatic vessels that are predominantly seen in the basal layer but sometimes also in the functional layer.

The spiral arteries and arterioles are hormonally responsive. Oestrogen and progesterone receptors have been demonstrated in the smooth muscle cells of these arteries although there is some heterogeneity in distribution and quantity of these receptors [5]. Oestrogen and progesterone receptors have been found also in the perivascular cells. It is unclear to what degree the actions of oestrogen and progesterone on endometrial blood vessel are mediated directly or indirectly via paracrine or autocrine factors.

The spiral arteries grow by hyperplasia and hypertrophy throughout the menstrual cycle as the endometrium grows in thickness. In the late proliferative and secretory phases and in early pregnancy, their growth exceeds that of the endometrium so that their natural coiled configuration is exaggerated further. Various factors are implicated in the cyclical regeneration of spiral arteries, including vascular endothelial growth factor (VEGF), angiopoietin-1 and -2 and receptors such as Flt-1, Flk1/KDR and Tie-1 and -2. It is not clear how steroids affect the growth process and the paracrine signals involved [6, 7].

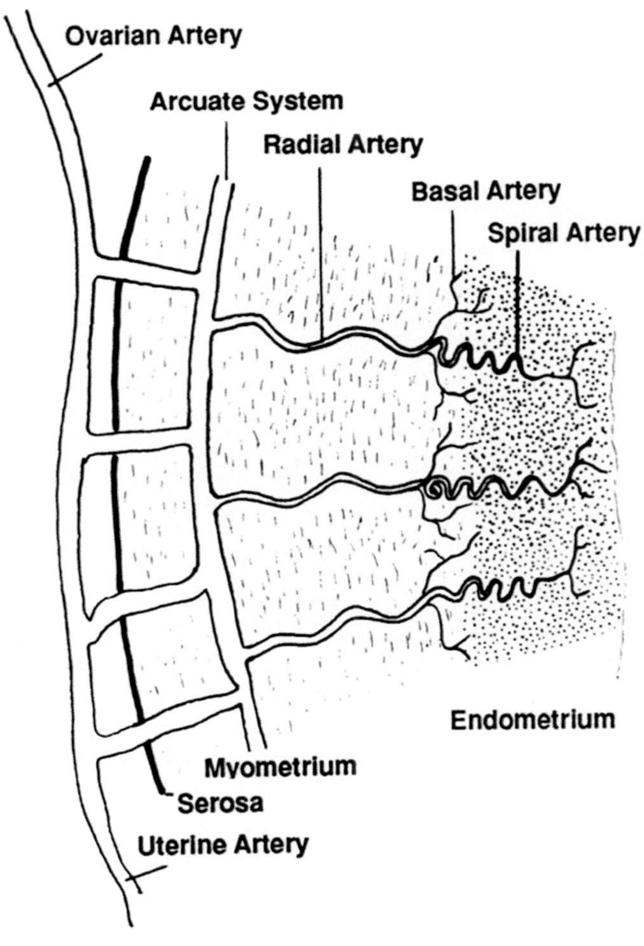

Fig. 15.10 Diagrammatic representation of the blood supply to the uterus. [adapted from Robertson WB. Uteroplacental vasculature. *J Clin Pathol 1972;29 (Suppl 10):9–17*]

15.2 Endometrial Changes During the Menstrual Cycle

These are summarized in Table 15.1.

15.2.1 Proliferative

The endometrium regenerates from the basal layer and the portion of the functional layer that remains after menstruation.

The usual duration of the proliferative phase is about 2 weeks. As the time required for development and maturation of follicles varies between cycles and differs in one woman to another, it is impossible to date the proliferative phase accurately. Accordingly, splitting the phase into early, middle and late proliferative is sufficient.

In the early proliferative phase, the glands show a straight, simple tubular morphology (Fig. 15.11) and are lined by low columnar epithelium with the nuclei arranged at different levels forming a pseudostratified appearance. At this instance, mitoses can be seen in the glands and in the stroma (Fig. 15.12). The stroma demonstrates minimal change throughout the proliferative phase. It appears dense and the stromal cells contain scant cytoplasm, thus having an appearance of naked nuclei on haematoxylin and eosin staining.

In the mid-proliferative phase, the endometrium thickens but elongation of glands gives rise to tortuosity of the glands, and stromal oedema develops (Fig. 15.13). Mitotic activity continues in the glands and stroma.

In the late proliferative phase, the glandular columnar epithelium is tall and becomes heaped to give a pseudostratified appearance (Fig. 15.14). The stromal oedema subsides

Table 15.1 Histological features of the endometrium through the menstrual cycle

	Glands	Stroma	Vessels
Proliferative—early	Small straight glands mitoses	Dense spindle cell stroma; mitoses	Relatively inconspicuous spiral arteries with thin walls
Proliferative—mid	Slightly tortuous glands	Loose, oedematous stroma with spindled cells	
Proliferative—late	Pseudostratified appearance; nuclei at various heights but most in basal half; smooth luminal surface; lumina sharp outline	Less oedematous stroma	
Secretory POD 1	Mitotic; subnuclear vacuolation;		
POD 2	Tortuous	No change	
POD 3			
POD 4	Less regular subnuclear vacuoles—secretory vacuoles on luminal side		
POD 5	Outline of glands irregular; widening diameter of and glands; papillary infoldings—Sawtooth No longer pseudostratified Apical surface of rough and indistinct Nuclei—round, vesicular and pale staining	Oedema starts; therefore can distinguish basal from functional Date 8 = max oedema	
POD 6			
POD 7			
POD 8			
POD 9		Oedema starts to regress	Spiral arteries appear more prominent
POD 10			Pre-decidual cuffing of spiral arteries
POD 11		Decidual change starts	
POD 12	Central—Sawtooth endometrium Secretions ++ Tall columnar epithelium Surface—may have flat to cuboidal cells; some luminal breakdown	Solid stroma; no oedema superficial still decidual change; granulated lymphocytes	
POD 13			
POD 14			
Menstrual	Glandular collapse; clumped epithelial glandular cells with secretory exhaustion	Crumbling stroma with compact balls of stromal cells overlying epithelial cells	Thrombosed spiral arteries

POD post-ovulatory day

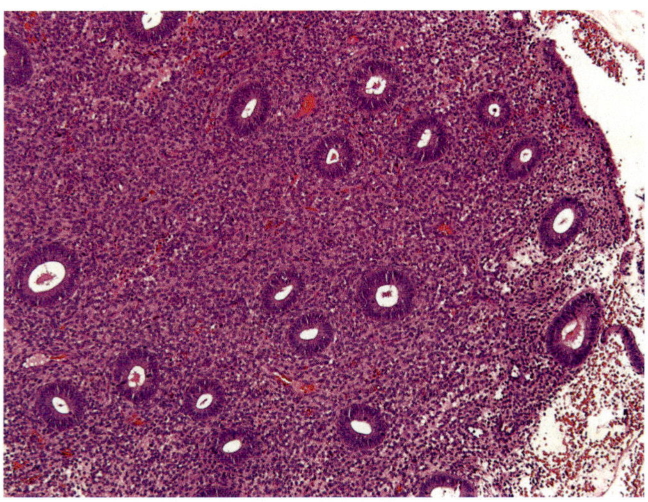

Fig. 15.11 Early proliferative phase endometrium: glands demonstrate a straight, simple tubular arrangement

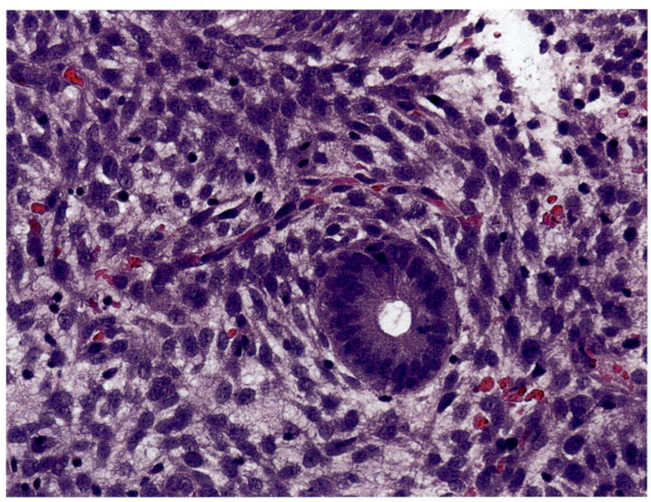

Fig. 15.12 Early proliferative phase endometrium: mitotic activity is seen in glands and stroma; the low columnar epithelium demonstrates elongated nuclei

resulting in further tortuosity of the glands. Mitotic activity is maximal in the glands and stroma, corresponding to the maximal pre-ovulation peak of oestrogen. During this period, the accumulation of glycogen and glycoproteins occurs before ovulation, but this is evident by electron microscopy or histochemistry only. The glandular lumina may also become distended with glycogen and glycoproteins.

During the proliferative phase, the endometrial spiral arteries are identifiable as thin-walled blood vessels that are relatively inconspicuous (Fig. 15.15).

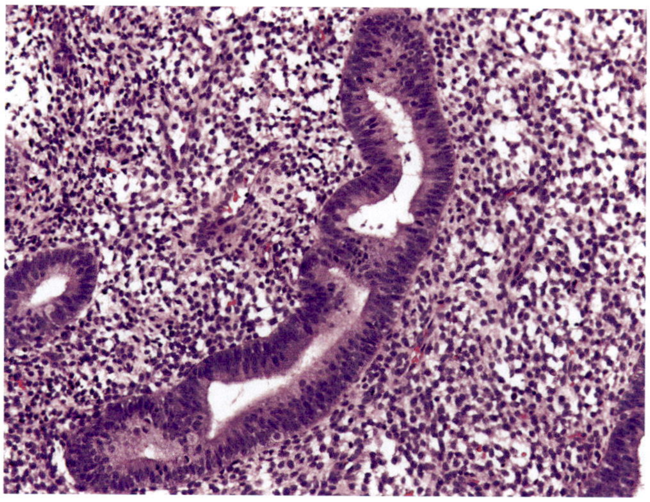

Fig. 15.13 Mid-proliferative phase endometrium: glands start becoming tortuous; the spiral arteries are thin-walled

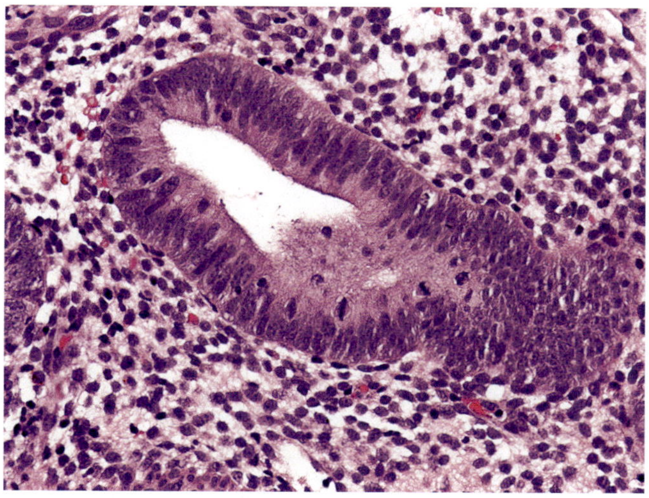

Fig. 15.14 Late proliferative phase endometrium: the tall columnar epithelium shows pseudostratification of nuclei

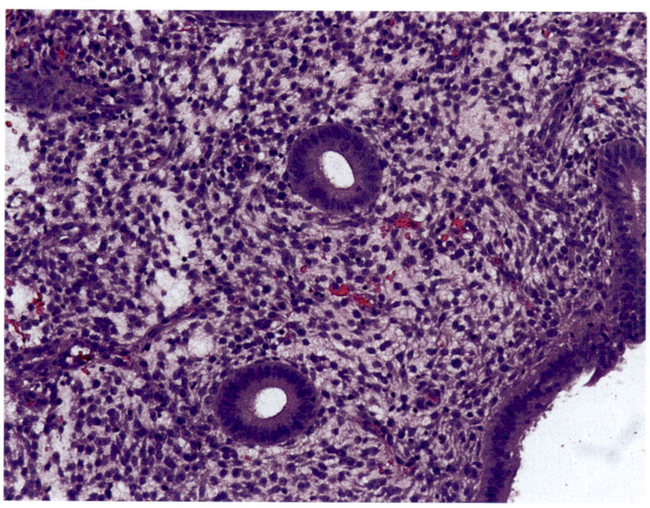

Fig. 15.15 Inconspicuous spiral arteries in proliferative phase endometrium

15.2.2 Secretory

The secretory phase is best divided into two stages, where glandular changes predominate in the first stage while stromal changes predominate in the second.

Endometrial biopsy cannot determine the exact day of ovulation due to a lag phase of about 36–48 h between ovulation and the appearance of histologic changes due to progestogenic effects on the endometrium. This can be determined only by daily plasma hormone measurements which can pinpoint the peak of the LH surge. This period is sometimes termed the interval phase with little change in the morphology of the endometrium except for increasing distension and tortuosity of the glands. There is gradual loss of the pseudostratification in the epithelium while mitotic activity is still readily evident.

Some 36–48 h following ovulation (Fig. 15.16), a clear vacuole made of glycogen and mucin is formed between the nucleus and the base of the cell. This subnuclear vacuolation may be focal or patchy initially and ovulation should be assumed to have taken place only when the majority of the endometrial glandular epithelial cells are vacuolated.

Taking Day 0 as the day of ovulation, on post-ovulatory day 2 (Day 16 of a 28 day "normal" menstrual cycle), the pseudostratification will have reduced. The epithelial nucleus will have moved upwards to the mid-region of the columnar cells, apparently pushed up by the accumulation of secretory material beneath them (Fig. 15.17). Mitotic activity continues in the glands and stroma but is much decreased.

At post-ovulatory day 3–4 (Day 17–18), the plasma progesterone levels rise, the secretory activity is maximal and increases to such an extent that the nucleus occupies the upper half of each cell (Fig. 15.18). As the secretory material

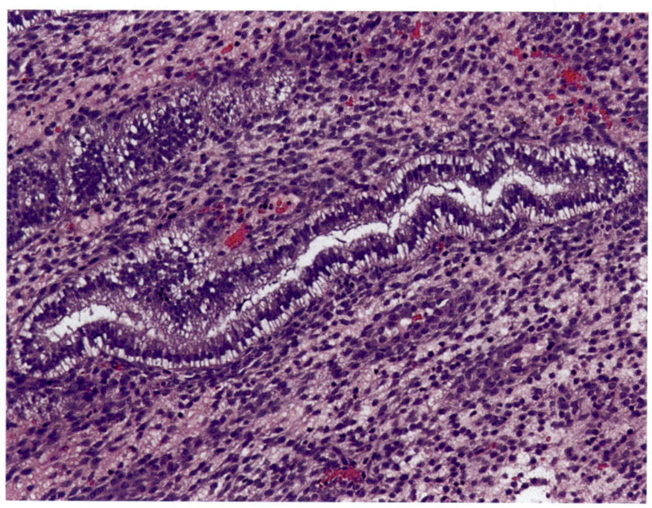

Fig. 15.16 Secretory phase endometrium (post-ovulatory day 1): the pseudostratified epithelium is almost smoothed out and the nuclei are now located in the mid-region of the epithelium; subnuclear vacuolation is almost uniform

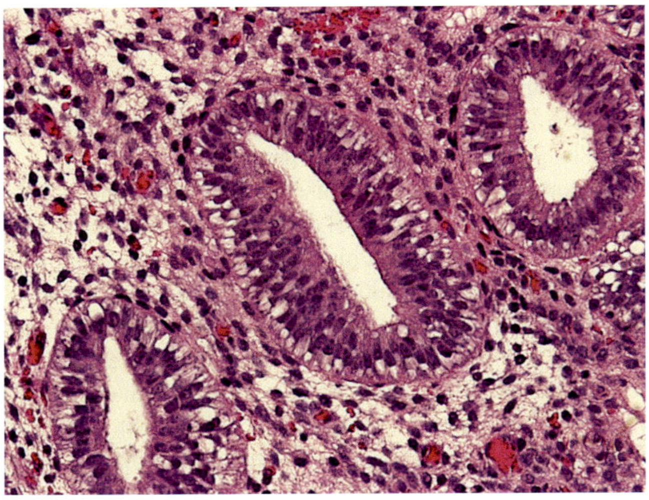

Fig. 15.17 Secretory phase endometrium (post-ovulatory day 3): nucleus is near to luminal border of the epithelial cells

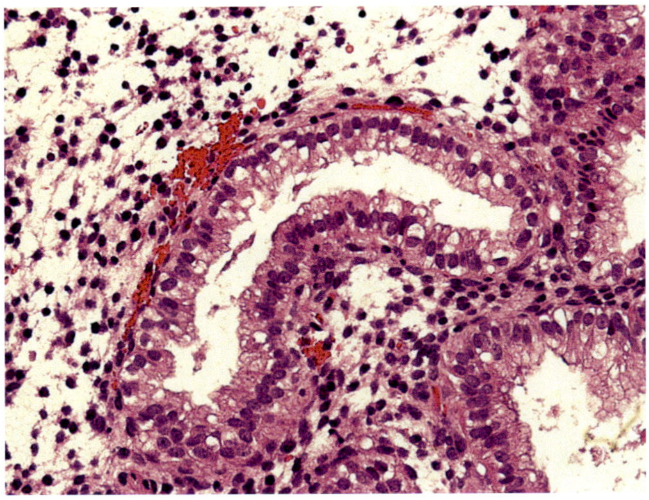

Fig. 15.19 Secretory phase endometrium (post-ovulatory day 4–5): the glandular epithelium shows supranuclear and subnuclear vacuolation

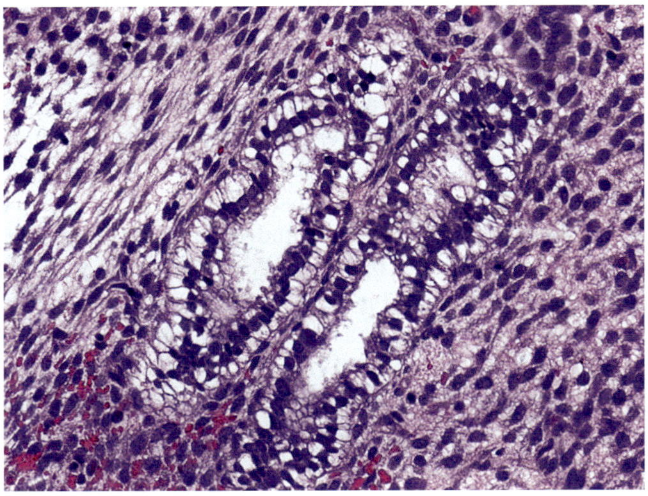

Fig. 15.18 Secretory phase endometrium (post-ovulatory day 3–4): the nuclei are pushed near to the luminal border and there is maximal subnuclear vacuolation

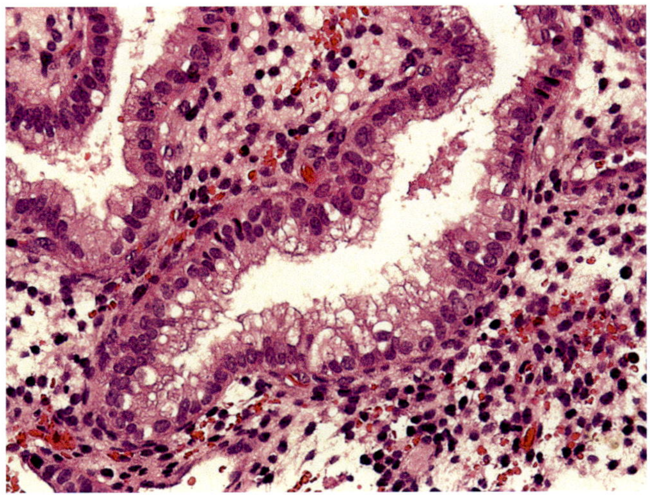

Fig. 15.20 Secretory phase endometrium (post-ovulatory day 6–7): the glands are dilated and demonstrate irregular border of the epithelial surface with secretory blebs on the luminal aspect

of the subnuclear vacuole moves to the apex of the cell, the nucleus starts to assume a more basal position and there is supra- and subnuclear vacuolation (Fig. 15.19). At this stage, the glands are distended and mitotic activity in the glands cease. There may still be occasional stromal mitoses.

By post-ovulatory day 6–7 (day 20–21), the nuclei assume basal position. The secretory blebs are apparent, and secretory material may protrude into the gland lumen. As it is shed by the apocrine method, the epithelial surface becomes irregular. The luminal secretory material results in prominent dilatation of the glands (Fig. 15.20). Meanwhile, the stroma starts becoming oedematous.

By post-ovulatory day 7–8 (day 21–22), if pregnancy does not ensue, the corpus luteum starts to involute and progesterone levels fall. Oestrogen levels, which have fallen following ovulation, reach a second lower peak. These hormonal changes coincide with a change in emphasis of the endometrial morphology from the glands to the stroma. Thus, secretory activity declines after day 22. The glands begin to involute and there is inspissation or gradual disappearance of the luminal secretions; the glandular nuclei are now basal (Fig. 15.21). Stromal oedema is maximal by day 22–23. The involuting glands collapse and show a sawtooth appearance (Fig. 15.22).

At post-ovulatory day 9–10 (day 23–24), as the stromal oedema begins to subside, the spiral arterioles become prominent. There is an increase in length of the arterioles and mitotic activity can be seen in them. Pre-decidual change of the stroma immediately around the spiral arterioles leads to a prominent cuffing appearance (Fig. 15.23).

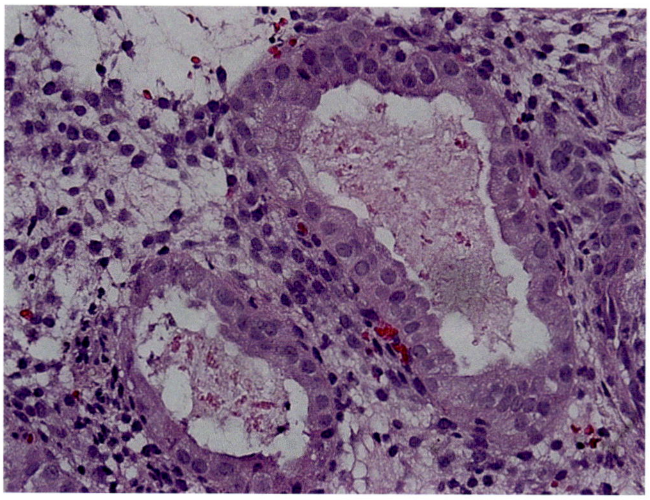

Fig. 15.21 Secretory phase endometrium (post-ovulatory day 8): the glands demonstrate basal nuclei with secretions in the lumen

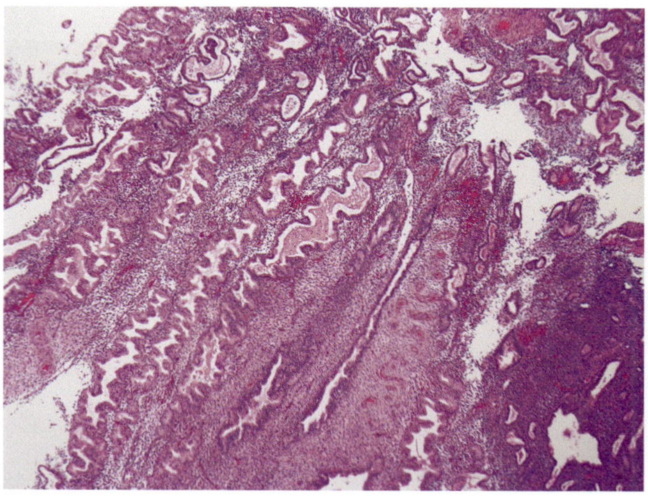

Fig. 15.22 Secretory phase endometrium (post-ovulatory day 8–9): glands show infolding of the epithelium to give a sawtooth appearance

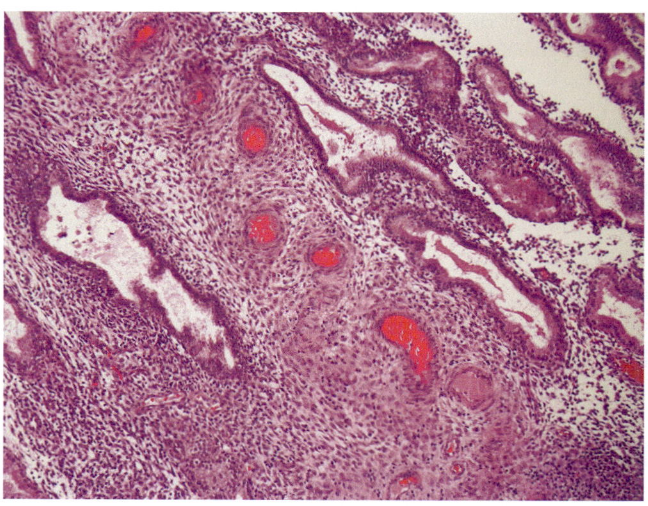

Fig. 15.23 Late secretory phase endometrium: spiral arteries are prominent with pre-decidua cuffing

Thereafter, from post-ovulatory day 12–14 (day 26–28), the stromal changes allow the endometrium to be divided into three separate zones or strata. The stromal cells enlarge and assume a polygonal shape with small rounded nuclei; the cytoplasm becomes abundant as a result of accumulation of glycogen and lipid. The area adjacent to the endometrial surface forms the stratum compactum in which the decidualized stromal cells predominate and the glands are inconspicuous, whether due to compression by the stroma or to a lack of secretions (Fig. 15.24). The intermediate layer or stratum spongiosum shows tortuous dilated glands with a sawtoothed appearance and separated by scant stroma. The spiral arterioles, with their pre-decidual cuff, course through the layer. The basal layer or stratum basale adjacent to the myometrium contains the deep portions of the glands set in a stroma that shows little change throughout the menstrual cycle. The glands progressively become effete. Granulated lymphocytes infiltrate the stroma, particularly the compact layer, during days 26 and 27 with a higher number on day 27 (Fig. 15.25).

The endometrial granulated lymphocytes are present throughout the secretory phase. They tend to aggregate

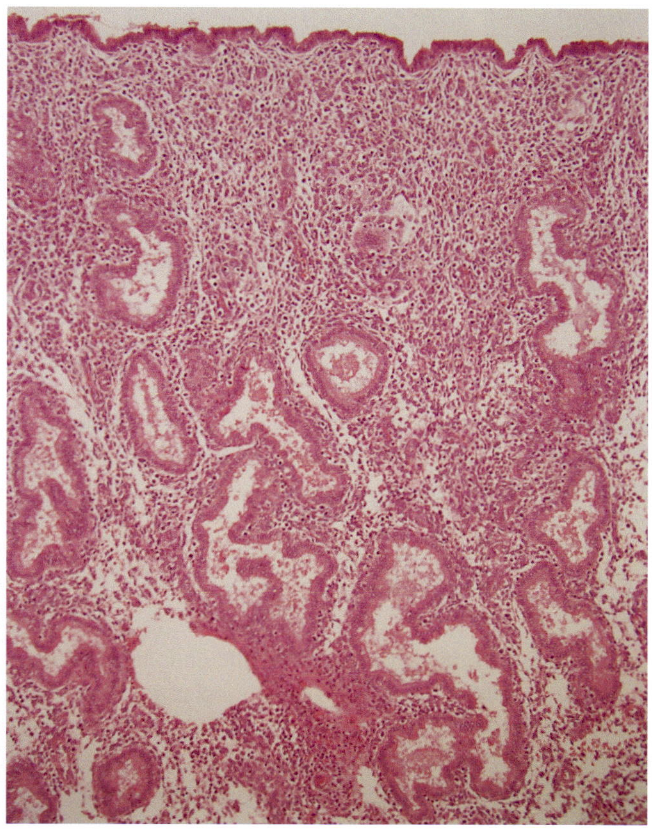

Fig. 15.24 Late secretory phase endometrium: the stratum compactum adjacent to the endometrial surface shows a relative absence of glands and the stroma is more compact compared with the subjacent stratum spongiosum which contains tortuous glands separated by sparse stroma

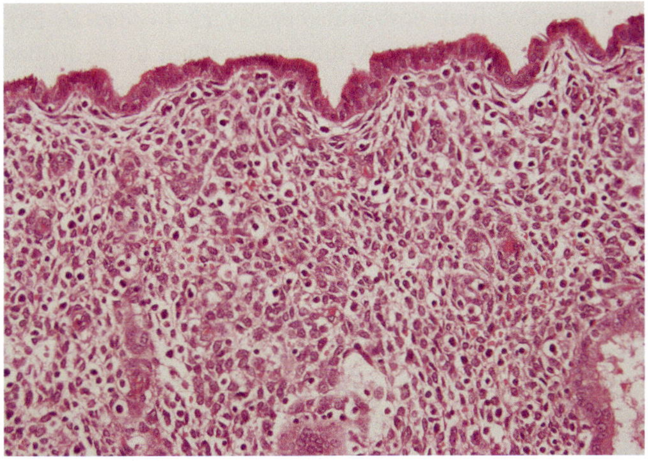

Fig. 15.25 Granulated lymphocytes in the stratum compactum in the late secretory phase

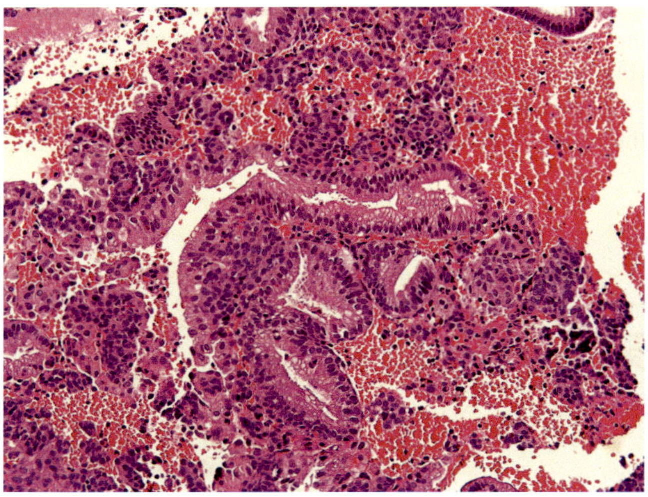

Fig. 15.26 Menstrual phase endometrium: the fully developed secretory endometrium shows characteristic disintegrating fragments

around the glands and spiral arteries, and proliferate between day 21 and 27. However, the stimulus for this proliferation is unclear.

15.2.3 Menstrual Phase

At the end of each menstrual cycle, the endometrial lining will start to shed if pregnancy has not occurred. Menstrual endometrium is characterized by break apart of fully developed secretory endometrium (Fig. 15.26). In addition, the glands show secretory exhaustion: there is disruption of the dilated glands which are lined by flattened cells showing a frayed border. Apoptosis is seen in the glandular epithelium (Fig. 15.27). There is a marked infiltration of the stroma by endometrial granulated lymphocytes and leucocytes (Fig. 15.28). Granulated lymphocytes contain lysosomes like

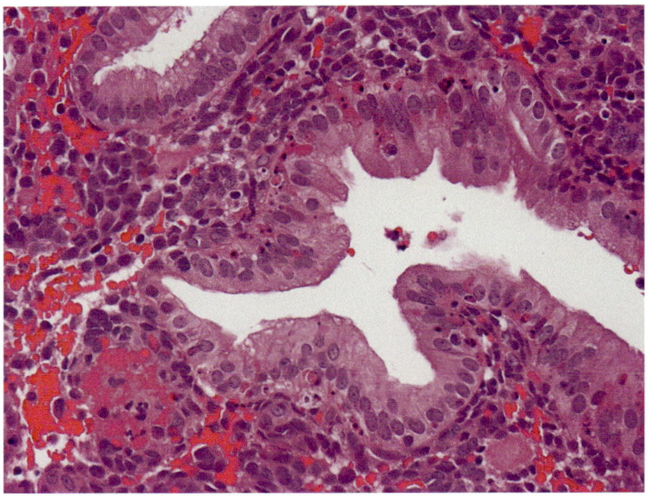

Fig. 15.27 Menstrual phase endometrium: there is secretory exhaustion; the dilated glands are disrupted and there is marked apoptotic activity

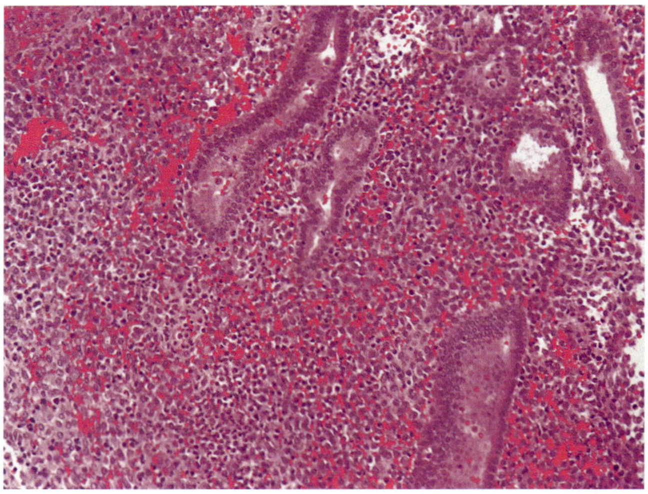

Fig. 15.28 Menstrual phase endometrium: early breakdown showing disruption of glands with some residual suprabasal vacuolation with condensation of stromal cells and infiltration of the stroma by leucocytes and granulocytes

perforin, granzyme A, T cell intracytoplasmic antigen granules and membrane type 1-matrix metalloproteinase. The release of lysosomes leads to the tissue breakdown while metalloproteinase leads to degradation of extracellular matrix. Coiling of the spiral arteries is accentuated due to collapse and the stroma is markedly condensed. As a consequence of a fall in progesterone and oestrogen, there is fluid loss that leads to stromal condensation and a sharp shrinkage in endometrial thickness (Fig. 15.29).

Increase in coiling of the arteries causes a further reduction in the already sluggish blood flow. Eventually, after red blood cells pass through the damaged walls of the ischaemic blood vessels for some time, small haematomas ensue. The shedding of blood occurs when the necrotic epithelium

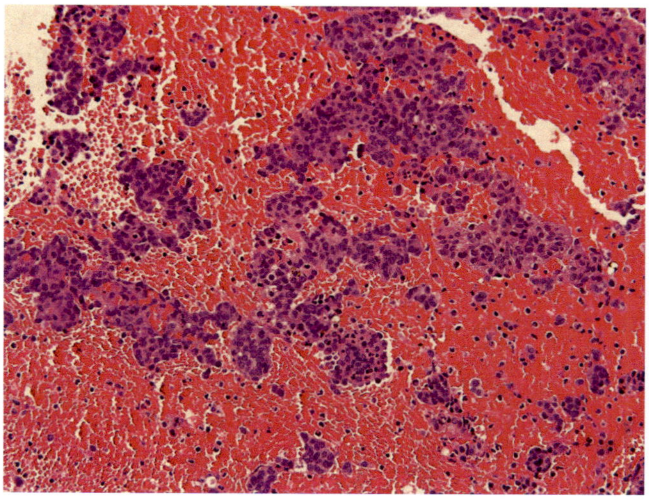

Fig. 15.29 Menstrual phase endometrium: markedly condensed stroma amidst haemorrhage

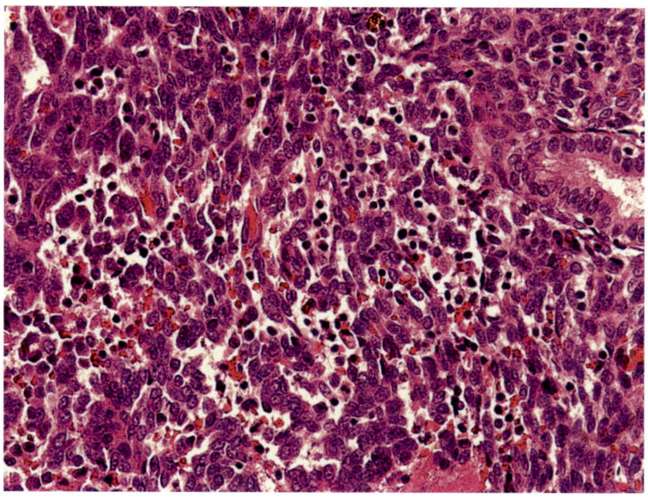

Fig. 15.30 Menstrual phase endometrium: marked infiltration by inflammatory cells

breaks down and shed directly into the uterine lumen. The process of endometrial shedding starts superficially and proceeds to the deeper layers. Shedding is along irregular lines of necrosis in the functional layer and rapid disintegration of the endometrium then takes place. The endometrium is usually shed in a piece-meal fashion but can be shed in larger fragments or even in the form of a uterine cast. At this stage, there is a heavy infiltration of the tissue by acute inflammatory cells (Fig. 15.30).

Haemostasis is achieved by the formation of fibrin and platelet plugs (Fig. 15.31). Regeneration starts well before cessation of obvious menstrual flow and is largely complete by the time that occurs. Menstruation usually lasts for 4 days although it can range from 3 to 5 days. Regeneration begins in the remnants of glands in the stratum basale and in those parts of the functional layer that are not shed in the menstrual process.

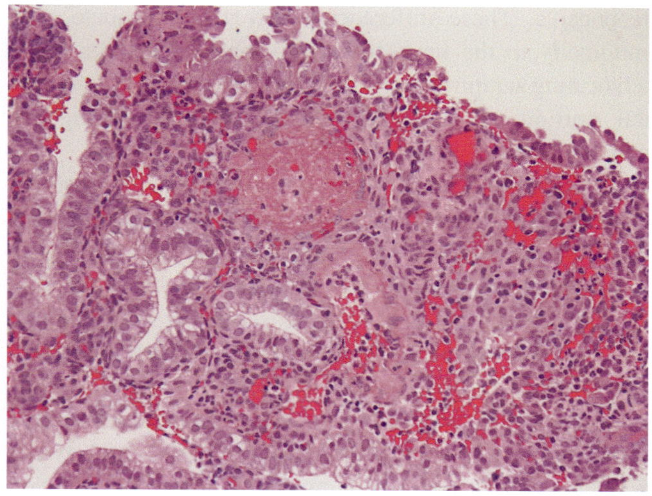

Fig. 15.31 Menstrual phase endometrium: fibrin plug within spiral arteriole and adjacent inflammation

15.2.4 Endometrial Dating

In an abnormal endometrium with pathologic lesions like endometrial polyps, endometrial hyperplasia and endometritis, one should not attempt to date the endometrium. Inactive or atrophic endometrium cannot be dated. Dating should be performed on endometrium from the functional layer since the basal endometrium does not respond to the hormonal changes to the same degree. Similarly, endometrium from the lower segment should not be dated as this area is relatively less responsive to hormonal changes. By convention, the biopsy is dated by the most advanced area dates.

The seminal observations of Noyes and his colleagues provided established criteria for the histological dating of the endometrium [8] but Noyes was cautionary about the imprecision of this method [9].

A theoretical contribution to the imprecision is that endometrial dating is discontinuous and arbitrary in that it is measured in days whereas the biological event of endometrial cycling is presumably continuous. The actual time difference between the day the biopsy was obtained and the biological date as predicated by the onset of the next menses may be 1 day more or less, and this can introduce an error of 1 day in about 15% of the biopsies.

At any stage of the cycle, there are regional variations in the histological date of the endometrium. The endometrium responds differently to the cyclical hormonal changes depending on its anatomical location within the uterus. The basal endometrium responds to oestrogen while the functional zone is responsive to progesterone; the superficial portion of the endometrium responds to both oestrogen and progesterone. Furthermore, the most reactive part of the endometrium is in the body and fundus whereas the lower uterine segment and isthmic endometrium are poorly responsive. These differences, however, contribute only minimally to the imprecision and there is little basis for advocating sampling from specific locations within the fundal portion of the uterus for purposes of dating the endometrium.

Imprecision can arise from the intra- and inter-observer variation. Discrepancy between two blinded readings by the same observer can be greater than 2 days in about 10% of observations, without any consistency in the direction of the discrepancy, while inter-observer agreement rate between two observers range from about 60% to 80% in most studies [9–11].

It is generally well known that the duration of the follicular phase can vary substantially between cycles and between women, rendering the ascertainment of the date of ovulation based on the date of the last menstrual period somewhat inaccurate. Dating of the endometrial biopsy generally assumes a 14-day luteal phase in women but what is less well known is that the duration of the luteal phase can also vary significantly. Only a small percentage of women ovulate 14 days before the onset of menses, even for women with regular 28-day cycles. The time from ovulation to the next menses ranges from 7 to 19 days (day 10 to day 22 of the menstrual cycle). Thus, the variability in the duration of the luteal phase adds further to the difficulty in ascertaining the date of ovulation based on the usual cycle length and duration of the menstrual period.

It has been proposed that dating of endometrium should be based upon time of serum LH surge, as histologic changes are most consistent during the period between 2–3 days pre-LH surge and 7–8 days post-LH surge [12].

15.2.4.1 Dating the Endometrium and Infertility

Uterine receptivity is defined as the state during the period of endometrial maturation when the blastocyst can be implanted. This so-called "window of implantation or receptivity" is only a short period of time [13]. Outside this time, the uterus is resistant to attachment by the embryo. The ovarian hormones, oestrogen and progesterone, primarily coordinate the regulation of endometrial receptivity [14]. Inadequate hormonal preparation of the endometrium, due to deficient production of progesterone by the corpus luteum or to a failure of the endometrium to respond, is thought by some to be a cause of recurrent spontaneous miscarriage and infertility. This condition, referred to as luteal phase defect, is defined as endometrial histology that is inconsistent with the chronological date of the menstrual cycle based on the woman's next menses. Thus, endometrial biopsy became commonly used as a tool in determining the presence of luteal phase defect in the investigation of the infertile woman although there is now greater reliance on hormone level measurements (see section on luteal phase defect).

The window of receptivity is defined histologically by the increase in epithelial secretory activity and glandular dilatation, prominence of subnuclear vacuoles and cessation of mitotic activity in the epithelial cells and coincides with the electron-microscopic appearances of transient epithelial cellular protrusions called pinopodes. These are flower-like membrane projections formed by transient fusion of hairy-like epithelial cell microvilli that appear about 1 week after ovulation and regress within just 2 days. Its appearances can vary up to 5 days between different individuals [15].

Several molecules involved in the development of the endometrium have been proposed as alternative non-histological markers for distinguishing receptive from non-receptive endometrium in clinical practice. These include integrins, adhesion molecules, [16] and gene-regulating micro-RNAs [17, 18]. These, and other candidate molecules, need to be assessed critically for reproducibility and relation to pregnancy outcome. It is possible that the presence or absence of these markers may be an epiphenomenon of abnormal endometrial development during the particular cycle of study. For example, although a lower number of CD56+ cells are seen in peri-implantation endometrium in women with luteal phase defect compared with in-phase endometrium, this finding could be due to the delayed or abnormal development of the endometrium in the first place. Furthermore, it is unclear whether aberrant expression of any of these molecules is a primary cause of reproduction failure, or whether some underlying endometrial pathology has a deleterious effect on embryo implantation and causes the aberrant molecule expression.

15.2.5 Postmenopausal Endometrium

The average age of menopause is 51 years, but this can vary between 45 and 55 years and, in extreme cases, may be as early as 30s to as late as 60s. As a result of involution of the ovaries, falling sex hormones mark the end of the reproductive phase. During the perimenopausal period, anovulatory cycles become more frequent and menstruation increasingly becomes irregular. There is a gradual reduction in size of the uterus: the endometrium becomes thinner and the glands are reduced in numbers and are lined by a cuboidal or low columnar epithelium and the stroma is rather dense (Fig. 15.32). Functional and basal layers cannot be distinguished. Occasionally, the glands become cystically dilated, are lined by a cuboidal or flattened epithelium, and are devoid of mitosis (Fig. 15.33). The stroma is fibrotic and less cellular. Benign cystic polyps may frequently co-exist with this atrophic postmenopausal endometrium.

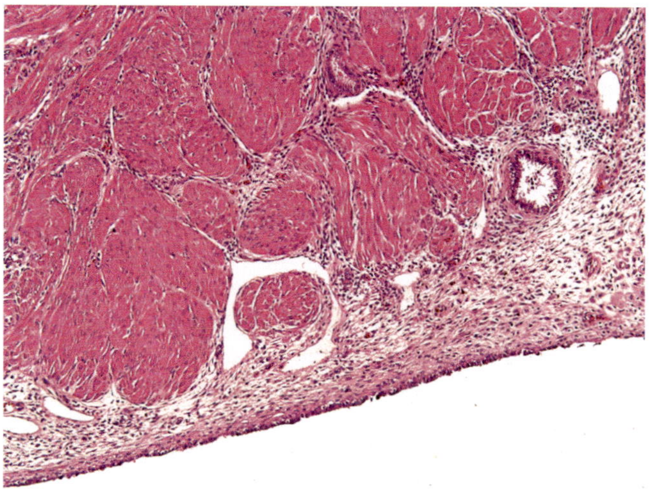

Fig. 15.32 Postmenopausal endometrium: the endometrium shows thinning with dense stroma and small numbers of glands

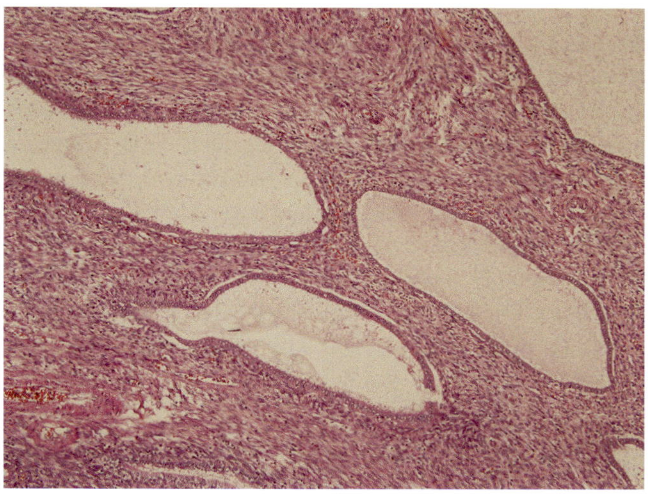

Fig. 15.33 Postmenopausal endometrium: cystically dilated glands lined by cuboidal epithelium

15.3 Pathologic Assessment of Endometrial Samples

15.3.1 Tissue Sources of the Endometrium

Endometrial samples submitted for pathological evaluation can be sourced as biopsies or as hysterectomy specimens. Biopsies are usually obtained in the workup for abnormal uterine bleeding, endometrial dating and evaluation of infertility. Regular endometrial sampling is carried out in asymptomatic women on postmenopausal hormone replacement or women with breast cancer receiving tamoxifen in order to exclude malignancy and premalignant changes. Histological evaluation of biopsy specimens obtained by dilatation and curettage, aspiration biopsy or by hysteroscopic-directed biopsy can provide guidance to the extent of definitive surgery, hence the term preoperative assessment.

Transvaginal ultrasonography [19] and hysteroscopy [20] are becoming more commonly used in conjunction with endometrial biopsy for the evaluation of women with abnormal uterine bleeding. The assessment of endometrial thickness by transvaginal ultrasonography may determine which women would benefit from an endometrial biopsy, both for symptomatic and asymptomatic women [21].

15.3.2 Preoperative Sampling of the Endometrium

15.3.2.1 Dilatation and Curettage

The history of endometrial curettage started in 1843 when a French gynaecologist named Joseph Recamier used a small scoop, or curette (small knife), attached to a long handle to remove what he believed was an intrauterine fungal growth that may have caused metrorrhagia. This procedure was termed curettage. With the introduction of antiseptics the procedure of cervical dilatation and endometrial curettage became widespread for diagnostic as well as for presumed therapeutic purposes. Modified versions of the devise that were lighter and more flexible began to appear after 1860.

This method of blind-sampling of the endometrium is traditionally considered as the gold standard. However, the number of specimens obtained from this method that were deemed adequate for histological interpretation varied from 77% to 94%. Furthermore, it was associated with a higher rate of perforation, infection and haemorrhage when compared with an aspiration sampling technique [22]. A study showed 22 of the 13,344 (0.16%) patients who underwent dilatation and curettage suffered uterine perforation (Fig. 15.34) [23].

There are few large studies evaluating the sensitivity and specificity of curettage. At a time when it was the practice to

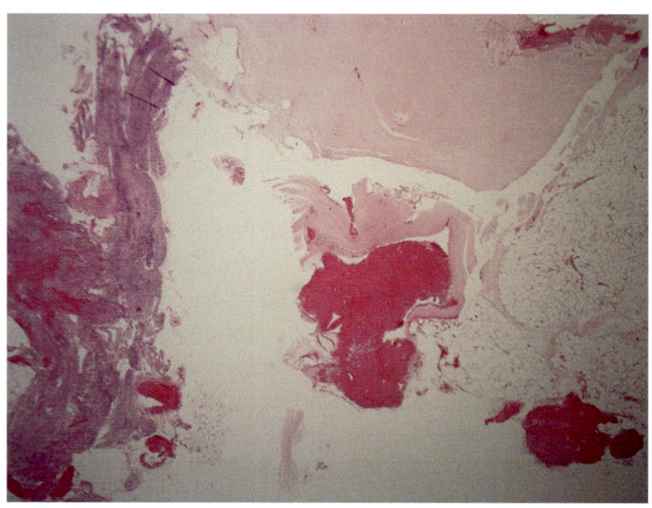

Fig. 15.34 Uterine perforation: mature adipose tissue (right) in curetting sample

perform a curettage prior to hysterectomy for ruling out unsuspected endometrial cancer, of the 50 consecutive curettage specimens performed prior to hysterectomy, in 16% less than a quarter of the uterine cavity had been curetted and in 60% less than half of the cavity was sampled [24]. The true incidence of lesions in uteri subjected to dilatation and curettage is unknown. Pathological examination of the surgically removed uteri provides the best approximation of the true incidence of disease. Endometrial and other lesions such as endometrial polyps, pedunculated submucous leiomyomas, endocervical polyps, placental polyps, and an undisturbed pregnancy were not identified in up to 10% of preoperative dilatations and curettages [25]. Historically, curettage has a sensitivity of about 20% in detecting endometrial cancer; in 181 women who had a pre-hysterectomy curettage, only 20% were found to have endometrial carcinoma in the excised uterus who had carcinoma diagnosed on curettage [26]. In another study, 163 women with abnormal uterine bleeding, the sensitivity of curettage in detecting endometrial pathology was only 49% [27].

The use of dilatation and curettage has been questioned because of the lack of accuracy in evaluating endometrial pathology, risk of infection and trauma, especially in nulliparous women, and the necessity of hospitalization and anaesthetic risk. Trauma can result in an incompetent cervix from excessive dilatation, perforation and haemorrhage.

15.3.2.2 Aspiration Biopsy Sampling

Monitoring of the endometrium nowadays is often performed as an outpatient or office procedure, with most instruments using either a suction mechanism or mechanical removal to sample the endometrial lining. These devices have been evaluated on the basis of operator and patient convenience, patient comfort, cost and their comparability with a formal curettage specimen. Others were evaluated by comparing the histological findings taken as endometrial biopsy and the subsequent hysterectomy specimen.

One of the most widely used devices is the Pipelle sampler and its variants. The Pipelle device is known to sample only 4.2% of the endometrial surface area. Arguably, the endometrium is not adequately sampled and the potential of missing some pathology exists [28]. The Tao brush, which relies on mechanical removal of the endometrium, is said to provide fewer insufficient specimens than the Pipelle method. Tissues obtained using the Tao brush can be interpreted by cytology using either smear examination or liquid-based techniques. A single study showed the Vabra aspirator could sample up to 41.6% of the endometrium [28]; however, it was found to be less effective than the Pipelle device in another study, with nearly a 50% inadequate sample rate which was nearly twice as much when compared to the Pipelle [29].

Comparison of these outpatient-sampling methods has an inherent drawback as the more complete the sampling of endometrium from the first procedure, the less likely a second procedure will obtain tissue that will lead to the similar diagnosis. Inevitably, the first procedure artificially reduces the diagnostic accuracy of the second. This is especially so for a localized lesion like an endometrial polyp or focal endometrial hyperplasia. Comparison of the different sampling techniques is dependent also on the diagnostic consideration being interrogated; a biopsy may be considered inadequate to reliably exclude hyperplasia but may be deemed sufficient to exclude malignancy.

Localized small endometrial lesions or polyps may go undetected using any outpatient endometrial biopsy method. Early well-differentiated endometrial carcinoma and minimal tumour volume were likely to be missed in women who were subjected to a pre-hysterectomy Pipelle biopsy. This may be due to sampling errors or diagnostic hindrance associated with minimal tissue biopsies. These observations call into question the role of these instruments as screening tools.

15.3.2.3 Hysteroscopic-Directed Sampling

Hysteroscopy allows direct visualization of the endometrium and its cavity. Thus, it may help identify pathological lesions missed by blind endometrial sampling, and enable a directed biopsy of abnormal areas. A comparison of hysteroscopy and directed biopsy with dilatation and curettage in 734 women with abnormal perimenopausal bleeding showed only four undiagnosed by hysteroscopy versus 23 undiagnosed by curettage [30]. Both transvaginal ultrasonography and hysteroscopy used in conjunction with endometrial biopsy can reassure the patient or physician that a negative biopsy is a valid result.

15.3.2.4 Comparison of Preoperative Sampling Methods

Endometrial cancer is staged surgically, but its management, including the extent of surgery, is dependent on the tumour type and degree of differentiation. A review of 45 studies showed that agreement on tumour grade was highest between hysterectomy and for preoperative tissue obtained by hysteroscopic biopsy (0.89, 95% CI 0.80–0.98) followed by office endometrial biopsy (0.73, 95% CI 0.60–0.86; $P = 0.08$) with dilatation and curettage (0.70, 95% CI 0.60–0.79; $P = 0.02$) significantly worse. Agreement on histologic subtypes was very good for endometrioid (0.95; 95% CI 0.94–0.97) and nonendometrioid carcinomas (0.81; 95% CI 0.69–0.92), respectively [31].

Histological subtyping and grading of endometrial carcinoma, particularly the endometrioid subtype, can have a discrepancy of up to 54% between curettage or outpatient endometrial sampling and hysterectomy specimens. Thus, treatment protocols based solely on pre-hysterectomy endometrial histology may result in inappropriate management as a result of moderate agreement on tumour grade.

15.3.3 When Is the Endometrial Sample Sufficient?

It is self-evident that there is a significant association between amount of endometrial tissue present for histologic evaluation and diagnostic accuracy. Yet, there are no published criteria defining an insufficient endometrial biopsy sample. Labelling minimal endometrial tissue as adequate risks a false negative report while calling it as inadequate may subject the patient to an unnecessary repeat procedure. Specimen adequacy is defined as sufficient size to determine the gland-to-stroma ratio and demonstrate endometrial morphologic features [32]. Some have considered a specimen to be inadequate when the aggregate size of all tissue fragments in a histological section are less than 1 mm^2 [33]. Others advocate a minimal endometrial tissue surface of 35 mm^2, as this cut-off demonstrates positive and negative predictive values for diagnosing atypical hyperplasia or endometrial carcinoma of 92.6% and 85.7%, respectively [34]. The quality of the specimen can be further assessed on two other factors: the quantity of the intact endometrium present and the lack of tissue fragmentation. Thus, an excellent sample was defined as tissue that completely covered at least 15 × 20 mm on a microscopic slide and contained intact endometrial tissue without fragmentation; a good specimen covered approximately 15 × 20 mm on a slide, with intact endometrium and minimal fragmentation; a fair sample contained a minimal amount of endometrial tissue while a poor sample consisted mainly of blood. A study of 1768 women found sampling of more than ten strips of endometrial tissue gave a near 100% negative predictive value, but this dropped to 81% when fewer than ten strips were sampled [35].

Inadequate specimens are often composed of blood, mucus, and fragmented pieces of surface or glandular epithelium with variable amount of stroma (Fig. 15.35). These samples are more often encountered when they are taken with the outpatient methods, such as the aspiration Pipelle device. It is also likely that this reflects the increasing use of these procedures in perimenopausal and postmenopausal women. The scanty material acquired with these methods should be carefully examined and not be dismissed as being inadequate for histological diagnosis. Close inspection to look for mitotic figures even if only one is present, and secretory vacuoles suggest proliferative and secretory endometrium, despite providing no architecture for evaluation.

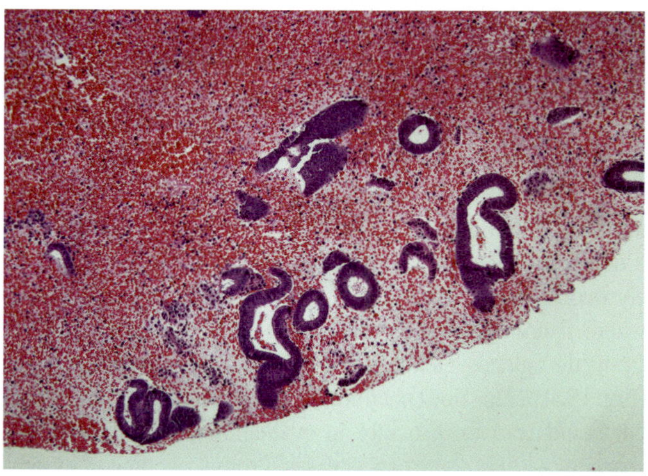

Fig. 15.35 Inadequate endometrial Pipelle specimen: there is insufficient material to assess gland-stroma ratio or endometrial morphological features

Some authors advocate descriptive reporting, including tissue that is non-endometrial in origin (i.e. endocervix), leaving the decision of follow-up to the gynaecologist [36].

15.3.4 Artefacts

15.3.4.1 Tissue Processing Artefacts

As endometrial tissue is soft and undergoes rapid autolysis, it has to be handled with care, with removal of clots and prompt fixation. The issue of a large quantity of blood or clots in the specimen may be resolved by application of a lysis buffer/ethanol solution before applying conventional fixation techniques.

15.3.4.2 Biopsy Artefacts

The use of biopsy bags for processing small impressionable pieces of tissue can result in artefacts. These may be seen as a tic-tac-toe pattern, elongated oval spaces in the tissue, or a serrated contour at the periphery of the tissue. These findings have been reported to be present in up to 60% of endometrial specimens, although it may be focal and not interfere with diagnosis. Placement on gauze or sponges may result in a checker box pattern with loss of significant portions of tissue.

15.3.4.3 Crush Artefact

Architectural artefacts can be created during the biopsy process. Telescoping of glands, or gland-within-gland configurations, and compression with crowding of glands due to fragmentation of stroma is commonly encountered in endometrial samples. These may cause confusion and be misinterpreted as hyperplasia or even malignancy (Figs. 15.36, 15.37, and 15.38). In glandular telescoping, each glandular structure is surrounded by a rim of normal glandular epithelium discounting the diagnosis of hyperplasia. In cases where stroma is lost, leading to epithelial crowding, the glands are separated by clear space or blood, and careful examination will often rule out an erroneous diagnosis of hyperplasia.

Pseudopapillary architecture is sometimes seen in highly disaggregated glandular epithelium without stroma which, by and large, is observed in atrophic endometrium. These samples should be carefully examined for nuclear atypia and

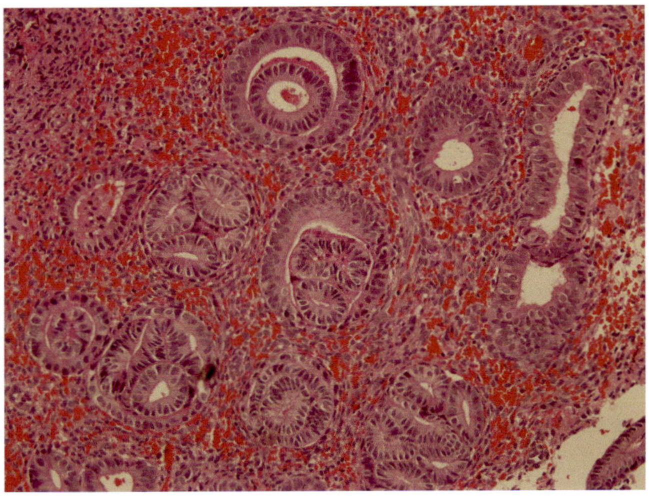

Fig. 15.36 Telescoping effect of glands simulates glandular hyperplasia

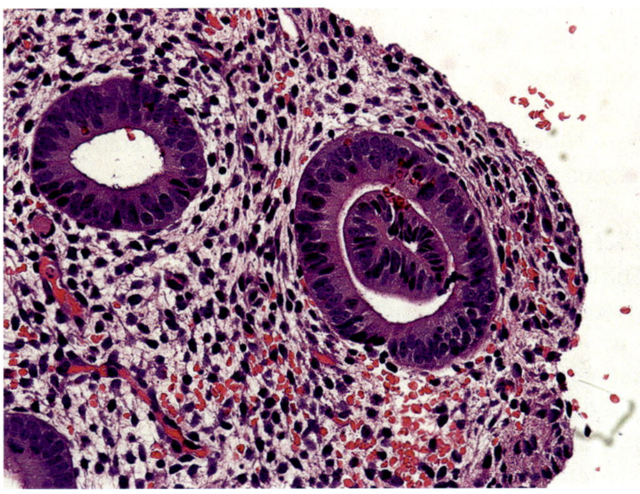

Fig. 15.37 Telescoping effect of glands creates a gland-within-gland appearance

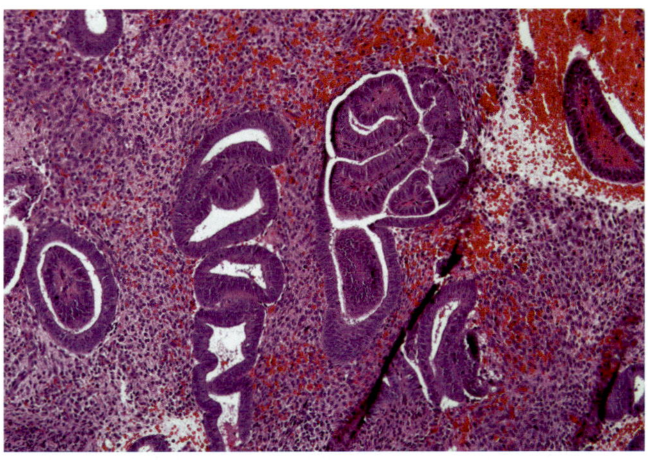

Fig. 15.38 Glands appearing crowded due to artefactual stromal fragmentation as shown by their separation by space and blood

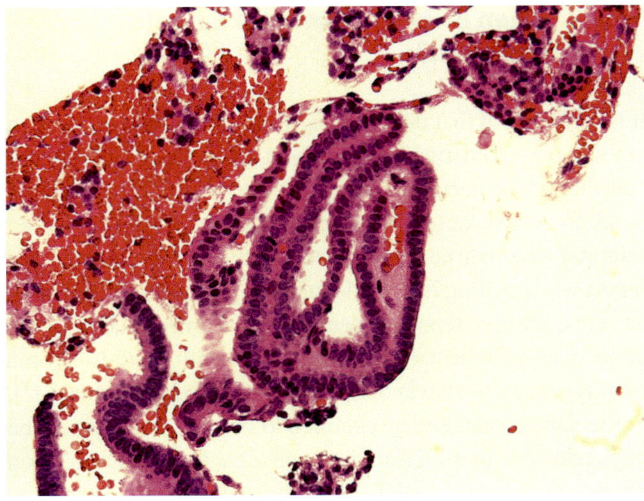

Fig. 15.39 Pseudopapillary architecture in disaggregated endometrium

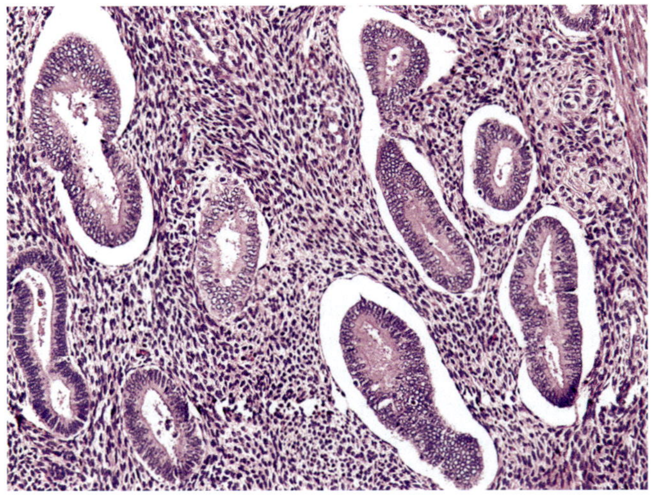

Fig. 15.40 Artefactual halo effect from retraction of stroma around glands

mitotic figures to rule out papillary neoplastic lesions and serous carcinoma (Fig. 15.39) [37].

15.3.4.4 Fixation Artefact

Formalin is the most widely used fixative. Some pathologists advocate Bouin's fixative as it gives great cytologic details, but it degrades DNA and prevents molecular testing if required. A common artefact encountered with hysterectomy specimens where fixation is poor or delayed is retraction of the stroma from the glands, leaving a halo-like space around them (Fig. 15.40). This does not normally create diagnostic difficulty, but could lead to difficulty in evaluation of lymph-vascular space invasion in some cancer cases. Prompt opening of hysterectomy specimen or injecting formalin through the external cervical os into the endometrial cavity has been shown to be effective in minimizing the autolysis of the endometrium.

15.4 Endometrial Changes Associated with Menstrual Cycle Disorders

15.4.1 Endometrial Glandular and Stromal Breakdown (Non-menstrual)

The difference between endometrial breakdown and breakdown in menstrual endometrium is that the latter is associated with a background of secretory phase changes. There is a heterogenous mixture of intact and breakdown endometrium. Other morphologic changes that may be observed are aggregation of stromal cells into clusters, nuclear debris in the stroma and base of glandular cells, [38] papillary syncytial metaplasia [39] and features of chronic bleeding such as haemosiderin deposition and aggregates of foamy histiocytes.

15.4.2 Functional Disorders and Dysfunctional Bleeding

The term "functional endometrial disorders" refers to abnormalities of endometrial morphology that have been attributed to ovarian dysfunction. Some of these "abnormalities" can be regarded as physiological, e.g. endometrial atrophy due to oestrogen deficiency. Alterations in tissue sensitivity to endogenous hormones around the time of menopause, which can differ in different parts of the endometrium in the same woman and between women, should also be regarded as physiological. Others, such as those attributed to luteal phase defect, are subtle and problematic because of observer variation, anatomical variation within the uterus and the influence of drugs/exogenous hormones. In the majority of cases, morphological features alone are inadequate for a definitive diagnosis. In these cases, accurate diagnosis requires a full clinical history, including a history of current and recent drug use/endocrine manipulation.

In a normal ovulatory cycle, menstruation follows the secretory phase and lasts for up to 5 days. When prolonged or excessive bleeding occurs in reproductive-age women in the setting of no known organic disease (such as polyps, hyperplasia or carcinoma for example), this is termed "dysfunctional uterine bleeding". It is the most common cause of abnormal uterine bleeding but remains a diagnosis of exclusion. There are no specific morphological features attributable to dysfunctional uterine bleeding and the cause of bleeding in these women remains obscure.

15.4.3 Anovulatory Cycles

Failure of ovulation can result from various factors that affect the hypothalamic-pituitary axis. Anovulatory cycles are common during the perimenopausal period and immediately after the onset of menarche. The frequency of its occurrence is unknown.

During an anovulatory cycle, there is follicular development without ovulation and subsequent corpus luteum formation. The follicle may persist for some time before eventually undergoing atresia. Consequently, the endometrium is subjected to the exposure of a relative oestrogen excess that is unopposed by progesterone. The endometrium will continue to demonstrate proliferative activity despite that at that time during the menstrual cycle, one would expect to see a secretory, or even a menstrual pattern. That being said, caution must be exercised as, in some women, the proliferative phase can be as long as 22 days. The endometrial glands are similar to those seen in the proliferative phase and there may be a mild degree of non-atypical hyperplasia that may be difficult to diagnose. This has led some to use the term disordered proliferative endometrium in this setting. This differs from endometrial hyperplasia without atypia, hitherto simple hyperplasia without atypia, [40] in the extent of involvement as crowded glands are focal in disordered proliferative endometrium, and diffuse in endometrial hyperplasia.

15.4.4 Luteal Phase Defect

Luteal phase defect, first described in 1949, [41] is reported in 3–5% of infertile women. This may occur spontaneously, or as a result of endocrine manipulation strategies such as those used for ovulation induction. The clinical significance of luteal phase defect is still debatable, as are the criteria used for diagnosing it.

It is unclear where and when the endometrial biopsy was first applied to the diagnosis of luteal phase defect. Chronological dating should be assigned prospectively, rather than retrospectively, to avoid inaccuracies caused by the variable length of the luteal phase, and the accelerated onset of menses induced by the procedure. Sampling performed during the window of implantation (i.e. 6–8 days post ovulation) is more sensitive for identifying altered patterns of endometrial maturation. The term "out-of-phase" endometrium is defined as a difference of "two or more days" or "more than two days". The consensus opinion is that luteal phase defect should be suspected when the endometrium is out of phase by at least 3 days, and the difference is present in two successive cycles [42]. It is unclear why the two-biopsy caveat is implicated as endometrial biopsies performed in two different menstrual cycles can be at variance. An out-of-phase biopsy followed by an in phase biopsy or vice versa can be seen in about 50% of women being investigated for infertility. A third biopsy must be taken in patients with divergent findings in the first two endometrial biopsies.

Following ovulation, affected women have a relative deficiency of progesterone relative to oestrogen. This results in a substandard response to progesterone by the endometrium [6], and the inability to maintain normal secretory endometrium and support embryo implantation. A general lag in glandular and stromal maturation in relation to the presumed day of ovulation is the most common histologic observation. In some cases, there may be an intimate admixture of proliferative and secretory phase endometrium, the so-called irregular ripening of the endometrium (Fig. 15.41). One should be aware that similar changes sometimes occur in the endometrium of otherwise normal women. A precise diagnosis can only be made if a full and accurate clinical history, including hormone profiles, and a detailed history of all recent drug treatment are available to the pathologist. Even in these cases, caution is advised in making this diagnosis given that there is significant inter-observer variation in endometrial dating and considerable anatomical variation in endometrial morphology. The precision of endometrial biopsy in predicting luteal phase defect has been questioned. A study demonstrated inconsistencies between findings in endometrial biopsy and LH surge [43], while another large study involving almost 600 fertile and infertile women found "out-of-phase" endometrium was more common in fertile women [44].

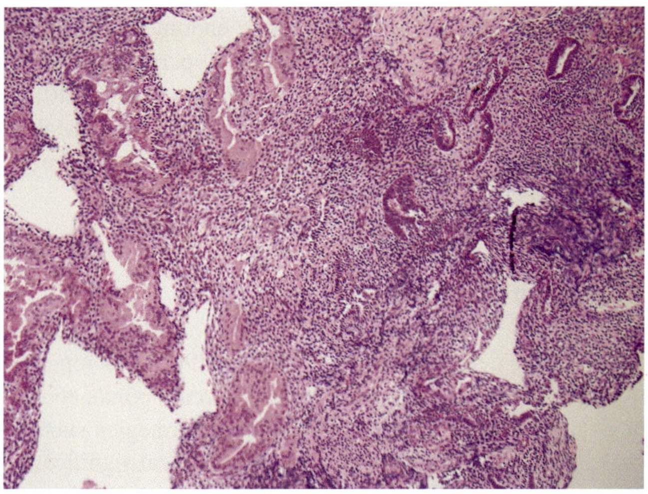

Fig. 15.41 So-called irregular ripening of the endometrium with intimate admixture of proliferative and secretory phase endometrium

15.4.5 Irregular Shedding

In irregular shedding, the morphology is of menstrual-type endometrium admixed with fragments displaying secretory and early proliferative patterns (Fig. 15.42). This is thought to be due to persistence of the corpus luteum with continued progesterone production resulting in delayed and prolonged menstrual bleeding. It has been suggested that many of these cases may be attributed to very early, missed abortions occurring during menstruation. Alternatively, this may be secondary to the loss of endometrium prepared for a blastocyst that did not implant, as the blastocyst is responsible for the luteotrophic maintenance of the corpus luteum.

15.4.6 Oestrogen Deficiency

The state of proliferation of the endometrium depends on a constant and adequate supply of oestrogen from the ovaries. The outcome of endometrial morphology is determined by

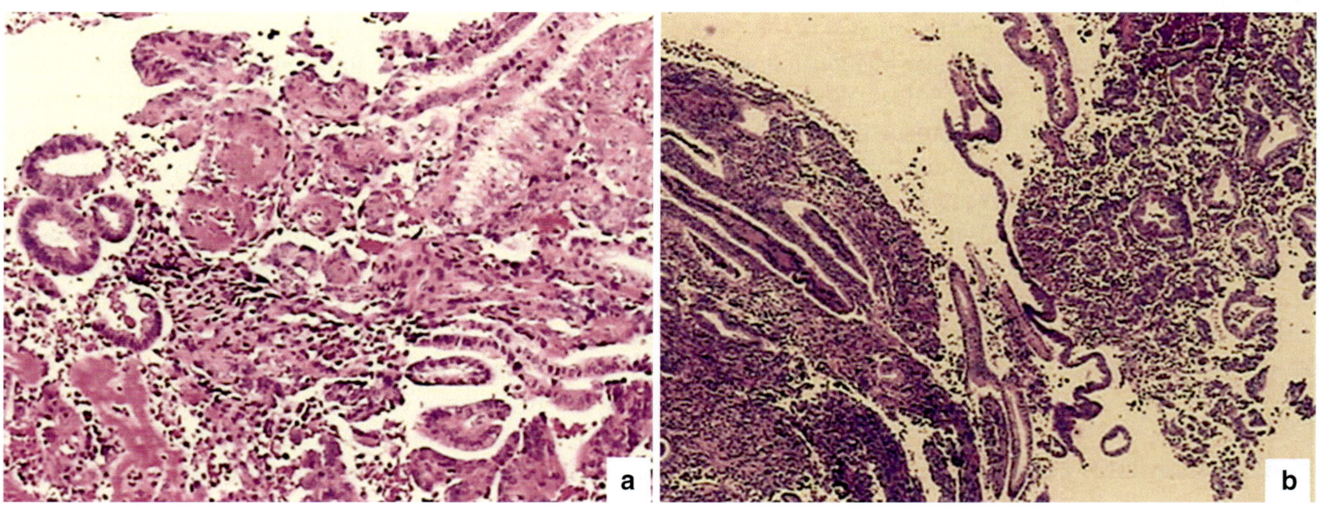

Fig. 15.42 Irregular shedding of the endometrium: there is a mixture of proliferative (**a**) and secretory (**b**) phase glands with condensed menstrual-type stroma

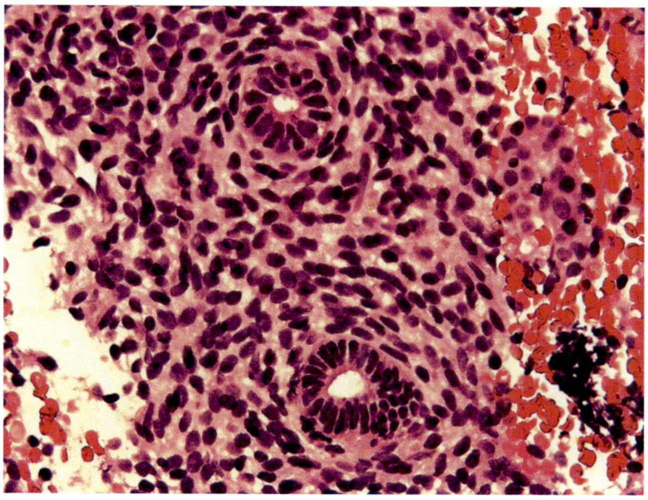

Fig. 15.43 Hypoplastic endometrium with narrow tubular glands set in a spindly stroma

the state of the endometrium when this oestrogen supply is compromised. If no oestrogen has been forthcoming since menarche, the result is a hypoplastic endometrium. On the other hand, a prolonged loss of oestrogen stimulus in a previously normal endometrium will result in an atrophic endometrium. If oestrogen levels are low, it may give rise to a weakly proliferative or inactive endometrium.

The cause of diminished oestrogen supply is abnormalities in the hypothalamus-pituitary-ovary axis. Women with Turner syndrome, for example, are born with non-functional ovaries. Primary ovarian disease such as premature ovarian failure, post-irradiation ovarian failure, or oophorectomy will also result in a lack of oestrogen. Hypopituitarism and other endocrine disorders such as hyperprolactinaemia, which leads to suppression of luteinizing hormone causing failure of rupture of ovarian follicles, even though mature, will also result in low oestrogen levels. Hypothalamic dysfunction can result from severe malnutrition, anorexia nervosa, severe stress, and other debilitating illness; athletes, particularly those involved in endurance events, have abnormal hypothalamic pulsatility. Depending on their age and extent of disease, these women may have different presentations. Commonly, they may have delayed puberty, delayed menarche, amenorrhoea, oligomenorrhoea or infertility.

The hypoplastic endometrium is morphologically indistinguishable from the atrophic endometrium. In both, the uterus may appear smaller. The endometrium is thinned with cuboidal or flattened surface epithelium and small sparse glands set in a spindly fibroblast-like stroma. Weakly proliferative or inactive endometrium resembles that seen in the immediate post-menstrual phase with narrow tubular glands showing occasional mitoses, set in a spindly stroma (Fig. 15.43).

15.5 Maturation Disorders Associated with Infertility and Treatment

15.5.1 Endometrial Changes Induced by Contraceptives

15.5.1.1 Combined Oral Contraceptive Pill

Modern oral contraceptives are composed of a combination of oestrogen (usually ethinylestradiol, 20 μg a day in low dose and 30–35 μg a day in standard dose preparations) and a progestogen (specifically a progestin, which is a synthetic progesterone preparation) given for 21 days, followed by a 7-day tablet-free interval during which withdrawal bleeding occurs. These combined oral contraceptive pills (COCP) suppress the release of gonadotropins leading to inhibition of follicular development and prevention of ovulation.

Oral contraceptive use results in endometrium with narrow, straight glands separated by pseudodecidualized stroma (Fig. 15.44). The glands are lined by cuboidal epithelial cells lacking nuclear pseudostratification and mitotic activity. Stromal blood vessels are thin-walled, dilated and sinusoid-like, and may contain thrombi [45].

15.5.1.2 Progestogen Contraception

Progestogen contraception is administered orally, as subdermal implants or as a medicated intrauterine device. The progestogen-only contraceptive pill (POP) contains a progestin, such as 30 μg levonorgestrel, and is taken continuously; the women experience light bleeds which may be irregular initially. Progestin-only contraceptive pills that

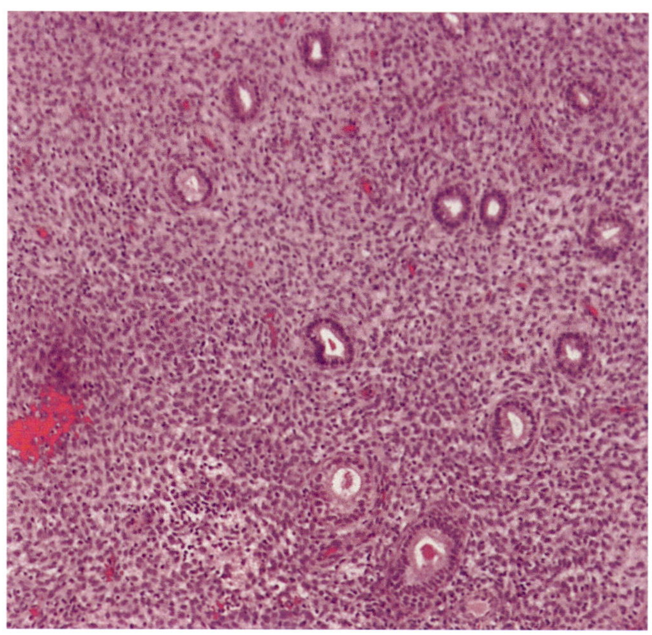

Fig. 15.44 Endometrium following oral contraceptive showing narrow, straight glands separated by pseudodecidualized stroma

contain 1.5 mg levonorgestrel ("morning after pill", emergency contraceptive pill, ECP) are taken within 3 days of unprotected sex. Progestin-containing subdermal implants can be left in situ for up to 3 years. Progestogen-only contraception can be delivered also through intramuscular injection of a higher dose of a progestin, such as medroxyprogesterone acetate. Progestin-medicated intrauterine contraceptive devices (IUCD), such as (Mirena®), release a daily low dose of progestin. Low dose progestogen-only contraceptives work mainly through thickening the cervical mucus and thinning the endometrium and are inconsistent in inhibiting ovulation. High-dose progestogen-only contraception, such as the injectable depot medication, inhibits follicular development and ovulation as well as having effects on cervical mucus and endometrial thickness. The effects of progestogen treatment on endometrium depend on duration, dose and partly on duration of treatment, partly on the dose and type of progestogen used.

Oral progestogen treatment is characterized by suppression of endometrial growth, variable endometrial stromal pseudodecidualization and increase in the number of granulated lymphocytes within the endometrium [46, 47]. In the early stages of treatment, endometrial glands show absence of mitotic activity and secretory features, while the stroma may be oedematous [45]. Prolonged use of oral progestogens leads to an atrophic pattern with glandular atrophy and abundant stromal pseudodecidualization [45–47]. The endometrial glands are widely spaced, lack tortuosity and are small and narrow, with a single layer of low cuboidal to flatlining epithelium. The stroma contains numerous, dilated, thin-walled blood vessels as well as numerous CD56+ granulated lymphocytes; there may be foci of stromal necrosis (Fig. 15.45).

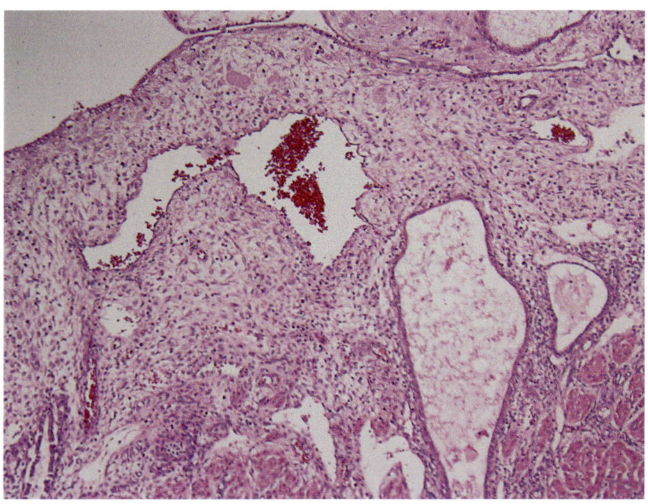

Fig. 15.45 Progestogen treatment: there is extensive stromal pseudodecidualization and increase in the number of granulated lymphocytes, and there are numerous dilated thin-walled blood vessels within the endometrium

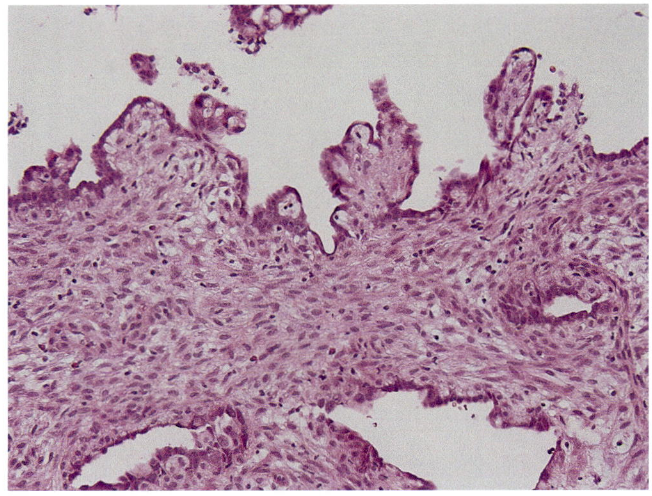

Fig. 15.46 Levonorgestrel-releasing intrauterine contraceptive device (Mirena®): pseudodecidualization of the stroma and papillary indentation of the surface epithelium

Studies on subdermal progestin implants have not focused on their effects on endometrial histology, but the changes appear to be non-specific. Atrophic, proliferative, pseudodecidualization and, less commonly, secretory changes have been described. Depomedroxyprogesterone acetate is an intramuscular progestogenic contraceptive. It results in a decrease in density of endometrial blood vessels and, after 6 months' use, endometrial atrophy.

The Mirena® coil is an intrauterine device, which consists of a plastic frame with a reservoir releasing levonorgestrel 20 µg/day directly into the endometrium, thereby avoiding systemic progestogenic side effects. Its morphological effects are those of a progestogen combined with those of an inert mechanical device [48–50]. Thus, the endometrial changes include stromal pseudodecidualization, glandular atrophy, increased numbers of CD56+ lymphocytes, an increase in stromal inflammatory cells including macrophages and a reactive (metaplastic) surface papillary pattern (Fig. 15.46). Less common findings are vacuolar stromal oedema, haemosiderin deposition, necrosis and calcifications (Fig. 15.47) [50].

15.5.2 Hormone Therapy

Hormone therapy, also referred to as hormone replacement therapy (HRT) or menopausal hormone therapy (MHT), has been used extensively in peri- and postmenopausal women to alleviate symptoms related to declining oestrogen and progesterone levels. Use of oestrogen as hormone therapy became popular following its introduction in the 1960s, as data suggested a decrease of diseases considered related to oestrogen deficiency such as osteoporosis and ischaemic heart disease. Later, in the mid-1970s, when unopposed

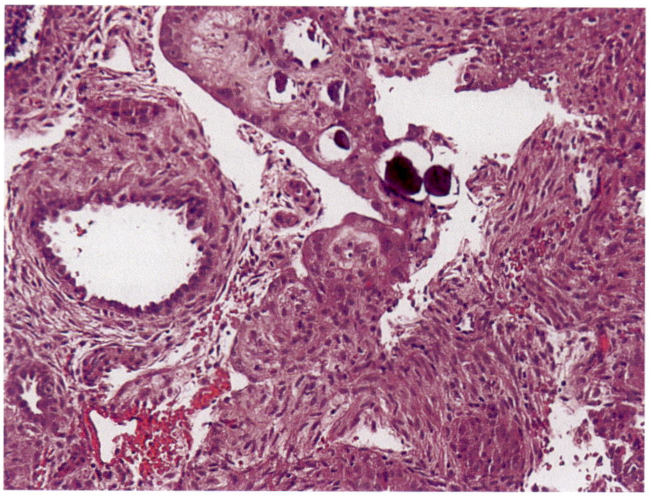

Fig. 15.47 Levonorgestrel-releasing intrauterine contraceptive device (Mirena®): calcification in the endometrium

oestrogen therapy was shown to increase the risk of endometrial carcinoma in women with an intact uterus, adding progestogen to the hormone replacement was found to minimize or eliminate that risk. The use of hormone replacement was widespread, but its use was abruptly curtailed in the early 2000s following the publication of the Women's Health Initiative (WHI) trials that reported an increased risk of invasive breast cancer, ischaemic heart disease, cerebrovascular disease and pulmonary embolism associated with hormone therapy [51]. A re-evaluation of the WHI trials did not show a long-term increase in either all-cause mortality or cause-specific mortality, including cardiovascular mortality, among 8506 postmenopausal women taking combined conjugated equine oestrogen with medroxyprogesterone acetate or 5310 postmenopausal women taking conjugated equine oestrogen alone [52]. The interplay between hormone therapy and health outcomes is complex and appears to also depend on age, time since menopause, when the therapy is commenced, dose, formulation, and duration of treatment.

15.5.2.1 Oestrogen-Only Hormone Therapy

Hormone therapy consisting of oestrogens alone has been shown to be associated with a significantly increased risk of endometrial hyperplasia. There is a direct relationship between the risk of developing endometrial hyperplasia and carcinoma and increasing daily dose and duration of oestrogen therapy [53]. Odds ratios for developing endometrial hyperplasia in oestrogen-only hormone therapy range from 5.4 for 6 months of treatment to 16.0 for 36 months of treatment with moderate dose oestrogen [54]. The reported risk ratios for endometrial carcinoma in oestrogen-treated women have ranged from 3.5 to 10 [55, 56]. The risk of endometrial cancer remains significantly elevated for 15 or more years after cessation of oestrogen treatment [56]. Endometrial carcinoma associated with oestrogen treatment demonstrates no specific morphological features. It does, however, have a relatively good prognosis. Affected women present at a younger age, with earlier stage, lower grade tumours and have higher survival rates when compared to non-oestrogen-treated women who develop endometrial carcinoma [57].

15.5.2.2 Combined Hormone Therapy

Combined progestogens and oestrogen therapy was introduced to minimize the undesirable endometrial effects of prolonged unopposed oestrogen treatment. Progestogen may be given continuously with oestrogen throughout the cycle (usually for postmenopausal women) or it may be added to the oestrogen in a sequential/cyclical fashion (usually for perimenopausal women). There is a vast number of combined hormone therapy preparations, in which the two active elements may be administered orally, topically, intradermally or a combination thereof; however, the hormones are most commonly administered orally, and the subsequent discussion refers to oral preparations alone.

In sequential hormone therapy regimes, oestrogen is given continuously and progestogen is added for 10–14 days per cycle or calendar month. In continuous combined hormone therapy regimes, a progestogen and an oestrogen are administered daily throughout the cycle.

Adding progestogens eliminates, at least for 3 years, the increased risk of endometrial hyperplasia associated with long-term oestrogen treatment [58]. A systematic review of 46 studies found no significant difference in the risk of endometrial hyperplasia between women on combined hormone therapy and placebo at 2 years [53]. The addition of progestogens also reduces the endometrial cancer risk associated with prolonged oestrogen treatment. One study described no significant increase in endometrial cancer risk between women who used continuous combined hormone therapy, or sequential moderate dose oestrogen combined hormone therapy, when compared to non-users, despite 3 years of therapy [53].

There are relatively few published studies detailing the effects of combined hormone therapy on endometrial morphology [59–62]. Combined hormone therapy results in a combination of proliferative and secretory changes both in endometrial glands and stroma [45, 63]. Thus, there is often an admixture of proliferative and secretory pattern glands separated by stroma showing varying degrees of stromal oedema, mitotic activity and pseudodecidualization (Fig. 15.48). In some cases, menstrual-type changes may be observed. Interpretation of these biopsies may be made more difficult by the co-existent finding of various epithelial metaplasias and hyperplasia features such as mitoses and glandular crowding.

Differences in endometrial response to continuous, compared with sequential combined, hormone therapy consisted

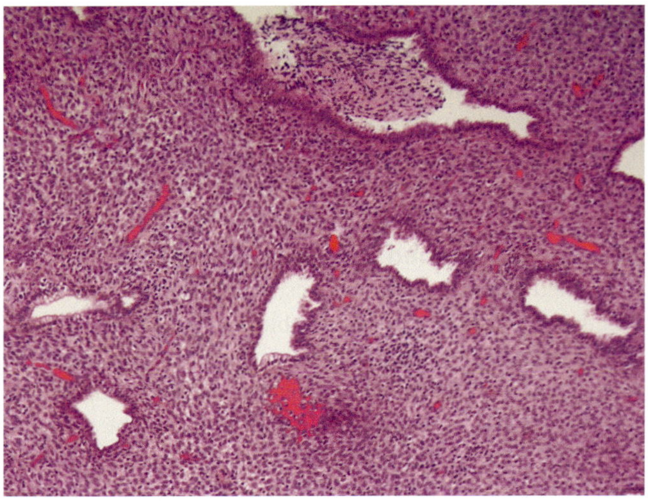

Fig. 15.48 Combined hormone therapy resulting in secretory changes in endometrial glands and pseudodecidualized stroma

of more unassessable, inactive or atrophic endometrium in the former group (59% vs. 21% respectively) [61]. Proliferative pattern endometrium was seen in 2% of the continuous combined hormone therapy group versus 17% of the sequential combined hormone therapy group, while secretory changes were present in 35% of the former and 50% of the latter.

Endometrial polyps are common among symptomatic and asymptomatic hormone therapy-treated women, particularly those receiving sequential hormone therapy. It is not clear whether hormone therapy confers an increased risk of endometrial polyps, although this would seem likely given its growth stimulating effects on the endometrium. BCL-2 expression was higher in endometrial polyps from women on combined continuous hormone therapy compared to those polyps from non-treated women, suggesting hormone therapy may inhibit apoptotic activity and may influence polyp growth [64]. Hormone therapy-associated endometrial polyps have a higher frequency of hyperplasia than non-hormone therapy-associated polyps [65].

15.5.2.3 Progestin-Only Hormone Therapy

Progestin only is used by women who prefer to avoid oestrogen during hormone therapy. This form of treatment is used for treating vasomotor symptoms [66]. It is administered as oral micronized progesterone, transdermal cream, vaginal gel or nasal spray. Large safety trials of progesterone as postmenopausal monotherapy are lacking and there is scant literature on the effects of progestin-only therapy on the endometrium. A small study showed that progesterone administered nasally did not induce secretory changes [67].

15.5.3 Endometrial Changes under the Influence of Hormone-Like Medicines

15.5.3.1 Selective Oestrogen Receptor Modulators

Selective oestrogen receptor modulators (SERMs) are competitive inhibitors of oestrogen binding to oestrogen receptors and can have mixed agonist and antagonist effects depending on the target tissue. The first-generation triphenylethylene derivatives, tamoxifen and toremifene, are used for treating premenopausal women with hormone receptor-positive breast cancer and, in the case of tamoxifen, in the prevention of breast cancer. Tamoxifen use can be extended, lasting up to 10 years. Clomiphene (clomifene) is also a first-generation triphenylethylene derivative and is indicated for ovulation induction. The second-generation benzothiophene derivative SERM, raloxifene, is indicated for the treatment and prevention of postmenopausal osteoporosis and for reducing the risk of breast cancer while bazedoxifene, a third-generation SERM, is indicated for the treatment of osteoporosis.

Unlike tamoxifen, which has an oestrogenic effect on the uterus, raloxifene, and bazedoxifene have an anti-oestrogenic effect on the uterus and thus can be used in combination with conjugated oestrogens as hormone therapy. Effects of SERMs on the endometrium have been studied most extensively with tamoxifen.

There is little information about the effects of tamoxifen on the endometrium of premenopausal women. In postmenopausal women, prolonged treatment with tamoxifen is associated with increased incidence of endometrial pathology that includes polyps, hyperplasia, metaplasia and cancer, of which polyp is the most common [68].

Endometrial polyps in postmenopausal women who receive prolonged treatment with tamoxifen can occur in a background of endometrial hyperplasia. They are often multiple, and considerably larger (mean diameter of 50 mm) than sporadic polyps (mean diameter 20 mm). Histologically, the polyps are composed of glands in abundant fibromyxoid connective tissue. Features that are characteristic of tamoxifen-related polyps are focal periglandular stromal condensation (Fig. 15.49) and diverse glandular epithelial metaplasia. Apocrine, mucinous, squamous, clear cell and papillary eosinophilic metaplasias may be seen. The glands may show polarization along the long axis of the polyp with focal branching or budding. Cystic dilatation of glands is also frequently observed [69, 70]. Proliferative activity is common in both the epithelial and stromal elements [69]. The rate of polyp formation appears to be similar for both toremifene and tamoxifen [71]. There is a relatively high prevalence of endometrial carcinoma developing within

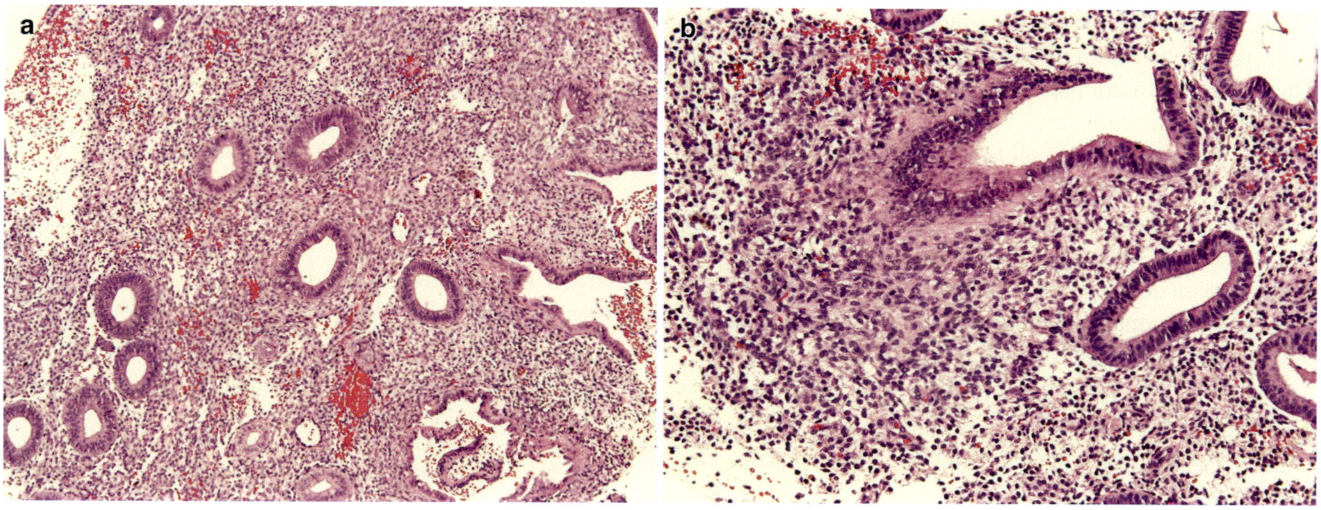

Fig. 15.49 Low (**a**) and high power (**b**) views of periglandular stromal condensation in tamoxifen-associated endometrial polyp

tamoxifen-related endometrial polyps, whereas this is rare in sporadic polyps. The precise risk of endometrial carcinoma developing in tamoxifen-related endometrial polyps remains uncertain as many studies are relatively small.

Hysterectomy specimens from tamoxifen-treated women with gynaecological symptoms demonstrate a variable degree of diffusely thickened endometrium. The cut surface of the endometrium may have a "Swiss cheese" appearance caused by cystic dilatation of endometrial glands [69]. On microscopic examination, features seen with tamoxifen-related polyps are complex glandular branching, focal glandular crowding, epithelial metaplasias and stromal fibrosis. Both the epithelial and stromal components of the endometrium show low mitotic activity [69], although the proliferation (MIB-1) index is higher in the epithelium of benign tamoxifen-treated endometrium than non-tamoxifen-treated endometrium [72, 73].

The increased risk of developing endometrial cancer for women taking tamoxifen is well established; this risk increases with cumulative dose and duration of treatment [74]. Many studies have found that the stage, grade, histology, and biology of tumours that develop in tamoxifen-treated women are no different from those that arise in the general population. Some smaller series studies have reported a poorer prognosis for tamoxifen-treated women with endometrial malignancies due to the finding of more aggressive subtypes such as endometrial stromal sarcomas, adenosarcoma, malignant mixed Mullerian tumours [75] or later stage endometrioid carcinomas [76]. Women using raloxifene [77] demonstrate a lower risk of endometrial cancer when compared with those who used tamoxifen and with SERM non-users, while women treated with bazedoxifene alone for postmenopausal osteoporosis had a lower rate of endometrial carcinoma and no increase in endometrial hyperplasia [78]. There may be an increased risk of endometrial cancer in subfertile women exposed to clomiphene, but the quality of evidence and the confounding factors underlying subfertility for which clomiphene is used render the association unclear [79].

15.5.3.2 Selective Progesterone Receptor Modulators

Selective progesterone receptor modulator (SPRM) is an agent that acts on the progesterone receptor but has mixed antagonistic and agonistic effects depending on the target tissue. Two SPRMs in use are mifepristone and ulipristal acetate, which are licensed for preoperative treatment of uterine leiomyomas. A variable spectrum of morphological changes in the endometrium, labelled as progesterone receptor modulator-associated endometrial changes (PAEC), have been described. The changes can be summarized as non-synchronous endometrium (mitotic activity and apoptosis in secretory glands), large cystic glands, and abnormal blood vessels [80]. There is dyssynchrony between glands and stroma: cystically dilated glands are seen with secretory epithelium but absent of stromal pre-decidualization, or cystic glands are seen admixed with weakly proliferative glands punctuated by apoptotic bodies. Clusters of thick-walled vessels, prominent anastomosing capillary networks or vascular ectasia can be present [81]. It has been suggested that the findings might differ by agent and dose over time. These changes appear to regress following ceasing treatment [82, 83].

15.5.3.3 Gonadotrophin-Releasing Hormone Agonists (Gnrh Agonists)

Gonadotrophin-releasing hormone agonists are used for short periods of time in the management of endometriosis [84], pre-surgery treatment of large leiomyomas [85], ovulation induction, and pre-endometrial ablation for heavy menstrual bleeding [86]. Commonly used drugs in this category include buserelin, goserelin, leuprorelin and nafarelin. These drugs are administered as once-monthly subcutaneous or intramuscular implants.

Treatment with GnRH agonists results in a fall in gonadotrophin levels within 10–14 days with consequent suppression of ovulation and ovarian hormone secretion. This results in marked hypo-oestrogenism and endometrial atrophy [87]. Amenorrhoea develops within 8 weeks. Cyclical endometrial changes are resumed in parallel with normal ovarian function, usually within 3 months of cessation of treatment [87].

15.5.3.4 Androgens

Drugs with androgenic effects include danazol, gestrinone and tibolone.

Danazol and gestrinone have combined androgenic, anti-oestrogenic and antiprogestogenic activity. Both are used in the treatment of endometriosis, and danazol is sometimes used for menorrhagia and other menstrual disorders. Both drugs cause endometrial atrophy, although danazol seems to induce atrophy earlier than gestrinone [88, 89].

Tibolone has oestrogenic and progestogenic activity, as well as weak androgenic activity. It is used for alleviation of menopausal symptoms, endometriosis and prevention of osteoporosis. Tibolone induces oestrogen-like changes in the lower genital tract but the endometrium remains inactive in over 90% women [90, 91]. One study reported a marginal increase in endometrial carcinoma risk, but not hyperplasia, over a 3-year period [92], while another showed no cases of endometrial hyperplasia or carcinoma over a 2-year period [93].

15.5.3.5 Phytoestrogens

Phytoestrogens are nonsteroidal plant compounds that are found in many fruits, vegetables and grains. The most common types of phytoestrogens are coumestans, lignans and isoflavones. These compounds are structurally or functionally similar to oestrogens and have been proposed a natural alternative to hormone therapy particularly for vasomotor symptoms. Phytoestrogen products do not appear to have an oestrogen agonistic effect on the endometrium when given for up to 1 year, and there is no evidence to suggest that phytoestrogens promote a proliferative endometrium [94].

References

1. Kitaya K, Yamaguchi T, Yasuo T, Okubo T, Honjo H. Post-ovulatory rise of endometrial CD16(−) natural killer cells: in situ proliferation of residual cells or selective recruitment from circulating peripheral blood? J Reprod Immunol. 2007;76:45–53.
2. Lee SK, Kim CJ, Kim DJ, Kang JH. Immune cells in the female reproductive tract. Immune Netw. 2015;15:16–26.
3. Manaster I, Mandelboim O. The unique properties of uterine NK cells. Am J Reprod Immunol. 2010;63:434–44.
4. Kammerer U, Rieger L, Kapp M, Dietl J, Ruck P. Immunocompetent cells in the endometrium of fetuses and children. Hum Reprod. 2003;18:969–75.
5. Perrot-Applanat M, Groyer-Picard MT, Garcia E, Lorenzo F, Milgrom E. Immunocytochemical demonstration of estrogen and progesterone receptors in muscle cells of uterine arteries in rabbits and humans. Endocrinology. 1988;123:1511–9.
6. Perrot-Applanat M, Ancelin M, Buteau-Lozano H, Meduri G, Bausero P. Ovarian steroids in endometrial angiogenesis. Steroids. 2000;65:599–603.
7. Rogers PA, Abberton KM. Endometrial arteriogenesis: vascular smooth muscle cell proliferation and differentiation during the menstrual cycle and changes associated with endometrial bleeding disorders. Microsc Res Tech. 2003;60:412–9.
8. Noyes RW, Hertig AT, Rock J. Dating the endometrial biopsy. Fertil Steril. 1950;1:3–25.
9. Noyes RW, Haman JO. Accuracy of endometrial dating: correlation of endometrial dating with basal body temperature and menses. Fertil Steril. 1953;4:504–17.
10. Duggan MA, Brashert P, Ostor A, Scurry J, Billson V, Kneafsey P, Difrancesco L. The accuracy and interobserver reproducibility of endometrial dating. Pathology. 2001;33:292–7.
11. Gibson M, Badger GJ, Byrn F, Lee KR, Korson R, Trainer TD. Error in histologic dating of secretory endometrium: variance component analysis. Fertil Steril. 1991;56:242–7.
12. Johannisson E, Landgren BM, Rohr HP, Diczfalusy E. Endometrial morphology and peripheral hormone levels in women with regular menstrual cycles. Fertil Steril. 1987;48:401–8.
13. Strowitzki T, Germeyer A, Popovici R, von Wolff M. The human endometrium as a fertility-determining factor. Hum Reprod Update. 2006;12:617–30.
14. Paulson RJ. Hormonal induction of endometrial receptivity. Fertil Steril. 2011;96:530–5.
15. Nikas G, Aghajanova L. Endometrial pinopodes: some more understanding on human implantation? Reprod Biomed Online. 2002;4(Suppl 3):18–23.
16. Kumar V, Soni UK, Maurya VK, Singh K, Jha RK. Integrin beta8 (ITGB8) activates VAV-RAC1 signaling via FAK in the acquisition of endometrial epithelial cell receptivity for blastocyst implantation. Sci Rep. 2017;7:1885.
17. Liu W, Niu Z, Li Q, Pang RT, Chiu PC, Yeung WS. MicroRNA and embryo implantation. Am J Reprod Immunol. 2016;75:263–71.
18. Zheng Q, Zhang D, Yang YU, Cui X, Sun J, Liang C, Qin H, Yang X, Liu S, Yan Q. MicroRNA-200c impairs uterine receptivity formation by targeting FUT4 and alpha1,3-fucosylation. Cell Death Differ. 2017;24:2161–72.
19. Campbell S. A short history of sonography in obstetrics and gynaecology. Facts Views Vis Obgyn. 2013;5:213–29.
20. Campo R, Van Belle Y, Rombauts L, Brosens I, Gordts S. Office mini-hysteroscopy. Hum Reprod Update. 1999;5:73–81.
21. Karlsson B, Granberg S, Wikland M, Ylostalo P, Torvid K, Marsal K, Valentin L. Transvaginal ultrasonography of the endometrium in women with postmenopausal bleeding-a Nordic multicenter study. Am J Obstet Gynecol. 1995;172:1488–94.
22. Grimes DA. Diagnostic dilation and curettage: a reappraisal. Am J Obstet Gynecol. 1982;142:1–6.
23. Ben-Baruch G, Menczer J, Shalev J, Romem Y, Serr DM. Uterine perforation during curettage: perforation rates and postperforation management. Isr J Med Sci. 1980;16:821–4.
24. Stock RJ, Kanbour A. Prehysterectomy curettage. Obstet Gynecol. 1975;45:537–41.
25. Word B, Gravlee LC, Wideman GL. The fallacy of simple uterine curettage. Obstet Gynecol. 1958;12:642–8.
26. Lerner HM. Lack of efficacy of prehysterectomy curettage as a diagnostic procedure. Am J Obstet Gynecol. 1984;148:1055–6.

27. Moradan S, Ghorbani R, Lotfi A. Agreement of histopathological findings of uterine curettage and hysterectomy specimens in women with abnormal uterine bleeding. Saudi Med J. 2017;38:497–502.
28. Rodriguez GC, Yaqub N, King ME. A comparison of the Pipelle device and the Vabra aspirator as measured by endometrial denudation in hysterectomy specimens: the Pipelle device samples significantly less of the endometrial surface than the Vabra aspirator. Am J Obstet Gynecol. 1993;168:55–9.
29. Naim NM, Mahdy ZA, Ahmad S, Razi ZR. The Vabra aspirator versus the Pipelle device for outpatient endometrial sampling. Aust N Z J Obstet Gynaecol. 2007;47:132–6.
30. Bedner R, Rzepka-Gorska I. Hysteroscopy with directed biopsy versus dilatation and curettage for the diagnosis of endometrial hyperplasia and cancer in perimenopausal women. Eur J Gynaecol Oncol. 2007;28:400–2.
31. Visser NCM, Reijnen C, Massuger L, Nagtegaal ID, Bulten J, Pijnenborg JMA. Accuracy of endometrial sampling in endometrial carcinoma: a systematic review and meta-analysis. Obstet Gynecol. 2017;130:803–13.
32. Koonings PP, Moyer DL, Grimes DA. A randomized clinical trial comparing Pipelle and tis-u-trap for endometrial biopsy. Obstet Gynecol. 1990;75:293–5.
33. Manganiello PD, Burrows LJ, Dain BJ, Gonzalez J. Vabra aspirator and pipelle endometrial suction curette. A comparison. J Reprod Med. 1998;43:889–92.
34. Reijnen C, Visser NCM, Bulten J, Massuger L, van der Putten LJM, Pijnenborg JMA. Diagnostic accuracy of endometrial biopsy in relation to the amount of tissue. J Clin Pathol. 2017;70:941–6.
35. Sakhdari A, Moghaddam PA, Liu Y. Endometrial samples from postmenopausal women: a proposal for adequacy criteria. Int J Gynecol Pathol. 2016;35:525–30.
36. Anderson MC, Robboy SJ, Russell P, Morse A. The normal endometrium. In: Robboy SJ, Anderson MC, Russell P, editors. Pathology of the female reproductive tract. London: Churchill Livingstone; 2002. p. 241–65.
37. McCluggage WG. My approach to the interpretation of endometrial biopsies and curettings. J Clin Pathol. 2006;59:801–12.
38. Stewart CJ, Campbell-Brown M, Critchley HO, Farquharson MA. Endometrial apoptosis in patients with dysfunctional uterine bleeding. Histopathology. 1999;34:99–105.
39. Zaman SS, Mazur MT. Endometrial papillary syncytial change. A nonspecific alteration associated with active breakdown. Am J Clin Pathol. 1993;99:741–5.
40. Emons G, Beckmann MW, Schmidt D, Mallmann P. New WHO classification of endometrial hyperplasias. Geburtshilfe Frauenheilkd. 2015;75:135–6.
41. Jones GE. Some newer aspects of the management of infertility. J Am Med Assoc. 1949;141:1123–9, illust.
42. McNeely MJ, Soules MR. The diagnosis of luteal phase deficiency: a critical review. Fertil Steril. 1988;50:1–15.
43. Murray MJ, Meyer WR, Zaino RJ, Lessey BA, Novotny DB, Ireland K, Zeng D, Fritz MA. A critical analysis of the accuracy, reproducibility, and clinical utility of histologic endometrial dating in fertile women. Fertil Steril. 2004;81:1333–43.
44. Coutifaris C, Myers ER, Guzick DS, Diamond MP, Carson SA, Legro RS, McGovern PG, Schlaff WD, Carr BR, Steinkampf MP, Silva S, Vogel DL, Leppert PC. Histological dating of timed endometrial biopsy tissue is not related to fertility status. Fertil Steril. 2004;82:1264–72.
45. Deligdisch L. Hormonal pathology of the endometrium. Mod Pathol. 2000;13:285–94.
46. Ludwig H. The morphologic response of the human endometrium to long-term treatment with progestational agents. Am J Obstet Gynecol. 1982;142:796–808.
47. Song JY, Fraser IS. Effects of progestogens on human endometrium. Obstet Gynecol Surv. 1995;50:385–94.
48. Silverberg SG, Haukkamaa M, Arko H, Nilsson CG, Luukkainen T. Endometrial morphology during long-term use of levonorgestrel-releasing intrauterine devices. Int J Gynecol Pathol. 1986;5:235–41.
49. Critchley HO, Wang H, Jones RL, Kelly RW, Drudy TA, Gebbie AE, Buckley CH, McNeilly AS, Glasier AF. Morphological and functional features of endometrial decidualization following long-term intrauterine levonorgestrel delivery. Hum Reprod. 1998;13:1218–24.
50. Phillips V, Graham CT, Manek S, McCluggage WG. The effects of the levonorgestrel intrauterine system (Mirena coil) on endometrial morphology. J Clin Pathol. 2003;56:305–7.
51. Rossouw JE, Anderson GL, Prentice RL, LaCroix AZ, Kooperberg C, Stefanick ML, Jackson RD, Beresford SA, Howard BV, Johnson KC, Kotchen JM, Ockene J, Writing Group for the Women's Health Initiative Investigators. Risks and benefits of estrogen plus progestin in healthy postmenopausal women: principal results from the Women's Health Initiative randomized controlled trial. JAMA. 2002;288:321–33.
52. Manson JE, Aragaki AK, Rossouw JE, Anderson GL, Prentice RL, LaCroix AZ, Chlebowski RT, Howard BV, Thomson CA, Margolis KL, Lewis CE, Stefanick ML, Jackson RD, Johnson KC, Martin LW, Shumaker SA, Espeland MA, Wactawski-Wende J, W.H.I. Investigators. Menopausal hormone therapy and long-term all-cause and cause-specific mortality: the women's health initiative randomized trials. JAMA. 2017;318:927–38.
53. Furness S, Roberts H, Marjoribanks J, Lethaby A. Hormone therapy in postmenopausal women and risk of endometrial hyperplasia. Cochrane Database Syst Rev. 2009;2:CD000402. https://doi.org/10.1002/14651858.CD000402.pub4.
54. Lethaby A, Farquhar C, Sarkis A, Roberts H, Jepson R, Barlow D. Hormone replacement therapy in postmenopausal women: endometrial hyperplasia and irregular bleeding. Cochrane Database Syst Rev. 2004;3:CD000402. https://doi.org/10.1002/14651858.
55. Shapiro S, Kelly JP, Rosenberg L, Kaufman DW, Helmrich SP, Rosenshein NB, Lewis JL Jr, Knapp RC, Stolley PD, Schottenfeld D. Risk of localized and widespread endometrial cancer in relation to recent and discontinued use of conjugated estrogens. N Engl J Med. 1985;313:969–72.
56. Paganini-Hill A, Ross RK, Henderson BE. Endometrial cancer and patterns of use of oestrogen replacement therapy: a cohort study. Br J Cancer. 1989;59:445–7.
57. Schwartzbaum JA, Hulka BS, Fowler WC Jr, Kaufman DG, Hoberman D. The influence of exogenous estrogen use on survival after diagnosis of endometrial cancer. Am J Epidemiol. 1987;126:851–60.
58. The writing group for the PEPI trial, effects of hormone replacement therapy on endometrial histology in postmenopausal women. The postmenopausal Estrogen/progestin interventions (PEPI) trial. JAMA. 1996;275:370–5.
59. Moyer DL, de Lignieres B, Driguez P, Pez JP. Prevention of endometrial hyperplasia by progesterone during long-term estradiol replacement: influence of bleeding pattern and secretory changes. Fertil Steril. 1993;59:992–7.
60. Piegsa K, Calder A, Davis JA, McKay-Hart D, Wells M, Bryden F. Endometrial status in post-menopausal women on long-term continuous combined hormone replacement therapy (Kliofem). A comparative study of endometrial biopsy, outpatient hysteroscopy and transvaginal ultrasound. Eur J Obstet Gynecol Reprod Biol. 1997;72:175–80.
61. Wells M, Sturdee DW, Barlow DH, Ulrich LG, O'Brien K, Campbell MJ, Vessey MP, Bragg A. Effect on endometrium of long term treatment with continuous combined oestrogen-progestogen replacement therapy: follow up study. BMJ. 2002;325:239–43.
62. Feeley KM, Wells M. Hormone replacement therapy and the endometrium. J Clin Pathol. 2001;54:435–40.

63. Whitehead MI, Townsend PT, Pryse-Davies J, Ryder T, Lane G, Siddle N, King RJ. Actions of progestins on the morphology and biochemistry of the endometrium of postmenopausal women receiving low-dose estrogen therapy. Am J Obstet Gynecol. 1982;142:791–5.
64. McGurgan P, Taylor LJ, Duffy SR, O'Donovan PJ. An immunohistochemical comparison of endometrial polyps from postmenopausal women exposed and not exposed to HRT. Maturitas. 2006;53:454–61.
65. Orvieto R, Bar-Hava I, Dicker D, Bar J, Ben-Rafael Z, Neri A. Endometrial polyps during menopause: characterization and significance. Acta Obstet Gynecol Scand. 1999;78:883–6.
66. Hitchcock CL, Prior JC. Oral micronized progesterone for vasomotor symptoms-a placebo-controlled randomized trial in healthy postmenopausal women. Menopause. 2012;19:886–93.
67. Cicinelli E, Petruzzi D, Scorcia P, Resta L. Effects of progesterone administered by nasal spray on the human postmenopausal endometrium. Maturitas. 1993;18:65–72.
68. Deligdisch L, Kalir T, Cohen CJ, de Latour M, Le Bouedec G, Penault-Llorca F. Endometrial histopathology in 700 patients treated with tamoxifen for breast cancer. Gynecol Oncol. 2000;78:181–6.
69. Ismail SM. Pathology of endometrium treated with tamoxifen. J Clin Pathol. 1994;47:827–33.
70. Kennedy MM, Baigrie CF, Manek S. Tamoxifen and the endometrium: review of 102 cases and comparison with HRT-related and non-HRT-related endometrial pathology. Int J Gynecol Pathol. 1999;18:130–7.
71. Zhou WB, Ding Q, Chen L, Liu XA, Wang S. Toremifene is an effective and safe alternative to tamoxifen in adjuvant endocrine therapy for breast cancer: results of four randomized trials. Breast Cancer Res Treat. 2011;128:625–31.
72. Mourits MJE, Ten Hoor KA, van der Zee AGJ, Willemse PHB, de Vries EGE, Hollema H. The effects of tamoxifen on proliferation and steroid receptor expression in postmenopausal endometrium. J Clin Pathol. 2002;55:514–9.
73. Dibi RP, Zettler CG, Pessini SA, Ayub AV, de Almeida SB, da Silveira GP. Tamoxifen use and endometrial lesions: hysteroscopic, histological, and immunohistochemical findings in postmenopausal women with breast cancer. Menopause. 2009;16:293–300.
74. American College of Obstetricians and Gynecologists. Committee opinion no. 601: Tamoxifen and uterine cancer. Obstet Gynecol. 2014;123:1394–7.
75. Bergman L, Beelen ML, Gallee MP, Hollema H, Benraadt J, van Leeuwen FE. Risk and prognosis of endometrial cancer after tamoxifen for breast cancer. Lancet. 2000;356:881–7.
76. Magriples U, Naftolin F, Schwartz PE, Carcangiu ML. High-grade endometrial carcinoma in tamoxifen-treated breast cancer patients. J Clin Oncol. 1993;11:485–90.
77. DeMichele A, Troxel AB, Berlin JA, Weber AL, Bunin GR, Turzo E, Schinnar R, Burgh D, Berlin M, Rubin SC, Rebbeck TR, Strom BL. Impact of raloxifene or tamoxifen use on endometrial cancer risk: a population-based case-control study. J Clin Oncol. 2008;26:4151–9.
78. Parish SJ, Gillespie JA. The evolving role of oral hormonal therapies and review of conjugated estrogens/bazedoxifene for the management of menopausal symptoms. Postgrad Med. 2017;129:340–51.
79. Skalkidou A, Sergentanis TN, Gialamas SP, Georgakis MK, Psaltopoulou T, Trivella M, Siristatidis CS, Evangelou E, Petridou E. Risk of endometrial cancer in women treated with ovary-stimulating drugs for subfertility. Cochrane Database Syst Rev. 2017;3:CD010931.
80. Fiscella J, Bonfiglio T, Winters P, Eisinger SH, Fiscella K. Distinguishing features of endometrial pathology after exposure to the progesterone receptor modulator mifepristone. Hum Pathol. 2011;42:947–53.
81. Mutter GL, Bergeron C, Deligdisch L, Ferenczy A, Glant M, Merino M, Williams AR, Blithe DL. The spectrum of endometrial pathology induced by progesterone receptor modulators. Mod Pathol. 2008;21:591–8.
82. Williams AR, Bergeron C, Barlow DH, Ferenczy A. Endometrial morphology after treatment of uterine fibroids with the selective progesterone receptor modulator, ulipristal acetate. Int J Gynecol Pathol. 2012;31:556–69.
83. Fauser BC, Donnez J, Bouchard P, Barlow DH, Vazquez F, Arriagada P, Skouby SO, Palacios S, Tomaszewski J, Lemieszczuk B, William AR. Safety after extended repeated use of ulipristal acetate for uterine fibroids. PLoS One. 2017;12:e0173523.
84. Bergqvist IA. Hormonal regulation of endometriosis and the rationales and effects of gonadotrophin-releasing hormone agonist treatment—a review. Hum Reprod. 1995;10:446–52.
85. Stjernquist M. Treatment of uterine fibroids with GnRH-analogues prior to hysterectomy. Acta Obstet Gynecol Scand Suppl. 1997;164:94–7.
86. Sowter MC, Lethaby A, Singla AA. Pre-operative endometrial thinning agents before endometrial destruction for heavy menstrual bleeding. Cochrane Database Syst Rev. 2002;3:CD001124.
87. West CP, Baird DT. Suppression of ovarian activity by Zoladex depot (ICI 118630), a long-acting luteinizing hormone releasing hormone agonist analogue. Clin Endocrinol. 1987;26:213–20.
88. Jeppsson S, Mellquist P, Rannevik G. Short-term effects of danazol on endometrial histology. Acta Obstet Gynecol Scand Suppl. 1984;123:41–4.
89. Marchini M, Fedele L, Bianchi S, Di Nola G, Nava S, Vercellini P. Endometrial patterns during therapy with danazol or gestrinone for endometriosis: structural and ultrastructural study. Hum Pathol. 1992;23:51–6.
90. Morris EP, Wilson PO, Robinson J, Rymer JM. Long term effects of tibolone on the genital tract in postmenopausal women. Br J Obstet Gynaecol. 1999;106:954–9.
91. Volker W, Coelingh Bennink HJ, Helmond FA. Effects of tibolone on the endometrium. Climacteric. 2001;4:203–8.
92. Ettinger B, Kenemans P, Johnson SR, Mol-Arts M, Van Os S, Seifert W, Verweij PJ, Cummings SR. Endometrial effects of tibolone in elderly, osteoporotic women. Obstet Gynecol. 2008;112:653–9.
93. Archer DF, Hendrix S, Gallagher JC, Rymer J, Skouby S, Ferenczy A, den Hollander W, Stathopoulos V, Helmond FA. Endometrial effects of tibolone. J Clin Endocrinol Metab. 2007;92:911–8.
94. Lethaby A, Marjoribanks J, Kronenberg F, Roberts H, Eden J, Brown J. Phytoestrogens for menopausal vasomotor symptoms. Cochrane Database Syst Rev. 2013;12:CD001395.

Endometrial Carcinogenesis

16

Wenxin Zheng, Oluwole Fadare,
and Charles Matthew Quick

Abstract

Endometrial cancer is the most common malignancy of the gynecological tract, with an estimated 61,380 new cases and 10,920 deaths reported by National Institutes of Health for the United States in 2017. Although the dualistic model of endometrial cancer development (types I and II) has been a popular analytic model for more than a generation, this model may be overly simplistic in routine practice, and may not adequately address the marked clinicopathologic heterogeneity that is now recognized to exist within the disparate group of neoplasms that are collectively classified as "endometrial cancer". A molecular-based classification of endometrial carcinoma from the Cancer Genome Atlas project (TCGA), based in part on a sequencing analysis of hundreds of endometrial cancers, generated four groups of endometrial carcinoma with corresponding molecular signatures. Thus far, this represents a promising classification scheme since it correlates better with prognosis and patient survival compared to all other available classifications. The TCGA study, as well as other molecular studies that have been published in the past two decades, have significantly improved our understanding of how endometrial cancers develop.

In this chapter, we summarize the most important advances in endometrial carcinogenesis by focusing on those advances with potential clinical implications for diagnosis and clinical management. Furthermore, we propose a unified pathologic classification for intraepithelial endometrial neoplasia.

W. Zheng (✉)
Department of Pathology, Obstetrics and Gynecology, University of Texas Southwestern Medical Center, Dallas, TX, USA
e-mail: Wenxin.Zheng@UTSouthwestern.edu

O. Fadare
Department of Pathology, University of California San Diego, San Diego, CA, USA

C. M. Quick
Department of Pathology, University of Arkansas for Medical Sciences, Little Rock, AR, USA

Keywords

Carcinogenesis · Endometrioid Carcinoma · Serous Carcinoma · Endometrium; · Molecular Subtypes · PTEN · CTNNB1 · beta-catenin · Microsatellie Instability · MSI · DNA MMR · mismatch repair proteins · TP53 · p53 · K-ras · PAX-2 · PIK3CA

16.1 Introduction

Current concepts of endometrial cancer successfully integrate traditional histopathology with pathogenetic mechanisms. Endometrial cancers have long been classified into two major subtypes (types I and II) based on light microscopic appearance, clinical behavior, and epidemiology [1]. Type I cancers, the prototype of which is endometrioid carcinoma, comprise approximately 75% of newly diagnosed endometrial cancers in North America. They are usually associated with unopposed estrogen exposure and are often preceded by precancerous lesions [2]. In contrast, type II endometrial cancers have non-endometrioid histology, typically endometrial serous carcinoma (ESC), and pursue a much more aggressive clinical course. Endometrial serous carcinoma is not associated with excess estrogen, but, similar to their endometrioid counterparts, have precancerous lesions that have been identified [2]. The morphologic and clinical differences are largely paralleled by the genetic distinctions with notably different types of gene mutations between endometrioid and serous cancers [3, 4].

Comparative studies that have utilized genome-wide methods such as expression profiling have further broadened our understanding of relevant genetic basis for the differences between these two different histologic types of endometrial cancers [5, 6]. As previously noted, such dualistic model has traditionally been popular because it accurately distinguishes the most disparately behaving histotypes; however, it has become progressively clear to both clinicians and pathologists that the model is inadequate. Based on the dualistic

W. Zheng et al. (eds.), *Gynecologic and Obstetric Pathology, Volume 1*, https://doi.org/10.1007/978-981-13-3016-2_16

model, patients with type I (endometrioid carcinoma) should have a very good prognosis; however, it is not an exceptionally rare event to see a low-stage, low-grade, ostensibly type I cancer with an aggressive pattern of recurrence that would be more expected in a type II cancer [7]. Endometrial clear cell carcinoma, which has traditionally been classified as one of the type II cancers, has a better prognosis than ESC and appears to be more prognostically heterogeneous [8, 9]. Diagnostic criteria to differentiate high-grade endometrioid carcinoma from ESC are suboptimal [10, 11], and in general the histotyping of high-grade endometrial carcinomas is associated with no more than moderate reproducibility. Furthermore, the spectrum of histotypes that are associated with a particular hormonal milieu evolves as the frequency of said milieu changes in patient subsets within the population. Advances in molecular technology have demonstrated areas of potential overlap between tumor histotypes that have traditionally been considered to be discordant. All of these factors have caused significant confusion in clinical practice, and has made clear that histologic based classification is far from perfect. Data from the Cancer Genome Atlas (TCGA), originally reported in 2013, has shifted the paradigm on how endometrial cancers are classified. It showed that a cohort of endometrioid and serous carcinomas can be classified into four molecular types based on their distinctive genetic characteristics [12]. More importantly, the molecular classification of these cancers appear to have a much better predictive value for patient survival than that the traditional dualistic model. In the following sections, we consider all available information to summarize the main molecular events that underlie the major histologic subtypes of endometrial cancers.

16.2 Endometrioid Carcinoma

16.2.1 The Role of Sex Steroid Hormone

- Estrogens and progestins act reciprocally on hormonally responsive endometrial tissue to regulate risk of endometrial cancer. Estrogens induce endometrial cells to grow, while progestin causes cellular differentiation and has the ability to oppose the biologic effects of coexisting estrogens through downregulation of the estrogen receptor within the endometrial cells. For this reason, the biologic effects of admixtures of circulating progestins and estrogens are dominated by progesterone or progestins. Women exposed to estrogens without opposing effects of progestins show a dose- and duration-dependent 2- to 10-fold increased cancer risk [13, 14]. It is apparent that progestins have a protective effect, which reduces risk for endometrial cancer. There are multiple cellular and molecular mechanisms by which sex hormones affect endometrial cancer risk. We summarize the relevant mechanisms here.
- Estrogen promotes cell proliferation and inhibits apoptosis through a complex downstream cascade of transcriptional changes including modulation of tumor suppressor function. One example is PTEN expression in normal endometrial glands, which is greatly elevated by estrogens and reduced by progestins during hormonal fluctuations of the normal menstrual cycle [15]. This reflects the role of *PTEN* as a regulator of mitosis and an inducer of apoptosis in the estrogen-stimulated proliferative endometrium; therefore, unopposed estrogen acts as a positive selection force for *PTEN* mutant cells. Apoptosis induced by progestins is partially mediated by increased expression of Bcl-2 and BAX. The ability of progestins to induce endometrial epithelial apoptotic cell death is extinguished after just a few days, but increases dramatically on withdrawal of progestins [16]. The relationship between hormones including exogenous hormones is summarized in Fig. 16.1.

16.2.2 Genetic Changes Involved in the Development of Endometrioid Carcinoma

Based on data from multiple genetic and clinicopathologic studies, we list here the common genetic changes in endometrioid endometrial cancers. These include, but are not limited to, specific mutations of *PTEN*, microsatellite instability (MSI), *K-ras*, and *β*-catenin (*CTNNB1*) genes.

PTEN Inactivation

Inactivation of the *PTEN* tumor suppressor gene (formerly known as *MMAC1*) is the most common genetic defect in endometrioid carcinoma and is seen in about 80% of tumors that are preceded by a histologically discrete precancerous lesion [17]. *PTEN* is a tumor suppressor gene encoding a lipid phosphatase which acts to maintain G1 arrest and enable apoptosis through three signal pathways: PI3K/AKT, FAK, and MAPK. The most commonly observed *PTEN* defect is inactivation of both alleles to generate a null expression of the protein, resulting in a complete loss of function. *PTEN* hemizygous inactivation may be still functionally significant when combined with abnormalities of other genes which converge on its downstream pathway. Additionally, *PTEN* promoter methylation is related with tumor metastasis and poor prognosis [18]. *PTEN* acts in opposition to phosphotidylinositol-3-kinase (*PIK3CA*) to

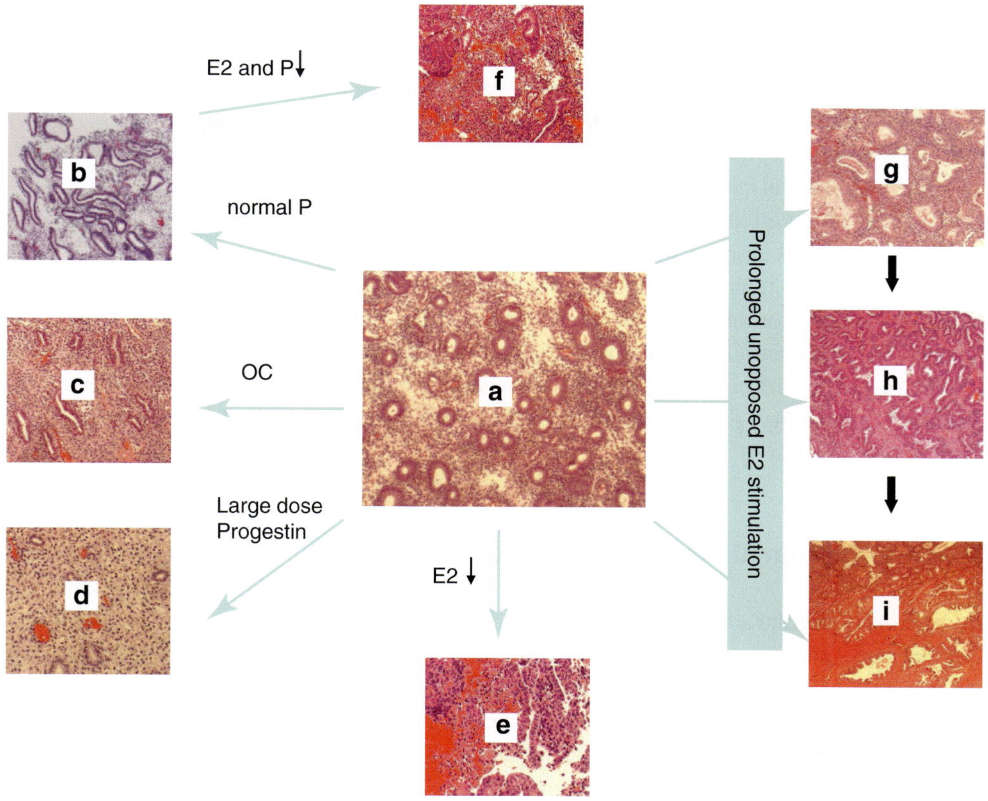

Fig. 16.1 A schematic depiction of the interrelationships between endogenous and exogenous hormones on endometrial physiology and neoplastic transformation

control levels of phosphorylated AKT. *PIK3CA* mutation can be present simultaneously with *PTEN* mutation in about 30% of endometrioid cancer cases, indicating these two genes possibly have a synergistic effect for the cancer development [19]. *PTEN* also is suggested to be a target of microsatellite instability (MSI)-driven mutagenesis, and it is interesting that deletion of >/=3 basepairs in *PTEN* is more common in MSI-positive cancers than those without MSI [20].

16.2.3 MSI and DNA Mismatch Repair Gene Dysfunction

Microsatellites are short segments of repetitive DNA bases that are scattered throughout the genome; they are found predominantly in noncoding DNA. MSI is the propensity to develop changes in the number of repeat elements as compared with normal tissue due to DNA repair errors made during replication. MSI is due to inactivation of any of a number of intranuclear proteins that comprise the mismatch repair system (MMR), leading to accumulation of structural changes in coding and noncoding repetitive elements of many genes. The MMR system is very important for gene stability, and represents the third type of mechanism for tumorgenesis next to oncogenes and tumor suppressor genes. So far, nine MMR genes have been successfully identified, including *hMSH2, hMSH3, hMSH4, hMSH5, hMSH6, hPMS1, hPMS2, hMLH1,* and *hMLH3*. Because simple repeat sequences are unstable in cells with MSI, and most commonly the observed mutation is secondary to defective *MLH1* expression (usually due to methylation). Since *MLH1* is important in repair of short segments (two to four bases), and *MSH2* and *MSH6* serve to repair larger insertion-deletion mutations, the combined defect of the mismatch repair system results in inhibition of both small and large insertion-deletion mismatch repair. MSI may specifically inactivate those genes which contain susceptible repeat elements, such as *PTEN*, transforming growth factor β-receptor type II (*TGF-βRII*), *BAX*, insulin-like growth factor II receptor (*IGFIIR*) and other genetic changes, resulting in secondary tumor subclones with an altered capacity of cancer development.

Due to menstrual cycling, the normal endometrium undergoes constant remodeling and proliferation and thus has an increased propensity for replicative errors; therefore, the endometrium is highly dependent on the MMR system. As a result, MMR mutation has been shown to be present in

25–30% of type I endometrial carcinoma [21, 22]. *MLH1* inactivation is the most common mechanism in MMR-related endometrial carcinoma and is accomplished by hypermethylation of CpG islands in the gene promoter, a process known as epigenetic silencing, which is related to sporadic endometrial carcinoma [23, 24]. Inherited or somatically acquired mutations of *MSH6*, another mismatch repair element, are also common in endometrial cancer patients with MSI-related tumors. A single nucleotide insertion (frameshift) mutation in *MSH2* has been described less frequently in endometrial cancers with MSI; this deletion occurs in a string of eight consecutive adenosine residues. All these features may guide us to screen patients with Lynch syndrome (see below).

16.2.4 *β*-Catenin *(CTNNB1)* Alteration

β-Catenin is a cellular adhesion component of the E-cadherin-catenin unit, and is essential for cell differentiation and maintenance of normal tissue architecture. It plays an important role in signal transduction. Increased nuclear levels of *β*-catenin produce transcriptional activation through the LEF/Tcf and the ubiquitin-proteasome pathways.

CTNNB1 mutation improves its protein stability, and leads to its accumulation in the cytoplasm and nuclei. Additionally, it activates its downstream target genes, such as transitional factors of wnt pathway. Abnormal *β*-catenin expression may be seen in endometrioid carcinoma (33–47%), and rarely non-endometrioid subtypes (1–3%) [25]. In all endometrioid carcinoma with *β*-catenin mutation, ER and most of PR are positive, suggestive of an intimate relationship between *β*-catenin and ER [26]. It may represent a pathway to endometrial carcinogenesis, which can be associated with squamous differentiation, a common finding in endometrioid cancers and atypical polypoid adenomyomas. Although MSI, *PTEN*, and *K-ras* mutations frequently coexist with each other, these molecular abnormalities are not usually seen in tumors with *β*-catenin alterations [27]. *CTNNB1* mutation can be seen in some atypical hyperplasia\EIN cases, indicating an early step of endometrial tumorigenesis. When mutation occurs, changes in *β*-catenin expression are usually seen throughout all tumor cells, suggesting a clonal expansion process. *β*-Catenin may also regulate the expression of the matrix metalloprotease-7, which would indicate a role in the establishment of the microenvironment necessary for initiation and maintenance of growth of the endometrioid cancers and their metastasis [28]. Of note, gain of function mutations in exon 3 of *CTNNB1* gene at 3p21 are seen in 25–40% of endometrioid cancers [29], resulting in stabilization of the protein. Mutations in exon 3 of the *CTNNB1* gene may identify low-grade, low-stage, endometrioid carcinomas at risk for recurrence [30, 31].

16.2.5 *K-ras* Mutation

K-ras mutations have been identified in 10–30% of endometrioid carcinomas as well as endometrial hyperplasia [32]. The latter suggests that *K-ras* mutation is an early event in carcinogenesis. Compared with endometrioid carcinoma, the rate of *K-ras* mutation in non-endometrioid cancers is relatively low. *K-ras* mutation may cause resistance to epidermal growth factor receptor (EGFR) inhibitors. There is a higher frequency of *K-ras* mutations in MSI cancers, and many of these are characterized as methylation-related GC → AT transitions. It has also recently found that *K-ras* mutations are more commonly seen in endometrioid carcinomas with mucinous differentiation or endometrial mucinous cancers [33, 34]. Accordingly, *K-ras* mutation analysis is not a suitable biomarker to differentiate endometrioid carcinoma from endometrial mucinous cancers. *K-ras* mutations have also been reported in associated with the microcystic elongated and fragmented (MELF) pattern of myometrial invasion in endometrioid carcinomas [35].

16.2.5.1 PAX 2

PAX2 is a gene that plays an important role in the embryonic development of the Mullerian and urogenital systems. It encodes a nuclear transcription factor, which is present in normal endometrium. Immunohistochemistry demonstrates nuclear staining in normal endometrial glands. Similar to PTEN, PAX2 does show loss in normal endometrium (36%), atypical hyperplasia or EIN (71%) and carcinoma (77%) as demonstrated by Monte et al. They suggest that a major mechanism of the development of atypical hyperplasia or EIN is the co-localization of PAX2 and PTEN within the same endometrial glands [36]. This “dual-hit” is thought to be the cause for the majority of sporadic endometrioid carcinomas, although the detailed molecular mechanisms are unclear. Many publications have sought to describe the relationship between *PAX2* loss, the immunohistochemical findings, and the diagnosis of atypical hyperplasia or EIN [17, 37, 38], the overall conclusion in this setting is that PAX2 has been found to be useful in the diagnosis of atypical hyperplasia or EIN.

16.2.6 PI3K/AKT Pathway

The PI3K/AKT pathway is activated in a broad range of malignant tumors. Stimulating signals through receptor tyrosine kinases (RTKs) activate *PI3K*, which phosphorylates PIP2 to generate PIP3. PIP3 binds to AKT triggering a complex cascade of signals that regulate growth, proliferation, survival, and motility. *PI3CA* mutation is often combined with other genetic abnormalities, such as mutations in c-erB2, *K-ras*, and *PTEN*. The lipid phosphatase, PTEN, antagonizes this process by dephosphorylating PIP3 to inhibit activation of AKT. About 28% endometrioid carcinomas have *PI3K* mutations [39], but ESCs also have these mutations at comparable frequencies.

16.2.7 FGFR2 Alterations

FGFR2 activation can promote cell proliferation, migration, and survival. *FGFR2* mutations are seen in 10–16% endometrioid cancers [40]. *FGFR2* mutation is often companied by PTEN loss, while *FGFR2* and *K-ras* mutations rarely coexist. Endometrioid carcinoma cell lines with *EGFR2* mutations have been reported as sensitive to pan-FGFR inhibitor PD173074, suggesting that FGFR2 could be a new therapeutic target [41].

16.2.8 MicroRNA (miRNA)

MiRNA is a small noncoding RNA (containing about 22 nucleotides), widely found in plants, virus, animals, and human beings, which functions in RNA silencing and post-transcriptional regulation of gene expression. Abnormal MiRNA expression is closely related to tumorigenesis and cancer development. In patients with endometrioid carcinomas, cancer tissues and blood plasma have a higher level of miRNAs (including miRNA-99a, -100, and -199b), which are able to suppress tumor growth through the mTOR pathway. Similarly, deletion of both miRNA-410 and -487, located on 14q32, is associated with a poor prognosis in patients with endometrioid cancers [42]. In contrast to the above miRNA species, miRNA-200 family (including miRNA-200a, -200b, -200c, and -429) are highly expressed in low-grade endometrioid cancers, which may promote tumor growth and recurrence [43–45].

16.2.9 The Model of Endometrioid Carcinoma Development

Endometrioid carcinoma is frequently preceded by estrogen-induced changes commonly referred to as hyperplasia, some of which are monoclonal proliferations of genetically altered endometrial glands presenting as a discrete lesion termed endometrioid intraepithelial neoplasia (EIN). The common term "hyperplasia" historically was applied to all entities, with the implication that non-atypical and atypical hyperplasia subgroups correspond to benign and precancerous groups, respectively. In the 2014 WHO classification, atypical hyperplasia is considered to be equivalent to EIN. Notably, the 2014 WHO classification termed it "endometrioid" rather than "endometrial" intraepithelial neoplasia to further clarify its role as an endometrioid carcinoma precursor. Somatic mutation of endometrial epithelium is very common in "normal" endometrium, and occurs in advance of any discernible histopathologic changes. The term "latent precancer" has been applied to this condition to emphasize that endometrial cancer risk is not necessarily increased at this stage. This preclinical phase of disease is recognizable only through genetic analysis of mutant cells or identified by biomarkers such as loss of PTEN expression and acquisition of microsatellite instability, not by routine microscopy. Based on this understanding, endometrioid carcinoma develops from a latent precancer to precancer (atypical hyperplasia or EIN), and to well-differentiated endometrioid carcinoma. The basic steps of cancer development as well as the main molecular alterations are summarized in Fig. 16.2.

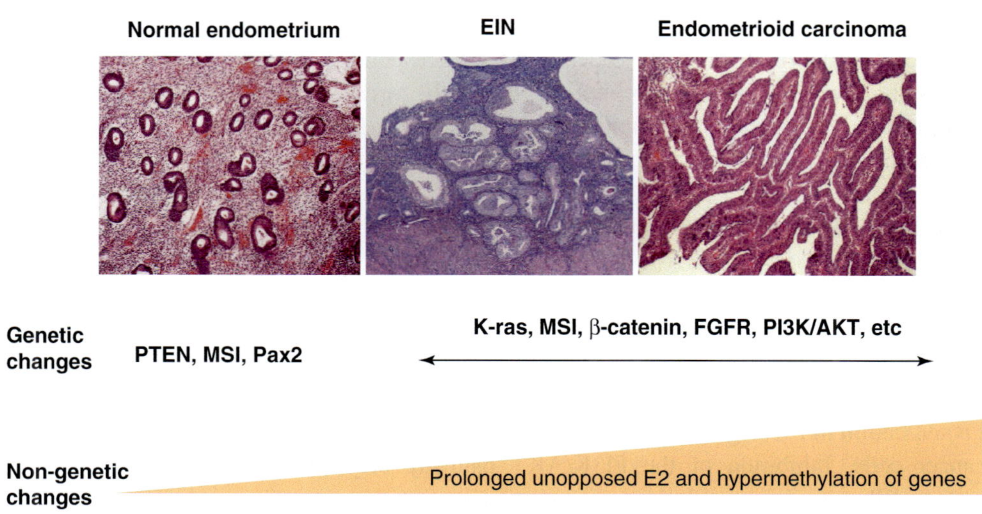

Fig. 16.2 Basic stages of endometrioid cancer evolution and major associated molecular alterations

16.2.10 Lynch Syndrome-Related Endometrial Cancer

In endometrial cancers, MSI is very common. There are two conditions which may result in MSI. One is hypermethylation of the *MLH1* gene promoter resulting in gene silencing. Hypermethylation is a common epigenetic event seen in 15–25% of corresponding sporadic cancers. The second condition is a germ line mutation of one or more of MMR genes (*MLH1, MSH2, MSH6,* or *PMS2*). Mutations of the above genes can induce MSI resulting in development of Lynch syndrome (LS), an autosomal dominant inherited cancer susceptibility syndrome, also known as hereditary non-polyposis colon cancer (HNPCC). Women with LS have a 40–60% chance of presenting with endometrial cancer, usually the endometrioid variant, as their first clinical manifestation. Among LS-related endometrial cancers, mutation of MSH2 is the most common (50–66%), and MLH1 (24–40%) and MSH6 (10–13%) are less frequent [46]. LS-related endometrial cancers have some special characteristics: the mean age is younger than the general population; there may be a lack of estrogen overstimulation; they have a tendency to involve the lower uterine segment (LUS); and they demonstrate mixed tumor histology, with increased tumor-infiltrating lymphocytes, and a Crohn-like inflammatory infiltrate at the tumor invading edge [47]. It should be noted that these morphologic findings are not specific and have a low predictive value for the presence of LS. This is the main reason universal screening by MMR immunohistochemistry is being employed in many medical centers.

16.2.11 Progestin-Resistant Endometrial Cancer

To preserve fertility, progestin has historically been administered to significant subsets of young patients with clinical stage I, grade 1 endometrial adenocarcinoma; however, a significant proportion of such cancers do not respond. Although the underlying mechanism of such resistance remain to be entirely clarified, some recently obtained insights are outlined below.

16.2.11.1 Progesterone Receptor (PR)

High-level expression of PRA and PRB has been associated with a decreased risk of persistence or progression, whereas low or absent PR in endometrial cancer cells is associated with a poor response to progesterone therapy. Moreover, progestin may activate the PI3K/AKT pathway independent of PR mediation in PR-negative or low-expression endometrial cancer cells. Inhibition of the PI3K/AKT pathway may restore PR expression and progestin sensitivity in some progestin-resistant endometrial cancer [48, 49]. From this perspective, manipulation of PI3K/AKT pathway remains a consideration for the clinical management of such patients after appropriate clinical validations.

16.2.12 Epidermal Growth Factor Receptor (EGFR) and Other Genes

High levels of EGFR expression have been reported in progestin-resistant endometrial cancer. Furthermore increased EGFR expression in endometrial cancer cell lines leads to reduced sensitivity to progestin treatment and decreased PR-B expression. As a result, the EGFR tyrosine kinase-specific inhibitor, Gefitib, may be useful in the treatment of endometrioid carcinoma [50]. Additionally, it has been found that Fas and FasL expression inhibits apoptosis [51]. The overexpression of Survivin through activation of Nrf2/AKR1C1 pathway may also contribute progestin resistance [52–54]. The clinical impact of these findings has yet to be determined as they are mostly in the research stage.

16.3 Endometrial Serous Carcinoma

Endometrial serous carcinoma (ESC) constitutes no more than 10% of all endometrial cancers, but frequently presents at an advanced stage and has a significantly worse prognosis than more common low- and intermediate-grade endometrioid cancers. ESC's potential for rapid tumor progression, as well as the high mortality that is associated with advanced stage disease, both underscore the importance of understanding endometrial serous carcinogenesis so that its precancers can be diagnosed, and effective therapeutic intervention can be administered.

Serous carcinoma arises predominantly in resting endometrium, manifesting first as p53 immunoreactive, morphologically normal endometrial cells (p53 signatures), evolving to endometrial glandular dysplasia (EmGD), which is the first morphologically identifiable precancerous lesion, then to serous endometrial intraepithelial carcinoma (SEIC, a carcinoma with a noninvasive growth pattern in the uterus but commonly associated extrauterine disease), and finally invasive ESC. This model of ESC development [2] has recently been recapitulated by a genetically engineered mouse model as well as in thoroughly described in other publications [55] (Figs. 16.3 and 16.4). Importantly, EmGD is a lesion that can be diagnosed by routine microscopic evaluation whose ablation or removal may potentially offer the opportunity to prevent the development of the associated malignancy.

Fig. 16.3 A comparison of the morphologic features of non-neoplastic, resting endometrium, EmGD and SEIC

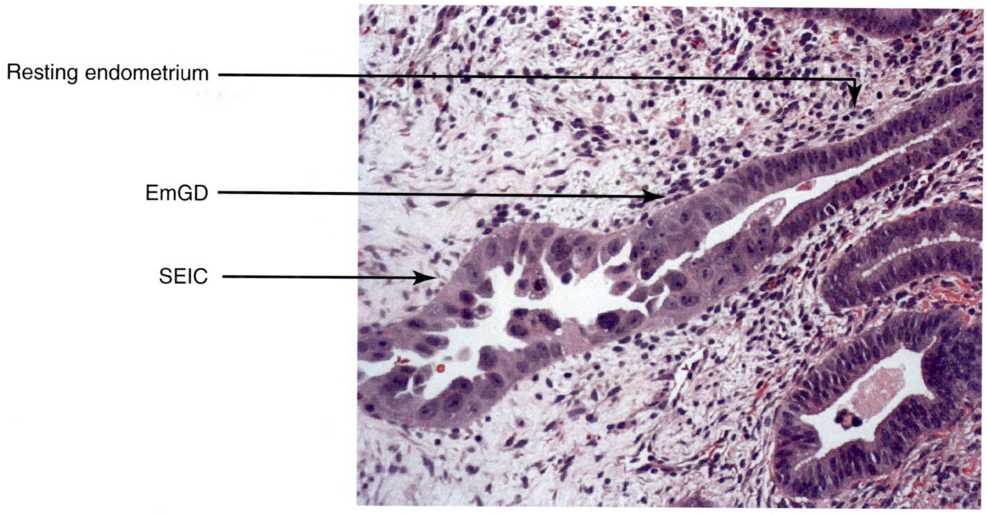

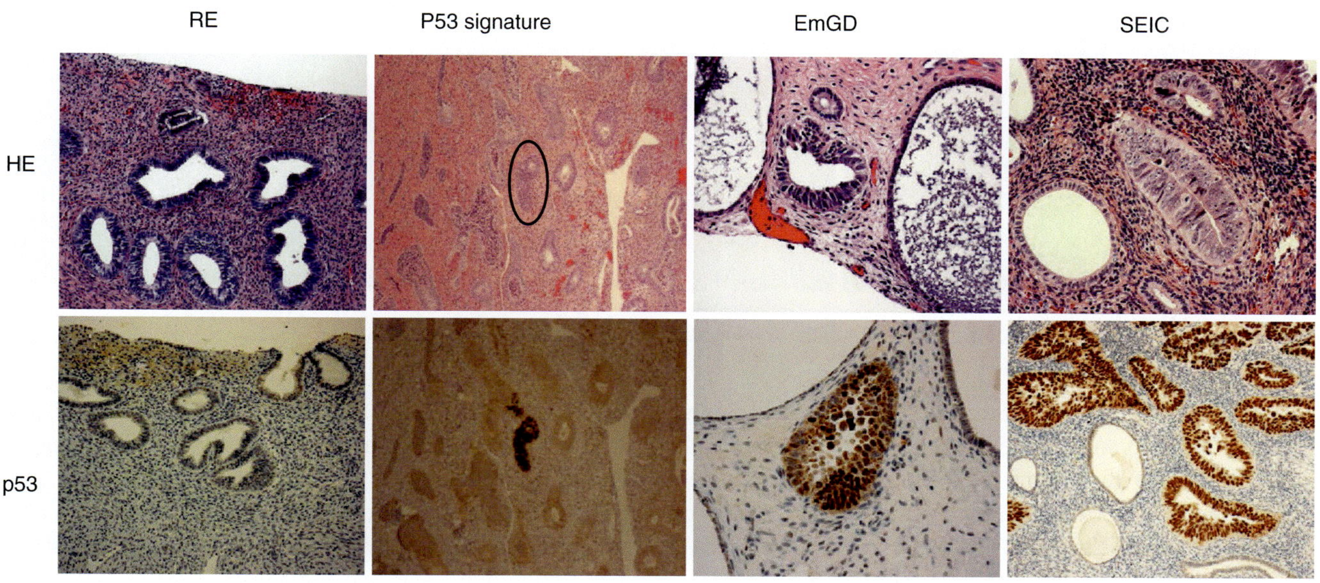

Fig. 16.4 p53 immunoreactivity patterns in resting, non-neoplastic endometrium, p53 signatures, EmGD and SEIC

16.3.1 Molecular Alterations in Endometrial Serous Neoplasia

There have been numerous studies on the molecular events underlying endometrial serous carcinogenesis. Some of these molecular events are also present in its precursor lesions, facilitating our understanding of the development of ESC. Whole exome sequencing of ESC cases has identified somatic mutations in *TP53* (81.6%), *PIK3CA* (23.7%), *FBXW7* (19.7%), and *PPP2R1A* (18.4%) among the 76 cases that were evaluated [56]. Zhao et al. found an increased mutational burden for *TP53, PIK3CA, PPP2R1A, KRAS, FBXW7,* and *CHD4/Mi2b*, along with amplification of chromosome segments containing *ERBB2* and *CCNE1* [57]. Comparable figures for Jones et al. included *TP53* (76%), *PIK3CA* (29%), *FBXW7* (12%), and *K-ras* (9.3%) [58], whereas Le Gallo et al. found somewhat different frequencies, with high frequency somatic mutations identified in the following genes: *CHD4* (17%), *EP300* (8%), *ARID1A* (6%), *TSPYL2* (6%), *FBXW7* (29%), *SPOP* (8%), *MAP3K4* (6%), and *ABCC9* (6%) [59].

16.3.1.1 Mutation of *TP53*

The p53 tumor suppressor gene, which is located on chromosome 17p 13.1, is the most commonly altered gene in human cancers [60, 61]. It is also the most important single gene for the generation of ESC [55]. Overexpression of the p53 protein, as assessed by immunohistochemistry, has been found in approximately 80–90% of ESC cases [62, 63], which is an extraordinarily high-rate supporting a significant role for

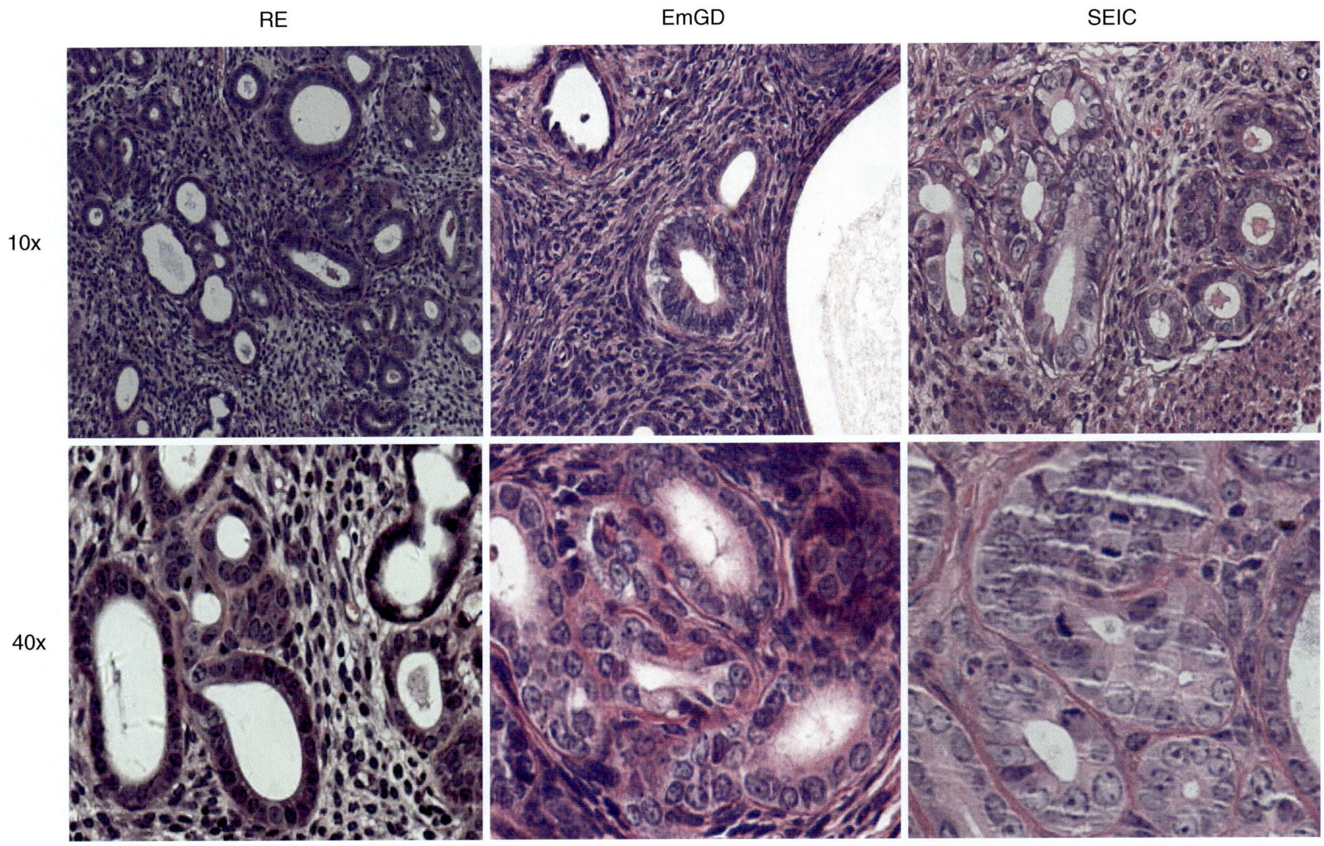

Fig. 16.5 Representative images of some key steps in the development of endometrial serous carcinoma

TP53 gene alterations in endometrial serous carcinogenesis. Based on previous studies, the frequency of *TP53* gene mutations in exons 5 to 8 from laser captured microdissected samples increases from p53 signature glands (42%), to EmGD (43%), to SEIC, (63–72%), and to ESC (96%) [64]. This is in contrast to the benign endometrial control uteri, where no *TP53* gene mutation is present in non-signature glands [64, 65]. From these studies, and others, the logical conclusion is that *TP53* gene mutation is a critical early step in endometrial serous carcinogenesis [2]. The importance of *TP53* mutation in the development of ESC is further supported by a *TP53* knockout mouse model, which recapitulates all the developmental processes observed in the humans [55]. Representative pictures of the ESC developmental model are illustrated in Fig. 16.5. This model recapitulates and confirms the process of ESC development in humans and is a useful foundation for further studies of ESC pathogenesis, early cancer detection, prevention, and clinical intervention.

Other non-*TP53* related molecular events that may be significant in the development of ESC are summarized below.

16.3.1.2 *PPP2R1A* Mutations

Somatic missense mutations in the Ser/Thr protein phosphatase 2A (PP2A) scaffold subunit gene *PPP2R1*A have been identified in 18–40% of ESC. *PPP2R1A* plays a critical role in diverse cellular functions, including negative regulation of cellular proliferation and potential tumor suppression [56, 66–68]. *PPP2R1A* mutations are also seen in subsets of carcinosarcomas, but are apparently uncommon in other histotypes. Accordingly, they may not only be directly involved in endometrial serous carcinogenesis but may also form a serous histotype-related molecular target.

16.3.1.3 Cyclin E/FBXW7 Oncogenic Pathways

Approximately 45% of ESC display amplification of the *CCNE1* gene as assessed by in situ hybridization [69]. The *CCNE1* gene encodes the cyclin E1 protein, which is overexpressed by IHC in approximately 90% of ESC [70]. Cyclin E is a downstream molecule of F-box and WD repeat domain-containing 7 (FBXW7), which is mutated in 10–30% of ESC. *CCNE1* amplifications have been identified in aggressive subsets of endometrioid carcinoma [71]; however, their significance in ESC is presently unclear.

16.3.1.4 *BRCA* Mutations

Some preliminary lines of evidence are suggestive of a relationship between the risk for breast cancers and endometrial cancers. One study from Sweden found that 7.28% of patients undergoing genetic counseling for an increased risk of breast cancer had family histories of both endometrial and breast cancer [72]. One large cohort study demonstrated that about 20% of women with ESC had a prior history of breast cancer and the ESC patients with breast cancer history tend to be younger than those patients without breast cancer history [73]. There are also reports suggesting a relationship between the germline *BRCA1* mutation and ESC [74, 75]. The risk for serous/serous-like endometrial carcinoma is increased in BRCA1+ women [75]. This risk should be considered when discussing the advantages and risks of hysterectomy at the time of RRSO in BRCA1+ women.

16.3.1.5 Alterations of Extracellular Adhesion Molecules

Overall, studies on role of extracellular adhesion molecules in ESC development are relatively rare compared to studies on oncogenes and tumor suppressor genes. Changes in extracellular adhesion molecules may be related to the easy detachment of neoplastic cells in ESC and SEIC which explains their very high-rate of extrauterine metastasis. E-cadherin and claudins are the two extracellular molecules that likely contribute to the ability of ESC to shed and spread to distant sites. It has been reported that the downregulation of E-cadherin is associated with the progression of endometrial cancers [76–79]. Additionally, the adhesion molecule CD44 may play a role. CD44 is a protein involved in cell adhesion and lymphocyte homing, and one of its isoforms, CD44v6, may be related to capillary lymphatic space invasion and metastasis. A significant loss of CD44 and its isoform CD44v6 has been found in ESC compared with that of endometrioid cancers [80].

Alterations in intercellular adhesion molecules likely facilitate the trans-tubal spread of endometrial serous cancer cells, which explains why these cancers frequently present at advanced stages. This has been demonstrated in a previous study where 6 (67%) of 9 SEIC cases demonstrated carcinomatous deposits in the pelvis or peritoneal cavity [81]. Among those cases, about half showed free-floating serous carcinoma in the tubal lumen. These findings suggest that at least some of the extrauterine diseases evolve via trans-tubal metastasis, a contention that is supported by identical clones that is found in ESC, SEIC, and serous carcinomas at extrauterine sites [82, 83].

16.3.1.6 Amplification of *HER2/neu*

HER2/neu, also known as C-erbB2, is a proto-oncogene that encodes the human epidermal growth factor receptor 2. Amplification of the *HER2/neu* gene and overexpression of the HER2/neu protein have been demonstrated in many tumors, including ESC. Although expression of *HER2/neu* is mainly seen in ESC and advanced stage disease, it has been observed that cases of EmGD and SEIC demonstrate overexpression of HER2/*neu* by immunohistochemistry. There is no clinical role for use of HER2/*neu* in the diagnosis of ESC or its precursors at this point.

16.3.1.7 *PIK3CA* Mutations

Possible driver mutations in the PIK3CA/AKT/mTOR pathway have been identified in 24–29% of ESC [56, 58]. *In vitro* studies have shown that oncogenic PIK3CA mutations are common in HER2/neu-amplified ESC, and that this may represent a mechanism of resistance to anti-HER2 treatment [84], which can be overcome by dual HER2/PIK3CA targeting [85].

16.3.1.8 Overexpression of p16

The tumor suppressor protein p16 is also known as CDKN2A. Studies on this molecule are mainly related to HPV-related cancers and precancers, but p16 overexpression has also been demonstrated in the majority of cases of ESC, with one report showing 92% of ESC cases (22/24) with p16 overexpression, as compared to less than 25% of endometrioid cases [86]. Interestingly, the mechanisms of p16 overexpression in ESC may be related to the inactivation of Rb gene rather than through a HPV E7 protein regulation as HPV DNA in situ hybridization was negative in all ESC cases in one study [87]. By gene expression profiling, p16 is significantly upregulated in ESC above normal endometrial cells and endometrioid carcinomas, all of which suggests dysregulation of the p16INKA/Cyclin D-CDK/pRb-E2F pathway [88, 89]. Additionally, it has been observed that p16 protein is overexpressed in lesions of EmGD and SEIC (Zheng et al., unpublished). In a clinical setting, diffuse, strong staining is usually supportive of a diagnosis of ESC or serous EIC.

16.3.1.9 Other Molecular Changes

Overexpression of Insulin-like growth factor II m-RNA binding protein 3 (IMP3) is typically expressed in embryonic tissues but rarely in adult tissue with the exception of placenta and gonads. IMP3 was found to be expressed in 3 (14%) of 21 EmGD, 16 (89%) of 18 serous EIC, and 48 (94%) of 51 ESC. In contrast, none of 35 EIN and only 5 (7%) of 70 endometrioid cancers exhibited IMP3 overexpression [90]. The findings suggest that IMP3 expression is more associated with endometrial serous cancer development and may contribute to its aggressive clinical behavior. The transcription factor NF-E2-related factor 2 (Nrf2) is thought to enhance resistance of cancer cells to chemotherapeutic drugs and was found to be expressed in 41 (89%) of 46 ESC cases, compared with marginal expression in endometrioid cancers and no expression in benign endometria [91]. Moreover, Nrf2 was also identified in EmGD and serous EIC in 40% and 75% of cases, respectively [91]. The relationship between Nrf2 and p53 mutation in latent precancer (p53 signature) and precancerous lesions has yet to be fully elucidated.

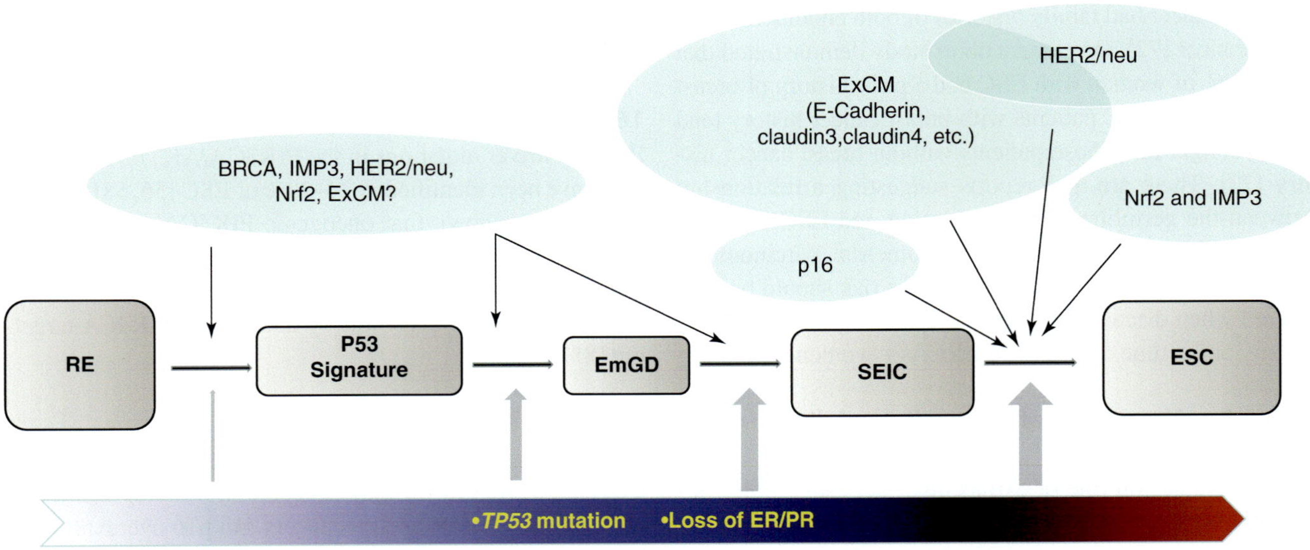

Fig. 16.6 Selected molecular events in endometrial serous carcinoma development

The molecular changes in the process of ESC development are summarized in Fig. 16.6.

16.3.2 The Model of Endometrial Serous Carcinogenesis

Previously, it was suggested that ESC arises from SEIC in atrophic endometria via an estrogen *independent* "de novo" process [3, 92]. It has been proposed that SEIC is a likely precursor lesion for ESC [3, 93, 94]. From a developmental and evolutionary point of view, this was probably correct, since the occurrence of the fully developed ESC typically appears later than the lesions of SEIC. However, this "precursor" concept is misleading as the "precursor" lesion of a given malignancy is not necessarily synonymous with its "precancer" lesion. Indeed, published data indicate that many observers, including gynecologists and pathologists, accepted SEIC as a precancer or, "noninvasive" cancer, controversially in the past. Many patients with SEIC experience recurrence or intra-abdominal serous carcinomatosis after simple hysterectomy without staging due to the limited understanding of this unusual "intraepithelial" carcinoma. It is now known that up to two-thirds of SEIC may be associated with extrauterine disease [2], the phenomenon is likely to be trans-tubal metastasis as discussed above.

There are several drawbacks of this "atrophic endometrium (AE) → SEIC → ESC" carcinogenesis model. First, this model does not incorporate the presence of dysplastic lesions bridging the gap between completely benign endometrium and frankly malignant SEIC. In the majority of other human organs, accepted models of epithelial carcinogenesis typically involve an evolution from benign epithelium → dysplasia (lesions in transition) → intraepithelial carcinoma or carcinoma in situ → invasive carcinoma. This is also supported by tubal serous carcinogenesis in which an intermediate lesion, termed "tubal lesions in transition (TILT)" links normal looking tubal mucosa to tubal intraepithelial carcinoma. Secondly, SEIC and/or ESC are not always associated with atrophic endometrium. Many gynecologic pathologists have identified ESC cases that mimicked endometrioid carcinoma partially because of the presence of non-atrophic background endometrium. One possibility is that ESC cases that were diagnosed more than 40 years ago were associated with an atrophic background more often because a limited number of women at that time were undergoing hormone replacement therapy. Hormone replacement therapy has become more popular in postmenopausal women in the recent past (although this practice is falling out of style due to its known side effects). The utilization of these hormones may help to explain why 40% of the background non-neoplastic endometrium in women diagnosed with ESC or SEIC were non-atrophic (34% proliferative, 6% hyperplastic) in one analysis [95]. These findings suggest that SEIC or ESC can derive not only from atrophic endometrium but also from resting or even hyperplastic endometrium depending on an individual woman's hormonal status. Finally, SEIC does not meet the criteria of "precancer" given its many shared features with ESC, including morphology, molecular biology, clinical behavior, and management [3, 63, 81, 95–98]. Accordingly, SEIC is best viewed as ESC with a noninvasive growth pattern in the uterus, rather than a precancerous lesion in the process of ESC development [2, 81]. Understanding the nature of SEIC—as an ESC without myometrial invasion but with a significant potential for extrauterine spread—will help to prevent the undertreatment of afflicted patients. The diagnostic term "SEIC" or "EIC" should not be used in the clinic without an explanatory comment in order to avoid management confusion [99]. Alternative terms such as ESC with a size description may suffice for diagnostic and management purposes.

In contrast to SEIC, EmGD meets the majority of criteria required to label a lesion as a precancer (as defined by a group of experts in the 2006 NCI consensus conference) [100]. This rationale may be summarized as follows: (1) EmGD lesions are morphologically identifiable (detailed diagnostic criteria are described in Chap. 17). (2) cytologically, direct transition between EmGD and SEIC, but not between EmGD and ESC, have been described [95]. (3) comparison of the extent, and range, of genomic damage between EmGD and ESC (including SEIC) explains their differing morphology and behavior [95, 101]. A p53 mutational analysis of laser capture microdissected endometrial samples demonstrated that *TP53* mutations increased in a progressive fashion from EmGD (16/37, 43%) to serous EIC (18/25, 72%) and ESC (21/23, 91%) [64]. In addition, IMP3 showed an increased level of expression from EmGD (3/21, 14%) to SEIC (16/18, 89%) and to ESC (48/51, 94%) [90]. (4) Identical *TP53* mutations have been found in EmGD and serous EIC or ESC [64]. (5) In a retrospective study, EmGD was found to be present and identifiable in endometrial biopsies taken prior to the development of ESC, indeed it has been estimated that a diagnosis of EmGD in an endometrial biopsy may confer up to a ninefold increased risk of developing ESC [102]. (6) A mouse model with p53 selectively knockout in the mullerian system has accurately recapitulated all of the processes detailed above [2]. Such findings at least partially indicate a lineage continuity between EmGD and ESC, therefore providing a reasonable evidence that ESC likely arises in EmGD [2].

Molecular changes typically occur prior to morphologic changes, which, in the case of serous carcinogenesis, has been identified as a group of benign-appearing endometrial glands/epithelia with intense p53 IHC staining, designated "p53 signatures" [65]. These p53 signatures were frequently found in the benign-appearing endometrium adjacent to ESC and only rarely in the endometrium adjacent to endometrioid carcinomas or in noncancerous uteri, and have been found to display a frequency of p53 gene mutation that is similar to lesions of EmGD.

Overall, the totality of available clinicopathologic and molecular evidence supports the concept of EmGD as the precancer for ESC, with p53 signatures representing a latent precancer in the process of endometrial serous carcinogenesis. This understanding begets the model of endometrial serous carcinogenesis from resting endometrium → p53 signature → EmGD → SEIC → ESC (Figs. 16.3–16.6).

16.4 Endometrial Clear Cell Carcinoma and Other Endometrial Cancers, Including Carcinosarcoma and Dedifferentiated Carcinoma

As listed in the 2014 WHO classification, endometrial cancers have multiple histologic types. Among them, knowledge of the carcinogenesis of endometrial clear cell carcinoma (ECCCs), carcinosarcoma, dedifferentiated/undifferentiated carcinoma, and other rare cancers of the endometrium are very much limited. This chapter will only briefly discuss a few key points of the genesis of these cancers.

16.4.1 Endometrial Clear Cell Carcinoma

Clear cell carcinoma of the endometrium is a rare type of endometrial cancer that has generally been considered to follow an aggressive course, although reported patient outcomes have been variable. Although ECCCs were not included in the original The Cancer Genome Atlas (TCGA) dataset [12], a few recent studies have established that ECCC is a molecularly heterogeneous histotype that may show features of ESC, endometrioid carcinoma, neither or both. TCGA-like molecular subsets are demonstrable in this tumor type [103, 104]. The variable biologic behavior of this tumor was highlighted in a recent genetic landscape study [105]. DeLair et al. performed a rigorous histopathological review, immunohistochemical analysis, and massively parallel sequencing targeting of 300 cancer-related genes of 32 pure ECCCs. Eleven (34%), seven (22%), and six (19%) ECCCs showed abnormal expression patterns for p53, ARID1A, and at least one DNA mismatch repair (MMR) protein, respectively. Targeted sequencing data were obtained from 30 of the 32 ECCs included in this study, and these revealed that two ECCCs (7%) were ultramutated and harbored mutations affecting the exonuclease domain of DNA polymerase epsilon (*POLE*). In *POLE* wild-type ECCCs, *TP53* (46%), *PIK3CA* (36%), *PPP2R1A* (36%), *FBXW7* (25%), *ARID1A* (21%), *PIK3R1* (18%), and SPOP (18%) were the genes most commonly affected by mutations. ECCCs less frequently harbored mutations affecting *CTNNB1* and *PTEN* but more frequently harbored PPP2R1A and TP53 mutations than non-POLE endometrioid carcinomas compared to the original TCGA—endometrial cancer study [12]. Compared to ESC results obtained by TCGA study, ECCCs less frequently harbored *TP53* mutations. When a surrogate model for the molecular-based TCGA classification [12] is used, all molecular subtypes previously identified in endometrioid and serous endometrial cancers are present in the studied cases of ECCCs. These include ultramutated , MMR-deficient, copy-number high with *TP53* mutation, and copy-number low (endometrioid-like) with wild-type *TP53* [105]. These ECCC cases, except those with copy-number high serous-like cancers, have had a significantly better prognosis than the authors expected [105]. Such findings show that ECCCs constitute a histologically and genetically heterogeneous group of tumors with varying outcomes. Accordingly, previous categorizations of ECCCs as type II or as being inherently aggressive cancers require a reevaluation.

16.4.2 Endometrial Carcinosarcoma

Carcinosarcoma of the endometrium is a rare gynecological neoplasm, which accounts for <3% of all uterine malignancies. Traditionally this tumor has been regarded as a subtype of uterine sarcoma, and its origin remains controversial. The exact nature and prognosis was not clear in the past.

The carcinomatous components may correspond to any Mullerian type, but the majority are high-grade, such as serous carcinoma. This type of tumor is broadly divided into two groups, homologous and heterologous, depending on the characteristics of the stroma or mesenchymal components. Both epithelial and mesenchymal components can be either intimately admixed or sharply demarcated, additionally, the components vary from relatively equal distribution to dramatically different proportions.

Traditionally, there have been four theories regarding the histogenesis of endometrial carcinosarcoma. (1) The collision theory suggests that the epithelial and mesenchymal elements have arisen independently and collide yielding a single mixed tumor; (2) the combination theory suggests that both components are derived from a single stem cell that has undergone divergent differentiation early in its evolution; (3) a composition tumor that is an endometrial carcinoma with reactive, atypical stroma; and (4) the conversion theory that suggests that the sarcomatous element is derived from carcinoma during the evolution of the tumor. It is believed that endometrial carcinosarcomas have a Mullerian duct origin and a capacity to differentiate into various mesenchymal and epithelial components. This "conversion theory" has been broadly accepted. Carcinosarcomas are mostly of monoclonal origin with the carcinomatous component being the driving force. At the molecular level, the conversion from epithelial to mesenchymal phenotype is likely through an epithelial-mesenchymal transition (EMT) process since the genetic changes in sarcoma are similar with the accompanied carcinomas [106, 107].

The pattern of metastasis in carcinosarcoma depends on dominancy of the type of tumor components. Most studies suggest that the behavior of carcinosarcomas is mainly governed by the carcinomatous component. Carcinoma typically spread through the lymphatic channels to nearby lymph nodes, while sarcomas frequently metastasize to the peritoneal cavity or hematogenously spread to distant organs. In sarcoma, lymph node metastasis is very uncommon. The majority of metastatic carcinosarcoma consist only of the carcinomatous component. Such observations suggest that the carcinomatous component is predominantly responsible for most metastasis and sarcomatous component plays only a minor role.

16.4.3 Endometrial Undifferentiated and Dedifferentiated Carcinoma

Undifferentiated endometrial carcinoma is a highly aggressive subtype of endometrial cancer. Histologically, undifferentiated endometrial carcinoma is composed of sheet-like monotonous and discohesive tumor cells, which typically possess scant to moderate amount of cytoplasm. These tumors lack any evidence of glandular formation or significant squamous differentiation. Because of this undifferentiated appearance, a definitive diagnosis may be difficult to impossible on biopsy specimens. Ancillary immunohistochemical analysis will essentially be negative for pankeratin, lymphoid markers, melanoma markers, epithelial membrane antigen (only rare cells), estrogen receptor, PAX8, and E-cadherin (relative to grade 3 endometrioid carcinomas) and can be used to support its diagnosis. Of note, CK18 may strongly stain rare cells. MMR protein immunohistochemistry may be useful as about half of undifferentiated endometrial carcinomas are MMR protein-deficient, whereas MMR protein deficiency is comparatively uncommon in other uterine malignancies [108].

Dedifferentiated endometrial carcinoma contains a component of undifferentiated carcinoma in addition to a component of typically low-grade endometrioid-type carcinoma. The undifferentiated component of dedifferentiated endometrial carcinoma exhibits similar histologic and immunophenotypic features to those seen in pure undifferentiated endometrial carcinomas. It is important to distinguish these tumors from other high-grade carcinoma as their behavior is significantly more aggressive.

It has been suggested that inactivation of core components of the switch/sucrose non-fermentable (SWI/SNF) chromatin remodeling complex proteins, specifically *ARID1A/ARID1B* (co-inactivation), BRG1 (encoded by *SMARCA4*), and INI1 (encoded by *SMARCB1*) as the likely molecular triggers underlying the apparent "dedifferentiation" of low-grade endometrioid carcinoma in about 70% of cases [109]. The loss of these core SWI/SNF complex proteins has been hypothesized to prevent müllerian epithelial differentiation, thereby arresting tumor cells in an undifferentiated state with significantly reduced level or even absent expression of Pax-8 and estrogen receptor, in contrast to that of the differentiated endometrioid component. Undifferentiated carcinomas with SWI/SNF complex-

Fig. 16.7 A proposed unified pathologic nomenclatural classification for endometrial preneoplasia

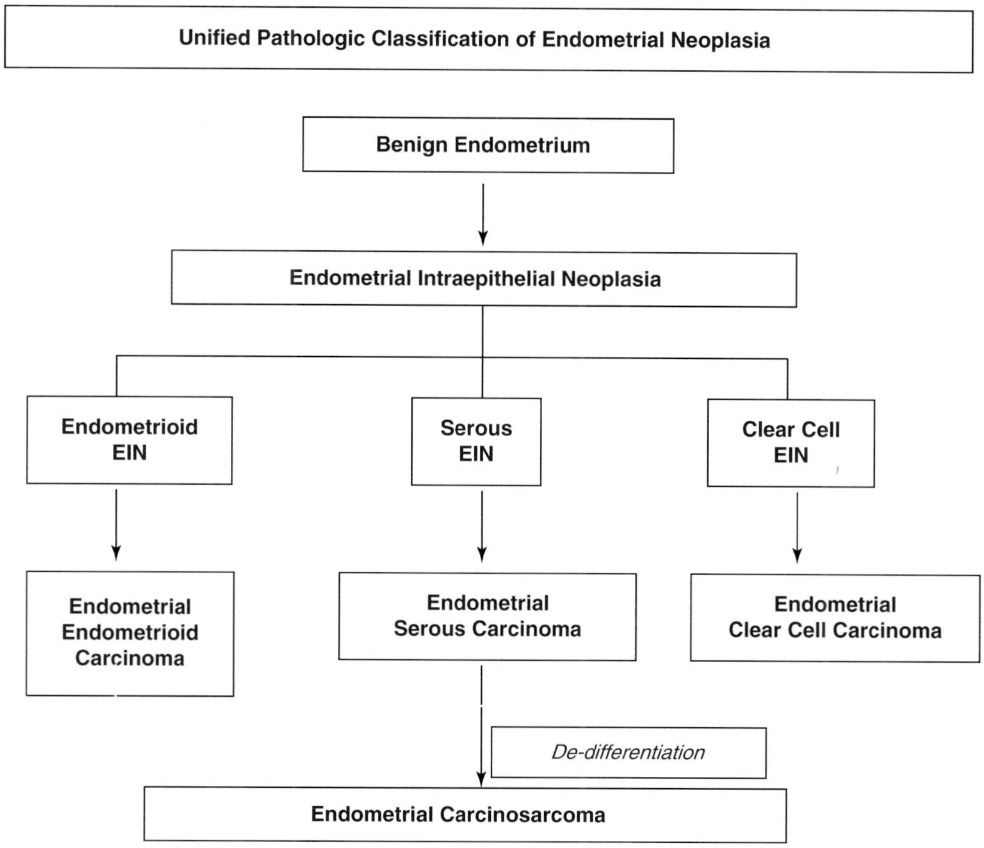

inactivation are more commonly associated with extrauterine disease and have a significantly worse prognosis [110]. Although dedifferentiated carcinomas behave badly in general, they do not universally behave poorly if associated with a *POLE* mutation [111]. Such findings further emphasize the importance of understanding the endometrial cancers at the molecular level.

16.5 A Proposed Unified Pathologic Nomenclatural Classification of Endometrial Preneoplasia

As discussed above, this chapter has primarily focused on the most common histologic types of endometrial cancer, including endometrioid and serous carcinomas, and briefly covered clear cell, undifferentiated, and dedifferentiated carcinoma. Diverse nomenclatures have been proposed for the various putative precursor lesions for these entities, the totality of which may potentially cause confusion in clinical practice. It has been suggested that an expanded definition of the term "endometrial intraepithelial neoplasia, EIN" that encompasses all the major histotypes should be included in each category as prefix. For endometrioid lesions, the proposal entails adoption of the EIN system advanced by Mutter and colleagues, in which a distinction is made between benign endometrial hyperplasia and strictly defined EIN; the latter would henceforth be referred to as "Endometrioid EIN." For serous lesions, the proposal entails discontinuation of the term "Endometrial Intraepithelial Carcinoma," as these lesions may metastasize and should be considered a special form of ESC. The precancerous lesion described previously as EmGD would be referred to as "Serous EIN" under the proposal. Similarly, the previously characterized putative precursor lesion for clear cell carcinomas will be designated "Clear cell EIN." This system is envisioned as one that can readily incorporate new information such as grading, or the description of precursors, for the other histotypes (Fig. 16.7). Much is unknown about the nature, morphologic spectrum, and clinical significance of endometrial precancers. It is hoped that the system proposed herein would provide a coherent nomenclatural framework in which candidate lesions can be investigated and reported in daily surgical pathology practice in a more uniformed manner.

References

1. Bokhman JV. Two pathogenetic types of endometrial carcinoma. Gynecol Oncol. 1983;15:10–7.
2. Zheng W, Xiang L, Fadare O, Kong B. A proposed model for endometrial serous carcinogenesis. Am J Surg Pathol. 2011;35:e1–e14.
3. Sherman ME, Bur ME, Kurman RJ. p53 in endometrial cancer and its putative precursors: evidence for diverse pathways of tumorigenesis. Hum Pathol. 1995;26:1268–74.

4. Coller HA, Grandori C, Tamayo P, et al. Expression analysis with oligonucleotide microarrays reveals that MYC regulates genes involved in growth, cell cycle, signaling, and adhesion. Proc Natl Acad Sci U S A. 2000;97:3260–5.
5. Risinger JI, Maxwell GL, Chandramouli GV, et al. Microarray analysis reveals distinct gene expression profiles among different histologic types of endometrial cancer. Cancer Res. 2003;63:6–11.
6. Zorn KK, Bonome T, Gangi L, et al. Gene expression profiles of serous, endometrioid, and clear cell subtypes of ovarian and endometrial cancer. Clin Cancer Res. 2005;11:6422–30.
7. Clarke BA, Gilks CB. Endometrial carcinoma: controversies in histopathological assessment of grade and tumour cell type. J Clin Pathol. 2010;63:410–5.
8. Fadare O, Zheng W, Crispens MA, et al. Morphologic and other clinicopathologic features of endometrial clear cell carcinoma: a comprehensive analysis of 50 rigorously classified cases. Am J Cancer Res. 2013;3:70–95.
9. Han G, Soslow RA, Wethington S, et al. Endometrial carcinomas with clear cells: a study of a heterogeneous group of tumors including interobserver variability, mutation analysis, and immunohistochemistry with HNF-1beta. Int J Gynecol Pathol. 2015;34:323–33.
10. Felix AS, Brasky TM, Cohn DE, et al. Endometrial carcinoma recurrence according to race and ethnicity: an NRG oncology/gynecologic oncology group 210 study. Int J Cancer. 2017;
11. Gilks CB, Oliva E, Soslow RA. Poor interobserver reproducibility in the diagnosis of high-grade endometrial carcinoma. Am J Surg Pathol. 2013;37:874–81.
12. Cancer Genome Atlas Research N, Kandoth C, Schultz N, et al. Integrated genomic characterization of endometrial carcinoma. Nature. 2013;497:67–73.
13. Potischman N, Hoover RN, Brinton LA, et al. Case-control study of endogenous steroid hormones and endometrial cancer. J Natl Cancer Inst. 1996;88:1127–35.
14. Effects of hormone replacement therapy on endometrial histology in postmenopausal women. The Postmenopausal Estrogen/Progestin Interventions (PEPI) Trial. The Writing Group for the PEPI Trial. JAMA. 1996;275:370–5.
15. Mutter GL, Lin MC, Fitzgerald JT, Kum JB, Eng C. Changes in endometrial PTEN expression throughout the human menstrual cycle. J Clin Endocrinol Metab. 2000;85:2334–8.
16. Zheng W, Baker HE, Mutter GL. Involution of PTEN-null endometrial glands with progestin therapy. Gynecol Oncol. 2004;92:1008–13.
17. Mutter GL, Lin MC, Fitzgerald JT, et al. Altered PTEN expression as a diagnostic marker for the earliest endometrial precancers. J Natl Cancer Inst. 2000;92:924–30.
18. Salvesen HB, MacDonald N, Ryan A, et al. PTEN methylation is associated with advanced stage and microsatellite instability in endometrial carcinoma. Int J Cancer. 2001;91:22–6.
19. Oda K, Stokoe D, Taketani Y, McCormick F. High frequency of coexistent mutations of PIK3CA and PTEN genes in endometrial carcinoma. Cancer Res. 2005;65:10669–73.
20. Cohn DE, Basil JB, Venegoni AR, et al. Absence of PTEN repeat tract mutation in endometrial cancers with microsatellite instability. Gynecol Oncol. 2000;79:101–6.
21. Burks RT, Kessis TD, Cho KR, Hedrick L. Microsatellite instability in endometrial carcinoma. Oncogene. 1994;9:1163–6.
22. Catasus L, Machin P, Matias-Guiu X, Prat J. Microsatellite instability in endometrial carcinomas: clinicopathologic correlations in a series of 42 cases. Hum Pathol. 1998;29:1160–4.
23. Esteller M, Catasus L, Matias-Guiu X, et al. hMLH1 promoter hypermethylation is an early event in human endometrial tumorigenesis. Am J Pathol. 1999;155:1767–72.
24. Duggan BD, Felix JC, Muderspach LI, et al. Microsatellite instability in sporadic endometrial carcinoma. J Natl Cancer Inst. 1994;86:1216–21.
25. Moreno-Bueno G, Hardisson D, Sanchez C, et al. Abnormalities of the APC/beta-catenin pathway in endometrial cancer. Oncogene. 2002;21:7981–90.
26. Koul A, Willen R, Bendahl PO, Nilbert M, Borg A. Distinct sets of gene alterations in endometrial carcinoma implicate alternate modes of tumorigenesis. Cancer. 2002;94:2369–79.
27. Palacios J, Gamallo C. Mutations in the beta-catenin gene (CTNNB1) in endometrioid ovarian carcinomas. Cancer Res. 1998;58:1344–7.
28. Brabletz T, Jung A, Dag S, Hlubek F, Kirchner T. beta-catenin regulates the expression of the matrix metalloproteinase-7 in human colorectal cancer. Am J Pathol. 1999;155:1033–8.
29. Fukuchi T. Pathology division NCCRITJSMHKSS. Beta-catenin mutation in carcinoma of the uterine endometrium. Cancer Res. 1998;58:3526.
30. Liu Y, Patel L, Mills GB, et al. Clinical significance of CTNNB1 mutation and Wnt pathway activation in endometrioid endometrial carcinoma. J Natl Cancer Inst. 2014;106
31. Kurnit KC, Kim GN, Fellman BM, et al. CTNNB1 (beta-catenin) mutation identifies low grade, early stage endometrial cancer patients at increased risk of recurrence. Mod Pathol. 2017;30:1032–41.
32. Engelsen IB, Akslen LA, Salvesen HB. Biologic markers in endometrial cancer treatment. APMIS. 2009;117:693–707.
33. Xiong J, He M, Jackson C, et al. Endometrial carcinomas with significant mucinous differentiation associated with higher frequency of k-ras mutations: a morphologic and molecular correlation study. Int J Gynecol Cancer. 2013;23:1231–6.
34. Xiong J, He M, Hansen K, et al. The clinical significance of *K-ras* mutation in endometrial "surface epithelial changes" and their associated endometrial adenocarcinoma. Gynecol Oncol. 2016;142:163–8.
35. Stewart CJ, Amanuel B, Grieu F, Carrello A, Iacopetta B. KRAS mutation and microsatellite instability in endometrial adenocarcinomas showing MELF-type myometrial invasion. J Clin Pathol. 2010;63:604–8.
36. Monte NM, Webster KA, Neuberg D, Dressler GR, Mutter GL. Joint loss of PAX2 and PTEN expression in endometrial precancers and cancer. Cancer Res. 2010;70:6225–32.
37. Quick CM, Laury AR, Monte NM, Mutter GL. Utility of PAX2 as a marker for diagnosis of endometrial intraepithelial neoplasia. Am J Clin Pathol. 2012;138:678–84.
38. Jeffus SK, Winham W, Hooper K, Quick CM. Secretory endometrial intraepithelial neoplasia. Int J Gynecol Pathol. 2014;33:515–6.
39. Yuan TL, Cantley LC. PI3K pathway alterations in cancer: variations on a theme. Oncogene. 2008;27:5497–510.
40. Byron SA, Gartside M, Powell MA, et al. FGFR2 point mutations in 466 endometrioid endometrial tumors: relationship with MSI, KRAS, PIK3CA, CTNNB1 mutations and clinicopathological features. PLoS One. 2012;7:e30801.
41. Byron SA, Pollock PM. FGFR2 as a molecular target in endometrial cancer. Future Oncol. 2009;5:27–32.
42. Torres A, Torres K, Pesci A, et al. Diagnostic and prognostic significance of miRNA signatures in tissues and plasma of endometrioid endometrial carcinoma patients. Int J Cancer. 2013;132:1633–45.
43. Lee JW, Park YA, Choi JJ, et al. The expression of the miRNA-200 family in endometrial endometrioid carcinoma. Gynecol Oncol. 2011;120:56–62.
44. Xiong H, Li Q, Liu S, et al. Integrated microRNA and mRNA transcriptome sequencing reveals the potential roles of miRNAs in stage I endometrioid endometrial carcinoma. PLoS One. 2014;9:e110163.
45. Karaayvaz M, Zhang C, Liang S, Shroyer KR, Ju J. Prognostic significance of miR-205 in endometrial cancer. PLoS One. 2012;7:e35158.

46. Bonadona V, Bonaiti B, Olschwang S, et al. Cancer risks associated with germline mutations in MLH1, MSH2, and MSH6 genes in Lynch syndrome. JAMA. 2011;305:2304–10.
47. Wang Y, Wang Y, Li J, et al. Lynch syndrome related endometrial cancer: clinical significance beyond the endometrium. J Hematol Oncol. 2013;6:22.
48. Upson K, Allison KH, Reed SD, et al. Biomarkers of progestin therapy resistance and endometrial hyperplasia progression. Am J Obstet Gynecol. 2012;207:36 e1–8.
49. Gu C, Zhang Z, Yu Y, et al. Inhibiting the PI3K/Akt pathway reversed progestin resistance in endometrial cancer. Cancer Sci. 2011;102:557–64.
50. Xu Y, Tong J, Ai Z, Wang J, Teng Y. Epidermal growth factor receptor signaling pathway involved in progestin-resistance of human endometrial carcinoma: In a mouse model. J Obstet Gynaecol Res. 2012;38:1358–66.
51. Wang S, Pudney J, Song J, et al. Mechanisms involved in the evolution of progestin resistance in human endometrial hyperplasia--precursor of endometrial cancer. Gynecol Oncol. 2003;88:108–17.
52. Chen X, Zhang Z, Feng Y, et al. Aberrant survivin expression in endometrial hyperplasia: another mechanism of progestin resistance. Mod Pathol. 2009;22:699–708.
53. Wang Y, Wang Y, Zhang Z, et al. Mechanism of progestin resistance in endometrial precancer/cancer through Nrf2-AKR1C1 pathway. Oncotarget. 2016;7:10363–72.
54. Fan R, Wang Y, Wang Y, Wei L, Zheng W. Mechanism of progestin resistance in endometrial precancer/cancer through Nrf2-survivin pathway. Am J Transl Res. 2017;9:1483–91.
55. Wild PJ, Ikenberg K, Fuchs TJ, et al. p53 suppresses type II endometrial carcinomas in mice and governs endometrial tumour aggressiveness in humans. EMBO Mol Med. 2012;4:808–24.
56. Kuhn E, Wu RC, Guan B, et al. Identification of molecular pathway aberrations in uterine serous carcinoma by genome-wide analyses. J Natl Cancer Inst. 2012;104:1503–13.
57. Zhao S, Choi M, Overton JD, et al. Landscape of somatic single-nucleotide and copy-number mutations in uterine serous carcinoma. Proc Natl Acad Sci U S A. 2013;110:2916–21.
58. Jones NL, Xiu J, Reddy SK, et al. Identification of potential therapeutic targets by molecular profiling of 628 cases of uterine serous carcinoma. Gynecol Oncol. 2015;138:620–6.
59. Le Gallo M, O'Hara AJ, Rudd ML, et al. Exome sequencing of serous endometrial tumors identifies recurrent somatic mutations in chromatin-remodeling and ubiquitin ligase complex genes. Nat Genet. 2012;44:1310–5.
60. Pietsch EC, Sykes SM, McMahon SB, Murphy ME. The p53 family and programmed cell death. Oncogene. 2008;27:6507–21.
61. Harris CC. p53: at the crossroads of molecular carcinogenesis and risk assessment. Science. 1993;262:1980–1.
62. Zheng W, Cao P, Zheng M, Kramer EE, Godwin TA. p53 overexpression and bcl-2 persistence in endometrial carcinoma: comparison of papillary serous and endometrioid subtypes. Gynecol Oncol. 1996;61:167–74.
63. Zheng W, Khurana R, Farahmand S, et al. p53 immunostaining as a significant adjunct diagnostic method for uterine surface carcinoma: precursor of uterine papillary serous carcinoma. Am J Surg Pathol. 1998;22:1463–73.
64. Jia L, Liu Y, Yi X, et al. Endometrial glandular dysplasia with frequent p53 gene mutation: a genetic evidence supporting its precancer nature for endometrial serous carcinoma. Clin Cancer Res. 2008;14:2263–9.
65. Zhang X, Liang SX, Jia L, et al. Molecular identification of "latent precancers" for endometrial serous carcinoma in benign-appearing endometrium. Am J Pathol. 2009;174:2000–6.
66. Nagendra DC, Burke J 3rd, Maxwell GL, Risinger JI. PPP2R1A mutations are common in the serous type of endometrial cancer. Mol Carcinog. 2012;51:826–31.
67. McConechy MK, Anglesio MS, Kalloger SE, et al. Subtype-specific mutation of PPP2R1A in endometrial and ovarian carcinomas. J Pathol. 2011;223:567–73.
68. Haesen D, Abbasi Asbagh L, Derua R, et al. Recurrent PPP2R1A mutations in uterine cancer act through a dominant-negative mechanism to promote malignant cell growth. Cancer Res. 2016;76:5719–31.
69. Kuhn E, Bahadirli-Talbott A, Shih IM. Frequent CCNE1 amplification in endometrial intraepithelial carcinoma and uterine serous carcinoma. Mod Pathol. 2014;27:1014–9.
70. Cocco E, Lopez S, Black J, et al. Dual CCNE1/PIK3CA targeting is synergistic in CCNE1-amplified/PIK3CA-mutated uterine serous carcinomas in vitro and in vivo. Br J Cancer. 2016;115:303–11.
71. Nakayama K, Rahman MT, Rahman M, et al. CCNE1 amplification is associated with aggressive potential in endometrioid endometrial carcinomas. Int J Oncol. 2016;48:506–16.
72. von Wachenfeldt A, Lindblom A, Gronberg H, et al. A hypothesis-generating search for new genetic breast cancer syndromes-a national study in 803 Swedish families. Hered Cancer Clin Pract. 2007;5:17–24.
73. Liang S, Pearl M, Liang S, et al. Personal history of breast cancer as a significant risk factor for endometrial serous carcinoma in women </= 55 years Old. Int J Cancer. 2011;128(4):763–70.
74. Hornreich G, Beller U, Lavie O, et al. Is uterine serous papillary carcinoma a BRCA1-related disease? Case report and review of the literature. Gynecol Oncol. 1999;75:300–4.
75. Shu CA, Pike MC, Jotwani AR, et al. Uterine cancer after risk-reducing salpingo-oophorectomy without hysterectomy in women with BRCA mutations. JAMA Oncol. 2016;2:1434–40.
76. Holcomb K, Delatorre R, Pedemonte B, et al. E-cadherin expression in endometrioid, papillary serous, and clear cell carcinoma of the endometrium. Obstet Gynecol. 2002;100:1290–5.
77. Mell LK, Meyer JJ, Tretiakova M, et al. Prognostic significance of E-cadherin protein expression in pathological stage I-III endometrial cancer. Clin Cancer Res. 2004;10:5546–53.
78. Nofech-Mozes S, Khalifa MA, Ismiil N, et al. Immunophenotyping of serous carcinoma of the female genital tract. Mod Pathol. 2008;21:1147–55.
79. Sakuragi N, Nishiya M, Ikeda K, et al. Decreased E-cadherin expression in endometrial carcinoma is associated with tumor dedifferentiation and deep myometrial invasion. Gynecol Oncol. 1994;53:183–9.
80. Soslow RA, Shen PU, Isacson C, Chung MH. The CD44v6-negative phenotype in high-grade uterine carcinomas correlates with serous histologic subtype. Mod Pathol. 1998;11:194–9.
81. Zheng W, Schwartz PE. Serous EIC as an early form of uterine papillary serous carcinoma: recent progress in understanding its pathogenesis and current opinions regarding pathologic and clinical management. Gynecol Oncol. 2005;96:579–82.
82. Kupryjanczyk J, Thor AD, Beauchamp R, et al. Ovarian, peritoneal, and endometrial serous carcinoma: clonal origin of multifocal disease. Mod Pathol. 1996;9:166–73.
83. Baergen RN, Warren CD, Isacson C, Ellenson LH. Early uterine serous carcinoma: clonal origin of extrauterine disease. Int J Gynecol Pathol. 2001;20:214–9.
84. Black JD, Lopez S, Cocco E, et al. PIK3CA oncogenic mutations represent a major mechanism of resistance to trastuzumab in HER2/neu overexpressing uterine serous carcinomas. Br J Cancer. 2015;113:1641.
85. Lopez S, Cocco E, Black J, et al. Dual HER2/PIK3CA targeting overcomes single-agent acquired resistance in HER2-amplified uterine serous carcinoma cell lines in vitro and in vivo. Mol Cancer Ther. 2015;14:2519–26.
86. Reid-Nicholson M, Iyengar P, Hummer AJ, et al. Immunophenotypic diversity of endometrial adenocarcinomas: implications for differential diagnosis. Mod Pathol. 2006;19:1091–100.

87. Chiesa-Vottero AG, Malpica A, Deavers MT, et al. Immunohistochemical overexpression of p16 and p53 in uterine serous carcinoma and ovarian high-grade serous carcinoma. Int J Gynecol Pathol. 2007;26:328–33.
88. Santin AD, Zhan F, Cane S, et al. Gene expression fingerprint of uterine serous papillary carcinoma: identification of novel molecular markers for uterine serous cancer diagnosis and therapy. Br J Cancer. 2005;92:1561–73.
89. Maxwell GL, Chandramouli GV, Dainty L, et al. Microarray analysis of endometrial carcinomas and mixed mullerian tumors reveals distinct gene expression profiles associated with different histologic types of uterine cancer. Clin Cancer Res. 2005;11:4056–66.
90. Zheng W, Yi X, Fadare O, et al. The oncofetal protein IMP3: a novel biomarker for endometrial serous carcinoma. Am J Surg Pathol. 2008;32:304–15.
91. Jiang T, Chen N, Zhao F, et al. High levels of Nrf2 determine chemoresistance in Type II endometrial cancer. Cancer Res. 2010;70(13):5486–96.
92. Lax SF, Kurman RJ. A dualistic model for endometrial carcinogenesis based on immunohistochemical and molecular genetic analyses. Verh Dtsch Ges Pathol. 1997;81:228–32.
93. Sherman ME, Bitterman P, Rosenshein NB, Delgado G, Kurman RJ. Uterine serous carcinoma. A morphologically diverse neoplasm with unifying clinicopathologic features. Am J Surg Pathol. 1992;16:600–10.
94. Ambros RA, Sherman ME, Zahn CM, Bitterman P, Kurman RJ. Endometrial intraepithelial carcinoma: a distinctive lesion specifically associated with tumors displaying serous differentiation. Hum Pathol. 1995;26:1260–7.
95. Zheng W, Liang SX, Yu H, et al. Endometrial glandular dysplasia: a newly defined precursor lesion of uterine papillary serous carcinoma. Part I: morphologic features. Int J Surg Pathol. 2004;12:207–23.
96. Liang SX, Chambers SK, Cheng L, et al. Endometrial glandular dysplasia: a putative precursor lesion of uterine papillary serous carcinoma. Part II: molecular features. Int J Surg Pathol. 2004;12:319–31.
97. Wheeler DT, Bell KA, Kurman RJ, Sherman ME. Minimal uterine serous carcinoma: diagnosis and clinicopathologic correlation. Am J Surg Pathol. 2000;24:797–806.
98. Tashiro H, Isacson C, Levine R, et al. p53 gene mutations are common in uterine serous carcinoma and occur early in their pathogenesis. Am J Pathol. 1997;150:177–85.
99. Fadare O, Zheng W. Insights into endometrial serous carcinogenesis and progression. Int J Clin Exp Pathol. 2009;2:411–32.
100. Berman JJ, Albores-Saavedra J, Bostwick D, et al. Precancer: a conceptual working definition-results of a Consensus conference. Cancer Detect Prev. 2006;30:387–94.
101. Liang SX, Cheng L, Chambers SK, et al. Endometrial glandular dysplasia, a newly defined precursor lesion of uterine papillary serous carcinoma: Part II, molecular features. Int J Surg Pathol. 2004;12:319–31.
102. Zheng W, Liang SX, Yi X, et al. Occurrence of endometrial glandular dysplasia precedes uterine papillary serous carcinoma. Int J Gynecol Pathol. 2007;26:38–52.
103. Hoang LN, McConechy MK, Meng B, et al. Targeted mutation analysis of endometrial clear cell carcinoma. Histopathology. 2015;66:664–74.
104. Le Gallo M, Rudd ML, Urick ME, et al. Somatic mutation profiles of clear cell endometrial tumors revealed by whole exome and targeted gene sequencing. Cancer. 2017;123:3261–8.
105. DeLair DF, Burke KA, Selenica P, et al. The genetic landscape of endometrial clear cell carcinomas. J Pathol. 2017;243:230–41.
106. Zhao S, Bellone S, Lopez S, et al. Mutational landscape of uterine and ovarian carcinosarcomas implicates histone genes in epithelial-mesenchymal transition. Proc Natl Acad Sci U S A. 2016;113:12238–43.
107. Cherniack AD, Shen H, Walter V, et al. Integrated Molecular Characterization of Uterine Carcinosarcoma. Cancer Cell. 2017;31:411–23.
108. Garg K, Leitao MM Jr, Kauff ND, et al. Selection of endometrial carcinomas for DNA mismatch repair protein immunohistochemistry using patient age and tumor morphology enhances detection of mismatch repair abnormalities. Am J Surg Pathol. 2009;33:925–33.
109. Karnezis AN, Hoang LN, Coatham M, et al. Loss of switch/sucrose non-fermenting complex protein expression is associated with dedifferentiation in endometrial carcinomas. Mod Pathol. 2016;29:302–14.
110. Kobel M, Hoang LN, Tessier-Cloutier B, et al. Undifferentiated endometrial carcinomas show frequent loss of core switch/sucrose nonfermentable complex proteins. Am J Surg Pathol. 2018;42(1):76–83.
111. Rosa-Rosa JM, Leskela S, Cristobal-Lana E, et al. Molecular genetic heterogeneity in undifferentiated endometrial carcinomas. Mod Pathol. 2016;29:1594.

Endometrial Precancers

17

Charles Matthew Quick, Oluwole Fadare, and Wenxin Zheng

Abstract

This chapter covers the precancerous lesions for endometrioid and serous carcinoma of the endometrium, with some additional coverage of the limited amount of available information on possible precancer for endometrial clear cell carcinoma. For endometrioid carcinoma, the precancerous lesion is atypical hyperplasia/endometrioid intraepithelial neoplasia, clinicopathologic features of which are discussed in detail. There is also coverage of the spectrum of endometrial alterations associated with prolonged unopposed estrogen exposure. For serous carcinoma, the precancer is endometrial glandular dysplasia (EmGD). The current state of knowledge on the latter is addressed, with an emphasis on practical diagnostic applications. Serous endometrial intraepithelial carcinoma (SEIC) may display extrauterine extension and cause patient mortality and is accordingly not considered to be a *precancerous* lesion. For endometrial clear cell carcinoma, intraepithelial growth patterns, which may be seen in isolation, have long been recognized; whether these are precursor lesions is unclear. A previously proffered precursor lesion for clear cell carcinoma requires additional evidentiary support.

C. M. Quick (✉)
Department of Pathology, University of Arkansas for Medical Sciences, Little Rock, AR, USA
e-mail: QuickCharlesM@uams.edu

O. Fadare
Department of Pathology, University of California San Diego, San Diego, CA, USA

W. Zheng
Department of Pathology, University of Texas Southwestern Medical Center, Dallas, TX, USA

Department of Obstetrics and Gynecology, University of Texas Southwestern Medical Center, Dallas, TX, USA

Keywords

Endometrial hyperplasia · Benign hyperplasia · Endometrial atypical hyperplasia · Endometrial intraepithelial neoplasia · Endometrioid intraepithelial neoplasia · Endometrial glandular dysplasia · Endometrial intraepithelial carcinoma · Endometrial precancer · Precursors of endometrial cancer

17.1 Introduction

Endometrial carcinoma is the most common malignancy of the female genital tract in Western countries. Endometrial carcinomas are recognized to be heterogeneous and to be classifiable into clinically distinct subsets at the morphologic, immunophenotypic, and molecular levels.

The pathologic identification of lesions that can be conclusively classified as "precancerous" offers the opportunity for such lesions to be ablated before their evolution into a cancer. On the other hand, the dynamic and hormone-sensitive microenvironment of the endometrium may result in benign epithelial alterations that may potentially be misclassified, or for clonal events whose natural history is to regress over time to be over-emphasized; overly aggressive clinical management in both of these scenarios may potentially have significant consequences for the patient. The challenge for the diagnostic pathologist is therefore to identify and to accurately report lesions that will directly inform patient management.

Precancerous lesions for endometrial cancer have predominantly been defined relative to the corresponding pathologically defined histotypes. Most of the published literature on endometrial precancers has centered on endometrioid and serous carcinomas, whereas a few papers have been published on putative precancers for clear cell carcinoma. This chapter will address the putative precancers for these three histotypes, with an emphasis on practical diagnostic applications. A detailed appraisal of endometrial carcinogenesis is outlined in Chap. 18.

W. Zheng et al. (eds.), *Gynecologic and Obstetric Pathology, Volume 1*, https://doi.org/10.1007/978-981-13-3016-2_17

17.1.1 Endometrioid (Type 1) Precancer

17.1.1.1 Clinical Features and Risk Factors

Patients suffering from endometrioid intraepithelial neoplasia/atypical hyperplasia (EIN/AH) typically present with abnormal, or postmenopausal, uterine bleeding, usually at prolonged intervals. In the vast majority of cases, these patients are obese; however, patients may have a family history of uterine cancer or other malignancies, especially in patients with hereditary nonpolyposis colorectal cancer syndrome (HNPCC/Lynch syndrome) or Cowden syndrome. In some cases the patient may have a historical exposure to exogenous estrogens or tamoxifen.

Risk of EIN/AH is multifactorial and may be due to endocrine imbalances (including obesity), genetic defects, or drug exposure. Obviously, the most common risk factor for type 1 precancerous lesions is excess estrogen, which, in many developed countries, directly correlates with obesity. Endometrial cancers and their precursors are known to be driven by increases in estrogen and dampened by relative increases in progestin [1]. Current formulations of hormonal contraceptives combine estrogen and progestins in low-dose forms, which when used in tandem have been shown to reduce the risk of development of cancer, and thus its precursor lesion, to levels below that of the general population [2, 3].

Sporadic cases of EIN/AH may be seen in the absence of obesity and excess estrogen. Recent emphasis has been placed on identification of germline mutations in a select group of patients, namely, those with Lynch syndrome. While the focus of most genetic testing is endometrial cancer, these lesions often do proceed through a histologically identifiable precancer, which may be seen adjacent to carcinoma in some cases. Indeed, precursor lesions have been evaluated in regard to their mismatch repair status, and the majority of cases are due to epigenetic inactivation of the MLH1 promoter region, which is consistent with trends noted in endometrial carcinoma [4, 5]. Currently, routine testing of premalignant lesions for mismatch repair deficiency is not warranted. Another syndrome which leads to increased risk of endometrioid precancers (and their subsequent carcinomas) is Cowden syndrome, which is a germline mutation of a mutant *PTEN* allele, which leads to a loss in normal *PTEN* tumor suppressor function [6, 7]. Loss of PTEN (and PAX2) function has been exploited clinically as an adjunctive immunohistochemical test for some precancers [8–10].

A well-described risk factor for development of precancerous lesions is tamoxifen therapy. In select patients, tamoxifen may be used as adjunct therapy or as a preventative measure in patients that have had, or are at high risk of developing breast cancer. While tamoxifen is an estrogen antagonist in the breast, it acts as an agonist in the endometrium. Patients on tamoxifen are prone to developing endometrial polyps, hyperplasia, and premalignant and malignant endometrioid lesions [11, 12].

17.1.1.2 Endometrial Hyperplasia

Prolonged exposure to estrogen, regardless of cause, exerts a proliferative effect on the endometrium. Commonly, the excess in estrogen relative to progestin is related to obesity, chronic anovulation, hormone replacement, or an estrogen-secreting ovarian tumor. Over time, this may lead to irregular endometrial cycles, retention of the endometrium, and sustained growth. This process can progress to so-called, benign, or non-atypical hyperplasias, which can set the stage for possible neoplastic transformation. Remodeling of the endometrium in this manner is a spectrum of disease, first manifesting in disordered (anovulatory) endometrium, followed by benign hyperplasia and finally EIN/AH [13]. The initial manifestation of this change is abnormal uterine bleeding, which typically prompts endometrial sampling and the histologic findings detailed in the sections below.

17.1.1.3 Disordered Proliferative Endometrium

The earliest histologic manifestation of relative estrogen excess is so-called disordered proliferative endometrium, or anovulatory endometrium. This pattern of endometrial growth is notable for its relative retention of a normal gland to stroma ratio at low magnification (Fig. 17.1). Occasional glands will display microcystic change in a background of otherwise unremarkable proliferative endometrium (Fig. 17.2). If time and estrogen exposure persist, the number and complexity of abnormal endometrial glands will increase to include microcysts, cysts, and sacculated and multilobular endometrial glands (Fig. 17.3). Patchy tubal metaplasia of the lining epithelium is usually present (Fig. 17.4).

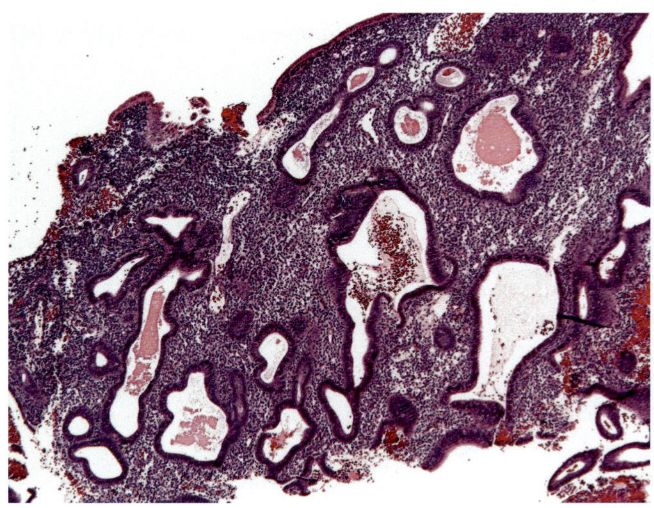

Fig. 17.1 Disordered proliferative (anovulatory) endometrium with a relatively preserved gland to stroma ratio

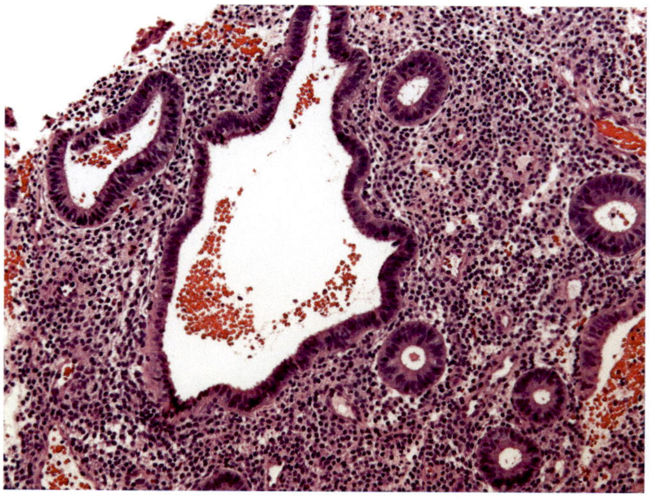

Fig. 17.2 Disordered proliferative (anovulatory) endometrium typically demonstrates enlarged, microcystic, or sacculated glands admixed with normal proliferative glands. Note the presence of tubal metaplasia within the enlarged glands

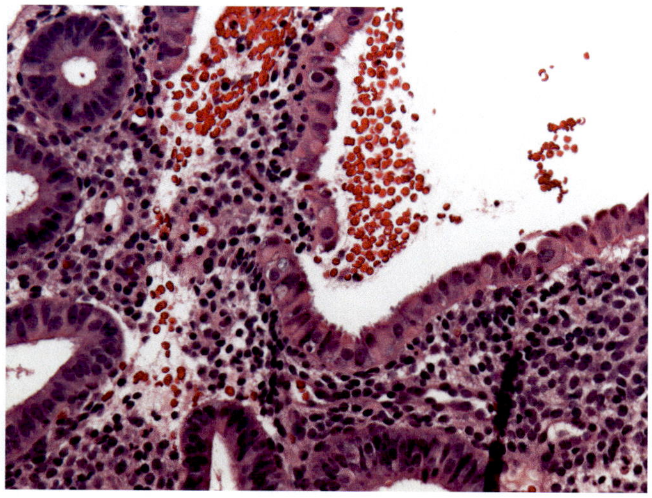

Fig. 17.4 The lining epithelium of glands in anovulatory endometrium frequently displays tubal metaplasia

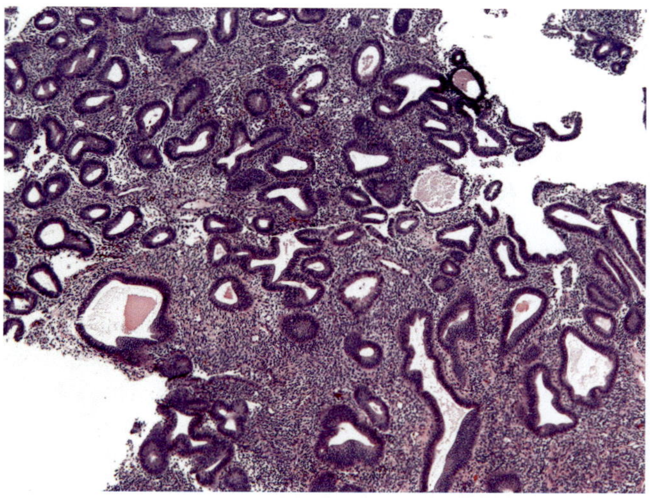

Fig. 17.3 Disordered proliferative endometrium with a slightly increased gland to stroma ratio. The glandular component consists of a mixture of normal proliferative glands and microcystic glands

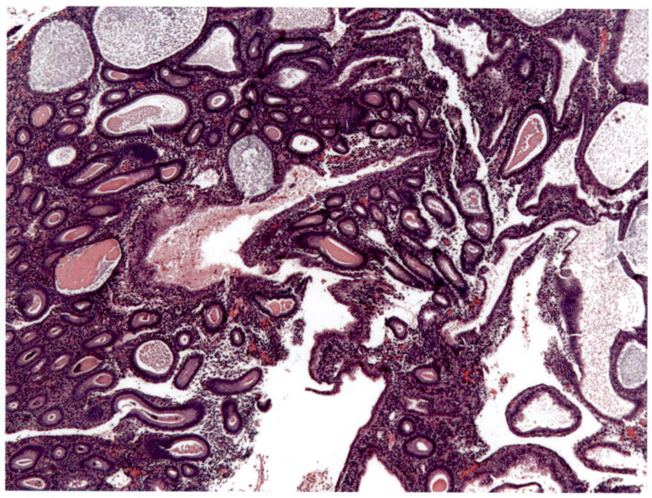

Fig. 17.5 Low-power image of non-atypical hyperplasia. Note the presence of small, closely apposed glands as well as scattered enlarged glands. The gland to stroma ratio should exceed 1:1

When these histologic features are present, a diagnosis of *disordered proliferative endometrium* or *proliferative endometrium with features of anovulation* is appropriate.

17.1.1.4 Benign Hyperplasia (Hyperplasia Without Atypia)

In patients with prolonged exposure to relative excesses in estrogen, endometrial remodeling will continue along the "disordered, hyperplastic, neoplastic" sequence. As this progression continues, the global gland to stroma ratio of the endometrium will increase, which is the cardinal difference between disordered proliferative and hyperplastic endometrium. Cases of benign hyperplasia are best identified at low power (2–4×) as a "regularly irregular" pattern of crowded, small, proliferative glands alternating with pockets of crowded, cystically dilated, or branched glands (Fig. 17.5). Importantly, higher magnification will reveal a lack of discernable cytologic changes in the glands throughout the entirety of the tissue. This lack of "cytologic demarcation" is the key histologic feature that sets benign hyperplasia apart from EIN/AH. In general, the nuclei resemble those seen in normal proliferative endometrium and are elongated and oriented perpendicular to the basement membrane (Fig. 17.6). Stromal and epithelial mitotic figures are readily apparent, but are not atypical. Stromal breakdown, hemorrhage, and associated reactive epithelial changes are not uncommon and are typically a consequence of microthrombi [14, 15].

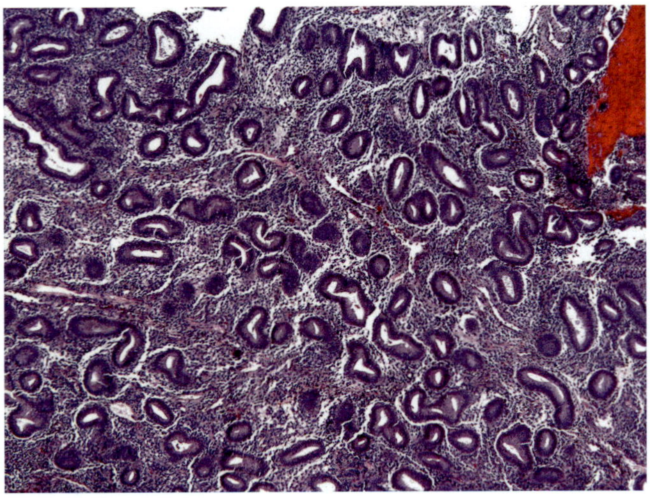

Fig. 17.6 Non-atypical hyperplasia lacks significant cytologic demarcation across the entire specimen. The glandular epithelium typically resembles that seen in otherwise normal proliferative endometrium

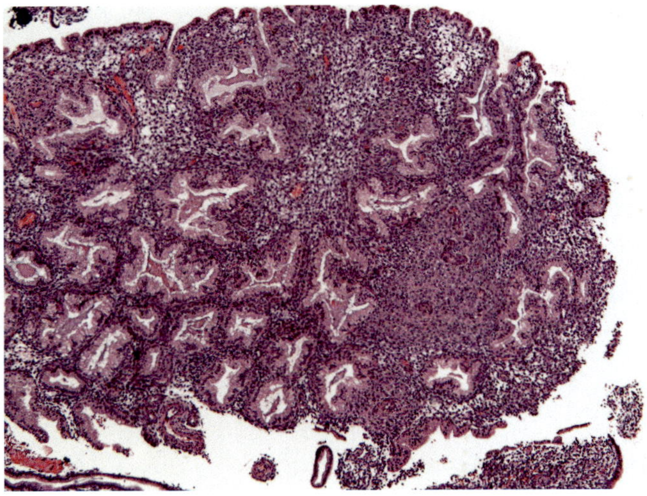

Fig. 17.7 Secretory endometrium will display a gland to stroma ratio that will often exceed 1:1. The presence of epithelial secretory vacuoles and stromal pseudo-decidualization can help to rule out a precancerous process

Patients with relative excesses in estrogen over long periods of time have an approximate two to tenfold increase in endometrial carcinoma risk [16, 17]. Previous studies in cases classified under previous schema (WHO 1994) demonstrated that untreated, non-atypical hyperplasias, which may be considered analogous to benign hyperplasia, had a minimal risk of progression based on their extent (1% for simple non-atypical hyperplasia and 3% for complex non-atypical hyperplasia) [18]. Treatment strategies consist of modulation of hormones, be it administration of progestins to counteract excess estrogen, or suppression of estrogen via weight loss or tumor removal (in the case of a functional ovarian tumor).

17.1.1.5 Differential Diagnosis

The differential diagnosis of benign hyperplasia includes disordered proliferative endometrium, secretory endometrium, and EIN/AH. Cases of disordered proliferative endometrium may contain small areas of glandular crowding, similar to that seen in benign hyperplasia; however, these areas are limited and will not be as widely distributed as in cases of hyperplasia. Secretory endometrium may display a global increase in the gland to stroma ratio throughout the specimen, causing concern for benign hyperplasia. Epithelial secretory vacuoles as well as stromal pseudo-decidualization can help to identify secretory endometrium (Fig. 17.7). Rare cases of secretory hyperplasia and EIN/AH may occur, and PAX2 loss in these cases can help to identify these subtle lesions (described in detail in the section on altered differentiation in EIN/AH). Finally, cases of overrun EIN/AH may lack discernable background endometrium, making it difficult to identify cytologic demarcation. These cases may closely resemble benign hyperplasia; however, EIN/AH typically displays a greater degree of glandular crowding and will generally lack the low-power "regularly irregular" pattern of benign hyperplasia. Careful application of PAX2 may be helpful in such cases [10].

17.1.1.6 Endometrial Intraepithelial Neoplasia/Atypical Hyperplasia

WHO 1994–2014

For 20 years the criteria set forth in the 1994 adaptation of the "WHO Blue Book" for tumors of the gynecologic tract provided a reliable method of classification of hyperplastic and precancerous lesions of the endometrium. This schema allowed endometrial lesions to be classified and assigned risk of development of carcinoma and was divided into four categories: simple hyperplasia with and without atypia and complex hyperplasia with and without atypia. The distinction of simple and complex hyperplasia, irrespective of atypia, was based on the overall gland to stroma ratio and the complexity of the glands in question. The presence of architectural (back to back glands) and epithelial complexity (epithelial tufts or buds) warranted a diagnosis of complex hyperplasia, whereas general increases in the gland to stroma ratio, without complex architecture, would be deemed "simple."

While the overall architecture of the lesions was an important facet of classification, the presence of "nuclear atypia" was widely considered to be the most important feature used to determine risk of progression. WHO 1994 described nuclear atypia as: loss of nuclear polarity, irregular shape and/or contours, vesicular and/or hyperchromatic chromatin, and the presence of prominent nucleoli. These features were relatively subjective and at times could be influenced by hormonal fluctuations and natural differences between patients.

That being said, the practice of using both cytologic and architectural features to classify hyperplastic and precancerous lesions proved powerful, hence the 20-year run of this classification scheme. While this method was positively received, there were problems with its application, namely, in the task of identifying nuclear atypia, which was detailed in multiple publications [19–22].

The most recent version of this classification scheme, released in 2014, builds upon our understanding of the underlying pathobiology of these endometrial lesions as well as several principles from the 1994 version of the diagnostic criteria. The 2014 adaptation endorses a two-tiered classification system with categories for non-atypical hyperplasia and EIN/atypical hyperplasia [14]. The category of EIN/AH represents a precancerous lesion with underlying molecular aberrations that set it apart from estrogen-driven hyperplasia (i.e., non-atypical hyperplasia). The implication of this diagnosis is that the patient has a precancerous lesion and is at significant risk of developing endometrioid adenocarcinoma. Alternatively, patients with hyperplasia that falls short of EIN/AH do not have a precancer and thus are at a lower, albeit increased relative to normal, risk of developing carcinoma. Non-atypical hyperplasia and EIN/AH are still linked due to the fact that non-atypical hyperplasias create the proper endometrial environment to allow for mutations to accumulate and for EIN/AH to develop.

The overlap of the 1994 and 2014 systems has been studied and shown that, as one would expect, the majority of complex atypical hyperplasias represent EIN/AH [23]. Perhaps more importantly, 44% of lesions classified as complex, non-atypical hyperplasia and 4% of lesions deemed simple, non-atypical hyperplasia were reclassified as EIN/AH [23]. This is striking, as these lesions would have been predicted to have little to no risk of progression to carcinoma under the 1994 classification system. This finding should not be surprising to many pathologists who utilized the four-tiered classification scheme and encountered difficulty in determining if nuclear atypia was present.

17.1.1.7 Atypical Hyperplasia/Endometrioid Intraepithelial Neoplasia and Cancer Risk

Patients with a diagnosis of EIN/AH carry a significant risk of progression to endometrioid adenocarcinoma. Within 1 year of an EIN/AH diagnosis, one-third of patients are found to be affected by carcinoma, which may be considered concurrent to their precancerous lesion in some cases [24]. Patients without carcinoma in their first year after diagnosis carry approximately a 45-fold increased risk of developing low-grade endometrioid carcinoma compared to those with a diagnosis of non-atypical hyperplasia [25]. These figures are in line with those described to be associated with the WHO 1994 classification system; however, the exact risk will likely never be known as most patients undergo hysterectomy shortly after their diagnosis of EIN/AH [26, 27].

17.1.1.8 Atypical Hyperplasia/Endometrioid Intraepithelial Neoplasia Diagnosis

The diagnosis of EIN/AH, as it is stated in the 2014 version of the WHO Blue Book, is similar to the "endometrial intraepithelial neoplasia" system put forth by Dr. George Mutter and colleagues. Of note, the name has been changed to endometri*oid* intraepithelial neoplasia in the WHO 2014 schema to avoid confusion with endometrial intraepithelial carcinoma, the precursor to uterine serous carcinoma. This classification scheme is unique in that a diagnosis of EIN/AH implies that the histology of the lesion is directly secondary to an underlying genetic defect.

The diagnostic criteria of EIN/AH include four components (Table 17.1):

1. Glandular crowding (volume percent stroma less than 55%, or simply glandular to stroma ratio > 1)
2. Cytologic demarcation from the background endometrium
3. Size greater than 1 mm
4. Exclusion of benign mimics and carcinoma

To diagnose EIN/AH all four of these criteria must be satisfied. In general, the first criterion—glandular crowding—is the first to be assessed when evaluating a biopsy. This assessment is best carried out at scanning magnification (Fig. 17.8). The overall gland to stroma ratio should be greater than 1:1.

Table 17.1 Diagnostic Criteria of Atypical Hyperplasia / Endometrioid Intraepithelial Neoplasia

Criteria	Definition	Tips for application
Gland crowding	The gland to stroma ratio should exceed 1:1	In practice, 55% of the tissue should be composed of glands vs. stroma. This is best determined at low power
Cytologic demarcation	Crowded glands should differ cytologically from the background endometrium	Once an area of crowded glands is noted, carefully analyze the cytology of the crowded focus to see if it differs from the adjacent normal. Best performed at 10–20×
Size	The size of the lesion should be greater than 1 mm	The 10× objective on most microscopes gives a field of view of approximately 2 mm; therefore, if the lesion is greater than 1/2 a 10× field, it is likely larger than 1 mm
Exclusion of mimics	Benign and malignant mimics should be excluded	Confirm that benign mimics such as endometrium with metaplasia, secretory endometrium, polyps, endometrial basalis, as well as carcinoma are not present

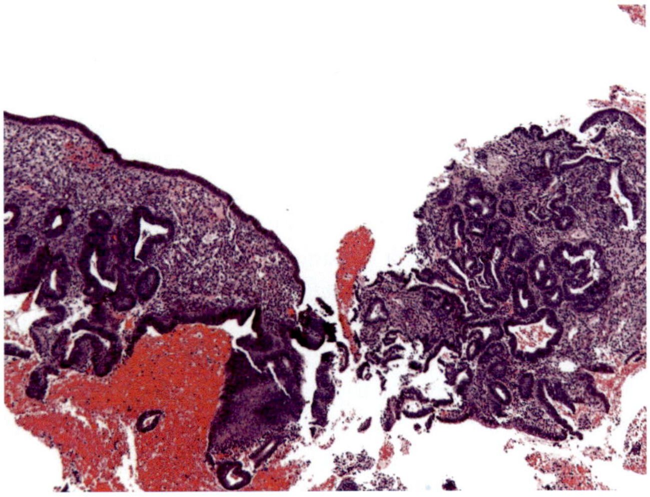

Fig. 17.8 Foci of endometrioid intraepithelial neoplasia/atypical hyperplasia are best recognized at low magnification as cluster of glands that are closely apposed relative to the surrounding background glands. The focus on the right side of this image demonstrates low-power glandular crowding

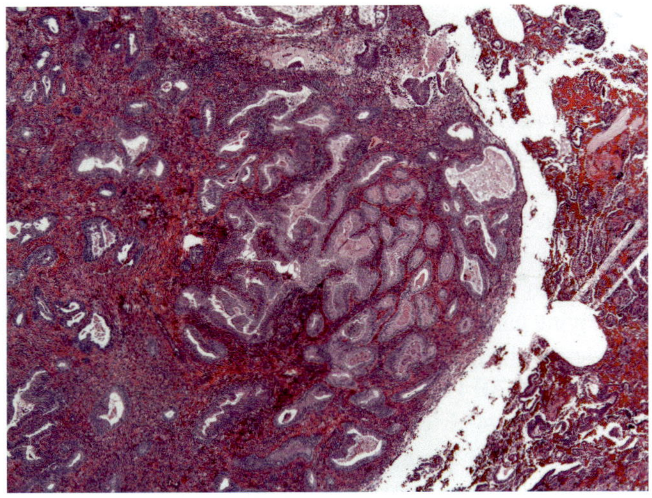

Fig. 17.9 A focus of EIN/AH which is recognizable as a cluster of cytologically demarcated glands with their greatest density in the center of the proliferation. The glandular density typically decreases toward the periphery of the lesion. Of note, the altered cytology of the crowded glands is noticeable even at low-power magnification in this image

Another way of stating this is that the volume of the stroma should be less than 55%. This quantification amounts to the impression that of the tissue composing the biopsy, a little less than half is made up of stroma. In typical cases of EIN/AH, about 10–30% of the volume of the tissue is composed of stroma. It is worth noting that glands should still be separated by stroma and that a diagnosis of focal adenocarcinoma should be entertained if this is not the case. The crowded glands are typically tubular or branching but occasionally may be dilated. The "epicenter" of the lesion will demonstrate a higher density of glands, which will decrease toward the periphery (Fig. 17.9). At the edges of the lesion, interspersed normal background glands may be seen admixed with precancerous glands (Fig. 17.10).

One of the most useful diagnostic criteria for diagnosing EIN/AH is the presence of cytologic demarcation between the precancerous lesion and the normal background endometrium. This demarcation may be due to both differences in cytology and/or nuclear features. The cytologic appearance of EIN/AH, and the background endometrium, may differ from patient to patient and may even be different in the same patient under the influences of varying levels of endogenous hormones. Cytologic demarcation becomes such a powerful histologic feature because these changes in cytology do not eliminate the difference in appearance between the precancer and normal. The presence of classically defined nuclear atypia (i.e., vesicular round nuclei, prominent nucleoli, anisonucleosis, and loss of polarity) does not need to be met for cytologic demarcation to be identified. Often cytologic demarcation can be identified at low magnification along with glandular crowding (Fig. 17.9), but in small samples, or samples with extensive glandular crowding, closer inspection for "orphan" background glands can be helpful (Fig. 17.11).

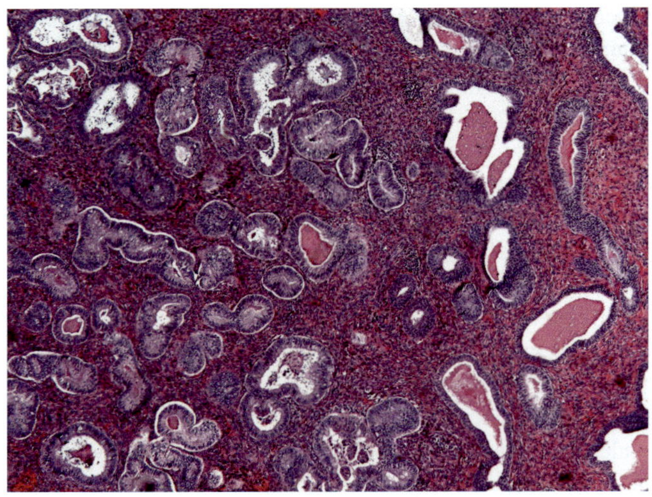

Fig. 17.10 The edge of an EIN/AH showing a mixture of precancerous glands (left) and normal background glands on the right

The minimum size of the crowded, cytologically altered focus should measure at least 1 mm. This is a historical criterion that was applied to the initial studies of computerized morphometry of endometrial lesions. One millimeter was determined to be the minimal size needed for accurate and reliable diagnosis of EIN. This size cutoff is retained in modern schema to prevent "overcalling" of small foci of compressed glands, artifactual crowding, or atypical glands as EIN/AH. Of note, separate foci of glandular crowding, spread across different tissue fragments, are not additive.

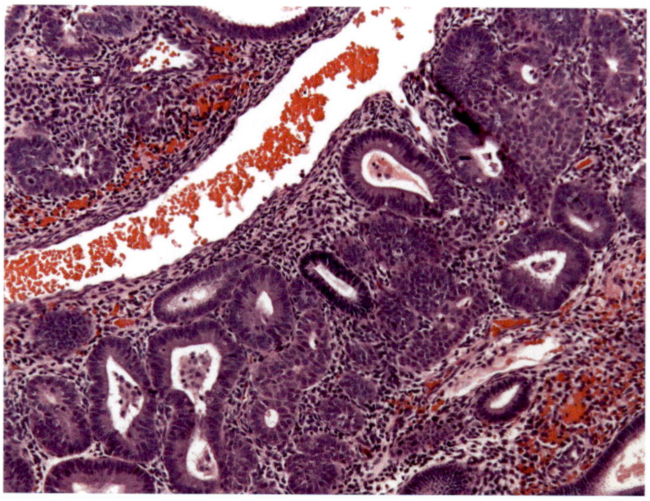

Fig. 17.11 An example of two "orphan" glands in a background of EIN/AH. These glands may not be seen at low power; therefore in overrun lesions a high-power search for them is the best plan of action

Lesions that demonstrate true cytologic demarcation and crowding, but are less than 1 mm in size, should be given a descriptive diagnosis with a comment recommending follow-up (discussed below).

The final step in diagnosing EIN/AH should consist of a systematic exclusion of potential mimics and adenocarcinoma. Some of the more common benign mimics include telescoping artifact (especially in pipelle biopsies), shearing of stroma leading to artifactual gland crowding, polyps, reactive epithelial changes (which may appear as cytologic demarcation), endometrial basalis, metaplastic epithelium, and non-atypical hyperplasia. Exclusion of adenocarcinoma, especially when focal, may be difficult. In general the presence of glandular fusion (creating cribriforming), luminal papillae, labyrinthine glandular lumen, solid growth, and back to back glands with thread-like intervening stroma are indicative of low-grade adenocarcinoma (Fig. 17.12a–d). As previously stated, when these features are focal, or the biopsy

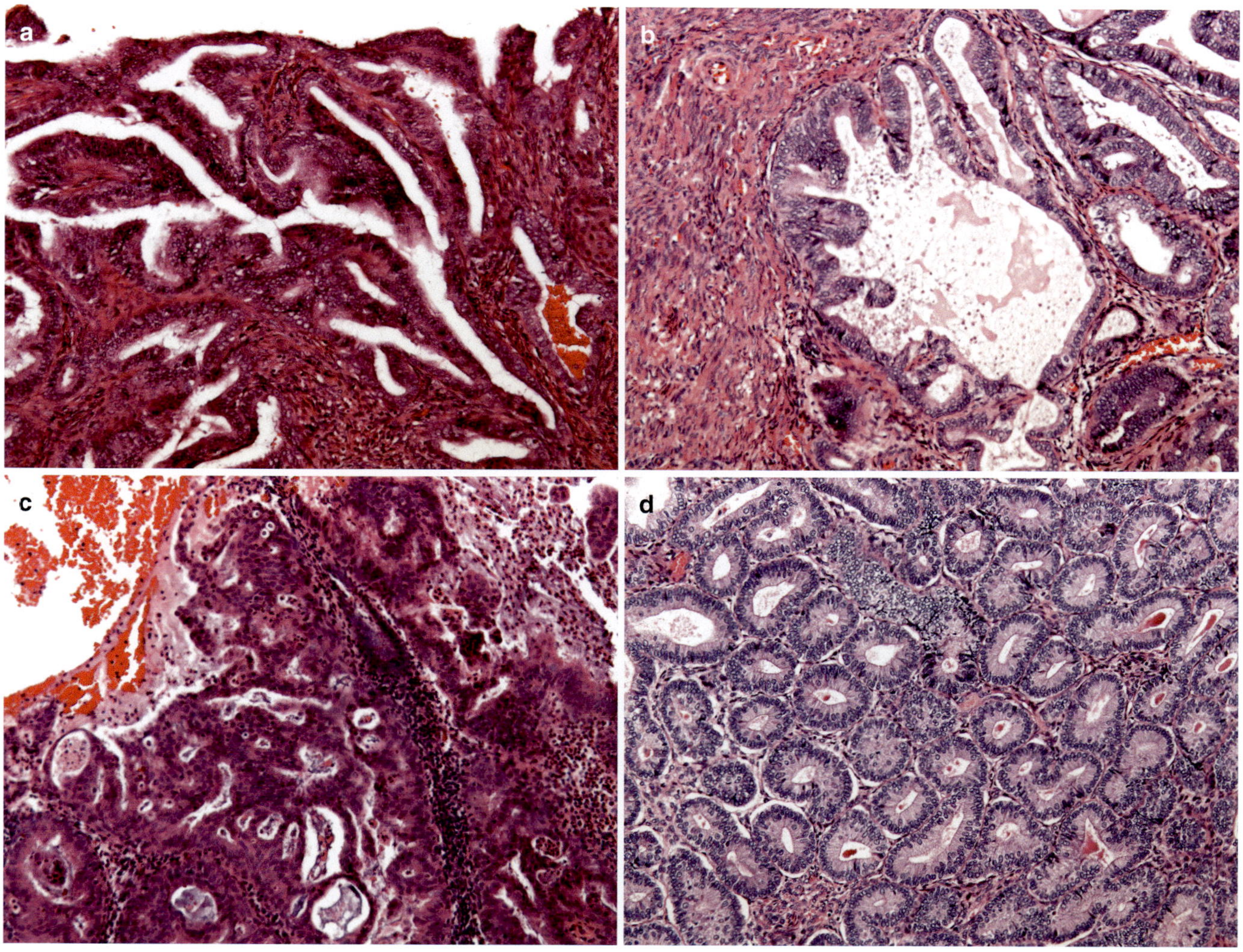

Fig. 17.12 The diagnosis of focal endometrioid adenocarcinoma may be difficult to distinguish in a background of EIN/AH. The presence of (**a**) maze-like endometrial glandular lumen, (**b**) intraglandular papillary tufts, (**c**) cribriforming, and (**d**) closely packed glands with thread-like intervening stroma are all diagnostic of low-grade endometrioid adenocarcinoma

is small, this distinction may be impossible to make. In this setting a diagnosis of "at least EIN/AH" with a comment describing the features and their limitations is appropriate. A descriptive diagnosis in this setting is preferable as it will allow the clinician and patient options regarding future treatment (i.e., additional sampling vs. hysterectomy).

17.1.1.9 Difficulties with Interpretation

Fragmentation and Sampling Artifacts

Unfortunately, fragmentation of endometrial samples is commonplace; however, in most cases the amount of specimen disruption is not sufficient to limit diagnosis. One of the more common sampling artifacts includes the shearing of glandular epithelium from stroma. This epithelium may then become compressed and give the false impression of true gland crowding (Fig. 17.13). Careful evaluation of these foci, looking for the absence of endometrial stroma, is necessary. Another common sampling artifact is gland telescoping. This occurs when gland epithelium prolapses into itself, creating a complex, gland-in-gland structure that may mimic neoplasia (Fig. 17.14). Often these telescoped glands are arranged singly and lack the traditional back to back arrangement of neoplastic lesions. Recognition of normal background endometrium surrounding the telescoped focus is helpful.

Fragmentation of the sample may directly interfere with the previously stated 1 mm minimum size needed to diagnose EIN/AH. It is important to remember that size of lesions is not additive across multiple fragments and that a single, contiguous 1 mm focus is needed. If a sub-1 mm focus of crowded, cytologically demarcated glands exists, the next best step is ordering levels. If levels do not help, then a descriptive diagnosis of the lesion (i.e., "small focus of atypical glands") with a comment describing them is warranted. In general it is appropriate to recommend follow-up sampling. If the lesion is at the edge of a tissue fragment, and there is concern for a larger lesion in the patient, a shorter interval (1 month) is advised. In most cases, repeat sampling in 3 months is appropriate.

Overrun AH/EIN

In some cases the precancerous process may occupy the entirety of the specimen, so-called overrun EIN/AH. When this occurs, it limits the evaluation of cytologic demarcation, which may give the false impression of a non-atypical hyperplasia, especially at low-power magnification. When this occurs the first step is careful examination of the proliferation for single, "orphan glands" surrounded by the EIN/AH (Fig. 17.15). These glands are typically more easily

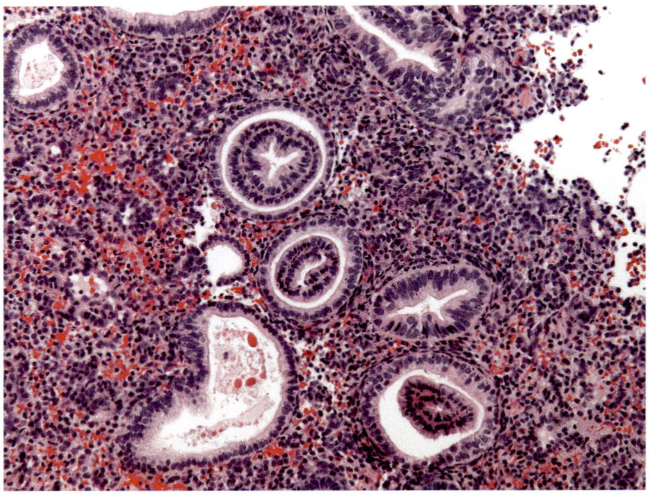

Fig. 17.14 Prolapse of the glandular epithelium into itself may mimic glandular complexity. The background architecture of the tissue fragment should be intact

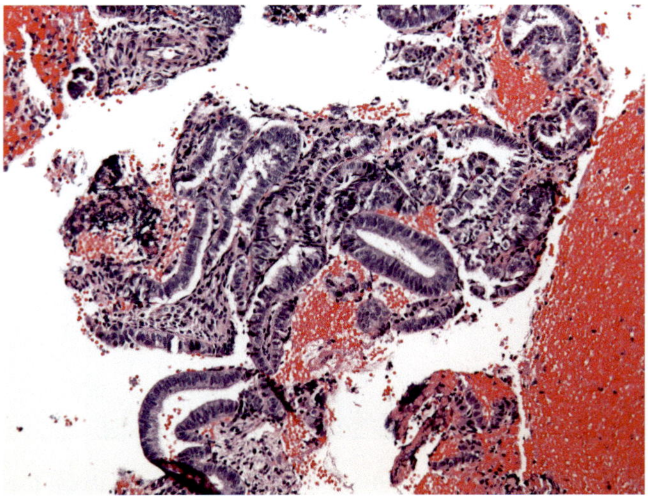

Fig. 17.13 Artifactual shearing of the endometrial glands out of the stroma may lead to the false impression of glandular crowding

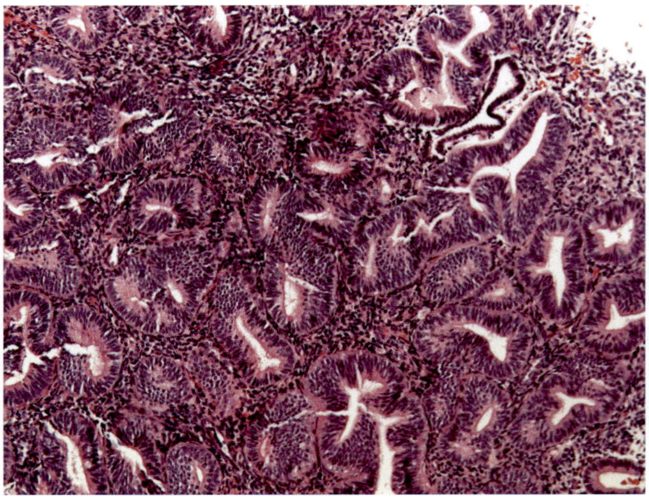

Fig. 17.15 Overrun EIN/AH. In this example a single, atrophic background endometrial gland is present in the upper right aspect of the image

identifiable at the periphery of the lesion. If no normal background glands can be identified, then the decision must be made based on the level of architectural complexity and the more classic definition of nuclear atypia (round, vesicular nuclei with nucleoli). Immunohistochemical staining with PAX2 may be helpful and is described in more detail in the "Genetic Profile and Immunohistochemistry" section of this chapter.

Polyps

Endometrial polyps may display many of the same features as EIN/AH. Glands in polyps may be crowded, appear different from the native endometrium, and be haphazardly arranged. Presence of fibrous, "polyp-like" stroma and thick-walled blood vessels can help to identify polyps, but they may be subtle in some cases. Around 20% of EIN/AH lesions arise in polyps, with postmenopausal women being disproportionally affected when compared to premenopausal women [28]. Because of the overlapping features, evaluation of a polyp for EIN/AH may be difficult. It is important to note that the level of glandular crowding of EIN/AH in a polyp may be highly variable. In general the degree of glandular crowding of the focus of EIN/AH will be greater than seen in the rest of the polyp (Fig. 17.16); however, in some cases the fibrous stroma appears to contain the proliferations and hold the glands apart, leading to a lower than normal ratio of glands to stroma. Additionally, the presence of cytologic demarcation should be evaluated only within the glands of the polyp, not including non-polyp endometrium, if present (Fig. 17.17) [28]. In suspicious lesions staining with PAX2 has been shown to be helpful [10].

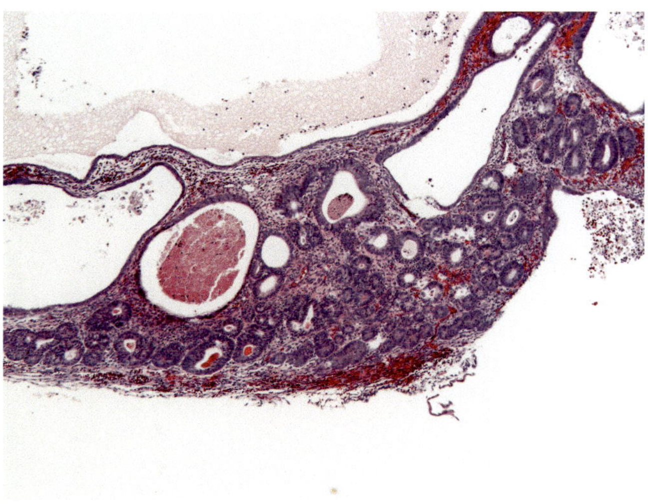

Fig. 17.16 An atrophic endometrial polyp with a focus of small, crowded, cytologically demarcated glands. This focus represents EIN/AH arising in an endometrial polyp

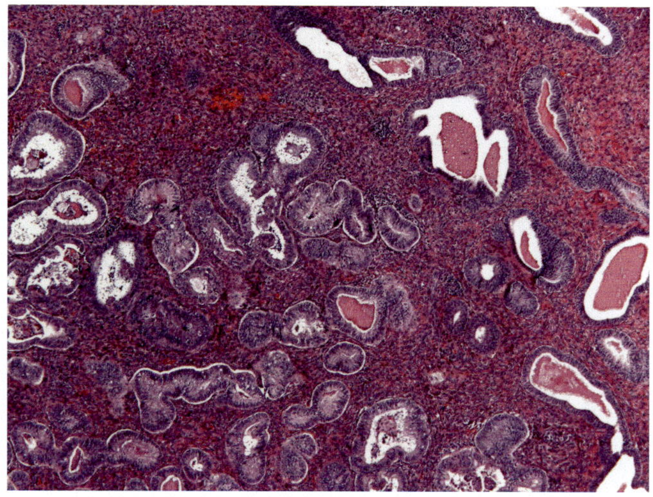

Fig. 17.17 Cytologic demarcation within an endometrial polyp. Only glands within the polyp should be compared for the purposes of determining if cytologic demarcation is actually present. Background, non-polypoid endometrium cannot be used

Metaplasia (Altered Differentiation)

Endometrial epithelium may undergo numerous shifts in phenotype or metaplasias. More common types include squamous/morular, mucinous, and tubular metaplasia. More rare variants include eosinophilic, secretory, and hobnail metaplasia. Papillary syncytial metaplasia is a unique type that displays both eosinophilic and hobnail metaplasia, along with a papillary growth pattern, and is usually reactive. These metaplasias may be seen in benign and malignant endometrium, and therefore the term "altered differentiation" has been proposed. Interestingly, altered differentiation has numerous causes, ranging from beta catenin mutations in morular metaplasia and inflammatory causes in eosinophilic and hobnail metaplasia to hormonal effects in secretory metaplasia [29–31].

One of the most commonly encountered types of altered differentiation is squamous. Squamous metaplasia may occur in two different forms, the common morular type and the much more rare laminar, superficial type termed ichthyosis uteri (Fig. 17.18). The more common, morular type, is composed of well-circumscribed, round aggregates of cells that appear to arise from the glandular epithelium, often filling the lumen (Fig. 17.19). These morules may occasionally involve multiple glands, leading to a wreath-like appearance of glands surrounding a central morula (Fig. 17.20). The glands surrounding these morules may appear to cribriform; however, this should not be considered diagnostic of carcinoma, and these areas should be avoided when evaluating glandular architecture. Occasionally clear cell change or necrosis may be seen associated with morules; these changes have no pathologic significance. Mutations in the *CTNNB1* gene are the most common molecular aberration, and morules usually demonstrate nuclear and cytoplasmic positivity

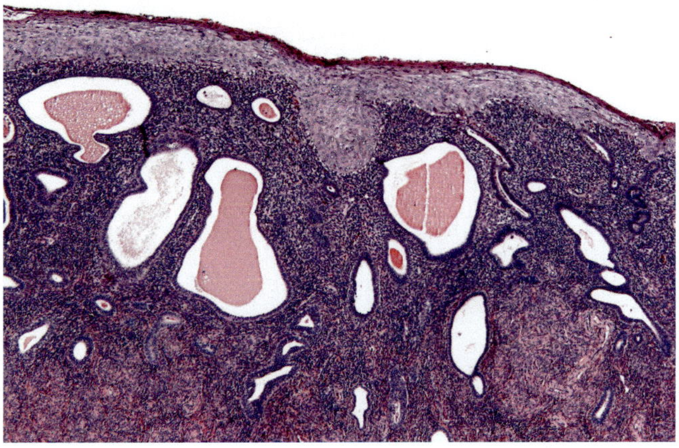

Fig. 17.18 Laminar squamous metaplasia of the endometrium (ichthyosis uteri)

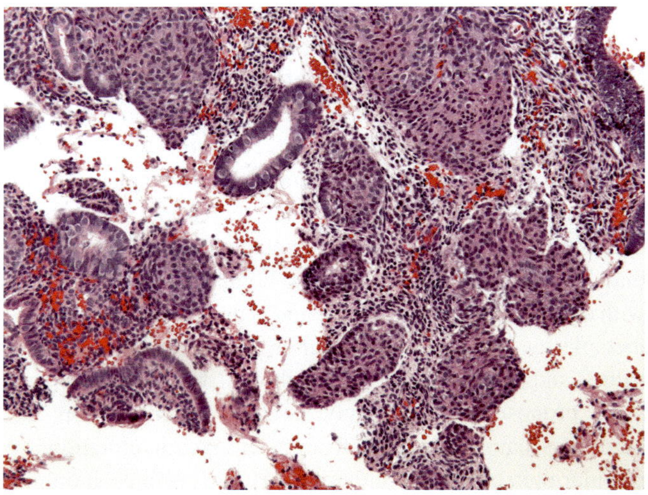

Fig. 17.19 Immature morular (squamous) metaplasia of the endometrium may often fill endometrial glands, obliterating the lumen

for beta catenin [32]. Squamous morules also demonstrate CDX2 and membranous CD10 staining, are typically negative for ER and PR, and have a low proliferative rate by Ki-67 [32]. Because morules have an association with EIN/AH and endometrioid adenocarcinoma, their presence should be documented, and a comment should be offered stating this association as well as the need for continued clinical observation [33].

Mucinous metaplasia may display two distinct phenotypes, endocervical type and intestinal type, of which endocervical type is much more common. Regardless of the type of metaplasia present, the prognosis is dependent wholly on the architecture of the metaplasia. This spectrum was best classified by Nucci et al., who subdivided mucinous metaplasia into Types A, B, and C [34]. Type A mucinous metaplasia consisted of simple mucinous epithelium that lacked stratification or atypia (Fig. 17.21). Type B metaplasias demonstrate epithelial tufting and pseudo-papillae but lack significant architectural distortion or atypia (Fig. 17.22). Type C mucinous metaplasia has the most significant clinical associations and contains cribriforming, microglandular growth, or villous architecture (Fig. 17.23). Type C metaplasia carried a 75% chance of being associated with adenocarcinoma and, as a result, should be considered analogous to EIN/AH [34]. This is contrasted with a very low rate of progression of Types A and B metaplasia, in which patients need clinical follow-up and periodic sampling.

Tubal metaplasia is a commonly encountered finding in many endometrial biopsies. This state of altered differentiation has been associated with increased levels of estrogen. It typically consists of glands lined by a combination of ciliated cells and enlarged, polygonal cells, similar to those seen in the fallopian tube (Fig. 17.24). It is frequently seen in association with cystic dilation of endometrial

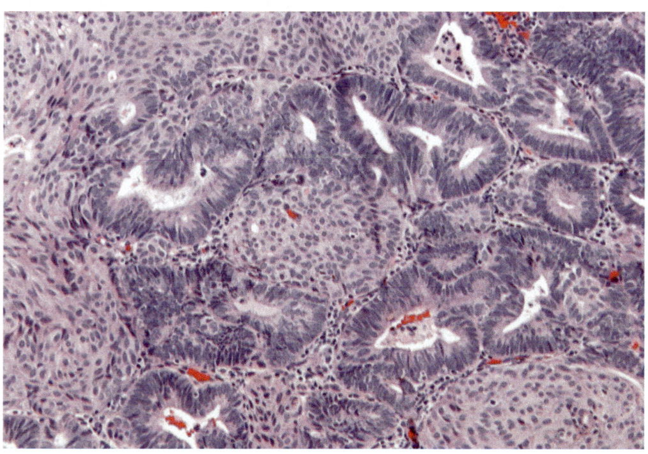

Fig. 17.20 Morular metaplasia may cause background glands to coalesce, leading to a wreath-like arrangement of glands around a central squamous morula. These glands may occasionally appear to cribriform; however, this is not diagnostic of adenocarcinoma

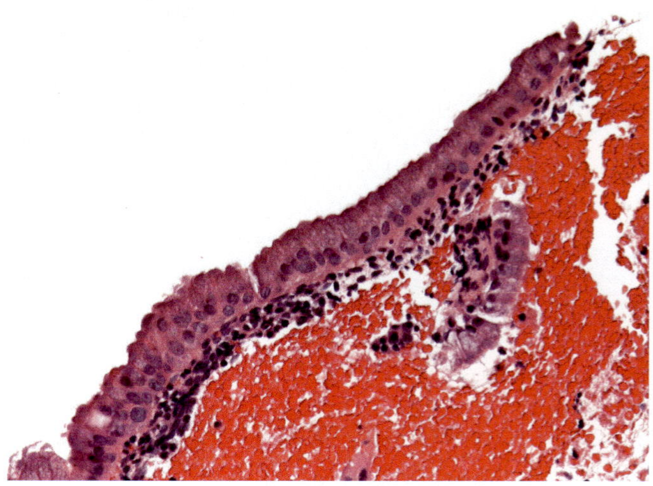

Fig. 17.21 Simple mucinous metaplasia (type A) consisting of a monolayer of mucinous epithelium with basally oriented nuclei and abundant apical cytoplasm

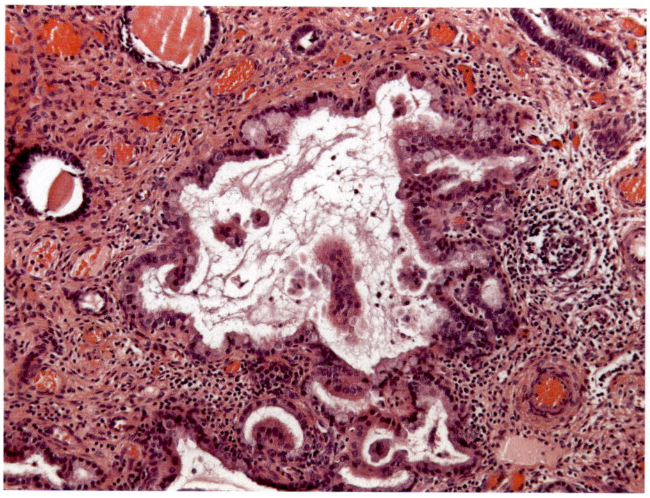

Fig. 17.22 Type-B mucinous metaplasia will display bland, mucinous epithelium; however, small epithelial tufts and papillae may be present. Nuclear atypia and complex architecture should be absent

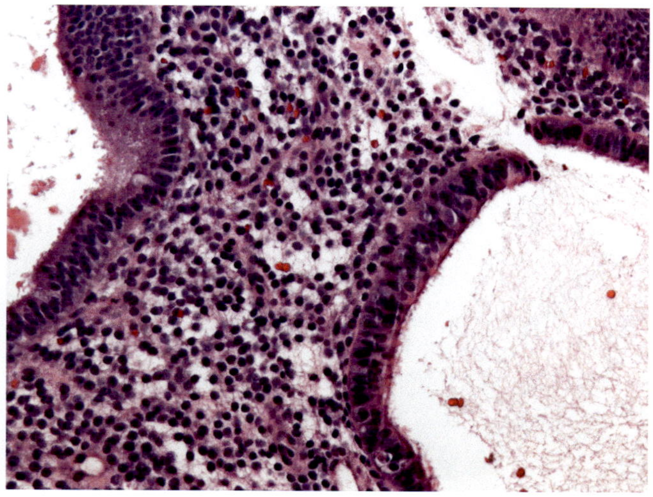

Fig. 17.24 Tubal metaplasia is frequently encountered in states of excess estrogenic stimulation. Close inspection of the epithelium will reveal ciliated and secretory tubal epithelial cells

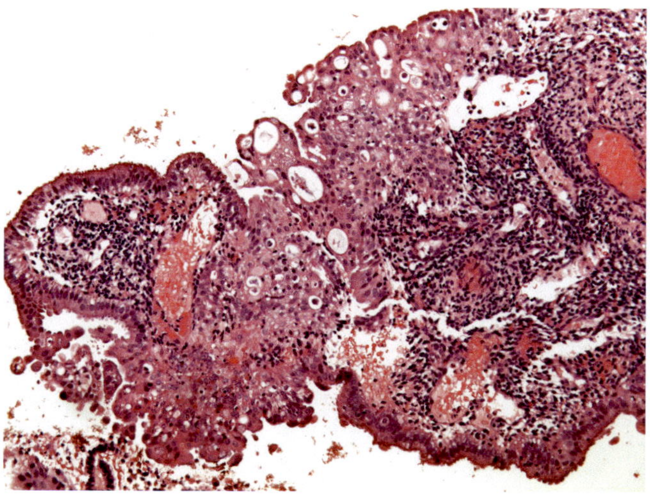

Fig. 17.23 Complex mucinous metaplasia often consists of sheets and cribriform growth of mucinous epithelium. Nuclear atypia may be present. This should be treated as analogous to EIN/AH

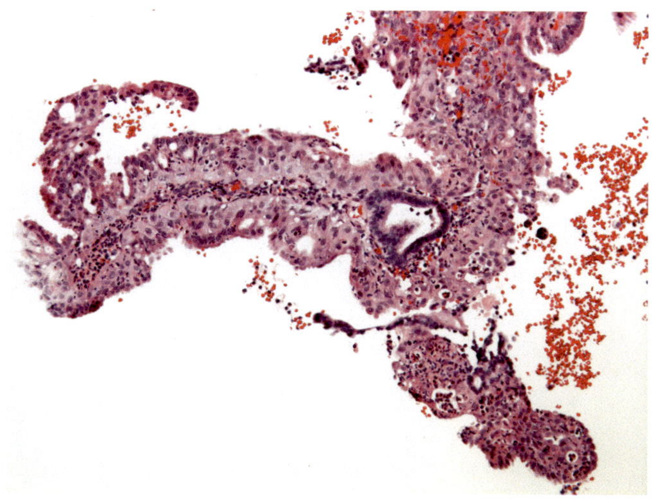

Fig. 17.25 Eosinophilic, syncytial (and sometimes papillary) metaplasia is often associated with inflammatory endometrial conditions and stromal breakdown. The presence of a brisk neutrophilic infiltrate is a helpful clue

glands in the setting of anovulatory endometrium/disordered proliferative endometrium. Rarely, EIN/AH or even "ciliated carcinomas" may be identified, but these lesions are defined by their architectural complexity and not by the presence of cilia.

Papillary syncytial metaplasia has long been considered a type of metaplasia; however, our current understanding is that this entity represents an exuberant reparative process. In most cases the superficial epithelium is composed of large, eosinophilic cells and may contain a neutrophilic infiltrate (Fig. 17.25). In some cases the epithelium may form pseudopapillae or colonize underlying endometrial glands (Fig. 17.26). Mild to moderate nuclear atypia may be present, and mitotic figures should be rare. It is usually seen in conjunction with stromal breakdown and hemorrhage (Fig. 17.27). The differential diagnosis of this lesion often includes endometrioid, serous, or clear cell carcinoma. Malignancy may be suspected in older patients with a background of atrophy. PAX2 loss may be suggestive of an endometrioid malignancy, while mutant p53 staining and diffuse p16 positivity can help to identify serous carcinoma. It should be noted that occasional cases of reactive atypia may display strong p53 staining; therefore p16 and Ki-67 stains may be helpful additions when considering this differential [35]. In cases where hobnail-type epithelium is present, a diagnosis of clear cell carcinoma or Arias-Stella effect may be entertained. Often clear cell carcinoma can be excluded by the lack of architectural complexity, mitotic activity, and severe nuclear atypia.

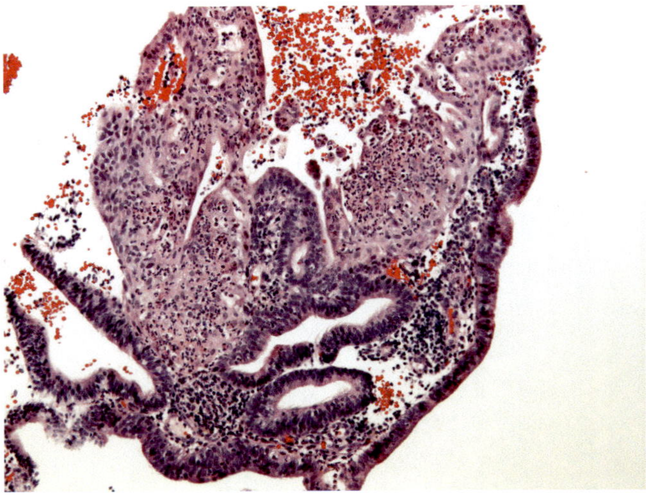

Fig. 17.26 Exuberant cases of eosinophilic metaplasia may colonize normal endometrial epithelium and even extend downward into endometrial glands

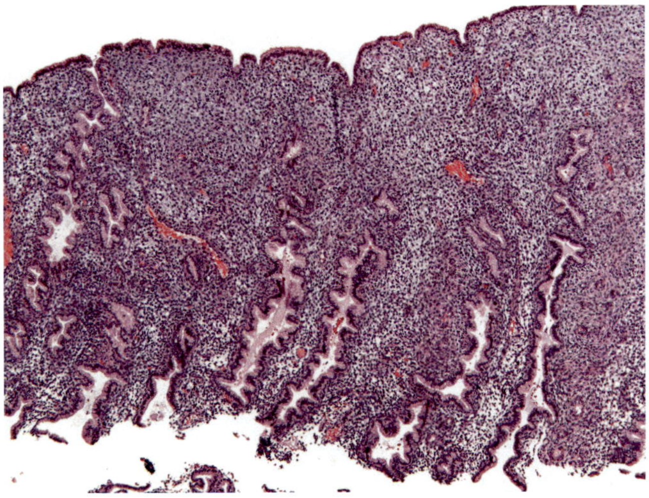

Fig. 17.28 Secretory endometrium often displays an orderly arrangement of glands at low magnification. Occasionally these glands may appear to line up, which is a clue to their benignity

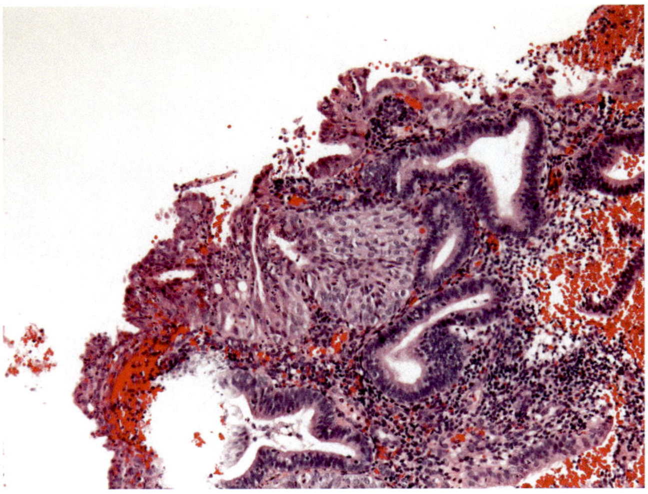

Fig. 17.27 Eosinophilic metaplasia often coexists with adjacent stromal hemorrhage and breakdown (upper center of image)

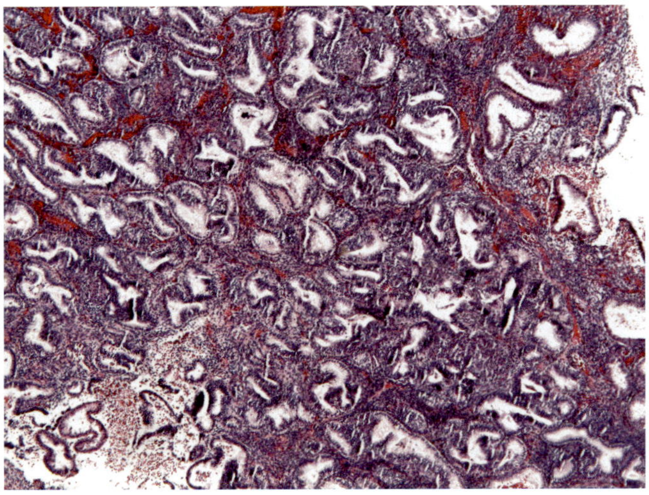

Fig. 17.29 So-called secretory EIN/AH displays a more haphazard arrangement of glands at low magnification

Secretory differentiation may be seen in both EIN/AH and low-grade adenocarcinomas. This state of altered differentiation is similar to that seen in normal secretory phase endometrium. Secretory endometrium may display some overlapping features with precancerous and cancerous endometrium, namely, glandular crowding and perceived glandular epithelial complexity (due to the torturous nature of the endometrial glands). At low-power magnification, secretory endometrium will display a more orderly and linear arrangement of glands than carcinoma with secretory differentiation (Fig. 17.28). Fortunately the diagnosis of secretory EIN/AH is rare, as it can be exceptionally challenging. In general, patients with secretory EIN/AH are premenopausal, with an average age of 45, and increased levels of progestin, whether it be from exogenous or endogenous sources [36]. Fortunately, these lesions have a greater tendency to regress when compared to traditional EIN/AH [36]. Glands in secretory EIN/AH tend to be larger, more complex, and haphazardly arranged than the surrounding normal secretory glands (Fig. 17.29). The cells will have abundant, vacuolated cytoplasm, a ruffled apical surface, and round vesicular nuclei (Fig. 17.30) [36, 37]. Unfortunately, these cytologic features are bland and not readily recognized as atypical; therefore low-power recognition of cytologic and architectural demarcation of the precancerous lesion is crucial. While the vast majority of EIN/AH arises in a background of proliferative pattern endometrium, there are rare cases that arise in a secretory background. These lesions will lack the luminal complexity of secretory EIN/AH and more closely resemble proliferative glands, which allow them to be easily identified at scanning magnification.

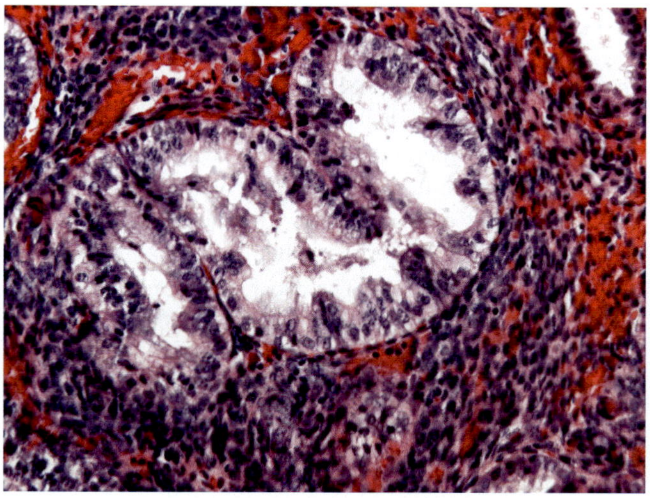

Fig. 17.30 The glandular epithelium of secretory EIN/AH often displays a ruffled border with abundant, vacuolated cytoplasm. The nuclei will be round and vesicular and typically lack significant atypia

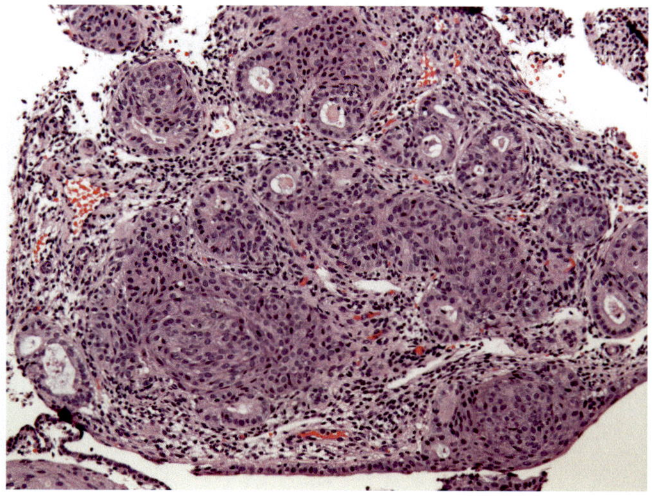

Fig. 17.31 Progestin-treated EIN/AH. Note the bland glandular epithelium and the persistence of morular metaplasia. The endometrial stroma is pseudo-decidualized

Progestin Effect

Surgical resection is the most common method of treatment of EIN/AH; however, a sizable number of patients opt for medical management with progestins. This may be due to a desire to maintain fertility, or because the patient is a poor surgical candidate. Progestins may be given continuously, in the form of intrauterine devices, or as interrupted therapy that allows for progestin withdrawal endometrial shedding. Regardless of the modality, routine surveillance biopsies of the endometrium (preferably after cessation of progestins and a withdrawal shed) necessitate familiarity with the features of progestin-treated EIN/AH. Correct interpretation of these specimens is critical to determine if the treatment is effective [38].

The most notable effect of exogenous progestins is pseudo-decidualization of the stroma, typically with a concurrent atrophy of the glandular component. The stromal cells appear eosinophilic and plump, while endometrial glands will decrease in size and density (Fig. 17.31). This decrease in glandular density may drive precancerous lesions below the normal threshold needed to trigger a diagnosis of EIN/AH (i.e.,~55% glands). The background glandular epithelium may range from atrophic to hypersecretory (Arias-Stella effect). Frequently the precancerous glands undergo metaplastic changes, most commonly consisting of eosinophilic and mucinous metaplasia (Fig. 17.32). Mitotic figures may be rare to absent. Squamous morules are typically not effected by progestin administration and may be present in otherwise unremarkable glands, serving as a histologic clue to the presence of progestin-treated EIN/AH (Fig. 17.33).

When evaluating biopsies from patients with known EIN/AH being treated with progestins, it is important to compare current and previous samples. Many patients may show a spectrum of response to progestin therapy, and it is critical to relay the presence of potentially non-responsive lesions to the treating physician [39]. In cases where no lesional glands are identified, a statement stating that no EIN/AH is present in the sample is appropriate; however, if atypical glands or frank EIN/AH is present, a diagnosis of "residual EIN/AH (with/without) progestin effect" is warranted. Avoid using the term "treated EIN/AH" in these cases, as it may falsely give the impression that the patient is cured.

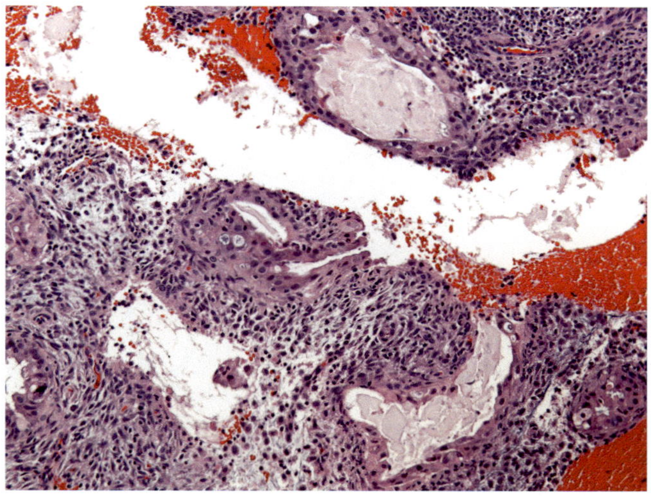

Fig. 17.32 Eosinophilic and mucinous metaplasia in an EIN/AH that has been treated with progestins

Sub-diagnostic Lesions

On occasion, biopsy material may contain a focus of glands with crowding, altered cytology, or both that fails to meet the other criteria for EIN/AH. Commonly, this consists of a minute focus of crowded glands that appear different from the background endometrium, yet are not 1 mm in size, or are

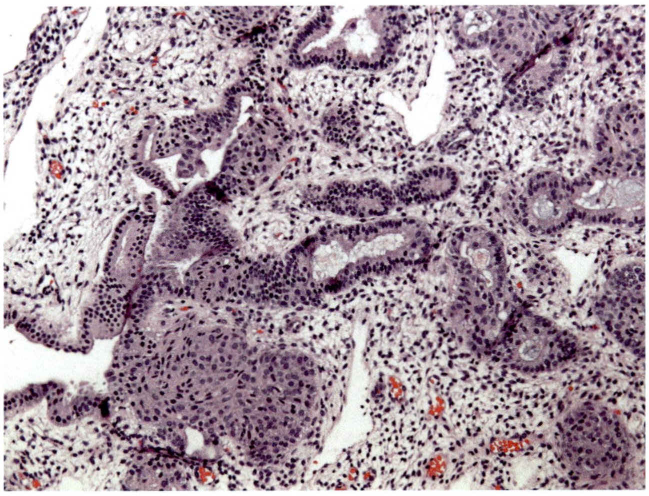

Fig. 17.33 Progestin-treated EIN/AH showing minimal glandular crowding. The presence of scattered squamous morules is a histologic clue to the presence of a precancerous lesion

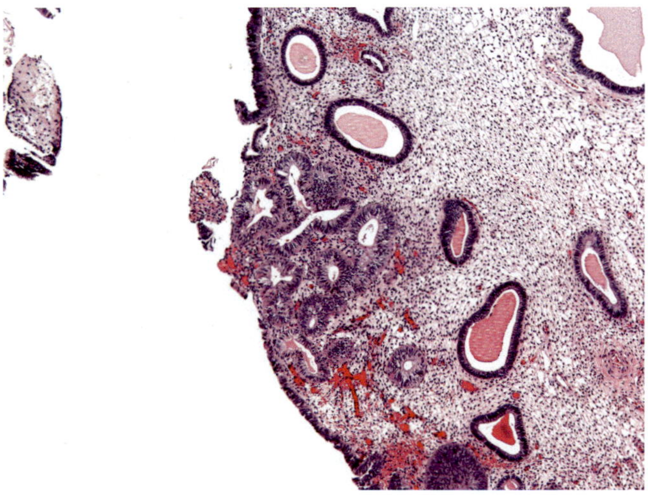

Fig. 17.34 A small area of crowded glands with cytologic demarcation. This focus measures slightly less than 1 mm and should be diagnosed descriptively with a recommendation of follow-up sampling

located at the edge of a tissue fragment (Fig. 17.34). When this occurs, the next best step is to order levels; however, if the lesion continues to be sub-diagnostic, then a descriptive diagnosis is appropriate. It is our practice to diagnose such lesions as "focal gland crowding (with/without) atypia" with a comment describing the features of the lesion and recommending follow-up in 2–3 (with atypia) or 6 (without atypia) months. These challenging lesions have been studied by Huang et al., who found that 33 of 143 (23%) of cases diagnosed as "gland crowding" contained a precancerous or cancerous lesion on follow-up [40]. It is worthwhile to note that these lesions are rare and are not felt to represent precursors to EIN/AH. Clear communication with the treating physician and recommendation of additional sampling is necessary to prevent the patient from being lost to follow-up.

17.1.1.10 Genetic Profile and Immunohistochemistry

The pathogenesis of EIN/AH, as well as its histologic features, demonstrates a step forward in our understanding of the endometrial hyperplasia/carcinoma sequence. EIN/AH is the histologic manifestation of underlying genetic aberrations, which not only allows us to better understand how these lesions form and progress, but utilize ancillary testing to aid in their diagnosis. The most commonly associated defects lie in *PTEN* and *PAX2* [8]. Corresponding immunohistochemical markers exist for both, and both have been shown to be potentially useful in a clinical setting.

PTEN

PTEN is a tumor suppressor gene that functions to regulate the cell cycle in the endometrium. It is expressed in normal endometrium in both a nuclear and cytoplasmic pattern. Normal endometrium may display patchy staining, with inactivation seen in up to 49% of glands. There is an increasing trend of inactivation seen in EIN/AH (44–63%) and adenocarcinoma (68–83%) [8, 41, 42]. Obviously inactivation of *PTEN* is a common event in the endometrium, and its detrimental effects are mitigated by menstrual shedding. This mechanism provides a regular shedding of damaged epithelium and helps to explain why anovulation is a risk factor for subsequent carcinoma. The diagnostic utility of *PTEN* is severely hampered by the frequency of inactivation seen in normal endometrium. Additionally, there are many technical and interpretative (nuclear and cytoplasmic staining) issues associated with *PTEN* use, which explains its limited role in a clinical setting.

PAX2

PAX2 is a gene that plays an important role in the embryonic development of the Mullerian and urogenital systems. It encodes a nuclear transcription factor, which is present in normal endometrium. Immunohistochemistry demonstrates nuclear staining in normal endometrial glands. Similar to *PTEN*, *PAX2* does show loss in normal endometrium (36%), EIN/AH (71%), and carcinoma (77%) as demonstrated by Monte et al. [8]. Apparent from the results of their work is that a major mechanism of the development of EIN/AH is the co-localization of *PAX2* and *PTEN* within the same endometrial glands [8]. This "dual hit" is thought to be the cause for the majority of sporadic endometrioid adenocarcinomas. As a diagnostic antibody, *PAX2* is much more robust and easy to interpret due to its nuclear staining pattern.

A myriad of papers have sought to describe the relationship between *PAX2* loss, the immunohistochemical findings, and the diagnosis of EIN/AH [8–10, 37, 43]. The general consensus is that in the right clinical setting, *PAX2* can be used to support a suspicion of EIN/AH. *PAX2* has been found to be lost in the majority of EIN/AH, which can be used to highlight suspicious foci (Fig. 17.35). Its most useful

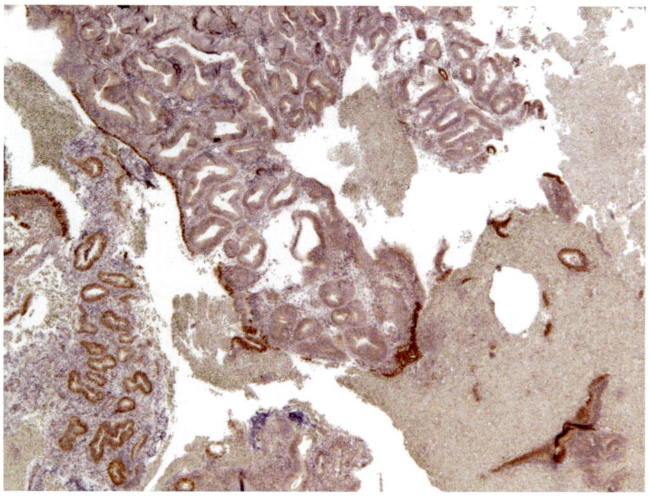

Fig. 17.35 A focus of crowded endometrial glands with *PAX2* loss. This cluster of glands was suspicious for EIN/AH on routine staining. Note the presence of a single "orphan" background gland in the upper right portion of this image

application is realized in fragmented samples, overrun EIN/AH, endometrial polyps, and secretory backgrounds (Fig. 17.36a–d) [10]. It has also been suggested that *PAX2* staining of precancerous lesions may be helpful in a training scenario to highlight subtle lesions and their H&E counterparts [10]. Interestingly, Joiner et al. described an uncommon, yet apparently altered, pattern of *PAX2* expression that consisted of increased intensity of the abnormal glands when compared to the background [9]. The significance of this pattern of staining has yet to be elucidated. It should be emphasized that care should be used when employing *PAX2* in a clinical setting as up to one-third of glands may be negative; however, multiple studies have shown that when correlated with suspicious H&E findings, loss of *PAX2* can be a valuable diagnostic aid.

17.1.1.11 Management and Prognosis

Most commonly, the standard treatment approach to a diagnosis of EIN/AH is total abdominal hysterectomy with

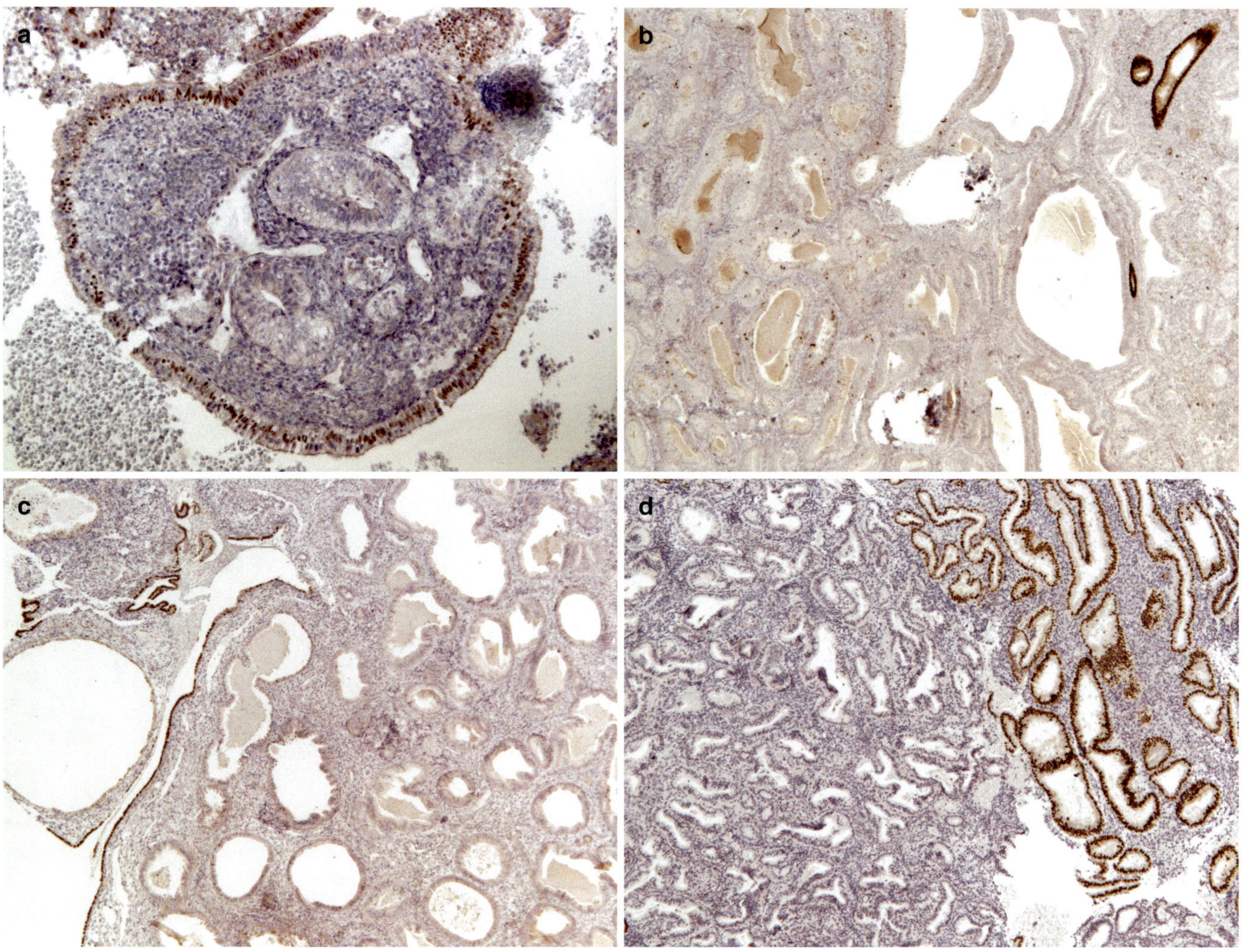

Fig. 17.36 Loss of *PAX2* by immunohistochemistry may be a helpful adjunct test in difficult cases. *PAX2* loss is most helpful in (**a**) small, suspicious lesions, (**b**) overrun lesions with scant background, (**c**) endometrial polyps, and (**d**) secretory backgrounds

bilateral salpingo-oophorectomy. Hormonal therapy with progestins remains a treatment option in patients who are poor surgical candidates, who desire to attempt to preserve fertility, or who are suspected of having small lesions or lesions limited to polyps (which may have been removed via polypectomy). One-third of patients with EIN/AH will suffer from occult/concurrent endometrioid adenocarcinoma within 1 year's time, and patients carry a 45-fold increase in risk of developing low-grade adenocarcinoma compared to those without EIN/AH [24, 25]. Increased risk of cancer aside, EIN/AH, represents a precancerous lesion and therefore the overall prognosis is excellent.

17.1.2 Endometrial Serous Precancer

Endometrial serous carcinomas (ESC) represent 10% of endometrial carcinomas but account for almost 40% of all patient mortality associated with uterine corpus cancer [44]. However, surgically staged patients with uterine corpus-confined ESC have relatively favorable outcomes [45–49], which highlights the significance of identifying the disease at an early stage, or more ideally, identifying it prior to its evolution into a true cancer with metastatic potential. Serous endometrial intraepithelial carcinoma (SEIC) has historically been considered the precancerous lesion of ESC, primarily based on its frequent association with conventional ESC, their shared cytological and immunophenotypical features, and its noninvasive growth pattern [48–51]. However, it is also well recognized that SEIC is not uncommonly associated with extrauterine, potentially fatal, tumor deposits that show the same morphological, immunophenotypical, and molecular properties as the intrauterine lesions from which they presumably originated [52–55]. Furthermore, overtly invasive ESC may show intraepithelial growth patterns outside of the uterine corpus, including in the endocervix, fallopian tube, and ovary, which limits the significance of intraepithelial growth patterns as an indicator of pre-invasiveness when such patterns are identified in the endometrium [48, 56]. For these reasons, SEIC is no longer considered a precancerous lesion, and current recommendations are for patients diagnosed with SEIC in a biopsy or curettage to undergo a surgical management that is similar in extent to their counterparts with the conventionally invasive disease [57].

The concept of endometrial glandular dysplasia (EmGD) as the most likely precancerous lesion to ESC was proposed in 2004 by Zheng et al. [58]. Several subsequent reports [58–64] have, in total, bolstered the conclusion that EmGD fulfils the definitional requirements of a precancer as established at a 2006 National Cancer Institute Consensus conference on the subject [65]. EmGD lesions likely reflect morphologic manifestations of key molecular events in endometrial serous carcinogenesis [66]. Clinicopathologic features of EmGD are described below.

17.1.2.1 Endometrial Glandular Dysplasia

EmGD was originally identified based on a detailed examination of the background endometrium in cases of SEIC, ESC, and endometrioid carcinoma [67]. Atypical glandular lesions that were ultimately classified as EmGD were identified 53% of the ESC cases and 1.7% of the endometrioid carcinoma cases [67]. As such, they have a significantly stronger association with the serous (compared to the endometrioid) carcinoma histotype. The average age of the patients with an EmGD lesion was 65 years (range 57–79) [67].

Pathologic Findings

EmGD lesions are not grossly evident. By definition, EmGD are endometrial glands or surface epithelia that show a degree of nuclear atypia that falls short of the level of anaplasia that is characteristic of SEIC or ESC but which are still notably distinct at the morphologic level from the background resting endometrium in which they are identified. Morphologic features are further described below:

- Nuclear features:
  - Shape: Nuclei of EmGD cells may be oval, round, or elongated (Figs. 17.37, 17.38, 17.39, and 17.40).
  - Size: Nuclei of EmGD cells are approximately 1.5–2-fold larger when compared to background resting endometrium; nuclei of SEIC are usually two- to four-fold larger.
  - Chromatin: Nuclei of EmGD cells may show hyperchromasia or an open chromatin pattern. However,

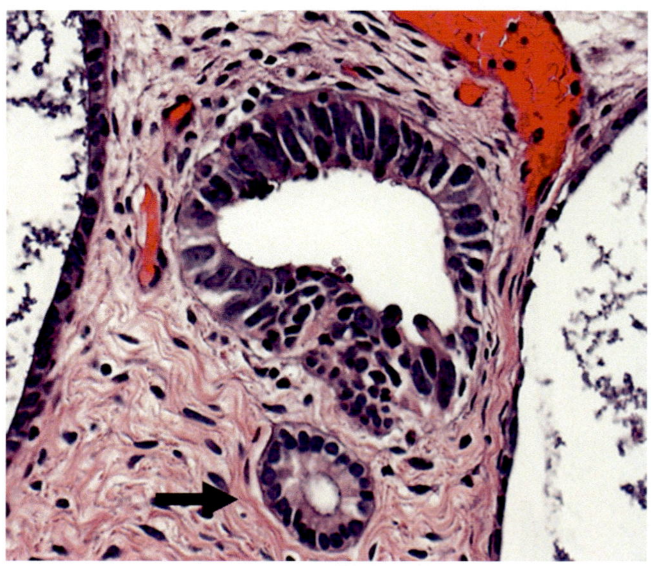

Fig. 17.37 Endometrial glandular dysplasia (EmGD) in a glandular pattern; compare nuclear size of constituent cells to those of the background endometrial resting/inactive epithelium (arrow)

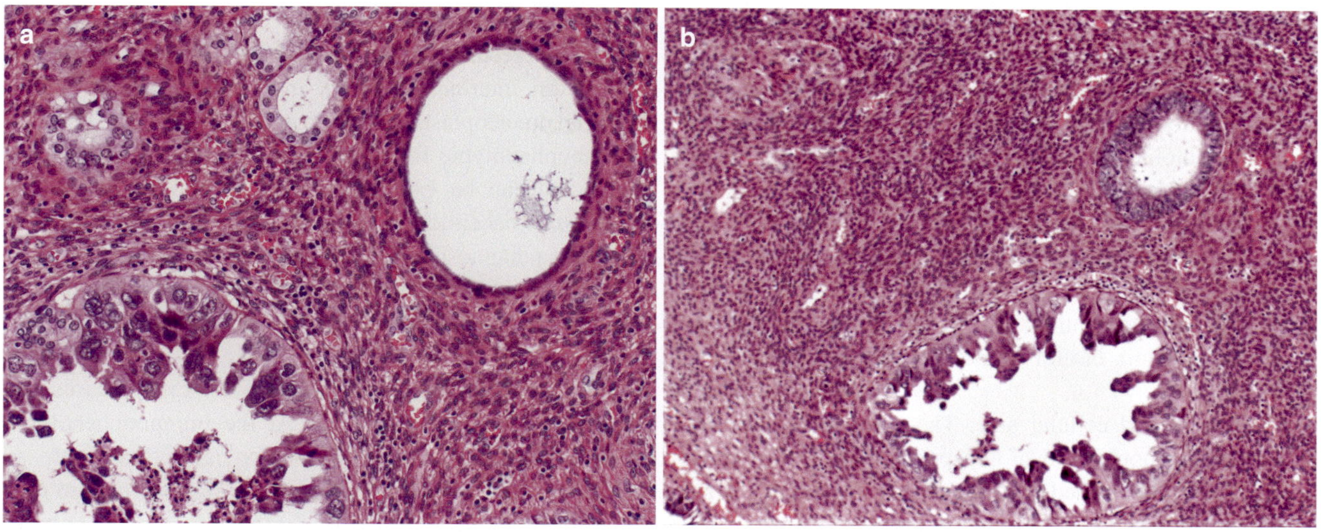

Fig. 17.38 Endometrial glandular dysplasia (EmGD) in a glandular pattern; (**a**) compare nuclear size of constituent cells to those of the background endometrial resting/inactive epithelium (right field) and serous EIC (lower field). This example of EmGD is comprised of glands with vaguely eosinophilic cytoplasm. (**b**) The EmGD gland (upper field) is atypical but less anaplastic than the glands of serous EIC (lower field)

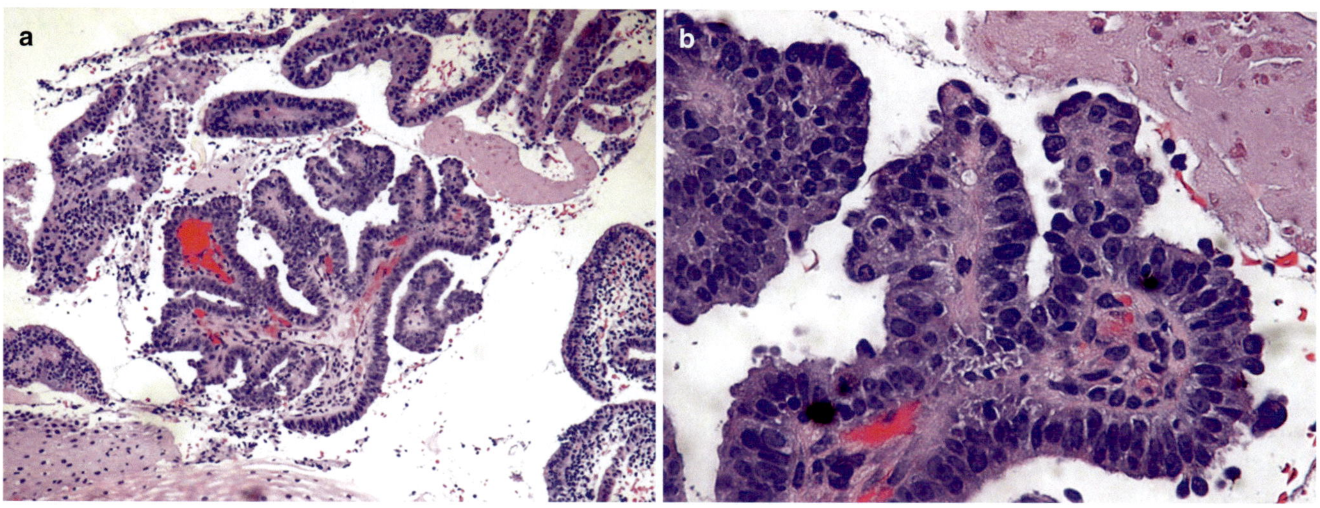

Fig. 17.39 Endometrial glandular dysplasia (EmGD) with papillary architecture. (**a**) Low-power magnification; (**b**) High-power magnification. Note the moderate nuclear atypia

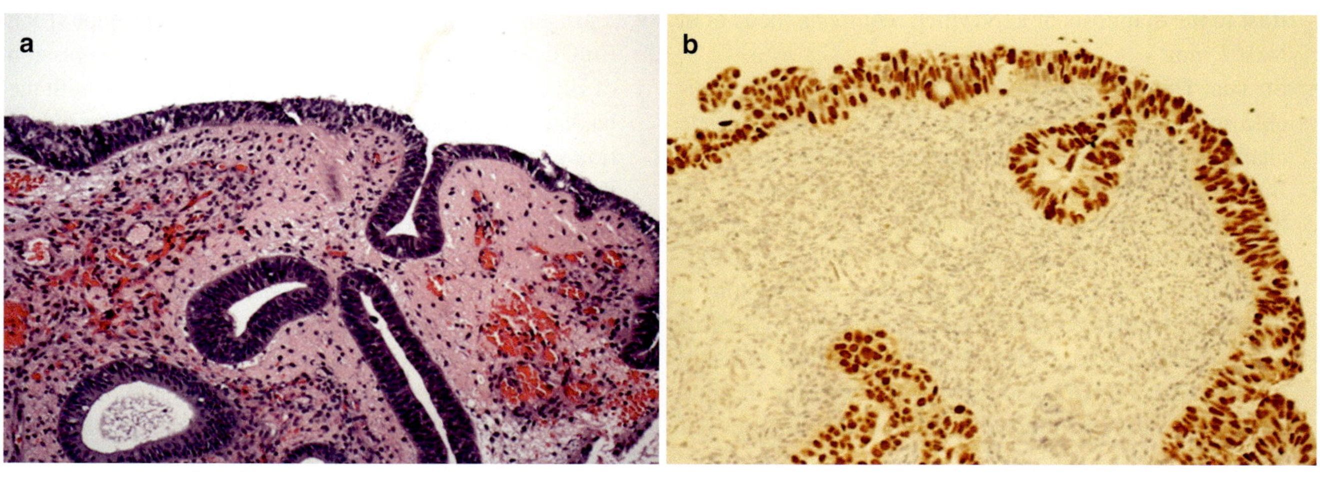

Fig. 17.40 Endometrial glandular dysplasia (EmGD) in a flat pattern involving the endometrial surface epithelia (**a**) and showing diffuse immunoreacticity for the p53 protein (**b**)

  when hyperchromatic, the level of hyperchromasia is less than what is seen in SEIC or ESC cells.
  - Nucleoli: Nucleoli of EmGD cells are visible at intermediate magnification, as compared with the overt nucleolomegaly (low-power visible macronucleoli) that is typical of SEIC or ESC.
  - Polarity: EmGD cells may show complete or partial loss of nuclear polarity, but this finding is not necessarily present.
  - Nuclear stratification: EmGD glands may show nuclear stratification, but this is rarely more than three layers thick.
- Cytoplasm and cellular size: The cytoplasm of EmGD may be eosinophilic or of nonspecific tincture. The combination of increased cytoplasm and increased nuclear size results in cells that are on average approximately two- to threefold greater than the cells of resting endometrium, as compared with SEIC cells, which are usually about four to five times larger.
- Mitotic figures and apoptotic bodies: EmGD glands typically do not show readily appreciable mitotic figures or apoptotic bodies; the presence of an isolated mitotic figure or apoptotic body does not exclude a diagnosis of EmGD.
- Architecture and topography: Foci of EmGD are usually in the form of glands. However, EmGD may also be configured in flat epithelial segments, or as small papillary intraglandular protrusions, each with thin fibrovascular cores (Figs. 17.37, 17.38, 17.39, and 17.40).
- Size: EmGD may be localized or extensive. Glands are typically scattered and non-confluent. When multifocal, it is very uncommon for the linear length of any individual focus to exceed 2 mm in greatest dimension. EmGD not uncommonly involves an endometrial polyp and may similarly involve the background endometrium within the same patient. Overall, there is no size limitation to qualify the diagnosis of EmGD, which is in contrast to the diagnosis of EIN which requires a focus of at least 1 mm.
- Stroma: The stroma around EmGD epithelia may be variable and is largely nonspecific. Overtly desmoplastic changes attributable to EmGD glands are not seen.
- Background endometrium: The functional state of the background endometrium is largely dependent on the hormonal state of an individual patient. The typical endometrium in which EmGD is identified is atrophic or weakly proliferative. Nonetheless, approximately 40% of patients with ESC or SEIC have a non-atrophic endometrial background [67], and this should be borne in mind when the aforementioned morphologic features of EmGD in a given case are being compared to the background endometrium.

Immunophenotype of EmGD

EmGD is presumed to represent a morphologic manifestation of an intermediate point in the neoplastic evolution between nonneoplastic endometrium and SEIC. The reported immunophenotypic features of EmGD reflect this intermediacy and can be exploited for diagnostic purposes. The immunohistochemical markers found to be most useful in reaching a diagnosis of EmGD are outlined below. The diagnostic value of each marker is maximized when used in combination with other markers:

- p53: As was previously noted, 43% of EmGD cases display a *TP53* mutation [60]. At the immunophenotypic level, lesions that are morphologically classifiable as EmGD have shown either a patchy staining pattern or a diffuse staining pattern. In the patchy staining pattern, more than half of the cells in an EmGD gland show strong and intense nuclear staining. This staining pattern will strike the observer as decidedly above the weak patchy staining that is characteristic of the wild-type pattern. The molecular correlates to this staining pattern are yet to be defined. In the diffuse staining pattern, the pattern of overexpression is similar to what is typically observed in SEIC and is indicative of a *TP53* mutation (Fig. 17.40b).
- Ki-67 (MIB-1): EmGD usually demonstrates a higher proliferative index than the background resting endometrium in which it is identified [67]. As such, the use of Ki67 is highly dependent on this comparison to the background endometrium since hormone levels of individual patients may vary. In those scenarios in which the background endometrium is of a proliferative pattern (or is hyperplastic), this marker is less useful.
- IMP3: IMP3 is frequently positive in ESC/SEIC and has similarly been found to be positive in EmGD [68]. The primary limitation of this marker regarding the diagnosis of EmGD is its low sensitivity. As with the other markers, IMP3 should be combined with others and should not be used in isolation.
- Estrogen receptor (ER) and progesterone receptor (PR): EmGD epithelia usually show a reduction in expression of ER and PR with more loss of PR as compared with the background glands [67], Fig. 17.41. This relative reduction encompasses both the intensity and extent of staining. As with Ki67, hormone receptors are less useful if the background endometrium is proliferative or hyperplastic.
- p16: p16 is diffusely immunoreactive in EmGD lesions, whereas background resting endometrium typically displays "mosaic" or patchy staining pattern for p16. Of note, metaplastic lesions, including papillary syncytial metaplasia and tubal metaplasia, are frequently immunoreactive for p16 [32, 35, 69]. As such, when deployed in the diagnosis of EmGD, p16 should be combined with other markers.

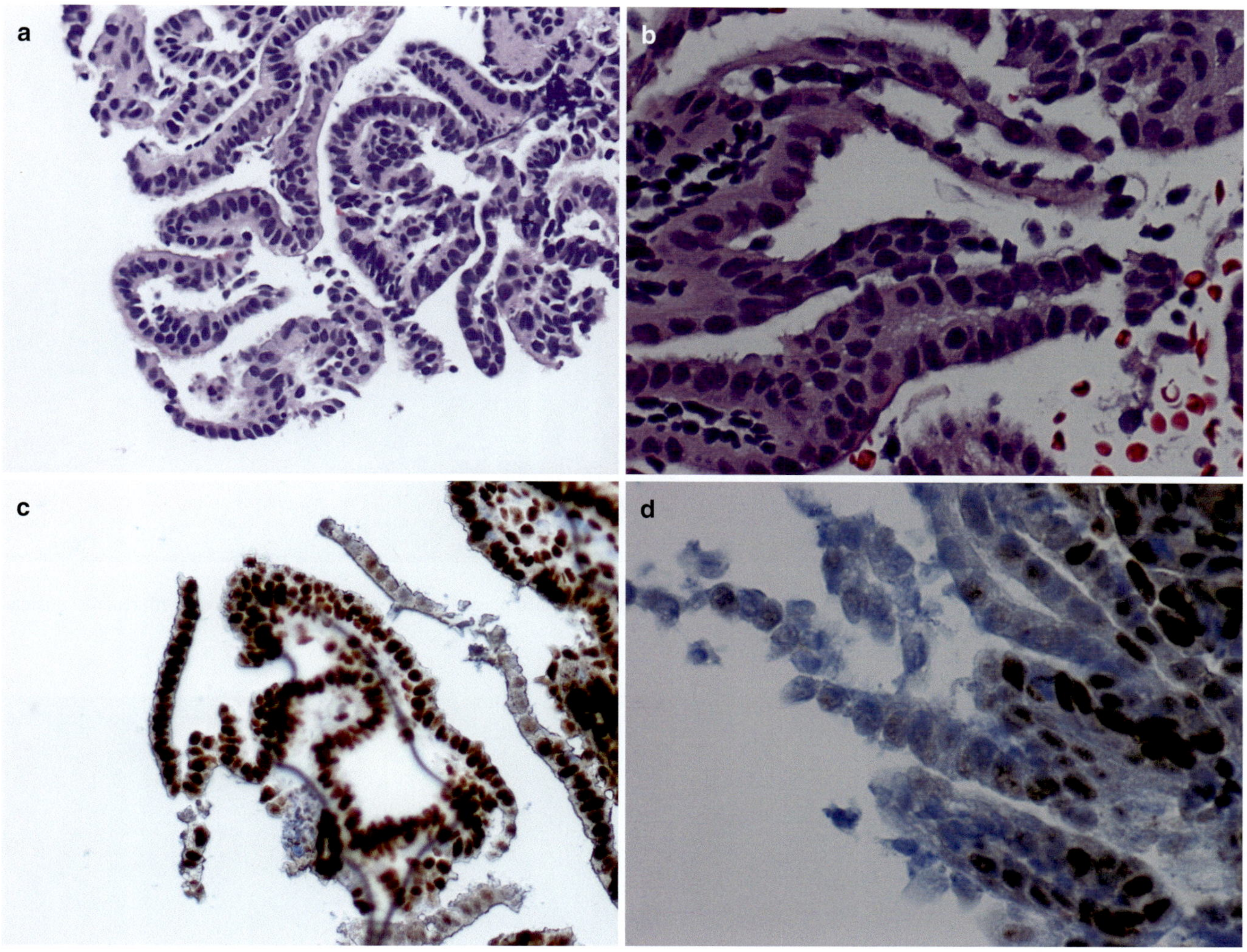

Fig. 17.41 Endometrial glandular dysplasia in a biopsy. In such cases with subtle atypia (**a**, **b**), immunohistochemistry for p53 (aberrant expression pattern) (**c**) and PR (reduction to loss of expression) (**d**) may be diagnostically useful

Molecular-Genetic Profile

Similar to ESC and SEIC, mutations of the *TP53* gene appear to play a significant role in the development of EmGD. In a previous analysis, Jia et al. found *TP53* mutations to be present in 43% of EmGD, compared with 0% in resting endometrium, 72% in SEIC, and 96% in ESC [60]. Most of the analyzed uteri showed at least one identical *TP53* mutant among lesions of EmGD, SEIC, and/or ESC [60]. In a separate analysis, loss of heterozygosity at the chromosomal region for *TP53* and 1p was noted in 31% and 18% of EmGD, respectively, compared to 78% and 47% of cancerous areas within the same uteri [58]. *TP53* gene homologue Trp53 knockout mice model clearly demonstrated lesions with characteristic features of EmGD, SEIC, and ESC [70]. These findings indicate that not all lesions that are morphologically recognizable as EmGD have a *TP53* mutation, and the frequency of *TP53* mutations in EmGD is notably lower than is typical of SEIC or ESC. It is unclear whether *TP53* wild-type and *TP53*-mutant cases of EmGD have differential patterns of regression, persistence, or progression. Other phenotypic alterations that have been demonstrated in EmGD include increased expression (relative to background endometrium) of IMP3, p16, and Nrf2, among others [66, 68, 71].

Differential Diagnosis

The differential diagnosis for EmGD includes reactive, reparative, and metaplastic changes in benign endometrium and SEIC (Figs. 17.42, 17.43, 17.44, 17.45, 17.46, and 17.47).

- Reactive, metaplastic, and reparative changes of the benign endometrium: Benign endometrium may show a variety of reactive, metaplastic, and reparative changes that may be related to bleeding, instrumentation, or unknown factors. The potential morphologic spectrum for these changes is wide and may include mild to moderate atypia. In general, the keys to their recognition include an awareness of the full morphologic spectrum of such

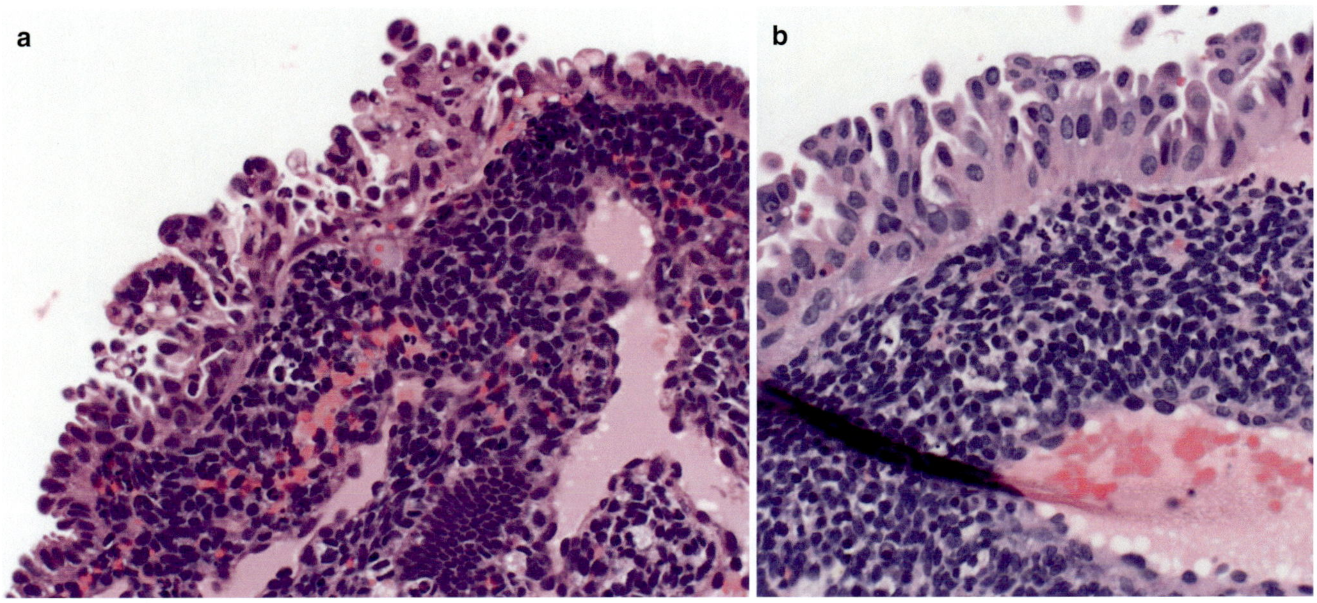

Fig. 17.42 Differential diagnosis of EmGD and serous EIC: papillary syncytial metaplasia (**a** - low power, **b** - high power) with reactive nuclear changes; note associated stromal breakdown

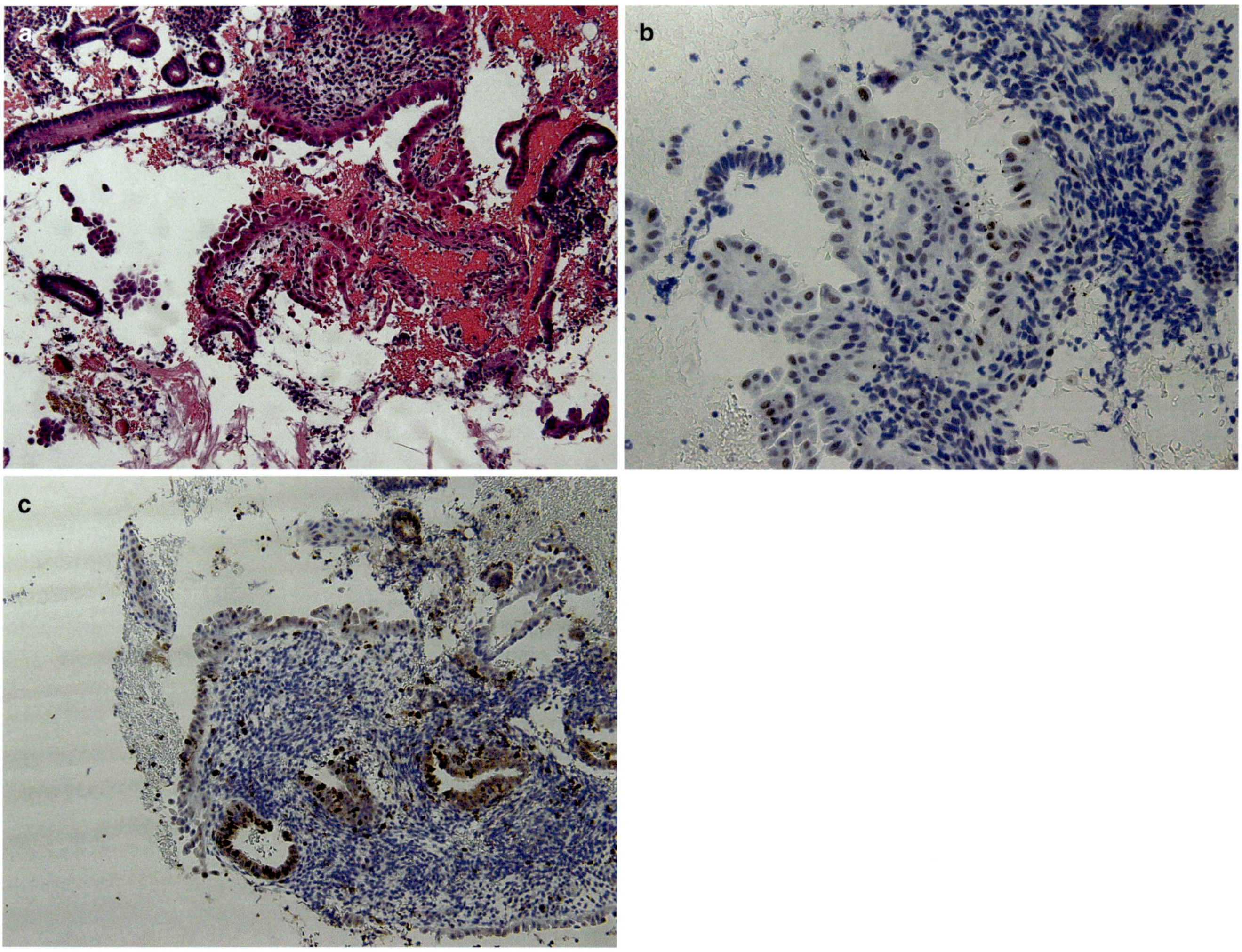

Fig. 17.43 Differential diagnosis of EmGD: metaplastic changes, including eosinophilic and hobnail change (**a**); note p53 wild-type staining pattern (**b**) and low proliferative index (**c**)

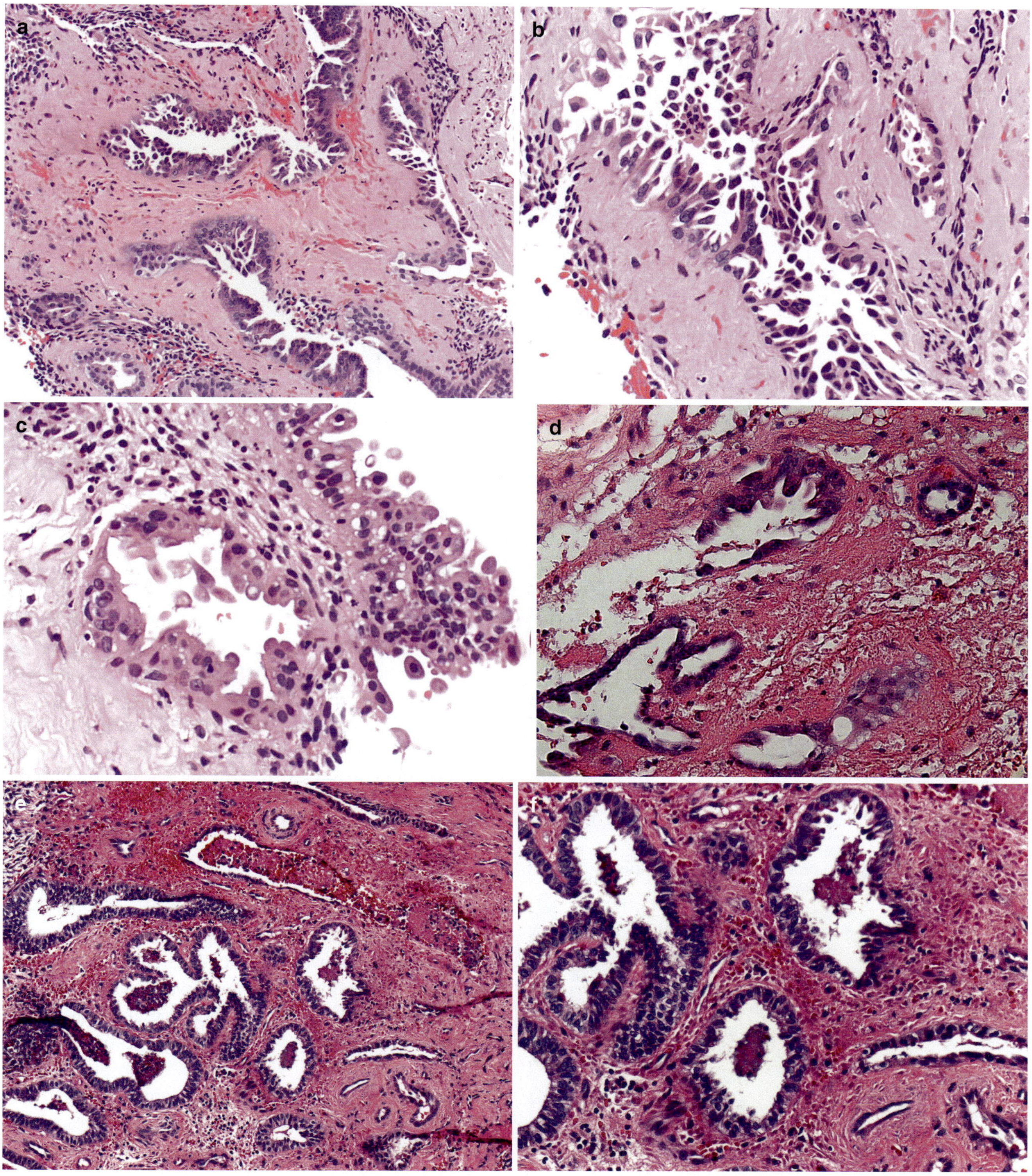

Fig. 17.44 The differential diagnosis for both EmGD and serous EIC includes epithelial changes associated with infarction in endometrial polyps. These may include florid pseudopapillary changes (**a**, **b**) and nuclear atypia (**c**–**f**)

changes [32, 72], morphology of the background in which the lesion is being identified, and the clinical context. Changes associated with prior instrumentation may include hyperchromasia and hobnail change (Fig. 17.47). The clinical history, as well as other morphologic changes associated with aforementioned instrumentation, will have the most diagnostic value, even prior to immunohistochemistry. Reactive changes associated with bleeding typically include eosinophilic and papillary syncytial change. Both may show nuclear enlargement and a variety

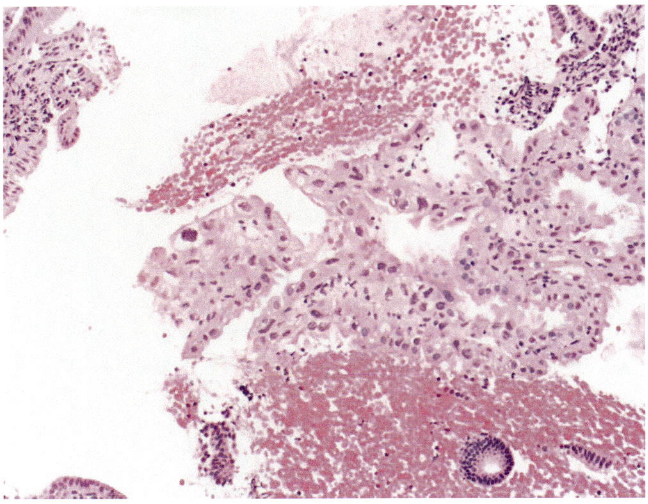

Fig. 17.45 Atypical changes in epithelium with eosinophilic and ciliated change, as well degenerative nuclear atypia

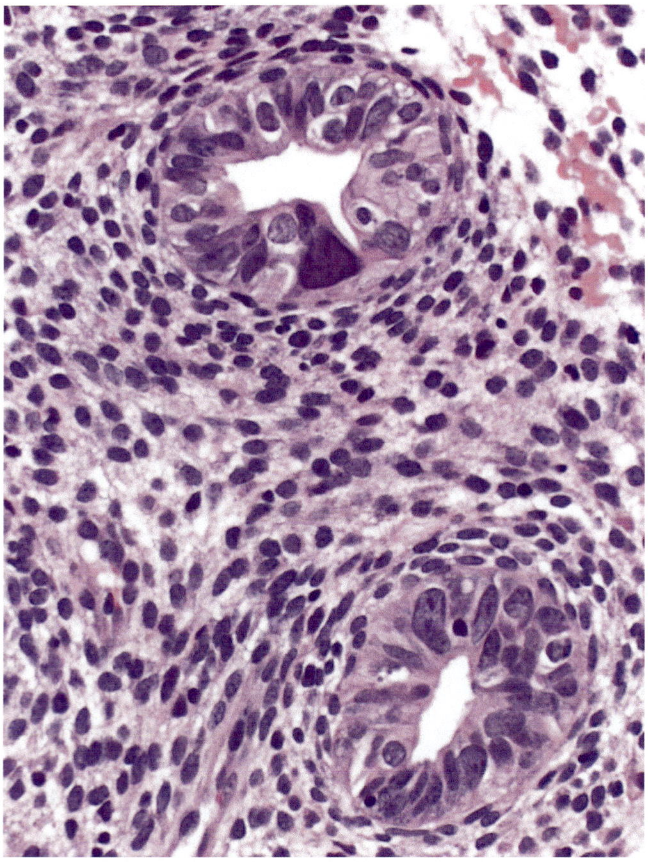

Fig. 17.46 Significant nuclear enlargement may be associated with exposure to cytotoxic chemotherapy. The involved nuclei are typically sporadic (non-diffuse)

of other mild atypical changes that most likely have a degenerative basis [73, 74]. Unlike EmGD, they show distinctive cytoplasmic syncytia, and their papillation is devoid of fibrovascular cores. Furthermore, these reactive

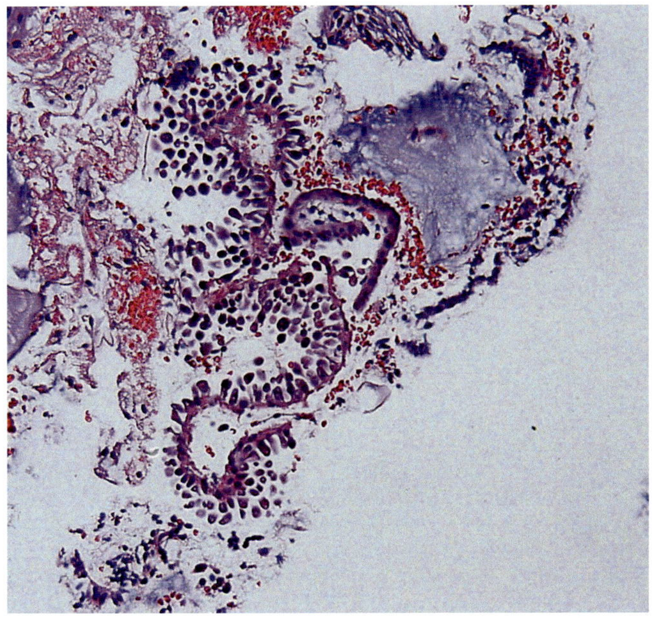

Fig. 17.47 Reactive hobnail change in a postmenopausal patient

changes are typically localized surface processes that are associated with breakdown and blood (Fig. 17.42). Immunohistochemically, they display a low proliferative index [73, 74], decreased expression of ER [35], and are non-immunoreactive for IMP3. p53 should be used with caution in this context, since epithelia of syncytial change may show increased p53 staining (albeit still at the wild-type level) [35]. Additionally, as was previously noted, these lesions may be p16 diffusely positive [35]. Some forms of tubal metaplasia show reactive form of nuclear atypia [75]. The changes may include pleomorphic, hyperchromatic, and enlarged nuclei with nucleolomegaly and increased nuclear to cytoplasmic ratios [75], Fig. 17.45. Paradoxically, these changes, which are also p16-immunoreactive, are more pronounced and atypical than would be allowable in EmGD, are typically in morphologic continuity with more conventional tubal metaplasia, and display a p53 and Ki-67 immunophenotype that is more consistent with background resting endometrium than EmGD [75]. Finally, significantly pleomorphic nuclei may be seen in the endometrium of patients with exposure to cytotoxic chemotherapy (Fig. 17.46). In the few reported cases, the pleomorphic nuclei have tended to be sporadic within individual glands and within the endometrium. Radiation-associated changes tend to be more diffuse.

- Endometrial polyps: The surface or body of an endometrial polyp may be involved by EmGD, and careful assessment of the glands of endometrial polyps is always warranted, especially in the postmenopausal patient population [76]. Nevertheless, as with non-polypoid endometrium, most alterations that stand out from the background

Table 17.2 Histopathological features of resting endometrium, EmGD and SEIC

	Resting endometrium[a]	EmGD	SEIC
Size	Normal	Two- to threefold-enlarged	Four- to fivefold-enlarged
Polarity of cells	Intact	Partial loss	Loss
Cytoplasm	Normal	Increased	Abundant
Nuclear features			
Size	Normal	1.5–2-fold-enlarged	2–4-fold-enlarged
Stratification	No	Present	Present
Hyperchromasia	Mild	Mild to moderate	Moderate to severe
Chromatin	Even distributed	Fine or granular	Coarse
Shape	Low columnar	Elongated/pencil shape; oval or round	Irregular
Nucleoli	Conspicuous	Inconspicuous	Prominent, like ESC
Mitotic figures	No	Occasional	Often
Apoptotic bodies	No	Often	Brisk
Growth pattern			
Surface	Nonspecific	Often	Often
Single gland	Nonspecific	Often	Often
Glandular clusters	No	Maybe present	Maybe present
Cribriforming	No	No	Maybe present
Polyp involvement	Occasional	Often	Often
Background endometrium	Resting endometrium[a]	Resting endometrium[a]	Resting endometrium[a]

[a]Resting endometrium including atrophic endometrium, weakly proliferative endometrium, and proliferative endometrium

in polyps are reactive in nature. Infarcted polyps may show a particularly distinctive spectrum of alterations that most likely represent exuberant iterations of the aforementioned reactive and metaplastic changes. These include a distinct intraglandular pseudopapillation, two- to threefold variation in nuclear size and/or shape, cellular syncytia, vesicular chromatin greater than background glands, and hobnail, clear, and eosinophilic cells [77] (Fig. 17.44). These are most easily recognized by paying careful attention to the background of hyalinization and infarction and any morphologic features that are diagnostic of metaplasia and by their p53 wild-type, Ki67-low immunophenotypic profile.

- SEIC: EmGD and SEIC are distinguished primarily based on the level of atypia. By definition, the atypia of SEIC is severe and is identical to the atypia of ESC. EmGD, by definition, does not show that level of atypia (Fig. 17.38). Similarly, SEIC displays brisk mitotic activity, whereas in EmGD, mitotic figures are inconspicuous. The morphologic features of EmGD, SEIC, and resting endometrium are compared and contrasted in Table 17.2.

Prognosis and Treatment

There are no published studies of patients diagnosed with EmGD in a biopsy or curettage and who were longitudinally followed without intervention. This may be related to the comparative rarity of the entity and/or the fact that immediate resection of the uterus is not an uncommon consideration on the rare occasions in which the diagnosis *is* made in isolation in a biopsy. Nonetheless, there is one retrospective analysis of endometrial biopsies that preceded an ultimate diagnosis of ESC [59]. In that analysis, the authors examined all available endometrial biopsies from a period of 3 months or earlier before hysterectomies that were ultimately diagnosed as bearing ESC or benign entities. Thirty-three percent of the biopsies from the ESC group had an EmGD lesion, as compared to 3.5% of the biopsies from the benign control group [59]. For the former group, the duration between the biopsy EmGD lesion and the hysterectomy ESC/SEIC tumor ranged from 16 to 98 months with an average of 33 months [59]. Although this retrospective analysis provided some valuable insights, the true regression, progression, and persistence rates of EmGD are unclear at present time. In our own experiences, isolated cases of EmGD (i.e., without SEIC and/or ESC) are not associated with extrauterine extension. This raises the possibility that an excisional or ablative intervention may be an effective way to prevent the development of ESC, although confirmatory studies are needed [63].

17.1.3 Putative Endometrial Clear Cell Precancer

17.1.3.1 Clinical Features

Clear cell carcinoma (CCC) is a rare histotype that in our experiences, and those of others, [78] represents less than 1% of endometrial carcinoma. The median age at diagnosis is 67 years, and approximately 48% of patients have extrauterine disease at presentation [79]. CCC is currently considered a "high-risk" histotype, and patients are managed accordingly [80]. Although the available data are not entirely congruent, there may be significant differences in prognosis, efficacy of adjuvant radiation, and risk of thromboembolic events between patients with CCC and those with other “high-risk” histotypes of endometrial carcinoma [80–84]. As such, CCC should be distinguished from these other histotypes.

Unlike their serous and endometrioid counterparts, there is a comparative dearth of published information on precursor lesions of CCC, possibly a function of the aforementioned rarity of the histotype. The currently available information is summarized below:

Clear Cell Endometrial Intraepithelial Carcinoma (Clear Cell EIC)

The concept of an in situ component for CCC was initially reported in a trio of reports of endocervical CCC in the 1970s [10–12]. In all the cases in those reports, the in situ carcinoma component was associated with a conventionally invasive or exophytic CCC [85–87]. In 2004, Moid and Berezowski reported an example of an isolated clear cell EIC that was unassociated with an invasive component [88]. This lesion was diagnosed in the hysterectomy specimen of a 70-year-old, was endometrium-confined, and was characterized by surface endometrial epithelium or non-myoinvasive endometrial glands that were partially or completely lined by atypical cells showing “clear cytoplasm, marked nuclear pleomorphism, coarse chromatin, irregular nuclear membranes, and prominent eosinophilic nucleoli,” occasional hobnail change, and no mitotic figures. The cells showed a wild-type p53 staining pattern and “moderate to high proliferative” indices [88]. The authors reported this lesion as “endometrial intraepithelial carcinoma, clear cell type.” In 2006, Fadare et al. [89] reported their findings from an evaluation of the background endometrium in 30 archived cases of pure CCC ($n = 14$) or mixed endometrial carcinomas with a >10% clear cell component ($n = 16$). Glands that displayed various degrees of a distinctive “atypical” cytologic alteration were identified in 90% of pure or mixed CCC cases and in none of the control group cases, the latter comprised of benign uteri or endometrioid carcinomas. Atypia was defined as “any gland or surface epithelial segment lined by cells that displayed nuclear enlargement, chromatin clumping, nucleolar prominence, pleomorphism, and/or hyperchromasia to a degree clearly above that of the adjacent normal glandular epithelia”; thus, “atypical” lesions encompassed a range of lesions [89]. The alterations at the most well-developed (i.e., most atypical) end of the spectrum are essentially analogous to the aforementioned clear cell EIC, i.e., they showed the cytological features of clear cell carcinoma but are nonconfluent and noninvasive (Fig. 17.48). Those that show lesser degrees of atypia were conceptualized as clear cell EmGD (described below) [89] (Figs. 17.49, 17.50, and 17.51). At present time, it is not entirely clear whether clear cell EIC simply represents a lepidic growth pattern from the adjacent malignancy, small foci of tubulocystic pattern CCC, or a precursor lesion. Given the rarity of reported clear cell EIC unassociated with the conventional cancer, their biologic behavior is uncertain.

17.1.3.2 Pathologic Findings

Clear cell EIC was defined in one report as “endometrial surface growth (over benign endometrium), isolated (from the main malignancy) glands lined partially or wholly by cells that were identical (cytologically and in mitotic indices) to the associated invasive malignancy, or rare clusters of glands that exhibited no significant confluence” [79]. So defined, clear cell EIC was identified in the adjacent endometrium in 41.7% of CCC cases and was not infrequently multifocal [79]. In one report from Ishida et al., conventional CCC was

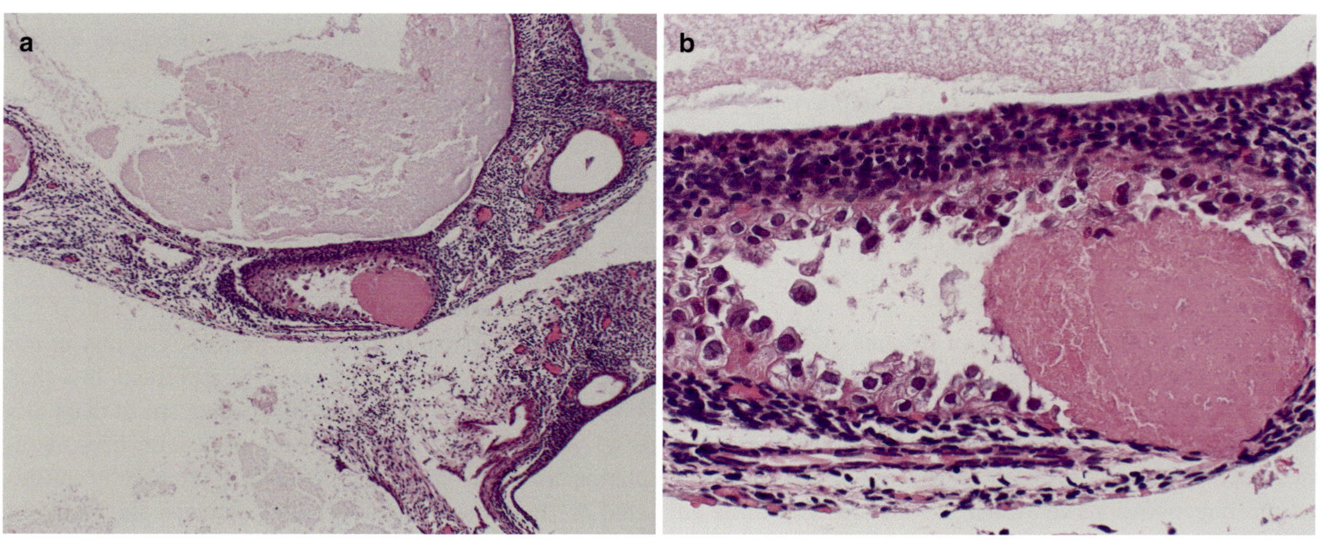

Fig. 17.48 Examples of isolated cases of clear cell intraepithelial carcinoma in a glandular pattern (**a**, **b**), flat pattern (**c**), or both (**d**, **e**)

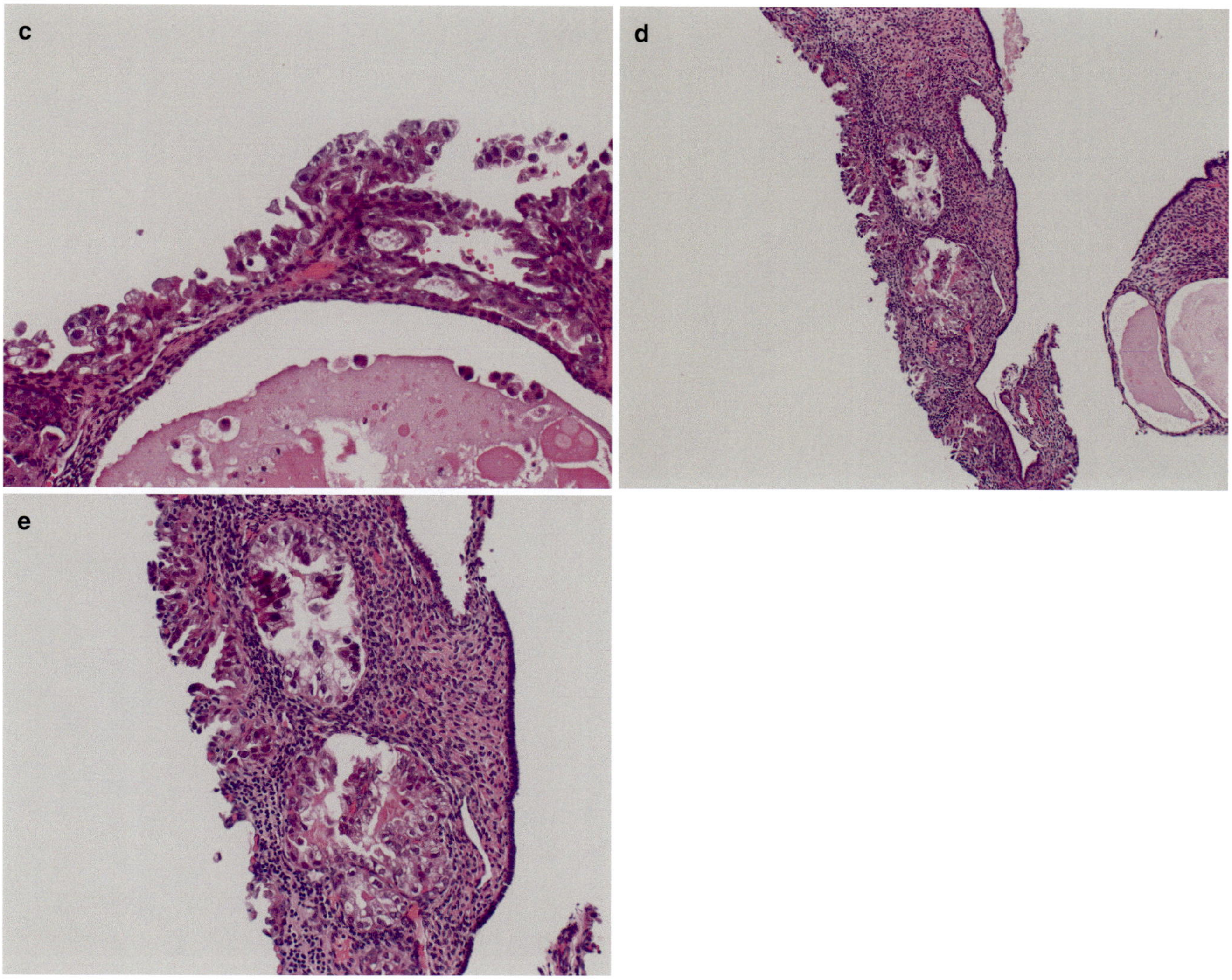

Fig.17.48 (continued)

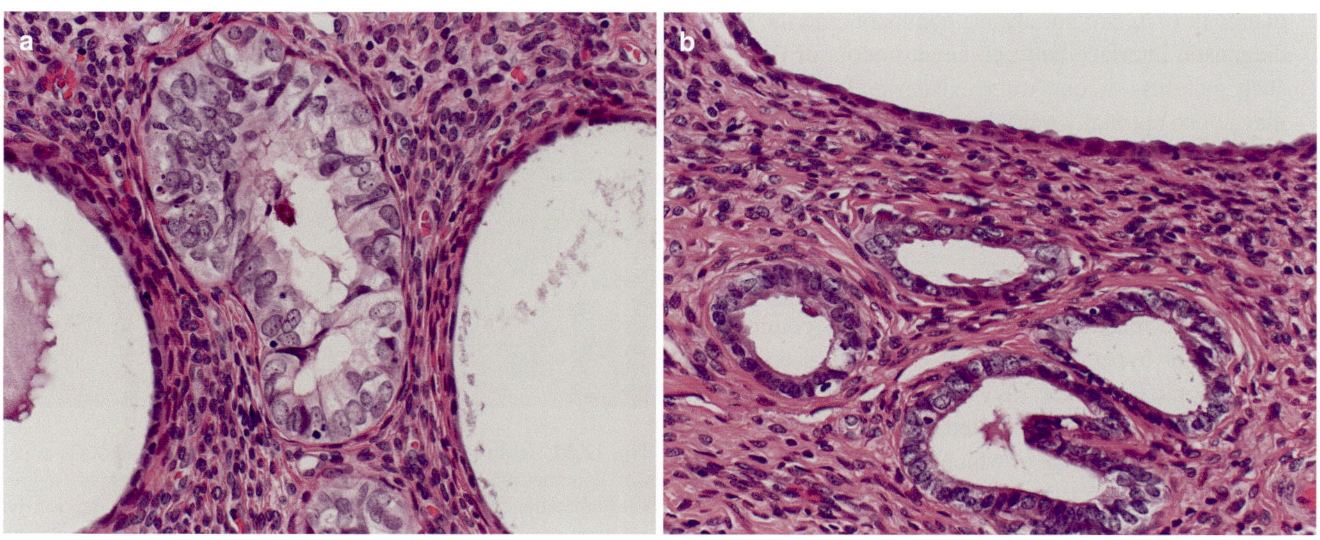

Fig. 17.49 This isolated gland (**a**) and cluster of glands (**b**) was identified in the non-tumoral endometrium associated with invasive clear cell carcinoma. They show nuclear changes that render them distinct from the background endometrium, as well as varying degrees of cytoplasmic clearing. Such lesions have been proffered to represent endometrial glandular dysplasia (EmGD) associated with clear cell carcinoma

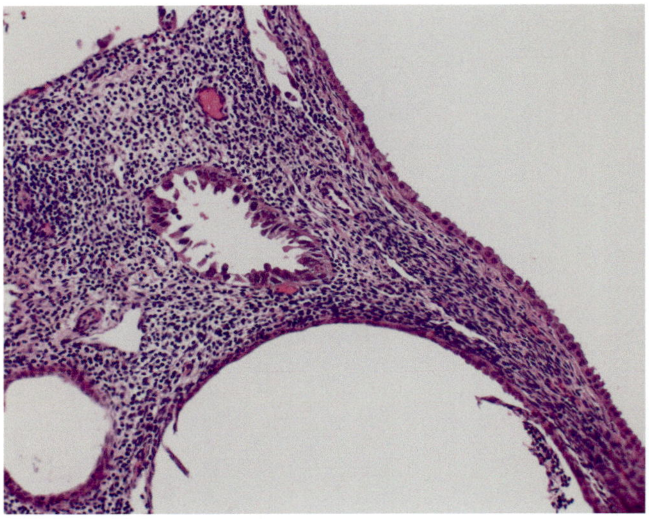

Fig. 17.50 This case showed hobnail change associated with hyperchromasia as the only abnormality in an endometrial polyp in a postmenopausal woman. Follow-up has been unremarkable

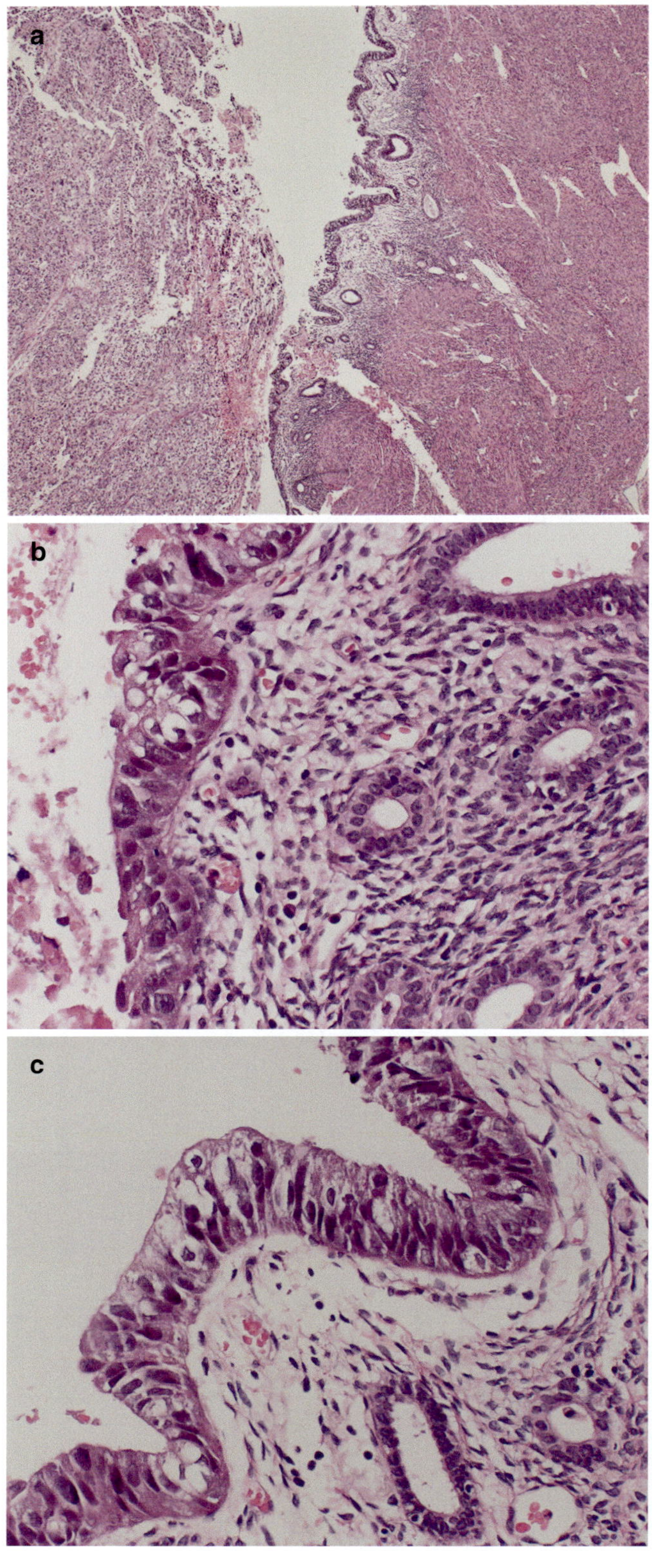

Fig. 17.51 In this case of clear cell carcinoma (**a**: left field), the adjacent endometrium (**a**: right field) showed a spectrum of variably atypical intraepithelial alterations, ranging from segments that were overtly carcinomatous (**b**) to those that displayed lesser degrees of atypia (**c**) that was nonetheless still more atypical than the background glands

identified in an endometrial polyp, whereas a small focus of clear cell EIC was identified in the background endometrium [90]. However, we have also encountered the reverse scenario wherein an intraepithelial pattern was present in a polyp, but a conventionally invasive carcinoma was in the non-polypoid endometrium. Clear cell EIC demonstrates the same immunophenotype as conventional CCC (Napsin A-positive/HNF1β-positive/ER-negative/PR-negative), although the data is limited.

17.1.3.3 Differential Diagnosis

- Clear cell carcinoma: A solid or true papillary pattern of CCC, no matter how small, should not be conceptualized as "intraepithelial" (Fig. 17.52). However, tubulocystic glands in CCC are not always confluent, and the precise diagnostic interface between small tumors of CCC with such patterns—if one truly exists—and clear cell EIC may not be optimally reproducible. To prevent undertreatment, we refrain from rendering an isolated diagnosis of clear cell EIC in biopsies and curettages and simply diagnose clear cell carcinoma with a comment about the lesional size and the fact the lesion exclusively displays an intraepithelial (in situ-like) growth pattern.
- Arias-Stella reaction: This alteration, most commonly a sequelae of hyperstimulation of endometrial epithelium by chorionic hormones, may be characterized by nucleomegaly, nucleolomegaly, hyperchromasia, and clear cell cytoplasmic change, all of which may raise the possibility of clear cell EIC [91], (Fig. 17.52). The background changes of gestation as well as the clinical history are the most important factors in contextualizing the observed

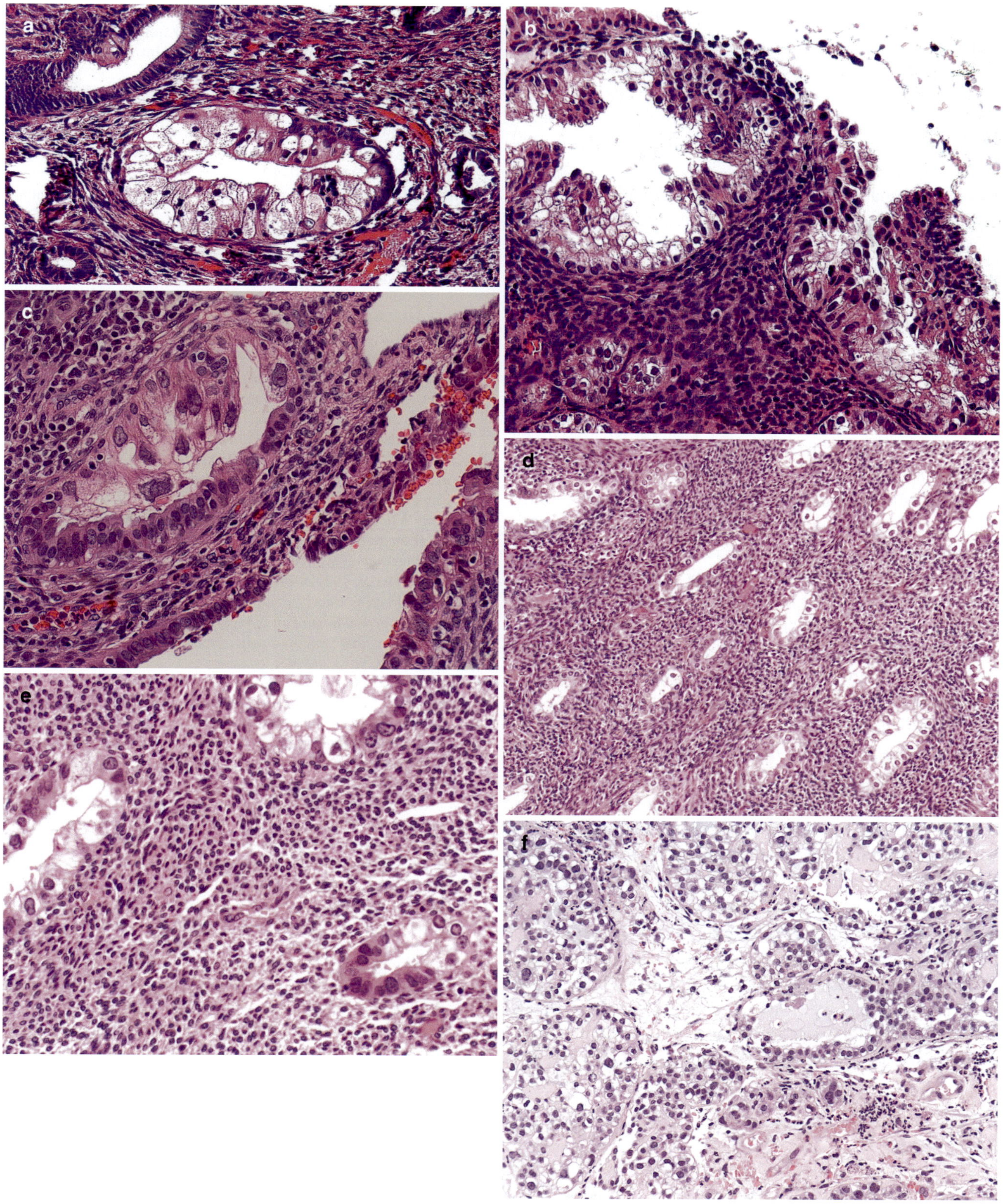

Fig. 17.52 The differential diagnosis of clear cell EmGD and clear cell intraepithelial carcinoma includes clear cell metaplasia, which is cytologically bland (**a**); Arias-Stella reaction, which is associated with a gestational-type background in most cases (**b**, **c**); radiation changes, which are diffuse within the endometrium (**d**, **e**); and clear cell carcinoma, which is more confluent and shows patterns of clear cell carcinoma (**f**)

changes. Immunohistochemistry using Ki67 and estrogen receptor (ER) may also be useful, since Arias-Stella reaction shows significantly lower proliferative index and higher estrogen receptor content than CCC [92]. Of note, Napsin A and HNF1β are expressed in Arias-Stella reaction, and both accordingly play a limited role in this differential diagnosis [93, 94].

- Therapy-related changes: Patients undergoing chemoradiation for cervical or other pelvic cancers may display distinctive endometrial changes that include nuclear enlargement and cytoplasmic clarity (Fig. 17.52). The diffuseness of the changes within the endometrium, the clinical history of treatment, and the absence of a CCC-like immunophenotype are all useful features to distinguish these treatment-related alterations from true clear cell EIC.

Clear Cell Endometrial Glandular Dysplasia (EmGD)

The concept of clear cell EmGD is based on the putative precursor lesions described in the aforementioned 2006 study [89]. These lesions were identified in the background endometrium of CCC or endometrial carcinomas with a >10% CCC component. By definition, they are atypical, in the sense that they stand out from the background endometrium (by virtue of nuclear enlargement, hobnail change, and/or hyperchromasia, typically in the setting of some degree of cytoplasmic clarity), but which nonetheless do not display the level of cytologic alteration that would be typical of clear cell EIC [89] detailed in Figs. 17.49, 17.50, and 17.51. There are no reported examples of clear cell EmGD in isolation (i.e., unassociated with a conventional CCC), although cases that raise the possibility have been seen, especially in polyps (Fig. 17.50). The true morphologic spectrum, immunophenotype, molecular profile, and biologic potential of clear cell EmGD have yet to be defined. Accordingly, this category is best considered provisional. Nonetheless, lesions that are worth considering in the differential diagnosis include the rare isolated clear cell change of the endometrium [cytologically bland and frequently with a progestational basis that is also reflected in the background endometrium [72]], radiation-associated clear cell change (Fig. 17.52: a more diffuse process), and secretory AH/EIN (discussed earlier).

References

1. Parazzini F, La Vecchia C, Bocciolone L, Franceschi S. The epidemiology of endometrial cancer. Gynecol Oncol. 1991;41:1–16.
2. Stanford JL, Brinton LA, Berman ML, et al. Oral contraceptives and endometrial cancer: do other risk factors modify the association? Int J Cancer. 1993;54:243–8.
3. Weiderpass E, Adami HO, Baron JA, et al. Use of oral contraceptives and endometrial cancer risk (Sweden). Cancer Causes Control. 1999;10(4):277–84.
4. Vierkoetter KR, Kagami LA, Ahn HJ, Shimizu DM, Terada KY. Loss of mismatch repair protein expression in unselected endometrial adenocarcinoma precursor lesions. Int J Gynecol Cancer. 2016;26(2):228–32.
5. Djordjevic B, Barkoh BA, Luthra R, Broaddus RR. Relationship between PTEN, DNA mismatch repair, and tumor histotype in endometrial carcinoma: retained positive expression of PTEN preferentially identifies sporadic non-endometrioid carcinomas. Mod Pathol. 2013;26(10):1401–12.
6. Mutter GL. PTEN, a protean tumor suppressor. Am J Pathol. 2001;158:1895–8.
7. Zhou XP, Kuismanen S, Nystrom-Lahti M, et al. Distinct PTEN mutational spectra in hereditary non-polyposis colon cancer syndrome-related endometrial carcinomas compared to sporadic microsatellite unstable tumors. Hum Mol Genet. 2002;11(4):445–50.
8. Monte NM, Webster KA, Neuberg D, Dressler GR, Mutter GL. Joint loss of PAX2 and PTEN expression in endometrial precancers and cancer. Cancer Res. 2010;70(15):6225–32.
9. Joiner AK, Quick CM, Jeffus SK. Pax2 expression in simultaneously diagnosed WHO and EIN classification systems. Int J Gynecol Pathol. 2015;34(1):40–6.
10. Quick CM, Laury AR, Monte NM, Mutter GL. Utility of PAX2 as a marker for diagnosis of endometrial intraepithelial neoplasia. Am J Clin Pathol. 2012;138(5):678–84.
11. Cheng WF, Lin HH, Torng PL, Huang SC. Comparison of endometrial changes among symptomatic tamoxifen-treated and nontreated premenopausal and postmenopausal breast cancer patients. Gynecol Oncol. 1997;66(2):233–7.
12. Cohen I, Perel E, Flex D, et al. Endometrial pathology in postmenopausal tamoxifen treatment: comparison between gynaecologically symptomatic and asymptomatic breast cancer patients. J Clin Pathol. 1999;52(4):278–82.
13. Mutter GL, Zaino RJ, Baak JPA, Bentley RC, Robboy SJ. The benign endometrial hyperplasia sequence and endometrial intraepithelial neoplasia (EIN). Int J Gynecol Pathol. 2007;26:103–14.
14. World Health Organization. WHO classification of tumors of female reproductive organs. Lyon: International Agency for Research on Cancer; 2014.
15. Mutter GL, The Endometrial Collaborative Group. Endometrial intraepithelial neoplasia (EIN): will it bring order to chaos? Gynecol Oncol. 2000;76:287–90.
16. Shapiro S, Kelly JP, Rosenberg L, Kaufman DW, Helmrich SP, Rosenshein NB, et al. Risk of localized and widespread endometrial cancer in relation to recent and discontinued use of conjugated estrogens. N Engl J Med. 1985;313:969–72.
17. Zeleniuch-Jacquotte A, Akhmedkhanov A, Kato I, Koenig KL, Shore RE, Kim MY, et al. Postmenopausal endogenous oestrogens and risk of endometrial cancer: results of a prospective study. Br J Cancer. 1985;84:975–81.
18. Kurman RJ, Kaminski PF, Norris HJ. The behavior of endometrial hyperplasia: a long term study of "untreated" hyperplasia in 170 patients. Cancer. 1985;56:403–12.
19. Allison KH, Reed SD, Voigt LF, Jordan CD, Newton KM, Garcia RL. Diagnosing endometrial hyperplasia: why is it so difficult to agree? Am J Surg Pathol. 2008;32(5):691–8.
20. Kendall BS, Ronnett BM, Isacson C, Cho KR, Hedrick L, Diener-West MKR. Reproducibility of the diagnosis of endometrial hyperplasia, atypical hyperplasia, and well-differentiated carcinoma. Am J Surg Pathol. 1998;22(8):1012–9.
21. Salman MC, Usubutun A, Boynukalin K, Yuce K. Comparison of WHO and endometrial intraepithelial neoplasia classifications in predicting the presence of coexistent malignancy in endometrial hyperplasia. J Gynecol Oncol. 2010;21(2):97–101.
22. Zaino RJ, Kauderer J, Trimble CL, Silverberg SG, Curtin JP, Lim PC, et al. Reproducibility of the diagnosis of atypical endome-

trial hyperplasia: a gynecologic oncology group study. Cancer. 2006;106(4):804–11.
23. Hecht JL, Ince TA, Baak JP, Baker HE, Ogden MW, Mutter GL. Prediction of endometrial carcinoma by subjective endometrial intraepithelial neoplasia diagnosis. Mod Pathol. 2005;18(3):324–30.
24. Mutter GL, Kauderer J, Baak JPA, Alberts DA. Biopsy histomorphometry predicts uterine myoinvasion by endometrial carcinoma: a Gynecologic Oncology Group Study. Hum Pathol. 2008;39(6):866–74.
25. Lacey JV, Mutter GL, Nucci MR, Ronnett BM, Ioffe OB, Rush BB, et al. Risk of subsequent endometrial carcinoma associated with endometrial intraepithelial neoplasia classification of endometrial biopsies. Cancer. 2008;113(8):2073–81.
26. Trimbel CL, Kaudener J, Zaino R, Silverberg S, Lim PC, Burke JJ, et al. Concurrent endometrial carcinoma in women with a biopsy diagnosis of atypical endometrial hyperplasia: a gynecologic oncology group study. Cancer. 2006;106(4):812–9.
27. Glede KC, Yen T, Chibbar R, Plerson R. Significance of concurrent endometrial cancer in women with a preoperative diagnosis of atypical endometrial hyperplasia. J Obstet Gynaecol Can. 2008;30(10):896–901.
28. Carlson JW, Mutter GL. Endometrial intraepithelial neoplasia is associated with polyps and frequently has metaplastic change. Histopathology. 2008;53:325–32.
29. Brachtel EF, Sanchez-Estevez C, Moreno-Bueno G, Prat J, Palacios J, Oliva E. Distinct molecular alterations in complex endometrial hyperplasia (CEH) with and without immature squamous metaplasia (squamous morules). Am J Surg Pathol. 2005;29:1322–9.
30. Saegusa M, Okayasu I. Frequent nuclear beta catenin accumulation and associated mutations in endometrioid-type endometrial and ovarian carcinomas with squamous differentiation. J Pathol. 2001;194:59–67.
31. Wheeler DT, Bristow RE, Kurman RJ. Histologic alterations in endometrial hyperplasia and well-differentiated carcinoma treated with progestins. Am J Surg Pathol. 2007;31:988–98.
32. Nicolae A, Preda O, Nogales F. Endometrial metaplasias and reactive changes: a spectrum of altered differentiation. J Clin Pathol. 2011;64:97–106.
33. Lin MC, Lomo L, Baak JPA, Eng C, Ince TA, Crum CP, et al. Squamous morules are functionally inert elements of premalignant endometrial neoplasia. Mod Pathol. 2009;22:167–74.
34. Nucci MR, Prasad CJ, Crum CP, Mutter GL. Mucinous endometrial epithelial proliferations: a morphologic spectrum of changes with diverse clinical significance. Mod Pathol. 1999;12:1137–42.
35. McCluggage WG, McBride HA. Papillary syncytial metaplasia associated with endometrial breakdown exhibits an immunophenotype that overlaps with uterine serous carcinoma. Int J Gynecol Pathol. 2012;31(3):206–10.
36. Parra-Herran CE, Monte NM, Mutter GL. Endometrial intraepithelial neoplasia with secretory differentiation: diagnostic features and underlying mechanisms. Mod Pathol. 2013;26(6):868–73.
37. Jeffus S, Winham W, Hooper K, Quick CM. Secretory endometrial intraepithelial neoplasia. Int J Gynecol Pathol. 2014;33:515–6.
38. Gultekin M, Diribas K, Dursan P, Ayhan A. Current management of endometrial hyperplasia and endometrial intraepithelial neoplasia (EIN). Eur J Gynaecol Oncol. 2009;30(4):396–401.
39. Mentrikoski MJ, Shah AA, Hanley KZ, Atkins KA. Assessing endometrial hyperplasia and carcinoma treated with progestin therapy. Am J Clin Pathol. 2012;138:524–34.
40. Huang EC, Mutter GL, Crum CP, Nucci MR. Clinical outcome in diagnostically ambiguous foci of "gland crowding" in the endometrium. Mod Pathol. 2010;23:1486–91.
41. Mutter GL, Ince TA, Baak JPA, Kust GA, Zhou XP, Eng C. Molecular identification of latent precancers in histologically normal endometrium. Cancer Res. 2001;61:4311–4.
42. Mutter GL, Lin MC, Fitzgerald JT, Kum JB, Baak JP, Lees JA, et al. Altered PTEN expression as a diagnostic marker for the earliest endometrial precancers. J Natl Cancer Inst. 2000;92:924–30.
43. Allison KH, Upson K, Reed SD, Jordan CD, Newton KM, Doherty J, et al. PAX2 loss by immunohistochemistry occurs early and often in endometrial hyperplasia. Int J Gynecol Pathol. 2012;31:151–9.
44. Hamilton CA, Cheung MK, Osann K, Chen L, Teng NN, Longacre TA, Powell MA, Hendrickson MR, Kapp DS, Chan JK. Uterine papillary serous and clear cell carcinomas predict for poorer survival compared to grade 3 endometrioid corpus cancers. Br J Cancer. 2006;94(5):642–6.
45. Kwon JS, Abrams J, Sugimoto A, Carey MS. Is adjuvant therapy necessary for stage IA and IB uterine papillary serous carcinoma and clear cell carcinoma after surgical staging? Int J Gynecol Cancer. 2008;18(4):820–4. Epub 2007 Sep 24
46. Huang CY, Tang YH, Chiang YC, Wang KL, Fu HC, Ke YM, Lau HY, Hsu KF, Wu CH, Cheng WF. Impact of management on the prognosis of pure uterine papillary serous cancer—a Taiwanese Gynecologic Oncology Group (TGOG) study. Gynecol Oncol. 2014;133:221–8.
47. Carcangiu ML, Tan LK, Chambers JT. Stage IA uterine serous carcinoma: a study of 13 cases. Am J Surg Pathol. 1997;21:1507–14.
48. Ambros RA, Sherman ME, Zahn CM, Bitterman P, Kurman RJ. Endometrial intraepithelial carcinoma: a distinctive lesion specifically associated with tumors displaying serous differentiation. Hum Pathol. 1995;26:1260–7.
49. Sherman ME, Bitterman P, Rosenshein NB, Delgado G, Kurman RJ. Uterine serous carcinoma. A morphologically diverse neoplasm with unifying clinicopathologic features. Am J Surg Pathol. 1992;16:600–10.
50. Spiegel GW. Endometrial carcinoma in situ in postmenopausal women. Am J Surg Pathol. 1995;19:417–32.
51. Zheng W, Khurana R, Farahmand S, Wang Y, Zhang ZF, Felix JC. p53 immunostaining as a significant adjunct diagnostic method for uterine surface carcinoma: precursor of uterine papillary serous carcinoma. Am J Surg Pathol. 1998;22:1463–73.
52. Hou JY, McAndrew TC, Goldberg GL, Whitney K, Shahabi S. A clinical and pathologic comparison between stage-matched endometrial intraepithelial carcinoma and uterine serous carcinoma: is there a difference? Reprod Sci. 2014;21:532–7.
53. Soslow RA, Pirog E, Isacson C. Endometrial intraepithelial carcinoma with associated peritoneal carcinomatosis. Am J Surg Pathol. 2000;24:726–32.
54. Baergen RN, Warren CD, Isacson C, Ellenson LH. Early uterine serous carcinoma: clonal origin of extrauterine disease. Int J Gynecol Pathol. 2001;20(3):214–9.
55. Yan Z, Hui P. Minimal uterine serous carcinoma with extrauterine tumor of identical morphology: an immunohistochemical study of 13 cases. Appl Immunohistochem Mol Morphol. 2010;18(1):75–9.
56. Kommoss F, Faruqi A, Gilks CB, Lamshang Leen S, Singh N, Wilkinson N, McCluggage WG. Uterine serous carcinomas frequently metastasize to the fallopian tube and can mimic serous tubal intraepithelial carcinoma. Am J Surg Pathol. 2017;41(2):161–70.
57. Zheng W, Schwartz PE. Serous EIC as an early form of uterine papillary serous carcinoma: recent progress in understanding its pathogenesis and current opinions regarding pathologic and clinical management. Gynecol Oncol. 2005;96:579–82.
58. Liang SX, Chambers SK, Cheng L, Zhang S, Zhou Y, Zheng W. Endometrial glandular dysplasia: a putative precursor lesion of uterine papillary serous carcinoma. Part II: molecular features. Int J Surg Pathol. 2004;12:319–31.

59. Zheng W, Liang SX, Yi X, Ulukus EC, Davis JR, Chambers SK. Occurrence of endometrial glandular dysplasia precedes uterine papillary serous carcinoma. Int J Gynecol Pathol. 2007;26:38–52.
60. Jia L, Liu Y, Yi X, Miron A, Crum CP, Kong B, Zheng W. Endometrial glandular dysplasia with frequent p53 gene mutation: a genetic evidence supporting its precancer nature for endometrial serous carcinoma. Clin Cancer Res. 2008;14:2263–9.
61. Fadare O, Zheng W. Endometrial Glandular Dysplasia (EmGD): morphologically and biologically distinctive putative precursor lesions of Type II endometrial cancers. Diagn Pathol. 2008;3:6.
62. Yi X, Zheng W. Endometrial glandular dysplasia and endometrial intraepithelial neoplasia. Curr Opin Obstet Gynecol. 2008;20:20–5.
63. Fadare O, Zheng W. Endometrial serous carcinoma (uterine papillary serous carcinoma): precancerous lesions and the theoretical promise of a preventive approach. Am J Cancer Res. 2012;2(3):335–9.
64. Zhang X, Liang SX, Jia L, Chen N, Fadare O, Schwartz PE, Kong B, Zheng W. Molecular identification of "latent precancers" for endometrial serous carcinoma in benign-appearing endometrium. Am J Pathol. 2009;174(6):2000–6.
65. Berman JJ, Albores-Saavedra J, Bostwick D, Delellis R, Eble J, Hamilton SR, Hruban RH, Mutter GL, Page D, Rohan T, Travis W, Henson DE. Precancer: a conceptual working definition—results of a Consensus Conference. Cancer Detect Prev. 2006;30:387–94.
66. Zheng W, Xiang L, Fadare O, Kong B. A proposed model for endometrial serous carcinogenesis. Am J Surg Pathol. 2011;35:e1–e14.
67. Zheng W, Liang SX, Yu H, Rutherford T, Chambers SK, Schwartz PE. Endometrial glandular dysplasia: a newly defined precursor lesion of uterine papillary serous carcinoma. Part I: morphologic features. Int J Surg Pathol. 2004;12:207–23.
68. Zheng W, Yi X, Fadare O, Liang SX, Martel M, Schwartz PE, Jiang Z. The oncofetal protein IMP3: a novel biomarker for endometrial serous carcinoma. Am J Surg Pathol. 2008;32:304–15.
69. Horree N, Heintz AP, Sie-Go DM, van Diest PJ. p16 is consistently expressed in endometrial tubal metaplasia. Cell Oncol. 2007;29(1):37–45.
70. Wild PJ, Ikenberg K, Fuchs TJ, Rechsteiner M, Georgiev S, Fankhauser N, Noske A, Roessle M, Caduff R, Dellas A, Fink D, Moch H, Krek W, Frew IJ. p53 suppresses type II endometrial carcinomas in mice and governs endometrial tumour aggressiveness in humans. EMBO Mol Med. 2012;4:808–24.
71. Chen N, Yi X, Abushahin N, Pang S, Zhang D, Kong B, Zheng W. Nrf2 expression in endometrial serous carcinomas and its precancers. Int J Clin Exp Pathol. 2010;4:85–96.
72. Hendrickson MR, Kempson RL. Endometrial epithelial metaplasias: proliferations frequently misdiagnosed as adenocarcinoma. Report of 89 cases and proposed classification. Am J Surg Pathol. 1980;4(6):525–42.
73. Shah SS, Mazur MT. Endometrial eosinophilic syncytial change related to breakdown: immunohistochemical evidence suggests a regressive process. Int J Gynecol Pathol. 2008;27(4):534–8. https://doi.org/10.1097/PGP.0b013e31817323b3.
74. Haley SL, Malhotra RK, Qiu S, Eltorky ME. The immunohistochemical profile of atypical eosinophilic syncytial changes vs serous carcinoma. Ann Diagn Pathol. 2011;15(6):402–6.
75. Simon RA, Peng SL, Liu F, Quddus MR, Zhang C, Steinhoff MM, Lawrence WD, Sung CJ. Tubal metaplasia of the endometrium with cytologic atypia: analysis of p53, Ki-67, TERT, and long-term follow-up. Mod Pathol. 2011;24(9):1254–61.
76. Hileeto D, Fadare O, Martel M, Zheng W. Age dependent association of endometrial polyps with increased risk of cancer involvement. World J Surg Oncol. 2005;3(1):8.
77. Fadare O, Renshaw IL, Parkash V. The Spectrum of morphologic alterations associated with infarction in endometrial polyps: a report of 41 cases. Int J Gynecol Pathol. 2017; https://doi.org/10.1097/PGP.0000000000000475. [Epub ahead of print]
78. Lewis GH, Folkins AK, Kong CS, Kempson RL, Longacre TA. Endometrial clear cell carcinoma: incidence and clinicopathologic features. Poster Session. United States and Canadian Academy of Pathology 101st Annual Meeting, Baltimore. 2013.
79. Fadare O, Zheng W, Crispens MA, Jones HW, Khabele D, Gwin K, Liang SX, Mohammed K, Desouki MM, Parkash V, Hecht JL. Morphologic and other clinicopathologic features of endometrial clear cell carcinoma: a comprehensive analysis of 50 rigorously classified cases. Am J Cancer Res. 2013;3(1):70–95.
80. Bernardini MQ, Gien LT, Lau S, Altman AD, Gilks B, Ferguson SE, Köbel M, Samouëlian V, Wesa M, Cameron A, Nelson G, Han G, Clarke B, Ho TC, Panzarella T, Atenafu EG, McAlpine JN. Treatment related outcomes in high-risk endometrial carcinoma: Canadian high risk endometrial cancer consortium (CHREC). Gynecol Oncol. 2016;141(1):148–54.
81. Altman AD, Ferguson SE, Atenafu EG, Köbel M, McAlpine JN, Panzarella T, Lau S, Gien LT, Gilks B, Clarke B, Cameron A, Nelson G, Han G, Samouëlian V, Ho TC, Louie K, Bernardini MQ. Canadian high risk endometrial cancer (CHREC) consortium: analyzing the clinical behavior of high risk endometrial cancers. Gynecol Oncol. 2015;139(2):268–74.
82. Fadare O. Clear cell carcinomas of the gynecologic tract and thromboembolic events: what do we know so far? Womens Health (Lond). 2014;10(5):479–81.
83. Abdulfatah E, Sakr S, Thomas S, Al-Wahab Z, Mutch DG, Dowdy S, Bandyopadhyay S, Munkarah A, Elshaikh M, Morris R, Ali-Fehmi R. Clear cell carcinoma of the endometrium: evaluation of prognostic parameters in a multi-institutional cohort of 165 cases. Int J Gynecol Cancer. 2017;27(8):1714–21.
84. Olawaiye AB, Boruta DM 2nd. Management of women with clear cell endometrial cancer: a Society of Gynecologic Oncology (SGO) review. Gynecol Oncol. 2009;113(2):277–83.
85. Hasumi K, Ehrmann RL. Clear cell carcinoma of the uterine endocervix with an in situ component. Cancer. 1978;42:2435–8.
86. Roth LM, Hornback NB. Clear-cell adenocarcinoma of the cervix in young women. Cancer. 1974;34(5):1761–8.
87. Parker JC, Van Ngell JR, Harralson JD. The mesonephroid (hypernephroid) carcinomatous pattern—a rare variant of primary endocervical adenocarcinoma. Cancer. 1973;32:259–65.
88. Moid F, Berezowski K. Pathologic quiz case: a 70-year-old woman with postmenopausal bleeding. Endometrial intraepithelial carcinoma, clear cell type. Arch Pathol Lab Med. 2004;128(11):e157–8.
89. Fadare O, Liang SX, Ulukus EC, Chambers SK, Zheng W. Precursors of endometrial clear cell carcinoma. Am J Surg Pathol. 2006;30(12):1519–30.
90. Ishida M, Iwai M, Yoshida K, Kagotani A, Okabe H. Clear cell adenocarcinoma present exclusively within endometrial polyp: report of two cases. Int J Clin Exp Pathol. 2014;7(4):1757–63.
91. Arias-Stella J. The Arias-Stella reaction: facts and fancies four decades after. Adv Anat Pathol. 2002;9(1):12–23.
92. Vang R, Barner R, Wheeler DT, Strauss BL. Immunohistochemical staining for Ki-67 and p53 helps distinguish endometrial Arias-Stella reaction from high-grade carcinoma, including clear cell carcinoma. Int J Gynecol Pathol. 2004;23(3):223–33.
93. Fadare O. Expression of Napsin A is common in Arias-Stella reaction. Hum Pathol. 2016;54:202.
94. Fadare O, Liang SX. Diagnostic utility of hepatocyte nuclear factor 1-beta immunoreactivity in endometrial carcinomas: lack of specificity for endometrial clear cell carcinoma. Appl Immunohistochem Mol Morphol. 2012;20(6):580–7.

18 Endometrial Carcinoma

Anne M. Mills

Abstract

Endometrial carcinoma is the most common type of gynecologic malignancy and has shown a steady rise in incidence over recent decades. Formerly, endometrial carcinomas were divided into type I and type II cancers; however, recent molecular advances have led to a more nuanced classification system that incorporates mismatch repair status, *POLE* mutations, and the overall burden of copy-number alterations. In this chapter, we review endometrial carcinoma histomorphologies and immunohistochemistry in the context of this new molecular understanding with attention to endometrioid, serous, clear cell, mucinous, undifferentiated/dedifferentiated, and neuroendocrine subtypes as well as carcinosarcomas. We address clinical variables such as epidemiology, individual risk factors, and hereditary predisposition syndromes and focus on current pathologic staging and grading recommendations, with emphasis on problematic areas. Finally, we discuss ancillary testing including Lynch syndrome screening approaches and emerging therapeutic biomarkers.

Keywords

Endometrial carcinoma · Endometrial cancer · Uterine cancer · Endometrioid carcinoma · Serous carcinoma
Clear cell carcinoma · Carcinosarcoma · Lynch syndrome

18.1 Introduction

Endometrial carcinomas encompass tumors with a range of morphologies which display a spectrum of clinical aggression. Historically, endometrial cancers were divided into two overarching categories: Type I and Type II carcinomas. This classification was first presented by Bokhman in 1983 and dominated thinking about the disease for the ensuing decades [1]. In this system, Type I carcinomas corresponded chiefly with low-grade, estrogen-driven endometrioid histology, whereas Type II carcinomas consisted predominantly of high-grade serous cancers unrelated to hormones [1, 2]. Type I cancers prototypically occurred in young women with increased estrogen exposure (often secondary to obesity), while Type II tumors were most often diagnosed in postmenopausal women without a history of increased steroid influence. Type I cancers tended to have a better prognosis with frequent response to progestin-based therapy, whereas Type II tumors were more aggressive and lacked a viable endocrine treatment option.

Despite the thorough extent to which the Type I/II labels permeated endometrial cancer literature and discussion among both pathologists and gynecologic oncologists, these designations never fully penetrated clinical practice. This was largely attributable to the poor alignment of many tumors with either of category. Carcinomas with mixed or ambiguous morphology, tumors with clear cell features, high-grade and dedifferentiated endometrioid tumors, carcinosarcomas, and undifferentiated endometrial cancers proved particularly problematic in this system. Binary classification of endometrial cancers was further confounded by poor diagnostic reproducibility among pathologists [3–7]. Over time, it became clear that the prevailing philosophy for approaching endometrial carcinoma was perhaps not fully aligned with tumor biology.

This problem has been addressed in recent years through the explosion of molecular testing and the advent of a genetically based understanding of endometrial cancer. In 2013, The Cancer Genome Atlas (TCGA) led to a new genomic classification schema for endometrial tumors [8]. This system divided endometrial malignancies into four categories: (1) ultramutated/polymerase ε (*POLE*); (2) hypermutated/mismatch repair-deficient/microsatellite unstable; (3) low copy-number abnormalities; and (4) high copy-number abnormalities. The first group is characterized by mutations in the exonuclease domain of DNA polymerase epsilon (*POLE*) and tends to display high histologic grade with paradoxically good outcomes. Mismatch repair-deficient cancers occur with both heritable

A. M. Mills (✉)
Department of Pathology, University of Virginia, Charlottesville, VA, USA
e-mail: AMM7R@hscmail.mcc.virginia.edu

W. Zheng et al. (eds.), *Gynecologic and Obstetric Pathology, Volume 1*, https://doi.org/10.1007/978-981-13-3016-2_18

(germline mutations in mismatch repair genes, e.g., Lynch syndrome) and somatic mechanisms (epigenetic *MLH1* promoter hypermethylation and sporadic mismatch repair gene mutations) and include both conventional endometrioid and dedifferentiated/undifferentiated histologies, as well as occasional other subtypes such as clear cell carcinoma. Low copy-number tumors most often show conventional endometrioid morphology, whereas high copy-number cases typically have serous or serous-like histology.

While this system has parallels with the old dualistic model, with many low copy-number and high copy-number cases aligning with the old Type I and Type II groups, respectively, the addition of the ultramutated/*POLE* and hypermutated/mismatch repair-deficient categories accounts for many previously difficult-to-classify tumors. Furthermore, some morphologically low-grade cases paradoxically fall into the high copy-number group and vice versa, further explaining the imperfect alignment between histologic grade and clinical aggression in endometrial carcinoma. The newly proposed Proactive Molecular Risk Classifier for Endometrial Cancer (ProMisE) attempts to incorporate the TCGA data into clinical practice [9–11]. This iterative system assesses tumors for mismatch repair deficiency, *POLE* mutation status, and p53 immunohistochemical pattern, respectively, and shows improved prognostic power relative to existing clinicopathologic stratifiers. TCGA-based risk assessment has proven particularly significant for patients with early-stage disease, and may ultimately inform treatment practices for these cases [12].

The improved molecular understanding of endometrial carcinoma is particularly relevant in the culture of precision medicine, wherein the impetus for individualized cancer prognostication and treatment increasingly exists both in academic and community medical care. Given this context, meaningful discussions of the histologic subtypes of endometrial carcinoma must now be embedded with consideration of the molecular underpinnings of these tumors. Thus, while this chapter is organized primarily according to histomorphology, molecular characteristics are discussed throughout. That said, pathologists must be mindful of the limits of current molecular data, particularly given the racial and ethnic disparities that exist in most large molecular datasets, including the TCGA [13]. The shortcomings of molecular datasets underscore the fact that microscopic assessment remains the cornerstone of endometrial carcinoma diagnosis, and is complemented, not supplanted, by molecular studies.

18.2 Epidemiology and Risk Factors

Endometrial carcinoma is the most common gynecologic malignancy. Cancer statistics from the United States reveal that more than 60,000 women in this country were diagnosed with endometrial carcinoma in 2016, and over 10,000 succumbed to the disease during that year [14]. This incidence reflects a steady increase since the early 1990s, likely attributable to the rise in obesity [15]. Five-year endometrial cancer survivorship is ~83% overall but shows marked racial disparities (85% for whites vs. 66% for blacks), which is a reflection of both the higher incidence of high-grade, non-endometrioid histotypes in black women as well as inadequate access to and quality of care [14, 16].

Endometrial cancers most often affect peri- and postmenopausal women, however, the age distribution is skewed younger for endometrioid cancers, particularly in the setting of increased estrogen exposure, whereas non-endometrioid histotypes more often occur in older women. The risk of developing endometrioid carcinoma has clearly been linked to elevated unopposed estrogen exposure. This increased exposure can occur through a variety of mechanisms including obesity, nulliparity, early menarche, late menopause, and Tamoxifen treatment [17, 18]. Historically non-endometrioid endometrial cancer subtypes such as serous carcinoma have been considered entirely unrelated to estrogen, although some recent evidence calls into question the presumed estrogen unresponsiveness of these tumors [19, 20].

Endometrial carcinoma risk is also informed by genetics, with several familial cancer syndromes imparting increased risk for tumors. The most common heritable risk factor for endometrial carcinoma is Lynch syndrome (hereditary nonpolyposis colorectal cancer syndrome), which occurs primarily in the setting of germline mutations in the mismatch repair genes *MSH2*, *MSH6*, *MLH1*, and *PMS2* [21–24]. Rare cases of Lynch syndrome are attributable to mutations in the MMR-related gene *EPCAM* and to heritable *MLH1* promoter hypermethylation [25–29]. Lynch syndrome underlies ~2–5% of all endometrial cancer cases and many centers have instituted universal tumor screening protocols to identify these patients [30–35]. Cowden syndrome, caused by germline defects in the *PTEN* gene, is associated with a far smaller proportion of endometrial cancers (well below 1%) [36–39]. Even more uncommon are Cowden-like syndromes which are characterized by mutations in the succinate dehydrogenase B/C/D (*SDHB-D*) gene and killen (*KLLN*) genes [37, 40]. Finally, although endometrial carcinoma has not traditionally been considered part of the *BRCA* mutation spectrum, recent evidence has challenged this teaching with some studies demonstrating increased rates of uterine serous and serous-like cancers among *BRCA*-mutated patients [41–44].

18.3 Clinical Presentation and Management

Endometrial cancers typically present with abnormal uterine bleeding and vaginal discharge. More advanced stage disease may result in diffuse pelvic pain and abdominal distention, as well as symptoms related to gastrointestinal and ureteral obstruction. Women with symptoms concerning for endometrial carcinoma are managed with a combination of pelvic ultrasonography, endometrial biopsy, and/or dilatation and curettage. Ultrasound is used to measure the endometrial stripe to assess for endometrial thickening. A thickness of ≥5 mm has been associated with 90% sensitivity and 54% specificity for endometrial carcinoma, while reducing the cutoff to 3 mm is associated with 98% sensitivity and 35% specificity [45]. Detection rates can further be maximized to ≥98% by performing a hysteroscopic-guided biopsy, which represents the gold standard for endometrial carcinoma diagnosis [46]. Dilatation and curettage is also an option; however, it has both lower accuracy and lower diagnostic yield relative to hysteroscopy with biopsy [47, 48].

Treatment of endometrial carcinoma is chiefly surgical and includes removal of the uterus with or without the adnexa. Surgical staging is also typically performed and includes removal of pelvic and sometimes para-aortic lymph nodes, although this can be avoided for low-grade, minimally invasive tumors. Adjuvant therapy is recommended in patients with advanced disease but has a less clear role in patients with low-stage tumors [49, 50]. Although endometrial carcinoma is primarily treated with surgery, select low-grade tumors may be managed exclusively with progestin-based hormonal therapy, such as medroxy-progesterone acetate (MPA) and megestrol acetate. Such conservative management should be reserved for well-differentiated endometrioid tumors without evidence of myometrial invasion or extrauterine spread. Hormonal treatment is most attractive for poor surgical candidates and women who strongly desire to preserve fertility. Finally, it is paramount that candidates for this nonsurgical approach appreciate that this is not the standard of care and accept the attendant risks.

18.4 Pathologic Features

18.4.1 Endometrial Carcinoma Grading

The first grading stratifier for endometrial carcinoma is histotype: serous carcinomas, clear cell carcinomas, carcinosarcomas, small/large cell neuroendocrine, and undifferentiated/dedifferentiated carcinomas are by definition high-grade tumors, as are mixed tumors with a ≥10% contribution of true serous or clear cell histology. The three-tiered International Federation of Gynecology and Obstetrics (FIGO) grading system does *not* apply to these cases; rather, FIGO grade should be designated as "not applicable" under the College of American Pathologists (CAP) synoptic reporting system.

In contrast, endometrioid carcinomas are classified as grade 1–3 using FIGO grading system, which is based on the proportion of non-squamous solid growth (Table 18.1, Fig. 18.1). The Gynecologic Oncology Group (GOG) released an updated clause to the system that allows for a one-step upgrade (e.g., grade 1 → 2, grade 2 → 3) on the basis of severe cytologic atypia irrespective of the percentage of solid growth [51, 52]. This work was spearheaded by Zaino and defined severe cytologic atypia includes large pleomorphic nuclei, course nuclear chromatin, and large irregular nucleoli; furthermore, the authors required that this atypia be present in the majority of the tumor cells. Subsequent work specified that severe atypia include nuclear pleomorphism visible from 10× and nuclear enlargement of

Table 18.1 International Federation of Gynecology and Obstetrics (FIGO) grading system for endometrioid carcinomas

Grade 1	≤5% non-squamous solid growth
Grade 2	6–50% non-squamous solid growth
Grade 3	>50% non-squamous solid growth

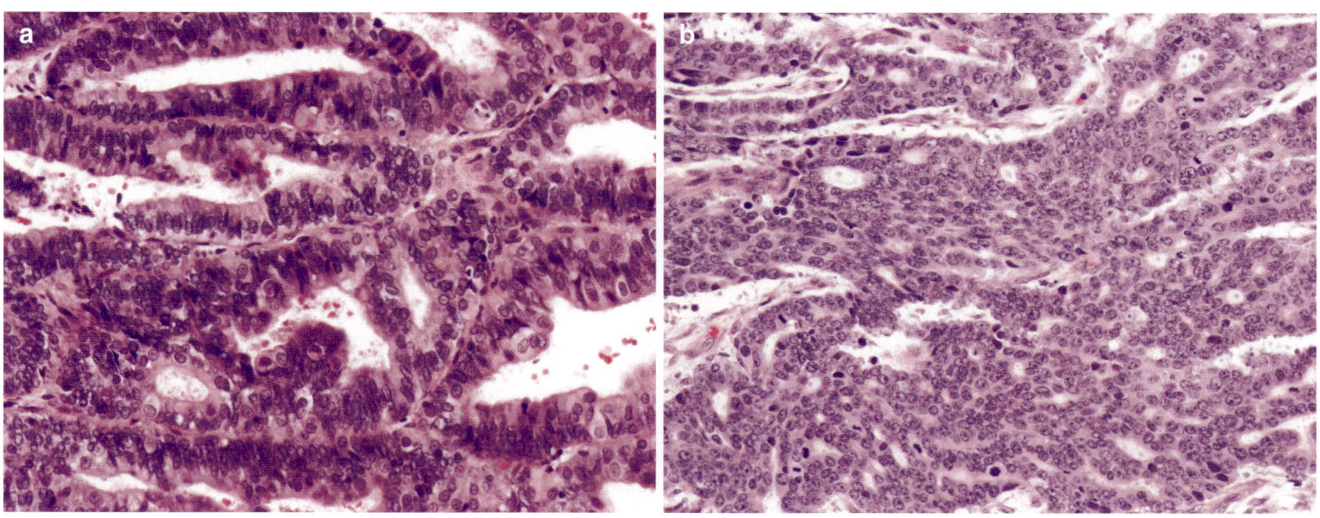

Fig. 18.1 FIGO grading in endometrioid carcinoma is based on the contribution of solid, non-squamous growth. Grade 1 carcinomas demonstrate ≤5% (**a**), Grade 2 carcinomas show 6–50% (**b**), and Grade 3 carcinomas show >50% (**c**)

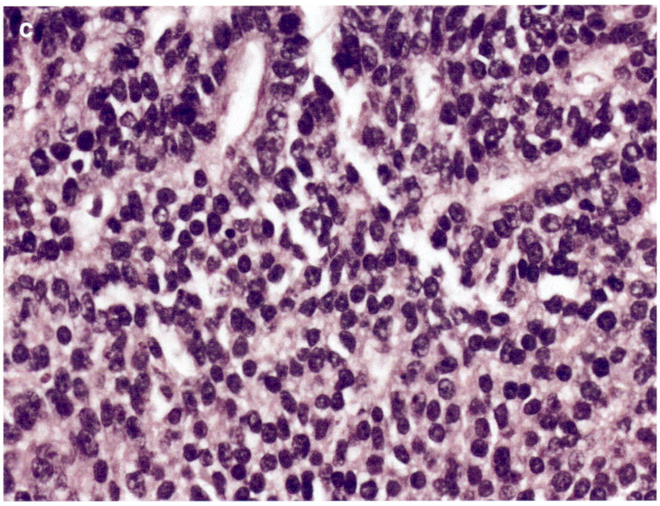

Fig. 18.1 (continued)

at least 1.5–2× normal [53]. The FIGO grading system also applies to mucinous endometrial carcinomas as they are considered close relatives of endometrioid carcinomas (and may indeed simply represent endometrioid tumors with diffuse mucinous metaplasia).

There has been some controversy over whether a binary grading system would be more appropriate for endometrioid carcinomas, as the current three-tiered system suffers from imperfect interobserver reproducibility and poor alignment with clinical decision tree branch points [5, 54–59]. A novel system proposed in 2005 combines papillary/solid growth, mitotic activity and nuclear atypia to divide endometrioid tumors into low-grade and high-grade [57]. This two-tiered system has shown robust interobserver reproducibility and, in some studies, improved correlation with outcome relative to the existing FIGO system. However, prognostic power of the binary system has not been retained on all studies [58] and, for now at least, the three-tiered FIGO grading system remains intact.

Table 18.2 International Federation of Gynecology and Obstetrics (FIGO) (2015) and American Joint Committee on Cancer (AJCC) (2017, 8th Edition) staging systems for endometrial carcinoma and carcinosarcoma

AJCC TNM stage	FIGO stage	Pathologic findings
Tumor		
pTX		Primary tumor cannot be assessed
pT0		No evidence of primary tumor
pTis		Carcinoma in situ (preinvasive carcinoma)
pT1	I	Tumor confined to the uterus, including endocervical glandular involvement
pT1a	IA	Tumor confined to the uterus; no or <1/2 myometrial invasion
pT1b	IB	Tumor confined to the uterus; ½ or more myometrial invasion
pT2	II	Cervical stromal invasion, but not beyond uterus
pT3a	IIIA	Tumor invades serosa or adnexa
pT3b	IIIB	Vaginal and/or parametrial involvement
	IIIC1	Pelvic node involvement
	IIIC2	Para-aortic involvement
pT4	IVA	Tumor invasion bladder and/or bowel mucosa
	IVB	Distant metastases including abdominal metastases and/or inguinal lymph nodes
Regional lymph nodes		
pNX		
pN0		
pN0(i+)		Isolated tumor cells in regional lymph nodes ≤0.2 mm
pN1	IIIC1	Regional lymph node metastases to pelvic lymph nodes
pN1mi	IIIC1	Regional lymph node metastases to pelvic lymph nodes >0.2 mm, ≤2.0 mm
pN1a	IIIC1	Regional lymph node metastases to pelvic lymph nodes >2.0 mm
pN2	IIIC2	Regional lymph node metastases to para-aortic lymph nodes, with or without positive pelvic nodes
pN2mi	IIIC2	Regional lymph node metastases to para-aortic lymph nodes >0.2 mm, ≤2.0 mm, with or without positive pelvic nodes
pN2a	IIIC2	Regional lymph node metastases to para-aortic lymph nodes >2.0 mm, with or without positive pelvic nodes
Distant metastases		
M0		No distant metastases
M1	IVB	Distant metastases (including metastases to inguinal lymph nodes, intraperitoneal disease, or lung, liver, or bone metastases; excludes metastases to para-aortic lymph nodes, vagina, pelvic serosa, or adnexa)

18.4.2 Endometrial Carcinoma Staging

Endometrial carcinoma is currently staged using both the 2015 International Federation of Gynecology and Obstetrics (FIGO) system and the 2017 American Joint Committee on Cancer Staging (AJCC) system [60, 61]. These two systems have considerable overlap, but diverge in several areas; therefore, inclusion of both is advisable for synoptic reporting purposes (Table 18.2).

The current iterations of these staging systems include several improvements to the prior versions. First, assessment for depth of invasion has been simplified so that pathologists need no longer differentiate between non-myoinvasive and <50% myometrial invasion. Second, pathologists are not required to distinguish between endocervical and endometrial mucosal involvement. Third, peritoneal washings are no longer incorporating into staging [54, 62]. Finally, the updated AJCC includes far more granularity regarding the extent of nodal involvement, with separate categories assigned for isolated tumor cells (<0.2 mm), micrometastases (0.2–2.0 mm), and macrometastases (>2.0 mm).

Despite these changes, there is persistent controversy about specific recommendations in the current staging schema. For instance, it remains debatable whether tumor emboli identified within ovarian vessels should independently upstage a patient to stage III, or whether cervical lymphovascular invasion should upstage to stage II. While the current guidelines dictate that tumor stage not be informed by lymphovascular involvement even in these locales, the biologic basis for this recommendation is questionable. Additionally, tumors confined to polyps are not specifically addressed. Furthermore, cervical stromal involvement remains inadequately defined and poorly reproducible [63]. Perhaps most problematic is the variability in prognosis for stage III A, B, and C tumors, attributable in large part to the contribution of grade and histotype on outcome. There have been proposals to enhance the clinical predictive power of this staging system by incorporating tumor grade and histology as well as the adequacy of nodal staging [55], and future refinements of the FIGO staging system are likely to integrate these elements.

18.4.2.1 Myometrial Invasion

One of the most problematic and clinically important areas of endometrial carcinoma pathology is assessment of invasion. Invasion of at least 50% of the myometrial thickness stratifies FIGO stage IB from IA tumors and is, for low-grade tumors, often a trigger for lymph nodal dissection at the time of frozen section. Invasion should be assessed by measuring the deepest point of tumor infiltration from the level of the endometrial-myometrial junction. This is ideally performed on a full-thickness section that includes the deepest point of invasion, adjacent normal endometrial-myometrial junction, and the uterine serosa. When endometrial thickness precludes submission of a full-thickness section in a single cassette, the section should be bisected and submitted in two separate cassettes.

There are a number of variables that can compound invasive assessment both on frozen and permanent sections, and this complexity is reflected in the relatively high interobserver variability in diagnosing endometrial cancer invasion (~30%) [54, 64, 65]. Gynecologic pathologists typically report lower depths of invasion than non-specialists, suggesting that overestimating invasion is a more significant problem than underestimating invasion. Difficulties in assessing the depth of myometrial involvement by endometrial carcinoma can be attributed to three broad categories: adenomyosis, problems visualizing the endometrial-myometrial junction, and challenging patterns of invasion.

Adenomyosis is straightforward when the glands are surrounded by evident endometrial stroma, but may become quite problematic when that stroma is sparse or indistinct (astroma adenomyosis) (Figs. 18.2 and 18.3). In particular, stroma that is hormonally altered can become eosinophilic and spindled, mimicking myometrium. Differentiating adenomyosis from invasion is often most challenging on frozen section, and can result in errors with both over-calling and under-calling the degree of invasion. It is important to assess for the overall milieu: if extensive adenomyosis is present, caution should be exercised before calling invasion in isolated astromal glands, particularly if they are cytologically indistinguishable from neighboring adenomyosis and show a similar geographic distribution. It is worth emphasizing that while benign cytology can help exclude invasion, the presence of atypical or frankly malignant cells within a focus of adenomyosis does not qualify as invasion. Indeed, this represents a situation analogous to endocervical gland extension of cervical squamous dysplasia wherein an otherwise superficial process populates preexisting glands. Thus, the crux of confirming adenomyosis is in assessing the overall distribution of glands and in proper evaluation of the stroma. Frustratingly, CD10 immunohistochemistry is of little utility in this setting because while it can highlight attenuated or indistinct stroma surrounding adenomyosis, it may also be

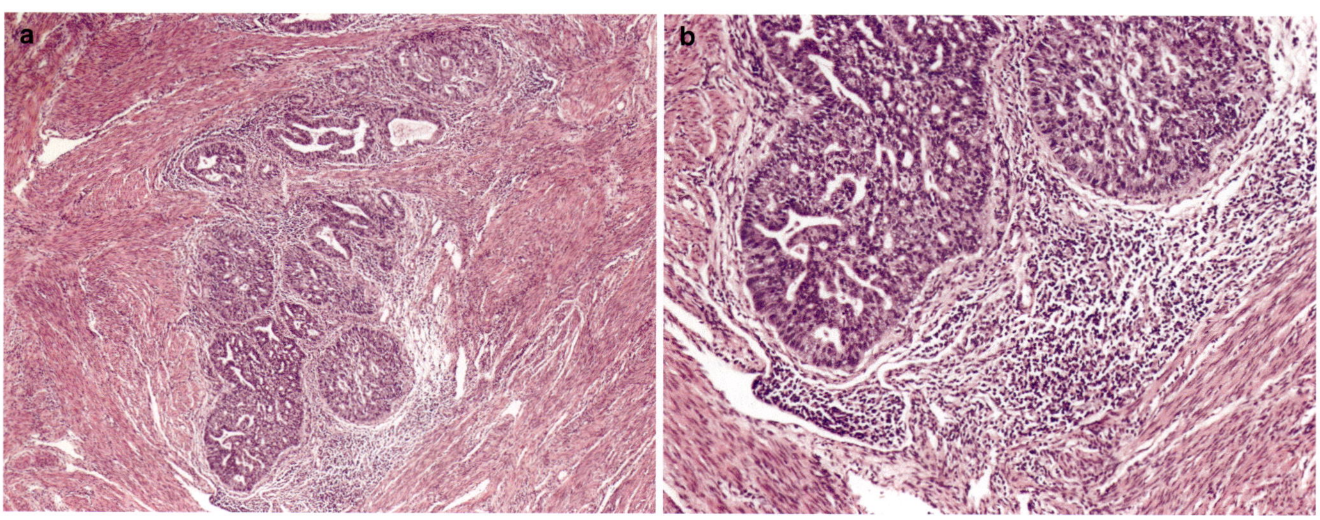

Fig. 18.2 Endometrioid endometrial carcinoma involving adenomyosis (**a**, **b**). This case demonstrates malignant glands surrounded by endometrial stromal tissue, compatible with extension into adenomyosis. All neoplastic glands show a circumferential stromal cuff without areas of infiltration into the myometrium. This finding can be seen in superficial cancers and does not upstage the tumor. It is important, and frequently challenging, to differentiate neoplastic involvement of adenomyosis from true invasion on intraoperative assessment

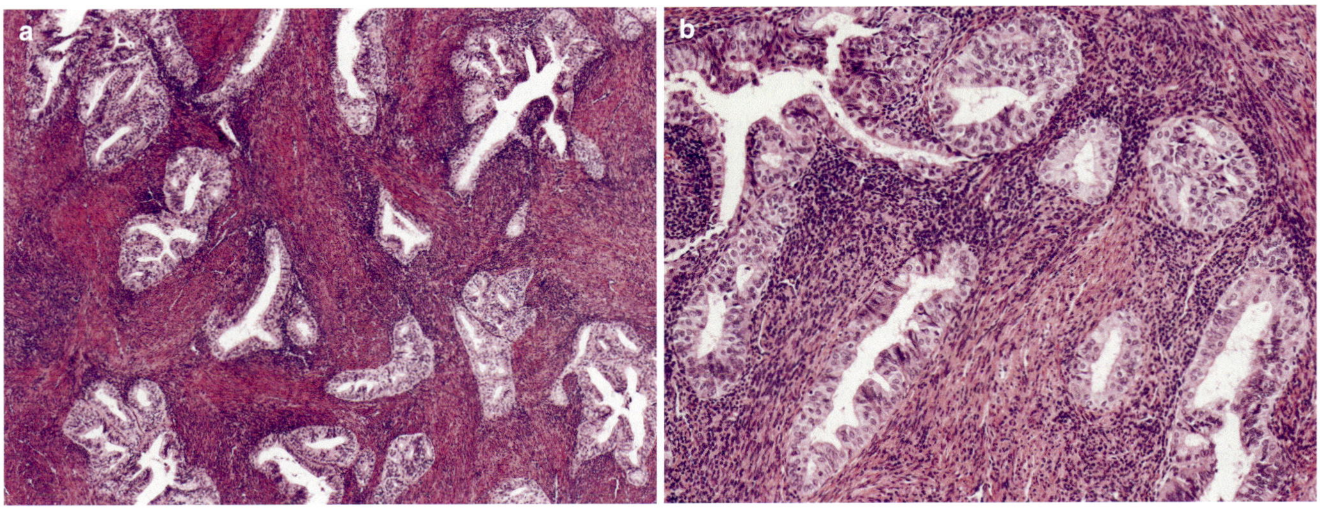

Fig. 18.3 Endometrioid endometrial carcinoma with focal myometrial invasion associated with adjacent adenomyosis (**a**, **b**). This case demonstrates extensive neoplastic involvement of adenomyosis, as well as foci of true myometrial invasion typified by infiltrative glands without a surrounding stromal cuff. This case is challenging because the invasive glands assume a subtle infiltration pattern without significant desmoplastic response, invoking the differential of stroma-poor adenomyosis. In this case, true myometrial invasion was ultimately confirmed based by the neoplastic glands' density and transmural distribution as well as the presence of multiple foci of lymphovascular invasion

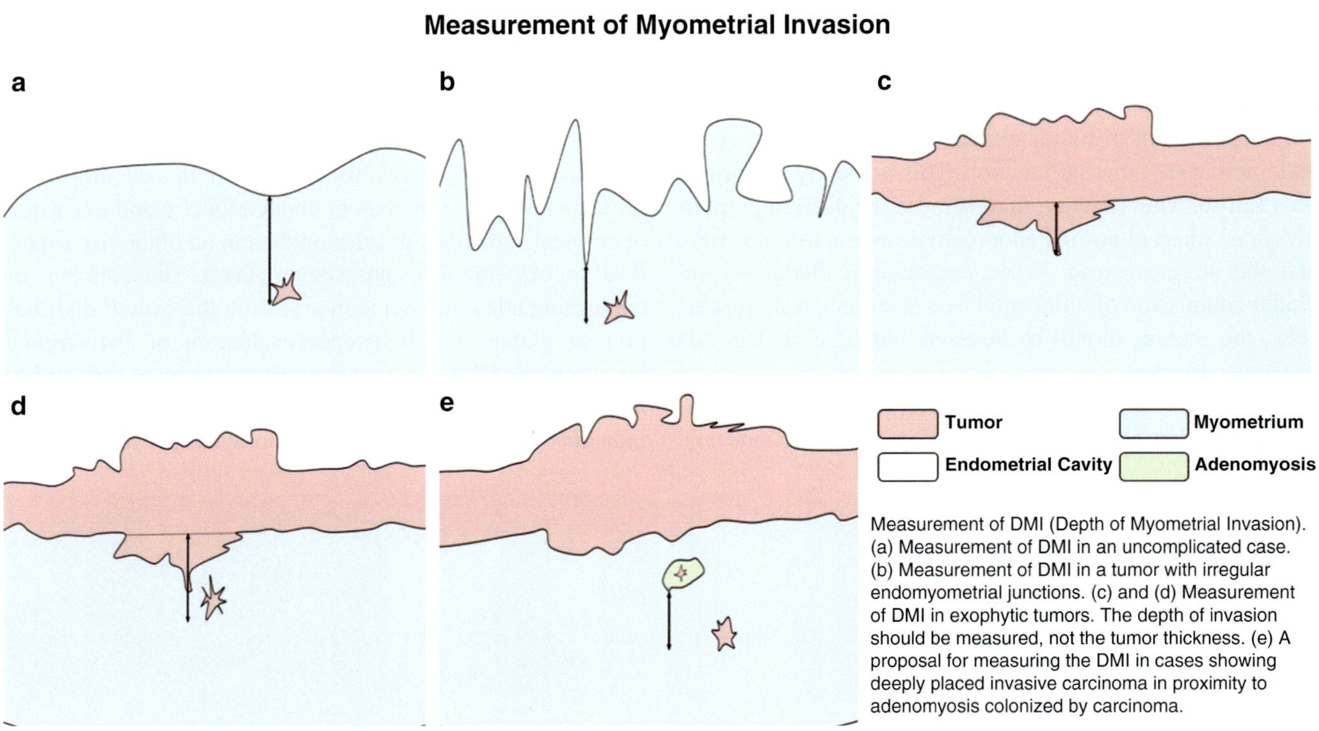

Fig. 18.4 Schematic demonstrating myometrial invasion. Figure courtesy of Dr. Wenxin Zheng

positive in myometrium surrounding invasive carcinoma. The issue can be compounded when invasive carcinoma arises within a focus of adenomyosis: that is, invasive tumor populating adenomyosis percolates beyond the boundaries of endometrial stroma and demonstrates true myometrial invasion. In these cases the invasive tumor typically shows a clear desmoplastic response that is distinct from the stroma surrounding the rest of the adenomyosis. Although management of such cases is not well codified, many gynecologic pathologists choose to measure depth of invasion from the point of intact adenomyosis, rather than the endometrial-myometrial junction [54, 64] (Fig. 18.4.).

Proper identification of the endometrial-myometrial junction is critical in order to accurately assess invasion. This junction is typically somewhat irregular in normal endometria and is therefore best evaluated from low power. An intact endometrial-myometrial junction should have stroma between the glands and the myometrium, be devoid of desmoplastic response, and have a relatively smooth and even border from low power. Localizing the endometrial-myometrial junction can be problematic when the normal architecture has been distorted by tumor. In such cases it is particularly important not to misinterpret exophytic growth (tumor thickness) as depth of invasion. Some pathologists suggest that proximity to thick-walled blood vessels can serve as a helpful clue that a tumor has strayed into the outer half of the myometrium, as such vessels are not typically present in the superficial myometrium. Conversely, one should be cautious calling >50% invasion for tumors that are distant from thick-walled blood vessels, as this may represent an exophytic tumor with only limited myometrial invasion. That said, this recommendation is not universally accepted and proximity to thick-walled vessels should best be treated only as a soft marker for deep invasion.

The pattern of infiltration can further complicate assessment (Table 18.3). Measuring invasion is easiest for conventional infiltrative tumors, which are typified by irregular, angulated glands that provoke a desmoplastic response (Fig. 18.5). More problematic is the broad or pushing pattern of invasion, which manifests as bulky, blunt tumor growth, often without an associated stromal

Table 18.3 Patterns of endometrial carcinoma invasion

	Description	Potential pitfalls
Conventional infiltrative	Invasion of irregular, angulated glands eliciting a desmoplastic response	Typically easy to recognize and measure correctly provided EMJ is appropriately identified
Pushing/broad	Invasion with a blunt, bulky edge rather than infiltrative tongues and individual glands; desmoplasia may be limited	Invasion may be underestimated (when depth is misinterpreted as thickness) or overestimated (in exophytic tumors when thickness is misinterpreted as depth)
Microcystic elongated and fragmented (MELF)	Invasive of single glands with paradoxically bland cells bearing attenuated cytoplasm and invoking a myxoinflammatory myometrial response	May be mistaken for vessels +/− lymphovascular involvement, leading to an underestimate of invasion
Adenoma malignum-like ("Melter/ melting")	Invasion with well-differentiated single glands and groups of glands without an associated stromal response	May be mistaken for adenomyosis, leading to an underestimate of invasion

EMJ endometrial-myometrial junction

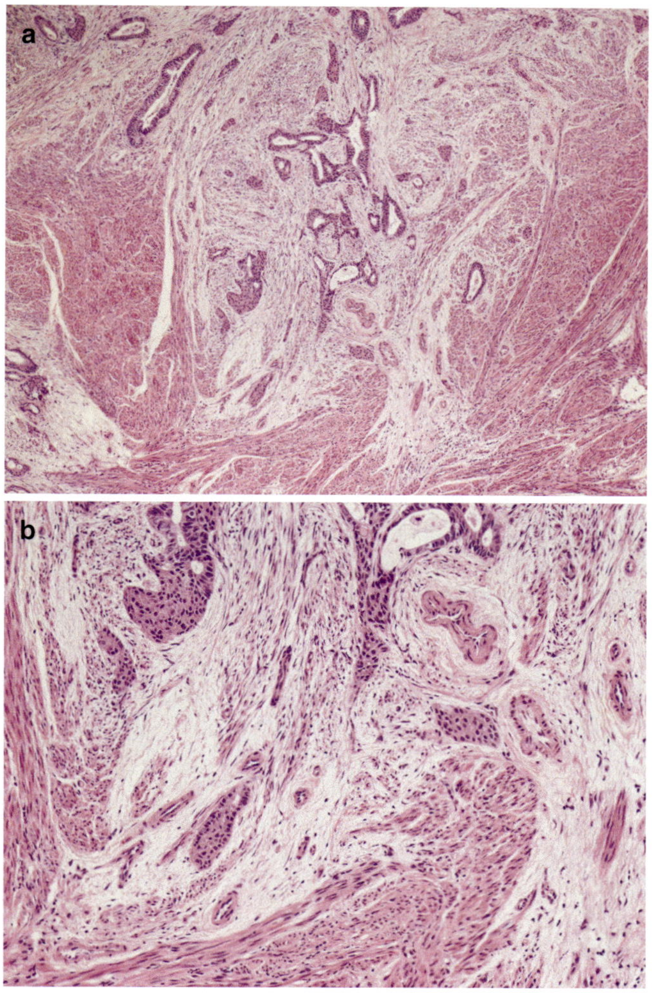

Fig. 18.5 Conventional invasion by endometrial carcinomas is typified by irregular glands embedded in desmoplastic stroma (**a**, **b**). This pattern is easily recognizable as invasion and can usually be recognized readily on frozen and permanent sections

response. It is this pattern that most commonly results in complete effacement of the normal endometrial-myometrial junction, necessitating reliance on other clues for orientation, such as proximity to thick-walled blood vessels as described above (Fig. 18.6). There are two less common patterns specific to the endometrioid subtype that can also pose particular difficulty in invasive assessments: the microcystic elongated and fragmented pattern (MELF) and the adenoma malignum-like pattern (so-called "melter" or "melting" pattern).

MELF invasion is characterized by paradoxically bland glands embedded in myxoinflammatory stroma (Fig. 18.7). The constituent gland lining cells often show squamous metaplasia or a histiocytoid appearance, marked attenuation, and low nuclear-to-cytoplasm ratios. More conventional atypical tumor cells can occasionally be seen within the gland lumen (Fig. 18.8). This pattern is seen in a small proportion of endometrioid carcinoma and readily mimics

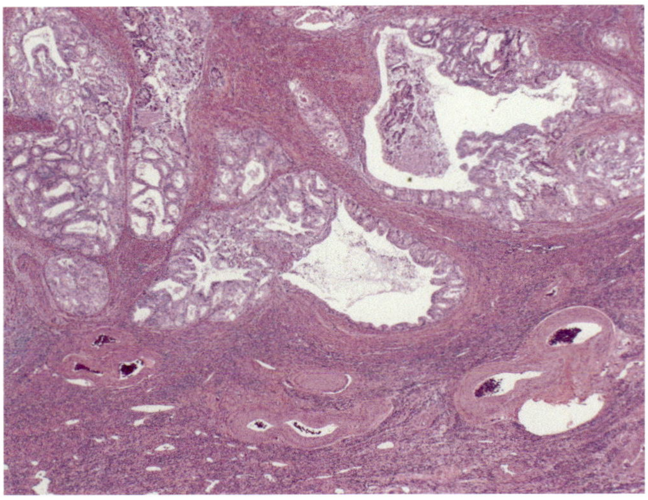

Fig. 18.6 Tumor proximity to thick-walled blood vessels helps confirm involvement of the outer-half of the myometrium when the tumor has effaced the endometrial-myometrial junction, as illustrated by this deeply infiltrative endometrioid carcinoma with pushing, broad-based infiltration

lymphovascular invasion. Interestingly, MELF is also associated with an increased incidence of true lymphovascular invasion, as well as increased rates of nodal metastases [66–70]. Independent prognostic significance has not been proven; however, in one large series cases with MELF showed a trend towards increased extravaginal recurrence [69]. MELF has been postulated to represent an early phase of epithelial-mesenchymal transition, with immunohistochemical analyses demonstrating an immunophenotype more typical of mesenchymal differentiation in the infiltrating MELF glands including decreased expression of hormone receptors and e-cadherin and positivity for Cycling D1 and fascin [71–73].

Adenoma malignum-like infiltration was described by Longacre & Hendrickson in 1999 and is also known as "diffusely infiltrative endometrial adenocarcinoma" or, colloquially, "melting" carcinoma (not to be confused with MELF!) [74] (Fig. 18.9). These subtly infiltrative endometrioid cancers are typified by round, regular glands situated

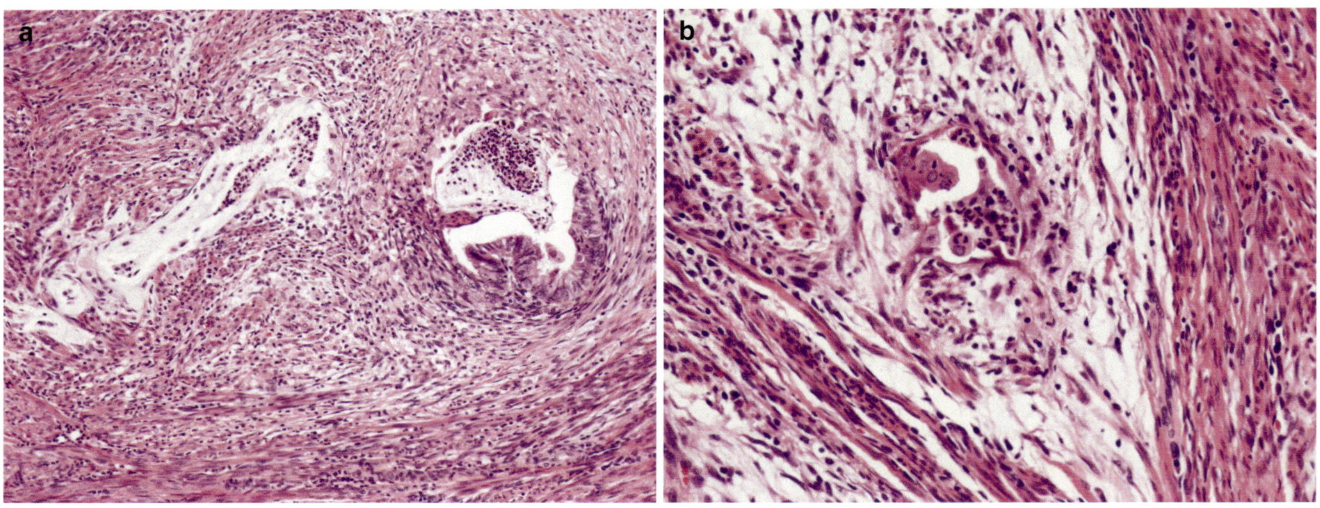

Fig. 18.7 The microcystic, elongated, and fragmented pattern (MELF) of infiltration is characterized by cytologically bland glands embedded in myxoinflammatory stroma (**a**, **b**)

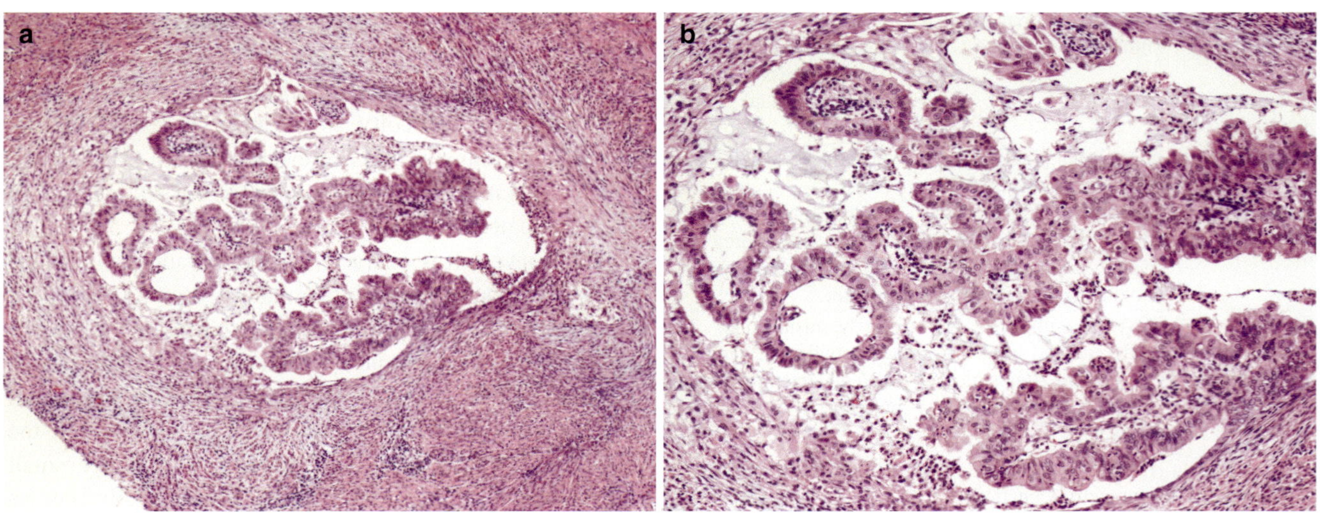

Fig. 18.8 In this example of MELF infiltration, atypical epithelial cells are seen within the glandular lumen, mimicking lymphovascular invasion. The surrounding myxoinflammatory stroma helps secure the diagnosis of myometrial—rather than lymphovascular—involvement (**a**, **b**)

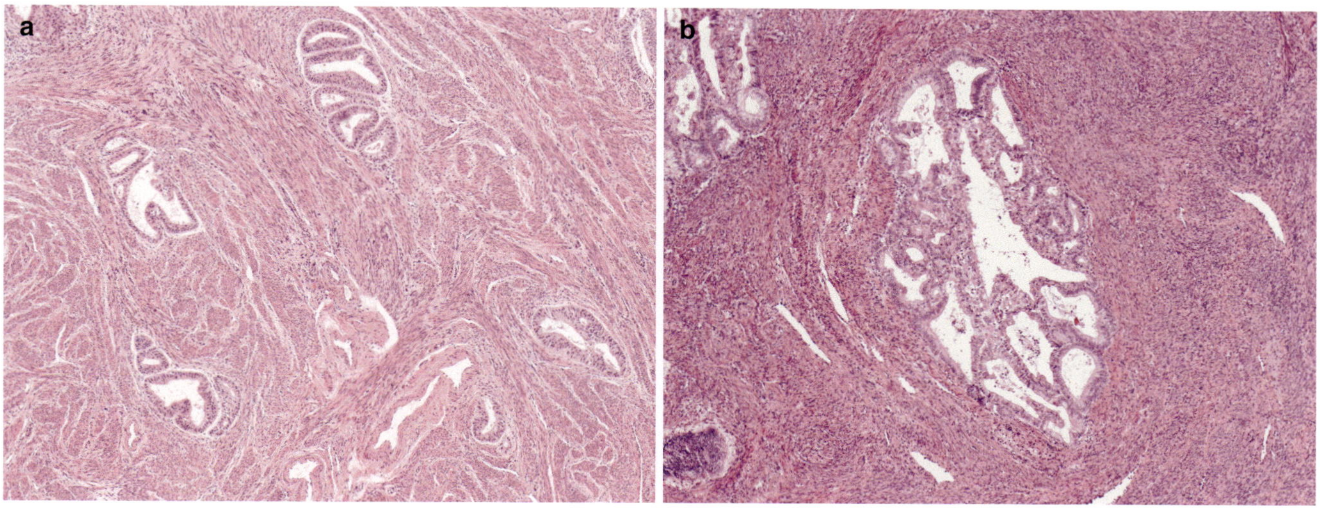

Fig. 18.9 Adenoma malignum-like infiltration (the so-called "melter" pattern) is characterized by subtly infiltrative, rounded glands percolating through the myometrium with no desmoplastic response (**a**, **b**). This pattern often results in an underestimate of invasive depth as the glands may be mistaken for stroma-poor adenomyosis, particularly at the time of frozen section. In the pictured case, the extensive transmural distribution of the neoplastic glands and complete lack of associated stroma throughout secured the diagnosis of true invasion

in a myometrium with little to no associated desmoplastic reaction. Invasion is frequently underestimated in these cases because the unapparent stromal reaction and cytologic banality of the glands can suggest adenomyosis with a paucity of stroma. The haphazard arrangement of the tumoral glands is a useful clue to the diagnosis, as adenomyosis more often shows a clustered pattern. Importantly, these endometrial tumors have no biologic or genetic relationship to adenoma malignum of the endocervix; the name is based purely on their subtle pattern of infiltration.

18.4.2.2 Intraoperative Evaluation

Intraoperative frozen sections are performed on endometrial carcinoma cases chiefly to determine whether staging should be performed. Staging is appropriate for all high-grade cancers including serous carcinomas, clear cell carcinomas, undifferentiated carcinomas, carcinosarcomas, and FIGO grade 3 endometrioid carcinomas given their increased propensity for extrauterine spread. For low- and intermediate-grade carcinomas, the depth of invasion and endocervical stromal involvement become critical factors in determining whether or not a staging procedure should be performed. Greater than 50% invasion of the myometrium is considered deep invasion and warrants staging even for FIGO Grade 1–2 endometrioid tumors; this is because tumors involving the outer half of the myometrium can potentially access the large, thick-walled blood vessels that provide conduits for extrauterine spread.

Although intraoperative assessments appropriately guide surgical management 95% of the time, occasionally the frozen section read varies significantly from the final assessment [75, 76]. Evaluating depth of invasion can be challenging for the reasons detailed in the preceding section "Assessing Endometrial Invasion." Difficulty identifying the endometrial/myometrial junction, stroma-poor adenomyosis, and MELF and melter patterns of invasion can all present challenges which can be augmented by frozen section artifacts. Sampling error can further compound the problem, as accurate microscopic assessment is contingent upon proper gross identification of the area of deepest invasion. Given sampling limitations, it is prudent to provide clinically actionable information and no more at the time of frozen section: an intraoperative assessment of "low- to intermediate-grade carcinoma limited to the inner half of the endometrium," for example, provides all the data needed to guide surgery and is less likely to be overturned than an unnecessarily specific read of "FIGO grade 1 endometrioid carcinoma with 3 of 20 mm of invasion."

18.4.2.3 Cervical Invasion

Under the current staging system, cervical invasion is defined as involvement of the cervical stroma and independently upstages the tumor to Stage II. Importantly, tumor growth limited to the endocervical mucosa does not constitute involvement. This can present interpretative problems when neoplastic cells colonize endocervical glands, as it can be difficult to ascertain whether true invasion is present (Fig. 18.10). In these instances, it is useful to assess the distribution of the background normal endocervical glands. If the tumor is distributed similar to the native endocervical glandular pattern, invasion is unlikely. However, true stromal invasion is present if tumor is seen infiltrating beyond this normal gland distribution. It is worth emphasizing that this area remains imperfectly reproducible and controversial.

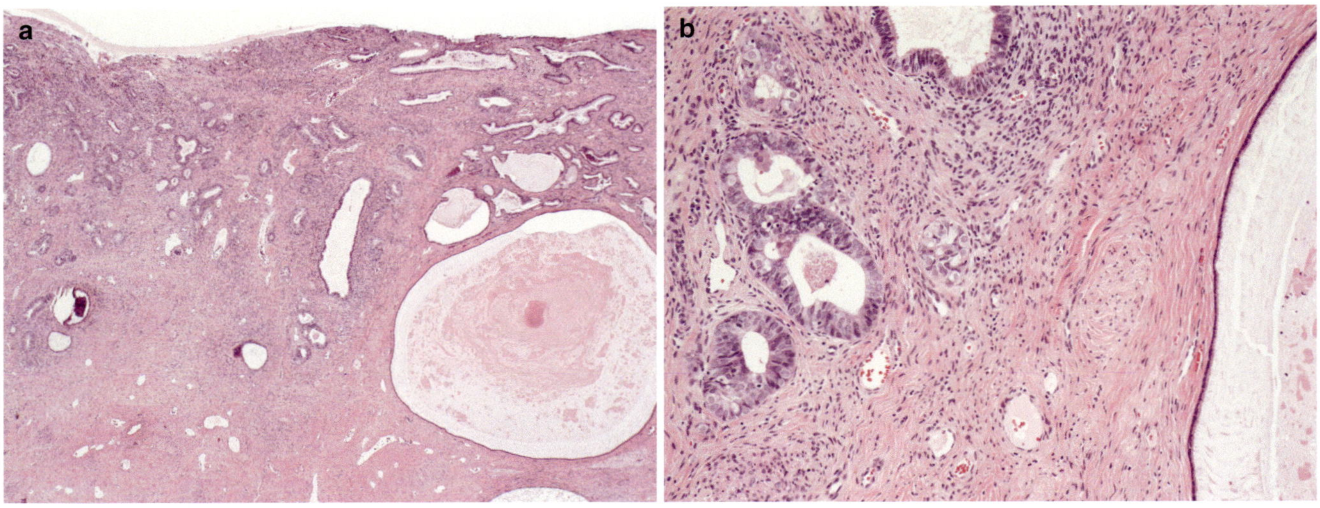

Fig. 18.10 Assessing cervical stromal invasion can be challenging for endometrial carcinomas, and remains an area of frequent controversy. This case demonstrates an endometrioid carcinoma extending through the lower uterine segment and into the endocervix (**a**, **b**). While the depth of the deepest neoplastic glands does not exceed that of the deepest native endocervical glands, this is in part due to the cystic dilation of some of the benign glands. Furthermore, the density of the malignant glands exceeds what one would expect for involvement limited to endocervical glandular extension. This tumor was therefore staged as involving the cervical stroma, with a comment that this involvement was relatively superficial

18.4.2.4 Parametrial Invasion

Parametrial invasion has been shown to be a poor prognostic factor in multiple studies [77–79]. The parametria are routinely assessed only in radical hysterectomies, which are primarily performed for cervical neoplasia but occasionally for other tumors such as endometrial carcinoma involving endocervix, and should be assessed completely in these cases. There is increasingly interest in submitting parametrial shavings on all malignant cases; however official recommendations on this remain pending.

18.4.2.5 Lymphovascular Invasion

Lymphovascular invasion is seen in up to 25% of endometrial cancers and is most common among high-grade tumors [59, 80, 81]. It has been shown to be an independent negative prognostic factor for low-stage cancers and can therefore guide treatment strategies, particularly for tumors that straddle treatment algorithms based on grade and stage [80, 82]. Lymphovascular invasion is defined by pathologic deposits of tumor within either blood vessels or lymphatic vessels. Helpful features include identification of an endothelial lining surrounding the tumor, associated hematopoietic elements within the vascular lumen, conformation of the tumor deposit to the vessel wall (with or without adherence to the wall), and proximity to thick-walled arteries (Fig. 18.11). The diagnosis of lymphovascular invasion can be complicated by technical artifacts (pseudoinvasion) as well as histologic mimics. Furthermore, intravascular menstrual or benign endometrial tissue must be excluded, particularly for benign hysterectomy specimens showing florid endometrial stromal breakdown.

Some sources of problematic artifact precede the specimen's arrival in surgical pathology. Laparoscopic hysterectomy is a well-documented cause of vascular pseudoinvasion [83, 84]. Another source of artifact occurs stems from the grossing bench: detached tumor fragments may occasionally be deposited in large vascular spaces by the grosser's knife, particularly when vessels are present at the cut edge of the specimen. Adherence to the vascular wall, along with associated fibrin thrombi, helps to exclude this possibility, although its absence doesn't exclude true vascular invasion. Caution should be exercised when involvement is limited to free-floating tumor fragments in large vessels, particularly at the cut specimen edge, as this often represent knife artifact. Lastly, retraction artifact around invasive nests of tumor can also mimic lymphatic invasion. Identification of an endothelial lining confirmed with immunohistochemical stains that highlight lymphatic channels (such as D2–40) can be helpful when the H&E appearance is ambiguous. Localization is also helpful: because lymphatics travel in parallel with veins, tumor juxtaposition near a vein supports true invasion over retraction artifact.

Histologic features are also important for differentiating lymphovascular invasion from its mimics. The MELF pattern of myometrial invasion, which is described in detail under the heading "Assessing Endometrial Invasion," is typified by detached tumor cells floating in angulated, infiltrative glands with attenuated lining. These flattened, cytologically banal lining cells masquerade as endothelium and may be misinterpreted as lymphovascular invasion. In such cases the presence of surrounding fibromyxoid stroma helps identify these as MELF glands rather than

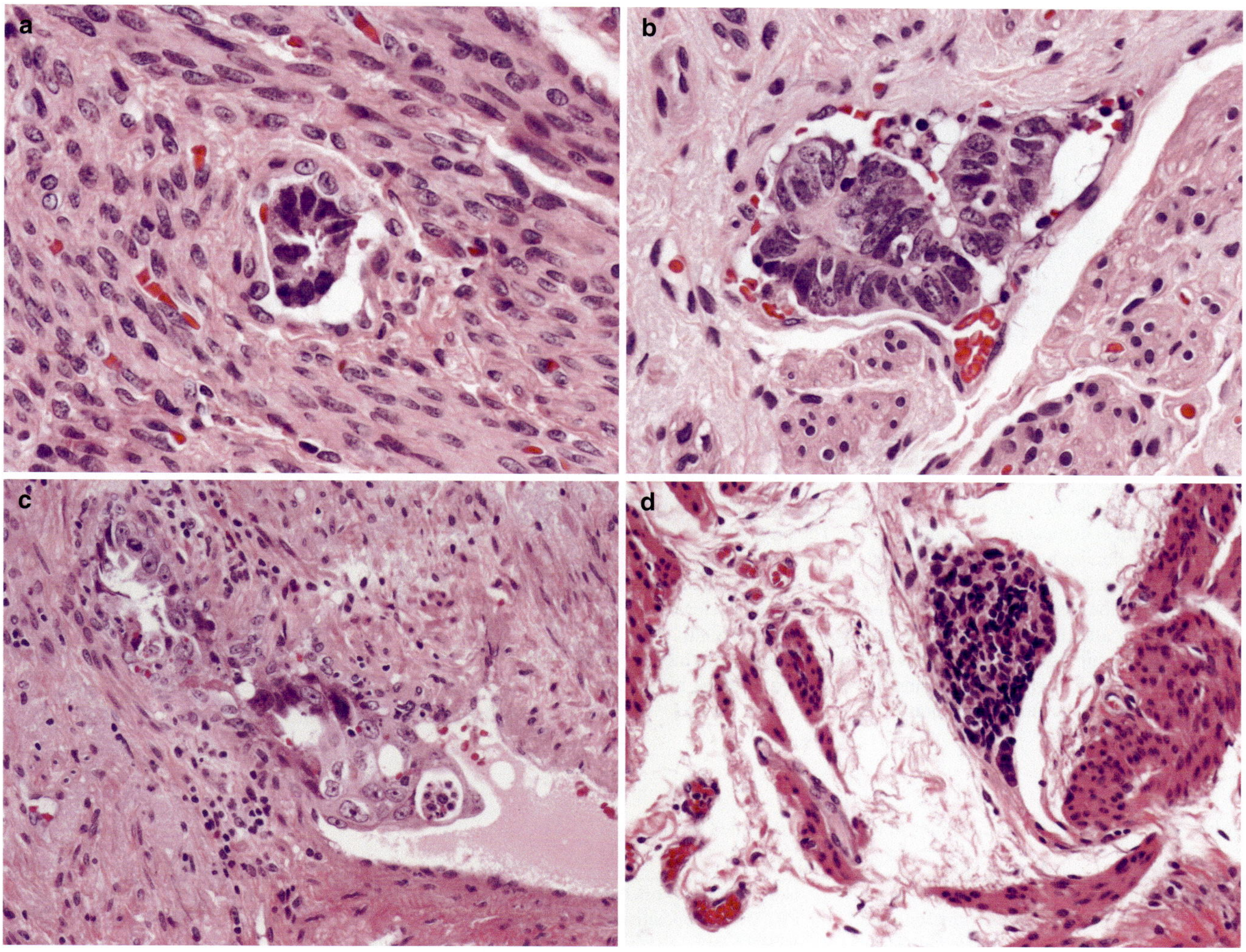

Fig. 18.11 Several features can aid in the diagnosis of lymphovascular invasion. Identification of an endothelial lining in the space (as seen in **a**) surrounding tumor deposits helps exclude retraction artifact, as does the presence of hematolymphoid elements within the lumen (illustrated in **b** and **c**) and adherence of the tumor deposit to the vascular wall (demonstrated in **b**–**d**)

vessels. Immunohistochemical staining for epithelial and lymphovascular markers is also useful for clarifying the epithelial nature of these glands. Conversely, a histologic feature that can lead to underestimating lymphovascular invasion is the he histiocytoid pattern of lymphovascular involvement. This pattern is characterized by dyshesive cells with eosinophilic cytoplasm admixed with normal blood components. Because these tumor cells appear singly, rather than in obvious clusters, they may be missed on casual review. In such cases appreciating nuclear atypia is critical for correctly identifying these malignant cells and cytokeratin staining can be enlisted to confirm their epithelial nature.

18.4.2.6 Peritoneal Washings

Peritoneal washing status is no longer incorporated in the FIGO or AJCC staging systems for endometrial carcinomas. This change derives from evidence that a positive peritoneal washing does not independently influence overall outcome [85–89]. That said the identification of neoplastic cells on cytology is considered a poor prognostic sign for non-endometrioid and high-grade endometrioid carcinomas [86]. The impact of positive cytology is less clear in low and intermediate-grade endometrioid cancers otherwise confined to the uterus. In these cases, neoplastic cells identified in washings are thought to often be biologically effete and, in many cases, artifactually displaced due to uterine manipulation [90] (Fig. 18.12).

18.4.2.7 Margin Status

The paracervical soft tissue represents the only true margin in total hysterectomy specimens, while radical hysterectomy specimens include a vaginal and parametrial margin. Reporting on these margins is optional.

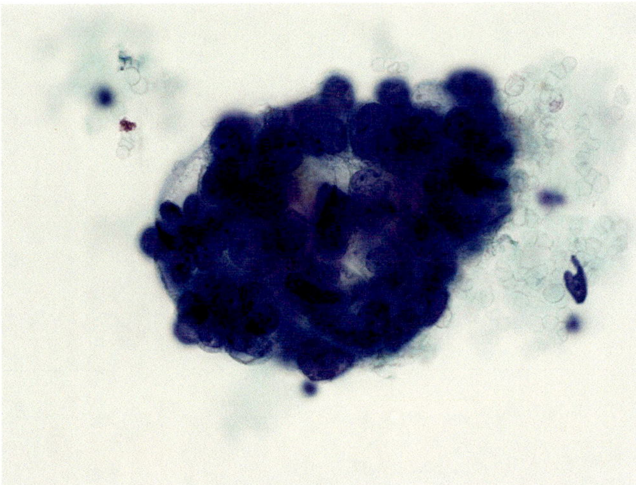

Fig. 18.12 Neoplastic cells are occasionally identified in peritoneal washings from endometrial carcinoma patients. The prognostic significance of this finding has not proven reproducible (particularly among low-grade endometrioid tumors) therefore current staging schema do not upstage on the basis of peritoneal fluid involvement alone. However, clinicians may alter treatment approach based on a positive fluid, particularly among high-grade tumors. This endometrial serous carcinoma showed abundant malignant cell clusters in the fluid as well as histologically confirmed peritoneal implants

18.4.3 Endometrial Carcinoma Histotypes

One of the most critical pieces of data about an endometrial carcinoma is its histologic subtype. Histologic type informs prognosis, surgical approach, vulnerability to endocrine therapy, and chemotherapeutic options. Correct assignment of histotype is therefore central to accurate diagnosis, and requires understanding of morphologic variants and mimics as well as molecular drivers. There are a range of endometrial histotypes which are associated with distinct molecular profiles and clinical outcomes (Table 18.4). The majority of endometrial carcinomas can be divided into endometrioid and serous carcinomas. Mucinous carcinomas are thought to represent a variant of endometrioid carcinoma and share both biologic behavior and management strategies with tumors bearing conventional endometrioid differentiation. Clear cell carcinoma is a rare subtype which is often overdiagnosed in endometrioid and serous cancers with clear cell features. The remaining cancers consist of high-grade malignancies which often derive from their better-differentiated counterparts: carcinosarcomas (malignant mixed müllerian tumors), dedifferentiated carcinomas, undifferentiated carcinomas, and neuroendocrine carcinomas.

Table 18.4 Endometrial carcinoma histotypes and associated features

Histotype	Microscopic	IHC	Molecular	Diagnostic pitfalls
Endometrioid	Glands resembling native endometrium with mild to moderate cytologic atypia and variable solid contributions	–Hormone receptors AR/PR/AR often positive –PTEN loss –Usually p53 wild type; subset of high-grades overexpressed or null –MMR loss 25–35%	–*PTEN*, *ARID1A, PIK3C* mutations –25–35% MMRd (majority epigenetic *MLH1* hypermethylation; remaining 5–10% germline and sporadic mutations) –*TP53* mutations in a subset of high-grade	–Abnormal p53 expression in a case which is morphologically endometrioid suggests serous-like behavior
Mucinous	>50% of tumor shows mucinous differentiation (defined by abundant intracytoplasmic mucin). Villoglandular and papillary common, but microacinar patterns also occur	–Similar to endometrioid carcinomas –Panel of ER (+), vimentin (+), p16 (wild type), and CEA (+/–) useful for differential of endocervical carcinoma	–Similar molecular profile to endometrioid carcinoma	–Typical endometrioid carcinomas often assume a mucinous phenotype after progestin therapy –Can be mistaken for endocervical adenocarcinoma in the lower uterine segment –Microacinar pattern can also mimic endocervical microglandular hyperplasia
Serous	Markedly atypical cells arranged in papillary, tubular, and solid arrangements. Prominent nucleoli and atypical mitotic figures common	–p53 abnormal (diffuse or null) –p16 overexpression –PR- –IMP3+ –PTEN intact –MMR intact	–*TP53*, *PIK3C* mutations; *HER2* amplification	–May be mistaken for villoglandular endometrioid carcinoma (p53 staining can confirm when null or diffusely positive)

Table 18.4 (continued)

Histotype	Microscopic	IHC	Molecular	Diagnostic pitfalls
Clear cell	Tubulocystic arrangements of clear or eosinophilic cells embedded in dense hyaline stroma. Nuclear hobnailing common	–HNF-β+ –Napsin+ –ER/PR/AR usually negative –p53 usually wild type –Ki67 at least 20–30%, often up to 50% –MMR loss ~10%	–*ARID1A, PIK3C, PTEN, KRAS, NRAS* mutations –MMRd common	–True endometrial clear cell carcinoma is extremely rare (<1% of endometrial cancers) –Clear cell morphology is more often attributable to secretory differentiation in endometrioid tumors or as an admixed component of serous carcinoma
Carcinosarcoma	Mixed malignant epithelial and mesenchymal tumors; sarcomatous component may have homologous or heterologous elements	-Varies with carcinoma component; p53 abnormalities common -Myogein and MyoD useful for confirming rhabdomyo-sarcomatous elements	-*TP53* mutations -EMT molecular signatures	-May mimic sarcoma on biopsy; important to note that differential includes carcinosarcoma to ensure appropriate staging
Dedifferentiated	Biphasic juxtaposition of well-differentiated endometrioid carcinoma with sheets of undifferentiated cells	–MMR, SMARCA4 (BRG1) loss common; SMARCB1 (INI) loss rare	–MMRd common –*POLE, TP53, SMARCA4* mutations common; rare *SMARCB1* mutations	–Often misclassified as Grade 2 or 3 endometrial carcinoma based on % glandular vs. solid
Undifferentiated	Confluent proliferation of undifferentiated cells without appreciable gland formation or mesenchymal differentiation	–Focal EMA/keratin positivity confirms epithelial origin –MMR, SMARCA4 (BRG1) loss common; SMARCB1 (INI) loss rare	–MMRd common –*POLE, TP53, SMARCA4* mutations common; rare *SMARCB1* mutations	–Morphologically indistinguishable from undifferentiated endometrial sarcoma; may also be mimic lymphoma
Neuroendocrine	Large cell or small cell neuroendocrine morphology; may occur alone or in concert with other histotypes	–Neuroendocrine marker (synaptophysin, chromogranin, CD56) staining in >10% of tumor cells –Dot-like keratin staining	–MMRd may be present	–Often under-recognized and classified as simply high-grade endometrial carcinoma

IHC immunohistochemistry, *MMRd* mismatch repair deficiency, *EMT* epithelial mesenchymal transition

18.4.3.1 Endometrioid Carcinoma

Clinical

Endometrioid carcinoma is the most common type of endometrial malignancy. It typically occurs in the context of increased estrogen levels with predisposing conditions including obesity, infertility, nulliparity, unopposed estrogen replacement therapy, tamoxifen exposure, and estrogen-producing ovarian tumors. It is also associated with heritable mismatch repair gene defects (Lynch syndrome) and in this setting isn't necessarily associated with increased estrogen exposure. The clinical presentation is typically of abnormal uterine bleeding in perimenopausal or postmenopausal women. Younger women may also be affected, however, particularly those with extremely high body-mass indexes. Women with Lynch syndrome present, on average, at a decade younger than women with sporadic endometrial tumors; however, older age at presentation does not exclude Lynch syndrome [31, 91].

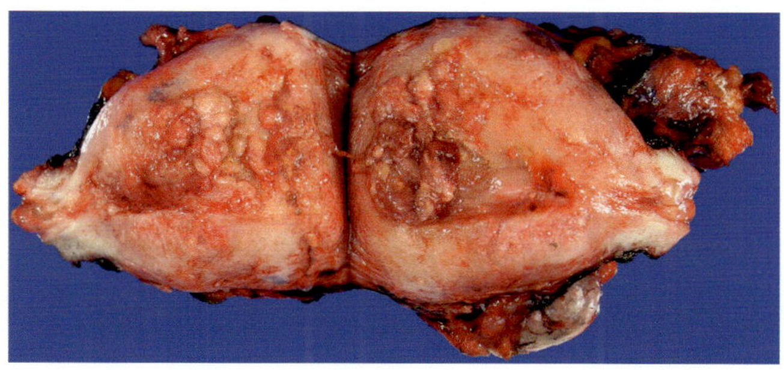

Fig. 18.13 Endometrioid carcinomas are often exophytic with a multinodular and fleshy appearance on gross exam, as is seen in this case carpeting the endometrial cavity. Other cases may be more subtle, which can present challenges when selecting the optimal section for intraoperative assessment

Gross

Endometrioid carcinomas have a gross presentation that ranges from exophytic, polypoid masses to flat, infiltrative plaques (Fig. 18.13). Tumors demonstrate light tan to light

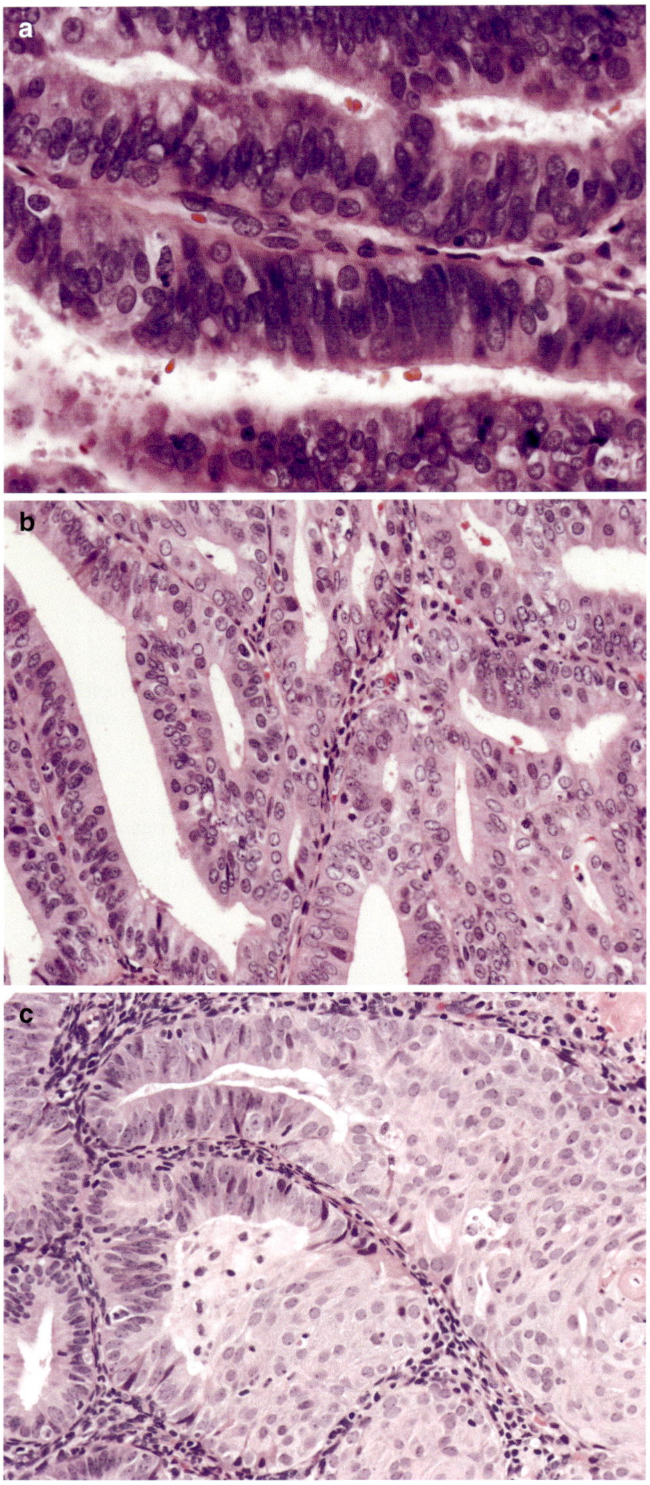

Fig. 18.14 Endometrioid carcinoma is defined by the neoplastic glands' cytologic resemblance to benign endometrium. The constituent cells typically bear hyperchromatic, elongate nuclei (**a**) but lack the marked cytologic atypia and prominent nucleoli typical of serous and other non-endometrioid histotypes. Superimposed metaplasias, such as ciliated metaplasia (**b**) and squamous metaplasia (**c**) are common

yellow coloring, sometimes with associated pinpoint or blotchy hemorrhages. The tumor surface is typically friable and soft, while the infiltrative portion often assumes a firm, rubbery texture. Infiltration of the myometrium can be difficult to appreciate grossly, particularly prior to formalin fixation,

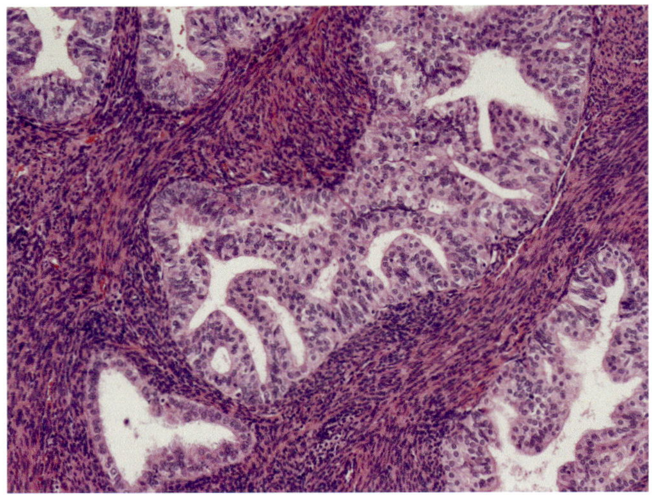

Fig. 18.15 Low-grade endometrioid carcinoma can be differentiated from hyperplasia on the basis of architecture, rather than atypia. The chief architectural feature warranting a diagnosis of malignancy is gland fusion. This endometrioid carcinoma shows banal cytology with prominent ciliated metaplasia. Despite this bland cytology, the extensive cribriform architecture is sufficient for a diagnosis of carcinoma

which can lead to challenges on frozen section assessment. Endometrioid carcinomas can involve any portion of the endometrial cavity from the fundus to the lower uterine segment. Lower uterine segment involvement has been related with Lynch syndrome-associated and *MLH1*-hypermethylated cancers; however, this anatomic localization is neither sensitive nor specific for mismatch repair deficiency [31].

Microscopic

Endometrioid carcinoma is fundamentally defined by the neoplastic glands' resemblance to normal endometrial epithelium (Fig. 18.14). Like benign endometrium, endometrioid carcinomas can take on a variety of metaplastic changes. This cytologic overlap with benign glands is illustrated by the fact that the diagnosis of low-grade endometrioid carcinoma is based first and foremost on architecture, rather than atypia (Fig. 18.15). Some degree of atypia is allowable and expected in endometrioid cancers; however, too much divergence from normal—extremely prominent nucleoli or marked anisocytosis, for example—undermines a diagnosis of endometrioid carcinoma and suggests possible serous or other non-endometrioid differentiation. The relationship between endometrioid carcinoma and benign endometrium is further demonstrated in the molecular underpinnings of these tumors: mutations in *PTEN* are quite common in endometrioid carcinoma, yet such mutations can also be seen in cycling endometrium [92–94]. Therefore, loss of PTEN expression has minimal utility in the diagnosis of endometrioid cancers.

18.4.3.2 Endometrioid Carcinoma vs. Atypical Hyperplasia/Endometrioid Intraepithelial Neoplasia (EIN)

Given that cytology and PTEN loss patterns may be shared across benign, hyperplastic, and malignant endometrial lesions [92–95], differentiating low-grade endometrial carcinoma from its precancers can be challenging. The most recent iteration of the World Health Organization classification (2014) system divides hyperplasias in a binary manner: those without atypia and those with atypia [96]. This latter category (atypical hyperplasia) is considered synonymous with endometrial intraepithelial neoplasia, a diagnostic classification conceived by Mutter and colleagues which was later modified to endometrioid intraepithelial neoplasia (EIN) [95]. The retention of the modifier "atypical" can generate some confusion among pathologists because cytologic atypia is not necessarily required for diagnosis: rather, atypical hyperplasia/EIN requires the presence of a "clonally distinct" (but not necessarily overtly atypical) population of glands. Importantly, this distinct appearance should not be attributable to metaplastic changes (ciliated/tubal, papillary, eosinophilic), which can be superimposed on benign glands without imparting risk of neoplastic progression. When one reflects back on the chief criterion for endometrioid carcinoma diagnosis—abnormalities in architecture, rather than cytologic atypia—the lack of a requirement for obvious atypia in a precancer lesion is sensible. It is also reasonable, however, to retain the term "atypical" in the diagnostic bottom line for the purposes of clinical care, as this term has long been the trigger for increased concern for our clinical colleagues and dropping it from the lexicon might result in their underestimation of risk.

The diagnosis and pathogenesis of atypical endometrial hyperplasia is discussed in detail in the preceding chapter. Here, we will discuss it briefly as it relates to the differential diagnosis of endometrial carcinoma. There can be a significant degree of interobserver variability at the interface between atypical hyperplasia and the low end of the endometrioid carcinoma spectrum. In general, the loss of single gland integrity—defined by some as glandular fusion of at least 2 mm in linear extent—is suggested to diagnose malignancy in endometrioid proliferations (Figs. 18.16 and 18.17).

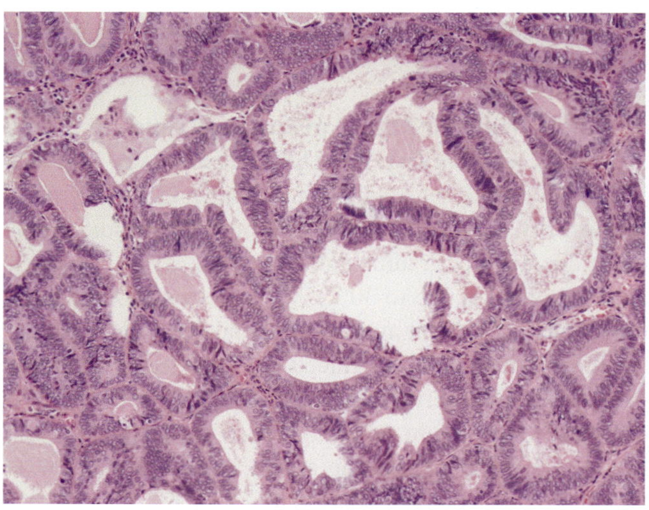

Fig. 18.16 There is considerable interobserver variability at the interface between atypical hyperplasia and low-grade endometrioid carcinoma. This field demonstrates predominantly hyperplasia with wisps of intervening stroma throughout. In the center of the field, possible gland fusion is noted focally. However, based on this area alone the proliferation fails to meet criteria for malignancy because the extent of gland fusion is <2 mm

It is worth emphasizing that in this location, invasion need not be seen directly as infiltrative glands percolating through endometrial stroma; rather, it is inferred by the loss of stroma between glands. This requirement derives from rigorous work from Kurman and Norris in 1982 [97]. They investigated nuclear atypia, mitotic activity, necrosis, cellular stratification, and stromal invasion in more than 200 endometrial curettings and determined that stromal invasion was the most predictive of carcinoma on subsequent hysterectomy. Stromal invasion is easily diagnosed when florid, expansile cribriform patterns are appreciated from low power, but becomes more challenging in cases small biopsies with closely packed individual glands showing minimal intervening stroma. Furthermore, the requirement for absolutely no stromal interruption can result in undercalling certain patterns. Longacre and Hendrickson addressed this problem in 1995 through pictorial galleries of architectural patterns

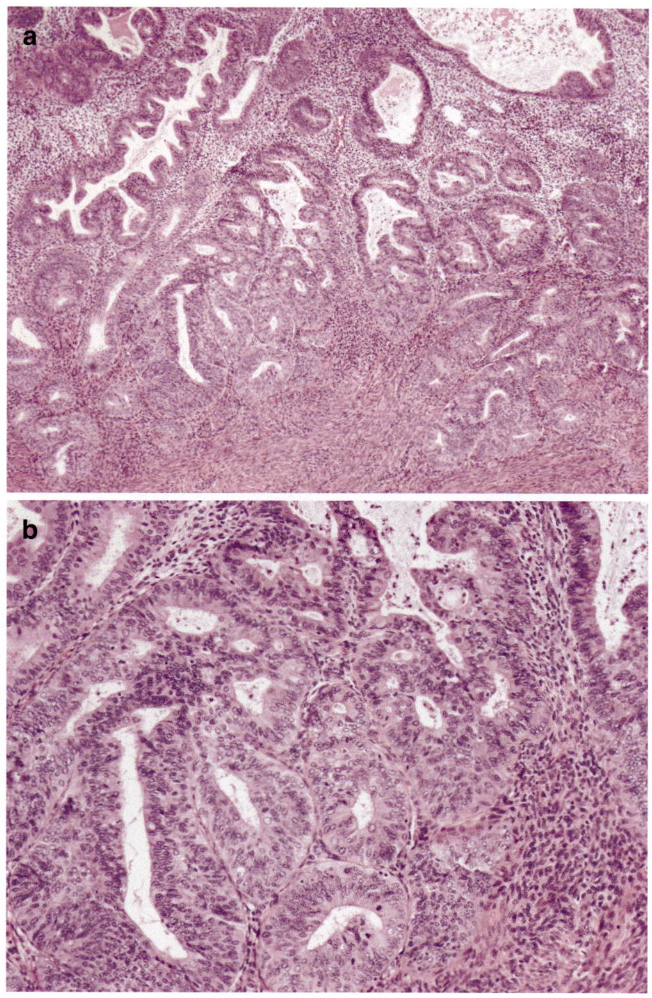

Fig. 18.17 Endometrial carcinoma most often arises in a background of atypical hyperplasia (**a**). The upper half of the field demonstrates hyperplasia while the lower half shows progression to low-grade endometrioid carcinoma. Higher power view of the invasive component reveals gland fusion and cribriforming (**b**). Cytologically, this proliferation is relatively bland and resembles the constituent cells of the background hyperplasia

associated with subsequent invasion, including extensive exophytic papillary patterns with delicate to broad cores, maze-like proliferations, and macroglands with significant internal complexity [98]. They also recommend that these patterns be present for the full span of a 10x objective field (using 15× eyepieces) [98, 99].

Even after decades of refinement of these morphologic criteria, the decision to upgrade to a malignant diagnosis remains challenging in some cases. This is particularly true for curettage specimens, when fragmentation can make it challenging to meet the 2 mm or 10× objective size requirements. Fortunately, our colleagues in gynecologic oncology often have a clear grasp of these challenges and usually understand when a biopsy or frozen section diagnosis is upgraded or downgraded based on the permanent resection material.

18.4.3.3 Endometrioid Carcinoma Grades

Endometrioid carcinomas are presently graded on three tiers according to the current FIGO classification system. Further discussion of this system, including its shortcomings and the argument for a binary system, can be found in the preceding section entitled "Endometrial Carcinoma Grading," and are summarized in Table 18.1. Briefly, endometrioid proliferations showing at least 2 mm of glandular fusion ≤5% solid non-squamous growth and without significant nuclear atypia can be classified Grade 1 (low-grade) endometrioid carcinomas (Fig. 18.18). Tumors with 6–50% solid formation (again, excluding squamous moralization) are classified as Grade 2 (intermediate grade) while those with >50% solid non-squamous growth are classified as Grade 3 (high grade).

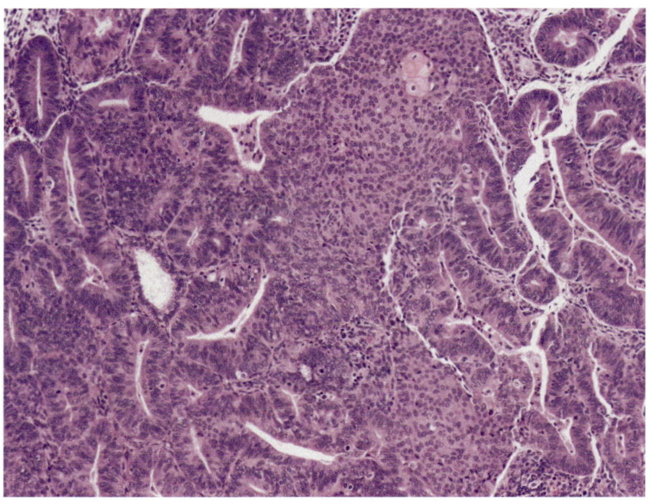

Fig. 18.18 It is critical that squamous metaplasia not be included in the contribution of solid components when FIGO grading endometrioid carcinomas. This is straightforward when the squamous metaplasia is brightly eosinophilic with evident intercellular bridges (as is seen focally in the upper right portion of this image), but is more challenging when metaplasia assumes a more basophilic appearance (as is seen in the majority of this image)

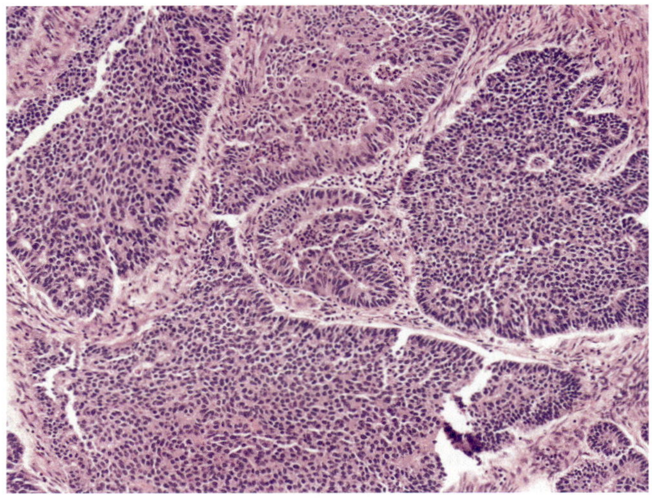

Fig. 18.19 Distinguishing between FIGO 2–3 endometrioid carcinomas and dedifferentiated carcinomas can be challenging. This case was diagnosed as grade 3 endometrioid carcinoma on the basis of >50% solid components with glandular contributions intimately admixed with the solid architecture; unlike dedifferentiated carcinoma, there is no abrupt transition to confluent sheet-like growth

Grade 1 endometrioid cancers are most diagnostically problematic when they mimic serous or clear cell neoplasia, particularly when papillary and villoglandular architecture is prominent. Challenges also arise when prominent metaplasia or other divergent differentiation raises the possibility of alternate sites-of-origin (for instance, tumors with marked mucinous or squamous differentiation may be mistaken for endocervical primaries). Grades 2 and 3 cancers, on the other hand, sometimes require distinction from dedifferentiated and undifferentiated cancers based on the presence, pattern, and distribution of the glandular component (Fig. 18.19). Guidance on addressing these differential diagnoses is in the ensuing sections.

18.4.3.4 Nuclear Atypia in Endometrioid Carcinoma: The Upgrade Clause

The issue of nuclear atypia in endometrioid carcinoma is nuanced. Historically, the criteria for endometrioid carcinoma diagnosis or grading did not include atypia, although a subset of cases (up to 30%) was expected to have more than moderate nuclear atypia. Subsequently, a caveat to the grading system was introduced in 1994 suggesting that cancers which otherwise qualified as Grade 1 endometrioid carcinomas ought to be upgraded to Grade 2 on the basis of significant nuclear atypia, while an otherwise Grade 2 tumor could be classified as Grade 3 for this reason [51, 52]. It is worth noting that application the nuclear upgrade clause may undergo further refinement as diagnosis is increasingly informed by ancillary studies (such as p53 immunostaining, discussed below) and molecular classifications.

18.4.3.5 p53 and Endometrioid Carcinomas

The nuclear upgrade clause may have its biologic foundation in mutation profiles that diverge from the conventional endometrioid genomic landscape. Although the old Type I vs. Type II approach to classification left little room for more aggressive subsets, data from the TCGA has revealed high copy number endometrioid cancers that cluster more closely with serous cancers than they do with their low copy number endometrioid counterparts [8]. *TP53* mutations were found in 15% of endometrioid cancers in the TGCA, and 22% of these were frameshift or nonsense mutations [100]. Furthermore, work from Oliva and colleagues shows that more than a third of grade 3 endometrioid cancers diffusely overexpress p53 [101]. Garg and Soslow also demonstrated that p53 overexpression correlates with adverse outcome in morphologically ambiguous endometrial tumors, including cases with predominantly endometrioid features [7, 102].

p53 immunoexpression is therefore postulated to mark a population of endometrioid cancers which can be expected to follow a clinical course commensurate with more conventionally "type II" histotypes. p53 immunohistochemistry also has utility in identifying serous cancers masquerading as villoglandular and papillary endometrioid tumors, a clinically significant and not entirely uncommon pitfall [103–105]. These two points raises questions as to whether p53 immunohistochemistry ought to be routinely performed on all tumors with apparent endometrioid morphology. While there is no consensus on this within the gynecologic pathology community, a low threshold for p53 immunohistochemistry is generally recommended, particularly given the growing interest in harmonizing microscopic interpretation with molecular data. p53 immunostaining is also recommended as a final step in the TCGA-informed ProMisE algorithm for classifying endometrial carcinomas, and may be more commonly enlisted should that risk classification system become more commonly utilized [11].

18.4.3.6 Endometrioid Carcinoma Variants and Associated Pitfalls

Within the endometrioid umbrella there are a host of architectural patterns including tumors comprised predominantly of macroglandular structures, tumors with broad villoglandular excrescences, and finely papillary tumors. Villous and papillary can be diagnostically problematic as they can be mistaken for other histotypes (chiefly serous carcinoma), particularly when significant atypia is present. Endometrioid carcinomas also include tumors with extensive mucinous, tubal, secretory, and squamous differentiation. Whether these non-endometrioid cell types represent metaplasia superimposed on endometrioid differentiation or a divergent neoplastic cell population becomes a somewhat academic question. Of greater clinical relevance is the fact that these histologies can invoke a variety of diagnostic challenges.

18.4.4 Endometrioid Carcinoma with Squamous Differentiation

Squamous differentiation occurs in approximately 25% of all endometrioid carcinomas; however, only those bearing >10% squamous contributions merit this diagnostic distinction [106, 107]. Squamous differentiation is defined by abundant eosinophilic cytoplasm, polygonal cell borders, and distinct cell membranes. Keratinization and intracellular bridges are helpful but not requisite features in this setting [107]. Squamous differentiation often manifests as discrete morules which are readily recognizable as metaplastic (Fig. 18.20). More problematic is squamatization which shows spindled morphology, central necrosis, or solid growth; these patterns can morphologically invoke concern about a high-grade tumor but do not actually impart any increased risk (Fig. 18.21). As is emphasized in the discussion on FIGO grading, it is critical to exclude squamous areas when calculating the overall solid components of tumors.

Historically the terms "adenocanthoma" and "adenosquamous carcinoma" were utilized to encompass endometrial cancers with significant squamous differentiation, with the former referring to cases with cytologically banal squamous metaplasia and the latter indicating high-grade squamous features. However, these categories proved neither reproduc-

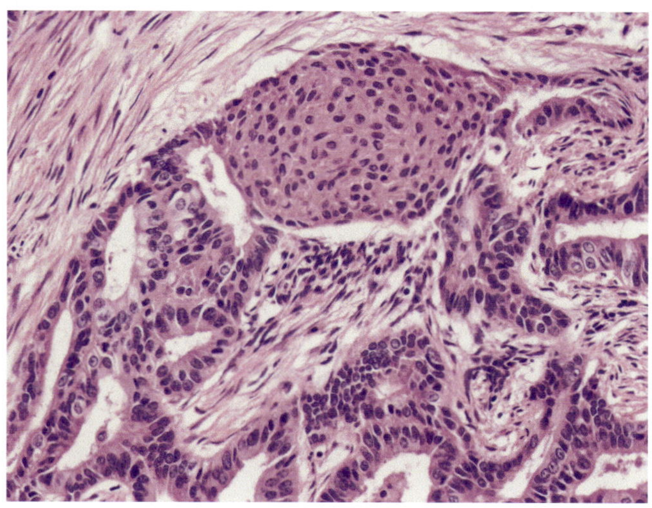

Fig. 18.20 Squamous morules are common in endometrioid carcinoma and are readily diagnosed when they demonstrate classic features such as eosinophilic cytoplasm, polygonal cell borders, and distinct cell membranes, as pictured in this case. Other cases display a more basophilic appearance which may be mistaken for solid endometrioid growth

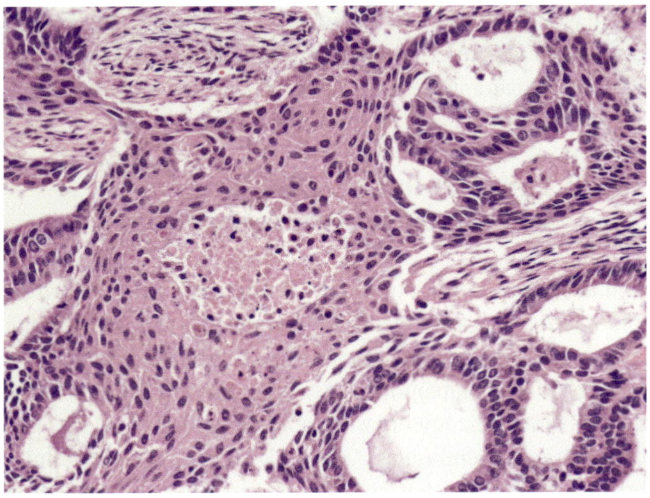

Fig. 18.21 Squamous metaplasia can show spindled architecture and central necrosis, which is of no prognostic significance. It is important not to mistake spindled squamous growth as evidence of a carcinosarcoma

ible nor clinically relevant when the background adenocarcinoma grade was considered, as squamous atypia tends to parallel the overall cancer grade (Fig. 18.22). These historical terms were therefore abolished in favor of the classifier "endometrioid carcinoma with squamous differentiation;" "adenosquamous carcinoma" of the endometrium is not a WHO-recognized entity [96, 106–108].

Extensive squamous differentiation can be diagnostically problematic when the tumor's site-of-origin is uncertain, as tumors with lower uterine segment involvement and significant squamous differentiation may be mistaken for cervical/endocervical primaries. This problem is compounded by the fact that p16 immunohistochemistry can be strongly positive in squamous metaplasia involving endometrioid glands (Fig. 18.23). Correlation with more specific human papillomavirus (HPV) testing, such as HPV DNA or RNA in situ hybridization, can be of utility in such cases. Immunohistochemical assessment of the glandular component can also aid in assign-

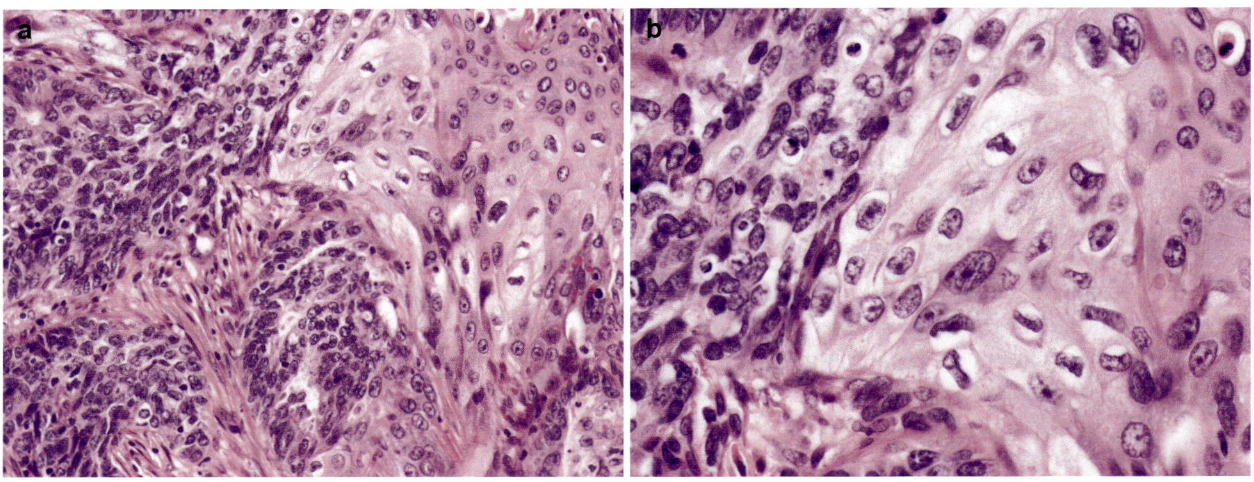

Fig. 18.22 The differentiation of squamous metaplasia typically parallels the overall tumor grade. This grade 3 endometrioid carcinoma displayed extensive squamous differentiation which shows moderate atypia paralleling the background endometrioid component (**a**, **b**). Cases like this were previously considered "adenosquamous carcinomas"; however, that classification is not an official designation under the current World Health Organization (WHO) classification system

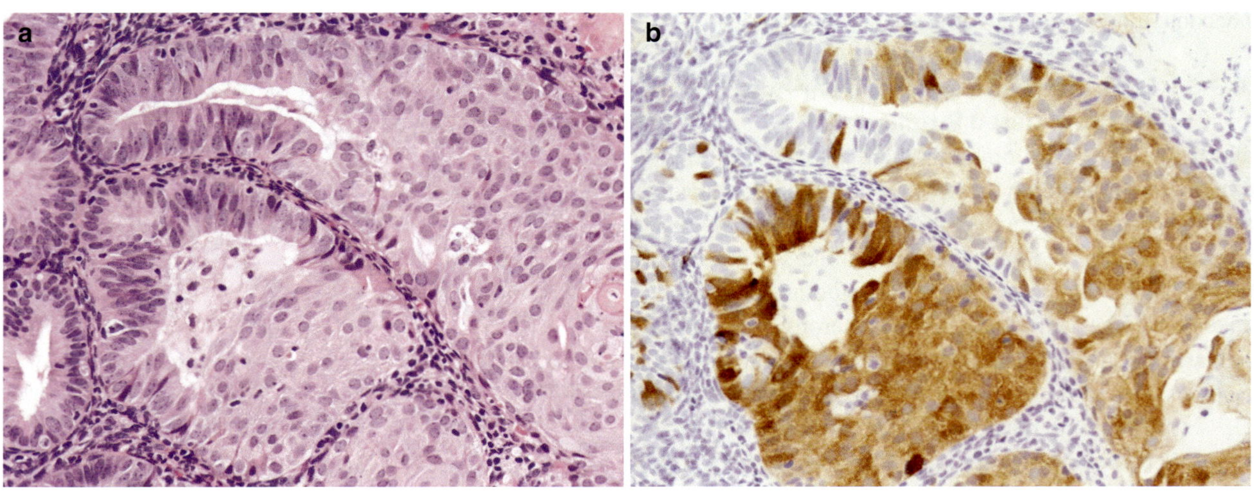

Fig. 18.23 Squamous metaplasia (**a**) is often diffusely positive for p16 (**b**), which can complicate assessment of cases with a differential diagnosis of endocervical carcinoma and potentially lead to misdiagnosis of an endocervical primary. Care should be taken to assess p16 expression only within the glandular component in such cases. The addition of other immunohistochemical studies (vimentin, estrogen receptor, CEA) and/or HPV in situ hybridization studies may be of utility in such cases

Table 18.5 Panel approach to ancillary testing for endometrial vs. endocervical primary

Ancillary test	Endometrial primary	Endocervical primary
ER	+++	+/–
Vimentin	+++	+/–
CEA	+/–	++/–
p16	+/–	+++
HPV RNA ISH	–	+++

ER estrogen receptor, *HPV* human papillomavirus, *ISH* in situ hybridization

ing origin: endometrioid tumors are typically strongly positive for estrogen receptor, progesterone receptor, and vimentin, whereas endocervical cancers show either absence or only weak expression of these markers [109, 110] (Fig. 18.24). Conversely, p16 should show strong, diffuse staining in endocervical carcinomas, while patchy staining is typically expected in low-grade tumors of endometrial origin, although occasional cases may show extensive positivity [111]. It is worth emphasizing that none of these immunohistochemical markers is entirely sensitive or specific in isolation, therefore a panel approach is recommended (Table 18.5). That said, p16 and ER are generally the most useful components of the panel approach, and vimentin and CEA results are sometimes not diagnostically additive. HPV DNA or RNA in situ hybridization can serve as an adjudicator for cases that remain challenging on immunohistochemical assessment. Correlation with prior Pap results and HPV DNA status is also prudent.

One final diagnostic pitfall surrounding endometrioid carcinomas with prominent squamous differentiation is confusion with clear cell carcinoma in cases wherein the squamous component has extensive cytoplasmic clearing. This is caused by abundant glycogenation of squamous cytoplasm and should not be mistaken for true clear cell differentiation. In these cases, the absence of significant cytologic atypia and hobnailing is useful, as is the absence of architectural features indicative of clear cell carcinoma (fibrous and hyalinized stroma, tubulocystic growth). Finally, the clear cells in these cases often merge with areas of more conventional squamous differentiation, further supporting clear cell change rather than true clear cell carcinoma. In this particular setting, immunohistochemistry by using squamous cell markers (CK5/6, p40 and sometimes p63) and clear cell carcinoma markers (Napsin A and P504S) can be helpful to differentiate squamous differentiation from clear cell carcinoma.

18.4.5 Endometrioid Carcinoma with Mucinous Differentiation

Endometrioid carcinomas frequently show focal mucinous differentiation (Fig. 18.25). This is typically thought to represent metaplasia and does not change the overall diagnosis when present in <50% of the tumor [112, 113]. Tumors showing a >50% mucinous phenotype are classified as "mucinous carcinomas," a distinct diagnostic category in the 2014 WHO which is discussed in greater detail in a subsequent section [96]. Prominent mucinous metaplasia is sometimes the result of prior progestin therapy, although this finding is by no means exclusively seen in this setting [114]. In cases with a prior diagnosis of endometrioid carcinoma, >50% mucinous morphology on a posttreatment therapy should not change the diagnosis to "mucinous carcinoma," although in the molecular level, the mucinous carcinoma or endometrioid carcinoma tends to have more K-ras mutations.

There is also evidence that tumors with *MLH1* hypermethylation show increased rates of mucinous differentiation relative to mismatch repair-intact and Lynch syndrome-associated counterparts [115]. Given these tumors' propensity to involve the lower uterine segment, this may lead to misdiagnosis of endocervical carcinoma [54, 115]. As with squamous metaplasia, the presence of a prominent mucinous component superimposed on endometrioid cancer can generate challenges related to assigning site-of-origin, particularly when the tumor is centered near the cervix. Difficult cases may require the previously mentioned immunohistochemical panel of estrogen receptor, vimentin, CEA, and p16 (Table 18.5). Correlation with Pap history is always prudent and HPV-specific assays, such as HPV DNA or RNA ISH, may be enlisted in cases that remain equivocal on immunohistochemistry.

18.4.6 Endometrioid Carcinoma with Secretory Differentiation

Secretory differentiation is encountered in endometrial carcinomas with some regularity and is defined by cells with subnuclear and/or supranuclear intracytoplasmic glycogen vacuoles, as are seen the early secretory phase of cycling endometria (Fig. 18.26). Most often this occurs only focally, in concert with overt endometrioid differentiation. It has been associated with endogenous or exogenous progestin stimulation [113, 116, 117]. Therefore, both mucinous and secretory differentiation are commonly associated with progestin usage.

Although the diagnosis of "secretory carcinoma" is not recognized as an independent entity, rare cases of endometrioid carcinoma show extensive secretory differentiation. Such cases have been shown to demonstrate clinical behavior on par with other well-differentiated endometrioid carcinomas, with only rare cases resulting in patient death [113, 116, 117]; however, these tumors can sometimes cause considerable diagnostic consternation.

Firstly, distinction from normal secretory endometrium may be challenging, as elevated glands-to-stroma ratios and

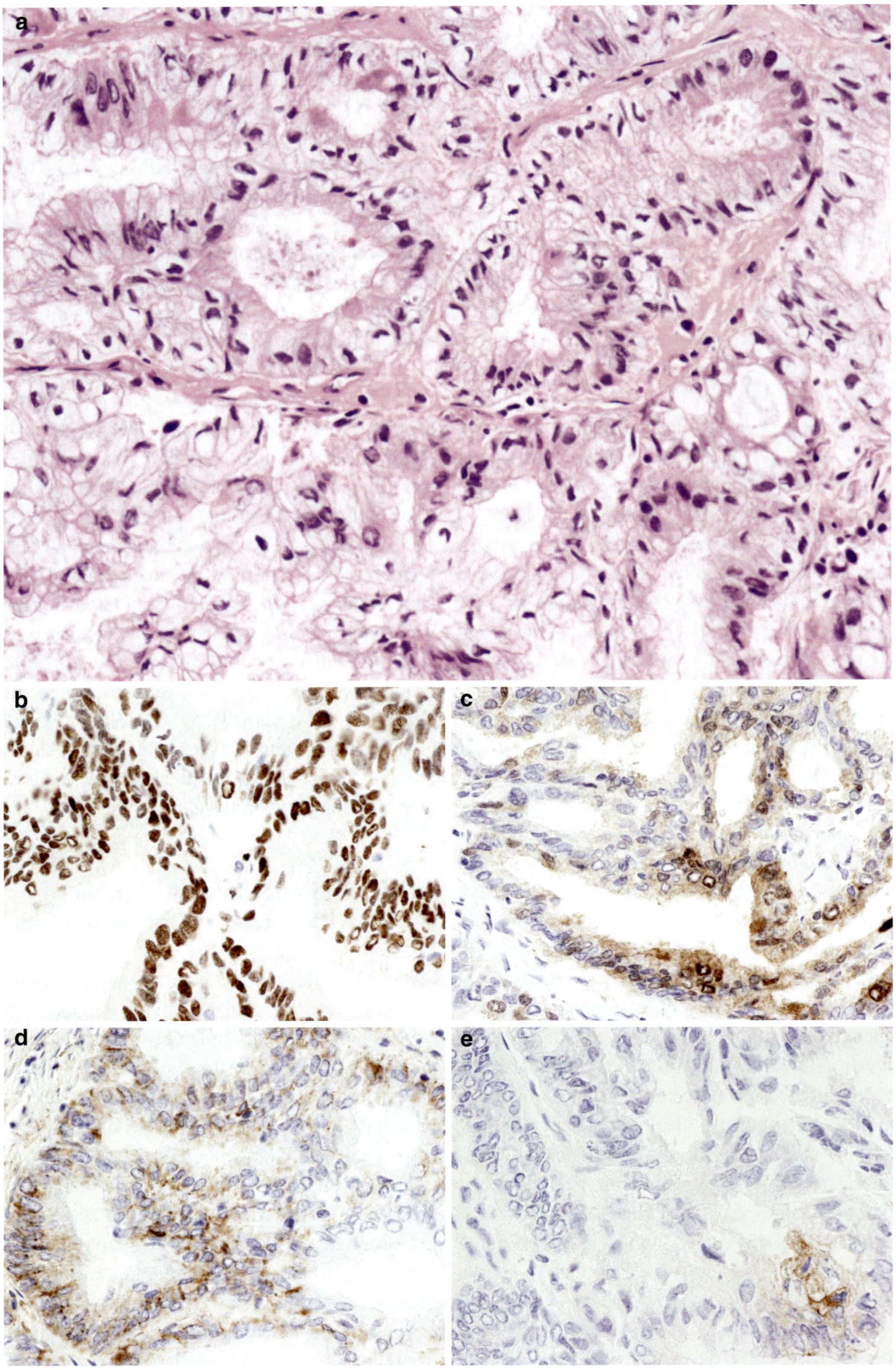

Fig. 18.24 A panel of immunostains can be helpful for assigning endometrial vs. endocervical origin in carcinomas with mucinous features. (**a**) Endometrial carcinomas are most often positive for estrogen receptor (ER) (**b**) and show only patchy p16 staining (**c**), whereas endocervical carcinomas are typically ER-negative and strongly, diffusely positive for p16. However, p16 expression may also be diffuse in occasional endometrioid cancers, particularly higher-grade tumors. Vimentin usually shows at least focal staining in endometrial carcinomas (**d**), and many cases are more extensively positive. In contrast, endocervical primaries are typically vimentin-negative. Finally, endometrial carcinomas usually have absent or only focal CEA expression (**e**), whereas strong diffuse positivity supports an endocervical primary. Unfortunately, in practice vimentin and CEA can often produce patchy results that do not contribute significantly to the diagnostic work-up. If the panel results remain equivocal, HPV-specific testing can be initiated

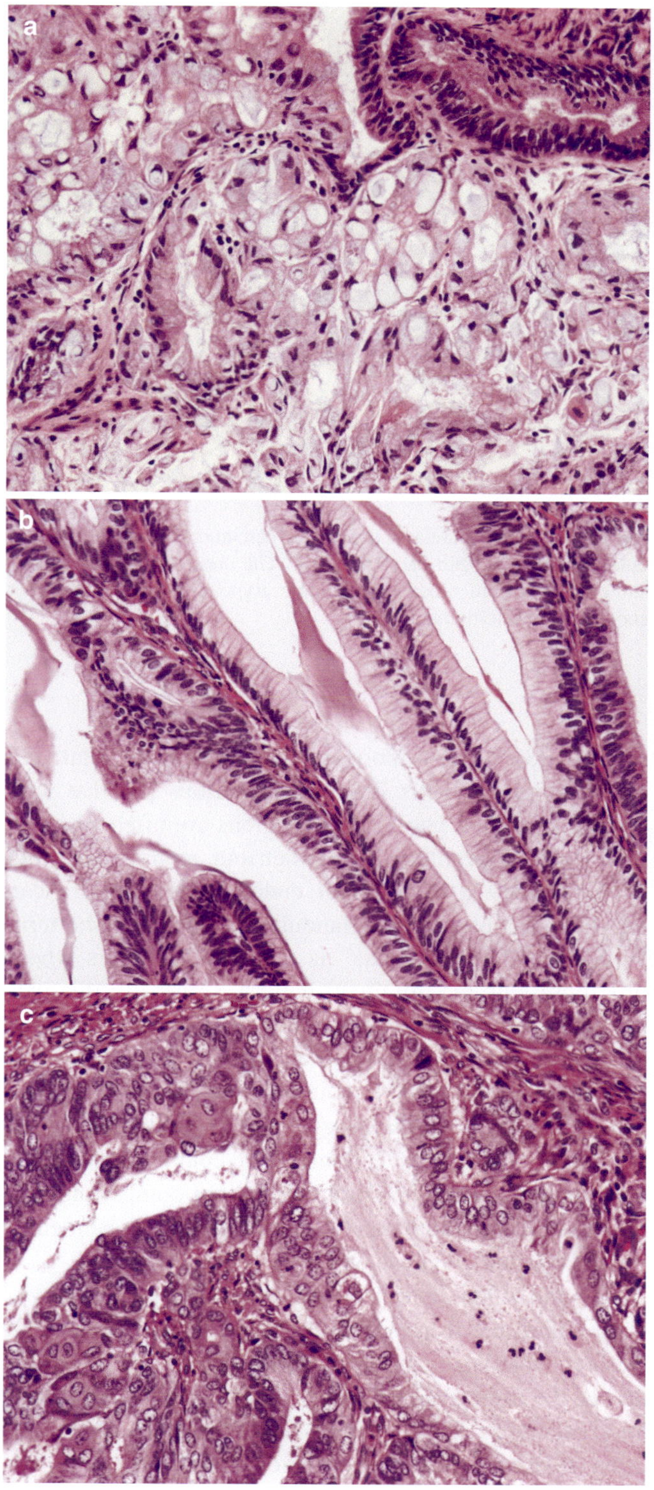

Fig. 18.25 Mucinous metaplasia is common in endometrioid carcinomas. When mucinous differentiation comprises >50% of the total volume, the tumor is classified as a "mucinous carcinoma." Mucinous morphology may manifest as signet-type cells (**a**) or as columnar cells reminiscent of endocervical epithelium (**b**). Some cases show only focal intracytoplasmic mucin with abundant intraluminal mucin, often with abundant associated neutrophils (**c**)

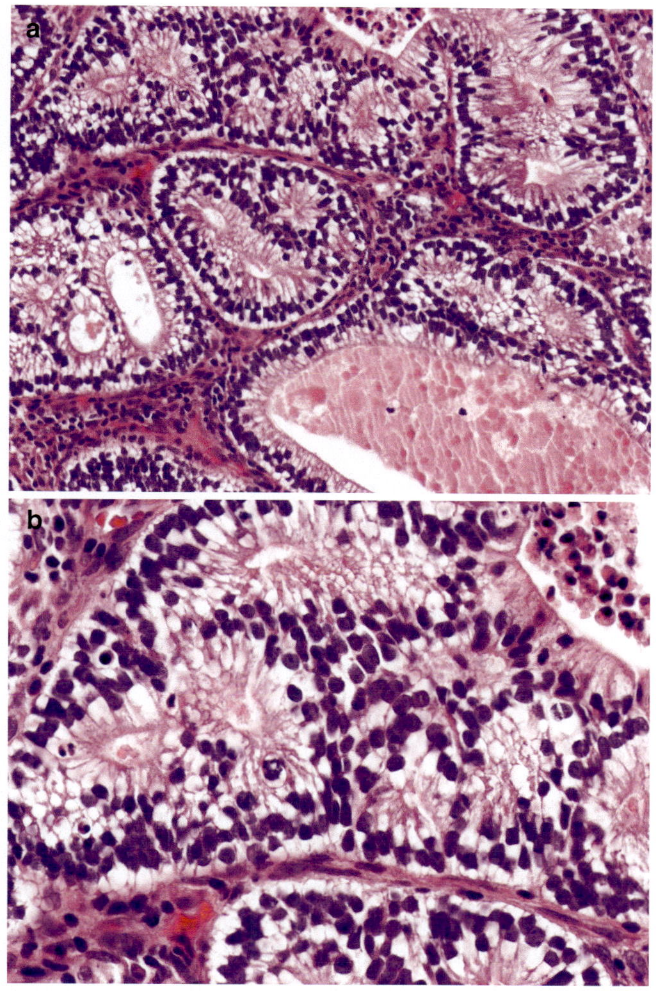

Fig. 18.26 Secretory differentiation may occur in endometrioid carcinomas and is characterized by subnuclear and/or supranuclear intracytoplasmic glycogen vacuoles. While often only focal and admixed with more conventional endometrioid differentiation, occasionally it can involve the majority of the tumor volume (**a**, **b**)

architectural complexity can be a normal feature of the secretory phase. That said, the degree of crowding and complexity and architectural irregularity remains much greater in secretory carcinomas and hyperplasias when compared to benign secretory change [118]. The presence of mitotic figures can also be extremely helpful, as mitotic activity is not a feature of the benign secretory phase. Ki67 may also be a useful ancillary study in this setting, as early secretory endometrium tends to have <3% Ki67 positivity whereas non-atypical and atypical hyperplasias show positivity in 17% and 36% of cells, respectively, and carcinomas demonstrate approximately 60% labeling [119].

The second diagnostic dilemma generated by endometrial carcinomas with extensive secretory differentiation is confu-

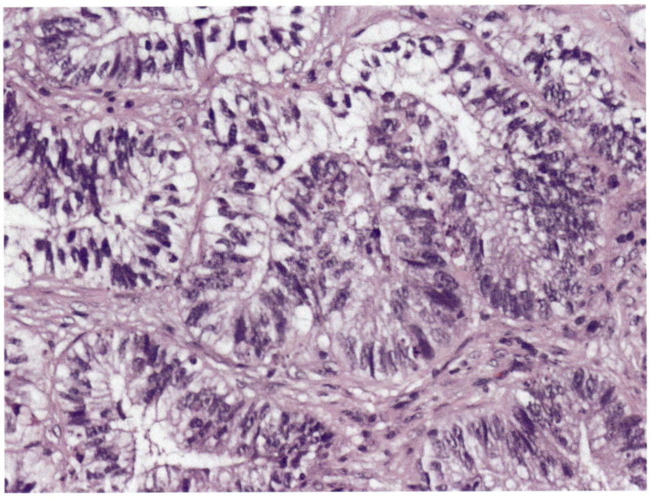

Fig. 18.27 Secretory differentiation in endometrioid carcinomas can generate confusion with clear cell carcinomas. This endometrioid carcinoma has areas with cytoplasmic clearing due to the presence of supranuclear and subnuclear vacuoles. This finding is consistent with secretory differentiation and does not impact the overall diagnosis. It is critical to not misinterpret this cytoplasmic clearing as evidence of a clear cell carcinoma component

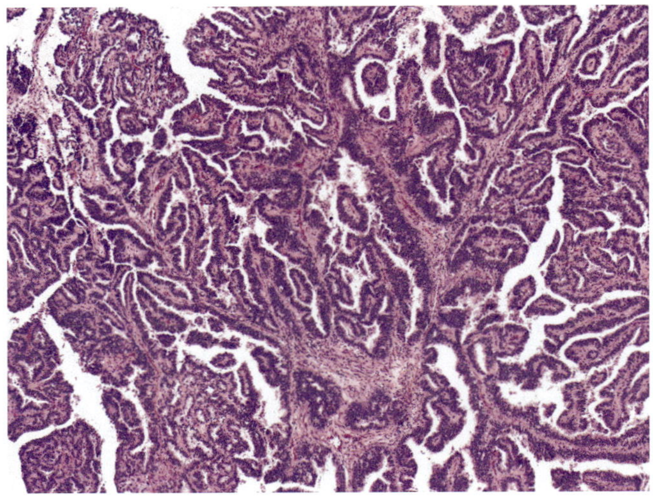

Fig. 18.28 Villoglandular endometrioid carcinomas demonstrate frondular growth with thin papillary cores. The constituent cells demonstrate only mild to moderate cytologic atypia consistent with other endometrioid carcinomas

sion with clear cell carcinoma (Fig. 18.27). The presence of clear cytoplasm is not sufficient for a clear cell carcinoma diagnosis: that entity is characterized by tubulocystic and papillary patterns with hobnail cells and prominent stromal hyalinization. Secretory differentiation superimposed on routine endometrioid carcinoma is far more common than true clear cell carcinoma of the endometrium, and cytoplasmic clearing should be interpreted in the context of the overall architecture, cytology, and stromal background [113, 120, 121]. Indeed, review of endometrial carcinomas originally classified as "clear cell carcinoma" resulted in the reclassification of 54% of cases after review by five experts [4]. Napsin A immunohistochemistry may also be of utility in this differential, as it shows relatively robust sensitivity (88%) and specificity (98%) for clear cell carcinoma in this location [122]. Hepatocyte nuclear factor-1β (HNF-1β) is also often positive and can be useful for excluding other histotypes [4]. Hormone receptor expression (including estrogen receptor, progesterone receptor, and androgen receptor) is also uncommon in clear cell carcinomas and strong, diffuse expression of these markers is more suggestive of endometrioid differentiation [4, 123].

18.4.7 Villoglandular Carcinoma

Villoglandular carcinoma is a variant of endometrioid carcinoma characterized by elongate, frondular growth reminiscent of a colonic villous adenoma [124, 125] (Fig. 18.28). These tumors are characterized by relatively bland neoplastic cells lining long, villous papillae with thin fibrovascular cores. These regions are often admixed with more conventional endometrioid architecture, and while roughly a third of all endometrioid cancers can show some areas of villoglandular architecture, the term "villoglandular carcinoma" is reserved for cases where this represents the dominant pattern. Generally this pattern is not thought to impart an increased clinical risk relative to other low-grade carcinomas, although some evidence suggests that myoinvasive villoglandular cancers may bear a worse prognosis that grade and stage-matched conventional endometrioid counterparts [125]. Nonetheless, at this juncture there is not compelling evidence that villoglandular features should independently impact clinical management.

The most important point related to villoglandular features relates not to prognosis, but to diagnosis. Confusion between villoglandular carcinomas and serous carcinomas is one of the most commonly encountered issues in gynecologic pathology, and may have contributed to the poor prognosis of some "villoglandular carcinomas" reported in the literature. Serous cancers frequently share the papillary architecture of villoglandular carcinomas, and misdiagnosis can occur in either direction if nuclear features are given insufficient attention. However, serous cancers tend to exhibit more complex papillae with epithelial buds and display prominent cytologic atypia including >3–4-fold nuclear variation in size, whereas villoglandular carcinomas should have low- to—at most—intermediate-grade nuclear features. The presence of prominent eosinophilic nucleoli and atypi-

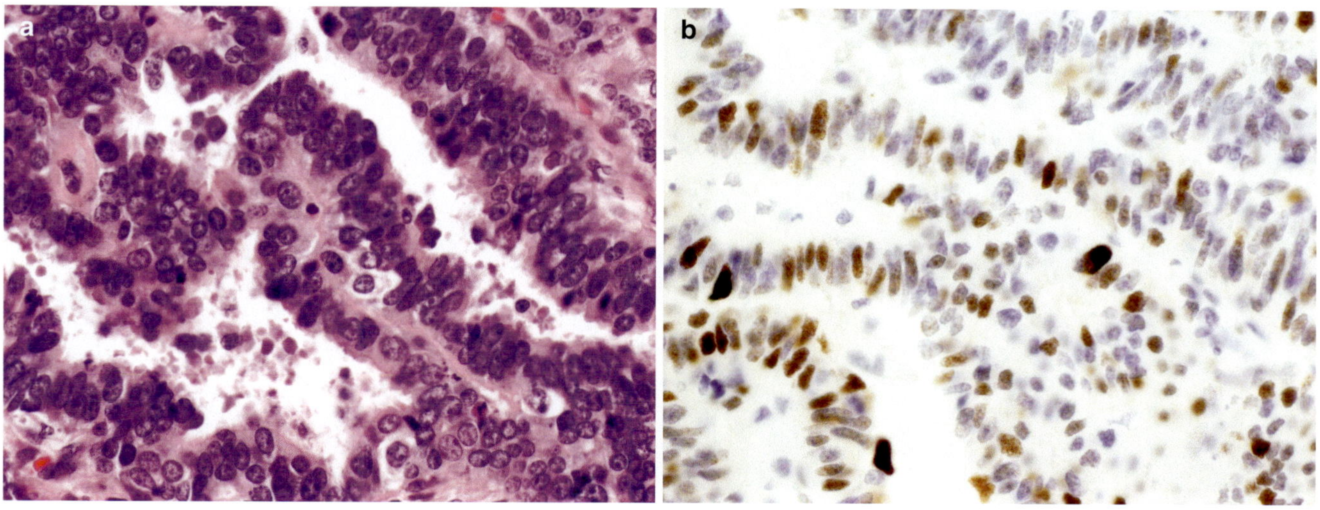

Fig. 18.29 Villoglandular endometrioid carcinomas can generate diagnostic confusion with serous carcinoma due to their prominent papillary growth. The absence of severe nuclear atypia is critical for confirming endometrioid differentiation in the context of this pattern (**a**). p53 immunohistochemical staining is also of utility as it is typically wild-type (**b**) in endometrioid cancers, whereas serous carcinomas show abnormal expression (most often diffuse overexpression)

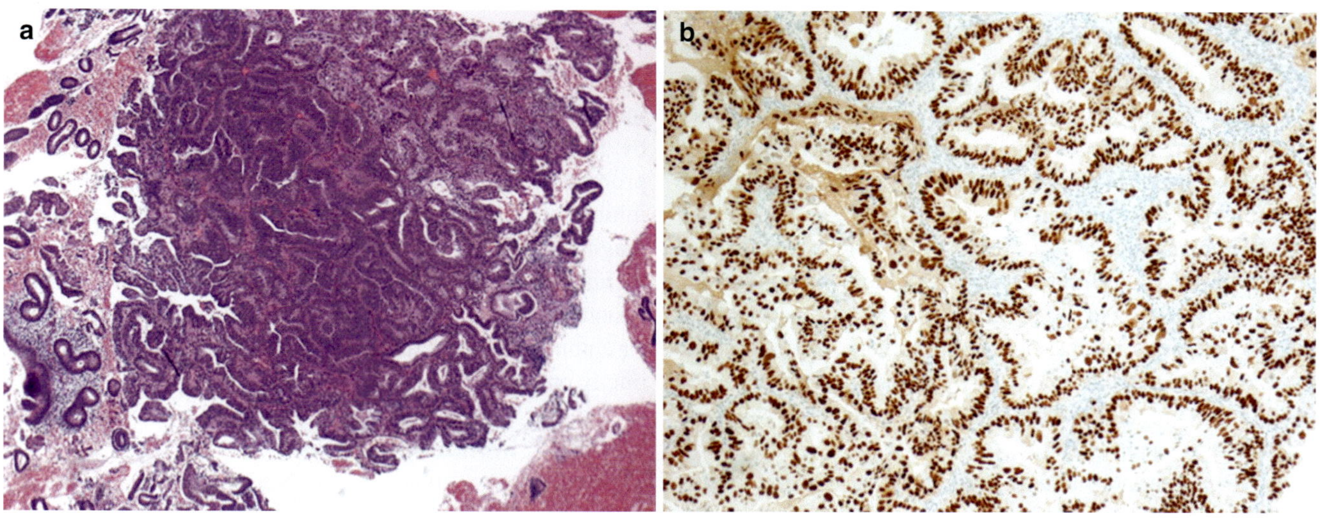

Fig. 18.30 Endometrial carcinomas with conventional endometrioid morphology (**a**) may occasionally demonstrate p53 mutational-type patterns (**b**). This finding corroborates evidence from the TCGA that some endometrioid cancers belong in the high copy-number subgroup along with serous carcinomas. Image courtesy of Drs. Dr. Wenxin Zheng and Charles Quick

cal mitotic figures is particularly suggestive of serous differentiation. p53 immunohistochemical staining can be extremely helpful in resolving this differential, as abnormal p53 expression (either diffuse or null pattern) is expected for serous cancers but is relatively uncommon in typical villoglandular carcinoma [126] (Fig. 18.29). Indeed, evidence suggests that endometrial carcinomas with villoglandular morphology, abnormal p53, and ambiguous nuclear features are likely to follow a clinical course comparable to serous carcinoma [102]. A very low threshold for p53 staining is therefore encouraged in the setting of villoglandular architecture, particularly in the context of the evolving molecular understanding of endometrial carcinoma wherein high-copy number cancers are not limited exclusively to those with conventional serous morphology [9–11, 100, 127, 128]. As illustrated by TCGA endometrial cancer data, a well-differentiated endometrioid carcinoma can show p53 mutational-type staining (Fig. 18.30).

18.4.8 Other Unique Morphologies

Endometrioid carcinomas can assume a variety of other appearances that can prove eye-catching and, occasionally,

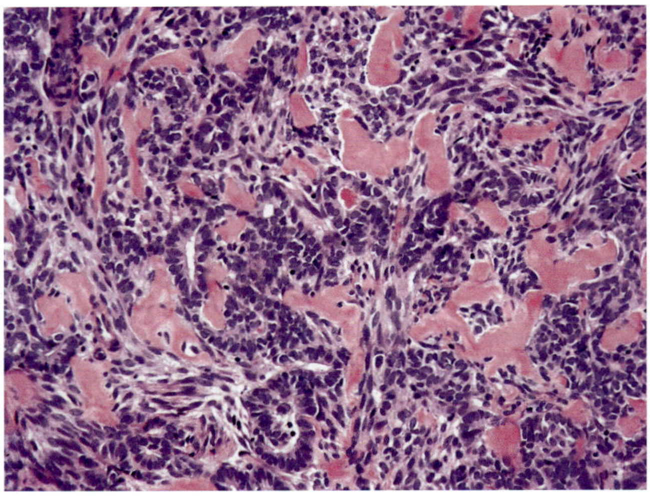

Fig. 18.31 The corded and hyalinized variant of endometrioid carcinoma shows neoplastic conventional endometrioid glands admixed with spindled and corded epithelium associated with dense hyalinized matrix material. It is important not to mistake the focally spindled morphology as evidence of a carcinosarcoma. Image courtesy of Dr. Robert Soslow

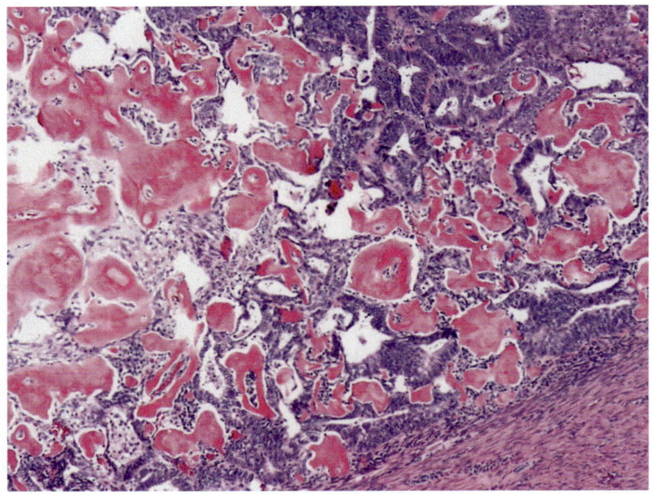

Fig. 18.32 Endometrioid carcinomas rarely demonstrate benign osseous metaplasia. Distinction from carcinosarcoma in these cases is critical, and is contingent on the benign nature of the osseous component. The tumor should be graded based exclusively on the glandular component and should not be mistaken for carcinosarcoma. Image courtesy of Dr. Robert Soslow

diagnostically challenging. Corded and hyalinized endometrioid carcinomas are characterized by regions of conventional endometrioid carcinoma admixed with swaths of dense, hyalinized matrix peppered with cords and trabeculae of epithelioid and spindled cells [113, 129] (Fig. 18.31). The biphasic appearance of these tumors may suggest carcinosarcoma; however, the limited atypia precludes this diagnosis. Immunohistochemistry can be useful in this setting and reveals negativity for mesenchymal markers such as smooth muscle actin, desmin, and CD10; furthermore, the corded components are inhibin-negative, arguing against a sex cord-stromal component [129].

Another rare morphologic variant demonstrates a prominent spindle cell component which may also invoke the differential of carcinosarcoma; however, on close review the spindle cell region is cytologically banal and mitotically inactive [113]. In contrast to the sharp epithelial-mesenchymal transitions that typify carcinosarcoma, the spindled cell component of such cases also merges imperceptibly with the glandular tissue. Both spindle and glandular components are positive for cytokeratins. Endometrioid carcinomas with metaplastic osseous differentiation may also be mistaken for carcinosarcomas (Fig. 18.32). In these cases, in contrast to carcinosarcomas, the osseous component is entirely benign and does not impact prognosis.

Uncommon endometrioid tumors may also display prominent tubular structures reminiscent of sex cord-like elements which can therefore invoke the possibility of a Sertoli cell tumor or an endometrial stromal sarcoma with sex cord-like elements; in both instances, the presence of a conventional endometrioid differentiation is helpful for excluding both these diagnoses, as is immunonegativity for inhibin [130]. Other cases can mimic granulosa cell tumors by forming Call-Exner-like structures and demonstrating prominent nuclear grooves; in these cases, negativity for inhibin and strong diffuse keratin staining helps secure the diagnosis [131].

Finally, the rare finding of abundant psammoma bodies in endometrioid carcinomas can spark confusion with serous carcinoma; however, the cytology of such cases remains distinctly endometrioid [132].

18.4.8.1 Immunophenotype

The immunophenotype of endometrioid endometrial carcinoma varies considerably based on grade. Low-grade endometrioid cancers are frequently strongly positive for estrogen receptor (ER) and progesterone receptor (PR), and often express androgen receptor (AR) [123, 133]. Expression of these markers can diminish, however, with increasing tumor grade. As discussed previously, low-grade endometrioid tumors are typically strongly vimentin-positive and CEA-negative with patchy p16 staining [110, 111]. This immunoprofile shifts somewhat with increasing grade with higher p16 expression being more common among less differentiated tumors. Finally, like other tumors of Müllerian origin, endometrioid cancers are typically PAX8-positive although high-grade cancers will occasionally lose expression of this marker [134, 135].

The molecular underpinnings of endometrioid cancers also influence their immunoexpression profiles. Loss of PTEN, for example, is typical of most conventional low-grade endometrioid cancers because *PTEN* mutations are

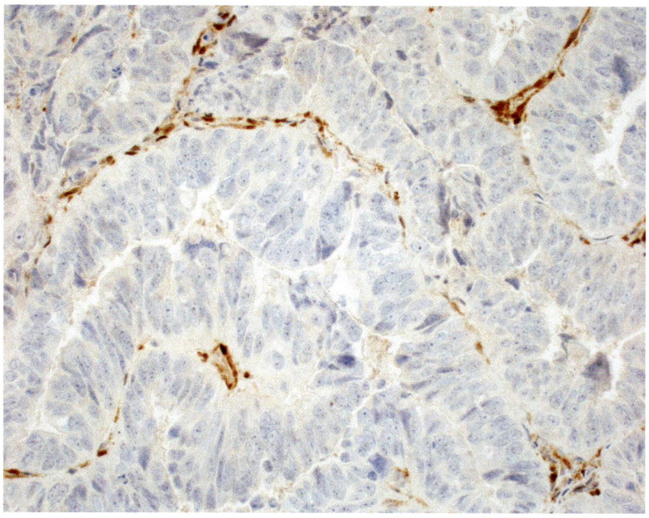

Fig. 18.33 Loss of PTEN expression is seen in many endometrioid carcinomas, as illustrated in this low-grade endometrioid case. This represents an early event in carcinogenesis, however, and is therefore of no utility in distinguishing hyperplasia from carcinoma. Image courtesy of Dr. Brooke Lane Howitt

common in this molecular subset [92, 93] (Fig. 18.33). However, PTEN immunohistochemistry has limited diagnostic value because isolated PTEN loss can also be seen in benign and hyperplastic endometrium [94]. Furthermore, abnormalities in PTEN expression can be seen even in the absence of *PTEN* gene mutations [136]. Similarly, p53 is invariability wild type among low-grade endometrioid tumors but shows abnormal expression (whether diffuse or null pattern) in a subset of high-grade cancers that correspond to the *TP53*-mutated, high copy-number molecular subset [7, 8, 101, 102, 104, 105]; this is discussed in detail in the preceding section "p53 and endometrioid carcinomas" and in the following section on molecular features. In general, p53 has diagnostic utility in differentiating between low-grade endometrioid carcinoma variants and its high-grade mimics, as in cases with a differential of villoglandular carcinoma vs. serous carcinoma [100, 105, 126, 137, 138].

In addition to p53, immunohistochemical staining for p16 has been shown to be of similar utility in differentiating between endometrioid and serous cancers, as serous cancers are typically strongly and diffusely p16-positive whereas endometrioid cancers display patchy, weak-to-moderate staining [138].

Complete loss of nuclear staining for one or more of the four mismatch repair (MMR) proteins MLH1, MSH2, MSH6, and PMS2 is found in 25–35% of endometrioid carcinomas [31]. The majority of these MMR-deficient cases show dual loss of MLH1 and PMS2 attributable to epigenetic hypermethylation of the *MLH1* promoter region [31–35, 91, 139, 140]. A smaller subset (~5–10%) demonstrates loss of PMS2, MSH2, and/or MSH6, *or* dual MLH1/PMS2 loss in the absence of hypermethylation, raising concern for heritable germline mutations associated with Lynch syndrome (Fig. 18.34). While these protein loss patterns were once considered essentially diagnostic of Lynch syndrome, it is now known that in a significant proportion of cases (perhaps up to 50% in universally screened populations) loss is attributable to somatic—rather than germline—mismatch repair gene mutations [91, 141]. The increased identification of somatic mutations is likely due to expanded Lynch syndrome screening practices, as the institution of universal screening has changed the tested population and, therefore, the positive predictive value of the test. Irrespective of somatic vs. germline etiology, loss of mismatch repair protein expression has been associated with increased PD-L1 expression and response to immunotherapy and is now therefore enlisted not only as a heritable cancer screening tool, but also as a therapeutic biomarker [142–145].

18.4.8.2 Molecular

Because endometrioid carcinomas encompass a broad range of cancers, the molecular signatures of these tumors vary considerably and span all four TGCA subsets [8]. A large proportion (~45–55%) of conventional endometrioid cancers fall into the low copy-number TCGA category. This subgroup includes the majority of low-grade endometrioid cancers as well as some intermediate and high-grade cancers. These tumors are relatively genetically "simple" and are typified by mutations in *PTEN* as well as genes involved in the PI3K pathway, including *PIK3CA* and *PIK3RI* [146–148]. *ARID1A* mutations are also identified in ~40% of endometrioid cancers, many of which reside in the low copy-number group [149].

The remaining endometrioid tumors with *ARID1A* mutations fall in the mismatch repair-deficient/microsatellite unstable TCGA category. Mismatch repair-deficient cancers account for another large subset (~25–35%) of endometrioid tumors and are characterized by abnormalities in the mismatch repair system attributable to germline mutations (e.g., Lynch syndrome), somatic gene mutations, or epigenetic hypermethylation [31, 32, 35, 91, 141]. Hypermethylation of the *MLH1* promoter is the most common cause of mismatch repair deficiency and is seen in up to a quarter of endometrial carcinomas [139, 150]. Unlike in the colon, this epigenetic change does not run in tandem with *BRAF* mutations [151–153]. The remaining mismatch repair-deficient cancers consist of an admixture of Lynch syndrome-associated tumors with associated germline defects and tumors with somatic mutations in one of the mismatch repair genes. Most often, germline and somatic mutations involve one of the four major mismatch repair proteins (*MLH1*, *PMS2*, *MSH2*, and *MSH6*). Rare cases are attributable to mutations in *EPCAM* which lead to *MSH2* silencing [26, 27, 29, 154, 155].The histology of this molecular subgroup ranges from uniformly low-grade,

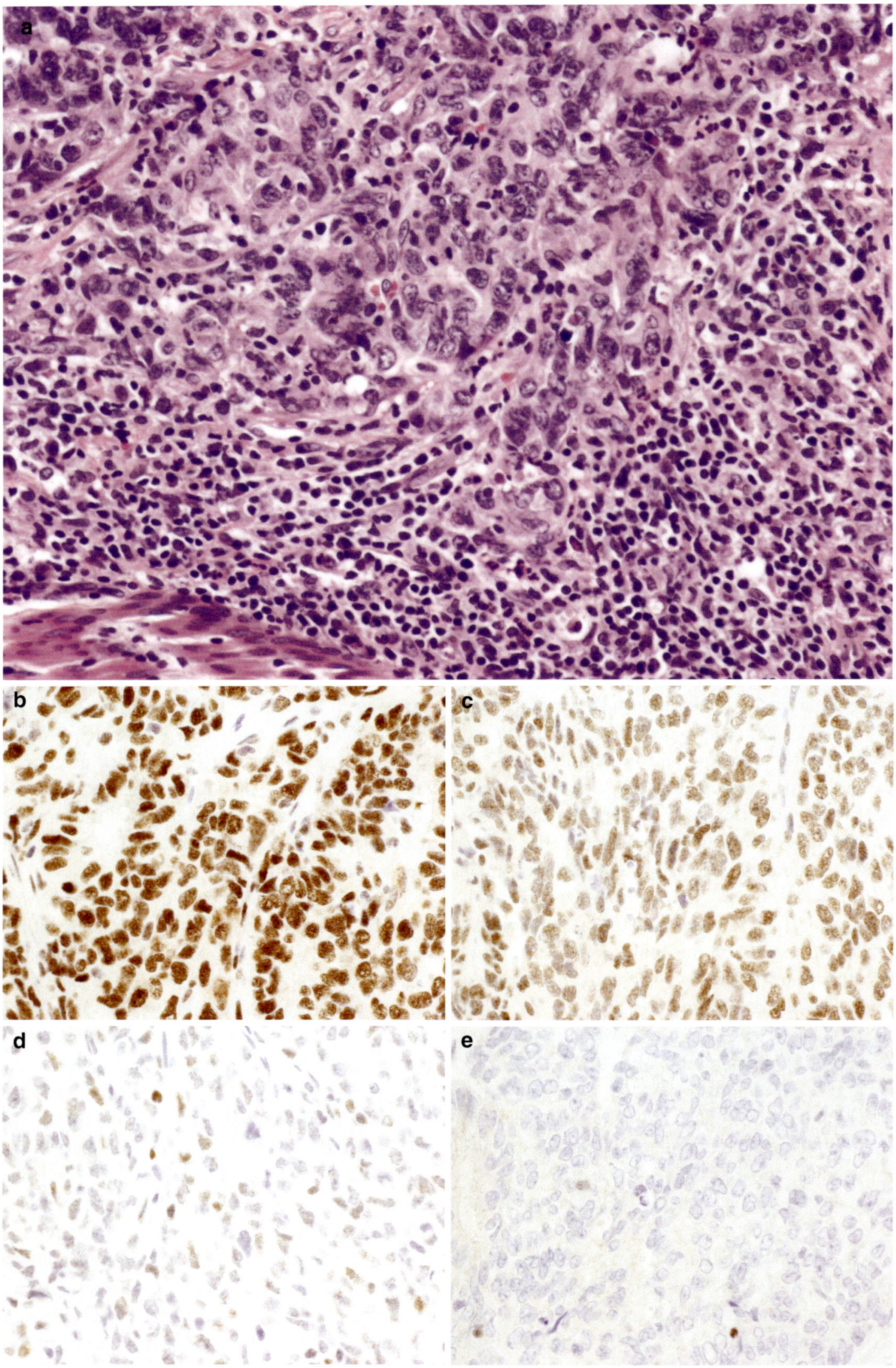

Fig. 18.34 Loss of mismatch repair protein expression is seen in over 25% of endometrioid carcinomas. This is most often attributable to epigenetic methylation of the *MLH1* promoter region leading to loss of MLH1 and PMS2 expression. In other cases, as in the endometrioid carcinoma illustrated here (**a**), loss is attributable to Lynch syndrome. This tumor demonstrates intact nuclear expression of MLH1 (**b**), PMS2 (**c**), and MSH2 (**d**) but shows loss of MSH6 (**e**). Scattered positive intratumoral lymphocytes provide a positive internal control. This patient demonstrated a germline *MSH6* mutation on further testing, confirming the diagnosis of Lynch syndrome. Notably, this tumor shows robust tumor-infiltrating lymphocytes, a common feature among mismatch repair-deficient cancers

conventional endometrioid carcinomas to high-grade, dedifferentiated tumors [30, 31, 156–158]. As a result of their capacity to rapidly accumulate mutations, these cancers are also associated with increased neoantigen loads, immunogenicity, and vulnerability to immunotherapy [142, 143, 159].

The *POLE*-mutated ("ultramutated") TCGA subset of cancers accounts for ~10% of endometrioid carcinomas and shares the mismatch repair-deficient group's propensity for high neoantigen production and immunogenicity [143, 159]. These tumors' capacity to rapidly accrue mutations is reflected in frequent biphasic and ambiguus morphology. This molecular subset is of clinical interest because they have a very good prognosis even in the context of relatively high-grade, high-stage malignancies. It is notable that while *POLE*-mutated cancers also bear *TP53* in 35% of cases, existing data suggests that it is the underlying *POLE*-mutation, rather than the superimposed *TP53*-mutation, that drives prognosis [160], although exact mechanism is unclear.

The final TCGA category seen among endometrioid tumors is the high copy-number subset. These tumors are genetically complex and frequently show *TP53* mutations. Although many of these are serous cancers, this category also includes occasional *TP53*-mutated, morphologically endometrioid carcinomas [8, 100–102, 104]. Indeed, this site likely encompasses many of the morphologically endometrioid but p53-overexpressing cancers that have been shown by Soslow and colleagues to follow a clinical course commensurate with their serous counterparts [7, 102].

The above findings have a significant impact in the diagnosis of endometrial serous carcinoma. Pathologists used to believe that endometrioid carcinoma rarely bear TP53 mutation, while finding a mutational-type p53 expression by immunohistochemistry is indicative of endometrial serous carcinoma, however this concept is no longer practical in the context of our improved molecular understanding of the disease.

18.4.8.3 Mucinous Carcinoma

Clinical

Mucinous carcinomas are recognized as a distinct tumor type by the 2014 WHO Classification System and comprise between 1 and 9% of all endometrial cancers, with variability in this rate attributable to differences in diagnostic criteria across studies [96, 112, 113]. Most of these tumors are restricted to the uterus and bear a prognosis comparable to grade-matched endometrioid counterparts [112].

Gross

Mucinous carcinomas often have grossly villous architecture with exophytic excrescences that may fill the endometrial cavity. In cases where mucinous differentiation is most pronounced, a mucoid cut surface may be appreciable on gross examination.

Microscopic

Mucinous endometrial carcinoma is defined by the presence of >50% mucinous differentiation, which is classified as cells showing abundant intracytoplasmic mucin [112, 113] (Fig. 18.35). On H&E stains mucin may appear as granular, palely eosinophilic, and/or finely vacuolated. Extracellular mucin may be abundant and often shows affiliated neutrophils [112]. Architecturally, mucinous carcinomas usually show significant glandular and papillary structures, although epithelial stratification is limited. Some cancers have a more microacinar pattern typified by small, closely packed glands with bland nuclear features. This pattern can be readily confused with benign endocervical hyperplasia [161, 162], particularly on limited samples. Caution should therefore be exercised when interpreting endometrial samples consisting exclusively of banal but abundant mucinous glands, with deference to a larger specimen for final diagnosis. Mucinous carcinomas may also be mistaken for endocervical carcinomas; an approach to this differential is discussed in detail in the preceding sections on endometrial carcinomas with squamous and mucinous differentiation, and is outlined in the accompanying table (Fig. 18.36 and Table 18.5). It is worth emphasizing that the vast majority of mucinous endometrial carcinomas demonstrate endocervical-type mucinous morphology, while intestinal-type mucinous morphology is extremely rare in endometrial primaries. Rare cases of intestinal differentiation have been reported, most recently in the setting of high-level microsatellite instability [163], but these cases constitute the exception rather than the rule. In contrast, intestinal features are appreciated in up to 10%

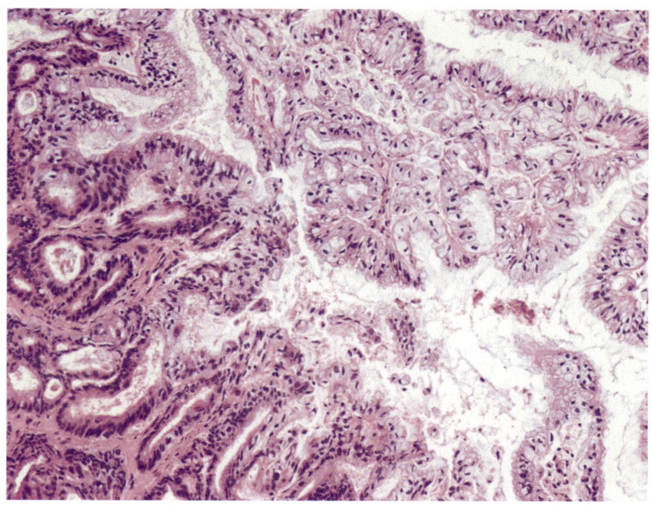

Fig. 18.35 Mucinous endometrial carcinomas are characterized by >50% mucinous differentiation manifesting as abundant intracytoplasmic mucin. Architectural arrangements range from papillary to microacinar. Often some components of conventional endometrioid carcinoma are present, as is illustrated in this case in the left-hand portion of the image

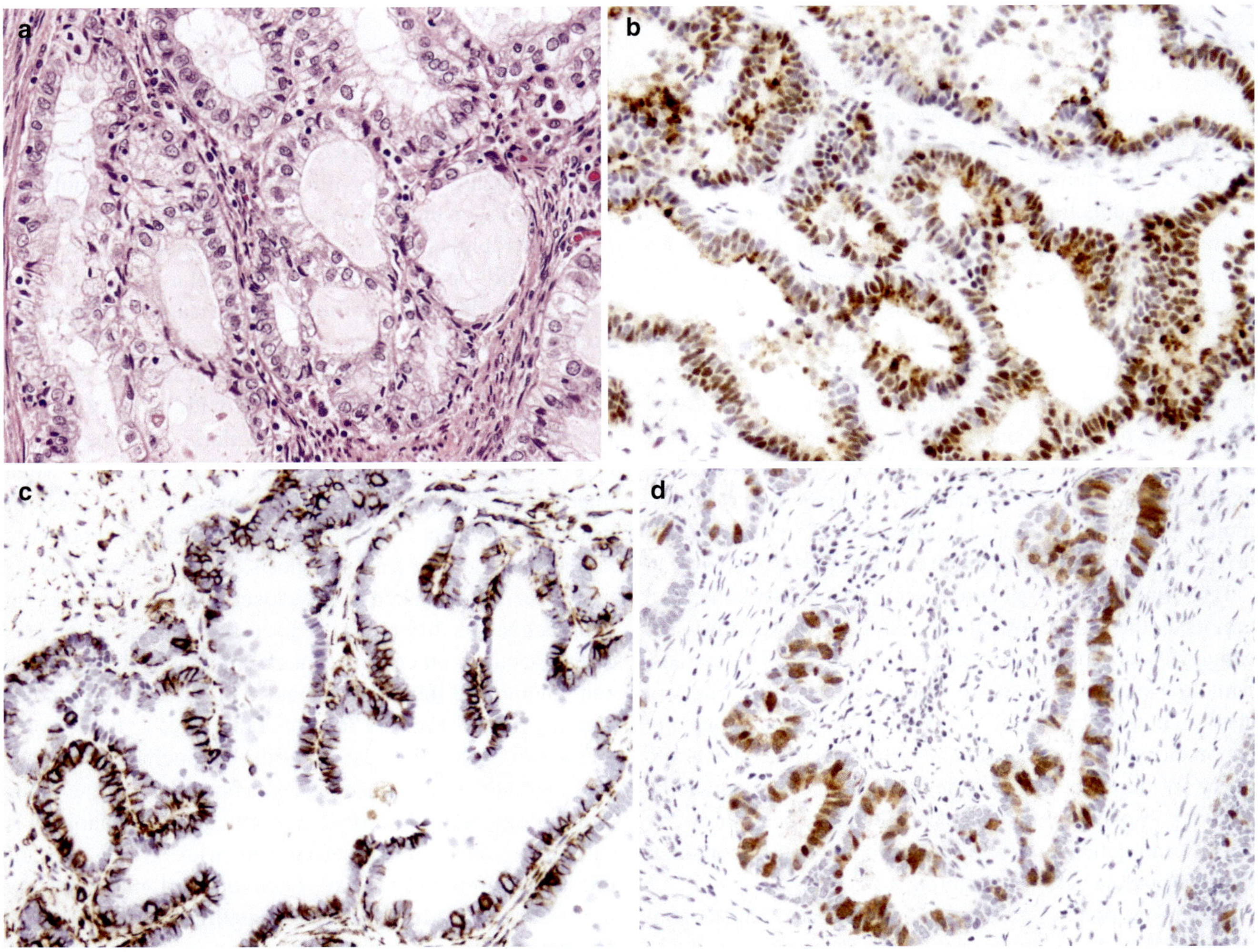

Fig. 18.36 Mucinous endometrial tumors may invoke the possibility of an endocervical primary, particularly when centered in the lower uterine segment. Immunohistochemistry can be useful for resolving this differential (Table 18.5). This mucinous carcinoma (**a**) shows strong estrogen receptor (ER) expression (**b**), strong vimentin expression (**c**), and only scattered p16 expression (**d**), supporting endometrial origin

of cancers arising from the endocervix [164, 165]. Thus, intestinal-type mucinous differentiation is far more likely to derive from an endocervical primary than from the endometrium.

Immunohistochemistry

The immunohistochemical features of mucinous endometrial carcinoma are similar to their conventional endometrioid counterparts, with positivity for vimentin and ER and negativity for CEA and p16 aiding in the distinction from endocervical carcinoma (Table 18.5).

Molecular

The molecular features of mucinous endometrial carcinoma are relatively similar to other endometrioid cancers, although *KRAS* mutations are more common whereas *PTEN* and *PAX2* mutations are less common [166]. There is also evidence that *MLH1* hypermethylated tumors may be disproportionately represented in this histologic group [115].

18.4.8.4 Serous Carcinoma

Clinical

Serous carcinomas comprise 5–10% of all endometrial cancers and constituted the prototypical "type II" cancers in the former binary classification system [113, 167]. Historically they were called "uterine papillary serous carcinomas (UPSC)"; however, this name has been abandoned as many cases display solid and glandular, rather than exclusively papillary architecture. When compared to their endometrioid counterparts, serous cancers occur in older women, are less likely to have a background hyperplasia, and are not clearly associated with increased estrogen [167, 168]. Presentation is typically in the sixth to seventh decade of life with postmenopausal bleeding.

Gross

Because endometrial serous carcinomas are not associated with increased estrogen, they often arise in atrophic uteri. However, such cancers can also be found in non-atrophic uteri. The uterine size or the endometrial status is mainly depending on the hormone (estrogen) levels of individual patients. These uteri can be significantly distorted by bulky tumor that appears exophytic and shaggy on cut section. Alternatively, serous carcinomas may be grossly inapparent when the disease volume is low. In some cases serous carcinoma rises focally in association with benign endometrial polyps; in these instances, the gross impression is indicative only of the benign polyp and does not yield clues as to the presence of a focal associated malignancy. Invasion is often grossly inapparent in serous cancers, and generous sampling is advisable to ensure appropriate representation of invasive depth for microscopy.

Microscopic

Serous carcinomas are comprised of high-grade cells arranged in papillae, sheets, and/or glands (Fig. 18.37). Most cases have a papillary predominance with slender to broad papillae arranged in complex, arborizing patterns. Other cases are characterized by confluent sheets of cells, while others assume prominent tubular architecture. The tumors frequently have a lavender tinctorial quality, a helpful clue to their diagnosis on low power. Both papillary and glandular arrangements classically show jagged "slit-like" spaces, an important clue that helps differentiate them from endometrioid tumors, which typically have more open and rounded glandular lumens (Fig. 18.38); however, some cases of serous carcinoma will also demonstrating a "gaping" glandular pattern of infiltration [167]. Although one study has reported that up to a third of cases show psammoma bodies, this feature is not specific for serous differentiation and is encountered only rarely in practice [132]. Many tumors show epithelial tufting into spaces, sometimes with nuclear "hobnailing" that can mimic clear cell carcinoma. Intraluminal papillation as well as sloughed atypical epithelial cells are also frequently present within gland lumens (Fig. 18.39).

Given the variability of serous carcinoma architecture and the frequent overlap between patterns seen in other tumor types, cytology is absolutely fundamental to the diagnosis: serous carcinoma is, by definition, a high-grade malignancy. This high cytologic grade manifests in enlarged, atypical cells with round to oval nuclei bearing irregular chromatin and prominent, often eosinophilic macronucleoli (Fig. 18.40). Occasional cells show smudgy hyperchromasia, and scattered wildly atypical "monster cells" may be identified. Brisk mitotic activity is expected (usually >12/10 HPFs) and atypical mitotic figures can be frequent

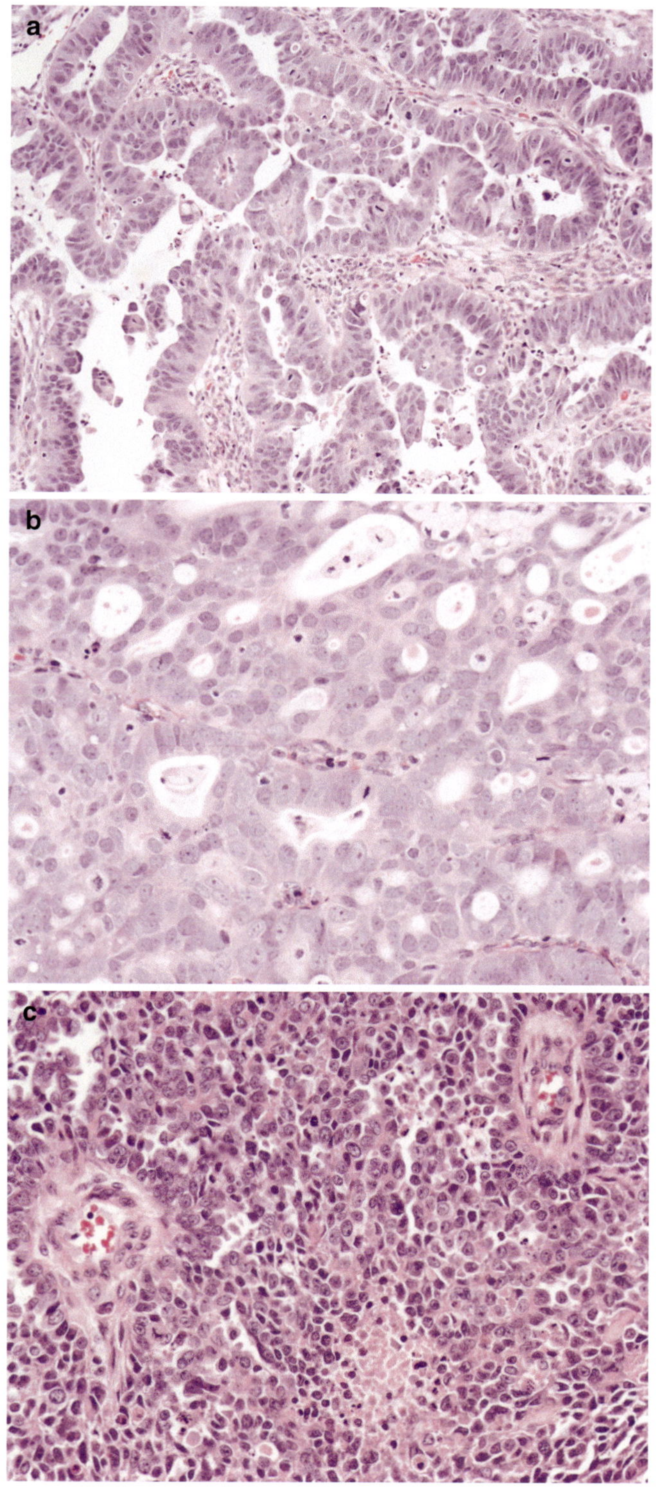

Fig. 18.37 Serous carcinomas are characterized by markedly atypical cells arranged in papillae (**a**), glands (**b**), or solid structures (**c**). Often the tumor cells have a lavender tinctorial quality, which serves as a helpful diagnostic clue from low power as it contrasts with the more densely basophilic staining of endometrioid cancers. Scattered fibrovascular cores can sometimes be appreciated even in cases with predominantly solid arrangements, as seen in **c**

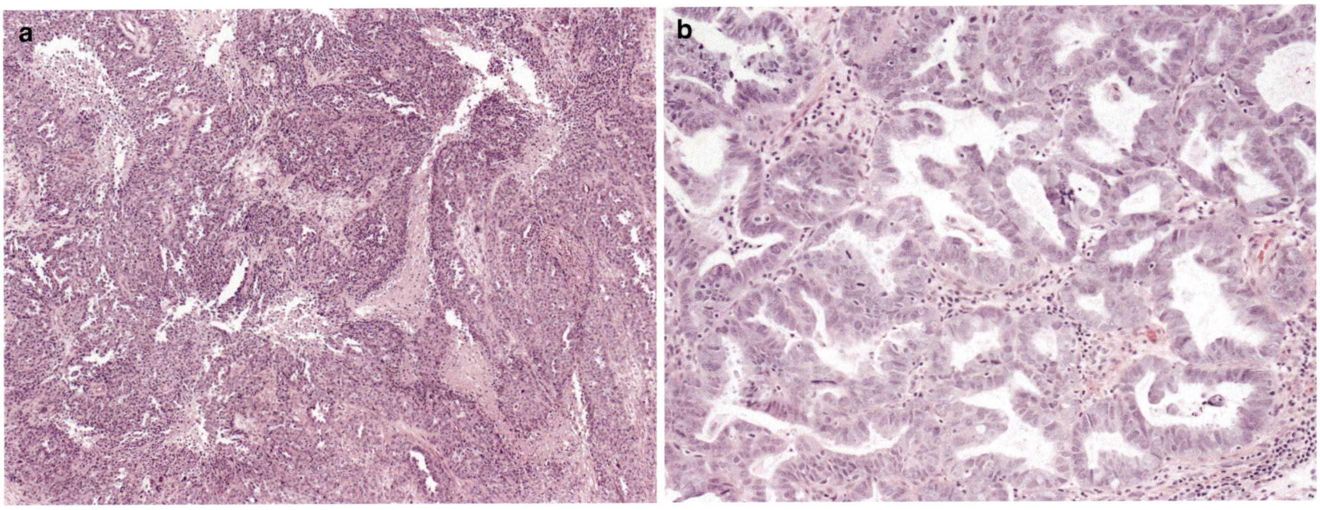

Fig. 18.38 Serous carcinomas often show slit-like spaces reflective of their underlying papillary architecture (**a**), although other cases have a gaping glandular pattern (**b**)

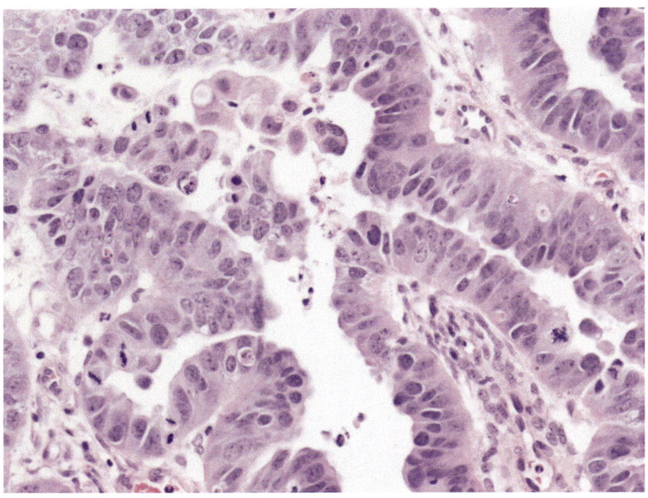

Fig. 18.39 Serous carcinomas with papillary and glandular structures frequently show atypical sloughed cells within lumens

(Fig. 18.41). The degree of nuclear atypia and proliferation is even more marked than is observed in clear cell carcinoma, a helpful point to consider in cases where prominent hobnailing invokes that differential (indeed, serous carcinoma with clear cell features is far more common than true clear cell carcinoma) (Fig. 18.42).

18.4.8.5 Serous Carcinoma Distinction from Mixed Endometrial Carcinoma

The possibility of a "mixed" carcinoma arises when areas of overt serous differentiation are associated with morphologies more reminiscent of endometrioid or clear cell carcinoma. Prior studies suggested that serous components comprising anywhere between 5 and 25% of a "mixed" cancer ultimately drove the tumor's prognosis [113, 169]. However, it is notable that many of the tumors classified as "mixed" in these studies would have been characterized as pure serous carcinomas using the updated criteria for serous carcinoma which allow for glandular and solid patterns of growth, as well as areas of clear cell differentiation [167, 170]. Further studies have suggested that morphologically mixed or ambiguous carcinomas with *TP53* mutations ultimately behave like serous cancers [7, 102], and most often demonstrate shared clonality across morphologies [171]. These findings are further corroborated by the TGCA's identification of a molecular subgroup defined by high copy-number alterations which includes both conventional serous cancers and occasional cancers with endometrioid and clear cell morphology, suggesting that morphologic distinctions are not as clean as the old type I/II classification schema suggested [9]. Ultimately, these data suggest that a diagnosis of "mixed" endometrial carcinoma should be approached with caution, and that in many instances a designation simply of serous carcinoma is appropriate when serous features are regionally present. This issue is discussed in further detail at the end of the chapter under the heading "Mixed Endometrial Carcinomas."

18.4.8.6 Minimal Serous Carcinoma and Serous Endometrial Intraepithelial Carcinoma (SEIC)

Although many serous carcinomas present with bulky disease, the diagnosis requires only >1 cm of invasive growth. Proliferations which meet morphologic criteria for serous carcinoma but which fall below the 1 cm cutoff are classi-

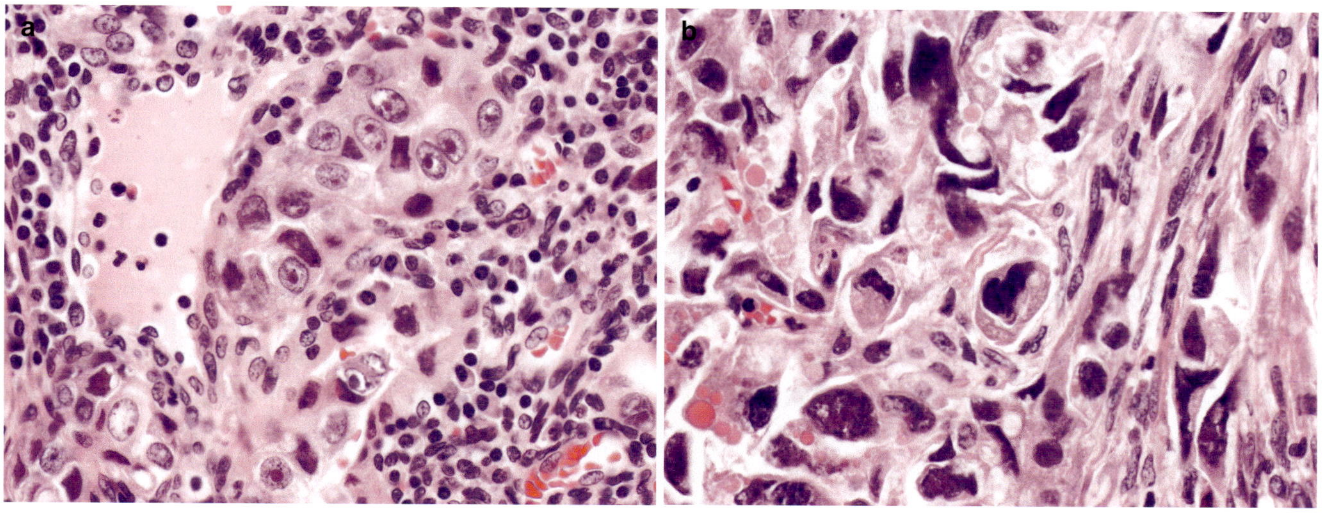

Fig. 18.40 Serous carcinomas are high-grade malignancies typified by marked cytologic atypia with prominent eosinophilic nuclei (**a**). Scattered smudgy, hyperchromatic nuclei are also often appreciated (**b**)

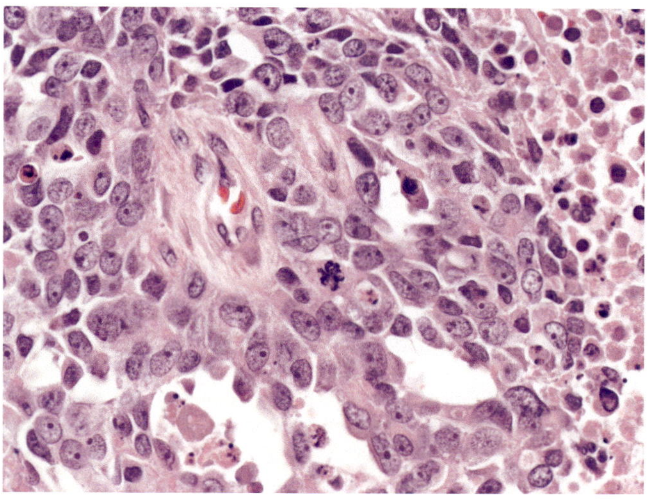

Fig. 18.41 Mitotic figures are readily identifiable in serous carcinomas and typically include atypical forms (center)

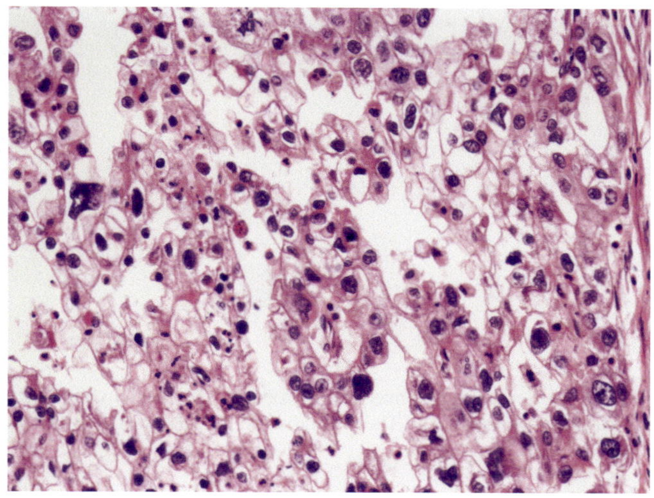

Fig. 18.42 Serous carcinomas can show areas of prominent clear cell differentiation, as seen in this case which elsewhere showed typical serous morphology. When conventional serous carcinoma differentiation is present elsewhere, these regions should not warrant a diagnosis of clear cell carcinoma. Whether such tumors ought to be classified as "mixed endometrial carcinomas" is debatable, and this diagnosis is approached by gynecologic pathologists with increasing caution

fied as "minimal serous carcinoma" [172]. This term includes both proliferations limited to the surface or to the glands [e.g., endometrial intraepithelial carcinoma (EIC)] and superficial carcinomas with ≤1 cm of invasion. EIC commonly shows serous differentiation; therefore, it is now designated as SEIC, which is discussed in detail in the preceding chapter; briefly, it is characterized by replacement of the surface epithelium or endometrial glands by high-grade cells morphologically comparable to those seen in serous carcinoma. It is identified in 90% of uterine serous carcinomas, supporting the thesis that it represents a precursor lesion [172–178]. SEIC shows elevated mitotic activity/Ki67 expression and displays abnormal p53 expression, important distinctions from its benign mimic, papillary syncytial metaplasia [20, 179]. Despite their low disease volume, SEICs and superficially invasive minimal serous carcinomas are commonly associated with extrauterine disease [20, 172, 177, 179, 180]. It is worth emphasizing that the term "minimal serous carcinoma" remains somewhat controversial, as no study has yet demonstrated a difference between SEIC and minimal serous carcinoma.

18.4.8.7 Staging Issues in Serous Carcinoma

Serous carcinomas have a predilection for deep myometrial invasion, which may not be appreciable on gross examination (Fig. 18.43). Importantly, depth of invasion has not been reproducibly linked to risk for extrauterine disease [20, 181]. This is in part because serous carcinomas deriving from the uterus, like those arising in the ovary, have a propensity for peritoneal spread. Careful staging, including assessment and directed biopsy of the omentum and peritoneal surfaces, is therefore advisable for endometrial serous carcinoma resections even when disease is only superficial (as with minimal serous carcinomas and SEICs, as discussed in the preceding section). Furthermore, fallopian tubes should be completely submitted for pathologic examination and carefully assessed as intraluminal cancer cells may be identified in cases with very focal/superficial endometrial serous carcinoma, and have been linked to peritoneal disease [182] (Fig. 18.44). This remains true even for tumors arising in and limited to polyps: serous carcinomas have a tendency to arise in otherwise benign endometrial polyps in postmenopausal women, and despite low disease volume and confinement to the polyp, extrauterine disease can occur in these cases [169, 183, 184] (Fig. 18.45). Nodal staging is also stan-

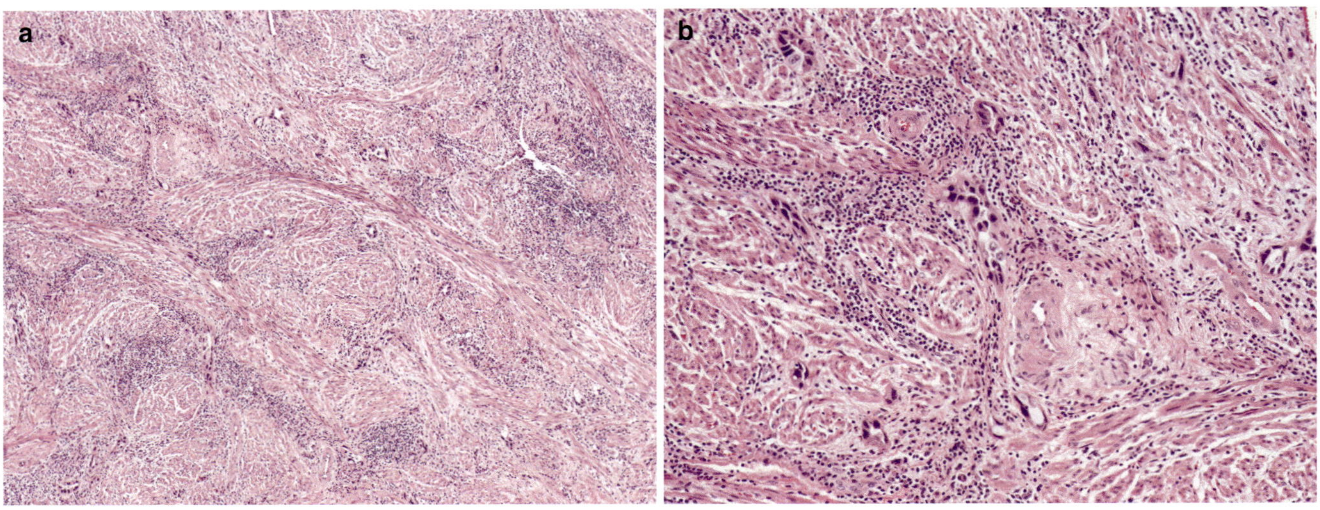

Fig. 18.43 Serous carcinomas have a propensity for deep myometrial invasion, which may be inappreciable on gross examination and subtle from low microscopic power (**a**). The infiltrative glands in this case are associated with robust inflammation but provoke little desmoplastic response (**b**)

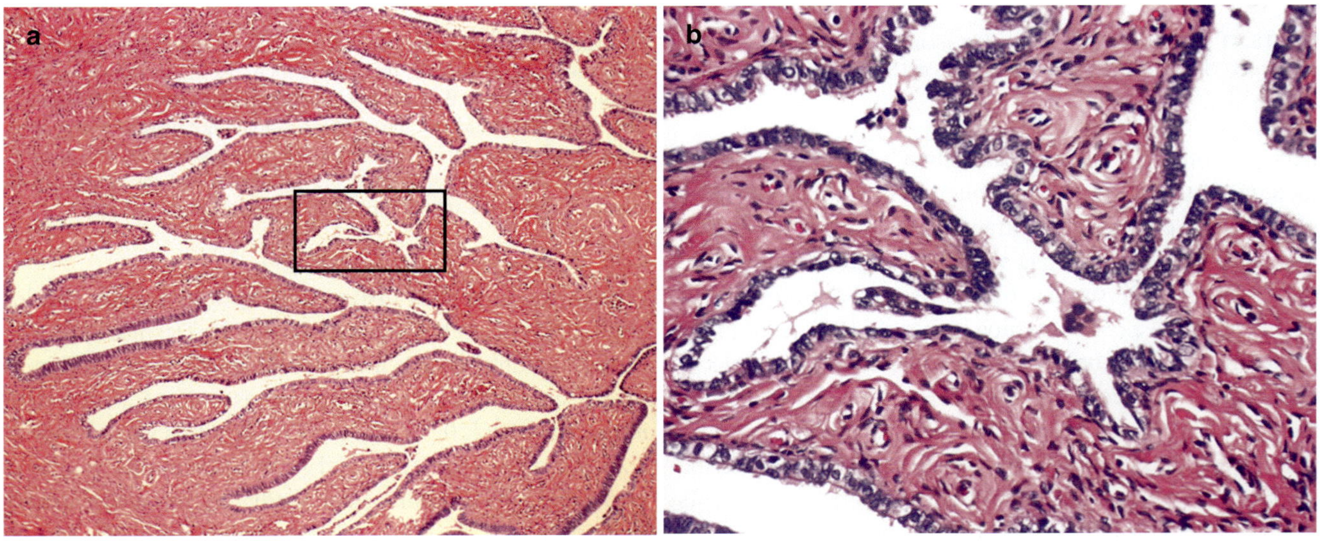

Fig. 18.44 Transtubal peritoneal spread may occur even with superficial serous endometrial carcinomas, therefore careful sectioning of the fallopian tubes is advisable even in cases with only superficial disease. In this case, intraluminal tumor cells were barely appreciable form low power (**a**), but can be identified on closer review of the area within the black box (**b**). Image courtesy of Dr. Wenxin Zheng

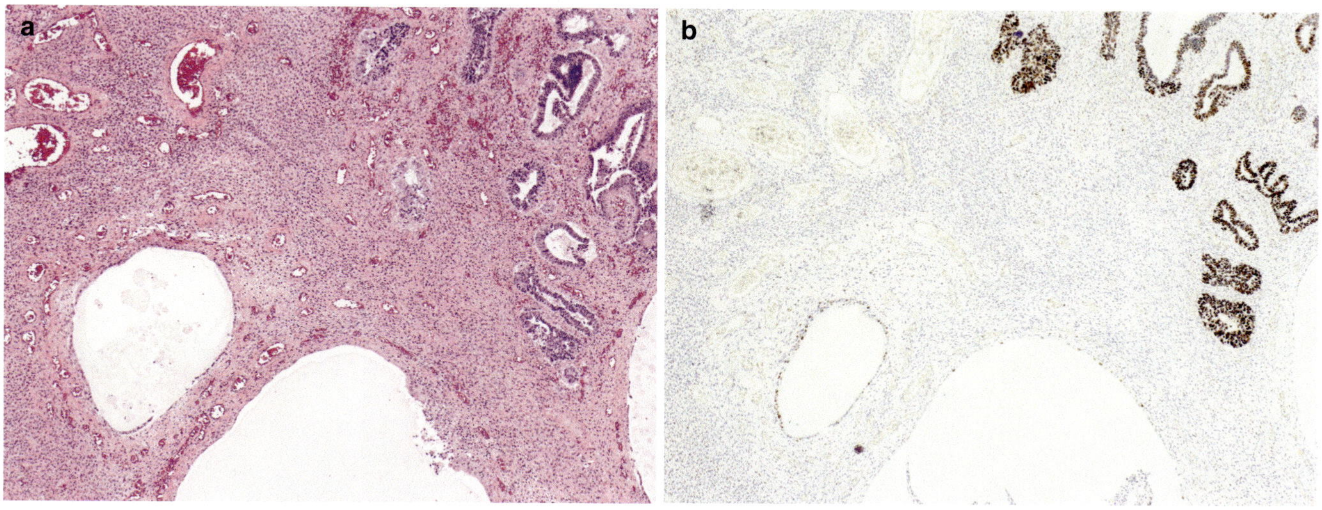

Fig. 18.45 Serous carcinomas often arise in endometrial polyps (a). The malignant glands are diffusely p53-positive in this case, which contrasts with the wild-type staining seen in the benign portions of the polyp (**b**)

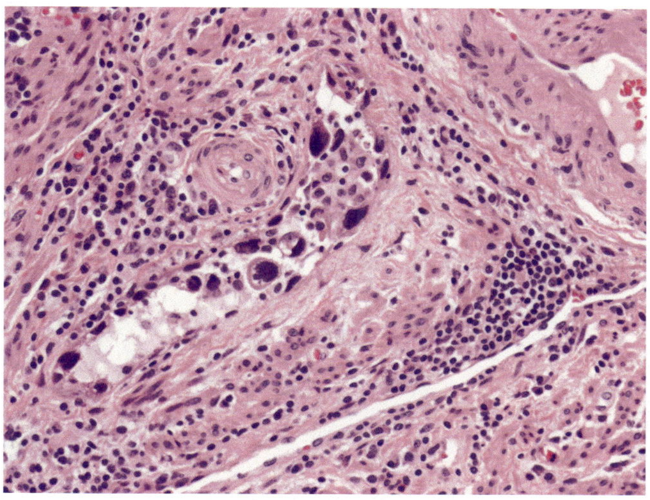

Fig. 18.46 Serous carcinomas have a propensity for lymphovascular invasion irrespective of depth of invasion. In this case, the proximity to a thick-walled vessel (upper right) supports lymphovascular involvement

dard for serous carcinoma given these tumors' propensity for lymphovascular involvement irrespective of tumor size or myometrial invasion (Fig. 18.46).

Immunohistochemistry

p53 is the most commonly enlisted immunostain in diagnosing serous carcinoma. Abnormal p53 expression is typical of serous carcinomas and is a relatively robust proxy for an underlying *TP53* mutation. Aberrant expression most commonly manifests as strong, diffuse nuclear staining consistent with overproduction of a dysfunctional protein [102, 104, 126] (Fig. 18.47). The required threshold for diffuse expression is the subject of some debate due in part to variability across laboratories; some authors advocate using a 50% cutoff but acknowledge that positive cases most often show far more extensive staining (>75%) [104]. Indeed, requiring only 50% staining raises considerable risk of serous carcinoma overdiagnosis. Many others therefore advocate an "all or nothing" approach to p53; that is, an abnormal interpretation should be rendered only in the presence of complete, diffuse positivity or total loss of expression. Given that interlaboratory variability exists, the identification of marked overexpression relative to internal control wild-type staining is helpful (and selection of sections for staining should contain adjacent normal whenever possible). The less common "null" pattern is seen in approximately 20% of cases with abnormal expression and corresponds with total loss of staining. As with overexpression, this pattern is easiest to diagnose when comparison normal/wild-type staining is present for comparison [102, 104, 126]. Extrapolation from literature in the ovary suggests that the overexpression pattern is most often attributable to missense mutations while the null pattern is due to frameshift, nonsense, and splice-site mutations which halt protein production altogether [185]. There is some indication that the null pattern carries a worse prognosis in the ovary; however, this has not been reproduced in the endometrium.

Serous carcinomas usually demonstrate strong p16 staining in the majority of tumor cells, which can be a worthwhile adjunct to p53 immunostaining when working up a tumor with a differential of low-grade endometrioid carcinoma [138] (Fig. 18.48). p16 can be particularly useful as a counterstain when dealing with very small samples with an apparent null p53 pattern. It is worth emphasizing that p16 loses its discriminatory utility for higher-grade cancers (as high-grade endometrioid cancers may also overexpress this marker), as well as cancers with a differential of endocervical origin (as p16 is used as a surrogate for human papillomavirus-associated carcinomas in this setting). Lack

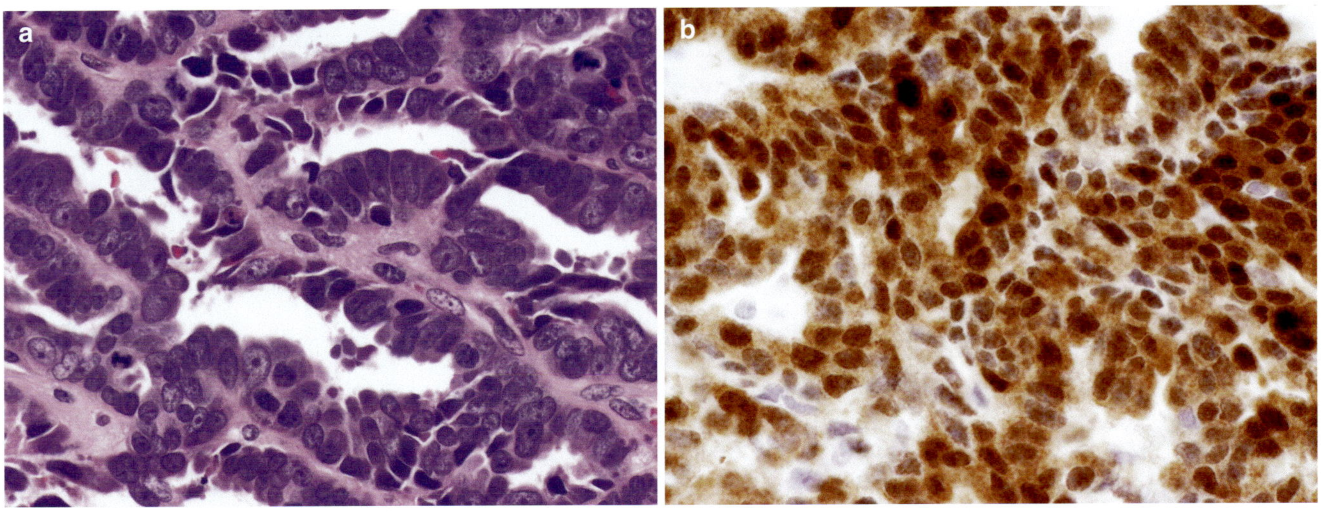

Fig. 18.47 p53 immunostaining is abnormal in serous carcinomas (**a**), and typically manifests as diffuse overexpression (**b**). The extent of staining required for "overexpression" is somewhat controversial; most advocate for a cutoff of at least 50% staining, although >75% staining (as seen in this case) is more typical

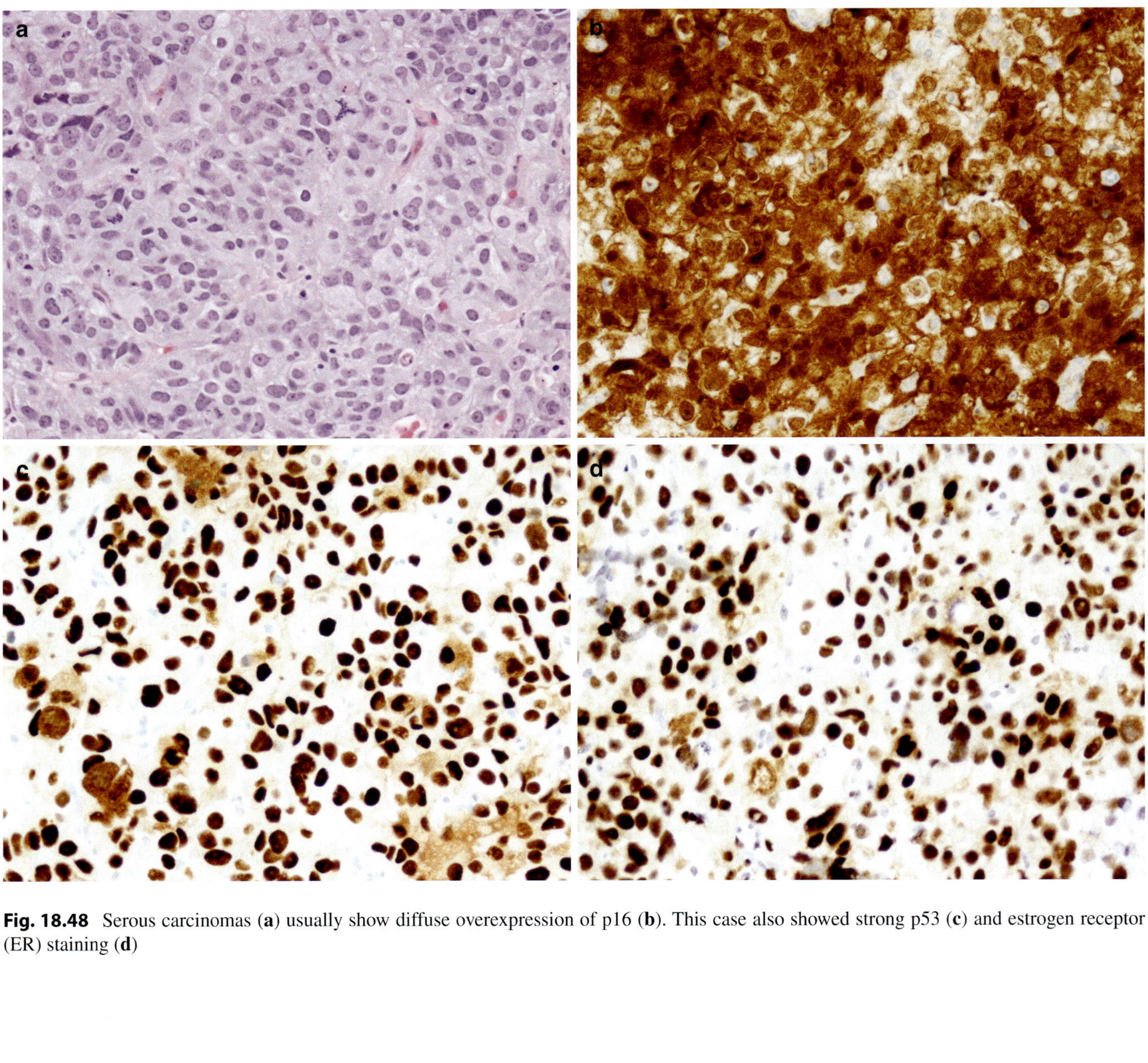

Fig. 18.48 Serous carcinomas (**a**) usually show diffuse overexpression of p16 (**b**). This case also showed strong p53 (**c**) and estrogen receptor (ER) staining (**d**)

of progesterone receptor (PR) staining is also of some value in differentiating serous carcinoma from endometrioid carcinoma, as is the presence of intact PTEN expression [186–188]. Finally, IMP3 is often positive in serous carcinoma and is useful for excluding endometrioid carcinomas, particularly when used in combination with p53, p16, PR, and PTEN [187–190].

Molecular

Serous carcinomas classically bear *TP53* mutations and reside within the copy number-high subgroup of the TCGA-based molecular endometrial carcinoma classification system [8]. Despite the strong association between *TP53* mutations and uterine serous carcinoma, this cancer type has not traditionally been included in the spectrum of Li-Fraumeni associated cancers. However, a recent study observed a 1.3% germline *TP53* mutation rate among endometrial serous carcinoma patients, which is considerably higher than expected in an unselected population [43].

HER2/*ERBB2* receptor tyrosine kinase amplification has also been identified in 17–80% of endometrial serous carcinomas and has been associated with advanced stage and decreased survival; however, unlike with breast and esophagogastric tumors, the therapeutic implications of this finding remain uncertain [191–193]. As is the case with endometrioid and clear cell carcinomas, *PIKC3* mutations are frequently encountered in uterine serous carcinomas [149]. In contrast to endometrioid and clear cell carcinomas, mutations involving *PTEN* and *ARID1A* are not typical of serous carcinomas. Additionally, abnormalities in mismatch repair genes are rarely encountered in these tumors, commensurate with the lack of association between serous carcinoma and Lynch syndrome [31, 35]. Furthermore, *POLE* mutations are not a feature of serous carcinomas.

Despite the strong association between ovarian serous carcinomas and heritable *BRCA* mutations, germline defects in *BRCA* genes have not been historically linked to an increased risk of uterine serous carcinoma. However, some recent evidence has challenged this tenant [41–43]. One study identified a 2% germline *BRCA1* mutation rate among patients with endometrial serous cancers, which is significantly higher than the rate in the general population (0.06%) and prompted the authors to recommend genetic screening in all endometrial serous carcinoma patients [43]. This suggestion was corroborated by a meta-analysis of 10 studies including 345 endometrial serous carcinoma patients, which revealed that the risk of carrying a germline *BRCA1/2* mutation was significantly increased among Ashkenazi Jewish women with endometrial serous carcinoma vs. Ashkenazi Jews without this diagnosis [42]. Somatic mutation status for *BRCA* genes is also of new interest in endometrial serous carcinomas given the role of poly ADP ribose polymerase (PARP) inhibitors in ovarian and breast cancers bearing *BRCA* mutations; however, this area has not yet been well-investigated in endometrial primaries.

18.4.8.8 Clear Cell Carcinoma

Clinical

True clear cell carcinoma of the endometrium is extremely rare, constituting <1–2% of all endometrial carcinomas. They typically present with postmenopausal bleeding with a mean age of diagnosis in the late 60s [108]. Estrogen does not appear to be a carcinogenic driver in this tumor type, and when compared to endometrioid carcinomas, they are less often associated with obesity and diabetes mellitus and more often associated with smoking and multiparity [117, 194, 195].

Gross

The gross appearance of clear cell carcinomas is similar to other endometrial carcinoma types. Tumors often appear as exophytic, irregular masses protruding into the endometrial cavity. On cut section they may be more solid than other endometrial cancers owing to the prominent contribution of dense stroma.

Microscopic

Clear cell carcinomas demonstrate hobnail or polygonal cells arranged in papillary, tubulocystic, and solid patterns (Fig. 18.49). Nuclear atypia is moderate to severe but typically falls short of the frank anaplasia and bizarre pleomorphism that can be observed in serous carcinomas; in their review of 50 cases, Fadare et al. identified only two tumors with grade 3 nuclei (Fig. 18.50). Scattered mitotic figures can be expected but overall the mitotic index is low in the majority of cases, another important distinction from serous carcinoma [170]. The cytoplasm is often clear, although eosinophilic cytoplasm may also be present in large areas of the tumor. As with its morphologic cousin clear cell renal carcinoma, intranuclear inclusions may be present in endometrial clear cell carcinoma. The presence of hyalinized stroma is an extremely useful diagnostic feature, as are brightly eosinophilic extracellular hyaline bodies which are seen in the majority—although not all—cases (Fig. 18.51). The identification of at least some regions of the tumor bearing this prototypic dense, hyalinized stroma is critical for accurate diagnosis, and its absence should raise the differential of another histologic subtype with superimposed clear cell features.

It is worth emphasizing that true clear cell carcinoma of the endometrium is rare, and that the presence of cells with clear cytoplasm is neither necessary nor sufficient for its diagnosis: in the series by Fadare et al., only 4% of cases

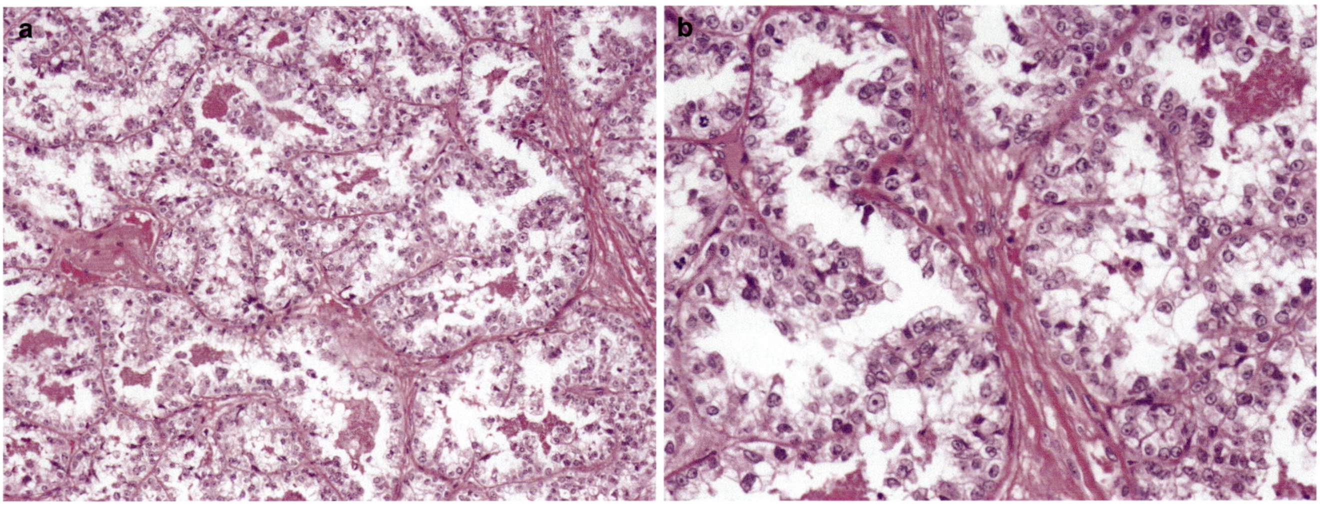

Fig. 18.49 Clear cell carcinomas can have solid, papillary, or tubulocystic arrangements of epithelial cells embedded in hyalinized stroma. This case shows a predominantly tubulocystic pattern of with strands of intercalating eosinophilic stroma. (**a**) The constituent cells show only moderate cytologic atypia and mitotic figures are not readily identified (**b**)

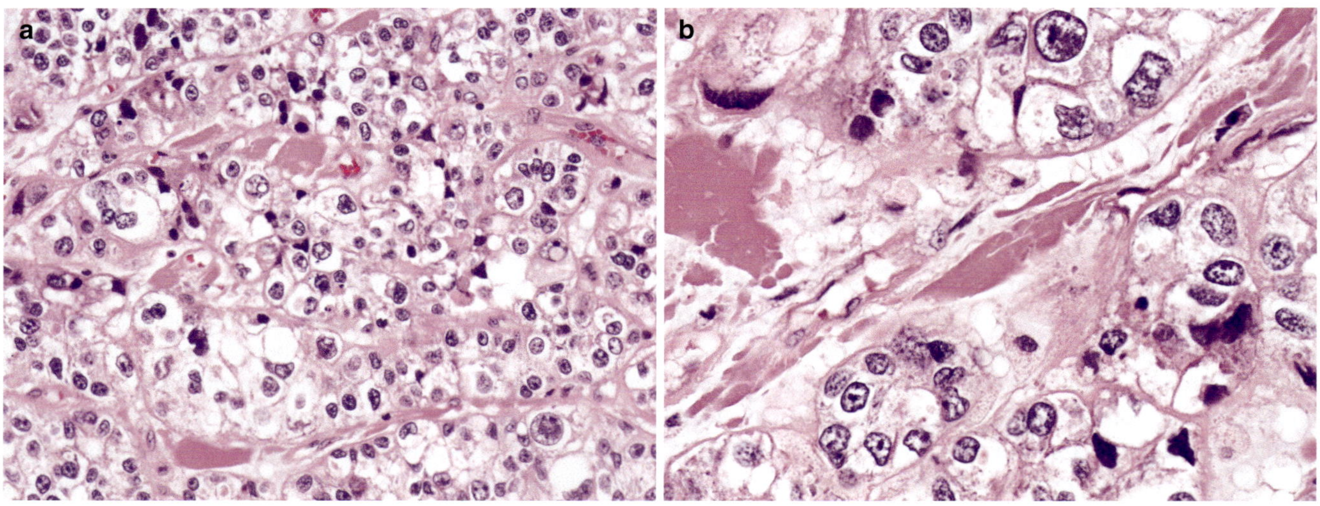

Fig. 18.50 Clear cell carcinomas only rarely show severe cytologic atypia. This case (**a**, **b**) shows regions of increased anaplasia and pleomorphism including occasional cells with smudgy hyperchromasia. The presence of dense hyaline material in the background provides support for the clear cell diagnosis, as does the absence of serous morphology elsewhere in the tumor

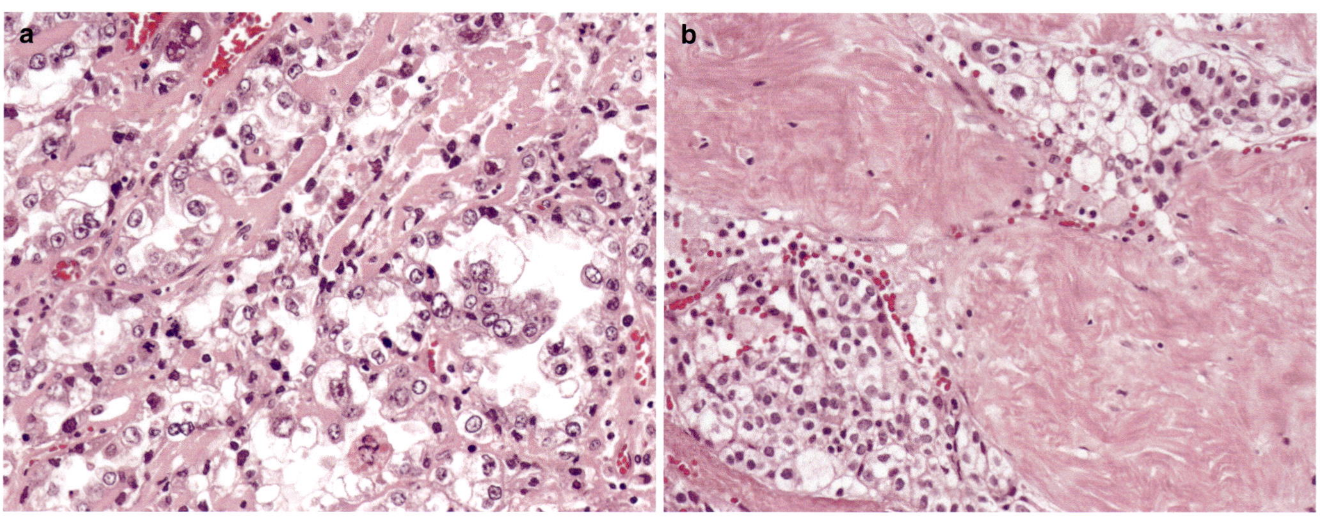

Fig. 18.51 Hyalinized stroma is critical for the diagnosis of clear cell carcinoma. This may manifest as strands and globules of eosinophilic material intimately admixed with tumor cells (**a**) or as broad swathes of stroma dividing epithelial areas (**b**)

were comprised exclusively of cytoplasmically clear cells and 10% had no clear cells at all [170]. Overdiagnosis of clear cell carcinoma is common: evaluation of 44 endometrial cancers originally interpreted as clear cell carcinoma by five experts lead to reclassification of 54% [4]. The most frequent cause of clear cytoplasm in endometrial tumors is secretory differentiation within an endometrioid carcinoma, followed by serous cancers with areas of cytoplasmic clearing. Only eliminating these other entities can a diagnosis of clear cell carcinoma be rendered with confidence.

Immunohistochemistry

Clear cell carcinomas tend to be negative for the hormone receptors ER, PR, and AR, which can be helpful when tackling a differential of endometrioid or serous carcinoma with clear cell features as these entities are more often hormone-receptor positive [123, 133]. Napsin A is positive in the majority of clear cell carcinomas and are not typical of other tumor types [4, 170, 196]. HNF-1β has also been proposed to be of utility, however work from Fadare et al. has shown that it has relatively low specificity for clear cell carcinoma [197]. Abnormal p53 expression is present in only a third of cases, therefore wild-type p53-staining can be helpful for excluding a serous carcinoma diagnosis (although abnormal p53 does not exclude clear cell) [198].

Loss of mismatch repair protein expression is seen in ~10% of endometrial clear cell carcinomas [199, 200], (Ketabi, Cai) and this staining should be performed routinely as part of Lynch syndrome screening [31]. PD-L1 expression is relatively common in this tumor type particularly (but not exclusively) in the setting of mismatch repair deficiency, suggesting possible vulnerability to checkpoint inhibitor therapies [201].

Molecular

Clear cell carcinomas are genotypically heterogenous and are present in all four TCGA subsets: copy-number high, copy-number low, mismatch repair-deficient, and even *POLE*-mutated [198]. Overall, the molecular profile of clear cell carcinomas shows more overlap with endometrioid carcinoma than with serous carcinoma, eroding the historical notion that clear cell carcinomas ought to be uniformly lumped with "type II"/serous cancers. Commonly mutated genes include *ARID1A*, *PTEN*, *PIK3A*, *KRAS*, and *NRAS* [4, 8, 198, 202]. Abnormalities in *TP53* also occur, but are less common than in serous carcinomas: just under half of clear cell carcinomas showing *TP53* mutations and even fewer cases (~one-third) show abnormal p53 expression [198]. Mutations involving the mismatch repair genes *MLH1*, *PMS2*, *MSH2*, and *MSH6* are identified in ~10%, and a subset of these will be attributable to germline mutations [199–201].

18.4.8.9 Undifferentiated and Dedifferentiated Carcinoma

Clinical

Undifferentiated and dedifferentiated endometrial carcinomas are considered rare, although they are often underdiagnosed as FIGO grade 2 or 3 endometrioid cancers therefore the true incidence may be significantly higher than is routinely reported [5, 203–205]. Correctly identifying these cases is clinically important, as evidence suggests that many of these tumors bear a worse prognosis than their FIGO 3 endometrioid counterparts [204]. Conversely, undifferentiated and dedifferentiated cases bearing *POLE* mutations demonstrate a paradoxically favorable clinical course [206]. The average age at presentation from one series of these tumors was 55 years, and many patients in this study fell below 40 years [207]; this likely reflects the association between undifferentiated/dedifferentiated morphology and Lynch syndrome [30, 156, 157]. Patients typically present with abnormal uterine bleeding [203].

Gross

Undifferentiated and dedifferentiated endometrial carcinomas most often manifest as large, polypoid intrauterine masses. The lower uterine segment is commonly involved [203–205, 207, 208].

The microscopically confluent areas may appear as grossly solid masses, whereas the well-differentiated components of dedifferentiated tumors may assume a shaggy or papillary macroscopic appearance. Necrosis is frequently present.

Microscopic

Undifferentiated endometrial carcinomas are comprised of relatively uniform, intermediate-sized cells arranged in poorly cohesive sheets without any evidence of epithelial architecture (Fig. 18.52). Gland formation is, by definition, entirely absent. Small amounts of keratinization are allowable, but uncommon. Mitotic figures are readily identified and can exceed 25 per 10 high-power fields. Necrosis is common. The morphologic differential includes lymphoma, melanoma, and high-grade endometrial stromal sarcoma, and epithelial assignment requires EMA and/or cytokeratin reactivity in at least a subset of cells.

Dedifferentiated endometrial carcinomas show regions morphologically identical to undifferentiated carcinoma which are juxtaposed with areas of FIGO grade 1 or 2 endometrioid carcinoma [203, 208] (Fig. 18.53). Often the gland-forming component lines the surface while the undifferentiated portion invades the underlying myometrium. Necrosis is common in the solid component (Fig. 18.54). Correct assignment as dedifferentiated

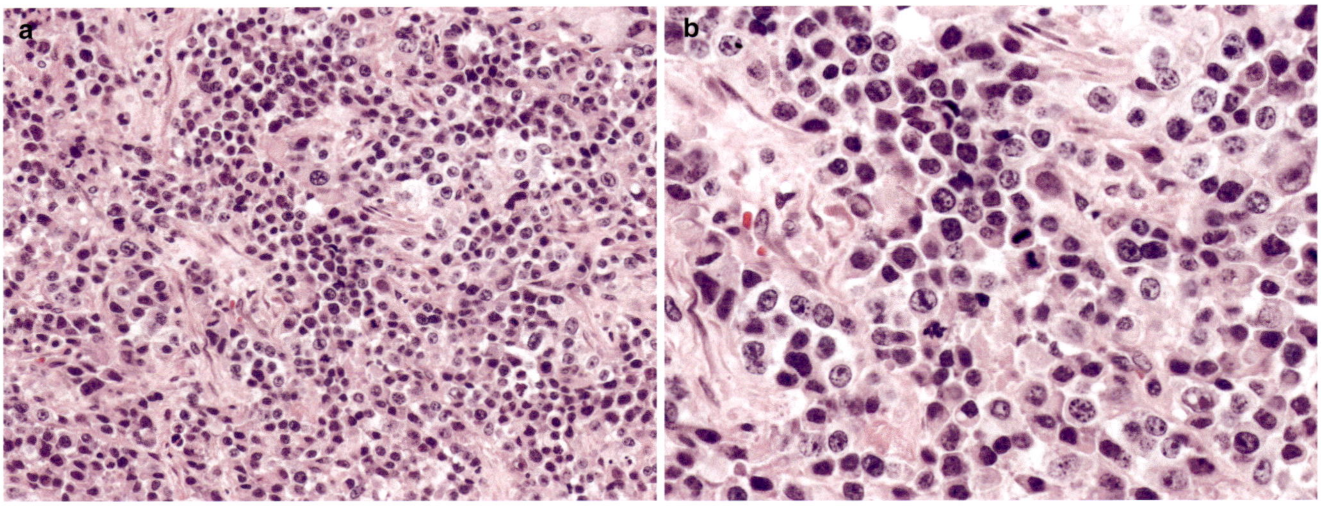

Fig. 18.52 Undifferentiated endometrial carcinoma is characterized by poorly cohesive sheets of homogenous, intermediate-sized cells without overt epithelial or mesenchymal differentiation. (**a**) Mitotic figures are abundant. (**b**) There is no morphologic evidence of epithelial differentiation on H&E staining, and diagnosis is contingent on immunohistochemical demonstrate of epithelial markers and exclusion of other malignancies (including stromal and hematopoietic tumors)

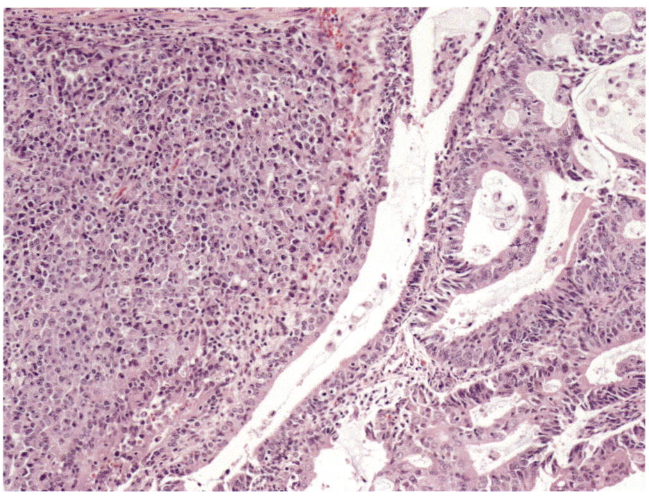

Fig. 18.53 Dedifferentiated endometrial carcinomas demonstrate an abrupt transition between conventional low- to intermediate-grade endometrioid carcinoma and solid, undifferentiated architecture. It is crucial that these tumors not be graded using the FIGO system based on the percentage of solid contributions, as this may result in an underestimation of their aggressive potential

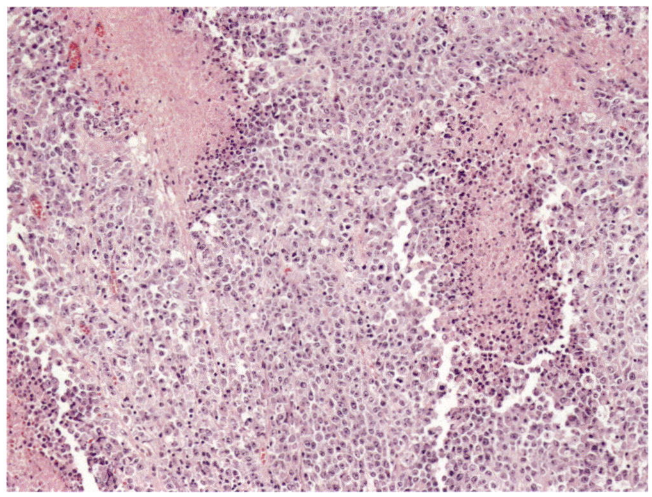

Fig. 18.54 Both dedifferentiated and undifferentiated endometrial carcinomas often show regions of zonal necrosis, as present in the right and upper left of this case of dedifferentiated carcinoma (areas with epithelial differentiation pictured in Fig. 18.43)

carcinoma requires identification of the abrupt transition between the well-differentiated and undifferentiated components. Erroneously applying the FIGO scoring system for endometrioid cancers can result in a dramatic underestimate of the aggressive potential of dedifferentiated carcinomas, particularly in cases that show <50% solid areas as these cancers may be misclassified as FIGO grade 2 lesions and, in the absence of deep myometrial invasion, managed quite conservatively.

Immunohistochemistry

Immunohistochemistry is required to assign epithelial differentiation to undifferentiated carcinomas. These tumors may be negative for most cytokeratins but should have at least focal immunopositivity for EMA and CK18 [203]. Vimentin is often positive, and staining with synaptophysin and chromogranin may be present in a minority of cells [203, 205]. PAX8 and estrogen receptor expression is often lost in undifferentiated tumors/areas of dedifferentiation, particularly among SMARCA4 (BRG1) and SMARCB1 (INI)-deficient cancers

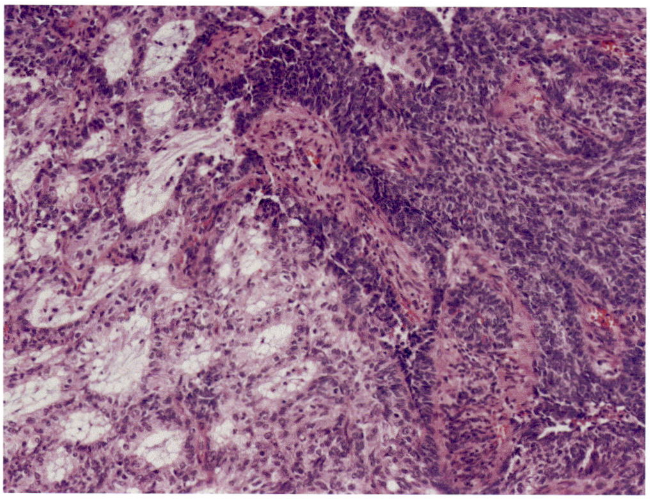

Fig. 18.55 Mismatch repair deficiency is common among dedifferentiated carcinomas. This case showed dual loss of MSH2 and MSH6 expression and had a *MSH2* germline mutation on germline testing, confirming Lynch syndrome

[209]. SMARCB1 (INI) deficiency is fairly uncommon in these cases, with a recent series of 21 cases identifying only one tumor with loss [206]. SMARCA4 (BRG1) loss was once thought to be similarly rare; however, recent work has demonstrated that nearly one-third of undifferentiated endometrial cancers lose SMARCA4 (BRG1) expression, and that rhabdoid histology often accompanies this finding [210, 211]. In contrast to their SMARCA4 (BRG1)-intact counterparts, dedifferentiated cancers with SMARCA4 (BRG1) loss do not typically demonstrate aberrant p53 immunostaining [209].

Finally, mismatch repair deficiency is associated with dedifferentiated morphology, with rapid accumulations of mutations presumably resulting in the abrupt morphologic transitions that define these cases [30, 31, 91, 156, 157] (Fig. 18.55).

Molecular

Undifferentiated and dedifferentiated endometrial cancers show considerable molecular heterogeneity and include the full spectrum of TCGA subsets [212]. One recent study of 18 cases revealed that 45% were mismatch repair-deficient/hypermutated, 11% were *POLE*/ultramutated, 11% were copy-number high, and 28% were copy-number low [212].Notably, some of the copy-number low cases showed *TP53* mutations suggestive of incipient progression to a copy-number high malignancy. That mismatch repair deficiency/hypermutation was the most common molecular feature reflects the known association between undifferentiated/dedifferentiated morphology and Lynch syndrome [30, 31, 91, 156, 157].

The presence of some *POLE*- mutated tumors is also unsurprising, given that like mismatch repair-deficient malignancies, ultramutated cancers rapidly accrue genetic changes that can lead to abrupt morphologic digressions. This swift mutation rate contributes to the immunogenicity of both the hypermutated and ultramutated subsets, leading to high neoantigen loads and PD-L1 overexpression [142, 143]. It is critical to note that the identification of *POLE* mutations in a subset of undifferentiated/dedifferentiated cancers has prognostic relevance, as these cases have been shown to demonstrate surprisingly favorable prognosis despite their high histologic grade, and even in the presence of concomitant *TP53* mutations [160, 206].

Molecular evidence also substantiates the immunohistochemical identification of SMARCA4 (BRG1) and, occasionally, SMARCB1 (INI) deficiency in a subset of undifferentiated/dedifferentiated endometrial cancers. Most often, this occurs in the context of mismatch repair deficiency [213]. SMARCA4 (BRG1) is a key ATPase in the switch/sucrose non-fermenting (SWI/SNF) complex, and recent work has implicated somatic frameshift/nonsense mutations affecting this complex in endometrial dedifferentiation [213]. Mutations affecting the related protein SMARCB1 (INI1) remain relatively uncommon among these tumors, with a single case out of 18 demonstrating a heterozygous *SMARCB1* mutation whole exome sequencing [212].

18.4.8.10 Carcinosarcoma (Malignant Mixed Müllerian Tumor)

Clinical

Carcinosarcomas [malignant mixed müllerian tumors (MMMT), malignant mixed mesodermal tumors, "Triple M Ts"] comprise 2–5% of all uterine malignancies and share predisposing risk factors with endometrial carcinoma, including increased estrogen exposure and obesity. Prior pelvic radiation has also been implicated as a risk factor [214]. Presentation is typically with postmenopausal bleeding, and many cases demonstrate a mass prolapsing through the cervix on pelvic exam [215, 216]. Evidence suggests that the vast majority of these tumors (80–90%) are epithelial in derivation [217–222], with a small minority representing malignant epithelial progression within/adjacent to adenosarcomas [223]. Indeed, recent evidence suggests that carcinosarcomas essentially represent a pure form of epithelial-to-mesenchymal transition (EMT) [224]. As such, carcinosarcomas should be staged using the FIGO system for endometrial carcinomas [225]. The rational for utilizing this staging system is underscored not only by molecular studies supporting epithelial origin, but also by metastatic spread patterns that parallel carcinomas, rather than sarcomas [222, 226]. These aggressive tumors often show pelvic and para-aortic lymph node involvement, and at 35% 5-year survival is worse than for other high-grade endometrial carcinomas [226].

Gross

Carcinosarcomas are typically bulky, exophytic masses with broad bases that expand the endometrial cavity. Protrusion through the cervical os is common. Cut section reveals firm, fleshy tissue with regions of hemorrhage and necrosis (Fig. 18.56).

Microscopic

Carcinosarcomas are biphasic tumors comprised of mixed malignant epithelial and mesenchymal components and are thought to represent metaplastic carcinomas in the majority of cases [217–222, 227] (Fig. 18.57). Both components are cytologically malignant and frequently demonstrate marked pleomorphism (Fig. 18.58). There is typically an abrupt transition between areas of carcinomatous and mesenchymal differentiation. The epithelial component may be endometrioid, serous, clear cell, undifferentiated, or mixed while the mesenchymal component can be either homologous (tissue types normally occurring in the uterus, e.g., malignant smooth muscle or endometrial stromal differentiation) or heterologous (e.g., tissue types not normally occurring in the uterus, such as malignant rhabdomyomatous, cartilaginous, osteoid, or lipomatous differentiation) (Figs. 18.59 and 18.60). Heterologous differentiation imparts a worse prognosis for stage I carcinosarcomas, therefore the character (homologous vs. heterologous) of the mesenchymal component is a required component of synoptic reporting for these tumors [228, 229]. The percentages of epithelial and mesenchymal tissue should also be reported. On rare occasions, an associated component of yolk sac tumor, melanocytic tumor, or primitive neuroectodermal tumor (PNET) may also be identified [230–232].

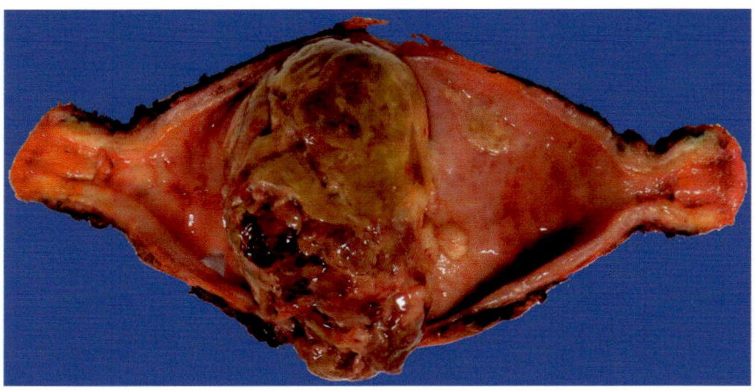

Fig. 18.56 Carcinosarcomas (MMMTs) often manifest as bulky, exophytic masses which expand the endometrial cavity. Necrosis and hemorrhage are commonly present. Image courtesy of Dr. Nicholas Jaeger

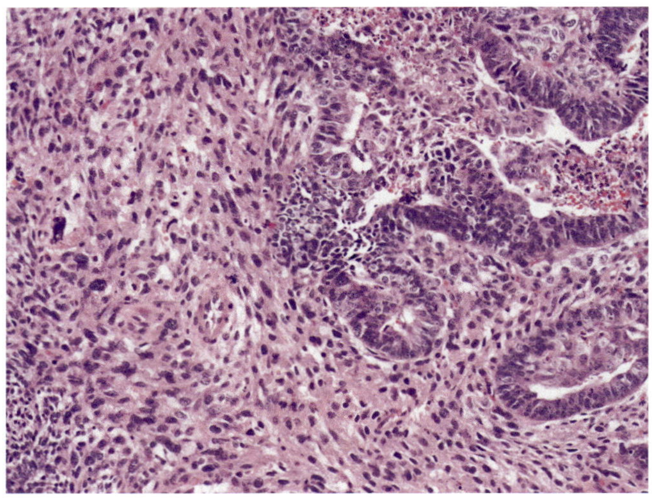

Fig. 18.57 Carcinosarcomas (MMMTs) are biphasic proliferations of malignant epithelial and mesenchymal tissue. This case demonstrates a non-descript sarcomatoid component compatible with homologous differentiation

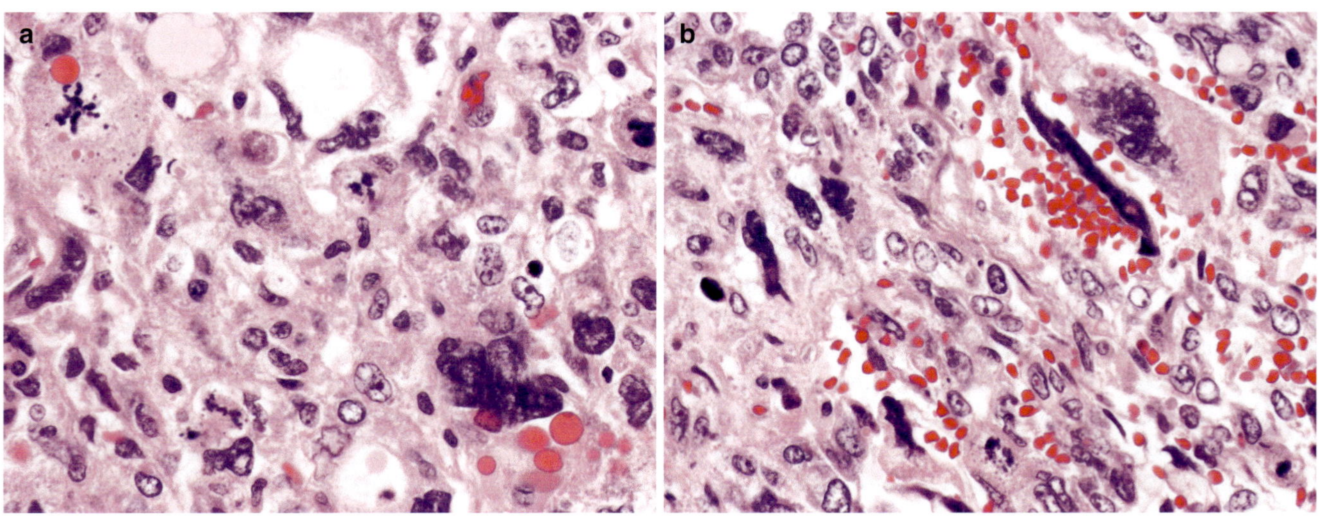

Fig. 18.58 Carcinosarcomas (MMMTs) typically show marked pleomorphism including atypical mitotic figures, multinucleate forms, and hyperchromatic, smudgy cells (**a**, **b**)

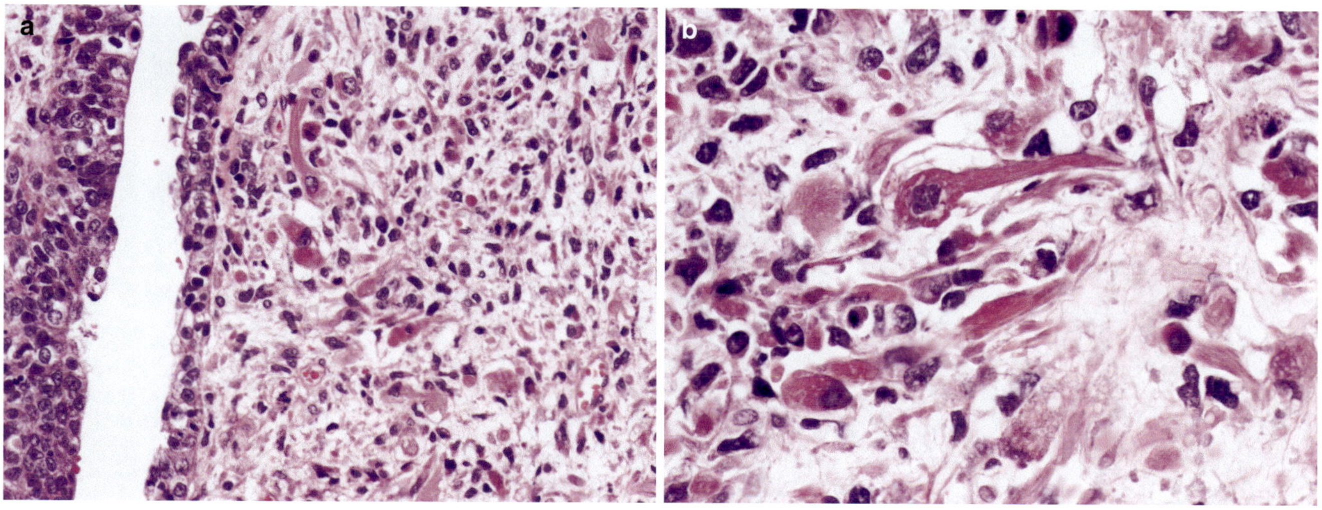

Fig. 18.59 Rhabdomyosarcomatous differentiation (**a**) is the most common type of heterologous differentiation in carcinosarcomas (MMMTs). Strap cells showing cytoplasmic striations are often appreciated (**b**)

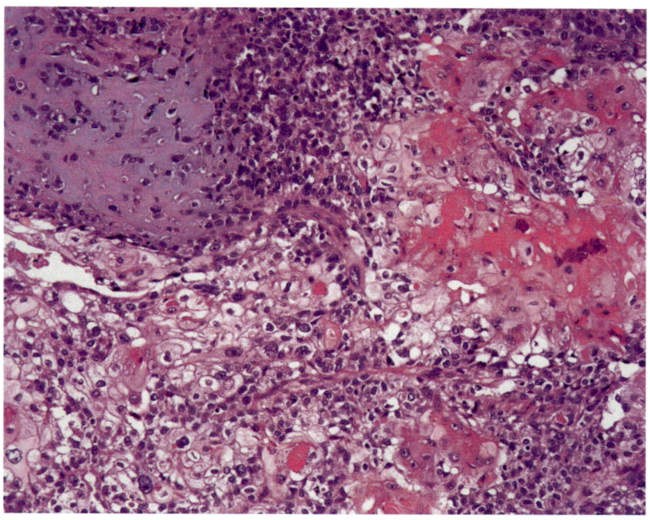

Fig. 18.60 Cartilaginous differentiation can be seen in the mesenchymal components of carcinosarcomas (MMMTs) (upper left). This constitutes heterologous differentiation and should be noted as such in the synoptic report. Image courtesy of Dr. Robert Soslow

Because the relative contributions of epithelial and mesenchymal tissues can vary considerably, diagnosis of carcinosarcoma is contingent on sampling and may not be possible at the time of original biopsy. The presence of a histologically heterogenous or difficult to classify carcinoma on biopsy should therefore prompt a comment that accounts for the possibility of a final diagnosis of carcinosarcoma. Similarly, caution should be exercised prior to rendering a diagnosis of sarcoma on a biopsy specimen alone, as this could result in improper staging. It is prudent to craft a comment that allows for the possibility of carcinosarcoma on any biopsy specimen consisting exclusively of malignant mesenchymal tissue. Carcinosarcomas may sometimes even mimic adenosarcomas, therefore even "Phyllodes-like" architecture with compressed, elongate glands and associated periglandular condensation does not preclude a final diagnosis of carcinosarcoma.

Immunohistochemistry

Immunohistochemistry is of limited value in carcinosarcoma diagnosis, although it can occasionally be of utility in confirming the presence of heterologous elements (for instance, the presence of myogenin and/or MyoD1 staining confirms rhabdomyoblastic differentiation). Because carcinosarcomas can derive from a variety of epithelial tumor types, immunoprofiles can vary considerably. Abnormal p53 expression is common and is usually shared across the epithelial and mesenchymal components, supporting the shared origin argument [233]. Mismatch repair protein loss is rare [30–32, 35, 156, 157, 234].

Molecular

The majority (80–90%) of carcinosarcomas are monoclonal tumors, arguing against the "collision tumor" theory of histogenesis for most cases [227, 233]. Molecular studies of epithelial mesenchymal transition (EMT) have shown upregulation of EMT-related markers in carcinosarcomas [235]. Mismatch repair deficiency/microsatellite instability is relatively uncommon when compared to other biphasic endometrial tumor types [30–32, 35, 156, 157, 234].

18.4.8.11 Neuroendocrine Carcinoma

Clinical

Neuroendocrine carcinomas have been reported in over 100 patients described in the English language literature and account for <1% of all endometrial malignancies [236–241]. Both small cell and large cell neuroendocrine carcinoma

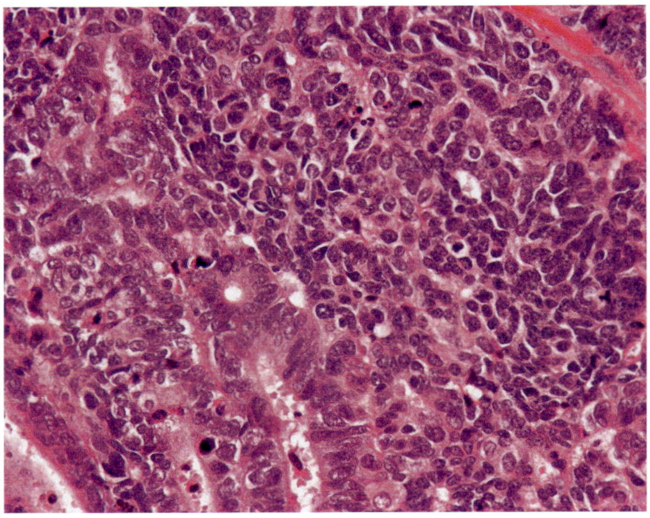

Fig. 18.61 Neuroendocrine endometrial tumors may be pure or mixed with conventional epithelial morphology, as is the case with this tumor showing an endometrioid component (lower left). Image courtesy of Dr. Robert Soslow

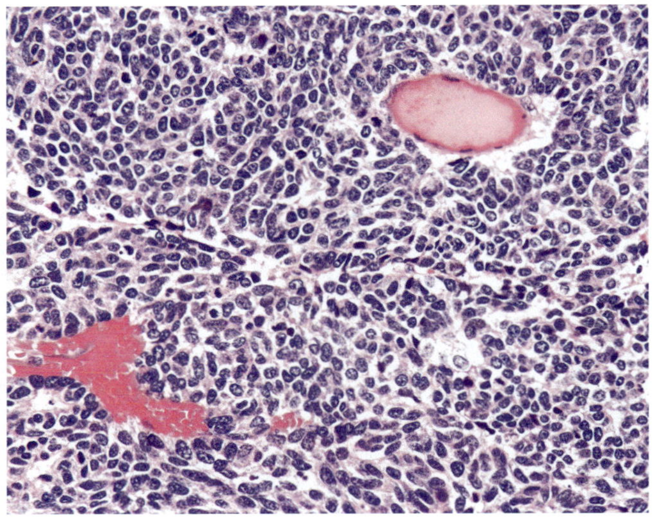

Fig. 18.62 Neuroendocrine endometrial tumors can assume a small cell morphology with cells bearing high nuclear:cytoplasm ratios and coarse chromatin. Image courtesy of Dr. Robert Soslow

variants typically occur in postmenopausal patients, with an average age of 60 years and 55 years, respectively [237, 242, 243]. As with other endometrial malignancies, these tumors typically present with abnormal uterine bleeding. Primary uterine carcinoid tumors are exceedingly uncommon, with only two cases reported in the literature; due to their extreme rarity, they will not be discussed further here [244, 245].

Histology

Endometrial neuroendocrine tumors may be pure, or they may occur in concert with other histologic subtypes including endometrioid and serous carcinoma [240, 241] (Fig. 18.61). The true incidence of endometrial carcinomas with neuroendocrine differentiation is unclear as this feature is commonly overlooked: a recent study of 25 cases reveals frequent under-recognition in the referral/consult setting [241]. The large cell subtype is more common and is characterized by large cells with vesicular to hyperchromatic nuclei and prominent nucleoli arranged in trabecular, nested, and corded arrangements. Peripheral palisading and geographic necrosis are common. The small cell subtype resembles small cell carcinoma of the lung and is comprised of poorly cohesive cells with condensed chromatin and scant cytoplasm (Fig. 18.62). Mitotic activity is typically brisk in both types.

Immunohistochemistry

Neuroendocrine carcinomas, by definition, must show positivity for at least one neuroendocrine marker (chromogranin, synaptophysin, and/or CD56) in >10% of cells. Cytokeratins classically show a perinuclear dot-like staining pattern. PAX8 expression is lost in two-thirds of cases [241]. p16 may be diffusely positive, as can be seen in neuroendocrine carcinomas elsewhere. CD117 and TTF1 can occasionally be positive. Mismatch repair protein loss is seen in over 40% [241].

Molecular

Defects in the mismatch repair system are common among endometrial cancers with neuroendocrine differentiation [241]. Rare *POLE*-mutated cancers show neuroendocrine differentiation [246].

18.4.9 Mixed Endometrial Carcinomas

According to the 2014 WHO, the term "mixed carcinoma" should be applied to endometrial cancers with two or more distinct histological patterns, each comprising a minimum of 5% of the tumor volume, one of which warrants a "Type II" designation (chiefly serous and clear cell carcinoma) under the old binary system [96] (Fig. 18.63). In general, the prognosis of these tumors is thought to be dictated by the higher-grade component. This definition of "mixed carcinoma" becomes somewhat problematic, however, in an era when the Type I/II classification system has fallen out of favor, and when abrupt digressions in histologic appearance can be explained by unifying molecular mechanisms, such as mismatch repair defects and *POLE* mutations. The International Society of Gynecologic Pathologists (ISGyP) has tackled this issue recently in through the Endometrial Carcinoma Project and has highlighted common problems surrounding the diagnosis of "mixed endometrial carcinomas" with serous and clear cell components; these findings are pending publication in 2018.

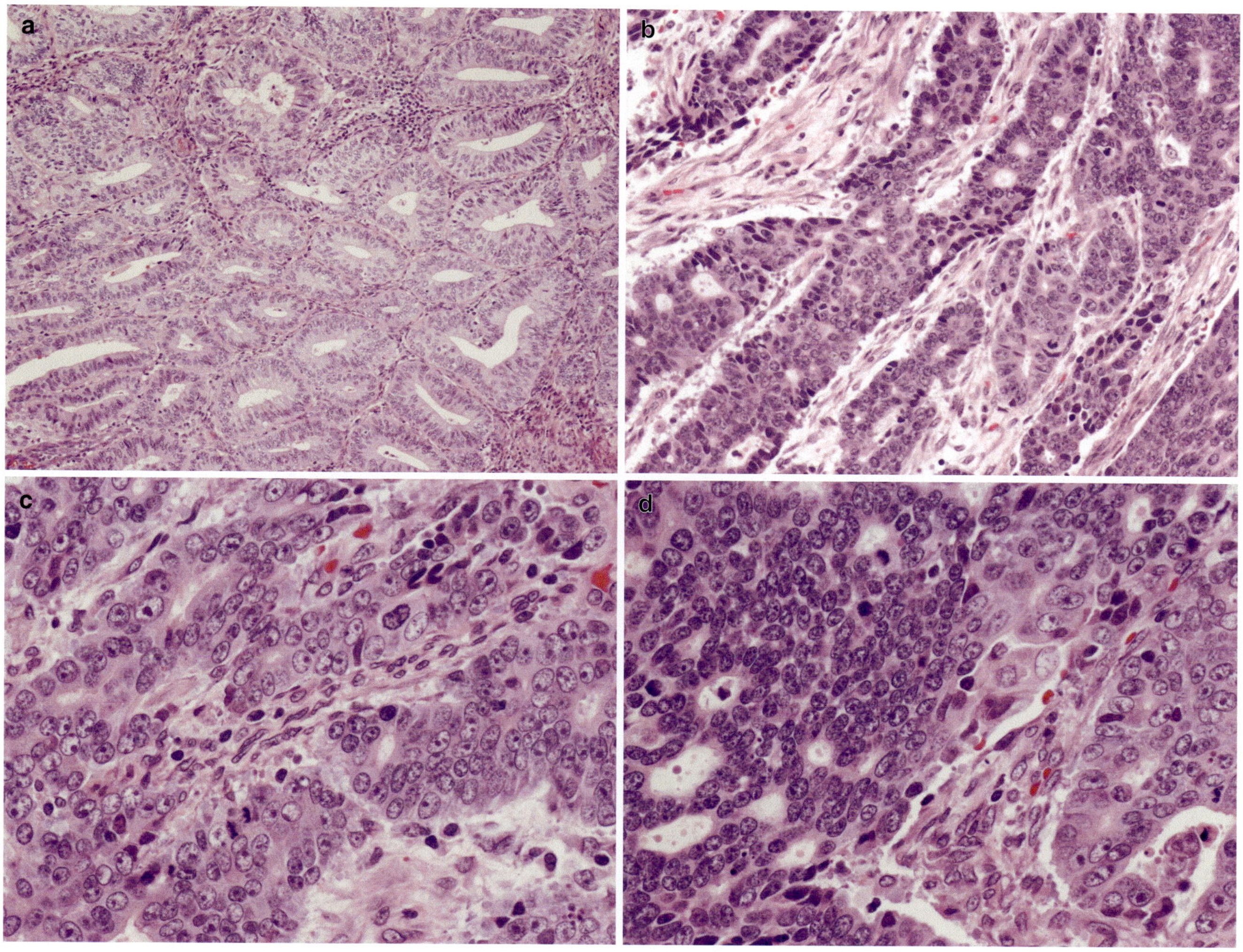

Fig. 18.63 Mixed carcinomas include cases with two or more distinct histological patterns, including at least a 5% contribution by a high-grade histotype. In practice, this category should be applied only sparingly. This tumor may have been classified as a "mixed carcinoma" by some, as low power examination revealed well-formed glands with possible endometrioid features (**a**) admixed with more atypical glands arranged in solid cords and glandular structures. (**b**) Some regions showed cytologic atypia with prominent nucleoli suggestive of serous differentiation (**c**), while others showed a dramatic juxtaposition of this morphology with a more basophilic, but still quite atypical, cell population (notably, this population lacked neuroendocrine marker expression) (**d**). Mismatch repair immunohistochemistry revealed loss of MSH2 and MSH6, suggesting that mismatch repair deficiency could help account for the ambiguous morphology

One potential complication with mixed carcinomas bearing apparent serous and endometrioid histologies is that much of the data on these cases predates routine use of p53 immunohistochemical staining as a diagnostic aid in cases with challenging morphology, suggesting that some cases previously identified as "mixed" might simply be classified as serous using modern classification approaches, particularly in serous cancers that display admixed papillary and glandular architecture. This is supported by multivariate analyses which have shown no significant survival differences between mixed and pure serous carcinomas [247–252]. On the other hand, other studies have shown that mixed serous carcinomas have an intermediate prognosis between endometrioid and serous carcinoma [253–255]. The "mixed" water is further muddied by the fact that the 5% cutoff is somewhat arbitrary, and there is no literature to suggest that serous cancer can be confidently excluded when the contribution falls beneath this threshold.

Cases with mixed clear cell components are similarly problematic. There is tremendous intraobserver variability in the diagnosis of clear cell components, and most instances apparent clear cell morphology represents a histologic variant of endometrioid or serous morphology [170]. Endometrioid tumors with at least 10% clear cell components have been shown, in one study, to bear a prognosis comparable to pure clear cell cancers; however, data on the prognostic implications of this finding are otherwise limited [256].

It bears emphasis that "mixed" is not synonymous with "ambiguous." Ambiguous morphologies are inherently difficult to classify and display overlapping histologic features of endometrioid, serous, and/or clear cell carcinoma within a single region [7]. In contrast, true mixed cancers have geographically separate areas with morphologically distinct differentiation. Similarly, dedifferentiated cancers should not be confused mixed cancers: these tumors show clear endometrioid morphology that abruptly degrades into undifferentiated malignancy, rather than juxtaposed regions with obvious differentiation in different directions. Excluding ambiguous and dedifferentiated cases from the "mixed endometrial carcinoma" umbrella further limits the scope of this tumor type.

In summary, a diagnosis of "mixed endometrial carcinoma" ought to be approached with caution, as current thinking suggests that, when appropriately applied, this is an extremely rare diagnosis. Based on the conclusions of the Endometrial Carcinoma Project, ISGyP recommends that this diagnosis be applied only to cases with spatially discrete, unequivocal serous and/or clear cell components. Given the uncertainty about where the clinically significant contribution threshold lies and the data to suggest that the high-grade component drives prognosis even when relatively low volume, *any* percentage of these tumor types should be reported (not just >5%). Utilizing immunohistochemistry (p53 for serous and Napsin A for clear cell) to confirm the presence of this component is advisable. Finally, the percentage of each tumor type and grade should also be provided in the bottom line diagnosis with the term "mixed endometrial carcinoma" applied parenthetically.

18.4.10 Endometrial Carcinoma Associated with Ovarian Carcinoma

Simultaneous endometrial and ovarian tumors are encountered with some frequency in gynecologic pathology, and often lead to diagnostic consternation regarding the question of synchronous primaries versus metastasis from one site to another. This issue is easily addressed when the morphology differs at each location, but becomes somewhat problematic when the tumors have shared histology. The diagnostic approach varies somewhat based upon whether the tumors are endometrioid or serous in differentiation.

18.4.10.1 Endometrial and Ovarian Endometrioid Tumors

Up to 20% of ovarian endometrioid cancers will also demonstrate endometrioid carcinoma in the uterus, and the majority of these cases are thought to represent dual primaries. Interestingly, <10% of these are attributable to Lynch syndrome; most synchronous primaries occur somatically [234, 257] and may be related to a hormonal "field effect," which is supported by the relatively young age, high body-mass-index, and frequent nulliparity of patients with synchronous endometrioid primaries [258]. Correctly identifying these as dual primaries is critical, because the individual tumors are typically low stage and the patients enjoy a favorable overall prognosis.

Several clinicopathologic features can be helpful in confirming independent origins for these tumors: dual primaries are usually low to intermediate grade and show no evidence of lymphovascular invasion. The presence of endometriosis adjacent to the ovarian component also supports in situ development, rather than metastasis. Conversely, a single uterine primary can be favored when the endometrial tumor shows deep invasion, high grade, and lymphovascular invasion while ovarian involvement is bilateral; this is a much more common scenario than ovarian spread to the uterus. When the ovary does represent the site-of-origin, metastasis exclusively to the endometrium is rare; therefore, an ovarian primary with endometrial spread should be favored only when peritoneal disease is also present. In these cases, spread to the uterus often occurs via the serosa so the distribution often favors the outer myometrium with little to no surface component.

MMR immunohistochemistry can occasionally be enlisted as a mechanism to help ascertain whether simultaneous ovarian and endometrial masses represent distinct primaries. Loss of MLH1 and PMS2 in one tumor but not the other, for example, favors independent primaries. Shared loss patterns are less readily interpreted: in a Lynch syndrome patient, for example, we would expect the same molecular signature in both tumors whether or not they represented independent primaries; on the other hand, in a germline-normal patient a shared tumoral loss pattern provides some support for a single site-of-origin. Retention of all mismatch repair markers across both tumors is essentially non-contributory to the work-up.

18.4.10.2 Endometrial and Ovarian Serous Tumors

The presence of synchronous serous tumors in the endometrium and ovary can be even more challenging, because short of molecular sequencing there is no ancillary study likely to be of utility in assigning site-of-origin: both tumors would be expected to show abnormal p53 expression, and only in the very rare scenario wherein one tumor showed a p53-null pattern and the other showed a p53-diffuse pattern would this be useful for suggesting dual primaries. We must therefore return to clinicopathologic basics when assessing these cases: bilateral ovarian involvement with a bulky, deeply invasive endometrial tumor strongly suggests uterine primary, whereas a large, unilateral ovarian tumor with only superficial endometrial involvement suggests ovarian origin.

18.4.11 Ancillary Testing in Endometrial Carcinoma

A diagnosis of endometrial carcinoma was once rendered exclusively on gross examination and H&E staining, and that assessment contained all the information needed to classify, stage, and prognosticate a tumor using the standards of the time. Tumors haven't changed, but times have, and we now have a host of ancillary techniques that expand the information we provide our patients and further guide clinical management. These tests allow us to screen patients for Lynch syndrome, classify tumors according to molecular understanding, and, increasingly, direct targeted therapy. The penetrance of these tests into clinical practice varies from routine (for mismatch repair testing for Lynch syndrome screening) to case-based utilization (p53 immunostaining) to scarcely employed outside of select academic centers (for *POLE* mutation testing). However, it's safe to assume that we will see expansion of ancillary testing in years to come, with the probable inclusion of studies that aren't even conceived of herein.

18.4.11.1 Lynch Syndrome Screening

Lynch syndrome is the most common heritable cancer syndrome and underlies roughly one in every 20 endometrial carcinomas. Often, the uterine tumor is the sentinel malignancy in these patients. The identification of Lynch syndrome patients at the time of endometrial cancer diagnosis therefore affords the opportunity to prevent associated malignancies not only in the patient, but also in affected family members. Although targeted screening of patients with strong clinical suspicion and/or suggestive tumor morphology can identify many Lynch syndrome patients, these methods have imperfect sensitivity [30–32, 35, 156, 157, 234].

Reflexive screening for Lynch syndrome is therefore now recommended for all endometrial carcinomas irrespective of tumor histology, patient age, and personal/family cancer history. Screening typically begins with immunohistochemistry to detect tumoral loss of expression for any of the four mismatch repair proteins MLH1, PMS2, MSH2, and MSH6, although initial screening with just PMS2 and MSH6 is a potential cost-effective alternative approach given that PMS2 and MSH6 degrade in the absence of their respective dimerization partners, MLH1 and MSH2 [35, 156] (Fig. 18.64).

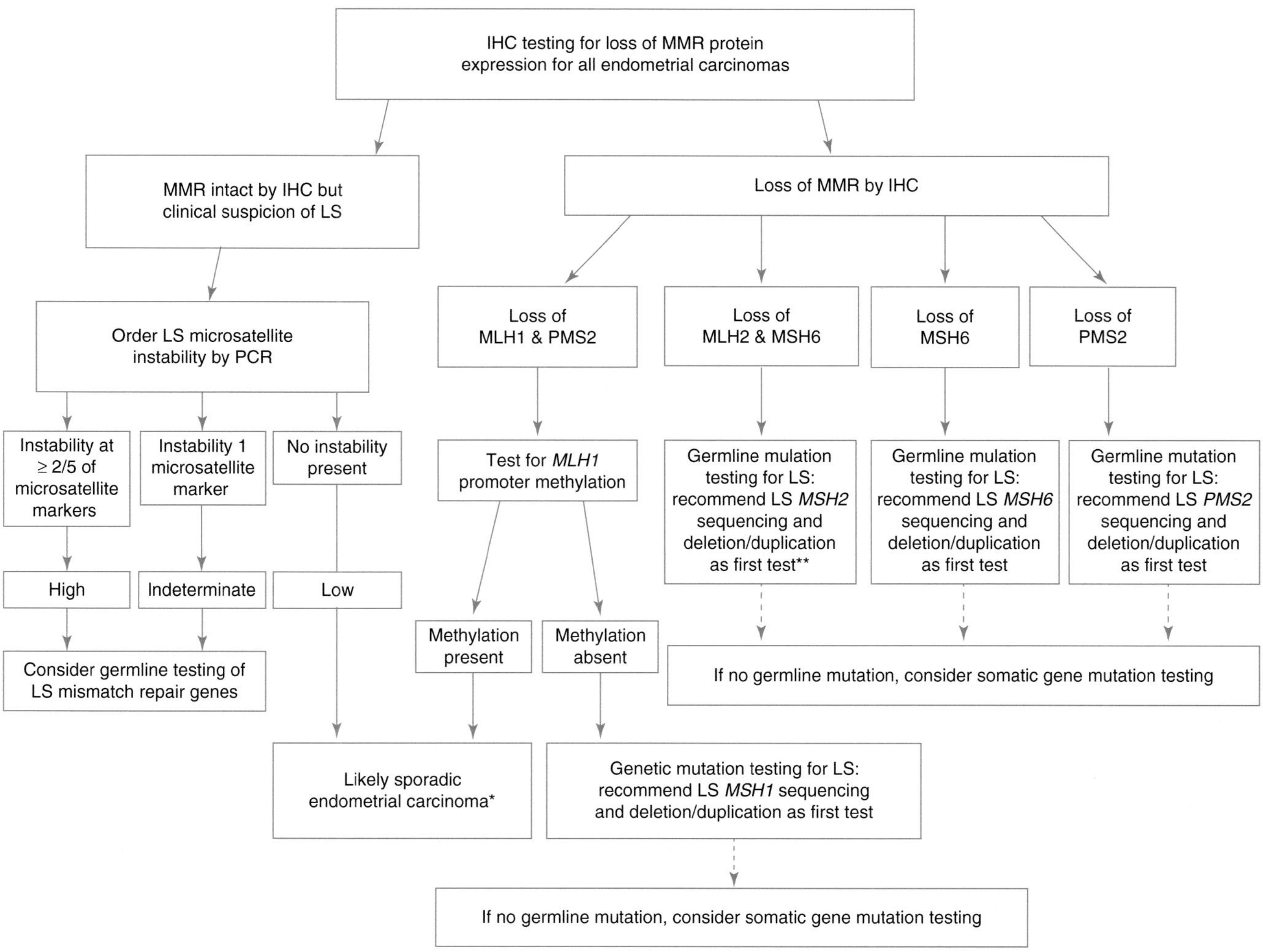

* If strong clinical suspicion for LS, consider *MLH1* promoter methylation analysis of non-neoplastic tissue/peripheral blood to evaluate for germline epigenetic *MLH1* promoter methylation .
** If *MSH2* and *MSH6* unmutated, consider LS *EPCAM* sequencing and deletion/duplication.

Fig. 18.64 Recommended Lynch syndrome screening algorithm for endometrial carcinomas. Figure courtesy of Dr. Teri Longacre

Loss of expression requires complete absence of nuclear staining throughout the tumor in the context of intact internal control lymphocyte and stromal staining. Care must be taken to evaluate only the carcinoma, not adjacent hyperplasia/endometrioid intraepithelial neoplasia. Staining heterogeneity and zonal absence of expression should not be classified as true loss as these are typically attributable to somatic, rather than germline, events [259]. Even faint, focal staining of tumor nuclei is considered positive, and these difficult-to-interpret patterns are encountered with some frequency, particularly with the PMS2 and MSH6 immunostains; indeed, this is why many centers elect to perform all four immunostains to facilitate comparison between the different markers.

Absence of MLH1 and PMS2 is the most commonly encountered loss pattern and is most often attributable to epigenetic hypermethylation of the *MLH1* promoter region, the presence of which excludes a heritable cancer syndrome in all but very rare scenarios [28, 151, 260] (Fig. 18.65). PCR-based testing for *MLH1* promoter hypermethylation is therefore recommended for all MLH1/PMS2-deficient cancers and effectively excludes Lynch syndrome in the vast majority of these cases. Unlike in the colon, *BRAF* mutation status does not parallel *MLH1* hypermethylation and therefore has no role in screening in the endometrium [151]. Hypermethylation testing may also play a role in a subset of cases with isolated PMS2 loss (chiefly those that have proven normal on germline testing), as somatic hypermethylation may sometimes lead to this pattern in the endometrium [261].

All other protein loss patterns warrant consideration for germline testing. Dual loss of MSH2/MSH6 is most suggestive of an *MSH2* mutation, while isolated MSH6 loss suggests an *MSH6* mutation (Fig. 18.66). When PCR testing proves hypermethylation is absent, loss of MLH1/PMS2 and isolated loss of PMS2 suggest mutations in *MLH1* and *PMS2*, respectively. The mutations underlying Lynch syndrome are heterogenous therefore whole gene sequencing is warranted; some companies begin by sequencing the gene implicated by the protein loss patterns, whereas others perform blanket testing of all four genes, plus the MSH2-related gene *EPCAM*, up front [26, 27, 154]. Not all patients will loss suggestive of Lynch syndrome will have constitutional mutations identified: in the past, this was often due to undetected germline mutations (such as *EPCAM* mutations and difficult-to-defect *MSH2* inversions), but expanded testing has made these false negative germline tests less common [25, 154, 262]. Instead, normal germline testing results now often represent truly normal germline status for all mismatch repair-associated genes. While loss of MSH2, MSH6, and/or PMS2 was once considered virtually diagnostic of an underlying germline mutation, we now know that as many as half of these cases can be explained by somatic mutations [91, 141]. It is unsurprising that the positive predictive value of mismatch repair testing has decreased since the advent of universal screening: when the tested population changes, so does the statistical characteristics of the test. It is critical to emphasize this point to clinical oncology colleagues and genetic counselors so that patients are appropriately apprised of the risk associated with mismatch repair protein loss and can guide their decisions about pursing germline testing accordingly.

The role for microsatellite instability testing in this algorithm is controversial. Microsatellite instability is a reliably proxy for underlying mismatch repair defects because it identifies replicative errors in areas of repeated nucleotides, which serve as veritable “canaries in the coal mine” for underlying mismatch repair problems. There is evidence that immunohistochemistry-based screening may miss up to 10% of Lynch syndrome-associated cancers, and that including microsatellite instability testing in the screening algorithm can capture these missed cases [263]. On the other hand, this test adds considerable expense, typically involves sending out material, and provides no information about the underlying mechanism of instability (therefore, methylation testing is still warranted to exclude epigenetic changes lest large numbers of patients be erroneously referred for germline testing. At present, microsatellite instability is therefore most often enlisted on a case-by-case basis when immunohistochemistry proves difficult to interpret, when intact mismatch repair staining fails to assuage a high clinical suspicion for familial disease, or when immunohistochemical and germline testing data provide conflicting results. Multi-gene hereditary cancel panel testing may ultimately bypass these tumor-based testing methods altogether [264], but are not yet widely clinically available or economically feasible.

18.4.11.2 Molecular Classification Testing

The TCGA-based understanding of endometrial carcinoma has prompted a shift from the old binary Type I/II system to a classification based on four molecular categories: ultramutated/*POLE*-mutated, hypermutated/mismatch repair-deficient/microsatellite unstable, copy number-low, and copy number-high [8]. Because category assignment can shift prognosis dramatically for some cancers (for example, high-grade, p53-overexpressing cancers that fall into the ultramutated/*POLE*-mutated group carry a paradoxically good prognosis), there has been a recent call to embed TCGA groupings into our routine diagnostic write-ups [9, 11]. This

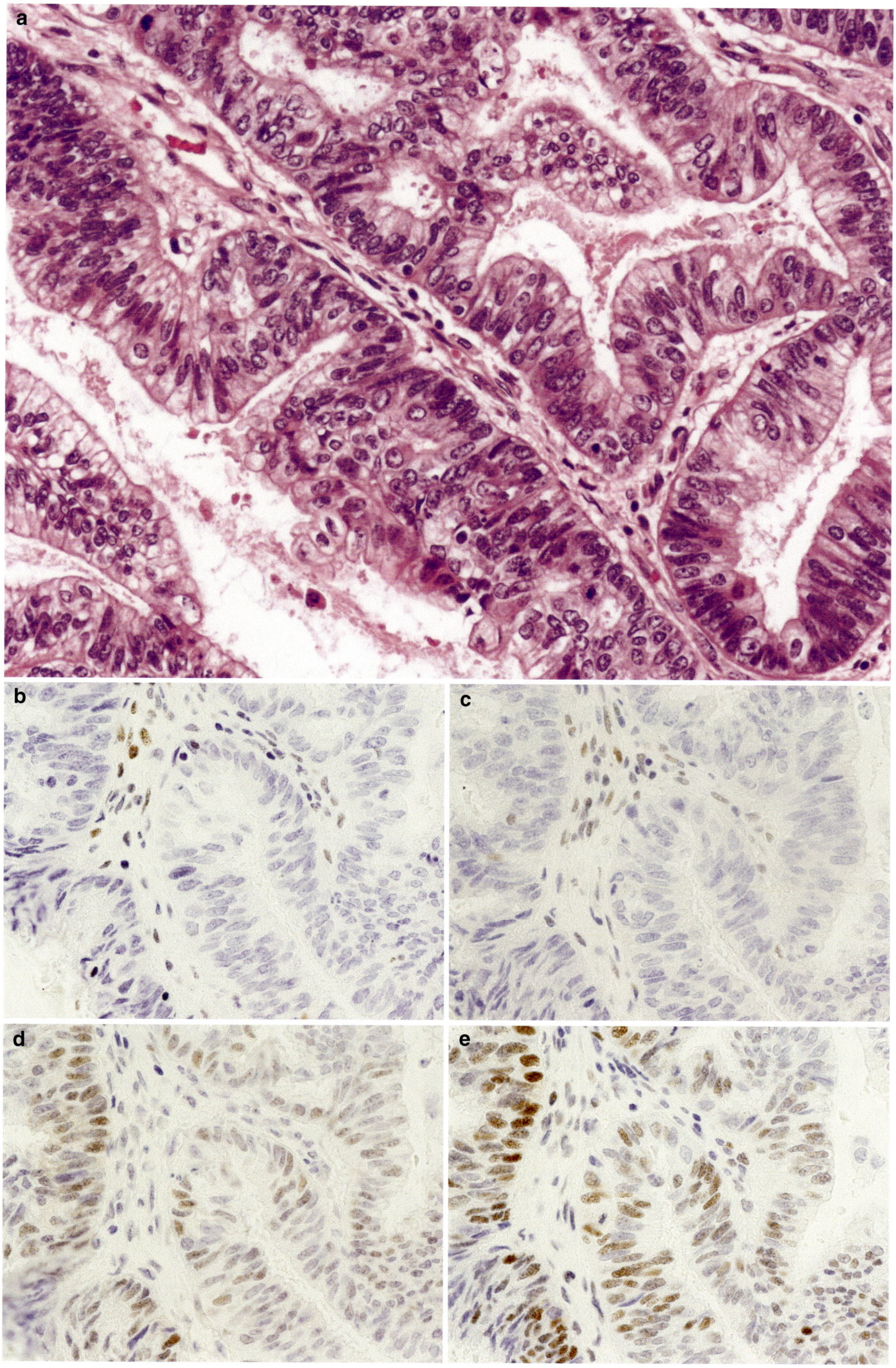

Fig. 18.65 This endometrial carcinoma (**a**) demonstrated PCR-confirmed hypermethylation of the *MLH1* promoter region, the most common cause of mismatch repair deficiency in endometrial cancers. Notably, mucinous features were prominent. Mismatch repair protein staining revealed dual loss of MLH1 (**b**) and PMS2 (**c**) within all tumor nuclei with preserved internal control positivity in stromal cells and tumor-associated lymphocytes. MSH2 (**d**) and MSH6 (**e**) were both intact

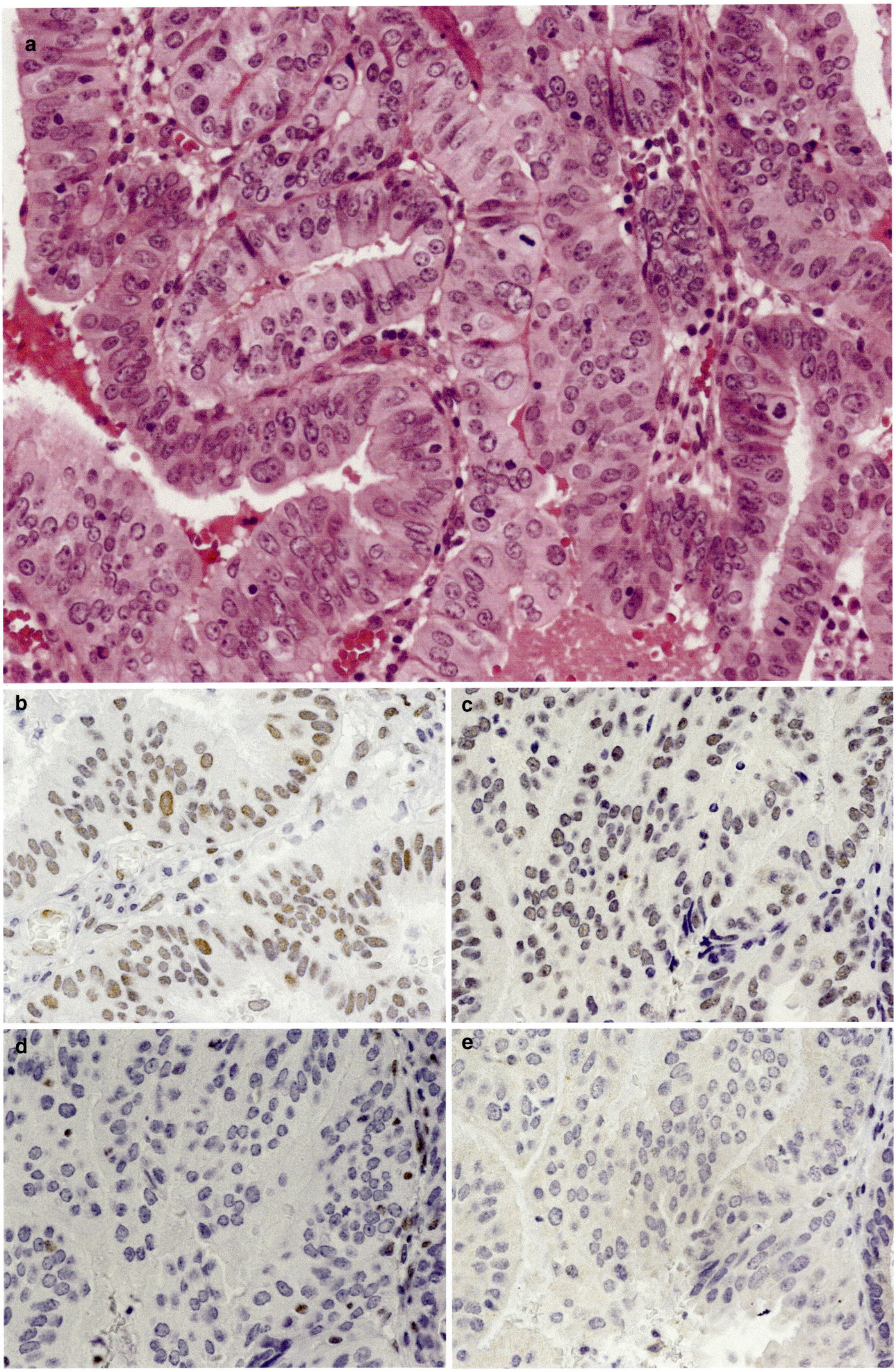

Fig. 18.66 This endometrial carcinoma (**a**) showed intact expression of MLH1 (**b**) and PMS2 (**c**), whereas MSH2 (**d**) and MSH6 (**e**) were lost in tumor nuclei with preserved internal control staining in stroma and inflammatory cells. This patient was referred for germline testing and an *MSH2* deletion was identified, confirming the diagnosis of Lynch syndrome

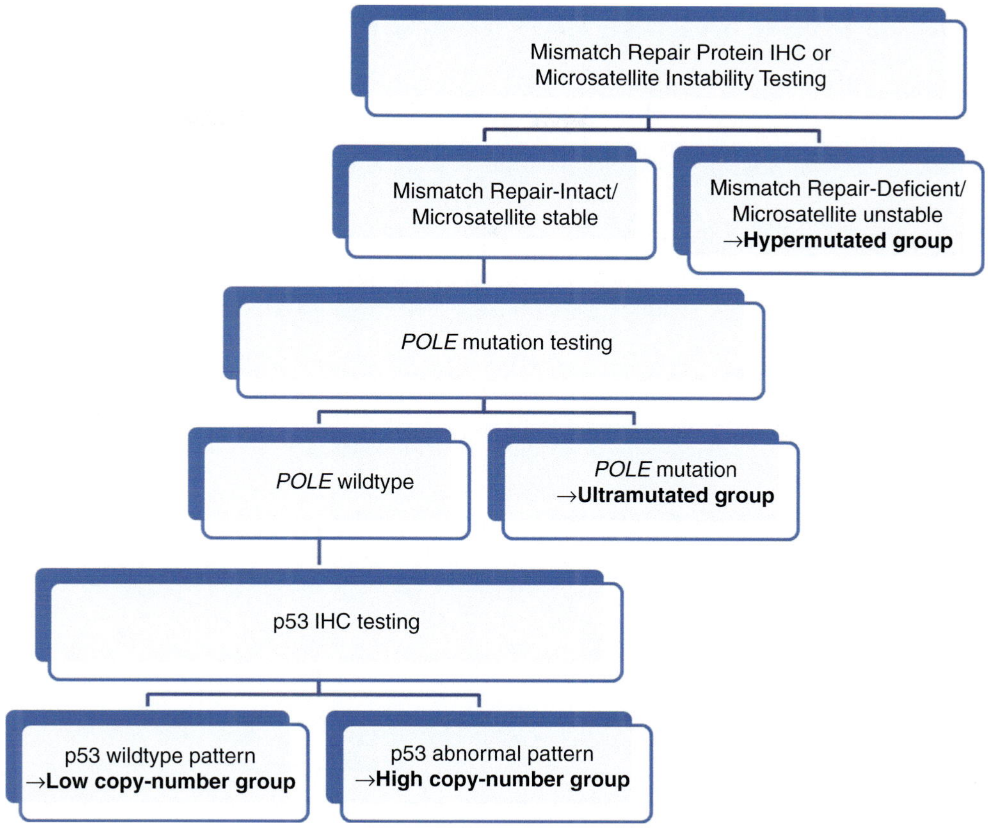

Fig. 18.67 Algorithm suggested in the Proactive Molecular Risk Classifier (ProMisE)

is codified in the Proactive Molecular Risk Classifier for Endometrial Cancer (ProMisE), which suggests an algorithm that begins with mismatch repair/microsatellite instability testing, progresses to *POLE* mutation testing for all mismatch repair-intact cases, and concludes with p53 immunohistochemistry to roughly divide the remaining cases into copy number-low vs. copy number-high [9, 11] (Fig. 18.67). The first step of this algorithm is straight-forward, as mismatch repair testing is now considered standard-of-care due to calls for universal Lynch syndrome screening from both the gynecologic oncology and pathology communities. p53 immunostaining is also routinely available and increasingly employed due to our growing appreciation of its role in cases endometrial cancers with challenging morphology [7, 102]. *POLE* mutation testing is not, however, readily accessible to most pathologists or their patients. At the moment, the absence of reflexive *POLE* mutation testing remains allowable: although evidence suggests that *POLE* status overrides other negative prognostic risk factors including high histologic grade and even superimposed *TP53* mutations, at this juncture gynecologic oncologists are not yet uniformly comfortable recommending more conservative management on the basis of this information. Whether the ProMisE system and the molecular testing that it entails become standard-of-care remains to be seen; for the moment, it is advisable to remain conversant in this topic, and to offer *POLE* mutation testing whenever clinicians suggest that it might influence their treatment approach.

18.4.11.3 Predictive Biomarker Testing

Historically, many of the ancillary tests that we applied to endometrial cancers served diagnostic and prognostic purposes only. Increasingly, however, tests are applied for their predictive power; that is, their ability to forecast whether a tumor will respond to a given treatment. Hormone receptor immunostaining is an old standby in predictive biomarker testing. Although reflexive staining of endometrial cancer has never permeated practice as it has in breast cancer care, estrogen and progesterone receptor staining is performed on clinicians' request with some regularity. However, the predictive value of estrogen and progesterone receptor staining as biomarkers for hormone therapy response remains somewhat dubious in this tumor type. There is some suggestion that cumulative assessment of estrogen receptor, progesterone receptor, androgen receptor, and Ki67 predicts response to oral medroxyprogesterone acetate [265]. There has been a recent wave of interest in androgen receptor expression in endometrial carcinomas as second-generation androgen antagonists have shown success in other tumor types including triple-negative breast carcinomas [123, 266–269]. The clinical utility of androgen receptor testing in this setting remains uncertain pending data on endometrial carcinoma responses to androgen antagonism.

The parallels with breast cancer biomarkers do not end with hormone receptors. There was considerable interest several years ago in a predictive role for HER2 testing in

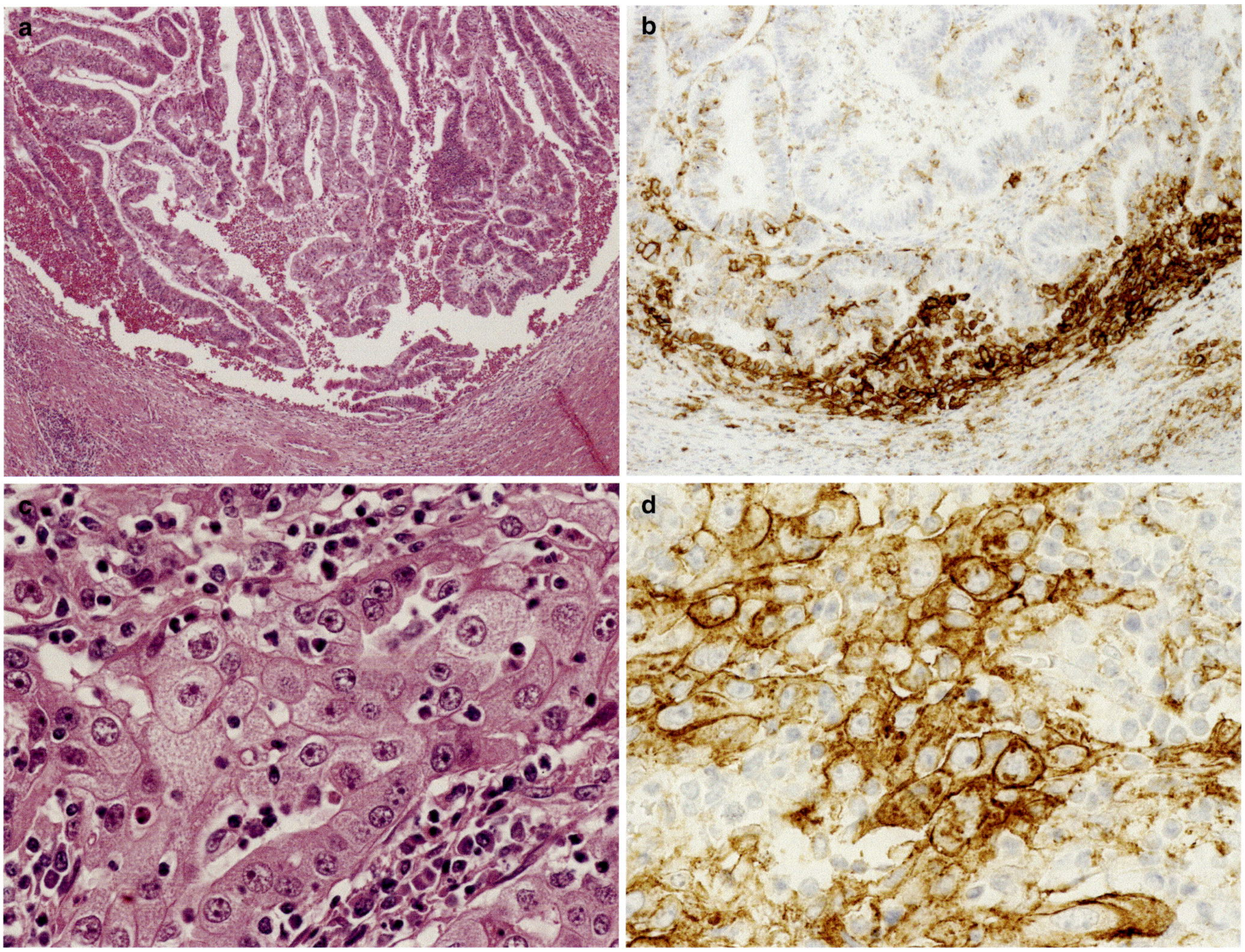

Fig. 18.68 PD-L1 expression is common among mismatch repair-deficient endometrial carcinomas. In some cases, expression is concentrated in tumor cells and tumor-associated macrophages at the infiltrating edge (A/B; this is the tumor with the germline *MSH2* mutation illustrated in Fig. 18.62). Other tumors show diffuse expression (C/D; this tumor bore a *MSH6* mutation)

endometrial carcinoma given the high frequency of HER2/*ERBB2* receptor tyrosine kinase amplification in endometrial serous carcinomas. However, clinical trials targeting HER2 in this tumor type have had fairly unimpressive results, and HER2 testing has therefore not permeated routine practice [191–193, 270].

Another potentially appealing target that has shown success in cancers from other locales is the PI3K-AKT pathway. Given that many endometrial carcinomas bear mutations in this pathway, there is growing interest in a possible role for AKT inhibitors in this tumor type [149, 271, 272]. If the success of preclinical models bears out in trials, testing for *PI3K* mutations may be warranted in a subset endometrial carcinoma cases.

A promising new development in predictive biomarker for endometrial carcinoma is the role of mismatch repair deficiency and *POLE* mutation status in predicting immunotherapeutic response [143, 144, 159, 273]. Hypermutated and ultramutated tumors have been shown to have elevated neoantigen loads, which in turn recruit robust cytotoxic T-cell infiltrates [143–145]. Many tumors escape immune attack by mounting evasive mechanisms such as PD-L1 expression [142, 143] and have in clinical trials have been shown to be vulnerable to PD-1/PD-L1 inhibition [144, 145] (Fig. 18.68). As more checkpoint inhibitors and immune modulatory molecule antagonists emerge, the menu of biomarker tests that predict immunotherapeutic response in endometrial carcinoma is sure to expand.

References

1. Bokhman JV. Two pathogenetic types of endometrial carcinoma. Gynecol Oncol. 1983;15(1):10–7.
2. Lax SF, Kurman RJ. A dualistic model for endometrial carcinogenesis based on immunohistochemical and molecular genetic analyses. Verh Dtsch Ges Pathol. 1997;81:228–32.

3. Gilks CB, Oliva E, Soslow RA. Poor interobserver reproducibility in the diagnosis of high-grade endometrial carcinoma. Am J Surg Pathol. 2013;37(6):874–81. https://doi.org/10.1097/PAS.0b013e31827f576a.
4. Han G, Soslow RA, Wethington S, et al. Endometrial carcinomas with clear cells: a study of a heterogeneous group of tumors including interobserver variability, mutation analysis, and immunohistochemistry with HNF-1beta. Int J Gynecol Pathol. 2015;34(4):323–33. https://doi.org/10.1097/PGP.0000000000000162.
5. Thomas S, Hussein Y, Bandyopadhyay S, et al. Interobserver variability in the diagnosis of uterine high-grade endometrioid carcinoma. Arch Pathol Lab Med. 2016;140(8):836–43. https://doi.org/10.5858/arpa.2015-0220-OA.
6. Murali R, Soslow RA, Weigelt B. Classification of endometrial carcinoma: more than two types. Lancet Oncol. 2014;15(7):e268–78. https://doi.org/10.1016/S1470-2045(13)70591-6.
7. Soslow RA. Endometrial carcinomas with ambiguous features. Semin Diagn Pathol. 2010;27(4):261–73.
8. Cancer Genome Atlas Research Network, Kandoth C, Schultz N, et al. Integrated genomic characterization of endometrial carcinoma. Nature. 2013;497(7447):67–73. https://doi.org/10.1038/nature12113.
9. Talhouk A, McConechy MK, Leung S, et al. A clinically applicable molecular-based classification for endometrial cancers. Br J Cancer. 2015;113(2):299–310. https://doi.org/10.1038/bjc.2015.190.
10. Talhouk A, Hoang LN, McConechy MK, et al. Molecular classification of endometrial carcinoma on diagnostic specimens is highly concordant with final hysterectomy: earlier prognostic information to guide treatment. Gynecol Oncol. 2016;143(1):46–53. https://doi.org/10.1016/j.ygyno.2016.07.090.
11. Talhouk A, McConechy MK, Leung S, et al. Confirmation of ProMisE: a simple, genomics-based clinical classifier for endometrial cancer. Cancer. 2017;123:802–13. https://doi.org/10.1002/cncr.30496.
12. Stelloo E, Nout RA, Osse EM, et al. Improved risk assessment by integrating molecular and clinicopathological factors in early-stage endometrial cancer-combined analysis of the PORTEC cohorts. Clin Cancer Res. 2016;22(16):4215–24. https://doi.org/10.1158/1078-0432.CCR-15-2878.
13. Spratt DE, Chan T, Waldron L, et al. Racial/ethnic disparities in genomic sequencing. JAMA Oncol. 2016;2(8):1070–4. https://doi.org/10.1001/jamaoncol.2016.1854.
14. Siegel RL, Miller KD, Jemal A. Cancer statistics, 2016. CA Cancer J Clin. 2016;66(1):7–30. https://doi.org/10.3322/caac.21332.
15. Ljungvall A, Zimmerman FJ. Bigger bodies: long-term trends and disparities in obesity and body-mass index among U.S. adults, 1960–2008. Soc Sci Med. 2012;75(1):109–19. https://doi.org/10.1016/j.socscimed.2012.03.003.
16. DeSantis CE, Siegel RL, Sauer AG, et al. Cancer statistics for African Americans, 2016: progress and opportunities in reducing racial disparities. CA Cancer J Clin. 2016;66(4):290–308. https://doi.org/10.3322/caac.21340.
17. Purdie DM, Green AC. Epidemiology of endometrial cancer. Best Pract Res Clin Obstet Gynaecol. 2001;15(3):341–54. https://doi.org/10.1053/beog.2000.0180.
18. McPherson CP, Sellers TA, Potter JD, Bostick RM, Folsom AR. Reproductive factors and risk of endometrial cancer. The Iowa women's health study. Am J Epidemiol. 1996;143(12):1195–202.
19. Setiawan VW, Yang HP, Pike MC, et al. Type I and II endometrial cancers: have they different risk factors? J Clin Oncol. 2013;31(20):2607–18. https://doi.org/10.1200/JCO.2012.48.2596.
20. Sherman ME, Sturgeon S, Brinton LA, et al. Risk factors and hormone levels in patients with serous and endometrioid uterine carcinomas. Mod Pathol. 1997;10(10):963–8.
21. Lynch HT, Lynch PM, Lanspa SJ, Snyder CL, Lynch JF, Boland CR. Review of the lynch syndrome: history, molecular genetics, screening, differential diagnosis, and medicolegal ramifications. Clin Genet. 2009;76(1):1–18. https://doi.org/10.1111/j.1399-0004.2009.01230.x.
22. Walsh MD, Cummings MC, Buchanan DD, et al. Molecular, pathologic, and clinical features of early-onset endometrial cancer: identifying presumptive lynch syndrome patients. Clin Cancer Res. 2008;14(6):1692–700. https://doi.org/10.1158/1078-0432.CCR-07-1849.
23. Hampel H, Frankel W, Panescu J, et al. Screening for lynch syndrome (hereditary nonpolyposis colorectal cancer) among endometrial cancer patients. Cancer Res. 2006;66(15):7810–7.
24. Barrow E, Robinson L, Alduaij W, et al. Cumulative lifetime incidence of extracolonic cancers in lynch syndrome: a report of 121 families with proven mutations. Clin Genet. 2009;75(2):141–9. https://doi.org/10.1111/j.1399-0004.2008.01125.x.
25. Ligtenberg MJ, Kuiper RP, Chan TL, et al. Heritable somatic methylation and inactivation of MSH2 in families with lynch syndrome due to deletion of the 3″ exons of TACSTD1. Nat Genet. 2009;41(1):112–7. https://doi.org/10.1038/ng.283.
26. Tutlewska K, Lubinski J, Kurzawski G. Germline deletions in the EPCAM gene as a cause of lynch syndrome—literature review. Hered Cancer Clin Pract. 2013;11(1):9. https://doi.org/10.1186/1897-4287-11-9.
27. Huth C, Kloor M, Voigt AY, et al. The molecular basis of EPCAM expression loss in lynch syndrome-associated tumors. Mod Pathol. 2012;25(6):911–6. https://doi.org/10.1038/modpathol.2012.30.
28. Hitchins MP, Ward RL. Constitutional (germline) MLH1 epimutation as an aetiological mechanism for hereditary non-polyposis colorectal cancer. J Med Genet. 2009;46(12):793–802. https://doi.org/10.1136/jmg.2009.068122.
29. Niessen RC, Hofstra RM, Westers H, et al. Germline hypermethylation of MLH1 and EPCAM deletions are a frequent cause of lynch syndrome. Genes Chromosomes Cancer. 2009;48(8):737–44. https://doi.org/10.1002/gcc.20678.
30. Clarke BA, Cooper K. Identifying lynch syndrome in patients with endometrial carcinoma: shortcomings of morphologic and clinical schemas. Adv Anat Pathol. 2012;19(4):231–8. https://doi.org/10.1097/PAP.0b013e31825c6b76.
31. Mills AM, Liou S, Ford JM, Berek JS, Pai RK, Longacre TA. Lynch syndrome screening should be considered for all patients with newly diagnosed endometrial cancer. Am J Surg Pathol. 2014;38(11):1501–9. https://doi.org/10.1097/PAS.0000000000000321.
32. Ring KL, Connor EV, Atkins KA, Ricketts W, Kashlan B, Modesitt SC. Women 50 years or younger with endometrial cancer: the argument for universal mismatch repair screening and potential for targeted therapeutics. Int J Gynecol Cancer. 2013;23(5):853–60. https://doi.org/10.1097/IGC.0b013e31828eed9c.
33. Moline J, Mahdi H, Yang B, et al. Implementation of tumor testing for lynch syndrome in endometrial cancers at a large academic medical center. Gynecol Oncol. 2013;130(1):121–6. https://doi.org/10.1016/j.ygyno.2013.04.022.
34. Ferguson SE, Aronson M, Pollett A, et al. Performance characteristics of screening strategies for lynch syndrome in unselected women with newly diagnosed endometrial cancer who have undergone universal germline mutation testing. Cancer. 2014;120(24):3932–9. https://doi.org/10.1002/cncr.28933.
35. Mills AM, Longacre TA. Lynch syndrome screening in the gynecologic tract: current state of the art. Am J Surg Pathol. 2016;40:e35–44. https://doi.org/10.1097/PAS.0000000000000608.
36. Pilarski R, Burt R, Kohlman W, Pho L, Shannon KM, Swisher E. Cowden syndrome and the PTEN hamartoma tumor syndrome: systematic review and revised diagnostic criteria. J Natl Cancer Inst. 2013;105(21):1607–16. https://doi.org/10.1093/jnci/djt277.

37. Mahdi H, Mester JL, Nizialek EA, Ngeow J, Michener C, Eng C. Germline PTEN, SDHB-D, and KLLN alterations in endometrial cancer patients with Cowden and Cowden-like syndromes: an international, multicenter, prospective study. Cancer. 2015;121(5):688–96. https://doi.org/10.1002/cncr.29106.
38. Folkins AK, Longacre TA. Hereditary gynaecological malignancies: advances in screening and treatment. Histopathology. 2013;62(1):2–30. https://doi.org/10.1111/his.12028.
39. Tan MH, Mester JL, Ngeow J, Rybicki LA, Orloff MS, Eng C. Lifetime cancer risks in individuals with germline PTEN mutations. Clin Cancer Res. 2012;18(2):400–7. https://doi.org/10.1158/1078-0432.CCR-11-2283.
40. Ni Y, Zbuk KM, Sadler T, et al. Germline mutations and variants in the succinate dehydrogenase genes in Cowden and Cowden-like syndromes. Am J Hum Genet. 2008;83(2):261–8. https://doi.org/10.1016/j.ajhg.2008.07.011.
41. Shu CA, Pike MC, Jotwani AR, et al. Uterine cancer after risk-reducing salpingo-oophorectomy without hysterectomy in women with BRCA mutations. JAMA Oncol. 2016;2(11):1434–40. https://doi.org/10.1001/jamaoncol.2016.1820.
42. de Jonge MM, Mooyaart AL, Vreeswijk MP, et al. Linking uterine serous carcinoma to BRCA1/2-associated cancer syndrome: a meta-analysis and case report. Eur J Cancer. 2017;72:215–25.
43. Pennington KP, Walsh T, Lee M, et al. BRCA1, TP53, and CHEK2 germline mutations in uterine serous carcinoma. Cancer. 2013;119(2):332–8. https://doi.org/10.1002/cncr.27720.
44. Liang SX, Pearl M, Liang S, et al. Personal history of breast cancer as a significant risk factor for endometrial serous carcinoma in women aged 55 years old or younger. Int J Cancer. 2011;128(4):763–70. https://doi.org/10.1002/ijc.25395.
45. Timmermans A, Opmeer BC, Khan KS, et al. Endometrial thickness measurement for detecting endometrial cancer in women with postmenopausal bleeding: a systematic review and meta-analysis. Obstet Gynecol. 2010;116(1):160–7. https://doi.org/10.1097/AOG.0b013e3181e3e7e8.
46. Dijkhuizen FP, Mol BW, Brolmann HA, Heintz AP. The accuracy of endometrial sampling in the diagnosis of patients with endometrial carcinoma and hyperplasia: a meta-analysis. Cancer. 2000;89(8):1765–72. https://doi.org/10.1002/1097-0142(20001015)89:8<1765::AID-CNCR17>3.0.CO;2-F.
47. Epstein E, Ramirez A, Skoog L, Valentin L. Dilatation and curettage fails to detect most focal lesions in the uterine cavity in women with postmenopausal bleeding. Acta Obstet Gynecol Scand. 2001;80(12):1131–6.
48. Lee DO, Jung MH, Kim HY. Prospective comparison of biopsy results from curettage and hysteroscopy in postmenopausal uterine bleeding. J Obstet Gynaecol Res. 2011;37(10):1423–6. https://doi.org/10.1111/j.1447-0756.2011.01558.x.
49. SGO Clinical Practice Endometrial Cancer Working Group, Burke WM, Orr J, et al. Endometrial cancer: a review and current management strategies: Part I. Gynecol Oncol. 2014;134(2):385–92. https://doi.org/10.1016/j.ygyno.2014.05.018.
50. SGO Clinical Practice Endometrial Cancer Working Group, Burke WM, Orr J, et al. Endometrial cancer: a review and current management strategies: Part II. Gynecol Oncol. 2014;134(2):393–402. https://doi.org/10.1016/j.ygyno.2014.06.003.
51. Zaino RJ, Silverberg SG, Norris HJ, Bundy BN, Morrow CP, Okagaki T. The prognostic value of nuclear versus architectural grading in endometrial adenocarcinoma: a gynecologic oncology group study. Int J Gynecol Pathol. 1994;13(1):29–36.
52. Zaino RJ, Kurman RJ, Diana KL, Morrow CP. The utility of the revised international federation of gynecology and obstetrics histologic grading of endometrial adenocarcinoma using a defined nuclear grading system. A gynecologic oncology group study. Cancer. 1995;75(1):81–6.
53. Winham WM, Lin D, Stone PJ, Nucci MR, Quick CM. Architectural versus nuclear atypia-defined FIGO grade 2 endometrial endometrioid adenocarcinoma (EEC): a clinicopathologic comparison of 154 cases with clinical follow-up. Int J Gynecol Pathol. 2014;33(2):120–6. https://doi.org/10.1097/PGP.0b013e31828bb4ed.
54. Soslow RA. Practical issues related to uterine pathology: staging, frozen section, artifacts, and lynch syndrome. Mod Pathol. 2016;29(Suppl 1):S59–77. https://doi.org/10.1038/modpathol.2015.127.
55. Barlin JN, Soslow RA, Lutz M, et al. Redefining stage I endometrial cancer: incorporating histology, a binary grading system, myometrial invasion, and lymph node assessment. Int J Gynecol Cancer. 2013;23(9):1620–8. https://doi.org/10.1097/IGC.0b013e3182a5055e.
56. Conlon N, Leitao MM Jr, Abu-Rustum NR, Soslow RA. Grading uterine endometrioid carcinoma: a proposal that binary is best. Am J Surg Pathol. 2014;38(12):1583–7. https://doi.org/10.1097/PAS.0000000000000327.
57. Alkushi A, Abdul-Rahman ZH, Lim P, et al. Description of a novel system for grading of endometrial carcinoma and comparison with existing grading systems. Am J Surg Pathol. 2005;29(3):295–304.
58. Guan H, Semaan A, Bandyopadhyay S, et al. Prognosis and reproducibility of new and existing binary grading systems for endometrial carcinoma compared to FIGO grading in hysterectomy specimens. Int J Gynecol Cancer. 2011;21(4):654–60. https://doi.org/10.1097/IGC.0b013e31821454f1.
59. Nofech-Mozes S, Ghorab Z, Ismiil N, et al. Endometrial endometrioid adenocarcinoma: a pathologic analysis of 827 consecutive cases. Am J Clin Pathol. 2008;129(1):110–4.
60. Amin MB, et al., editors. AJCC cancer staging manual. 8th ed. New York: Springer; 2017.
61. Amant F, Mirza MR, Koskas M, Creutzberg CL. Cancer of the corpus uteri. Int J Gynaecol Obstet. 2015;131(Suppl 2):S96–104. https://doi.org/10.1016/j.ijgo.2015.06.005.
62. Zaino RJ. FIGO staging of endometrial adenocarcinoma: a critical review and proposal. Int J Gynecol Pathol. 2009;28(1):1–9. https://doi.org/10.1097/PGP.0b013e3181846c6d.
63. Zaino RJ, Abendroth C, Yemelyanova A, et al. Endocervical involvement in endometrial adenocarcinoma is not prognostically significant and the pathologic assessment of the pattern of involvement is not reproducible. Gynecol Oncol. 2013;128(1):83–7. https://doi.org/10.1016/j.ygyno.2012.09.035.
64. Ali A, Black D, Soslow RA. Difficulties in assessing the depth of myometrial invasion in endometrial carcinoma. Int J Gynecol Pathol. 2007;26(2):115–23. https://doi.org/10.1097/01.pgp.0000233165.56385.0b.
65. Kir G, Kir M, Cetiner H, Karateke A, Gurbuz A. Diagnostic problems on frozen section examination of myometrial invasion in patients with endometrial carcinoma with special emphasis on the pitfalls of deep adenomyosis with carcinomatous involvement. Eur J Gynaecol Oncol. 2004;25(2):211–4.
66. Hertel JD, Huettner PC, Pfeifer JD. Lymphovascular space invasion in microcystic elongated and fragmented (MELF)-pattern well-differentiated endometrioid adenocarcinoma is associated with a higher rate of lymph node metastasis. Int J Gynecol Pathol. 2014;33(2):127–34. https://doi.org/10.1097/PGP.0b013e318285657b.
67. Pavlakis K, Messini I, Vrekoussis T, et al. MELF invasion in endometrial cancer as a risk factor for lymph node metastasis. Histopathology. 2011;58(6):966–73. https://doi.org/10.1111/j.1365-2559.2011.03802.x.
68. Quick CM, May T, Horowitz NS, Nucci MR. Low-grade, low-stage endometrioid endometrial adenocarcinoma: a clinicopathologic analysis of 324 cases focusing on frequency and pattern of myoinvasion. Int J Gynecol Pathol. 2012;31(4):337–43. https://doi.org/10.1097/PGP.0b013e31823ff422.
69. Joehlin-Price AS, McHugh KE, Stephens JA, et al. The microcystic, elongated, and fragmented (MELF) pattern of

invasion: a single institution report of 464 consecutive FIGO grade 1 endometrial endometrioid adenocarcinomas. Am J Surg Pathol. 2017;41(1):49–55. https://doi.org/10.1097/PAS.0000000000000754.
70. Dogan Altunpulluk M, Kir G, Topal CS, Cetiner H, Gocmen A. The association of the microcystic, elongated and fragmented (MELF) invasion pattern in endometrial carcinomas with deep myometrial invasion, lymphovascular space invasion and lymph node metastasis. J Obstet Gynaecol. 2015;35(4):397–402. https://doi.org/10.3109/01443615.2014.960827.
71. Stewart CJ, Brennan BA, Leung YC, Little L. MELF pattern invasion in endometrial carcinoma: association with low grade, myoinvasive endometrioid tumours, focal mucinous differentiation and vascular invasion. Pathology. 2009;41(5):454–9. https://doi.org/10.1080/00313020903041135.
72. Stewart CJ, Little L. Immunophenotypic features of MELF pattern invasion in endometrial adenocarcinoma: evidence for epithelial-mesenchymal transition. Histopathology. 2009;55(1):91–101. https://doi.org/10.1111/j.1365-2559.2009.03327.x.
73. Zaino RJ. Unusual patterns of endometrial carcinoma including MELF and its relation to epithelial mesenchymal transition. Int J Gynecol Pathol. 2014;33(4):357–64. https://doi.org/10.1097/PGP.0000000000000137.
74. Longacre TA, Hendrickson MR. Diffusely infiltrative endometrial adenocarcinoma: an adenoma malignum pattern of myoinvasion. Am J Surg Pathol. 1999;23(1):69–78.
75. Noumoff JS, Menzin A, Mikuta J, Lusk EJ, Morgan M, LiVolsi VA. The ability to evaluate prognostic variables on frozen section in hysterectomies performed for endometrial carcinoma. Gynecol Oncol. 1991;42(3):202–8.
76. Quinlivan JA, Petersen RW, Nicklin JL. Accuracy of frozen section for the operative management of endometrial cancer. BJOG. 2001;108(8):798–803.
77. Yura Y, Tauchi K, Koshiyama M, et al. Parametrial involvement in endometrial carcinomas: its incidence and correlation with other histological parameters. Gynecol Oncol. 1996;63(1):114–9.
78. Watanabe Y, Satou T, Nakai H, et al. Evaluation of parametrial spread in endometrial carcinoma. Obstet Gynecol. 2010;116(5):1027–34. https://doi.org/10.1097/AOG.0b013e3181f80a49.
79. Sato R, Jobo T, Kuramoto H. Parametrial spread is a prognostic factor in endometrial carcinoma. Eur J Gynaecol Oncol. 2003;24(3-4):241–5.
80. Nofech-Mozes S, Ackerman I, Ghorab Z, et al. Lymphovascular invasion is a significant predictor for distant recurrence in patients with early-stage endometrial endometrioid adenocarcinoma. Am J Clin Pathol. 2008;129(6):912–7. https://doi.org/10.1309/CP3HGX7H753QQU8T.
81. Creasman WT, Morrow CP, Bundy BN, Homesley HD, Graham JE, Heller PB. Surgical pathologic spread patterns of endometrial cancer. a gynecologic oncology group study. Cancer. 1987;60(8 Suppl):2035–41.
82. Prat J. Prognostic parameters of endometrial carcinoma. Hum Pathol. 2004;35(6):649–62.
83. Krizova A, Clarke BA, Bernardini MQ, et al. Histologic artifacts in abdominal, vaginal, laparoscopic, and robotic hysterectomy specimens: a blinded, retrospective review. Am J Surg Pathol. 2011;35(1):115–26. https://doi.org/10.1097/PAS.0b013e31820273dc.
84. Kitahara S, Walsh C, Frumovitz M, Malpica A, Silva EG. Vascular pseudoinvasion in laparoscopic hysterectomy specimens for endometrial carcinoma: a grossing artifact? Am J Surg Pathol. 2009;33(2):298–303. https://doi.org/10.1097/PAS.0b013e31818a01bf.
85. Fadare O, Mariappan MR, Hileeto D, Wang S, McAlpine JN, Rimm DL. Upstaging based solely on positive peritoneal washing does not affect outcome in endometrial cancer. Mod Pathol. 2005;18(5):673–80.
86. Haltia UM, Butzow R, Leminen A, Loukovaara M. FIGO 1988 versus 2009 staging for endometrial carcinoma: a comparative study on prediction of survival and stage distribution according to histologic subtype. J Gynecol Oncol. 2014;25(1):30–5. https://doi.org/10.3802/jgo.2014.25.1.30.
87. Kadar N, Homesley HD, Malfetano JH. Positive peritoneal cytology is an adverse factor in endometrial carcinoma only if there is other evidence of extrauterine disease. Gynecol Oncol. 1992;46(2):145–9.
88. Ebina Y, Hareyama H, Sakuragh N, et al. Peritoneal cytology and its prognostic value in endometrial carcinoma. Int Surg. 1997;82(3):244–8.
89. Kasamatsu T, Onda T, Katsumata N, et al. Prognostic significance of positive peritoneal cytology in endometrial carcinoma confined to the uterus. Br J Cancer. 2003;88(2):245–50. https://doi.org/10.1038/sj.bjc.6600698.
90. Sonoda Y, Zerbe M, Smith A, Lin O, Barakat RR, Hoskins WJ. High incidence of positive peritoneal cytology in low-risk endometrial cancer treated by laparoscopically assisted vaginal hysterectomy. Gynecol Oncol. 2001;80(3):378–82. https://doi.org/10.1006/gyno.2000.6079.
91. Mills AM, Sloan EA, Thomas M, et al. Clinicopathologic comparison of lynch syndrome-associated and "lynch-like" endometrial carcinomas identified on universal screening using mismatch repair protein immunohistochemistry. Am J Surg Pathol. 2016;40(2):155–65. https://doi.org/10.1097/PAS.0000000000000544.
92. Monte NM, Webster KA, Neuberg D, Dressler GR, Mutter GL. Joint loss of PAX2 and PTEN expression in endometrial precancers and cancer. Cancer Res. 2010;70(15):6225–32. https://doi.org/10.1158/0008-5472.CAN-10-0149.
93. Baak JP, Van Diermen B, Steinbakk A, et al. Lack of PTEN expression in endometrial intraepithelial neoplasia is correlated with cancer progression. Hum Pathol. 2005;36(5):555–61.
94. Mutter GL, Monte NM, Neuberg D, Ferenczy A, Eng C. Emergence, involution, and progression to carcinoma of mutant clones in normal endometrial tissues. Cancer Res. 2014;74(10):2796–802. https://doi.org/10.1158/0008-5472.CAN-14-0108.
95. Jarboe EA, Mutter GL. Endometrial intraepithelial neoplasia. Semin Diagn Pathol. 2010;27(4):215–25.
96. Kurman RJ, International Agency for Research on Cancer, World Health Organization. WHO classification of tumours of female reproductive organs. 4th ed. Lyon: International Agency for Research on Cancer; 2014. p. 307. http://firstsearch.oclc.org/WebZ/DECRead?standardNoType=1&standardNo=9283224353&sessionid=0&srcdbname=worldcat&key=717c2894fe3e657660a8a5f0444e4218db82da7f6820cabd06e06df832401f0c&ectype=TOC
97. Kurman RJ, Norris HJ. Evaluation of criteria for distinguishing atypical endometrial hyperplasia from well-differentiated carcinoma. Cancer. 1982;49(12):2547–59.
98. Longacre TA, Chung MH, Jensen DN, Hendrickson MR. Proposed criteria for the diagnosis of well-differentiated endometrial carcinoma. A diagnostic test for myoinvasion. Am J Surg Pathol. 1995;19(4):371–406.
99. McKenney JK, Longacre TA. Low-grade endometrial adenocarcinoma: a diagnostic algorithm for distinguishing atypical endometrial hyperplasia and other benign (and malignant) mimics. Adv Anat Pathol. 2009;16(1):1–22. https://doi.org/10.1097/PAP.0b013e3181919e15.
100. Schultheis AM, Martelotto LG, De Filippo MR, et al. TP53 mutational spectrum in endometrioid and serous endometrial cancers. Int J Gynecol Pathol. 2016;35(4):289–300. https://doi.org/10.1097/PGP.0000000000000243.
101. Alvarez T, Miller E, Duska L, Oliva E. Molecular profile of grade 3 endometrioid endometrial carcinoma: is it a type I or type II endometrial carcinoma? Am J Surg Pathol. 2012;36(5):753–61. https://doi.org/10.1097/PAS.0b013e318247b7bb.

102. Garg K, Leitao MM Jr, Wynveen CA, et al. P53 overexpression in morphologically ambiguous endometrial carcinomas correlates with adverse clinical outcomes. Mod Pathol. 2010;23(1):80–92. https://doi.org/10.1038/modpathol.2009.153.
103. McCluggage WG. Ten problematical issues identified by pathology review for multidisciplinary gynaecological oncology meetings. J Clin Pathol. 2012;65(4):293–301. https://doi.org/10.1136/jclinpath-2011-200352.
104. McCluggage WG, Soslow RA, Gilks CB. Patterns of p53 immunoreactivity in endometrial carcinomas: 'all or nothing' staining is of importance. Histopathology. 2011;59(4):786–8. https://doi.org/10.1111/j.1365-2559.2011.03907.x.
105. Malpica A. How to approach the many faces of endometrioid carcinoma. Mod Pathol. 2016;29(Suppl 1):S29–44. https://doi.org/10.1038/modpathol.2015.142.
106. Zaino RJ, Kurman R, Herbold D, et al. The significance of squamous differentiation in endometrial carcinoma. Data from a gynecologic oncology group study. Cancer. 1991;68(10):2293–302.
107. Zaino RJ, Kurman RJ. Squamous differentiation in carcinoma of the endometrium: a critical appraisal of adenoacanthoma and adenosquamous carcinoma. Semin Diagn Pathol. 1988;5(2):154–71.
108. Abeler VM, Kjorstad KE. Endometrial adenocarcinoma with squamous cell differentiation. Cancer. 1992;69(2):488–95.
109. Castrillon DH, Lee KR, Nucci MR. Distinction between endometrial and endocervical adenocarcinoma: an immunohistochemical study. Int J Gynecol Pathol. 2002;21(1):4–10.
110. McCluggage WG, Sumathi VP, McBride HA, Patterson A. A panel of immunohistochemical stains, including carcinoembryonic antigen, vimentin, and estrogen receptor, aids the distinction between primary endometrial and endocervical adenocarcinomas. Int J Gynecol Pathol. 2002;21(1):11–5.
111. Kong CS, Beck AH, Longacre TA. A panel of 3 markers including p16, ProExC, or HPV ISH is optimal for distinguishing between primary endometrial and endocervical adenocarcinomas. Am J Surg Pathol. 2010;34(7):915–26. https://doi.org/10.1097/PAS.0b013e3181e3291e.
112. Ross JC, Eifel PJ, Cox RS, Kempson RL, Hendrickson MR. Primary mucinous adenocarcinoma of the endometrium. A clinicopathologic and histochemical study. Am J Surg Pathol. 1983;7(8):715–29.
113. Clement PB, Young RH. Non-endometrioid carcinomas of the uterine corpus: a review of their pathology with emphasis on recent advances and problematic aspects. Adv Anat Pathol. 2004;11(3):117–42.
114. Wheeler DT, Bristow RE, Kurman RJ. Histologic alterations in endometrial hyperplasia and well-differentiated carcinoma treated with progestins. Am J Surg Pathol. 2007;31(7):988–98. https://doi.org/10.1097/PAS.0b013e31802d68ce.
115. Sloan EA, Moskaluk CA, Mills AM. Mucinous differentiation with tumor infiltrating lymphocytes is a feature of sporadically methylated endometrial carcinomas. Int J Gynecol Pathol. 2017;36:205–16. https://doi.org/10.1097/PGP.0000000000000315.
116. Tobon H, Watkins GJ. Secretory adenocarcinoma of the endometrium. Int J Gynecol Pathol. 1985;4(4):328–35.
117. Christopherson WM, Alberhasky RC, Connelly PJ. Carcinoma of the endometrium: I. A clinicopathologic study of clear-cell carcinoma and secretory carcinoma. Cancer. 1982;49(8):1511–23.
118. Truskinovsky AM, Lifschitz-Mercer B, Czernobilsky B. Hyperplasia and carcinoma in secretory endometrium: a diagnostic challenge. Int J Gynecol Pathol. 2014;33(2):107–13. https://doi.org/10.1097/PGP.0b013e3182a2945d.
119. Gurda GT, Baras AS, Kurman RJ. Ki-67 index as an ancillary tool in the differential diagnosis of proliferative endometrial lesions with secretory change. Int J Gynecol Pathol. 2014;33(2):114–9. https://doi.org/10.1097/PGP.0000000000000092.
120. Silva EG, Young RH. Endometrioid neoplasms with clear cells: a report of 21 cases in which the alteration is not of typical secretory type. Am J Surg Pathol. 2007;31(8):1203–8. https://doi.org/10.1097/PAS.0b013e3180339ed7.
121. Cochrane DR, Tessier-Cloutier B, Lawrence KM, et al. Clear cell and endometrioid carcinomas: are their differences attributable to distinct cells of origin? J Pathol. 2017; https://doi.org/10.1002/path.4934.
122. Fadare O, Desouki MM, Gwin K, et al. Frequent expression of napsin A in clear cell carcinoma of the endometrium: potential diagnostic utility. Am J Surg Pathol. 2014;38(2):189–96. https://doi.org/10.1097/PAS.0000000000000085.
123. Zadeh SL, Duska LR, Mills AM. Androgen receptor expression in endometrial carcinoma. Int J Gynecol Pathol. 2017; https://doi.org/10.1097/PGP.0000000000000401.
124. Zaino RJ, Kurman RJ, Brunetto VL, et al. Villoglandular adenocarcinoma of the endometrium: a clinicopathologic study of 61 cases: a gynecologic oncology group study. Am J Surg Pathol. 1998;22(11):1379–85.
125. Ambros RA, Ballouk F, Malfetano JH, Ross JS. Significance of papillary (villoglandular) differentiation in endometrioid carcinoma of the uterus. Am J Surg Pathol. 1994;18(6):569–75.
126. Garg K, Soslow RA. Strategies for distinguishing low-grade endometrioid and serous carcinomas of endometrium. Adv Anat Pathol. 2012;19(1):1–10. https://doi.org/10.1097/PAP.0b013e318234ab36.
127. Hoang LN, Kinloch MA, Leo JM, et al. Interobserver agreement in endometrial carcinoma histotype diagnosis varies depending on the cancer genome atlas (TCGA)-based molecular subgroup. Am J Surg Pathol. 2017;41(2):245–52. https://doi.org/10.1097/PAS.0000000000000764.
128. Piulats JM, Guerra E, Gil-Martin M, et al. Molecular approaches for classifying endometrial carcinoma. Gynecol Oncol. 2017;145:200–7.
129. Murray SK, Clement PB, Young RH. Endometrioid carcinomas of the uterine corpus with sex cord-like formations, hyalinization, and other unusual morphologic features: a report of 31 cases of a neoplasm that may be confused with carcinosarcoma and other uterine neoplasms. Am J Surg Pathol. 2005;29(2):157–66.
130. Eichhorn JH, Young RH, Clement PB. Sertoliform endometrial adenocarcinoma: a study of four cases. Int J Gynecol Pathol. 1996;15(2):119–26.
131. Fujibayashi M, Aiba M, Iizuka E, Igarashi A, Muraoka M, Takagi K. Granulosa cell tumor-like variant of endometrioid carcinoma of the ovary exhibiting nuclear clearing with biotin activity: a subtype showing close macroscopic, cytologic, and histologic similarity to adult granulosa cell tumor. Arch Pathol Lab Med. 2005;129(10):1288–94.
132. Parkash V, Carcangiu ML. Endometrioid endometrial adenocarcinoma with psammoma bodies. Am J Surg Pathol. 1997;21(4):399–406.
133. Lax SF, Pizer ES, Ronnett BM, Kurman RJ. Comparison of estrogen and progesterone receptor, ki-67, and p53 immunoreactivity in uterine endometrioid carcinoma and endometrioid carcinoma with squamous, mucinous, secretory, and ciliated cell differentiation. Hum Pathol. 1998;29(9):924–31.
134. Brunner AH, Riss P, Heinze G, Meltzow E, Brustmann H. Immunoexpression of PAX 8 in endometrial cancer: relation to high-grade carcinoma and p53. Int J Gynecol Pathol. 2011;30(6):569–75. https://doi.org/10.1097/PGP.0b013e31821ac6c3.
135. Yemelyanova A, Gown AM, Wu LS, Holmes BJ, Ronnett BM, Vang R. PAX8 expression in uterine adenocarcinomas and mesonephric proliferations. Int J Gynecol Pathol. 2014;33(5):492–9. https://doi.org/10.1097/PGP.0b013e3182a54afa.

136. Djordjevic B, Hennessy BT, Li J, et al. Clinical assessment of PTEN loss in endometrial carcinoma: immunohistochemistry outperforms gene sequencing. Mod Pathol. 2012;25(5):699–708. https://doi.org/10.1038/modpathol.2011.208.
137. Chiang S, Soslow RA. Updates in diagnostic immunohistochemistry in endometrial carcinoma. Semin Diagn Pathol. 2014;31(3):205–15. https://doi.org/10.1053/j.semdp.2014.03.002.
138. Yemelyanova A, Ji H, Shih I, Wang TL, Wu LS, Ronnett BM. Utility of p16 expression for distinction of uterine serous carcinomas from endometrial endometrioid and endocervical adenocarcinomas: immunohistochemical analysis of 201 cases. Am J Surg Pathol. 2009;33(10):1504–14. https://doi.org/10.1097/PAS.0b013e3181ac35f5.
139. Newton K, Jorgensen NM, Wallace AJ, et al. Tumour MLH1 promoter region methylation testing is an effective prescreen for lynch syndrome (HNPCC). J Med Genet. 2014;51(12):789–96. https://doi.org/10.1136/jmedgenet-2014-102552.
140. Heald B, Plesec T, Liu X, et al. Implementation of universal microsatellite instability and immunohistochemistry screening for diagnosing lynch syndrome in a large academic medical center. J Clin Oncol. 2013;31(10):1336–40. https://doi.org/10.1200/JCO.2012.45.1674.
141. Haraldsdottir S, Hampel H, Tomsic J, et al. Colon and endometrial cancers with mismatch repair deficiency can arise from somatic, rather than germline, mutations. Gastroenterology. 2014;147(6):1308–1316.e1. https://doi.org/10.1053/j.gastro.2014.08.041.
142. Sloan EA, Ring KL, Willis BC, Modesitt SC, Mills AM. PD-L1 expression in mismatch repair-deficient endometrial carcinomas, including lynch syndrome-associated and MLH1 promoter hypermethylated tumors. Am J Surg Pathol. 2016; https://doi.org/10.1097/PAS.0000000000000783.
143. Howitt BE, Shukla SA, Sholl LM, et al. Association of polymerase e-mutated and microsatellite-instable endometrial cancers with neoantigen load, number of tumor-infiltrating lymphocytes, and expression of PD-1 and PD-L1. JAMA Oncol. 2015;1(9):1319–23. https://doi.org/10.1001/jamaoncol.2015.2151.
144. Le DT, Durham JN, Smith KN, et al. Mismatch-repair deficiency predicts response of solid tumors to PD-1 blockade. Science. 2017;357(6349):409–13.
145. Le DT, Uram JN, Wang H, et al. PD-1 blockade in tumors with mismatch-repair deficiency. N Engl J Med. 2015;372(26):2509–20. https://doi.org/10.1056/NEJMoa1500596.
146. Rudd ML, Price JC, Fogoros S, et al. A unique spectrum of somatic PIK3CA (p110alpha) mutations within primary endometrial carcinomas. Clin Cancer Res. 2011;17(6):1331–40. https://doi.org/10.1158/1078-0432.CCR-10-0540.
147. Oda K, Stokoe D, Taketani Y, McCormick F. High frequency of coexistent mutations of PIK3CA and PTEN genes in endometrial carcinoma. Cancer Res. 2005;65(23):10669–73.
148. Urick ME, Rudd ML, Godwin AK, Sgroi D, Merino M, Bell DW. PIK3R1 (p85alpha) is somatically mutated at high frequency in primary endometrial cancer. Cancer Res. 2011;71(12):4061–7. https://doi.org/10.1158/0008-5472.CAN-11-0549.
149. O'Hara AJ, Bell DW. The genomics and genetics of endometrial cancer. Adv Genomics Genet. 2012;2012(2):33–47. https://doi.org/10.2147/AGG.S28953.
150. Gausachs M, Mur P, Corral J, et al. MLH1 promoter hypermethylation in the analytical algorithm of lynch syndrome: a cost-effectiveness study. Eur J Hum Genet. 2012;20(7):762–8. https://doi.org/10.1038/ejhg.2011.277.
151. Metcalf AM, Spurdle AB. Endometrial tumour BRAF mutations and MLH1 promoter methylation as predictors of germline mismatch repair gene mutation status: a literature review. Fam Cancer. 2014;13(1):1–12. https://doi.org/10.1007/s10689-013-9671-6.
152. He M, Breese V, Hang S, Zhang C, Xiong J, Jackson C. BRAF V600E mutations in endometrial adenocarcinoma. Diagn Mol Pathol. 2013;22(1):35–40. https://doi.org/10.1097/PDM.0b013e31826c7fe0.
153. Parsons MT, Buchanan DD, Thompson B, Young JP, Spurdle AB. Correlation of tumour BRAF mutations and MLH1 methylation with germline mismatch repair (MMR) gene mutation status: a literature review assessing utility of tumour features for MMR variant classification. J Med Genet. 2012;49(3):151–7. https://doi.org/10.1136/jmedgenet-2011-100714.
154. Ligtenberg MJ, Kuiper RP, Geurts van Kessel A, Hoogerbrugge N. EPCAM deletion carriers constitute a unique subgroup of lynch syndrome patients. Fam Cancer. 2013;12(2):169–74. https://doi.org/10.1007/s10689-012-9591-x.
155. Rumilla K, Schowalter KV, Lindor NM, et al. Frequency of deletions of EPCAM (TACSTD1) in MSH2-associated lynch syndrome cases. J Mol Diagn. 2011;13(1):93–9. https://doi.org/10.1016/j.jmoldx.2010.11.011.
156. Rabban JT, Calkins SM, Karnezis AN, et al. Association of tumor morphology with mismatch-repair protein status in older endometrial cancer patients: implications for universal versus selective screening strategies for lynch syndrome. Am J Surg Pathol. 2014;38(6):793–800. https://doi.org/10.1097/PAS.0000000000000177.
157. Garg K, Soslow RA. Lynch syndrome (hereditary non-polyposis colorectal cancer) and endometrial carcinoma. J Clin Pathol. 2009;62(8):679–84. https://doi.org/10.1136/jcp.2009.064949.
158. Chui MH, Ryan P, Radigan J, et al. The histomorphology of lynch syndrome-associated ovarian carcinomas: toward a subtype-specific screening strategy. Am J Surg Pathol. 2014;38(9):1173–81. https://doi.org/10.1097/PAS.0000000000000298.
159. Eggink FA, Van Gool IC, Leary A, et al. Immunological profiling of molecularly classified high-risk endometrial cancers identifies POLE-mutant and microsatellite unstable carcinomas as candidates for checkpoint inhibition. Oncoimmunology. 2016;6(2):e1264565. https://doi.org/10.1080/2162402X.2016.1264565.
160. Hussein YR, Weigelt B, Levine DA, et al. Clinicopathological analysis of endometrial carcinomas harboring somatic POLE exonuclease domain mutations. Mod Pathol. 2015;28(4):505–14. https://doi.org/10.1038/modpathol.2014.143.
161. Young RH, Scully RE. Uterine carcinomas simulating microglandular hyperplasia. A report of six cases. Am J Surg Pathol. 1992;16(11):1092–7.
162. Zaloudek C, Hayashi GM, Ryan IP, Powell CB, Miller TR. Microglandular adenocarcinoma of the endometrium: a form of mucinous adenocarcinoma that may be confused with microglandular hyperplasia of the cervix. Int J Gynecol Pathol. 1997;16(1):52–9.
163. Trippel M, Imboden S, Papadia A, et al. Intestinal differentiated mucinous adenocarcinoma of the endometrium with sporadic MSI high status: a case report. Diagn Pathol. 2017;12(1):39. https://doi.org/10.1186/s13000-017-0629-0.
164. Stolnicu S, Barsan I, Hoang L, et al. International endocervical adenocarcinoma criteria and classification (IECC): a new pathogenetic classification for invasive adenocarcinomas of the endocervix. Am J Surg Pathol. 2017; https://doi.org/10.1097/PAS.0000000000000986.
165. McCluggage WG, Shah R, Connolly LE, McBride HA. Intestinal-type cervical adenocarcinoma in situ and adenocarcinoma exhibit a partial enteric immunophenotype with consistent expression of CDX2. Int J Gynecol Pathol. 2008;27(1):92–100. https://doi.org/10.1097/pgp.0b013e31815698e7.
166. Yoo SH, Park BH, Choi J, et al. Papillary mucinous metaplasia of the endometrium as a possible precursor of endometrial mucinous adenocarcinoma. Mod Pathol. 2012;25(11):1496–507. https://doi.org/10.1038/modpathol.2012.113.

167. Hendrickson M, Ross J, Eifel P, Martinez A, Kempson R. Uterine papillary serous carcinoma: a highly malignant form of endometrial adenocarcinoma. Am J Surg Pathol. 1982;6(2):93–108.
168. Suarez AA, Felix AS, Cohn DE. Bokhman Redux: endometrial cancer "types" in the 21st century. Gynecol Oncol. 2017;144(2):243–9.
169. Carcangiu ML, Radice P, Casalini P, Bertario L, Merola M, Sala P. Lynch syndrome-related endometrial carcinomas show a high frequency of nonendometrioid types and of high FIGO grade endometrioid types. Int J Surg Pathol. 2010;18(1):21–6. https://doi.org/10.1177/1066896909332117.
170. Fadare O, Zheng W, Crispens MA, et al. Morphologic and other clinicopathologic features of endometrial clear cell carcinoma: a comprehensive analysis of 50 rigorously classified cases. Am J Cancer Res. 2013;3(1):70–95.
171. Kobel M, Meng B, Hoang LN, et al. Molecular analysis of mixed endometrial carcinomas shows clonality in most cases. Am J Surg Pathol. 2016;40(2):166–80. https://doi.org/10.1097/PAS.0000000000000536.
172. Rabban JT, Zaloudek CJ. Minimal uterine serous carcinoma: current concepts in diagnosis and prognosis. Pathology. 2007;39(1):125–33.
173. Ambros RA, Sherman ME, Zahn CM, Bitterman P, Kurman RJ. Endometrial intraepithelial carcinoma: a distinctive lesion specifically associated with tumors displaying serous differentiation. Hum Pathol. 1995;26(11):1260–7.
174. Zheng W, Xiang L, Fadare O, Kong B. A proposed model for endometrial serous carcinogenesis. Am J Surg Pathol. 2011;35(1):e1–e14. https://doi.org/10.1097/PAS.0b013e318202772e.
175. Zheng W, Liang SX, Yi X, Ulukus EC, Davis JR, Chambers SK. Occurrence of endometrial glandular dysplasia precedes uterine papillary serous carcinoma. Int J Gynecol Pathol. 2007;26(1):38–52. https://doi.org/10.1097/01.pgp.0000228138.56222.4e.
176. Zheng W, Schwartz PE. Serous EIC as an early form of uterine papillary serous carcinoma: recent progress in understanding its pathogenesis and current opinions regarding pathologic and clinical management. Gynecol Oncol. 2005;96(3):579–82.
177. Zheng W, Khurana R, Farahmand S, Wang Y, Zhang ZF, Felix JC. P53 immunostaining as a significant adjunct diagnostic method for uterine surface carcinoma: precursor of uterine papillary serous carcinoma. Am J Surg Pathol. 1998;22(12):1463–73.
178. Fadare O, Zheng W. Insights into endometrial serous carcinogenesis and progression. Int J Clin Exp Pathol. 2009;2(5):411–32.
179. Wheeler DT, Bell KA, Kurman RJ, Sherman ME. Minimal uterine serous carcinoma: diagnosis and clinicopathologic correlation. Am J Surg Pathol. 2000;24(6):797–806.
180. Soslow RA, Pirog E, Isacson C. Endometrial intraepithelial carcinoma with associated peritoneal carcinomatosis. Am J Surg Pathol. 2000;24(5):726–32.
181. Goff BA, Kato D, Schmidt RA, et al. Uterine papillary serous carcinoma: patterns of metastatic spread. Gynecol Oncol. 1994;54(3):264–8.
182. Snyder MJ, Bentley R, Robboy SJ. Transtubal spread of serous adenocarcinoma of the endometrium: an underrecognized mechanism of metastasis. Int J Gynecol Pathol. 2006;25(2):155–60. https://doi.org/10.1097/01.pgp.0000179614.47838.82.
183. Trahan S, Tetu B, Raymond PE. Serous papillary carcinoma of the endometrium arising from endometrial polyps: a clinical, histological, and immunohistochemical study of 13 cases. Hum Pathol. 2005;36(12):1316–21.
184. Silva EG, Jenkins R. Serous carcinoma in endometrial polyps. Mod Pathol. 1990;3(2):120–8.
185. Yemelyanova A, Vang R, Kshirsagar M, et al. Immunohistochemical staining patterns of p53 can serve as a surrogate marker for TP53 mutations in ovarian carcinoma: an immunohistochemical and nucleotide sequencing analysis. Mod Pathol. 2011;24(9):1248–53. https://doi.org/10.1038/modpathol.2011.85.
186. Darvishian F, Hummer AJ, Thaler HT, et al. Serous endometrial cancers that mimic endometrioid adenocarcinomas: a clinicopathologic and immunohistochemical study of a group of problematic cases. Am J Surg Pathol. 2004;28(12):1568–78.
187. Mhawech-Fauceglia P, Yan L, Liu S, Pejovic T. ER+/PR+ TFF3+/IMP3− immunoprofile distinguishes endometrioid from serous and clear cell carcinomas of the endometrium: a study of 401 cases. Histopathology. 2013;62(7):976–85. https://doi.org/10.1111/his.12096.
188. Gatius S, Matias-Guiu X. Practical issues in the diagnosis of serous carcinoma of the endometrium. Mod Pathol. 2016;29(Suppl 1):S45–58. https://doi.org/10.1038/modpathol.2015.141.
189. Alkushi A, Kobel M, Kalloger SE, Gilks CB. High-grade endometrial carcinoma: serous and grade 3 endometrioid carcinomas have different immunophenotypes and outcomes. Int J Gynecol Pathol. 2010;29(4):343–50. https://doi.org/10.1097/PGP.0b013e3181cd6552.
190. Zheng W, Yi X, Fadare O, et al. The oncofetal protein IMP3: a novel biomarker for endometrial serous carcinoma. Am J Surg Pathol. 2008;32(2):304–15. https://doi.org/10.1097/PAS.0b013e3181483ff8.
191. Diaz-Montes TP, Ji H, Smith Sehdev AE, et al. Clinical significance of her-2/neu overexpression in uterine serous carcinoma. Gynecol Oncol. 2006;100(1):139–44.
192. Konecny GE, Santos L, Winterhoff B, et al. HER2 gene amplification and EGFR expression in a large cohort of surgically staged patients with nonendometrioid (type II) endometrial cancer. Br J Cancer. 2009;100(1):89–95. https://doi.org/10.1038/sj.bjc.6604814.
193. Santin AD, Bellone S, Gokden M, et al. Overexpression of HER-2/neu in uterine serous papillary cancer. Clin Cancer Res. 2002;8(5):1271–9.
194. Brinton LA, Trabert B, Anderson GL, et al. Serum estrogens and estrogen metabolites and endometrial cancer risk among postmenopausal women. Cancer Epidemiol Biomarkers Prev. 2016;25(7):1081–9. https://doi.org/10.1158/1055-9965.EPI-16-0225.
195. Brinton LA, Felix AS, McMeekin DS, et al. Etiologic heterogeneity in endometrial cancer: evidence from a gynecologic oncology group trial. Gynecol Oncol. 2013;129(2):277–84. https://doi.org/10.1016/j.ygyno.2013.02.023.
196. Ju B, Wang J, Yang B, et al. Morphologic and immunohistochemical study of clear cell carcinoma of the uterine endometrium and cervix in comparison to ovarian clear cell carcinoma. Int J Gynecol Pathol. 2017; https://doi.org/10.1097/PGP.0000000000000430.
197. Fadare O, Liang SX. Diagnostic utility of hepatocyte nuclear factor 1-beta immunoreactivity in endometrial carcinomas: lack of specificity for endometrial clear cell carcinoma. Appl Immunohistochem Mol Morphol. 2012;20(6):580–7. https://doi.org/10.1097/PAI.0b013e31824973d1.
198. DeLair DF, Burke KA, Selenica P, et al. The genetic landscape of endometrial clear cell carcinomas. J Pathol. 2017; https://doi.org/10.1002/path.4947.
199. Ketabi Z, Bartuma K, Bernstein I, et al. Ovarian cancer linked to lynch syndrome typically presents as early-onset, non-serous epithelial tumors. Gynecol Oncol. 2011;121(3):462–5. https://doi.org/10.1016/j.ygyno.2011.02.010.
200. Cai KQ, Albarracin C, Rosen D, et al. Microsatellite instability and alteration of the expression of hMLH1 and hMSH2 in ovarian clear cell carcinoma. Hum Pathol. 2004;35(5):552–9.
201. Willis BC, Sloan EA, Atkins KA, Stoler MH, Mills AM. Mismatch repair status and PD-L1 expression in clear cell carcinomas of the ovary and endometrium. Mod Pathol. 2017; https://doi.org/10.1038/modpathol.2017.67.
202. Allo G, Bernardini MQ, Wu RC, et al. ARID1A loss correlates with mismatch repair deficiency and intact p53 expression in

high-grade endometrial carcinomas. Mod Pathol. 2014;27(2):255–61. https://doi.org/10.1038/modpathol.2013.144.
203. Tafe LJ, Garg K, Chew I, Tornos C, Soslow RA. Endometrial and ovarian carcinomas with undifferentiated components: clinically aggressive and frequently underrecognized neoplasms. Mod Pathol. 2010;23(6):781–9. https://doi.org/10.1038/modpathol.2010.41.
204. Al-Loh S, Al-Hussaini M. Undifferentiated endometrial carcinoma: a diagnosis frequently overlooked. Arch Pathol Lab Med. 2013;137(3):438–42. https://doi.org/10.5858/arpa.2011-0461-RS.
205. Altrabulsi B, Malpica A, Deavers MT, Bodurka DC, Broaddus R, Silva EG. Undifferentiated carcinoma of the endometrium. Am J Surg Pathol. 2005;29(10):1316–21.
206. Espinosa I, Lee CH, D'Angelo E, Palacios J, Prat J. Undifferentiated and dedifferentiated endometrial carcinomas with POLE exonuclease domain mutations have a favorable prognosis. Am J Surg Pathol. 2017;41(8):1121–8. https://doi.org/10.1097/PAS.0000000000000873.
207. Tafe LJ. Targeted next-generation sequencing for hereditary cancer syndromes: a focus on lynch syndrome and associated endometrial cancer. J Mol Diagn. 2015;17(5):472–82. https://doi.org/10.1016/j.jmoldx.2015.06.001.
208. Silva EG, Deavers MT, Bodurka DC, Malpica A. Association of low-grade endometrioid carcinoma of the uterus and ovary with undifferentiated carcinoma: a new type of dedifferentiated carcinoma? Int J Gynecol Pathol. 2006;25(1):52–8.
209. Hoang LN, Lee YS, Karnezis AN, et al. Immunophenotypic features of dedifferentiated endometrial carcinoma—insights from BRG1/INI1-deficient tumours. Histopathology. 2016;69(4):560–9. https://doi.org/10.1111/his.12989.
210. Ramalingam P, Croce S, McCluggage WG. Loss of expression of SMARCA4 (BRG1), SMARCA2 (BRM) and SMARCB1 (INI1) in undifferentiated carcinoma of the endometrium is not uncommon and is not always associated with rhabdoid morphology. Histopathology. 2017;70(3):359–66. https://doi.org/10.1111/his.13091.
211. Strehl JD, Wachter DL, Fiedler J, et al. Pattern of SMARCB1 (INI1) and SMARCA4 (BRG1) in poorly differentiated endometrioid adenocarcinoma of the uterus: analysis of a series with emphasis on a novel SMARCA4-deficient dedifferentiated rhabdoid variant. Ann Diagn Pathol. 2015;19(4):198–202. https://doi.org/10.1016/j.anndiagpath.2015.04.001.
212. Rosa-Rosa JM, Leskela S, Cristobal-Lana E, et al. Molecular genetic heterogeneity in undifferentiated endometrial carcinomas. Mod Pathol. 2016;29(11):1390–8. https://doi.org/10.1038/modpathol.2016.132.
213. Karnezis AN, Hoang LN, Coatham M, et al. Loss of switch/sucrose non-fermenting complex protein expression is associated with dedifferentiation in endometrial carcinomas. Mod Pathol. 2016;29(3):302–14. https://doi.org/10.1038/modpathol.2015.155.
214. Seidman JD, Kumar D, Cosin JA, Winter WE 3rd, Cargill C, Boice CR. Carcinomas of the female genital tract occurring after pelvic irradiation: a report of 15 cases. Int J Gynecol Pathol. 2006;25(3):293–7. https://doi.org/10.1097/01.pgp.0000189240.03780.b1.
215. D'Angelo E, Prat J. Pathology of mixed mullerian tumours. Best Pract Res Clin Obstet Gynaecol. 2011;25(6):705–18. https://doi.org/10.1016/j.bpobgyn.2011.05.010.
216. McCluggage WG. A practical approach to the diagnosis of mixed epithelial and mesenchymal tumours of the uterus. Mod Pathol. 2016;29(Suppl 1):S78–91. https://doi.org/10.1038/modpathol.2015.137.
217. McCluggage WG. Uterine carcinosarcomas (malignant mixed mullerian tumors) are metaplastic carcinomas. Int J Gynecol Cancer. 2002;12(6):687–90.
218. de Brito PA, Silverberg SG, Orenstein JM. Carcinosarcoma (malignant mixed mullerian (mesodermal) tumor) of the female genital tract: immunohistochemical and ultrastructural analysis of 28 cases. Hum Pathol. 1993;24(2):132–42.
219. Bitterman P, Chun B, Kurman RJ. The significance of epithelial differentiation in mixed mesodermal tumors of the uterus. A clinicopathologic and immunohistochemical study. Am J Surg Pathol. 1990;14(4):317–28.
220. Silverberg SG, Bolin MG, DeGiorgi LS. Adenoacanthoma and mixed adenosquamous carcinoma of the endometrium. A clinicopathologic study. Cancer. 1972;30(5):1307–14.
221. Voutsadakis IA. Epithelial to mesenchymal transition in the pathogenesis of uterine malignant mixed mullerian tumours: the role of ubiquitin proteasome system and therapeutic opportunities. Clin Transl Oncol. 2012;14(4):243–53. https://doi.org/10.1007/s12094-012-0792-4.
222. Sreenan JJ, Hart WR. Carcinosarcomas of the female genital tract. A pathologic study of 29 metastatic tumors: further evidence for the dominant role of the epithelial component and the conversion theory of histogenesis. Am J Surg Pathol. 1995;19(6):666–74.
223. Seidman JD, Chauhan S. Evaluation of the relationship between adenosarcoma and carcinosarcoma and a hypothesis of the histogenesis of uterine sarcomas. Int J Gynecol Pathol. 2003;22(1):75–82.
224. Zhao S, Bellone S, Lopez S, et al. Mutational landscape of uterine and ovarian carcinosarcomas implicates histone genes in epithelial-mesenchymal transition. Proc Natl Acad Sci U S A. 2016;113(43):12238–43.
225. Pecorelli S. Revised FIGO staging for carcinoma of the vulva, cervix, and endometrium. Int J Gynaecol Obstet. 2009;105(2):103–4.
226. de Jong RA, Nijman HW, Wijbrandi TF, Reyners AK, Boezen HM, Hollema H. Molecular markers and clinical behavior of uterine carcinosarcomas: focus on the epithelial tumor component. Mod Pathol. 2011;24(10):1368–79. https://doi.org/10.1038/modpathol.2011.88.
227. Jin Z, Ogata S, Tamura G, et al. Carcinosarcomas (malignant mullerian mixed tumors) of the uterus and ovary: a genetic study with special reference to histogenesis. Int J Gynecol Pathol. 2003;22(4):368–73. https://doi.org/10.1097/01.pgp.0000092134.88121.56.
228. Ferguson SE, Tornos C, Hummer A, Barakat RR, Soslow RA. Prognostic features of surgical stage I uterine carcinosarcoma. Am J Surg Pathol. 2007;31(11):1653–61. https://doi.org/10.1097/PAS.0b013e3181161ba3.
229. McCluggage WG, Colgan T, Duggan M, et al. Data set for reporting of endometrial carcinomas: recommendations from the international collaboration on cancer reporting (ICCR) between united kingdom, united states, canada, and australasia. Int J Gynecol Pathol. 2013;32(1):45–65. https://doi.org/10.1097/PGP.0b013e31825d808b.
230. Shokeir MO, Noel SM, Clement PB. Malignant mullerian mixed tumor of the uterus with a prominent alpha-fetoprotein-producing component of yolk sac tumor. Mod Pathol. 1996;9(6):647–51.
231. Amant F, Moerman P, Davel GH, et al. Uterine carcinosarcoma with melanocytic differentiation. Int J Gynecol Pathol. 2001;20(2):186–90.
232. Euscher ED, Deavers MT, Lopez-Terrada D, Lazar AJ, Silva EG, Malpica A. Uterine tumors with neuroectodermal differentiation: a series of 17 cases and review of the literature. Am J Surg Pathol. 2008;32(2):219–28. https://doi.org/10.1097/PAS.0b013e318093e421.
233. Wada H, Enomoto T, Fujita M, et al. Molecular evidence that most but not all carcinosarcomas of the uterus are combination tumors. Cancer Res. 1997;57(23):5379–85.
234. Broaddus RR, Lynch HT, Chen LM, et al. Pathologic features of endometrial carcinoma associated with HNPCC: a comparison with sporadic endometrial carcinoma. Cancer. 2006;106(1):87–94. https://doi.org/10.1002/cncr.21560.

235. Chiyoda T, Tsuda H, Tanaka H, et al. Expression profiles of carcinosarcoma of the uterine corpus-are these similar to carcinoma or sarcoma? Genes Chromosomes Cancer. 2012;51(3):229–39. https://doi.org/10.1002/gcc.20947.
236. Estruch A, Minig L, Illueca C, Romero I, Guinot JL, Poveda A. Small cell neuroendocrine tumour of the endometrium and the importance of pathologic diagnosis. Ecancermedicalscience. 2016;10:668. https://doi.org/10.3332/ecancer.2016.668.
237. Huntsman DG, Clement PB, Gilks CB, Scully RE. Small-cell carcinoma of the endometrium. A clinicopathological study of sixteen cases. Am J Surg Pathol. 1994;18(4):364–75.
238. Bahig H, Portelance L, Legler C, Gilbert L, Souhami L. Small cell carcinoma of the endometrium: report of a case and review of the literature. Minerva Ginecol. 2009;61(4):365–9.
239. Bige O, Saatli B, Secil M, Koyuncuoglu M, Saygili U. Small cell neuroendocrine carcinoma of the endometrium and laparoscopic staging: a clinicopathologic study of a case and a brief review of the literature. Int J Gynecol Cancer. 2008;18(4):838–43.
240. Howitt BE, Kelly P, McCluggage WG. Pathology of neuroendocrine tumours of the female genital tract. Curr Oncol Rep. 2017;19(9):59. https://doi.org/10.1007/s11912-017-0617-2.
241. Pocrnich CE, Ramalingam P, Euscher ED, Malpica A. Neuroendocrine carcinoma of the endometrium: a clinicopathologic study of 25 cases. Am J Surg Pathol. 2016;40(5):577–86. https://doi.org/10.1097/PAS.0000000000000633.
242. Taraif SH, Deavers MT, Malpica A, Silva EG. The significance of neuroendocrine expression in undifferentiated carcinoma of the endometrium. Int J Gynecol Pathol. 2009;28(2):142–7. https://doi.org/10.1097/PGP.0b013e3181895539.
243. van Hoeven KH, Hudock JA, Woodruff JM, Suhrland MJ. Small cell neuroendocrine carcinoma of the endometrium. Int J Gynecol Pathol. 1995;14(1):21–9.
244. Chetty R, Clark SP, Bhathal PS. Carcinoid tumour of the uterine corpus. Virchows Arch A Pathol Anat Histopathol. 1993;422(1):93–5.
245. Gonzalez-Bosquet E, Gonzalez-Bosquet J, Garcia Jimenez A, Gil A, Xercavins J. Carcinoid tumor of the uterine corpus. A case report. J Reprod Med. 1998;43(9):844–6.
246. Church DN, Stelloo E, Nout RA, et al. Prognostic significance of POLE proofreading mutations in endometrial cancer. J Natl Cancer Inst. 2014;107(1):402. https://doi.org/10.1093/jnci/dju402.
247. Fader AN, Starks D, Gehrig PA, et al. An updated clinicopathologic study of early-stage uterine papillary serous carcinoma (UPSC). Gynecol Oncol. 2009;115(2):244–8. https://doi.org/10.1016/j.ygyno.2009.07.030.
248. Faratian D, Stillie A, Busby-Earle RM, Cowie VJ, Monaghan H. A review of the pathology and management of uterine papillary serous carcinoma and correlation with outcome. Int J Gynecol Cancer. 2006;16(3):972–8.
249. Lim P, Al Kushi A, Gilks B, Wong F, Aquino-Parsons C. Early stage uterine papillary serous carcinoma of the endometrium: effect of adjuvant whole abdominal radiotherapy and pathologic parameters on outcome. Cancer. 2001;91(4):752–7. https://doi.org/10.1002/1097-0142(20010215)91:4<752::AID-CNCR1061>3.0.CO;2-E.
250. Patsavas K, Woessner J, Gielda B, et al. Optimal surgical debulking in uterine papillary serous carcinoma affects survival. Gynecol Oncol. 2011;121(3):581–5. https://doi.org/10.1016/j.ygyno.2010.11.048.
251. Rauh-Hain JA, Growdon WB, Schorge JO, et al. Prognostic determinants in patients with stage IIIC and IV uterine papillary serous carcinoma. Gynecol Oncol. 2010;119(2):299–304. https://doi.org/10.1016/j.ygyno.2010.07.010.
252. Slomovitz BM, Burke TW, Eifel PJ, et al. Uterine papillary serous carcinoma (UPSC): a single institution review of 129 cases. Gynecol Oncol. 2003;91(3):463–9.
253. Coenegrachts L, Garcia-Dios DA, Depreeuw J, et al. Mutation profile and clinical outcome of mixed endometrioid-serous endometrial carcinomas are different from that of pure endometrioid or serous carcinomas. Virchows Arch. 2015;466(4):415–22. https://doi.org/10.1007/s00428-015-1728-5.
254. Goldberg H, Miller RC, Abdah-Bortnyak R, et al. Outcome after combined modality treatment for uterine papillary serous carcinoma: a study by the rare cancer network (RCN). Gynecol Oncol. 2008;108(2):298–305.
255. Roelofsen T, van Ham MA, Wiersma van Tilburg JM, et al. Pure compared with mixed serous endometrial carcinoma: two different entities? Obstet Gynecol. 2012;120(6):1371–81. https://doi.org/10.1097/AOG.0b013e318273732e.
256. Hsu KF, Chou HH, Huang CY, et al. Prognostic factors and treatment outcomes for patients with surgically staged uterine clear cell carcinoma focusing on the early stage: a Taiwanese gynecologic oncology group study. Gynecol Oncol. 2014;134(3):516–22. https://doi.org/10.1016/j.ygyno.2014.07.005.
257. Soliman PT, Broaddus RR, Schmeler KM, et al. Women with synchronous primary cancers of the endometrium and ovary: do they have lynch syndrome? J Clin Oncol. 2005;23(36):9344–50.
258. Jain V, Sekhon R, Pasricha S, et al. Clinicopathological characteristics and prognostic factors of synchronous endometrial and ovarian cancers—a single-institute review of 43 cases. Int J Gynecol Cancer. 2017;27(5):938–46. https://doi.org/10.1097/IGC.0000000000000971.
259. Watkins JC, Nucci MR, Ritterhouse LL, Howitt BE, Sholl LM. Unusual mismatch repair immunohistochemical patterns in endometrial carcinoma. Am J Surg Pathol. 2016;40(7):909–16. https://doi.org/10.1097/PAS.0000000000000663.
260. Suter CM, Martin DI, Ward RL. Germline epimutation of MLH1 in individuals with multiple cancers. Nat Genet. 2004;36(5):497–501. https://doi.org/10.1038/ng1342.
261. Kato A, Sato N, Sugawara T, et al. Isolated loss of PMS2 immunohistochemical expression is frequently caused by heterogenous MLH1 promoter hypermethylation in lynch syndrome screening for endometrial cancer patients. Am J Surg Pathol. 2016;40(6):770–6. https://doi.org/10.1097/PAS.0000000000000606.
262. Rhees J, Arnold M, Boland CR. Inversion of exons 1-7 of the MSH2 gene is a frequent cause of unexplained lynch syndrome in one local population. Fam Cancer. 2014;13(2):219–25. https://doi.org/10.1007/s10689-013-9688-x.
263. Bartley AN, Luthra R, Saraiya DS, Urbauer DL, Broaddus RR. Identification of cancer patients with lynch syndrome: clinically significant discordances and problems in tissue-based mismatch repair testing. Cancer Prev Res (Phila). 2012;5(2):320–7. https://doi.org/10.1158/1940-6207.CAPR-11-0288.
264. Ring KL, Bruegl AS, Allen BA, et al. Germline multi-gene hereditary cancer panel testing in an unselected endometrial cancer cohort. Mod Pathol. 2016;29(11):1381–9. https://doi.org/10.1038/modpathol.2016.135.
265. Yunokawa M, Yoshida H, Watanabe R, et al. Allred score is a promising predictor of prognosis and medroxyprogesterone acetate efficacy in patients with endometrial cancer. Cancer Chemother Pharmacol. 2017;80(1):127–34. https://doi.org/10.1007/s00280-017-3342-5.
266. Chia K, O'Brien M, Brown M, Lim E. Targeting the androgen receptor in breast cancer. Curr Oncol Rep. 2015;17(2):4-014-0427-8. https://doi.org/10.1007/s11912-014-0427-8.
267. Gucalp A, Tolaney S, Isakoff SJ, et al. Phase II trial of bicalutamide in patients with androgen receptor-positive, estrogen

receptor-negative metastatic breast cancer. Clin Cancer Res. 2013;19(19):5505–12. https://doi.org/10.1158/1078-0432.CCR-12-3327.

268. Munoz J, Wheler JJ, Kurzrock R. Androgen receptors beyond prostate cancer: an old marker as a new target. Oncotarget. 2015;6(2):592–603.

269. Tangen IL, Onyango TB, Kopperud R, et al. Androgen receptor as potential therapeutic target in metastatic endometrial cancer. Oncotarget. 2016; https://doi.org/10.18632/oncotarget.10334.

270. Engelsen IB, Stefansson IM, Beroukhim R, et al. HER-2/neu expression is associated with high tumor cell proliferation and aggressive phenotype in a population based patient series of endometrial carcinomas. Int J Oncol. 2008;32(2):307–16.

271. Chen J, Zhao KN, Li R, Shao R, Chen C. Activation of PI3K/Akt/mTOR pathway and dual inhibitors of PI3K and mTOR in endometrial cancer. Curr Med Chem. 2014;21(26):3070–80.

272. Slomovitz BM, Coleman RL. The PI3K/AKT/mTOR pathway as a therapeutic target in endometrial cancer. Clin Cancer Res. 2012;18(21):5856–64. https://doi.org/10.1158/1078-0432.CCR-12-0662.

273. Santin AD, Bellone S, Buza N, et al. Regression of chemotherapy-resistant polymerase epsilon (POLE) ultra-mutated and MSH6 hyper-mutated endometrial tumors with nivolumab. Clin Cancer Res. 2016;22(23):5682–7. https://doi.org/10.1158/1078-0432.CCR-16-1031.

19 Endometritis and Tumor-Like Lesions

Bojana Djordjevic, Isabel Alvarado-Cabrero, and Simona Stolnicu

Abstract

A wide variety of benign endometrial conditions may involve the endometrium. These include infectious and noninfectious forms of endometritis, endometrial metaplasias, endometrial polyps, and iatrogenically induced endometrial conditions. Careful microscopic examination, correlation with clinical findings, and in some instances the use of ancillary testing are required to attain the correct diagnosis.

Keywords

Endometrial polyps · Endometritis · Endometrial metaplasia

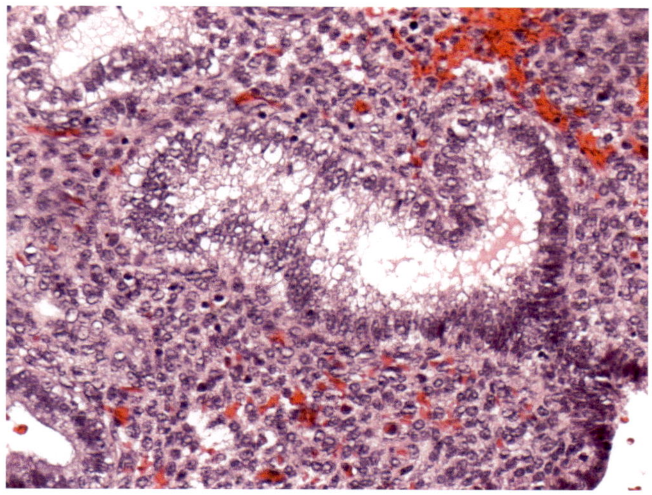

Fig. 19.1 Secretory phase endometrium. Lymphocytes in the endometrial stroma are considered a normal finding. They fluctuate in number and density throughout the menstrual cycle

19.1 Endometritis

A variety of immunocompetent cells, including T cells, macrophages, neutrophils, and natural killer cells infiltrates the endometrium. These cell subpopulations fluctuate in density during the different phases of the menstrual cycle (Fig. 19.1) [1] and are thought to play a crucial role in the dynamic endometrial tissue remodeling essential for conception and/or menstruation. By contrast, antibody-bearing lymphocytes such as B cells and plasmacytes are rare immunocompetent cells in this mucosal tissue [2].

Endometritis is a disorder that affects women of reproductive age, although it may also occur in postmenopausal patients. Patients typically present with abnormal vaginal bleeding, most commonly intermenstrual bleeding or menorrhagia. Endometritis may have both an infectious and noninfectious etiology [3, 4].

Endometritis may be acute, chronic, nonspecific, or specific such as tuberculosis, sarcoidosis, or coccidioidomycosis. These latter forms are uncommon, but acute and chronic nonspecific endometritis are frequent. The most common causes of endometritis are the following:

1. Ascending infection involving the vagina and cervix, frequently following instrumentation
2. Insertion of foreign material in an attempt to induce abortion
3. Insertion of intrauterine devices
4. Retained products of conception

B. Djordjevic
Division of Anatomic Pathology, Sunnybrook Health Sciences Centre, Toronto, ON, Canada

Department of Laboratory Medicine and Pathobiology, University of Toronto, Toronto, ON, Canada

I. Alvarado-Cabrero
Department of Pathology, Mexican Oncology Hospital, Mexico City, Mexico

S. Stolnicu (✉)
Department of Pathology, University of Medicine and Pharmacy of Targu Mures, Targu Mures, Romania

W. Zheng et al. (eds.), *Gynecologic and Obstetric Pathology, Volume 1*, https://doi.org/10.1007/978-981-13-3016-2_19

19.1.1 Acute Endometritis

Acute endometritis is usually characterized by abundant neutrophilic infiltration in the endometrial stroma. Glandular lumina may also be filled with polymorphonuclear leukocytes (Fig. 19.2). It may be frequently found following abortion or childbirth when products of conception and/or decidua are retained.

19.1.2 Chronic Endometritis

Chronic endometritis is usually the result of acute endometritis that either has not been treated or has been treated inadequately. The presence of plasma cells, most numerous in the periglandular and subepithelial stroma and around lymphoid aggregates, is the most important histologic feature of endometritis [5] (Fig. 19.3). The number of plasma cells does not appear to correlate with the severity of endometritis [6].

19.1.3 Specific Forms of Endometritis

19.1.3.1 *Actinomyces israelii*

Infection with *Actinomyces israelii* is another cause of endometritis. This organism is most commonly found in endometritis in association with the presence of an intrauterine device (Fig. 19.4) and accompanied by an intense inflammatory response, with many plasma cells, lymphocytes, and neutrophils throughout the endometrial tissue (Fig. 19.5). The organism shows sulfur granules, which can be stained by Gram and methenamine silver stains [7, 8].

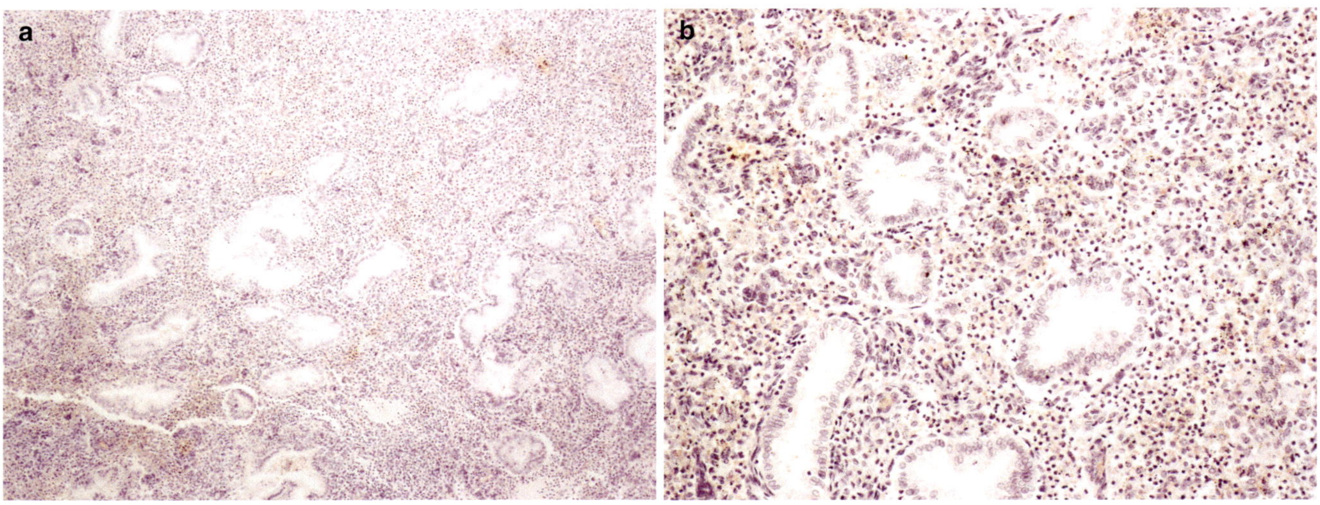

Fig. 19.2 Acute endometritis. Polymorphonuclear leukocytes are present throughout the stroma. (**a**) Low- and (**b**) high-power view

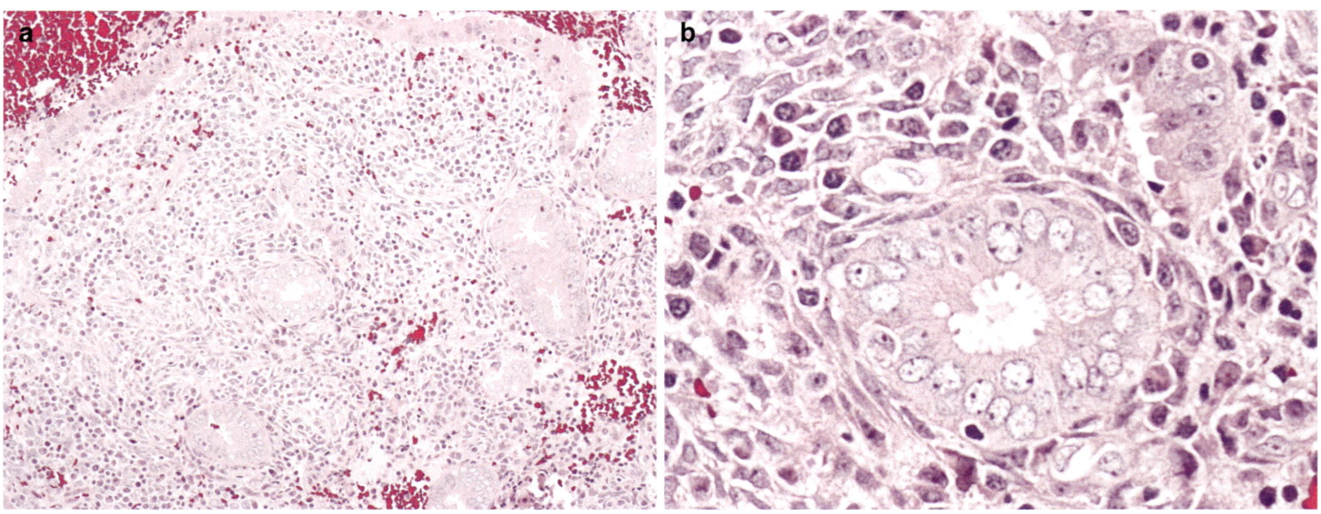

Fig. 19.3 Chronic endometritis. (**a**) Low-power view illustrates increased stromal cellularity associated with a mononuclear infiltrate; (**b**) high-power view shows plasmacytic infiltrate

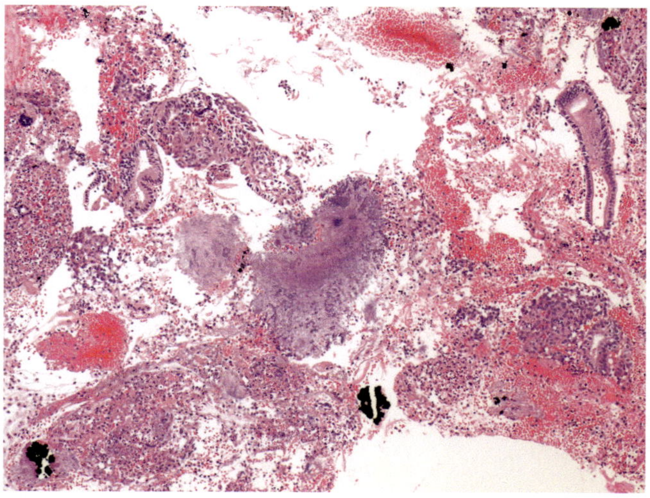

Fig. 19.4 Intrauterine device. Actinomyces sulfur granule surrounded by multifragmented endometrium

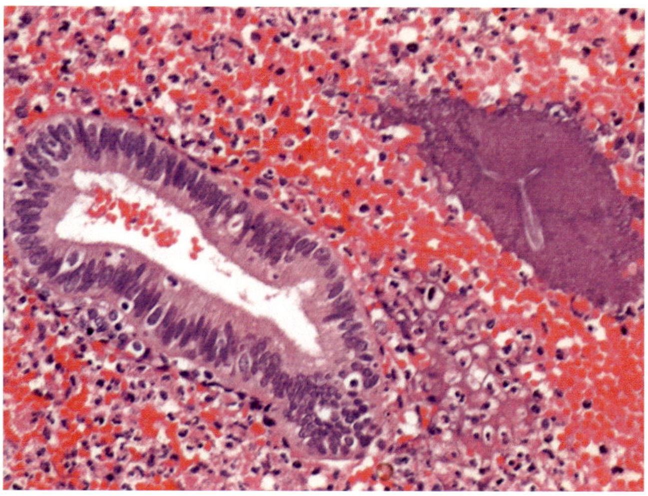

Fig. 19.5 Actinomyces infection. Endometrial gland and actinomycotic granule with associated acute inflammatory infiltrate

19.1.3.2 *Chlamydia trachomatis*

Chlamydia trachomatis is a relatively common cause of infection in both the upper and lower female genital tract, and as a consequence, the patients may develop pelvic inflammatory disease and infertility, although it is not clear whether the organism is the only one responsible for the disease or it may be accompanied by other pathogenic agents. *Chlamydia trachomatis* endometritis does not have specific histological features, although stromal necrosis, reactive atypia of the epithelial cells, and numerous plasma cells may be seen, and a definitive diagnosis requires culture in most cases [9, 10] (Fig. 19.6).

19.1.3.3 Tuberculosis Endometritis

The majority of tuberculosis endometritis are found in women who are being investigated for infertility. The patient may present without any gynecological symptoms or with irregular bleeding or amenorrhea [11].

The principal histological features of tuberculous endometritis are epithelioid cell granulomata (Fig. 19.7). The granulomata may be sparse in distribution and tend to be small and central. Caseation is unusual. Confirmation of the diagnosis of endometrial tuberculosis is best done by culture of the endometrial tissue. Staining the section with Ziehl-Neelsen stain is unlikely to be helpful [12].

19.1.3.4 Cytomegalovirus

Cytomegalovirus (CMV) infection of the endometrium has been rarely reported. It may be associated in some patients with pregnancy and immunosuppression [13]. The infection is accompanied by the characteristic viral cytopathic effects in epithelial and sometimes in endothelial cells (Fig. 19.8). The affected cells contain a usually large single, basophilic intranuclear inclusion, surrounded by a narrow clear space separating it from the nuclear membrane.

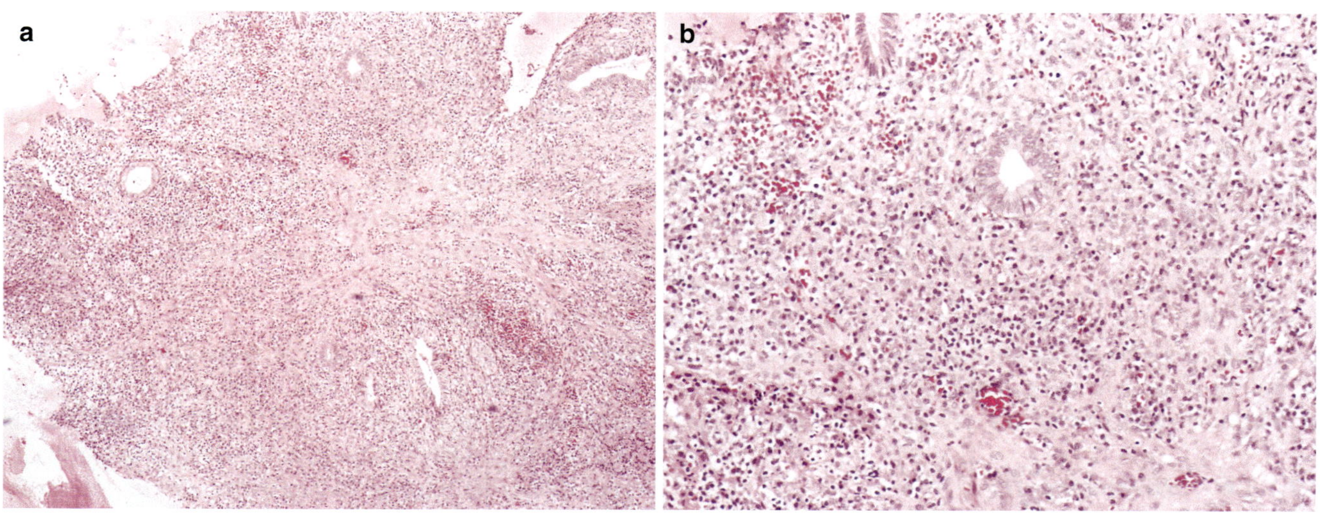

Fig. 19.6 Endometritis consisting with *Chlamydia trachomatis*. (**a**) Lower-power view shows increased stromal cellularity; (**b**) high-power view shows dense infiltrates of plasma cells within the stroma. Endometrial culture for *Chlamydia trachomatis* was positive

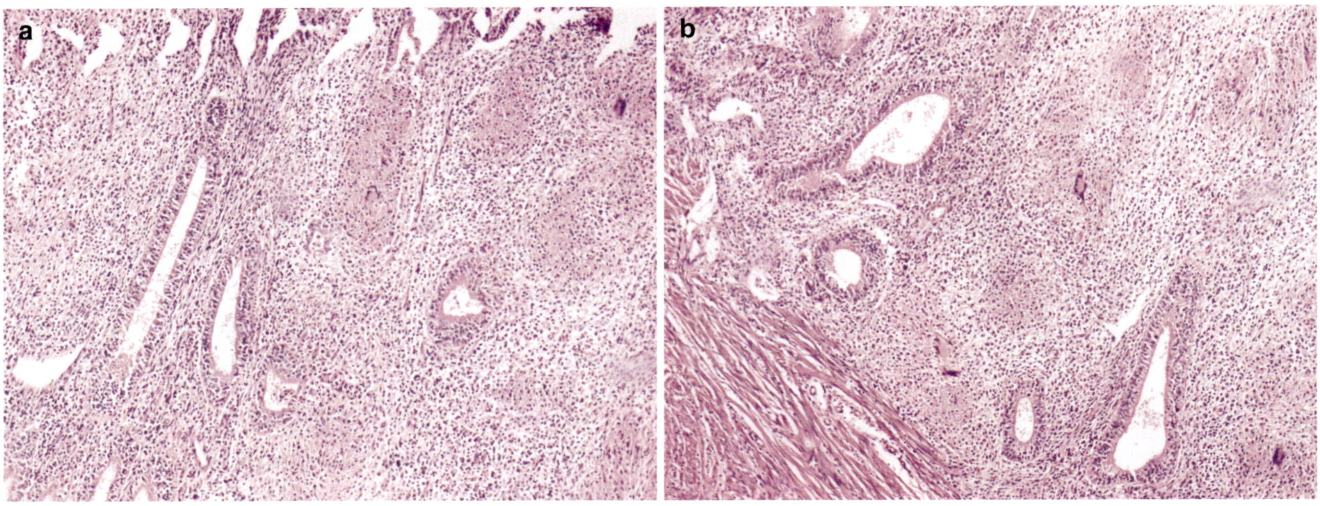

Fig. 19.7 Tuberculous endometritis. (**a**, **b**) Several noncaseating granulomas are scattered throughout the endometrial stroma

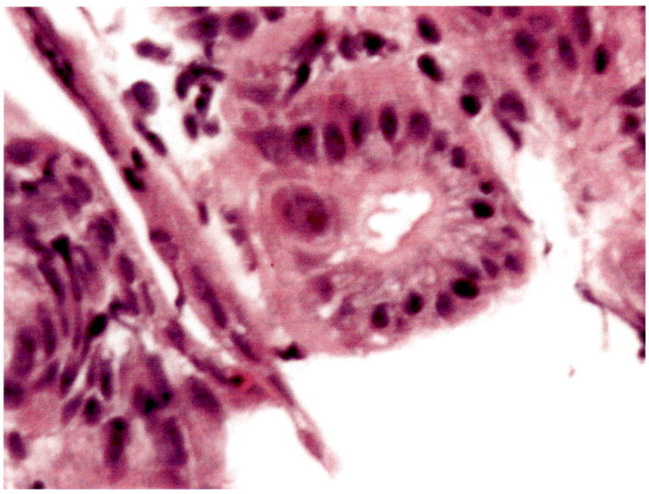

Fig. 19.8 Cytomegalovirus infection of the endometrial cell characterized by a large basophilic intranuclear inclusion

19.1.3.5 Herpetic Endometritis

Endometrial infection by herpes simplex virus (HSV) is rare [14]. It has been shown that more than 95% of genital herpes infections are caused by HSV type II. The infections may represent dissemination of the virus in immunocompromised patients, or ascending infections in women with lower genital tract disease. Symptoms include abnormal uterine bleeding and malodorous vaginal discharge [14]. Histologic features of herpetic endometritis are represented by nuclear inclusions and ground glass nuclei found in epithelial glands, as well as in stromal and endothelial cells. Necrosis of the endometrial glands and stroma may also occur [15].

19.1.3.6 Schistosomiasis

Schistosoma haematobium is a parasite that may cause diseases of the urinary tract but also of the female genital tract [16, 17]. In fact, up to 75% of women excreting *S. haematobium* ova in the urine may have schistosoma ova in the uterine cervix, vagina, or vulva [18]. Ova are most commonly found in the cervix, followed by the vagina, ovaries, and less commonly found in the fallopian tubes, vulva, and uterus. There are several reports of schistosomiasis of the female genital tract due to *S. mansoni* from Puerto Rico and Brazil [19].

Gynecologic *S. haematobium* has been associated with a range of lesions in the female genital tract such as ulcers, malignant tumors, and polyps [17, 18].

The histological diagnosis of schistosomiasis is often based on the finding of ova in the tissue. The morphologic findings associated to the presence of the ova are represented by the following five different types of changes [17]:

1. Ill-defined epithelioid granulomata and diffuse infiltration of the tissues by eosinophils, plasma cells, lymphocytes, and macrophages, while the ova are not present
2. Circumscribed granulomata represented by epithelioid cells, lymphocytes, eosinophils and fibroblasts in the presence of degenerating ova.
3. Foreign body giant cells associated with shell fragments in the presence of rare inflammatory cells
4. Large numbers of shell fragments surrounded by fibrous tissue with little or no inflammatory response
5. Sparse shell fragments without the presence of fibrosis

19.1.3.7 Malakoplakia

Malakoplakia is an uncommon and unusual type of granulomatous inflammation more often developing in the urinary tract, while the female genital tract is rarely interested [20]. In the female genital tract however, organs involved by malakoplakia are the vagina, endometrium, ovaries, fallopian tubes, and vulva. Genital malakoplakia is infrequent before menopause. The most common presenting symptom is

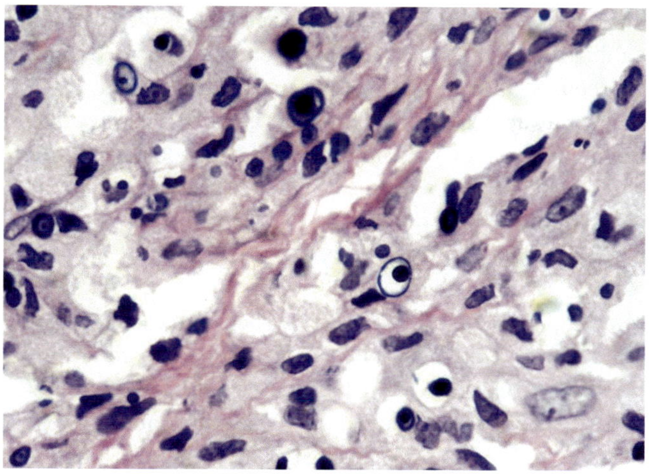

Fig. 19.9 Endometrium malakoplakia. Endometrial histiocytic infiltrate with Michaelis-Gutmann bodies

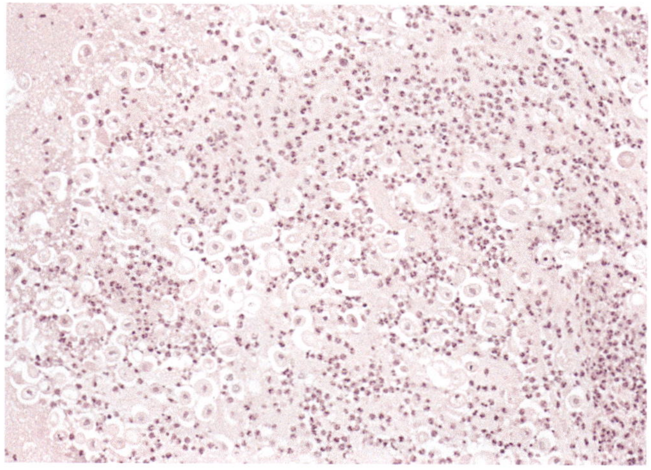

Fig. 19.10 Postpartum endometritis (acute endometritis). Abundant polymorphonuclear leukocytes infiltrate the decidua

vaginal bleeding, while menstrual irregularities, discharge, and dyspareunia are rarely reported [21].

Microscopically, endometrial tissue is diffusely involved by a mixed inflammatory infiltrate consisting of plasma cells, lymphocytes, and neutrophilic granulocytes. A large number of von Hansemann histiocytes characterized by an eosinophilic granular cytoplasm are also present. In the cytoplasm of some of these macrophages, round-basophilic bull's eye-like structures, known as Michaelis-Gutmann bodies (Fig. 19.9), are easily recognized. Endometrial glands are few and atrophic [22].

19.1.3.8 Mycoplasma and Endometritis

Pelvic inflammatory disease (PID) is the most frequently diagnosed severe gynecological infectious disorder, with serious sequelae in some cases. Although *Mycoplasma genitalium* has not been identified through serologic investigations in most cases, molecular studies have shown an association between *Mycoplasma genitalium* and nongonococcal cervicitis or acute endometritis [23].

Infection with a related pathogen, *Ureaplasma urealyticum*, produces subtle changes in the endometrium that may be easily missed at microscopic examination. The inflammatory cells are usually represented by lymphocytes, histiocytes with few neutrophils, and plasma cells [24].

19.1.3.9 Toxoplasma

Based on serological studies, *Toxoplasma gondii* is one of the most prevalent protozoan parasites in humans [25]. High prevalence of the infection has been reported affecting pregnant women and women of childbearing age in Latin America, Eastern Central Europe, the Middle East, Asia, and Africa [26].

Human infection is acquired through ingestion of food or water contaminated with oocytes shed in the feces of cats or viable tissue cysts in undercooked or raw meat. Primary infection during pregnancy may cause spontaneous abortion or stillbirth, while in utero infection may cause congenital abnormalities.

Toxoplasmosis has been linked to infertility and nonspecific inflammatory reaction in the endometrium. The microorganism can be identified by immunofluorescence [27].

19.1.3.10 Postpartum Endometritis

Postpartum endometritis refers to infection of the decidua, which is typically polymicrobial. It may also extend into the myometrium or involve the parametrium. Postpartum endometritis is a common cause of postpartum morbidity. The main pathogens involved are aerobic gram-positive cocci (group B streptococcus, enterococci, and staphylococcal species), anaerobic gram-positive cocci (*Peptococcus*), aerobic gram-negative bacilli (*E. coli*), and anaerobic gram-negative bacilli (*Bacteroides*) [28].

Fever is often the first sign, in association with uterine tenderness, uterine bleeding, and foul-smelling lochia. The histopathologic examination of the endometrium reveals prominence of neutrophils and tissue necrosis, signs of an acute infection (Fig. 19.10) [29].

19.1.3.11 "Senile" Endometritis

During menopause, the endometrium becomes thin and inactive. The vascular supply is diminished, and endometritis can occur. Plasma cells and increased numbers of lymphocytes are seen in the stroma [30].

19.1.3.12 Sarcoidosis

Sarcoidosis is a systemic disease that predominantly affects women of premenopausal age. Thirty to fifty percent of cases exhibit extrapulmonary involvement, which occurs in the genital tract in less than 1% of the cases [31–33]. Endometrial sarcoidosis may present as menometrorrhagia,

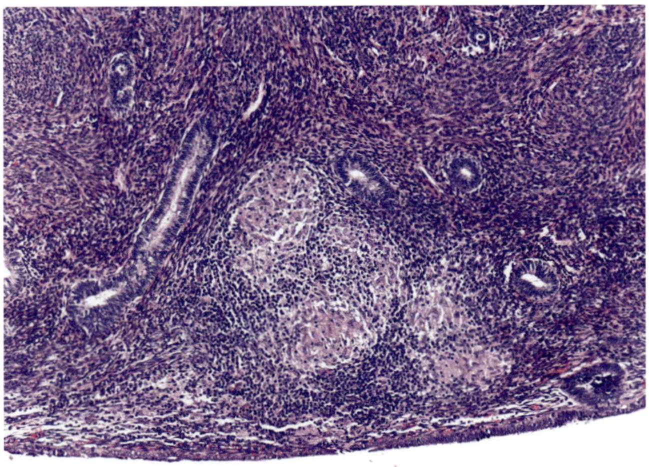

Fig. 19.11 Sarcoidosis involving the endometrium. Multiple noncaseating epithelioid cell granulomata (Courtesy of Dr. Francisco F. Nogales)

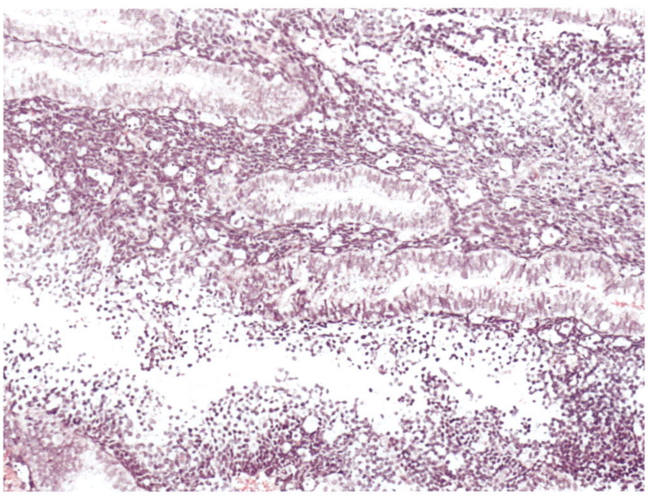

Fig. 19.12 Histiocytic endometritis. Endometrium with a sheet of histiocytic cells

postmenopausal bleeding, or rarely as a polypoid lesion or serometra [34–36]. Microscopically, sarcoidosis appears in the endometrium as noncaseating epithelioid granulomata (Fig. 19.11). Diagnosis of sarcoidosis should not be made without correlation with clinical history, exclusion of infectious (as described in the text above), and other noninfectious conditions. Focal noncaseating granulomata most commonly occur in the setting of previous endometrial instrumentation or bleeding [33, 37].

19.1.3.13 Histiocytic Endometritis

Histiocytic endometritis is a process seen following conditions like hematometra or pyometra, characterized by replacement of the endometrial layer by sheets of lipid containing histiocytic cells (Fig. 19.12). Histiocytic inflammation is an unusual condition that involves organs such as the kidney and gallbladder, which are subject to chronic obstruction with subsequent infection. Involvement of the uterus is rare. Greater awareness of this condition is needed because it can mimic malignancy with infiltration of the endometrium [38].

19.2 Endometrial Polyps

The endometrial polyp is a common benign tumor-like lesion that is considered to be a benign neoplasm according to the latest World Health Organization (WHO) classification [39, 40]. It represents the second most common cause of abnormal uterine bleeding. The lesion develops more frequently in patients during late reproductive (usually after 40 years of age) or postmenopausal years. Endometrial polyps occur frequently in patients receiving tamoxifen treatment for breast cancer or patients receiving hormonal replacement therapy. Thus, hormonal influences may play a role in endometrial polyp pathogenesis. Different studies have demonstrated a correlation between the development of an endometrial polyp and various chromosomal anomalies (involving chromosomes 6 and 12) [41]; polyps arise as a monoclonal neoplastic proliferation of genetically altered stromal cells, and while some authors believe that the glandular component is secondarily incorporated, others contend that the stromal proliferation induces the polyclonal proliferation of benign glands through a yet poorly understood mechanism [39, 42]. Hypertension, obesity, and late menopause are associated with the development of endometrial polyps.

19.2.1 Clinical Presentations

Clinically, a polyp is associated with intermenstrual or postmenopausal uterine bleeding and infertility, but in about 25% of cases, the diagnosis is an incidental finding, especially when the polyp is of small size. In about 15–25% of patients have multiple polyps [43].

19.2.2 Gross Findings

On ultrasound examination and macroscopically, an endometrial polyp has a characteristically round to oval shape and protrudes into the uterine cavity. It can be sessile (broad base) or pedunculated (narrow base), with size ranging from less than 1 cm to as large as the uterine cavity itself (Figs. 19.13, 19.14, and 19.15). Since the polyp frequently occupies the uterine cavity, biopsy with a Pipelle device may be challenging, especially while trying to obtain tissue from the non-polypoid areas of the endometrium. If it is too large or pedunculated, the tumor can protrude through the

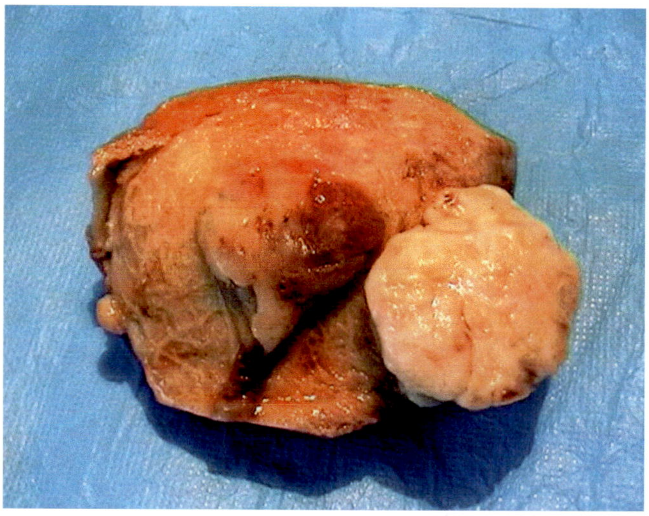

Fig. 19.13 Endometrial polyp: macroscopic examination reveals the presence of a polyp within the uterine fundus and a leiomyoma in the uterine wall; the polyp has a round shape, a broad base, a gray color, and the external surface is smooth and shiny

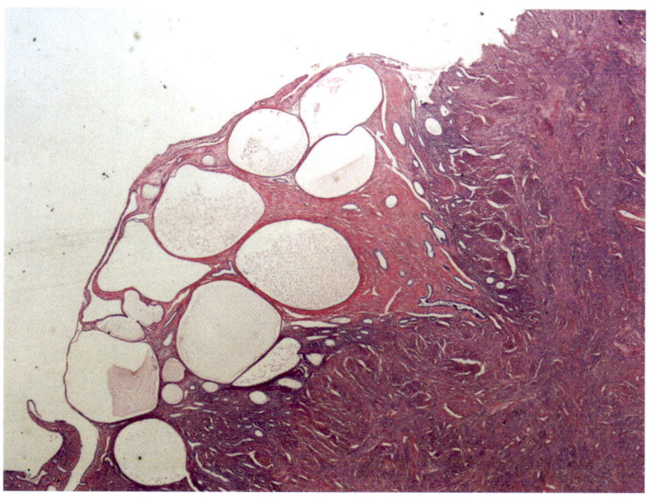

Fig. 19.14 Endometrial polyp of small size

endocervical canal and reach the external cervix mimicking a cervical lesion. The polyp can be located anywhere in the uterine cavity, but it is most commonly found in the uterine fundus. The external surface is smooth and shiny. On cross section, the polyp is of gray-white color and contains multiple cystic cavities of variable diameter due to cystic dilatation of the glandular elements. There may be infarction areas resembling hemorrhage, secondary to torsion.

19.2.3 Microscopic Findings and Biomarkers

Microscopically, the lesion consists of (1) irregularly distributed glands within a (2) hypocellular stroma that contains (3) thick-walled vessels (Fig. 19.16). In general, two out of the three abovementioned criteria should be met within a region of endometrial functionalis for a diagnosis of endometrial polyp in a curettage sample. The glandular and stromal components usually differ in appearance from glands in the adjacent normal endometrium in the vicinity (Figs. 19.17, 19.18, and 19.19). The base of the polyp can be broad or thin and can be examined within a surgical specimen (Figs. 19.20, 19.21, 19.22, and 19.23). Within a polyp, the glands can be of small size and round shape or have a branched irregular outline. They are and sometimes cystically dilated. Other times, due to the elongation of the polypoid mass, glands located in the stalk of a polypoid mass may also look elongated (Fig. 19.24). Usually, the glands are oriented in parallel to the surface epithelium. The epithelium may show weak secretory or proliferative activity, or a variety of metaplastic changes (discussed later), depending on the age of the patients and the hormonal influence (Figs. 19.25, 19.26, 19.27, 19.28, 19.29, and 19.30). Areas of necrosis and thrombosis can occur followed by regeneration of the epithelium, which may sometimes present with reactive atypia. Regenerative changes

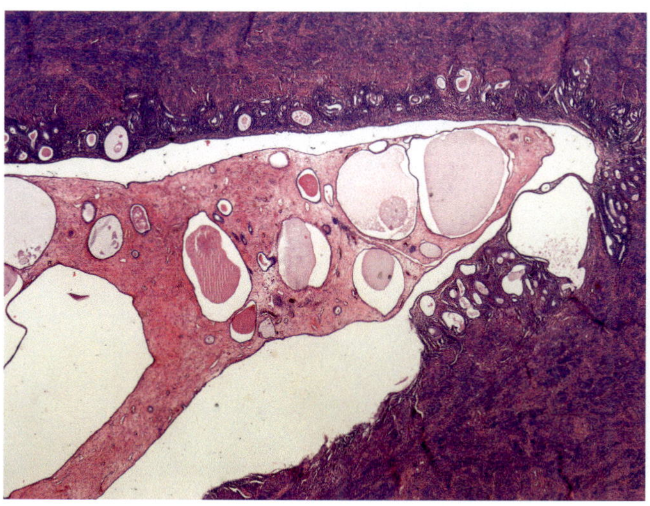

Fig. 19.15 Endometrial polyp of larger size occupying the uterine cavity

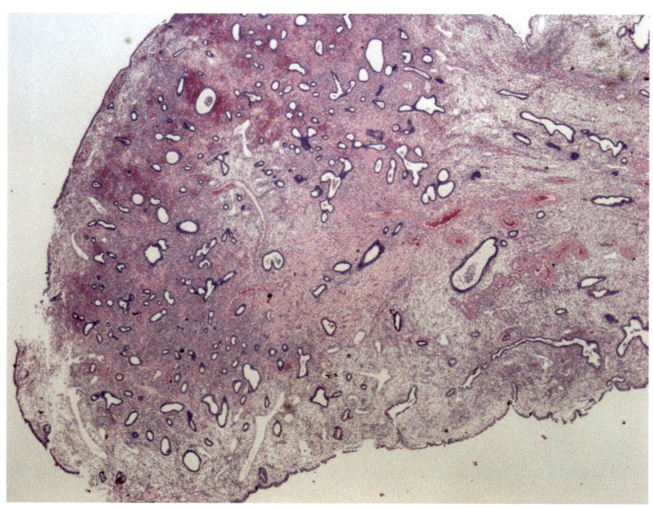

Fig. 19.16 Endometrial polyp represented by glandular component, within a fibrous stroma containing thick-walled vessels

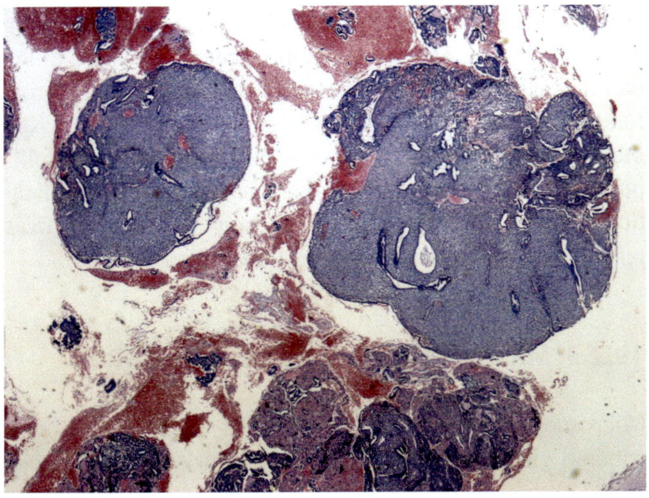

Fig. 19.17 Endometrial polyp: the appearance differs from the one of the fragments of endometrial mucosa in the vicinity

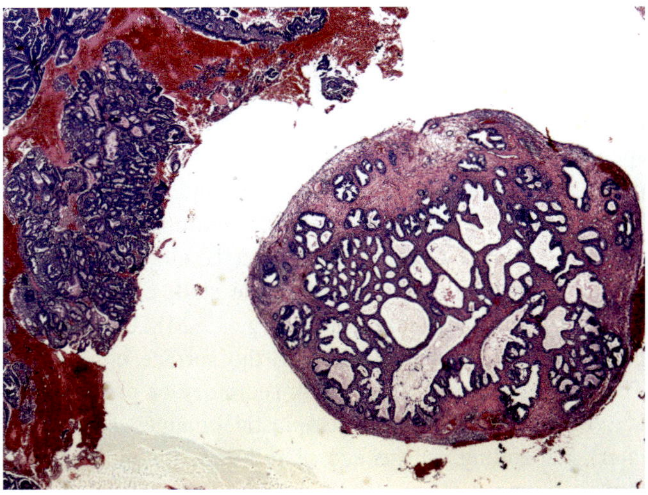

Fig. 19.18 Endometrial polyp: the appearance differs from the one of the fragments of endometrial mucosa with endometrioid-type adenocarcinoma in the vicinity

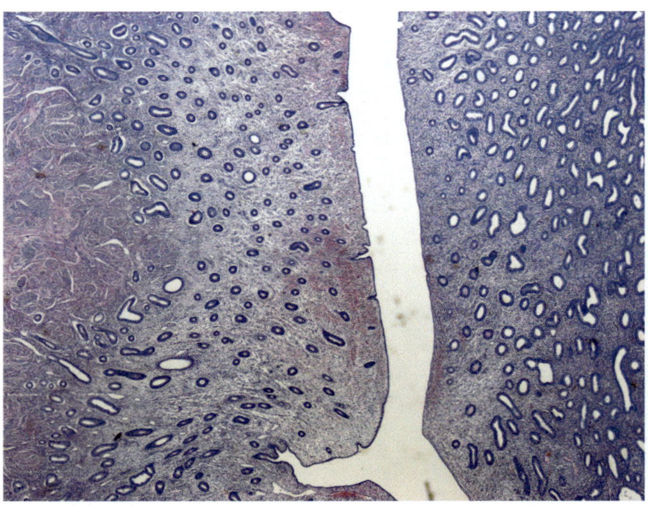

Fig. 19.19 Endometrial polyp: the appearance is very similar to the one of the normal mucosa (left side) except the more numerous glands within the polyp which are more disoriented (right side)

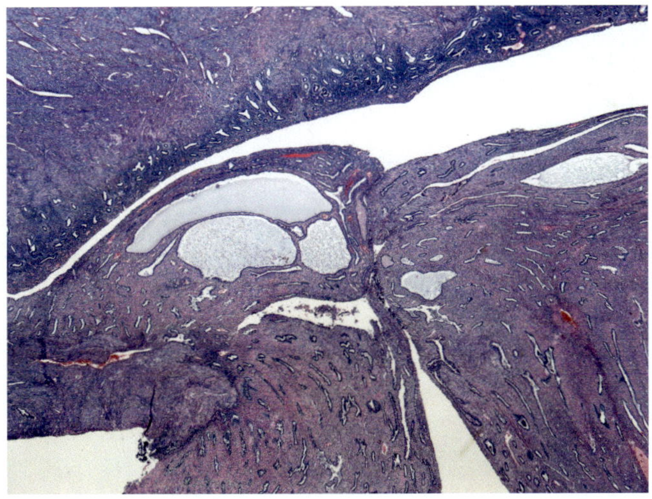

Fig. 19.20 Endometrial polyp with a thin base of implantation

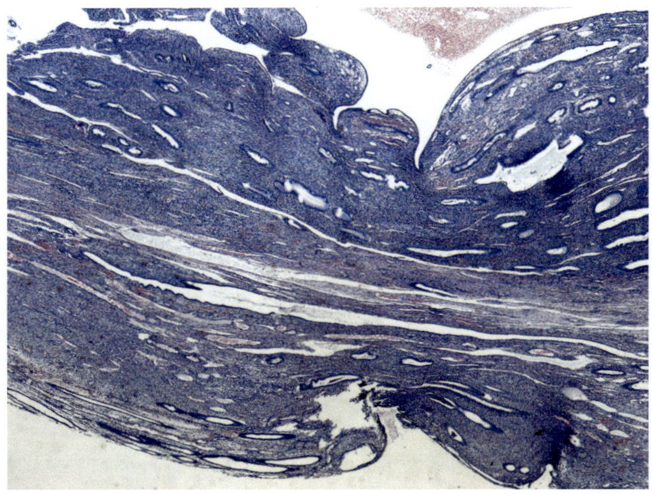

Fig. 19.21 The base of a pediculate polyp has a similar appearance with the rest of the polyp, but the glands are more elongated

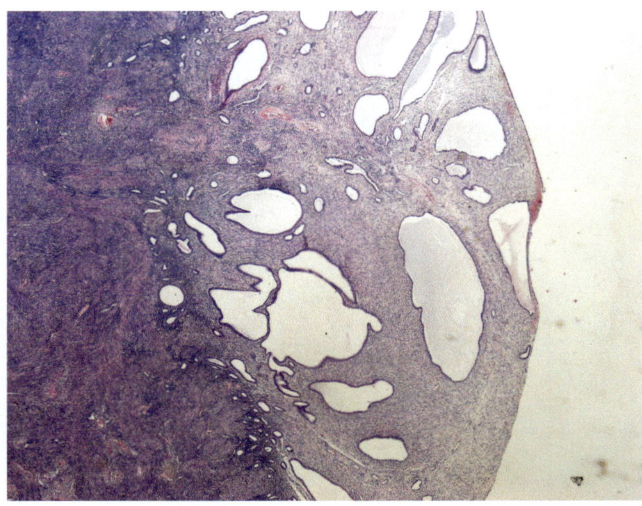

Fig. 19.22 Atrophic endometrial polyp of small size but with broad base

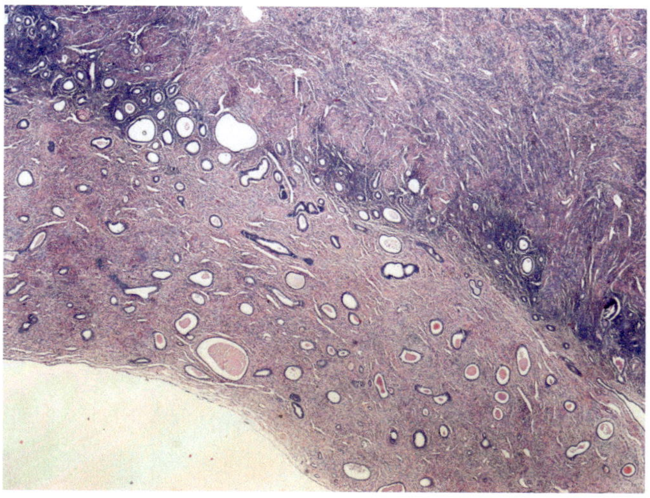

Fig. 19.23 Atrophic endometrial polyp with broad base (sessile)

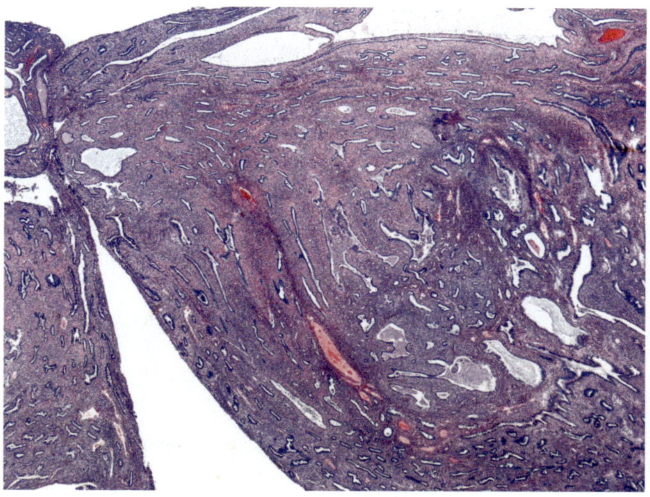

Fig. 19.24 Endometrial polyp: due to the elongation of the polypoid mass, the glands may be elongated as well

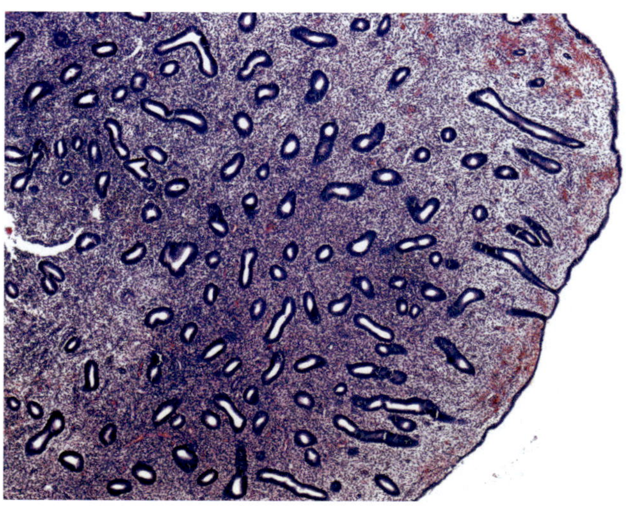

Fig. 19.25 Within an endometrial polyp, the glands can be of small size and round shape

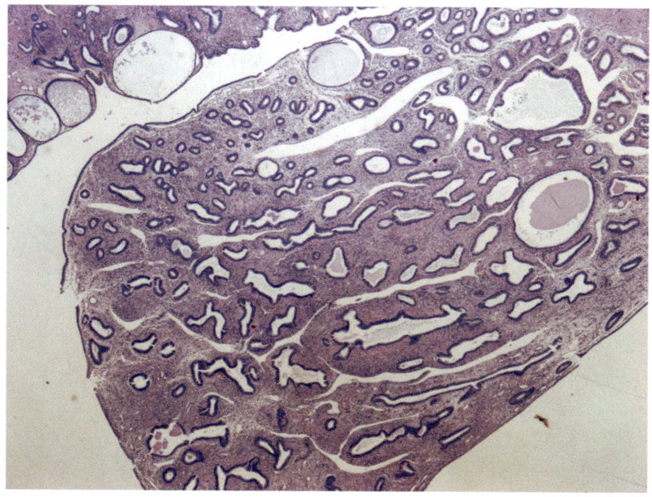

Fig. 19.26 Endometrial polyp with glands that are small and round but admixed with larger size glands and glands of various size and shape

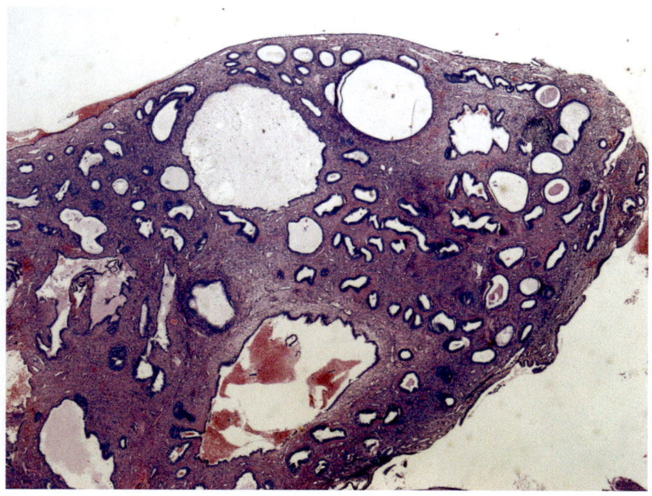

Fig. 19.27 Endometrial polyp with cystically dilated glands

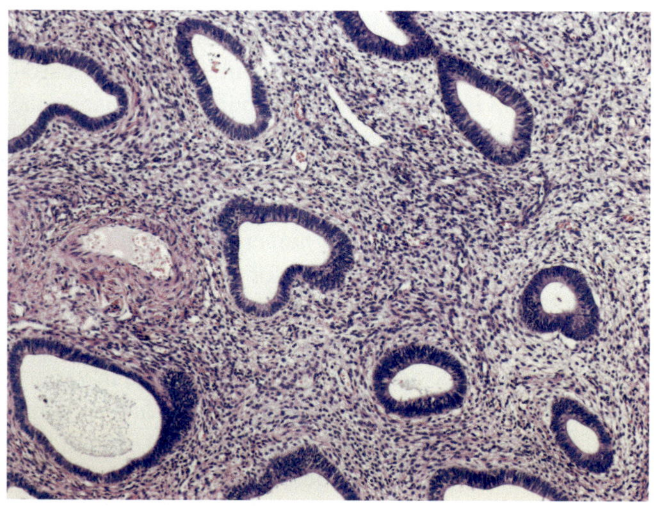

Fig. 19.28 Endometrial polyp: glands are lined by pseudostratified epithelium lacking atypia

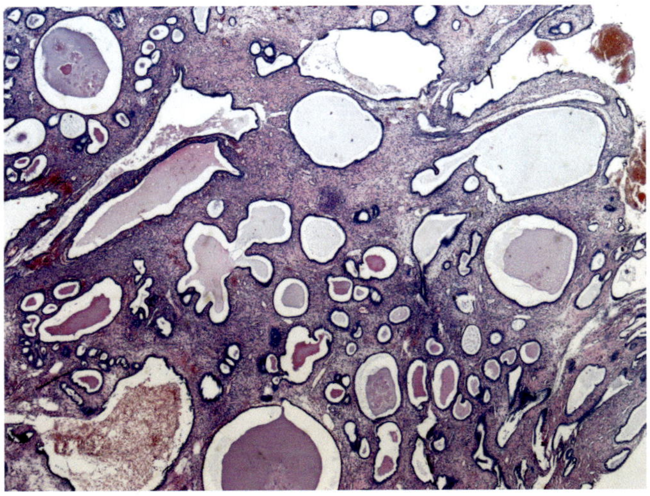

Fig. 19.29 Endometrial polyp containing various size and shape glands

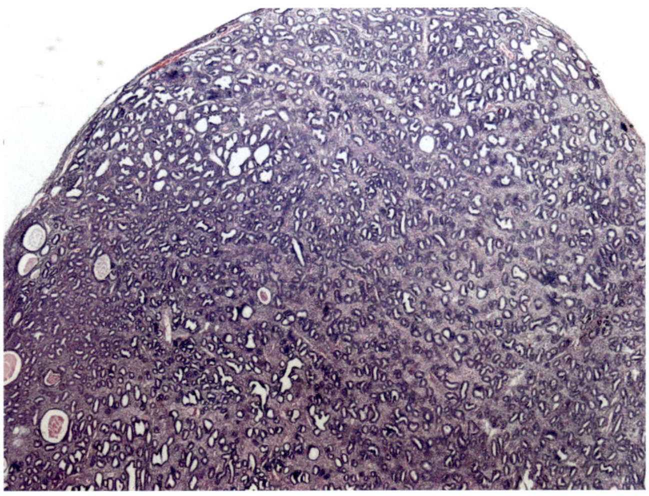

Fig. 19.30 Sometimes the polyp can present numerous glands

can occur especially in older patients, and these changes should not be interpreted as intraepithelial serous carcinoma. The p53 immunostain can help in differentiating the two lesions since the regenerative changes would be focally positive for this marker only (Figs. 19.31, 19.32, 19.33, 19.34, 19.35, 19.36, and 19.37). In an endometrial polyp, thick-walled vessels are more numerous than in a normal endometrium, another clue for correct diagnosis (Figs. 19.38 and 19.39). The stroma is composed of spindle-shaped fibroblasts, and, in rare cases, atypical bizarre cells can be encountered, similar to the one described in various polypoid lesions of the vulva, vagina, cervix, and endometrium and with unclear etiology (Figs. 19.40, 19.41, and 19.42) [44]. These cells can be focal or multifocal. Their nuclei are stellate in shape, hyperchromatic, and may be multilobulated and contain prominent nucleoli. It is important that these nuclear features are not misinterpreted as a

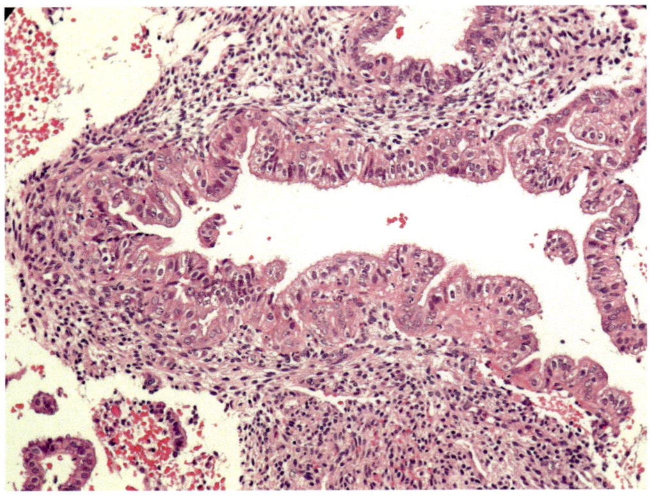

Fig. 19.31 Ciliated metaplasia within a polyp (Courtesy of Dr. Francisco F. Nogales)

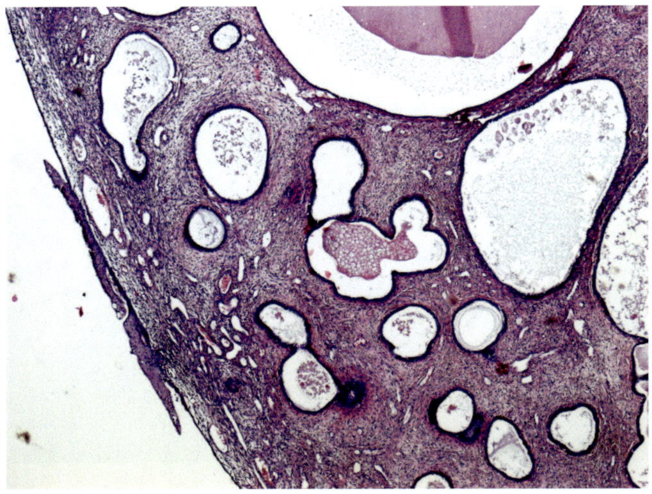

Fig. 19.32 Area of squamous metaplasia involving the surface epithelium of a polyp

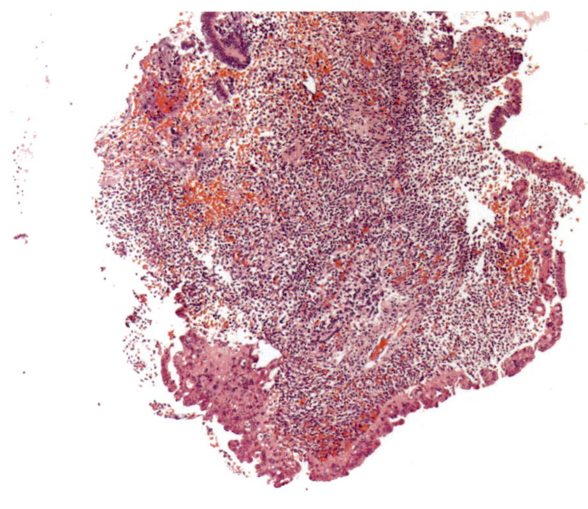

Fig. 19.33 Extensive areas of papillary syncytial metaplasia in a polyp of a patient of 89 years old (Courtesy of Dr. Francisco F. Nogales)

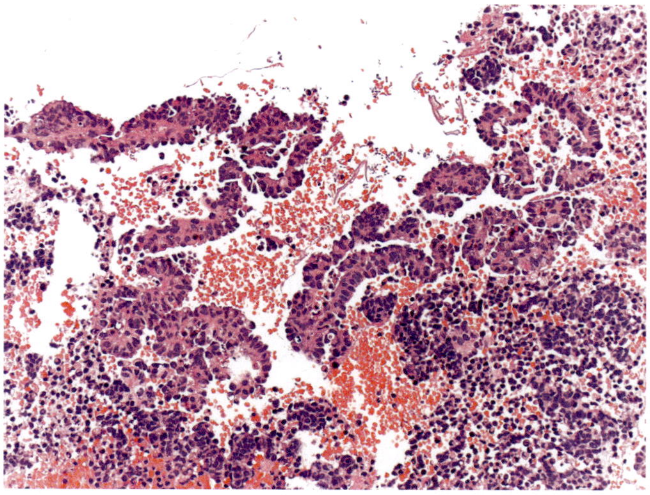

Fig. 19.34 Regenerative changes within a polyp should not be interpreted as intraepithelial serous carcinoma (Courtesy of Dr. Francisco F. Nogales)

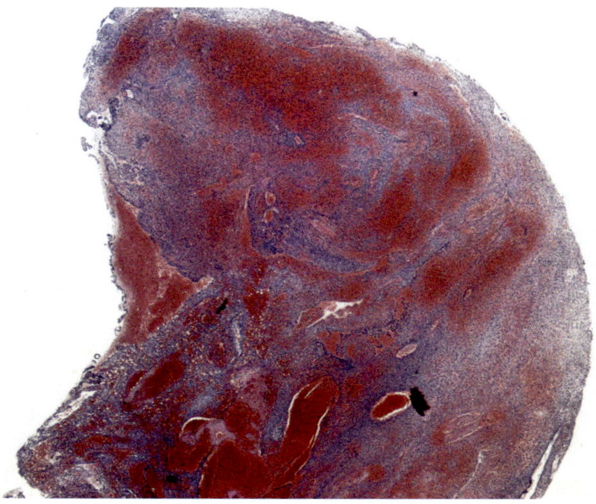

Fig. 19.35 Massive hemorrhage due to the torsion of a polyp

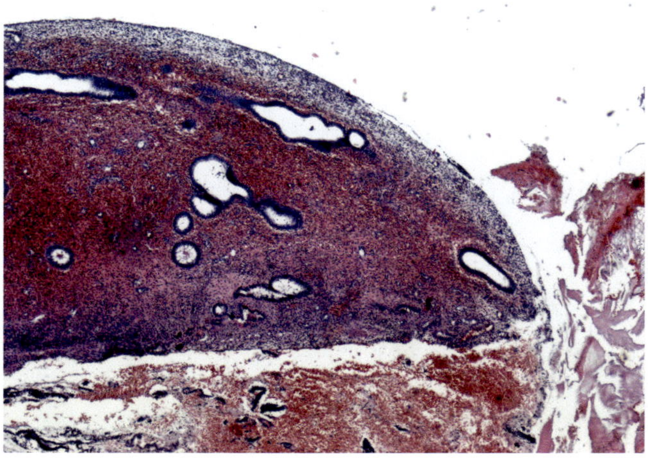

Fig. 19.36 Endometrial polyp with torsion: areas of glandular and stromal component are difficult to detect

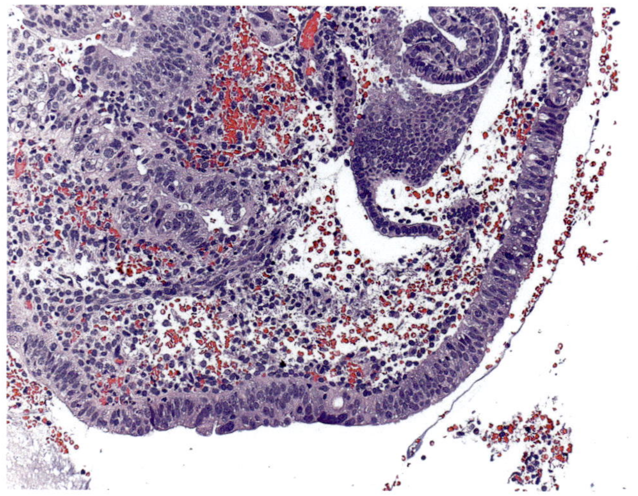

Fig. 19.37 Due to torsion or necrosis, areas of regeneration can occur especially involving the surface epithelium with cells presenting larger amount of eosinophilic cytoplasm and enlarged hyperchromatic nuclei; however, the mitotic figures are absent

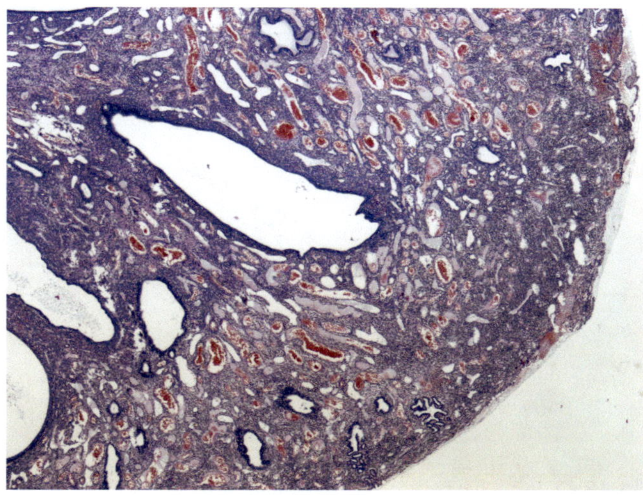

Fig. 19.38 Endometrial polyp with numerous thick-walled vessels

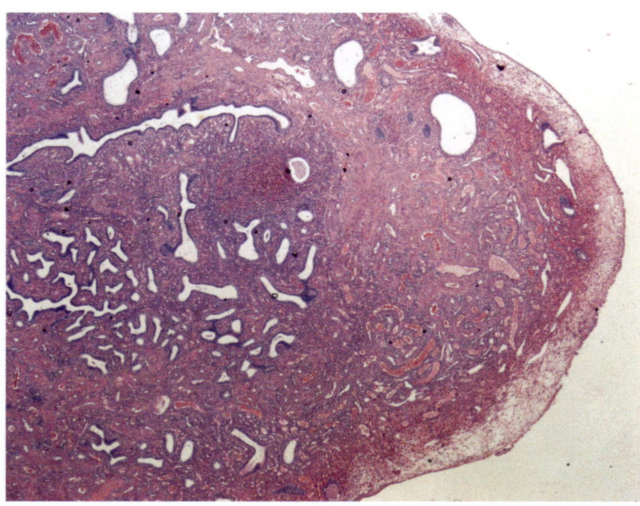

Fig. 19.39 The thick-walled vessels are more numerous in an endometrial polyp than in a normal endometrium, which is a clue for correct diagnosis

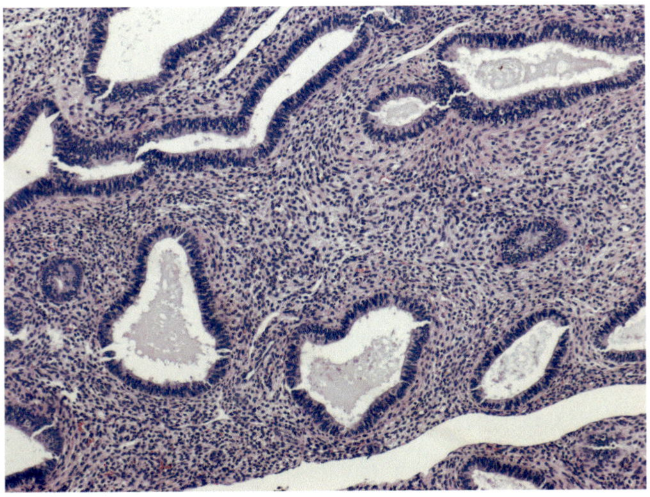

Fig. 19.40 The stroma of a polyp is composed of spindle-shaped fibroblasts

malignant feature. In these particularly difficult situations, ancillary immunohistochemical stains are helpful, since these cells are invariably positive for vimentin, estrogen receptor (ER), progesterone receptor (PR), and androgen receptor (AR), and occasionally and focally for CD10, for smooth muscle markers such as actin, desmin, and h-caldesmon. However, atypical stromal cells are consistently negative for cytokeratins, epithelial membrane antigen, myogenin, CD34, factor VIII, and macrophage markers [44]. On some occasions, a nonspecific inflammatory infiltrate represented by lymphocytes and plasma cells can be encountered within a polyp. When polyp stroma exhibits increased mitotic activity (up to five mitotic figures/10HPF) or is more cellular, this is very unusual and is more characteristic for either adenosarcoma (as a cambium layer) or hyperplasia (if this is a diffuse phenomenon) [45] (Figs. 19.43, 19.44, 19.45, 19.46, and 19.47). Also, some

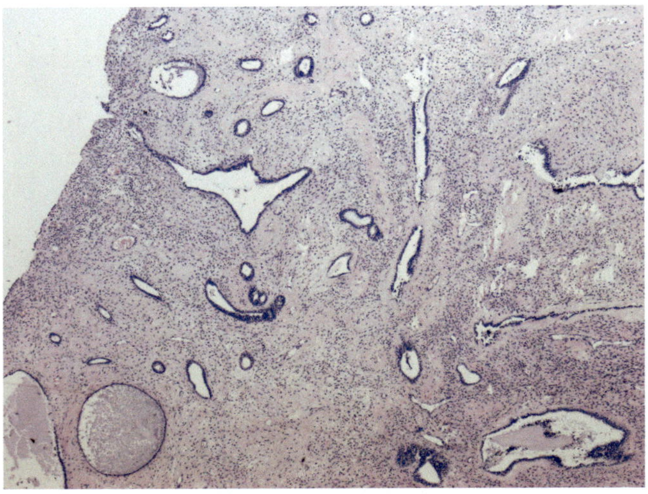

Fig. 19.41 Atrophic polyp with less cellular stroma

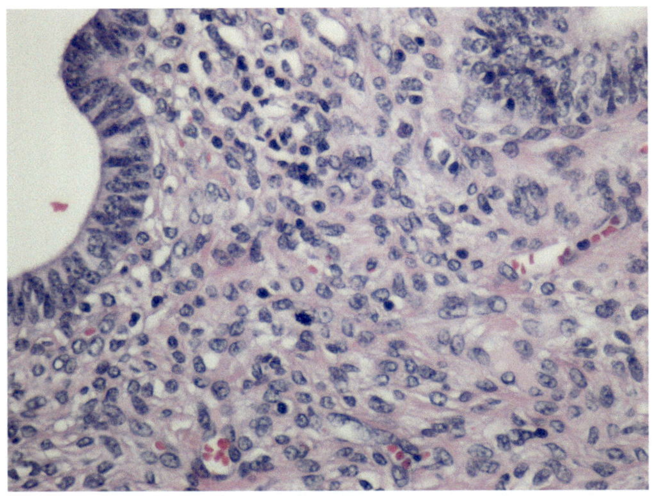

Fig. 19.43 Endometrial polyp with increased mitotic activity within the stroma

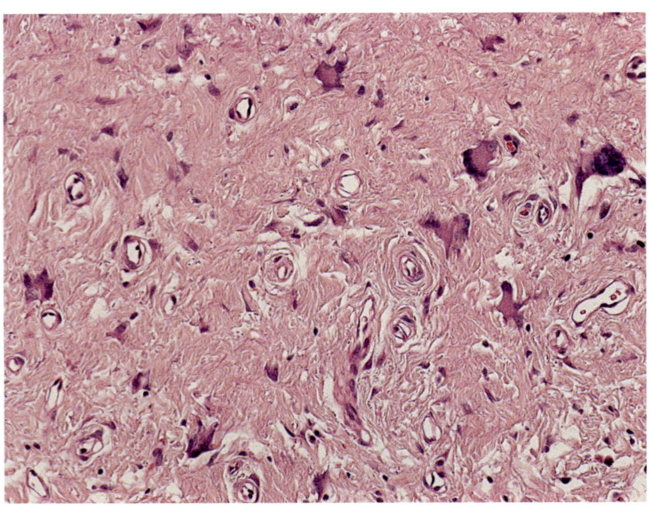

Fig. 19.42 Atypical stromal cells: enlarged cells of stellate or bizarre shape, with moderate to severe atypical hyperchromatic, and no mitoses

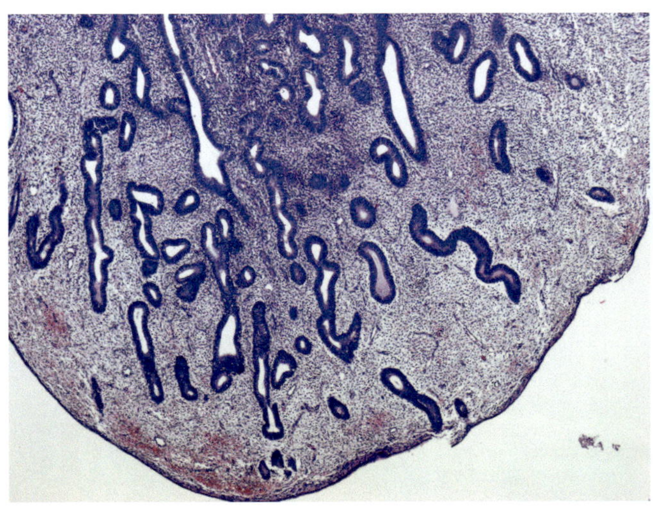

Fig. 19.44 Endometrial polyp with stromal edema

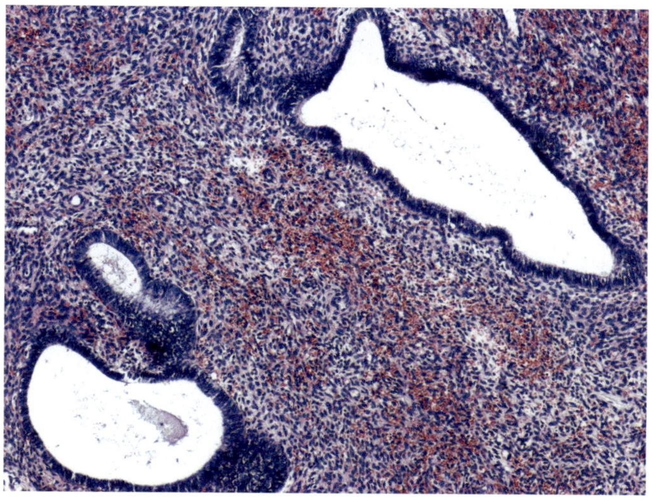

Fig. 19.45 Endometrial polyp with numerous erythrocytes within the stroma

polyps can present areas of smooth muscle differentiation as well as decidual areas. Very rarely, polyps can present areas of hyperplasia or endometrial intraepithelial neoplasia (EIN) as well as areas of invasive endometrioid adenocarcinoma. Polyps occurring especially in postmenopausal patients have a higher risk of associated EIN in about 5% of cases [46]. Also, areas of in situ or invasive serous carcinoma can occur in polyps especially in elderly women (Figs. 19.48, 19.49, 19.50, 19.51, 19.52, and 19.53). Since in some cases, very small microscopic foci of serous carcinoma may occur, these areas can be overlooked in a large polyp. In rare cases, metastasis occurs within a polyp, most of the times from a primary breast carcinoma (Fig. 19.54).

There are several types of endometrial polyps such as hyperplastic, atrophic, functional (with secretory or proliferative glands), and mixed. The hyperplastic polyp is the most frequent and consists of glands resembling those

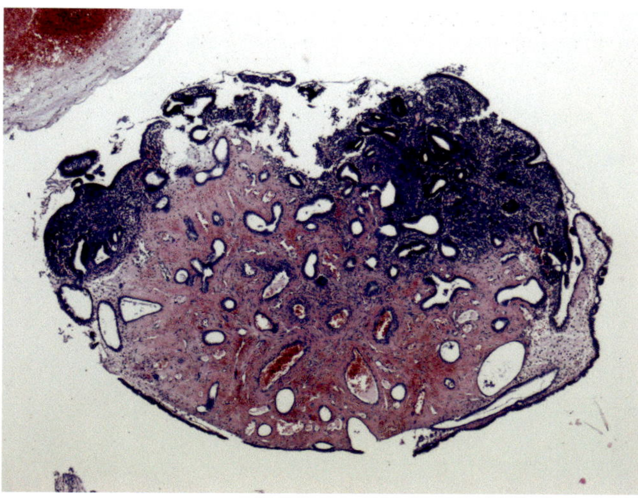

Fig. 19.46 Endometrial polyp with areas of more cellular stroma

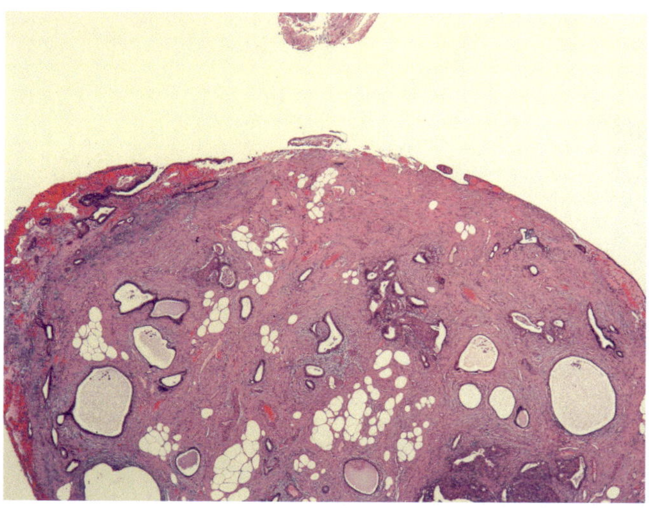

Fig. 19.47 Endometrial polyp with areas of lipomatous metaplasia (Courtesy of Dr. Francisco F. Nogales)

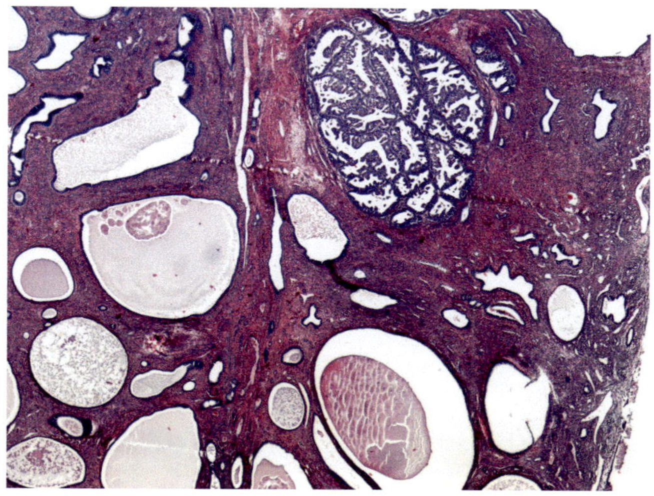

Fig. 19.48 Endometrial polyp with a small area of endometrial hyperplasia

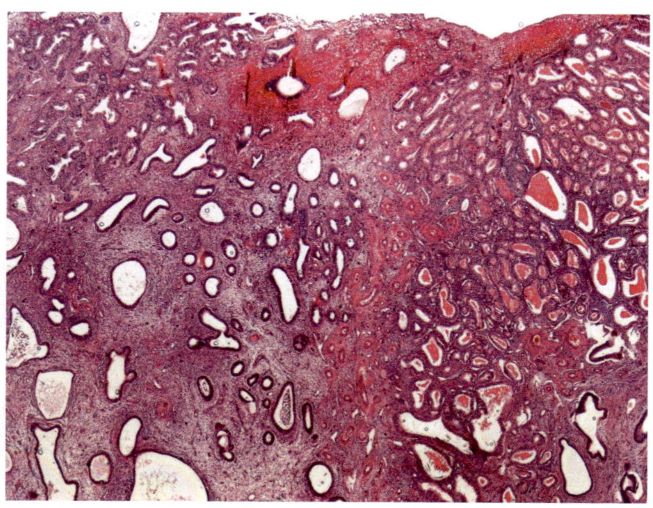

Fig. 19.49 Endometrial polyp with endometrial hyperplasia

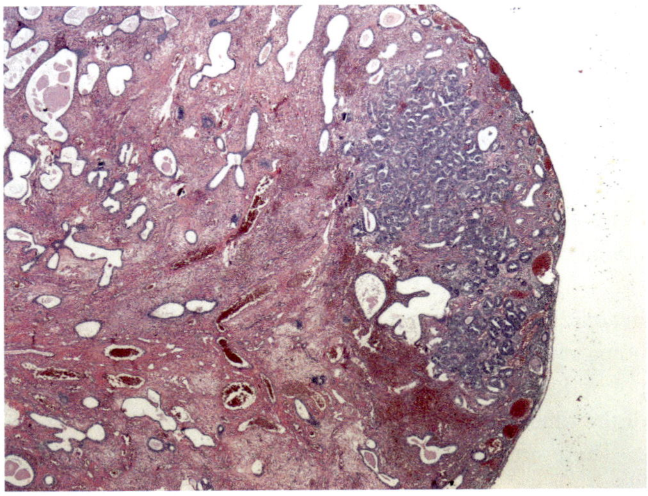

Fig. 19.50 Endometrial polyp with area of EIN (endometrial intraepithelial neoplasia)

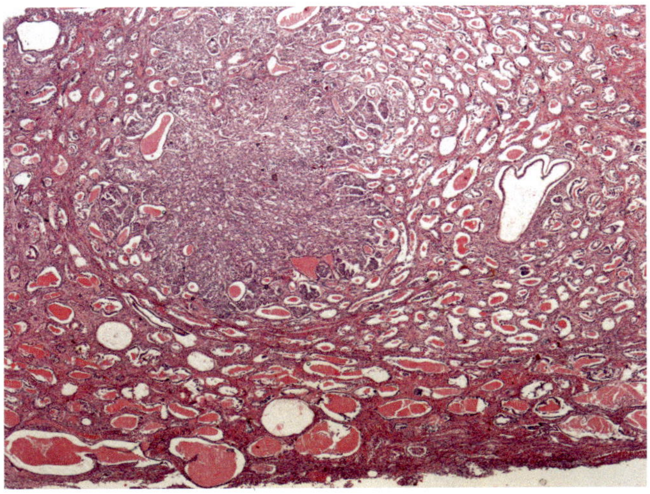

Fig. 19.51 Endometrial polyp with area of endometrioid-type adenocarcinoma

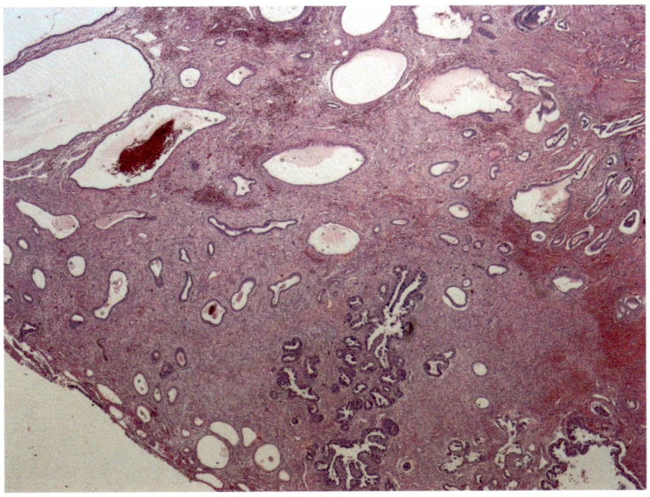

Fig. 19.52 Endometrial polyp with a small area of in situ serous carcinoma in an old patient; these areas can be overlooked especially within in a large polyp

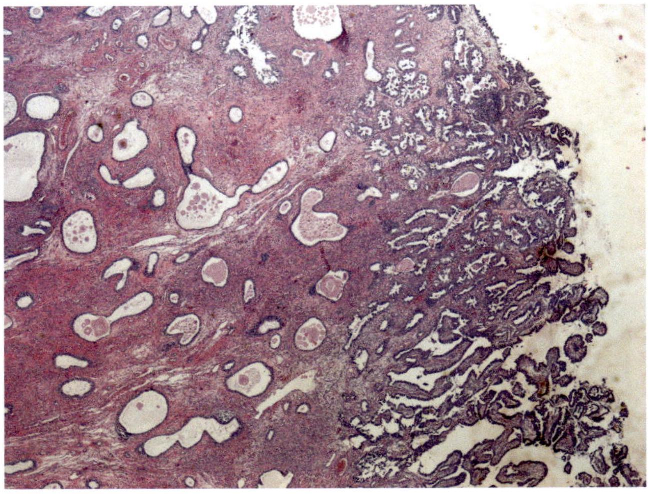

Fig. 19.53 Endometrial polyp with an area of serous carcinoma

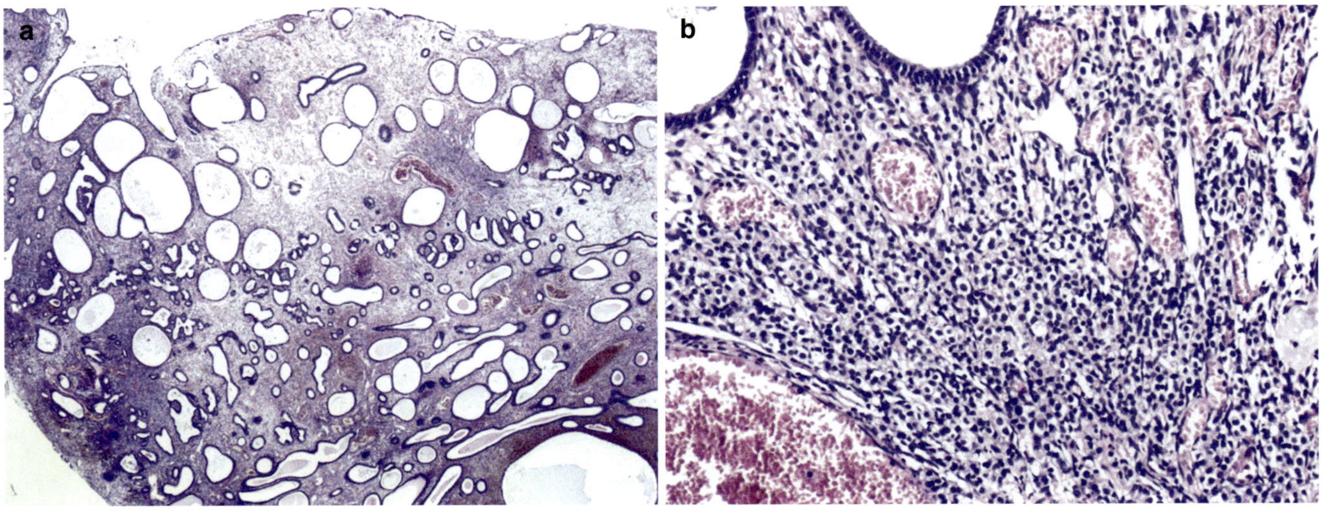

Fig. 19.54 Endometrial polyp with metastasis of primary breast carcinoma in a 65-year-old patient with history of breast carcinoma: (**a**) the polyp contains areas of small cells within the stroma; (**b**) the cells are small and uniform, and some of them present intracytoplasmic lumina resembling a lobular carcinoma of the breast; (**c**) the cells are positive for cytokeratin 7; (**d**) ER; (**e**) mammaglobin; (**f**) GCDFP15; (**g**) HMW cytokeratin; and (**h**) are negative for E-cadherin

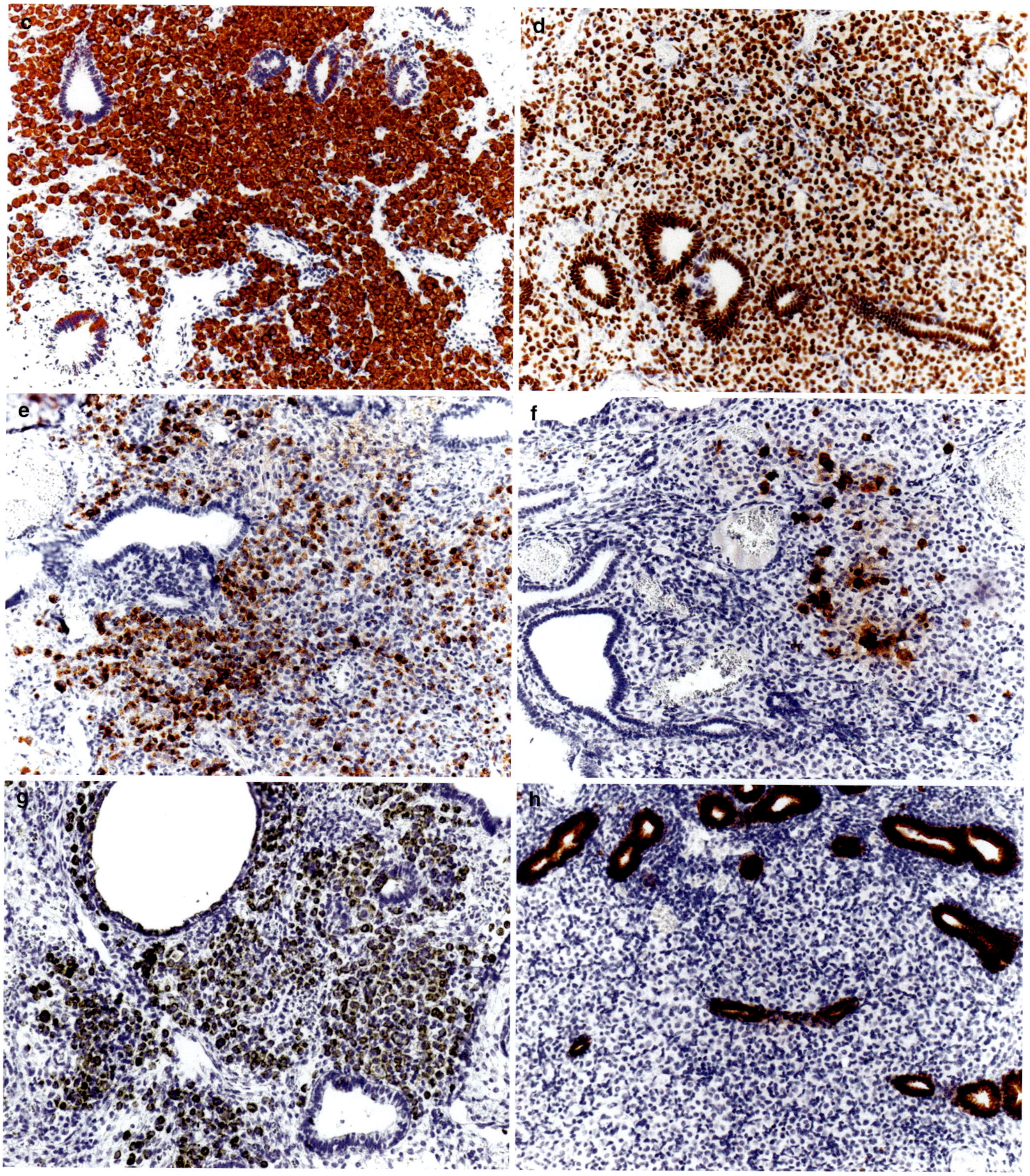

Fig. 19.54 (continued)

identified in endometrial hyperplasia or proliferative-type endometrium. It contains glands of various shapes and sizes, with irregular distribution and having proliferative or secretory activity. This type of polyp occurs under the estrogenic stimulation during the reproductive period and is frequently encountered. An atrophic polyp consists of small or cystically dilated glands, lined by a usually attenuated and atrophic, sometimes cuboid and rarely cylindrical epithelium. This type of polyp appears more frequently in postmenopausal patients and, according to some authors, is a variant of a hyperplastic or functional polyp, which has undergone regressive changes. The functional polyp is a rarer lesion and consists of glands with a similar appearance to that of the adjacent endometrium, thus suggesting that this type of polyp responds to hormonal stimulation during the menstrual cycle. Sometimes the glands may be indistinguishable from those in the rest of the endometrium, but most often the glands within the polyp are different from the ones within the mucosa. The mixed polyp usually occurs in the lower uterine segment and is represented by endometrial and endocervical glands; however, some authors mention that this type of polyp may occur within the fundus of the uterine body where endometrial glands have undergone mucinous metaplasia [47] (Figs. 19.55, 19.56, 19.57, 19.58, 19.59, and 19.60).

While the diagnosis of an endometrial polyp is straightforward on a hysterectomy sample, it is more difficult on endometrial curettage where the polyp is removed piecemeal. In this context, curettage fragments will consist of irregularly shaped glands of various sizes and haphazardly

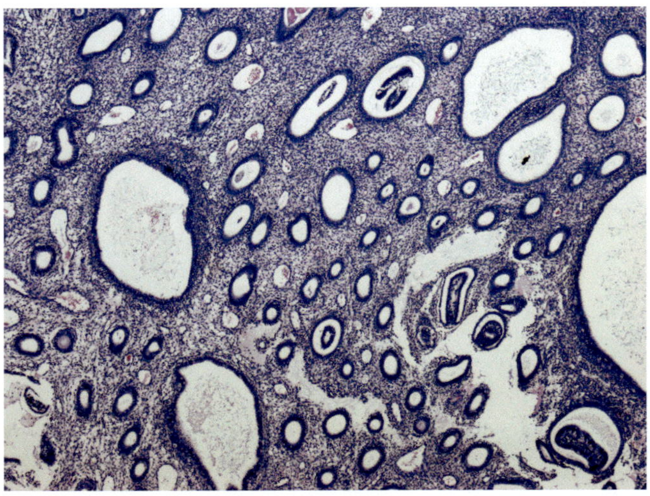

Fig. 19.55 Hyperplastic polyp: the glands resembling those identified in endometrial hyperplasia or proliferative-type endometrium; note the telescoping phenomenon

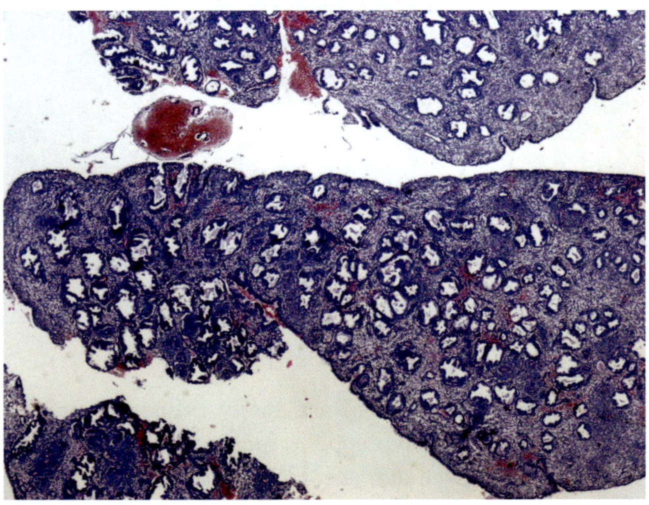

Fig. 19.56 Functional polyp within a curettage sampling

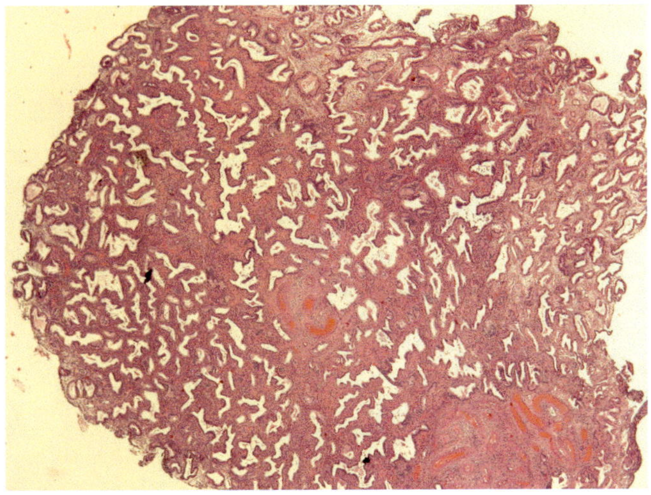

Fig. 19.57 Functional polyp in which the glands respond to hormonal stimulation (Courtesy of Dr. Francisco F. Nogales)

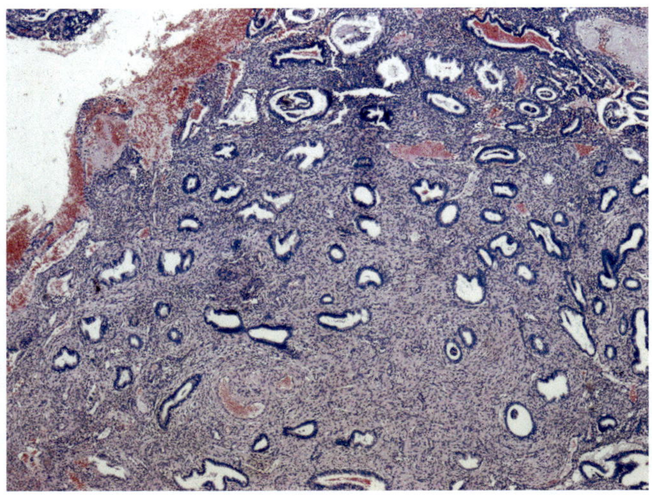

Fig. 19.58 Mixed polyp: glands of endometrial and endocervical type within the same lesion

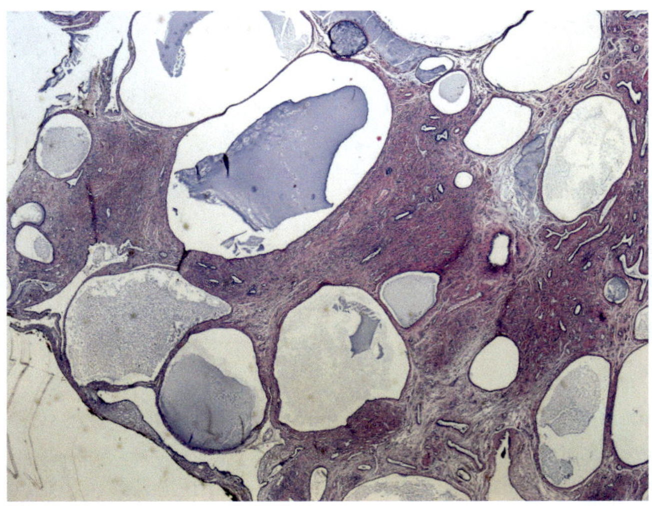

Fig. 19.59 Atrophic polyp: small or cystically dilated glands within a hypocellular stroma

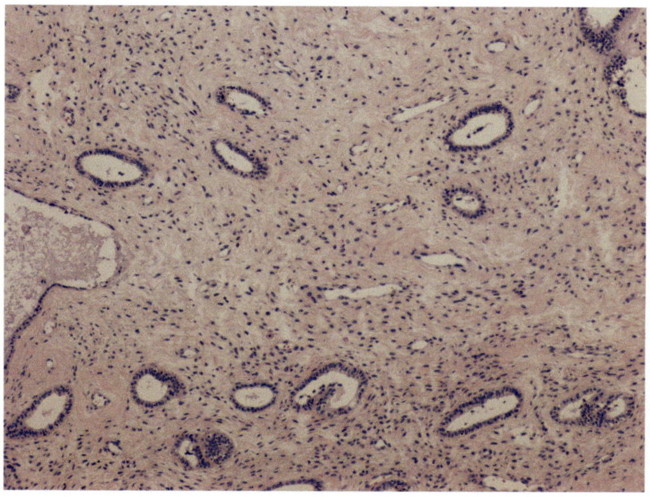

Fig. 19.60 Atrophic polyp: the epithelium lining the glands is very attenuated, and the stroma is very hypocellular

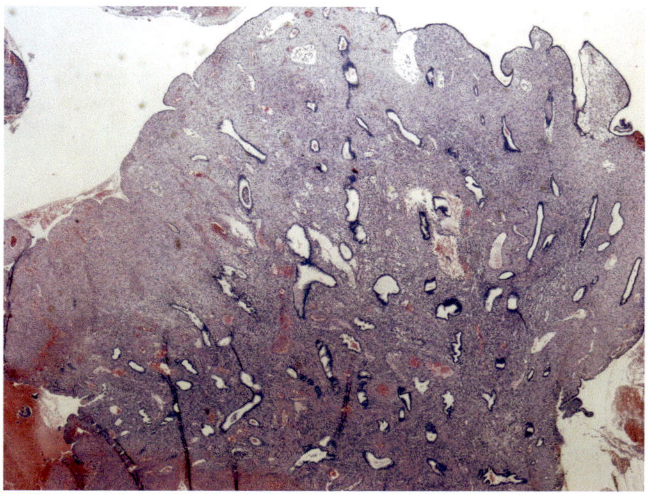

Fig. 19.61 On a curettage sample, the characteristic appearance of a polyp is represented by fragments almost entirely covered by the epithelium

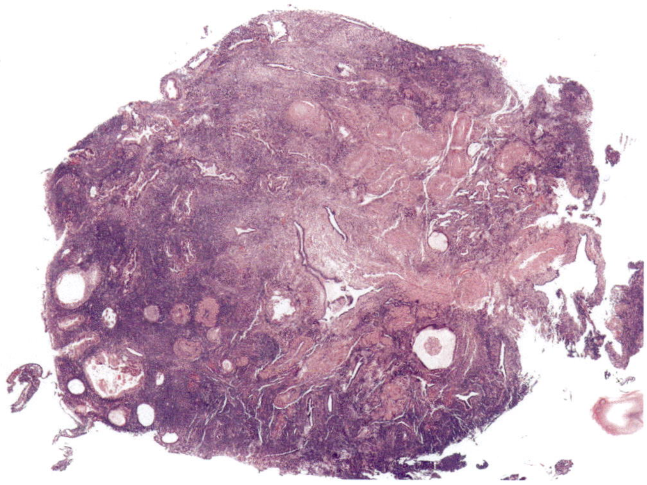

Fig. 19.62 Endometrial polyp with hypercellular stroma can be mistaken with endometrial hyperplasia; however, the presence of numerous thick-walled vessels is very helpful

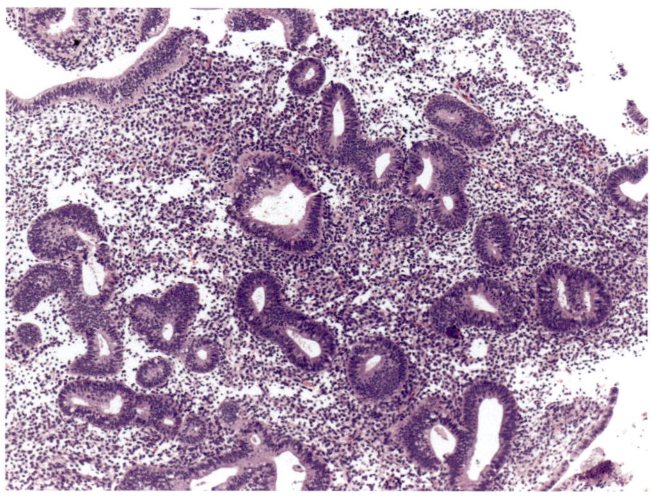

Fig. 19.63 Endometrial hyperplasia has a stroma represented by active stromal cells, while the thick-walled vessels are absent

oriented and surrounded by a fibrous or collagenized stroma with thick-walled vessels (Fig. 19.61). The appearance of the hyperplastic glands should be different from background endometrium. Central vessels, surface lining epithelium, and a connecting stalk may not be seen in all specimens.

19.2.4 Differential Diagnosis

Differential diagnosis of an endometrial polyp includes endometrial hyperplasia, endometrial intraepithelial neoplasia (EIN), adenofibroma, adenosarcoma, submucosal leiomyoma, polypoid adenomyoma (see below), atypical polypoid adenomyoma (see below), endometrial stromal nodule, endometrial carcinoma with polypoid configuration, lower uterine segment/basalis, and normal endometrium fragments. Endometrial hyperplasia may sometimes have a polypoid appearance, but the stroma is represented by active stromal cells with large vesicular nuclei and mitotic activity, while the vessels have a thin-walled appearance (Figs. 19.62 and 19.63). Immunohistochemical stain with p16 can be helpful in differentiating between the two lesions, since most of the polyps show stromal p16 positivity, while this marker is negative in stromal hyperplasia (stromal p16 expression might be a reflection of p16-induced cellular senescence within a polyp) [48, 49] (Fig. 19.64). Atypical hyperplasia/endometrial intraepithelial neoplasia (EIN) can also sometimes present a polypoid configuration; however, the glands are lined by atypical epithelium. On the other hand, EIN can also occur within a

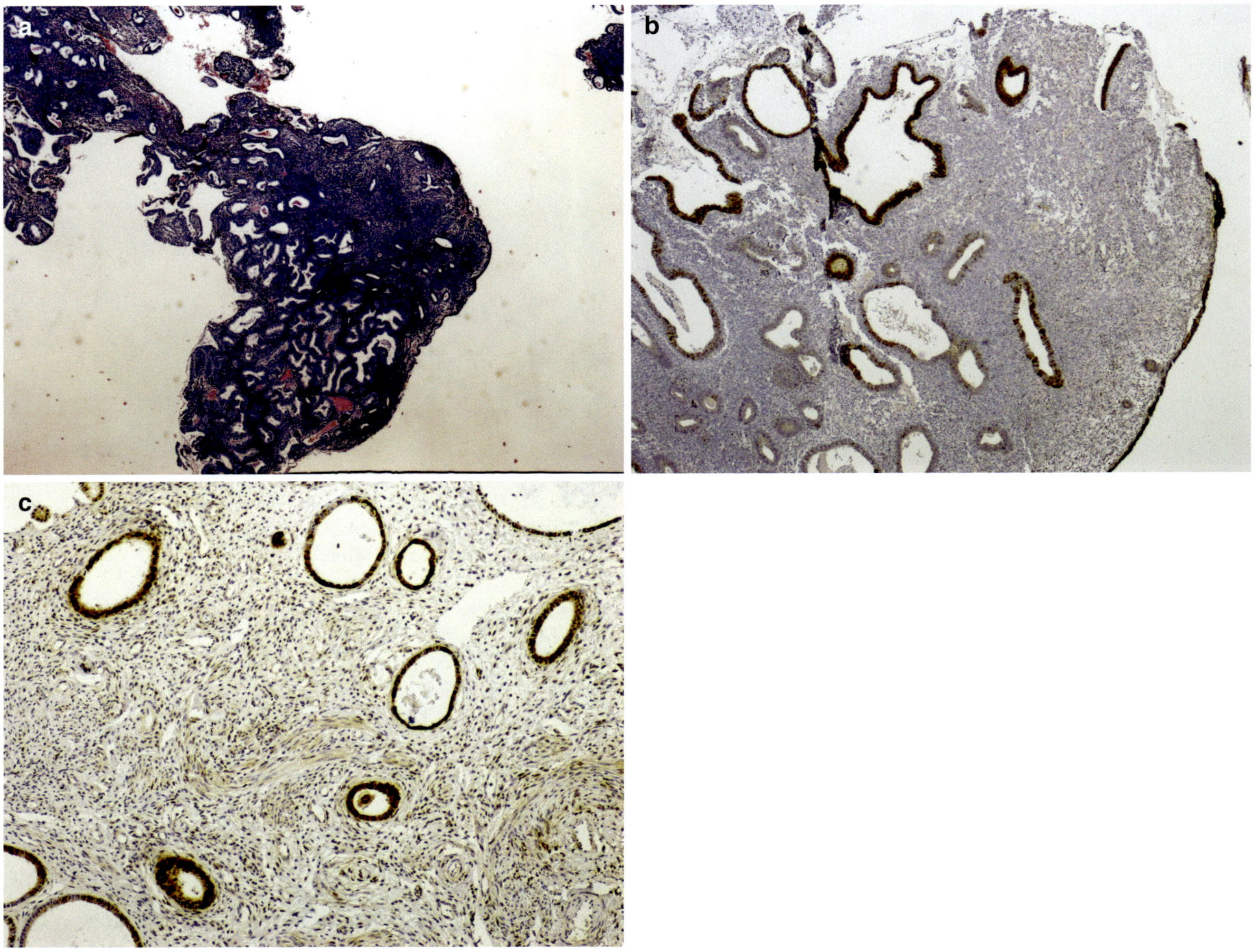

Fig. 19.64 (**a**) Endometrial hyperplasia can have a polypoid appearance; (**b**) to differentiate from a true polyp, p16 is a good marker being negative within the stroma of hyperplasia; and (**c**) positive (nuclear staining) in the stroma of a polyp

polyp, characterized as a focal area of crowded glands with an atypical cytology that differs from that of the glands within the background polyp. In adenofibroma, a very rare tumor and macroscopically similar to an adenosarcoma, a phyllode-like architecture is characteristic, while this is absent in a polyp (Fig. 19.65). In the case of endometrial polyps with bizarre stromal cells as well as in polyps with cystically dilated glands and focal areas of stromal condensation, differential diagnosis is made with adenosarcoma (in which phyllode-like architecture is characteristic, with cystically dilated glands presenting stromal polypoid intrusions together with cytologically atypical stroma, mitotic figures, and sometimes heterologous elements) (Fig. 19.66). A study of 29 uterine polyps with features such as phyllode-like architecture, intraglandular polypoid projections, altered periglandular stroma, stromal cytological atypia, and increased mitotic figures revealed however that uterine pol-

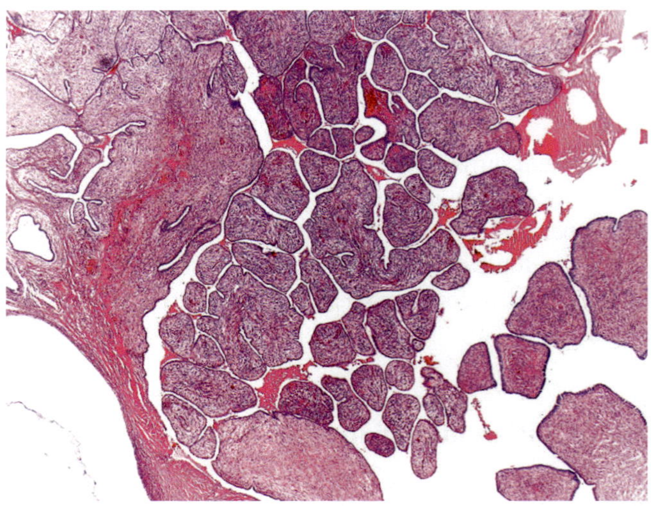

Fig. 19.65 In adenofibroma, a phyllode-like architecture is characteristic, while this is absent in a polyp

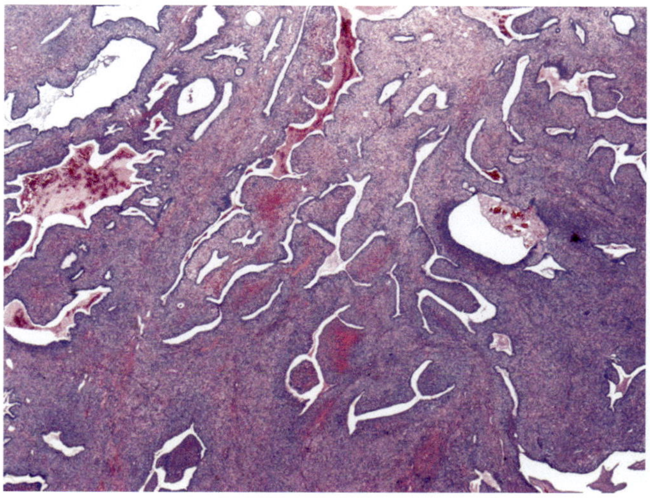

Fig. 19.66 Uterine adenosarcoma which phyllode-like architecture, cystically dilated glands presenting stromal polypoid intrusions together with cytologically atypical stroma, mitotic figures

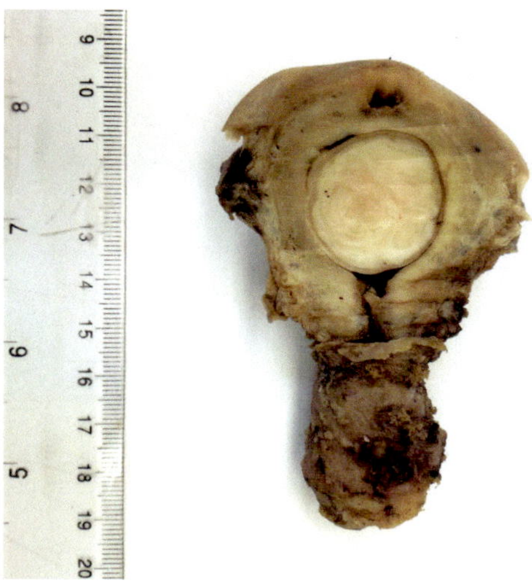

Fig. 19.67 Submucosal leiomyoma protruding within the uterine cavity and mimicking the appearance of a polyp but has harder consistency

yps with features overlapping with those of Müllerian adenosarcoma have a benign clinical course even with conservative management no cases showing progression or malignant transformation [45]. In submucosal leiomyoma, the nodule is protruding within the uterine cavity and may grossly mimic the appearance of a polyp but has harder consistency and a fascicular pattern on the cut surface. Microscopically, the submucosal leiomyoma is easily distinguished from an endometrial polyp. Attenuated endometrium typically covers the leiomyoma surface (Figs. 19.67 and 19.68). Endometrial stromal nodule can grossly have a polypoid appearance but usually has a yellow color. Microscopically, it is composed of cytologically bland ovoid endometrial stromal cells with indistinct cytoplasm and supported by small arterioles and does not contain glandular elements (Figs. 19.69 and 19.70). Endometrial carcinoma (of any histological type) can also have a polypoid

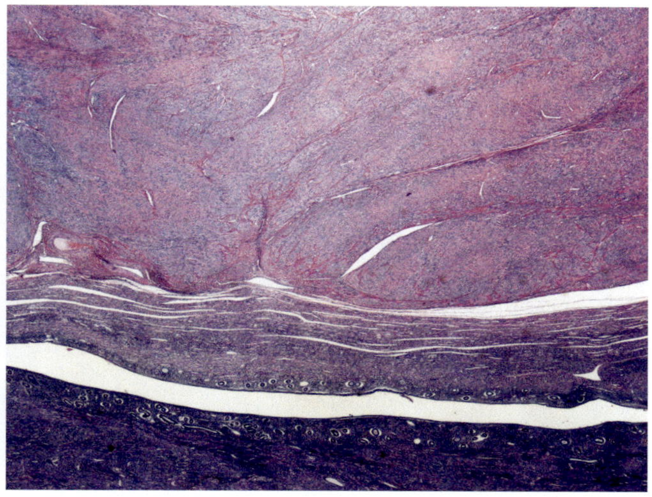

Fig. 19.68 Submucosal leiomyoma: on microscopic examination, the nodule consists of a proliferation of smooth muscle cells arranged in fascicles, while the mucosa only covers the surface of the nodule

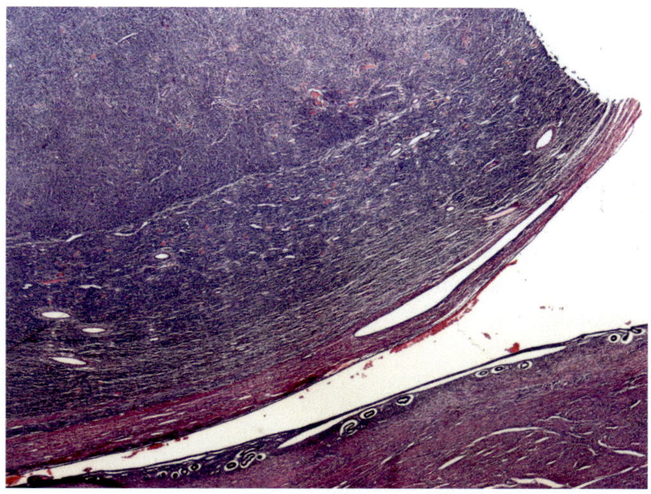

Fig. 19.69 Endometrial stromal nodule can have a polypoid appearance filling the uterine cavity

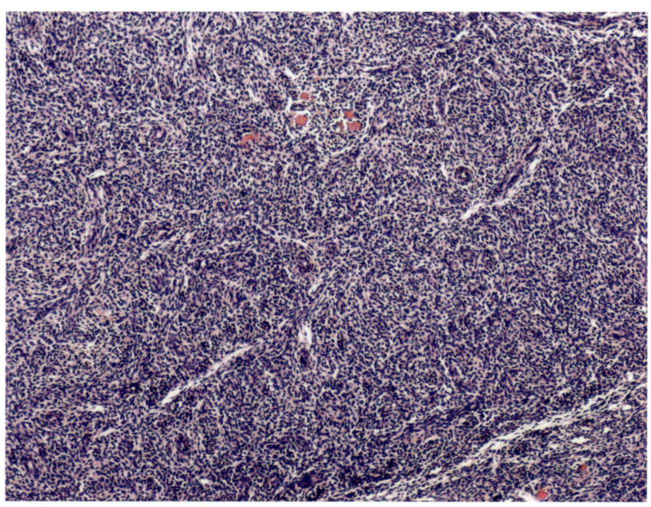

Fig. 19.70 On microscopic examination, n is composed of cytologically bland ovoid cells with indistinct cytoplasm and supported by small arterioles

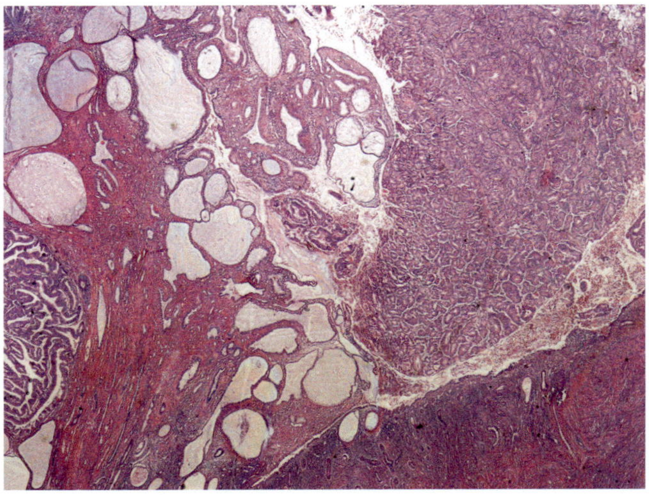

Fig. 19.71 Endometrial adenocarcinoma of endometrioid-type developed on a polyp

configuration especially when it develops within a polyp, but it is represented by atypical glands as well as more solid areas associated with other signs of invasion (Figs. 19.71 and 19.72). Other entities in the differential diagnosis of a polyp are represented by lower uterine segment and deep endometrial basalis and can display fibrous or collagenous stroma. Finally, fragments of true polyps may be confused with fragments of normal endometrium covered on three sides by surface epithelium due to fixation and tangential sectioning.

19.2.5 Prognosis

Treatment of a polyp consists of polypectomy. If the polyp is associated with areas of atypical hyperplasia (EIN), hysterectomy or management with progestin agents (in poor surgical candidates or patients interested fertility preservation) is advised. Recurrence rate after resection of a polyp is low.

19.2.6 Tamoxifen-Related Polyp

Tamoxifen is a drug used in treatment of patients with breast carcinoma in whom estrogen and/or progesterone receptors have been found positive. The treatment lasts 5–10 years according to recent international guidelines [50]. Some of these patients can develop endometrial polyps [51]. Polyps related to tamoxifen therapy tend to be larger than non-tamoxifen polyps, with a wide implantation base within the fundus; they are usually multiple and have cysts on the cut surface (Fig. 19.73). Tamoxifen polyps may harbor foci of

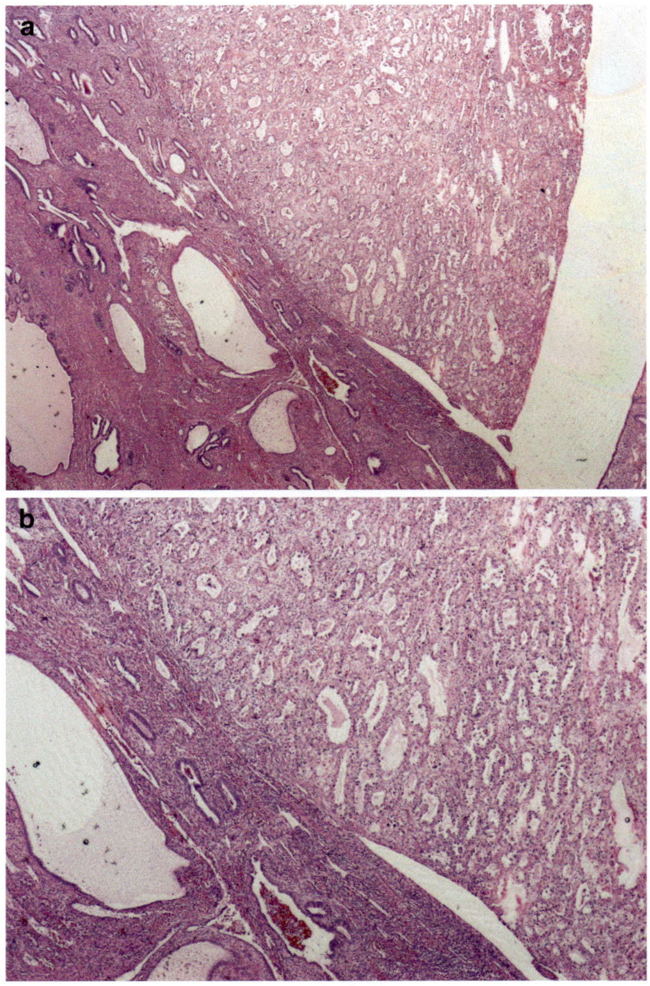

Fig. 19.72 (**a**) Clear cell carcinoma developed within a polyp; (**b**) tubules and cysts lined by clear cell with hobnail appearance and atypical nuclei

mucinous, squamous, and tubal glandular metaplasia as well as stromal smooth muscle metaplasia. A distinct cambium layer can be detected in some cases. Malignant transformation on the form of endometrioid adenocarcinoma or carcinosarcoma (Müllerian mixed mesenchymal tumor) can occur (Fig. 19.74). Polyps related to tamoxifen are more likely to recur after surgical excision [52].

19.2.7 Polypoid Adenomyoma of Endometrioid Type

19.2.7.1 Clinical Presentation

Polypoid adenomyoma is a benign biphasic lesion that occurs in women of both reproductive and postmenopausal age, who typically present with abnormal uterine bleeding [53]. Some of these lesions may develop from areas of adenomyosis.

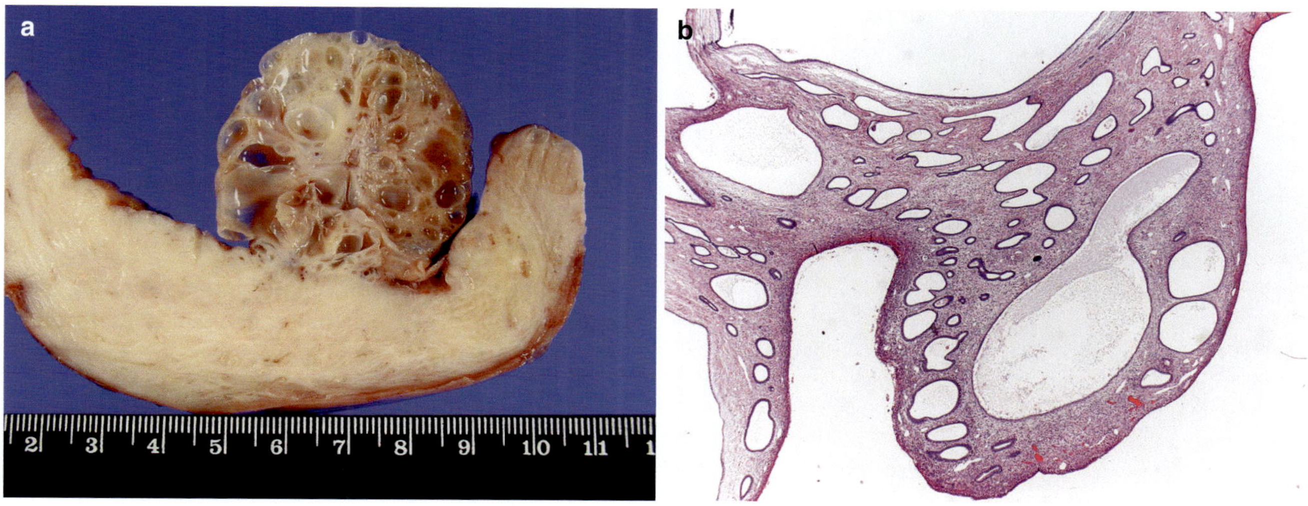

Fig. 19.73 (**a**) Tamoxifen-related polyp has larger size, a wide implantation base, and cysts on the cut surface and (**b**) on microscopic examination (Courtesy of Dr. Francisco F. Nogales)

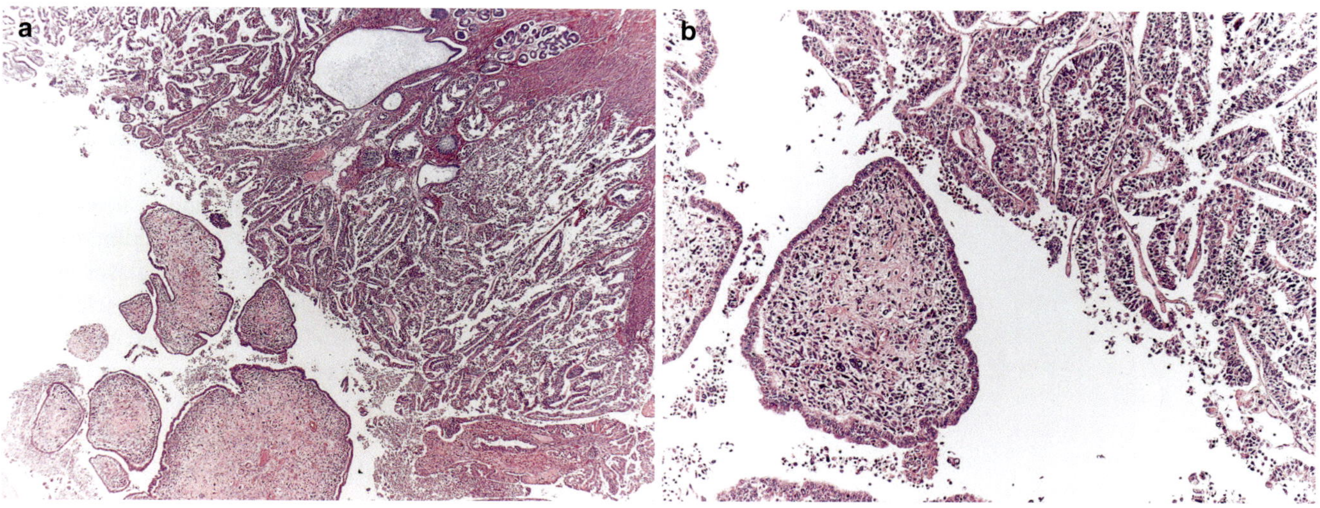

Fig. 19.74 (**a**, **b**) Malignant transformation on the form of carcinosarcoma can occur within a polyp after tamoxifen treatment

19.2.7.2 Gross Findings

Macroscopically, polypoid adenomyoma appears as an exophytic polypoid growth within the endometrium or superficial myometrium. On the cut surface, it is solid and has a white color, reminiscent of leiomyoma, or may have small cystic areas resembling an endometrial polyp.

19.2.7.3 Microscopic Findings

Microscopically, the lesion has well-demarcated margins, and it is composed of fascicles of smooth muscle fibers containing areas of small and round endometrial-like glands. The glands are usually of proliferative type and may or may not be surrounded by areas of endometrial-type stroma (Figs. 19.75 and 19.76). The proportion between the glandular and smooth muscle component is very variable from one polypoid adenomyoma to another, and even within the same lesion, but in general, the smooth muscle component is more prominent than the glandular component. Neither the glands nor the stroma exhibit cellular atypia. Morular, tubal, and mucinous metaplasia can occasionally occur.

19.2.7.4 Differential Diagnosis

Differential diagnosis includes adenosarcoma, especially when the polypoid adenomyoma presents with increased mitotic stromal activity. Key differentiating features are the absence of smooth muscle differentiation (except very rare cases) and the presence of cytologic atypia and periglandular cuffing together with the phyllodes-like architecture in the adenosarcoma. Another differential diagnosis is with adenomyosis, which in contrast to the polypoid adenomyoma does not form a mass but diffusely and multifocally involves the

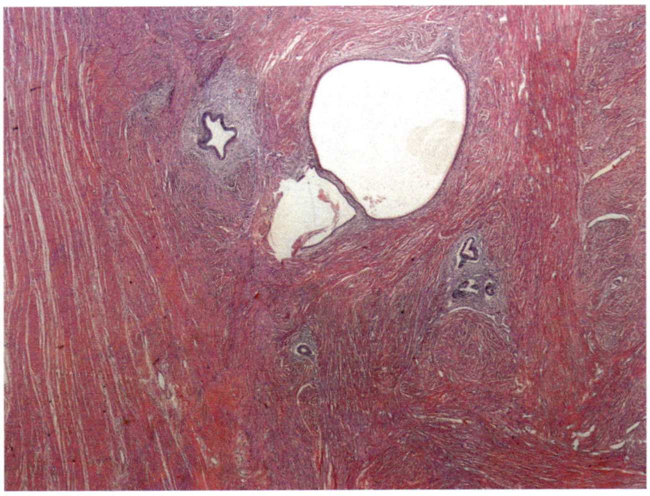

Fig. 19.75 Polypoid adenomyoma of endometrioid type: the lesion has well-demarcated margins, and it is composed of fascicles of smooth muscle fibers containing areas of small and round endometrial-like glands usually of proliferative type surrounded by areas of endometrial-type stroma

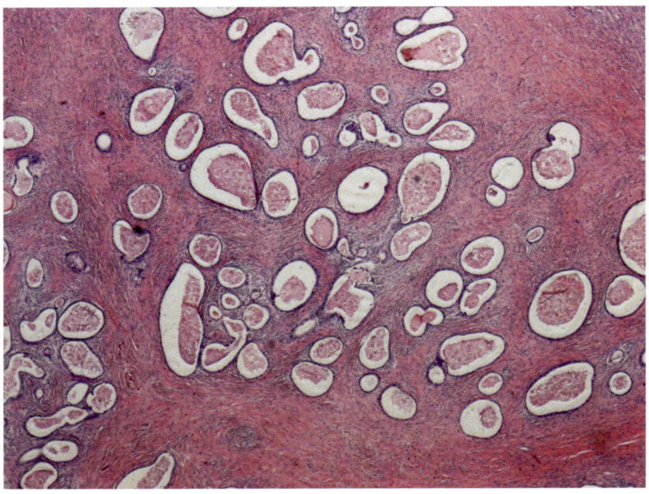

Fig. 19.76 Polypoid adenomyoma of endometrioid type: the endometrioid stroma can be absent in some of these lesions or reduced to a very thin rim around the glandular component

uterine wall. Submucosal leiomyomas can have entrapped rare glands, but these are very superficial and not randomly distributed through the lesion like in the polypoid adenomyoma. Endometrial polyps with smooth muscle metaplasia differ from endometrioid-type polypoid adenomyoma by the fact that in the former lesion, the metaplastic smooth muscle areas are usually centrally located and not distributed throughout, while the remaining stroma is fibrotic and has thick-walled vessels. In polypoid adenomyoma of endocervical type, the appearance is similar except the location (within the cervix) and the epithelium lining the glands (of cylindrical endocervical type while the rim of endometrial stroma is absent).

19.2.7.5 Prognosis

Polypoid adenomyoma of endometrioid type is benign, and surgical resection is curative.

19.2.8 Atypical Polypoid Adenomyoma

19.2.8.1 Clinical Presentation

Atypical polypoid adenomyoma is a lesion occurring more frequently in the premenopausal or perimenopausal women (mean age is 38 years old). It has been also reported in patients with Turner syndrome who received estrogen replacement therapy and in nulliparous patients [54]. 25% of patients have a history of infertility.

Atypical polypoid adenomyoma is clinically associated with abnormal uterine bleeding.

19.2.8.2 Gross Findings

Macroscopically, the appearance is similar to that of the endometrial polyp, with the exception that it is more frequently located in the lower part of the uterine body. It is a round, polypoid, sessile, or pedunculated formation with a smooth, solid, white-gray surface with an average diameter of 2 cm. Multiple lesions can occur.

It was described in 1981 by Mazur and is a particular focal polypoid lesion, represented by a proliferation of irregular endometrial glands with squamous metaplasia associated with a prominent stroma with smooth muscle fibers [55]. Although extensively studied, the pathogenesis of the lesion is still controversial, and most authors consider that it arises from an endometrial stromal precursor cell following prolonged estrogenic stimulation. Recent studies show abnormalities including MLH-1 promoter hypermethylation, *PTEN* and *KRAS* mutations, and microsatellite instability, similar to endometrial atypical hyperplasia and endometrioid-type adenocarcinoma. This may provide an explanation for why atypical polypoid adenomyoma is commonly associated with these lesions and suggests a biological connection between them [56, 57].

19.2.8.3 Microscopic Findings

Microscopically, the tumor has a lobulated architecture on low-power examination, the lobules being represented by hyperplastic endometrial glands of irregular shape and with various degrees of architectural complexity and haphazardly arranged in a collagenous fibrous stroma, which typically contains stromal endometrial cells as well as short smooth muscle fiber bundles (the bundles are shorter than those in the normal myometrium) and myofibroblasts. Rarely, stromal cells may have moderate atypia or mitotic activity (up to 3–5 mitoses/10HPF). Some tumors may have necrotic foci. The epithelium of the glands may exhibit cytologic atypia, mitotic activity, and eosinophilic cytoplasm. Areas

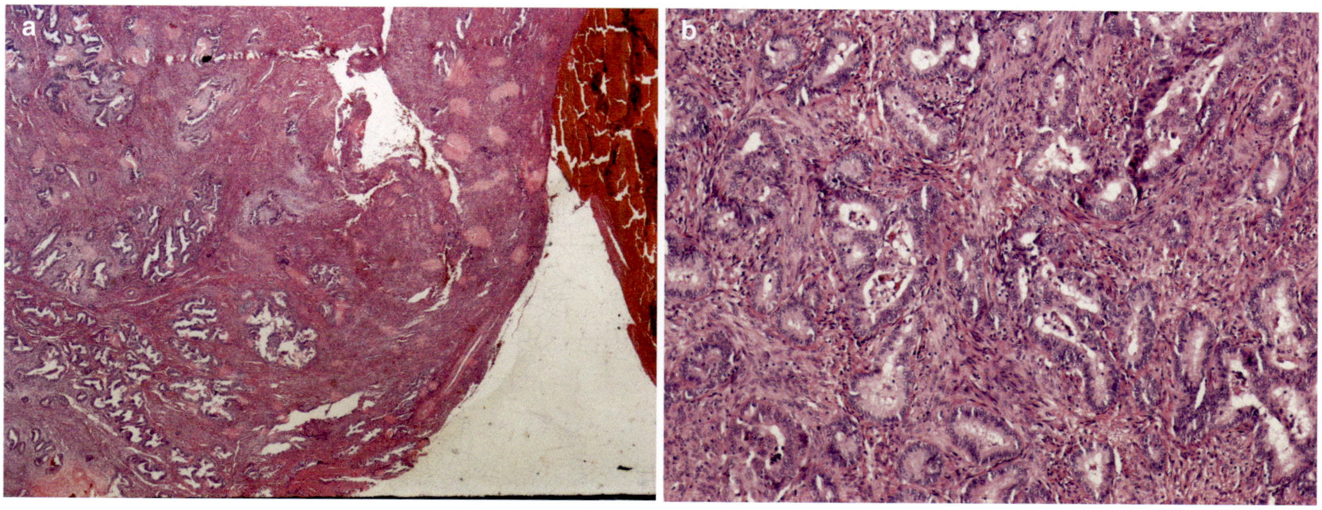

Fig. 19.77 Atypical polypoid adenomyoma on curettage: (**a**) areas of blood mixed with fragment with a lobulated architecture on low-power examination; (**b**) represented by hyperplastic endometrial glands of irregular shape arranged in a collagenous fibrous stroma with smooth muscle fibers

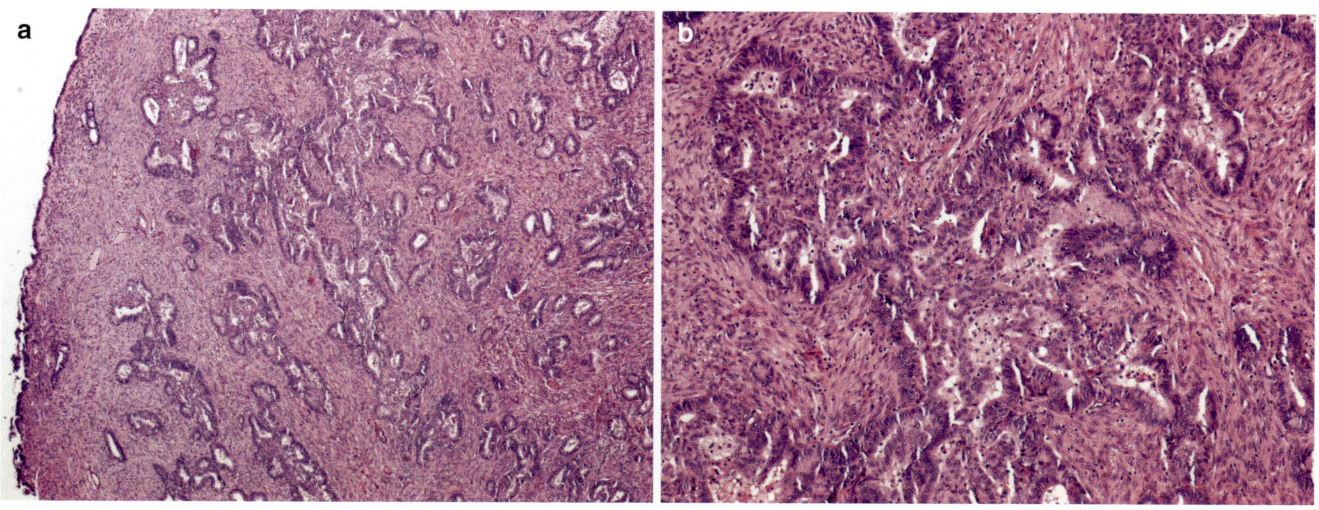

Fig. 19.78 Atypical polypoid adenomyoma: (**a**) hyperplastic endometrial glands of irregular shape and with various degrees of architectural complexity; (**b**) with foci of squamous metaplasia within a stroma with bundles of smooth muscle fibers

of squamous metaplasia in the form of morules, with central or focal necrosis and keratinization and obliterating the glandular lumina, occur in about 90% of the cases (Figs. 19.77, 19.78, and 19.79). The glands may sometimes have complex architecture including cribriform or solid areas and are lined by an atypical epithelium such that confusion with endometrial carcinoma may arise. In some cases, the lesion may be associated with the superficial invasion of the adjacent myometrium as well as areas of atypical hyperplasia or grade 1 endometrioid-type adenocarcinoma in the adjacent endometrium. Therefore, some authors suggest that lesions containing complex glands and meeting the diagnostic criteria for a well-differentiated endometrioid-type carcinoma should be called atypical polypoid adenomyoma with a low malignancy potential, precisely to suggest their ability to have a more aggressive local behavior, extrauterine disease, or metastasis [58]. These features are more likely to be observed in the setting of an excisional specimen, rather than endometrial biopsy or curettage.

19.2.8.4 Differential Diagnosis

Differential diagnosis includes endometrial hyperplasia, polypoid adenomyoma, endometrial carcinoma of endometrioid type, adenofibroma, and adenosarcoma. With regard to endometrial hyperplasia, the lesion very rarely has a polypoid configuration and does not contain smooth muscle bundles. Polypoid adenomyoma is represented by glands without signs of atypia, and the presence of squamous morules is a rare finding. Endometrial carcinoma is a malignant tumor which is treated differently, and, as a consequence, differen-

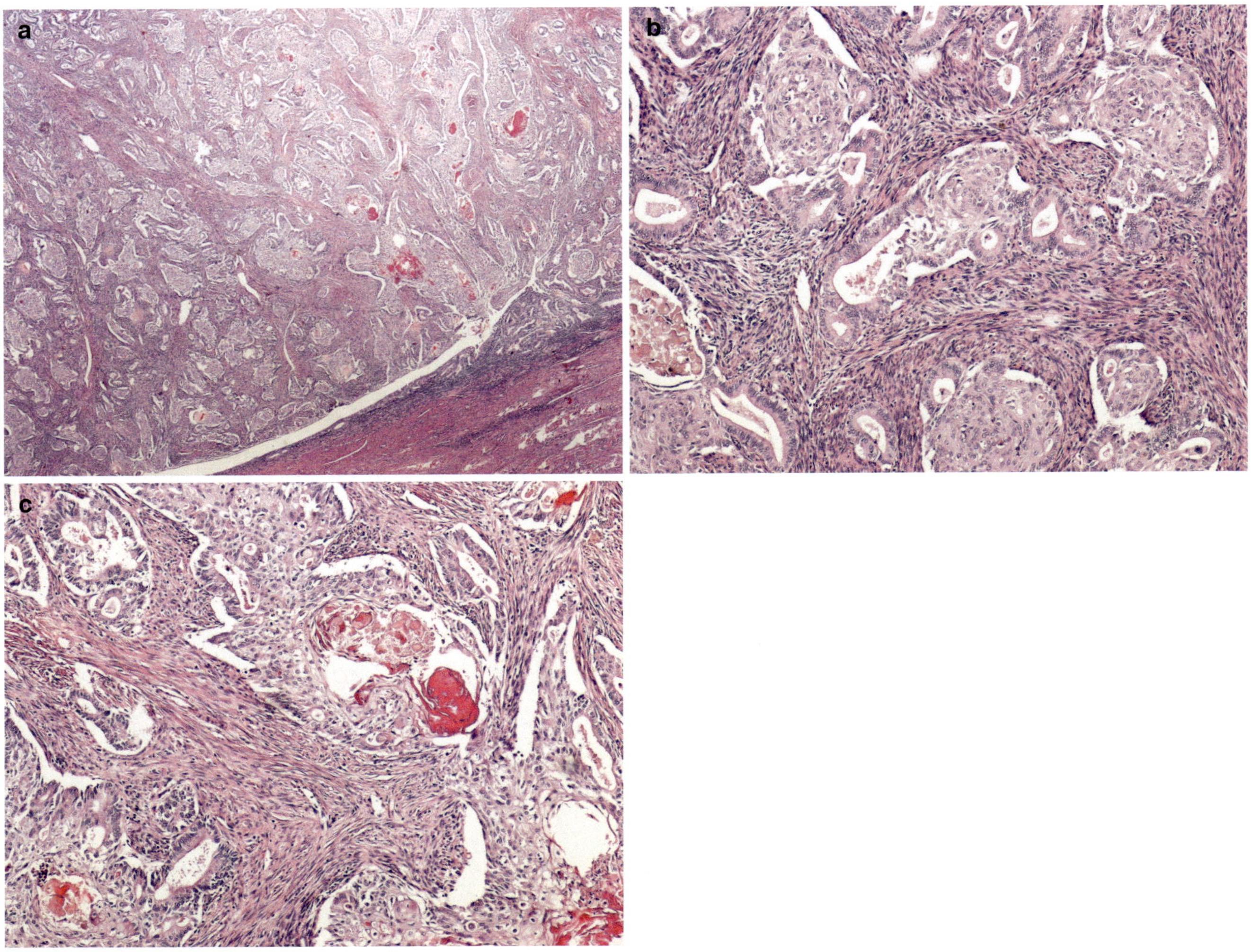

Fig. 19.79 Atypical polypoid adenomyoma: (**a**) another case with a polypoid configuration, very complex glandular architecture; (**b**) the glands presenting extensive areas of squamous metaplasia in the form of morules and necrotic areas; (**c**) while the squamous metaplasia with central keratinization is obliterating the glandular lumina in some areas

tial diagnosis from an atypical polypoid adenomyoma is of great importance. In endometrial carcinoma of endometrioid type, the atypical glands invade the stroma and are surrounded by a stromal desmoplasia. Also, solid areas may appear in addition to atypical glands in higher grade tumors. When the diagnosis is performed on a curettage sample, the myometrium invaded by the atypical glands is less cellular and has a more ordered appearance than in atypical polypoid adenomyoma. However, in cases in which differentiation between the two lesions is not possible on a curettage sample, procurement of additional tissue is recommended. Immunohistochemistry is not helpful in the context of this differential. In adenofibroma, the glandular structures are benign, while the stroma does not contain smooth muscle fibers, and the lesion has characteristic papillary projections and a phyllodes-like architecture. In the case of adenosarcoma, although sometimes smooth muscle component may occur within the mesenchymal component, in additions to adenofibromatous features, there is typical periglandular stromal cuffing, atypia, and mitotic activity.

19.2.8.5 Prognosis

Atypical polypoid adenomyoma is considered to be a benign lesion. It is associated with a less than 2% risk of developing a carcinoma due to the fact that some lesions have a proliferation of atypical glands, especially in postmenopausal patients [59]. Therefore, surgical excision or curettage of the uterine cavity and follow-up is the therapeutic indication especially if the patient wants to maintain the reproductive function, while hysterectomy is indicated in patients with malignant lesions who no longer wish to maintain fertility. In some cases, local recurrences may occur more frequently, especially in low malignant potential lesions (lesions containing complex glands and are indistinguishable from well-differentiated endometrioid adenocarcinoma) treated conservatively [58, 60].

19.3 Endometrial Metaplasias

Endometrial cells may undergo transformation into a variety of epithelial types not present in normal endometrium. These metaplastic changes may occur in the setting of inflammation, repair, endogenous or exogenous hormonal changes, and neoplastic and preneoplastic conditions. Some metaplasias, such as tubal, mucinous, or squamous, involve transformation of the endometrium into epithelial types found elsewhere in the Müllerian tract, a transformation mediated by the *HOX* gene family [61]. Although the metaplastic changes are generally not considered to be of clinical significance in their own right, it is important to recognize them in the context of pathological lesions or conditions with which they may be associated. They should also be accurately distinguished from true pathological entities; some metaplasias, such as tubal and hobnail metaplasia, may exhibit nuclear features that mimic neoplasia. On the other hand, mucinous and secretory type of clear cell metaplasia, when superimposed on preneoplastic or neoplastic endometrial proliferations, may make them appear deceptively bland.

19.3.1 Squamous and Morular Metaplasia

Endometrial glands with squamous metaplasia feature prominent cell borders and abundant eosinophilic keratinizing or nonkeratinizing cytoplasm (Figs. 19.80 and 19.81). In nonneoplastic epithelium, squamous metaplasia is thought to be a reactive change, due to endometrial mechanical irritation (from earlier generation intrauterine devices) [62] or from chronic infections. When appearing in association with endometrioid adenocarcinoma, squamous metaplasia itself may have cytologically malignant features, including nuclear atypia and enlargement. In some endometrioid adenocarcinomas, squamous metaplasia may be rather extensive, obscuring the true solid tumor component and making it difficult to accurately determine the tumor grade.

A form of diffuse endometrial squamous metaplasia with or without keratinization [63, 64], ichthyosis uteri, is believed to be preceded by long-term chronic endometritis and is relatively rare in countries with ready access to antibiotics. Ichthyosis uteri may be associated with an even more rare form of endometrial squamous carcinoma.

Morular metaplasia is characterized by cells with eosinophilic to amphophilic cytoplasm and indistinct cell borders (Figs. 19.82 and 19.83). Morular metaplasia may involve glands partially or completely, with little to no preservation of the glandular lumen. Morular metaplasia is frequently associated endometrial atypical hyperplasia /EIN and with endometrial endometrioid adenocarcinoma [65, 66]. Thus,

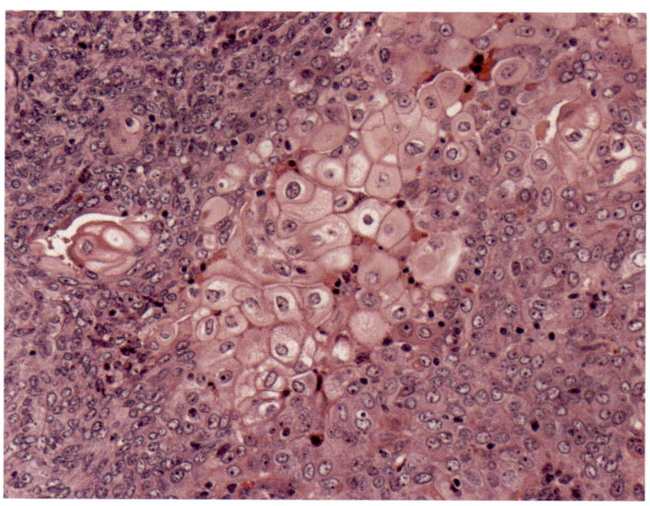

Fig. 19.80 Nonkeratinizing squamous metaplasia in endometrial endometrioid adenocarcinoma. Note the glassy eosinophilic cytoplasm with areas of clearing, as well as prominent cell membranes

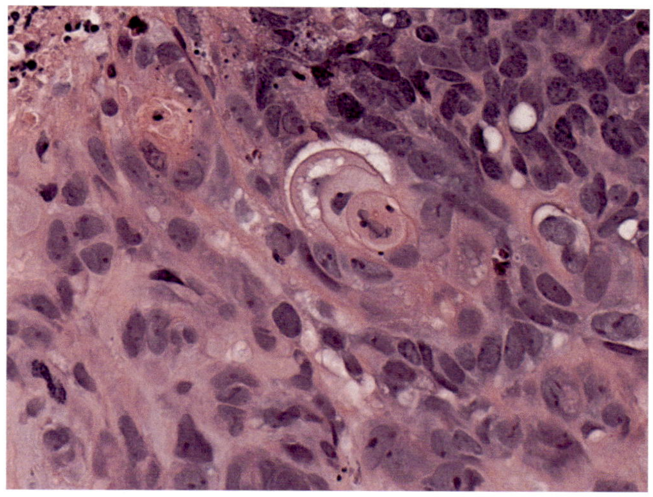

Fig. 19.81 Squamous metaplasia with keratin formation in endometrial endometrioid adenocarcinoma

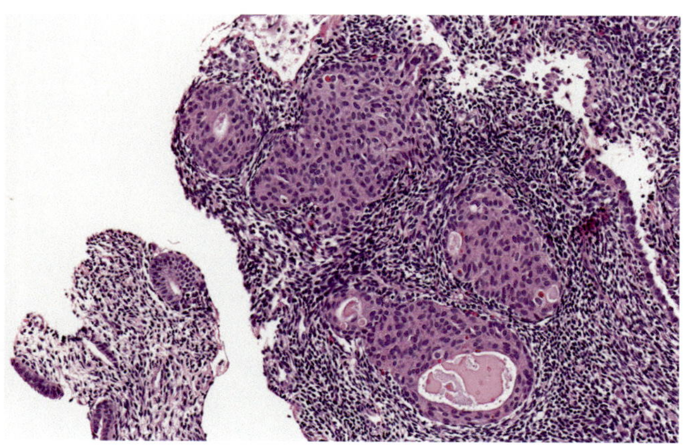

Fig. 19.82 Morular metaplasia with partial to complete glandular involvement

when encountering morular metaplasia in isolation on endometrial biopsy, particularly when tissue is limited, this association should be mentioned in the diagnostic comment. Morular metaplasia may differentiate into squamous metaplasia, but the two have distinct immunophenotypes. Morular metaplasia expresses CD10, β-catenin (nuclear), and CDX2, while ER, PR, and p63 may be focally positive. In contrast, squamous metaplasia expresses ER, PR, and p63, while it may be focally positive for CD10 and CDX2 and shows rarely positive nuclei for b-catenin [67].

19.3.2 Mucinous Metaplasia

Mucinous metaplasia is characterized by variable amounts of intracytoplasmic mucin in endometrial glands. The mucin is of endocervical type or pyloric type but rarely of intestinal type (Fig. 19.84). Mucinous metaplasia may be seen in association with chronic endometritis or in post-pregnancy endometritis. It may also be encountered in progestin-treated endometrial hyperplasia or carcinoma, particularly in lesions that have shown partial or complete response to progestin therapy [68] (Fig. 19.85). Endometrial endometrioid adenocarcinoma also frequently exhibits areas of mucinous metaplasia (Fig. 19.86). In all of the above examples, mucinous metaplasia is a focal finding and occurs in the context of other lesions. However, diffuse and complex mucinous endometrial proliferations, which consist of

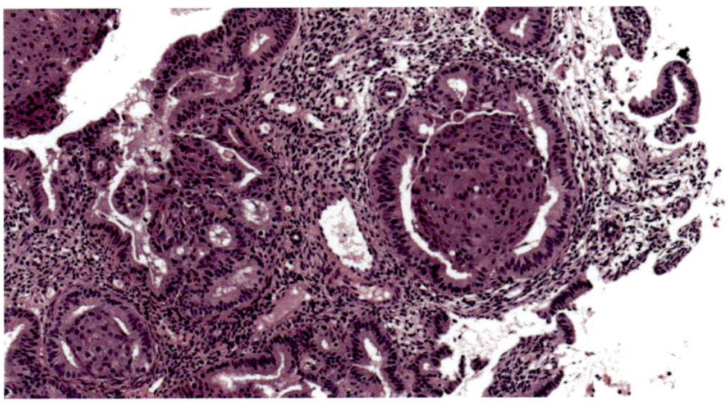

Fig. 19.83 Mucinous metaplasia in an otherwise non-pathologic endometrium

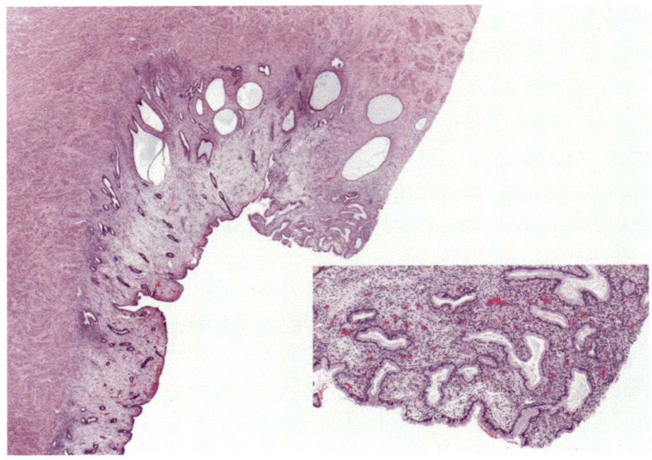

Fig. 19.84 Mucinous metaplasia in progestin-treated atypical endometrial hyperplasia/EIN

Fig. 19.85 Mucinous metaplasia in endometrial adenocarcinoma

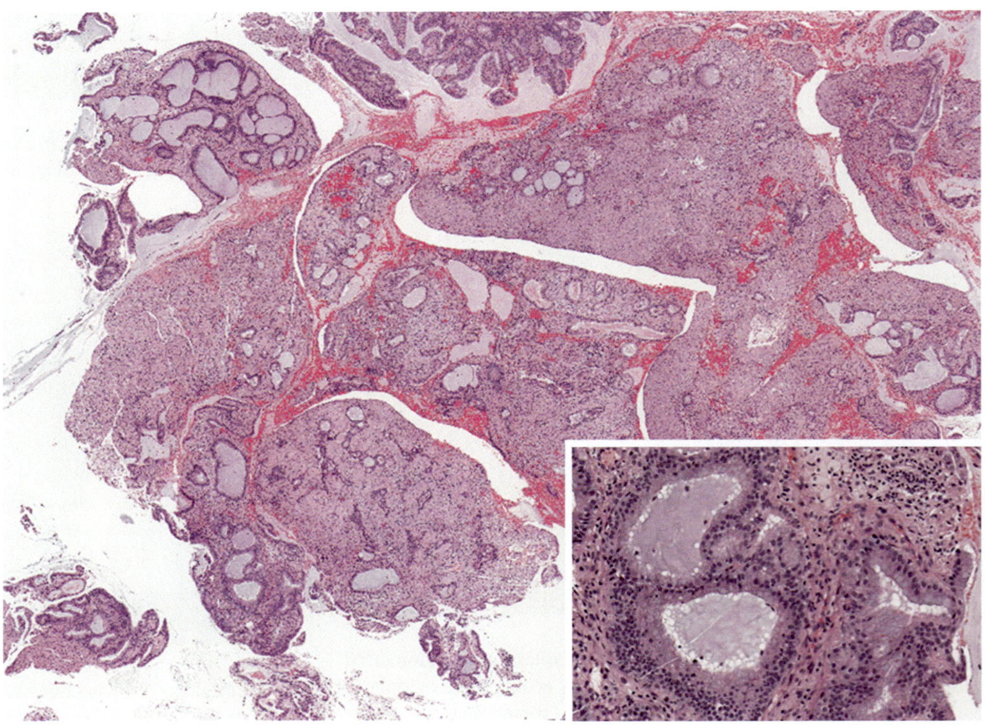

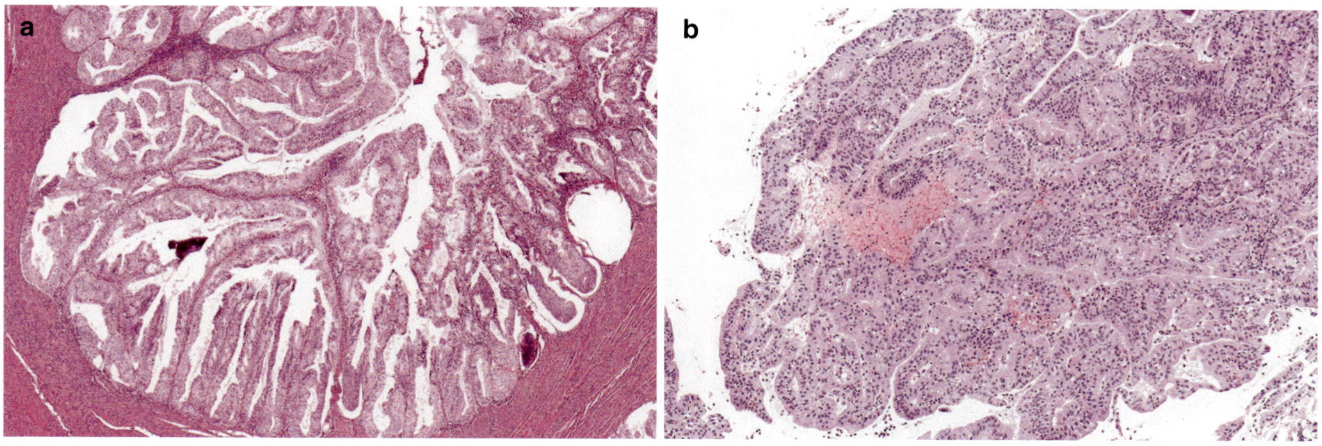

Fig. 19.86 (**a**, **b**) Complex glandular proliferation with mucinous metaplasia. When seen on biopsy, this entity should not be confused with benign endocervical tissue. Despite bland nuclear features, the architectural complexity here is worrisome. Mucinous endometrial carcinoma was present in the excisional specimen

cribriform or complex papillary formations, confer a high risk of endometrial carcinoma on subsequent excisional specimen. They must not be mistaken for benign endocervical tissue, nor for benign endometrial glands when encountered on endometrial biopsy [69]. Despite their architectural complexity, such proliferations have deceptively bland nuclear features (Fig. 19.86).

19.3.3 Ciliated (Tubal) Metaplasia

Tubal metaplasia is a common finding in endometrium, particularly in the proliferative phase [70] or in conditions of unopposed estrogen [71]. Endometrial cells recapitulate the appearance of tubal epithelium, including ciliated cells, secretory cells, and peg cells (Fig. 19.87). In some tubal metaplasias, the secretory cells may exhibit small but prominent nucleoli. Secretory cells can be highlighted by the bcl-2 immunostain [72]. Tubal metaplasia may be on occasion occur in foci of atypical endometrial hyperplasia/EIN or endometrial adenocarcinoma [46, 48] (Fig. 19.88).

19.3.4 Eosinophilic Metaplasia

Eosinophilic and oncocytic metaplasias are nonspecific cytoplasmic changes that may occur in benign or neoplastic endometrium [73–75] (Fig. 19.89). The key differential diagnosis is endometrial adenocarcinoma with oncocytic changes, which may have deceptively bland nuclei, but nevertheless displays marked architectural complexity and/or infiltrative pattern [76, 77].

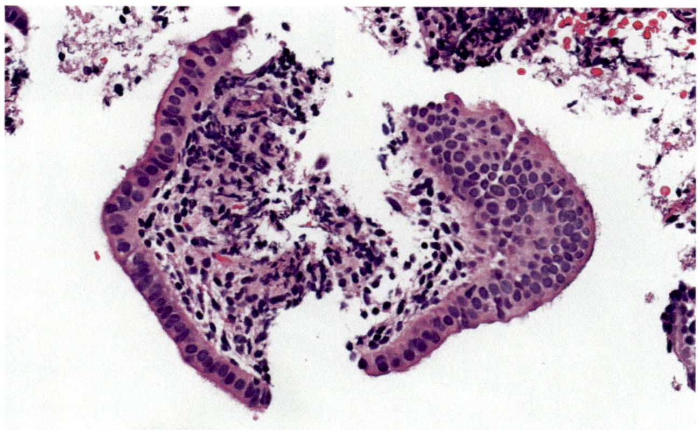

Fig. 19.87 Tubal metaplasia. Ciliated cells, secretory cells, and peg cells are present

19.3.5 Syncytial Metaplasia

Syncytial metaplasia is considered to be a reparative change which occurs frequently in the setting of dysfunctional uterine bleeding (due to a variety of menstrual cycle abnormalities or due to the presence of myometrial leiomyomata). As such, this change may be seen in association with glandular-stromal breakdown. Strips of eosinophilic endometrial glands which lack discernible cell borders (syncytial appearance) typically appear draped over balls of endometrial stromal cells. Polymorphonuclear cells frequently infiltrate the epithelium (Fig. 19.90).

19.3.6 Hobnail Cell Metaplasia

Another reparative endometrial change may take the form of hobnail cell metaplasia. The change is usually focal and may

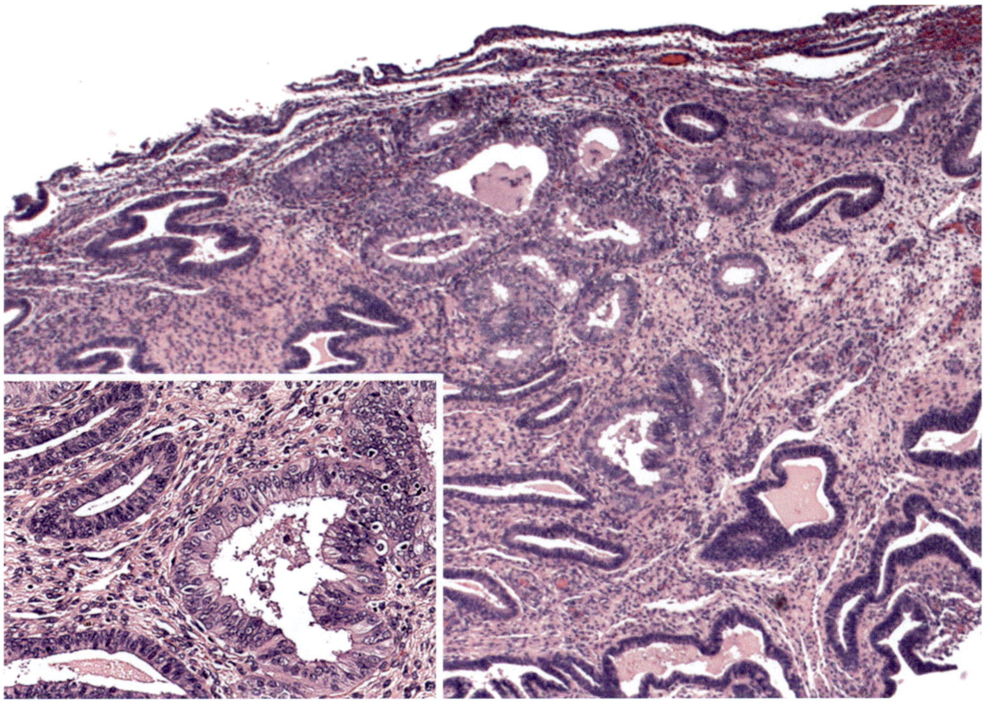

Fig. 19.88 Tubal metaplastic changes superimposed on a focus of atypical in endometrial hyperplasia/EIN

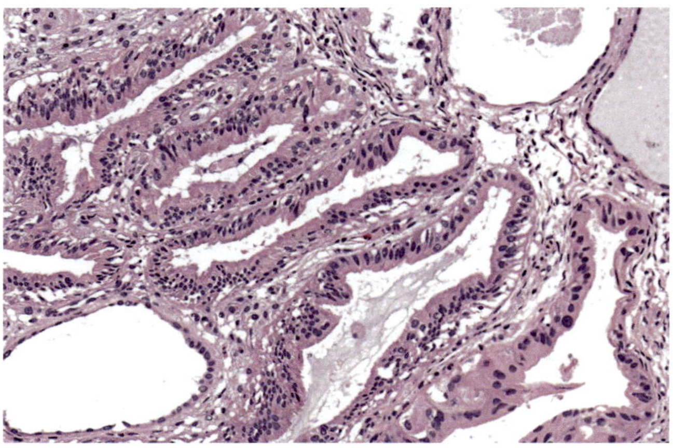

Fig. 19.89 Eosinophilic metaplasia. Cuboidal to columnar cells with eosinophilic cytoplasm and bland nuclei are present

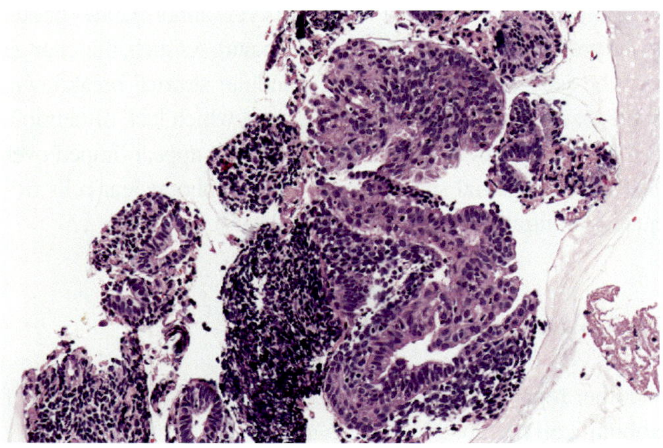

Fig. 19.90 Syncytial metaplasia. The cell boundaries between endometrial gland cells are indistinct. The epithelium is draped over clusters of endometrial stromal cells, consistent with glandular-stromal breakdown

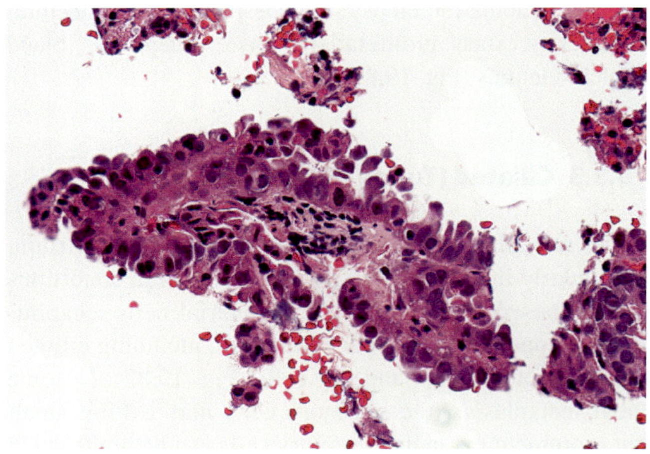

Fig. 19.91 Hobnail cell metaplasia. Hobnailed eosinophilic cytoplasm. The nuclei have a smudged appearance

be accompanied by syncytial metaplasia. Hobnail cell metaplasia may be evocative of intraepithelial serous carcinoma or clear cell carcinoma. Key differentiating features from these lesions include the absence of mitotic activity in hobnail cell metaplasia. Some of the nuclei have a smudged appearance with indistinct nucleoli. Although the nuclei may be somewhat enlarged, the nuclear to cytoplasmic ratio remains low (Fig. 19.91).

19.3.7 Clear Cell Metaplasia

Clear cell metaplasia is characterized by clearing of endometrial cell cytoplasm without evidence of mucin accumulation. Clear cell change may occur in nonneoplastic endometrium (Fig. 19.92) or in endometrioid hyperplasia and carcinoma (Figs. 19.93 and 19.94), sometimes in the setting of endogenous hormonal changes or exogenous hormonal therapy. Of particular relevance is secretory-type clear cell change, which may be superimposed on neoplastic or preneoplastic endometrial proliferations and may obscure their usual nuclear atypia, thus mimicking normal secretory endometrium. When encountering these entities on biopsy, it may be difficult to recognize them, especially in premenopausal patients in the secretory phase of the menstrual cycle. Application of Ki-67 immunohistochemistry may be useful, as the neoplastic proliferations with secretory change have been reported to have a higher proliferative signal than the surrounding secretory endometrium [78, 79]. Procurement of additional tissue during the proliferative phase may be suggested in the diagnostic comment.

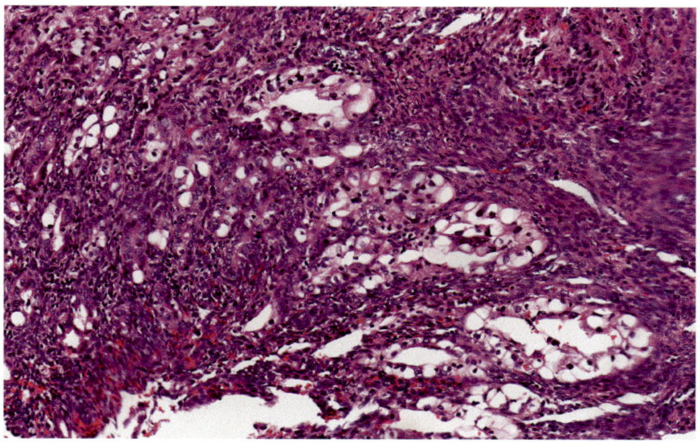

Fig. 19.92 Clear cell change in inactive endometrium of a postmenopausal patient. Note the bland nuclei with a somewhat haphazard placement of within the cell

19.3.8 Metaplasia of Endometrial Stromal Cells

Metaplasia of stromal endometrial cells is a relatively infrequent phenomenon. Cartilaginous [80], osseous [81], adipose [82], and smooth muscle tissue metaplasias may occur. The latter formations are referred to as plexiform tumorlets, which appear as sex cord-like trabeculae that co-express smooth muscle markers such as desmin, smooth muscle antigen, and caldesmon [83] (Fig. 19.95). Mesenchymal metaplasias of the endometrium are usually an incidental diagnosis and do not have much clinical significance. The key differential diagnosis includes retention of fetal tissue post pregnancy termination, more commonly

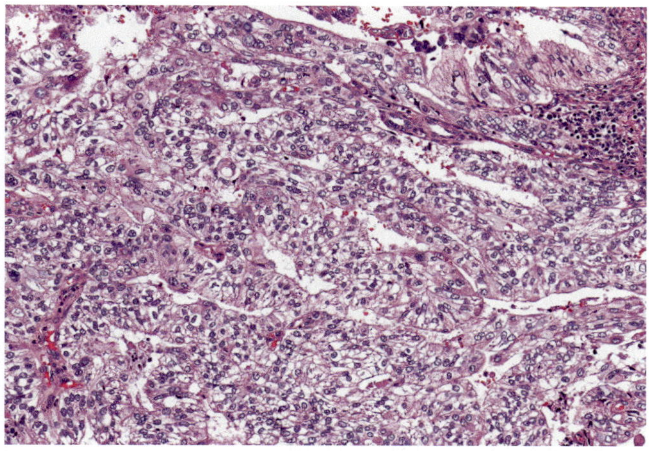

Fig. 19.94 Endometrioid adenocarcinoma with clear cell change. The appearance of clear cytoplasm prompts consideration of clear cell carcinoma in the differential diagnosis; however, the relative nuclear size uniformity and the absence of other clear cell carcinoma features make this possibility unlikely

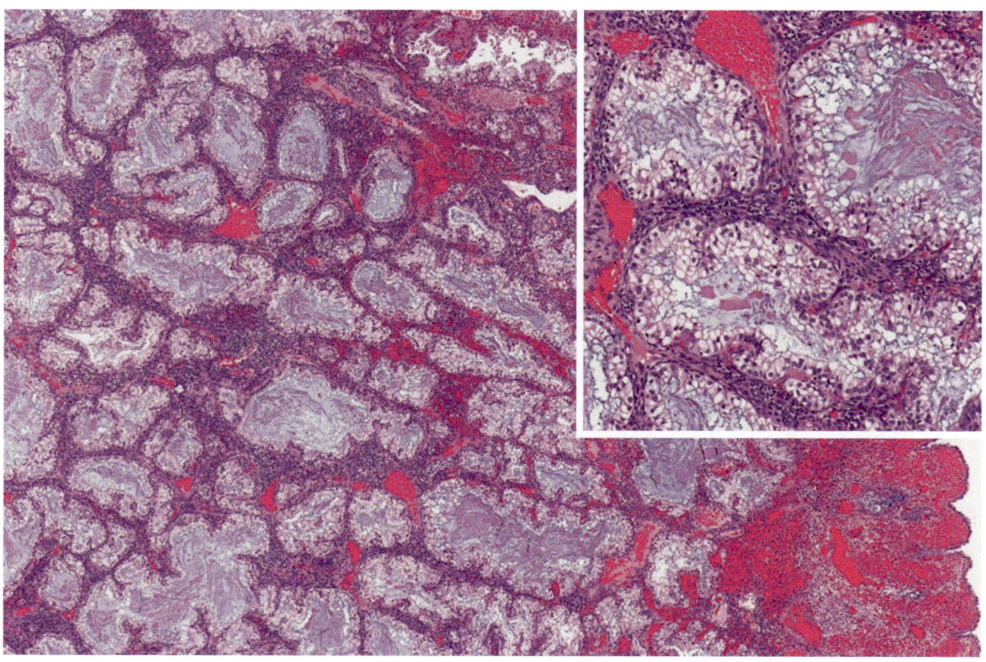

Fig. 19.93 Endometrial hyperplasia with superimposed clear cell metaplasia in a premenopausal patient in a secretory phase of the menstrual cycle. Although the nuclei are bland, the endometrial glands appear crowded within intact endometrial stroma. A repeat biopsy during the proliferative phase of the menstrual cycle was recommended in order to rule out the possibility of atypical endometrial hyperplasia/EIN

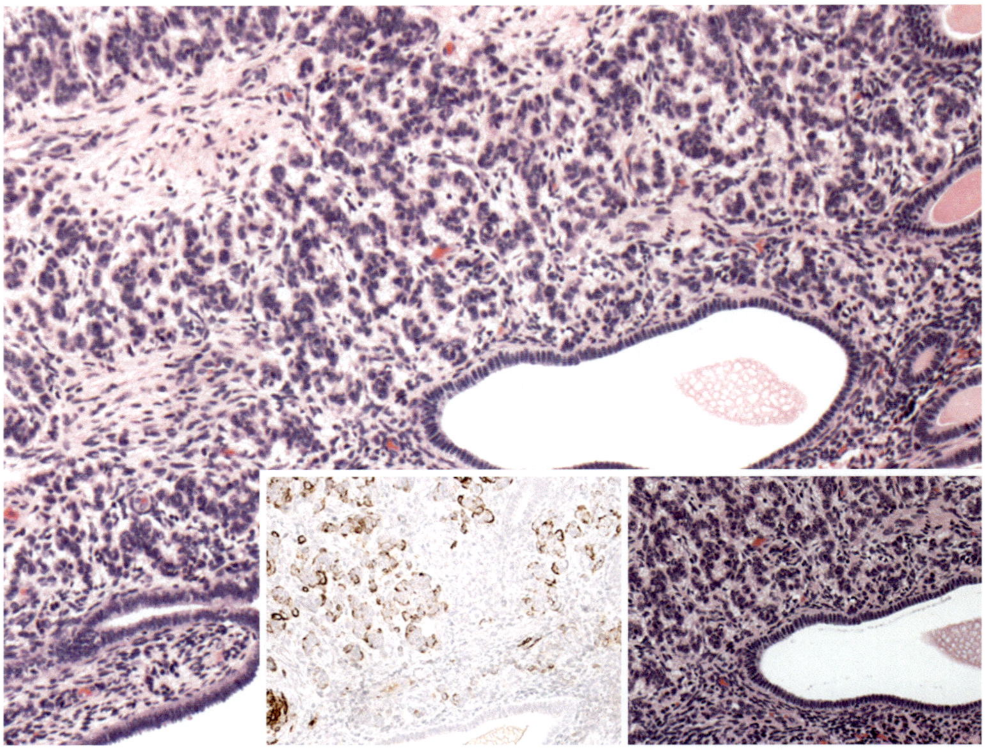

Fig. 19.95 Smooth muscle metaplasia of endometrial stromal cells. Cell formations appear as sex cord-like trabeculae and show immunoreactivity with caldesmon (inset)

bone [84] and rarely glial tissue [85]. Endometrial extramedullary hematopoiesis is an unusual finding and should raise concern for systemic hematologic disease [86].

19.4 Other Benign Lesions of the Endometrium

19.4.1 Endometrial Changes Influenced by Intrauterine Device

In recent decades, intrauterine devices (IUDs) have been widely adopted as a contraceptive device, particularly in Asia and South America. Depending on the type of IUD and duration of time of exposure, different endometrial changes may arise in the endometrium. The mechanical effect is represented by the compression of the mucosa which can gain a wavy instead of a linear pattern with slight indentations of the surface (similar to the shape of the IUD). In addition, near the area of contact to the IUD, the surface of the mucosa may become fibrotic and form adhesions to the device. Squamous and hobnail metaplasia can also develop (see section on endometrial metaplasias). The surface epithelium as well as the epithelium lining the glands may present focal atypia without mitotic figures. Chronic endometritis is a common finding in the presence of IUDs. With IUDs containing progestin agents, the endometrial glands adopt an inactive or sometimes weakly secretory pattern, while the stroma exhibits pseudodecidual changes (Fig. 19.96). A well-recognized infection due to the IUD effect, although rare, is *Actinomyces israelii* infection of the uterine cavity, as well as fallopian tubes and ovaries. Actinomyces organisms may frequently present on a routine Papanicolaou smear. The diagnosis is based on the finding of neutrophilic infiltrate associated with gram-positive colonies (sulfur granules), with a dense finely granular core and thin radiating filaments at the periphery. Pseudo-actinomycotic radiate granules have been also described in response to the IUD. Unlike

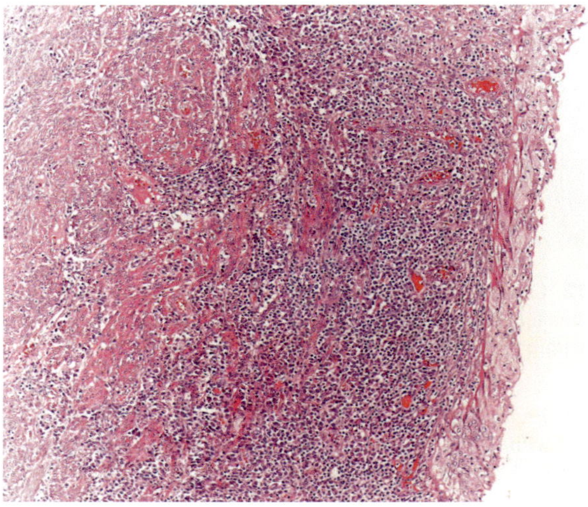

Fig. 19.96 Endometrial changes influenced by intrauterine device: the surface of the mucosa developed areas of squamous metaplasia within the surface epithelium, while the stroma presents inflammatory infiltrate

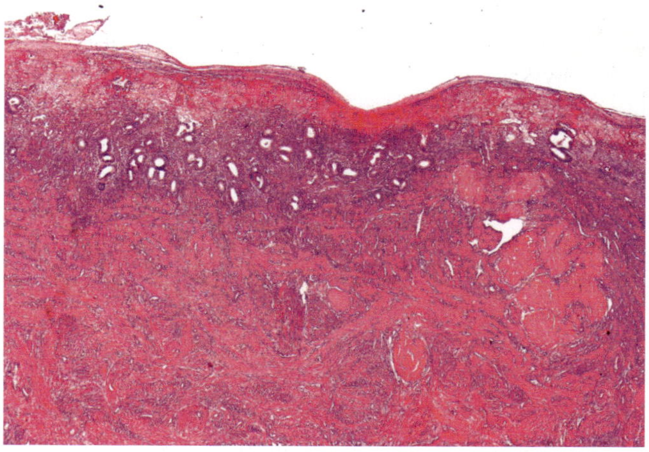

Fig. 19.97 Endometrial changes influenced by endometrial curettage: thin mucosa represented only by basalis layer, with edema, hemorrhage, and inflammatory infiltrate within the endometrial stroma

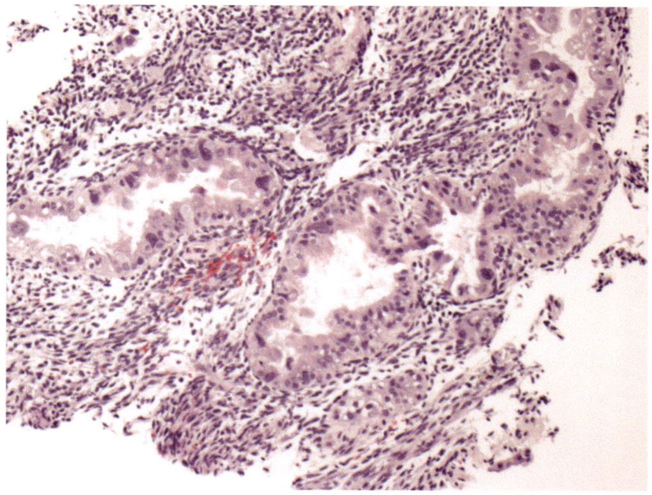

Fig. 19.98 Radiation change: on microscopic examination, one can detect glands of normal shape and architecture that are lined by epithelial cells with irregular and hyperchromatic nuclei, smudged chromatin, but no mitotic activity

Actinomyces israelii colonies, the pseudo-actinomycotic granules are composed of calcium, lipid material, and glycoproteins lacking the filaments [7].

19.4.2 Endometrial Changes Influenced by Endometrial Curettage

Endometrial curettage is commonly performed for diagnosis and treatment of uterine bleeding. It may produce changes in the endometrium, but also within the endocervical mucosa during the passage [87]. In the endometrium, the changes are represented by artefactual crowding of the endometrial glands, fragmentation of the glands, telescoping (glands within glands), papillary pattern, edema, hemorrhage, and inflammatory infiltrate within the endometrial stroma (Fig. 19.97). Cellular atypia characterized by enlarged and hyperchromatic nuclei, sometimes with a hobnail appearance, involving both the surface epithelium and endometrial glands may occur. Taken together, these changes can be misinterpreted as pathological lesions especially when mimicking the endometrial hyperplasia, particularly on endometrial biopsy. Notably, atypical mitoses are absent in endometria with reactive changes [87].

19.4.3 Radiation Changes

Patients undergoing radiotherapy for cervical carcinoma or other pelvic malignant tumors may exhibit radiation changes that may last for years or decades in the endometrial mucosa. These changes do not usually produce macroscopic lesions. However, in rare cases, after radiotherapy, the uterus becomes smaller and fibrotic. On microscopic examination within a very thin and atrophic mucosa, surface epithelium and glands of normal shape and architecture are lined by epithelial cells with irregular and hyperchromatic nuclei, smudged chromatin, but no mitotic activity (Fig. 19.98). The cytoplasm of these cells can be either eosinophilic or can present vacuoles. The endometrial stroma can be fibrotic but can also present cellular atypia. On some occasions, similar to the cervical stroma after radiotherapy, it may contain areas of xanthogranulomatous reaction with foreign body cells, hemosiderin deposits, inflammatory cells, and psammoma bodies. Rarely, the hobnail appearance of the cells may be confused with Arias-Stella phenomenon; however, the clinical history of the patients facilitates the diagnosis.

19.4.4 Other Benign Endometrial Disorders

19.4.4.1 Endometrial Psammoma Bodies

Psammoma bodies are rarely encountered within the endometrium and are usually not related to a malignant process of the uterine cavity or adnexa, but rather to a benign condition such as endometrial polyps, endometriosis, endosalpingiosis, and mature cystic teratoma [88]. However, further evaluation of the endometrial cavity with hysteroscopy and adnexal assessment is recommended to exclude a malignant process, such as serous borderline tumor of the ovary, for example, whenever endometrial psammoma bodies are found during microscopic examination (Fig. 19.99).

19.4.4.2 Asherman Syndrome

This is a rare pathological process, also known as *synechiae*, and may present on infertility workup. Although relatively rare, typically occurs after endometrial curettage for

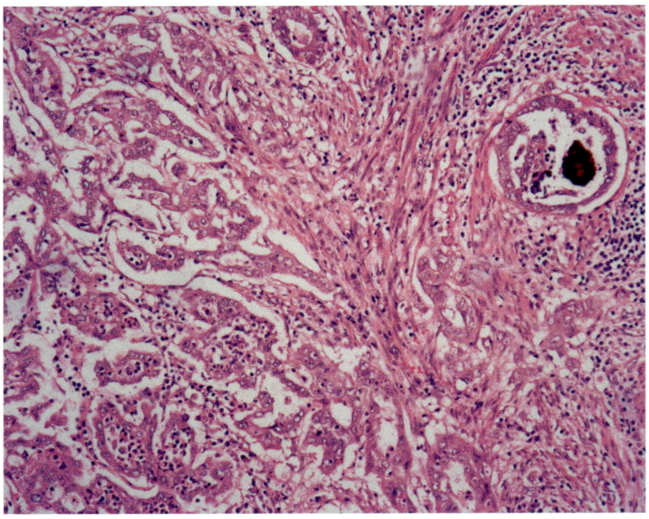

Fig. 19.99 Endometrioid-type adenocarcinoma of the endometrium: psammoma body associated with atypical glands infiltrating the myometrium (Courtesy of Dr. Robert A. Soslow)

therapeutic abortion or miscarriage or for uterine bleeding during the puerperium. The lesion may also occur after genital tuberculosis as a complication of the disease. It is represented by various amounts of fibrous tissue occupying the uterine cavity and involving the endometrial mucosa. The correct diagnosis is only made by hysteroscopy, and the treatment consists of removing those areas in order to allow the patient to become pregnant. In some patients, the Asherman syndrome may produce the obliteration and obstruction of the inner endocervical canal and may result in hematometra or pyometra.

19.4.4.3 Intravascular Endometrial Tissue

Endometrial tissue fragments can be displaced into uterine blood vessels during menses or during surgical procedures [89]. The endometrial fragments can consist of glands or stromal cells or both and do not have atypia (Fig. 19.100). Very rarely, intravascular endometrial tissue can be detected

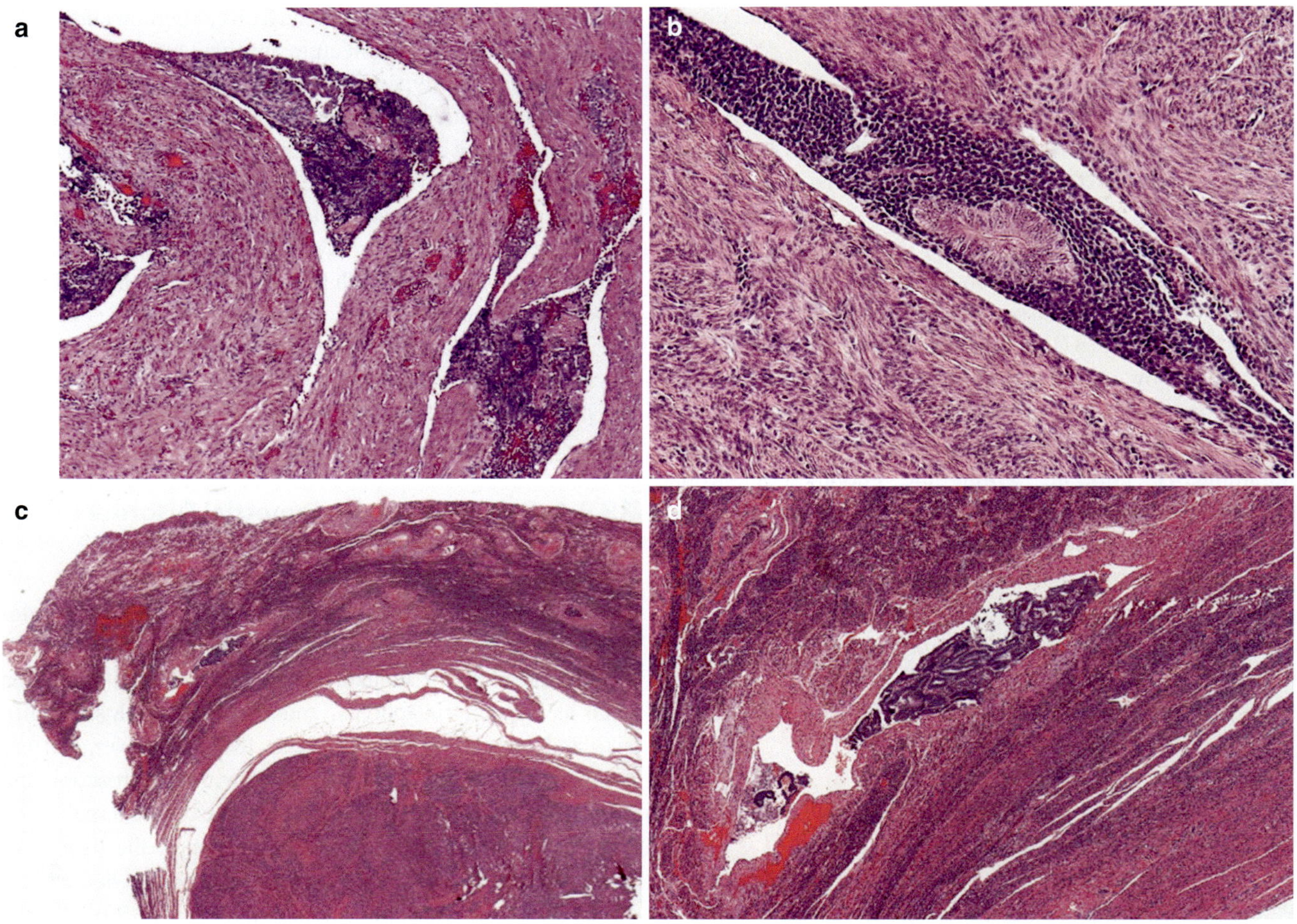

Fig. 19.100 Endometrial tissue fragment composed of (**a**, **b**) glands and stroma without atypia within uterine blood vessels; (**c**, **d**) in contrast to endometrial carcinoma tissue artifactually displaced into large-walled vessels in the myometrium remote from the tumor, after robotic surgery (Courtesy of Dr. Robert A. Soslow)

not only in the uterine vessels but also outside the uterus (such as within the ovarian vessels) not related to menses but to other pathologic conditions [90, 91]. Pathologists should be aware of this phenomenon in order to avoid interpreting the cells within vessels as being neoplastic.

References

1. Kitaya K. Accumulation of uterine CD16(−) natural killer (NK) cells: friends, foes, or Jekyll-and-Hyde relationship for the conceptus? Immunol Investig. 2008;37:467–81.
2. Kitaya K, Yasuo T, Tada Y, et al. Current understanding of chronic endometritis. Diagn Histopathol. 2013;19:231–7.
3. Cicinelli E, Ballini A, Marinaccio M, et al. Microbiological findings in endometrial specimen: our experience. Arch Gynecol Obstet. 2012;285:1325–9.
4. Kasius JC, Broekmans FJ, Sie-Go DM, et al. The reliability of the histological diagnosis of endometritis in asymptomatic IVF cases: a multicenter observer study. Hum Reprod. 2012;27:153–8.
5. Cicinelli E, De Ziegler D, Nicoletti R, et al. Chronic endometritis: correlation among hysteroscopic, histologic, and bacteriologic findings in a prospective trial with 2190 consecutive office hysteroscopies. Fertil Steril. 2008;89:677–84.
6. Kitaya K, Yasuo T. Inter-observer and intra-observer variability in immunohistochemical detection of endometrial stromal plasmacytes in chronic endometritis. Exp Ther Med. 2013;5:485–8.
7. Boyle DP, McCluggage WG. Combined actinomycotic and pseudoactinomycotic radiate granules in the female genital tract: description of a series of cases. J Clin Pathol. 2009;62:1123–6.
8. Sharma S, Valiathan M, Rao L, et al. Endometrial actinomycosis in post menopausal female in the absence of an intrauterine contraceptive device: a rare cause of bleeding per vaginum. J Clin Diagn Res. 2012;6:1062–3.
9. Ingerslev HJ, Moller BR, Mardh PA. Chlamydia trachomatis in acute and chronic endometritis. Scand J Infect Dis Suppl. 1982;32:59–63.
10. Winkler B, Reumann W, Mitao M, et al. Chlamydial endometritis. A histological and immunohistochemical analysis. Am J Surg Pathol. 1984;8:771–8.
11. Dwivedi K, Prasad M. Tuberculous endometritis—an unusual cause of postmenopausal bleeding in the United Kingdom. J Obstet Gynaecol. 2016;36:124–5.
12. Rivasi F, Curatola C, Garagnani L, et al. Detection of Mycobacterium tuberculosis DNA by polymerase chain reaction from paraffin samples of chronic granulomatous endometritis. Histopathology. 2007;51:574–8.
13. Frank TS, Himebaugh KS, Wilson MD. Granulomatous endometritis associated with histologically occult cytomegalovirus in a healthy patient. Am J Surg Pathol. 1992;16:716–20.
14. Giraldo-Isaza MA, Jaspan D, Cohen AW. Postpartum endometritis caused by herpes and cytomegaloviruses. Obstet Gynecol. 2011;117:466–7.
15. McGill AL, Bavaro MF, You WB. Postpartum herpes simplex virus endometritis and disseminated infection in both mother and neonate. Obstet Gynecol. 2012;120:471–3.
16. Madden F. A case of bilharzia of the vagina. Lancet. 1899;153:1716.
17. Wright ED, Chiphangwi J, Hutt MS. Schistosomiasis of the female genital tract. A histopathological study of 176 cases from Malawi. Trans R Soc Trop Med Hyg. 1982;76:822–9.
18. Poggensee G, Kiwelu I, Weger V, et al. Female genital schistosomiasis of the lower genital tract: prevalence and disease-associated morbidity in northern Tanzania. J Infect Dis. 2000;181:1210–3.
19. Arean VM. Manson's schistosomiasis of the female genital tract. Am J Obstet Gynecol. 1956;72:1038–53.
20. Dong H, Dawes S, Philip J, et al. Malakoplakia of the urogenital tract. Urol Case Rep. 2015;3:6–8.
21. Chadha S, Vuzevski VD, ten Kate FJ. Malakoplakia of the endometrium: a rare cause of postmenopausal bleeding. Eur J Obstet Gynecol Reprod Biol. 1985;20:181–9.
22. Chalvardjian A, Picard L, Shaw R, et al. Malacoplakia of the female genital tract. Am J Obstet Gynecol. 1980;138:391–4.
23. Cohen CR, Manhart LE, Bukusi EA, et al. Association between Mycoplasma genitalium and acute endometritis. Lancet. 2002;359:765–6.
24. Chaim W, Horowitz S, David JB, et al. Ureaplasma urealyticum in the development of postpartum endometritis. Eur J Obstet Gynecol Reprod Biol. 2003;109:145–8.
25. Kijlstra A, Jongert E. Control of the risk of human toxoplasmosis transmitted by meat. Int J Parasitol. 2008;38:1359–70.
26. Pappas G, Roussos N, Falagas ME. Toxoplasmosis snapshots: global status of Toxoplasma gondii seroprevalence and implications for pregnancy and congenital toxoplasmosis. Int J Parasitol. 2009;39:1385–94.
27. El-Tantawy N, Taman A, Shalaby H. Toxoplasmosis and female infertility: is there a co-relation? Am J Epidemiol Infect Dis. 2014;2:29–32.
28. Yokoe DS, Christiansen CL, Johnson R, et al. Epidemiology of and surveillance for postpartum infections. Emerg Infect Dis. 2001;7:837–41.
29. Dalton E, Castillo E. Post partum infections: a review for the non-OBGYN. Obstet Med. 2014;7:98–102.
30. Blaustein A. Endometritis. In: Interpretation of endometrial biopsies., 2nd. New York: Raven Press; 1985. p. 88–116.
31. Judson MA, Baughman RP, Teirstein AS, et al. Defining organ involvement in sarcoidosis: the ACCESS proposed instrument. ACCESS Research Group. A Case Control Etiologic Study of Sarcoidosis. Sarcoidosis Vasc Diffuse Lung Dis. 1999;16:75–86.
32. Porter N, Beynon HL, Randeva HS. Endocrine and reproductive manifestations of sarcoidosis. QJM. 2003;96:553–61.
33. Almoujahed MO, Briski LE, Prysak M, et al. Uterine granulomas: clinical and pathologic features. Am J Clin Pathol. 2002;117:771–5.
34. Romer T, Schwesinger G, Foth D. Endometrial sarcoidosis manifesting as recurrent serometra in a postmenopausal woman. Acta Obstet Gynecol Scand. 2001;80:482–3.
35. Pearce KF, Nolan TE. Endometrial sarcoidosis as a cause of postmenopausal bleeding. A case report. J Reprod Med. 1996;41:878–80.
36. Rosa e Silva JC, de Sa Rosa e Silva AC, Aguiar FM, et al. Isolated endometrial polypoid sarcoidosis in a post-menopausal patient: case report. Maturitas. 2006;53:489–91.
37. Hoff E, Prayson RA. Incidental granulomatous inflammation of the uterus. South Med J. 2002;95:884–8.
38. Wader JV, Jain A, Kumbhar SS, et al. Histiocytic endometritis. Am J Case Rep. 2013;14:329–32.
39. Kurman RJ. WHO classification of tumours of female reproductive organs. Lyon: IARC; 2014. p. 133.
40. Soslow RA, Longacre T. Uterine pathology: Cambridge illustrated surgical pathology. Cambridge: Cambridge University Press; 2012. p. 97.
41. Tallini G, Vanni R, Manfioletti G, et al. HMGI-C and HMGI(Y) immunoreactivity correlates with cytogenetic abnormalities in lipomas, pulmonary chondroid hamartomas, endometrial polyps, and uterine leiomyomas and is compatible with rearrangement of the HMGI-C and HMGI(Y) genes. Lab Investig. 2000;80:359–69.
42. Fletcher JA, Pinkus JL, Lage JM, et al. Clonal 6p21 rearrangement is restricted to the mesenchymal component of an endometrial polyp. Genes Chromosomes Cancer. 1992;5:260–3.

43. Reslova T, Tosner J, Resl M, et al. Endometrial polyps. A clinical study of 245 cases. Arch Gynecol Obstet. 1999;262:133–9.
44. Rodrigues MI, Goez E, Larios K, et al. Atypical stromal cells as a diagnostic pitfall in lesions of the lower female genital tract and uterus: a review and presentation of some unusual cases. Patol Rev Latinoam. 2009;47:103–7.
45. Howitt BE, Quade BJ, Nucci MR. Uterine polyps with features overlapping with those of Mullerian adenosarcoma: a clinicopathologic analysis of 29 cases emphasizing their likely benign nature. Am J Surg Pathol. 2015;39:116–26.
46. Lee SC, Kaunitz AM, Sanchez-Ramos L, et al. The oncogenic potential of endometrial polyps: a systematic review and meta-analysis. Obstet Gynecol. 2010;116:1197–205.
47. Malpica A, Deavers MT, Euscher E. Biopsy interpretation of the uterine cervix and corpus. Philadelphia: Lippincot Williams and Wilkins; 2010. p. 136.
48. Barsan I, Moncea D, Chira L, et al. p16—A new marker for differentiating between endometrial polyps and endometrial hyperplasia on curettage and Pipelle biopsy, 27th European Congress of Pathology, Belgrade. Virchows Arch. 2015;467(Suppl 1):1–279.
49. Moritani S, Ichihara S, Hasegawa M, et al. Stromal p16 expression differentiates endometrial polyp from endometrial hyperplasia. Virchows Arch. 2012;461:141–8.
50. National Comprehensive Cancer Network. NCCN clinical practice guidelines in oncology. Breast Cancer (Version 2.2017). https://www.nccn.org/professionals/physician_gls/. Accessed 22 Dec 2017.
51. Hachisuga T, Miyakawa T, Tsujioka H, et al. K-ras mutation in tamoxifen-related endometrial polyps. Cancer. 2003;98:1890–7.
52. Biron-Shental T, Tepper R, Fishman A, et al. Recurrent endometrial polyps in postmenopausal breast cancer patients on tamoxifen. Gynecol Oncol. 2003;90:382–6.
53. Gilks CB, Clement PB, Hart WR, et al. Uterine adenomyomas excluding atypical polypoid adenomyomas and adenomyomas of endocervical type: a clinicopathologic study of 30 cases of an underemphasized lesion that may cause diagnostic problems with brief consideration of adenomyomas of other female genital tract sites. Int J Gynecol Pathol. 2000;19:195–205.
54. Clement PB, Young RH. Atypical polypoid adenomyoma of the uterus associated with Turner's syndrome. A report of three cases, including a review of "estrogen-associated" endometrial neoplasms and neoplasms associated with Turner's syndrome. Int J Gynecol Pathol. 1987;6:104–13.
55. Mazur MT. Atypical polypoid adenomyomas of the endometrium. Am J Surg Pathol. 1981;5:473–82.
56. Ota S, Catasus L, Matias-Guiu X, et al. Molecular pathology of atypical polypoid adenomyoma of the uterus. Hum Pathol. 2003;34:784–8.
57. Nemejcova K, Kenny SL, Laco J, et al. Atypical polypoid adenomyoma of the uterus: an immunohistochemical and molecular study of 21 cases. Am J Surg Pathol. 2015;39:1148–55.
58. Longacre TA, Chung MH, Rouse RV, et al. Atypical polypoid adenomyofibromas (atypical polypoid adenomyomas) of the uterus. A clinicopathologic study of 55 cases. Am J Surg Pathol. 1996;20:1–20.
59. Anastasiadis PG, Koutlaki NG, Skaphida PG, et al. Endometrial polyps: prevalence, detection, and malignant potential in women with abnormal uterine bleeding. Eur J Gynaecol Oncol. 2000;21:180–3.
60. Mittal KR, Peng XC, Wallach RC, et al. Coexistent atypical polypoid adenomyoma and endometrial adenocarcinoma. Hum Pathol. 1995;26:574–6.
61. Cheng W, Liu J, Yoshida H, et al. Lineage infidelity of epithelial ovarian cancers is controlled by HOX genes that specify regional identity in the reproductive tract. Nat Med. 2005;11:531–7.
62. Risse EK, Beerthuizen RJ, Vooijs GP. Cytologic and histologic findings in women using an IUD. Obstet Gynecol. 1981;58:569–73.
63. Bewtra C, Xie QM, Hunter WJ, et al. Ichthyosis uteri: a case report and review of the literature. Arch Pathol Lab Med. 2005;129:e124–5.
64. Crum CP, Richart RM, Fenoglio CM. Adenoacanthosis of endometrium: a clinicopathologic study in premenopausal women. Am J Surg Pathol. 1981;5:15–20.
65. Jovanovic AS, Boynton KA, Mutter GL. Uteri of women with endometrial carcinoma contain a histopathological spectrum of monoclonal putative precancers, some with microsatellite instability. Cancer Res. 1996;56:1917–21.
66. Mutter GL. Diagnosis of premalignant endometrial disease. J Clin Pathol. 2002;55:326–31.
67. Nicolae A, Preda O, Nogales FF. Endometrial metaplasias and reactive changes: a spectrum of altered differentiation. J Clin Pathol. 2011;64:97–106.
68. Wheeler DT, Bristow RE, Kurman RJ. Histologic alterations in endometrial hyperplasia and well-differentiated carcinoma treated with progestins. Am J Surg Pathol. 2007;31:988–98.
69. Nucci MR, Prasad CJ, Crum CP, et al. Mucinous endometrial epithelial proliferations: a morphologic spectrum of changes with diverse clinical significance. Mod Pathol. 1999;12:1137–42.
70. Masterton R, Armstrong EM, More IA. The cyclical variation in the percentage of ciliated cells in the normal human endometrium. J Reprod Fertil. 1975;42:537–40.
71. Mazur MT, Kurman RJ. Diagnosis of endometrial biopsies and curettings: a practical approach. New York: Springer-Verlag; 1995. p. 1–260.
72. Cameron RI, Maxwell P, Jenkins D, et al. Immunohistochemical staining with MIB1, bcl2 and p16 assists in the distinction of cervical glandular intraepithelial neoplasia from tubo-endometrial metaplasia, endometriosis and microglandular hyperplasia. Histopathology. 2002;41:313–21.
73. Hendrickson MR, Kempson RL. Endometrial epithelial metaplasias: proliferations frequently misdiagnosed as adenocarcinoma. Report of 89 cases and proposed classification. Am J Surg Pathol. 1980;4:525–42.
74. Kaku T, Silverberg SG, Tsukamoto N, et al. Association of endometrial epithelial metaplasias with endometrial carcinoma and hyperplasia in Japanese and American women. Int J Gynecol Pathol. 1993;12:297–300.
75. Mai KT, Yazdi HM, Boone SA. 'Minimal deviation' endometrioid carcinoma with oncocytic change of the endometrium. Arch Pathol Lab Med. 1995;119:751–4.
76. Mai KT, Yazdi HM, Boone SA. Minimal deviation' endometrioid carcinoma with oncocytic change of the endometrium. Arch Pathol Lab Med. 1995;119:751–4.
77. Kajiwara H, Kumaki N, Hirabayashi K, et al. A case of oncocytic carcinoma of the endometrium. Arch Gynecol Obstet. 2009;279:733–8.
78. Truskinovsky AM, Lifschitz-Mercer B, Czernobilsky B. Hyperplasia and carcinoma in secretory endometrium: a diagnostic challenge. Int J Gynecol Pathol. 2014;33:107–13.
79. Gurda GT, Baras AS, Kurman RJ. Ki-67 index as an ancillary tool in the differential diagnosis of proliferative endometrial lesions with secretory change. Int J Gynecol Pathol. 2014;33:114–9.
80. Roth E, Taylor HB. Heterotopic cartilage in the uterus. Obstet Gynecol. 1966;27:838–44.
81. Courpas AS, Morris JD, Woodruff JD. Osteoid tissue in utero. Report of 3 cases. Obstet Gynecol. 1964;24:636–40.
82. Nogales FF, Gomez-Morales M, Raymundo C, et al. Benign heterologous tissue components associated with endometrial carcinoma. Int J Gynecol Pathol. 1982;1:286–91.
83. Nogales FF, Nicolae A, Garcia-Galvis OF, et al. Uterine and extrauterine plexiform tumourlets are sex-cord-like tumours with myoid features. Histopathology. 2009;54:497–500.
84. Tyagi SP, Saxena K, Rizvi R, et al. Foetal remnants in the uterus and their relation to other uterine heterotopia. Histopathology. 1979;3:339–45.

85. Russell P, de Costa C, Yeoh G. Fetal glial allograft in the endometrium: case report of a recurrent pseudo-tumor. Pathology. 1993;25:247–9.
86. Creagh TM, Bain BJ, Evans DJ, et al. Endometrial extramedullary haematopoiesis. J Pathol. 1995;176:99–104.
87. Scott M, Lyness RW, McCluggage WG. Atypical reactive proliferation of endocervix: a common lesion associated with endometrial carcinoma and likely related to prior endometrial sampling. Mod Pathol. 2006;19:470–4.
88. Fausett MB, Zahn CM, Kendall BS, et al. The significance of psammoma bodies that are found incidentally during endometrial biopsy. Am J Obstet Gynecol. 2002;186:180–3.
89. Krizova A, Clarke BA, Bernardini MQ, et al. Histologic artifacts in abdominal, vaginal, laparoscopic, and robotic hysterectomy specimens: a blinded, retrospective review. Am J Surg Pathol. 2011;35:115–26.
90. Sahin AA, Silva EG, Landon G, et al. Endometrial tissue in myometrial vessels not associated with menstruation. Int J Gynecol Pathol. 1989;8:139–46.
91. Ooi K, Valentine R. Intravascular endometrial tissue in an ovary of a patient with abnormal endometrial histology. Pathology. 1994;26:212–4.

Index

W. Zheng et al. (eds.), *Gynecologic and Obstetric Pathology, Volume 1*, https://doi.org/10.1007/978-981-13-3016-2

F

G

H

I

K

L

M

N

O

P

R

S

MIX
Papier aus verantwortungsvollen Quellen
Paper from responsible sources
FSC® C105338

If you have any concerns about our products,
you can contact us on
ProductSafety@springernature.com

In case Publisher is established outside the EU,
the EU authorized representative is:
Springer Nature Customer Service Center GmbH
Europaplatz 3, 69115 Heidelberg, Germany

Printed by Libri Plureos GmbH
in Hamburg, Germany